Computational Modeling of Neural Activity

Computational Modeling of Neural Activity

Editor: Emerson Gibson

AMERICAN
MEDICAL PUBLISHERS
www.americanmedicalpublishers.com

AMERICAN
MEDICAL PUBLISHERS
www.americanmedicalpublishers.com

Cataloging-in-Publication Data

Computational modeling of neural activity / edited by Emerson Gibson.
p. cm.
Includes bibliographical references and index.
ISBN 979-8-88740-018-1
1. Computational neuroscience. 2. Neurology--Models. 3. Neurology--Data processing. 4. Neurosciences--Data processing. 5. Neuroinformatics. 6. Information storage and retrieval systems--Neurology. I. Gibson, Emerson.
QP357.5 .C66 2023
612.8--dc23

American Medical Publishers,
41 Flatbush Avenue,
1st Floor, New York,
NY 11217, USA

ISBN 979-8-88740-018-1 (Hardback)

Contents

Preface

Computational modeling for neural activity refers to the use of computers to simulate and study complex systems using mathematics, computer science, and physics. In biology, these models integrate different data sets in a coherent and unified computational framework in order to explain certain neuroscience phenomena including neurological disorders such as dyslexia, depression, post-traumatic stress disorder (PTSD), and schizophrenia. Computation models predict disease progression through the study of molecular processes, cell to cell interactions, and the manner in which these changes affect tissues and organs. In recent years, a number of computational tools including NEURON, BRIAN, NEST, and the virtual brain (TVB), have been developed to create, validate, and investigate models of brain networks. This book is a compilation of chapters that discuss the most vital concepts and emerging trends in computational modeling for neural activity. It is a collective contribution of a renowned group of international experts. The book, with its detailed analyses and data, will prove immensely beneficial to professionals and students involved in this area at various levels.

Various studies have approached the subject by analyzing it with a single perspective, but the present book provides diverse methodologies and techniques to address this field. This book contains theories and applications needed for understanding the subject from different perspectives. The aim is to keep the readers informed about the progresses in the field; therefore, the contributions were carefully examined to compile novel researches by specialists from across the globe.

Indeed, the job of the editor is the most crucial and challenging in compiling all chapters into a single book. In the end, I would extend my sincere thanks to the chapter authors for their profound work. I am also thankful for the support provided by my family and colleagues during the compilation of this book.

Editor

1

The anesthetic propofol shifts the frequency of maximum spectral power in EEG during general anesthesia: Analytical insights from a linear model

Axel Hutt*

INRIA CR Nancy - Grand Est, Team CORTEX, Villers-les-Nancy, France

The work introduces a linear neural population model that allows to derive analytically the power spectrum subjected to the concentration of the anesthetic propofol. The analytical study of the power spectrum of the systems activity gives conditions on how the frequency of maximum power in experimental electroencephalographic (EEG) changes dependent on the propofol concentration. In this context, we explain the anesthetic-induced power increase in neural activity by an oscillatory instability and derive conditions under which the power peak shifts to larger frequencies as observed experimentally in EEG. Moreover the work predicts that the power increase only occurs while the frequency of maximum power increases. Numerically simulations of the systems activity complement the analytical results.

Keywords: general anesthesia, propofol, neural fields, power spectrum, EEG

***Correspondence:**
Axel Hutt, INRIA CR Nancy - Grand Est, Team CORTEX, 615 rue du Jardin Botanique, 54602 Villers-les-Nancy, France.
e-mail: axel.hutt@inria.fr

1. INTRODUCTION

General anesthesia (GA) is an important medical application in today's hospital surgery. Although GA is omnipresent in recent medicine, its underlying neural interactions have been a long-standing mystery. In the last decades, the anesthetic phenomena have attracted theoreticiens, e.g., (Steyn-Ross et al., 1999; Bojak and Liley, 2005; Hutt, 2011), who aim to describe mathematically some major experimental phenomena by population models (Steyn-Ross et al., 2004, 2012; Bojak and Liley, 2005; Hutt and Longtin, 2009; Hindriks and van Putten, 2012), or spiking-neuron models (McCarthy et al., 2008; Ching et al., 2010). Most theoretical studies aim to explain signal features of electroencephalographic (EEG) data observed during anesthesia. Such features comprise the diminution of α-activity accompanied by a subsequent enhancement of δ-activity while increasing anesthetic concentration (Gugino et al., 2001; Cimenser et al., 2011; Murphy et al., 2011) and the power enhancement of activity induced by some anesthetics (McCarthy et al., 2008; Ching et al., 2010). Another example is the increase of the frequency of maximum EEG-power to higher values as observed experimentally in several studies (Gugino et al., 2001; Ching et al., 2010; Murphy et al., 2011; Boly et al., 2012; Hindriks and van Putten, 2012). The current work focusses on the power enhancement and the frequency shift of maximum power while increasing the anesthetic concentration and gives insights into its origin by the analytical treatment of a linear neural field model.

One of the major objectives of this work is to answer the question whether it is possible to explain spectral EEG-features observed during GA by a low-dimensional linear model. The advantage of such a reduced model is the analytical tractability and an identification of underlying neural interactions or even the origin of the spectral feature. Here the difficulty is to find a simple model, that, however, still involves important, i.e., realistic and neural interactions. We are convinced that such a model has been found in a previous work (Hutt and Longtin, 2009). The present work will simplify further this spatio-temporal model while taking into account the biophysical effects of the anesthetic propofol on synaptic receptors and hence retaining the neurobiological plausibility.

The simplicity of the model will allow to reveal the effect of different actions of the anesthetic propofol on synaptic receptors on the frequency of maximum spectral power. Moreover, the work gives criteria under which conditions the frequency of maximum power increases with increasing propofol concentration and when it may decreases. In the analytical treatment, we will see that the power enhancement for larger propofol concentrations may be explained by an oscillatory instability and we predict that it always occurs while the frequency of maximum power increases.

2. METHODS

2.1. THE MODEL

The neural field model under study (Hutt and Longtin, 2009) describes the evolution of the mean membrane potential of a neural population in a small spatial patch at spatial location x and at time t. Similar models have been derived and studied before (Wilson and Cowan, 1972; Amari, 1977; Ermentrout, 1998) and applied successfully to explain spatio-temporal neural activity observed experimentally (Ermentrout and Cowan, 1979; Huang et al., 2004; Angelucci and Bressloff, 2006; Schwabe et al., 2006). The population includes both excitatory and inhibitory neurons and takes into account excitatory and inhibitory synapses. Assuming that excitatory and inhibitory neurons exhibit identical effective membrane potentials, i.e., an identical difference between excitatory and inhibitory post-synaptic potentials, the mean excitatory and inhibitory post-synaptic potentials $V_e(x, t)$ and $V_i(x, t)$, respectively, obey

$$\hat{L}_e V_e(x,t) = a_e \int_{\mathcal{D}} K_e(x-y) S_e[V_e(y,t) - V_i(y,t)]dy + I(x,t)$$
$$\hat{L}_i V_i(x,t) = a_i \int_{\mathcal{D}} K_i(x-y) S_i[V_e(y,t) - V_i(y,t)]dy \quad (1)$$

with the circular spatial population domain $\mathcal{D}$ of length L, i.e., assuming periodic boundary conditions. The model under study differs from some other previous models, e.g., by Liley and Bojak (2005), by the implementation of synaptic action, generation of action potentials or axonal connectivity [see also the work of Coombes et al. (2007) for a comparison of the current model and other models]. The functionals $S_e[\cdot]$ and $S_i[\cdot]$ are continuously increasing and represent the population firing rate of excitatory and inhibitory neurons, respectively. In the population the single neurons are connected by a complex system of axons from neuron somata to synapses. The kernels $K_e(x)$ and $K_i(x)$ are the probability density of such connections in the population. Here axonal transmission delay is neglected for simplicity although it is straightforward to include it in this type of model (Hutt and Longtin, 2009). In addition, the model considers excitatory and inhibitory synapses, $\hat{L}_e = \hat{L}_e(d/dt)$ and $\hat{L}_i = \hat{L}_i(d/dt)$ denote functional operators describing the corresponding temporal synaptic response phase and the factors a_e, a_i represent the corresponding synaptic efficacies.

Mathematically, the differential operators are the inverse of the integral operators in

$$V(t) = \int_{-\infty}^{t} h(t-\tau)P(\tau)\, d\tau \quad (2)$$

where $h(t)$ is the synaptic response function, or more precisely the electric current response in the synaptic receptor to an impact of binding neurotransmitters (Koch, 1999). The function $P(\tau) > 0$ is the mean pulse activity arriving at the synapses. In a reasonable approximation, the response function reads

$$h(t) = \frac{a}{\tau} e^{-t/\tau}$$

with the decay time constant τ and the synaptic efficacy $a > 0$. Then the response amplitude is $h(0) = a/\tau$ and the charge transferred in the receptor $\rho = a$ is the time integral over the current flow. The corresponding differential operator stipulates $\hat{L}V(t) = aP(t)$ leading to

$$\hat{L}\left(\frac{\partial}{\partial t}\right) = \tau\frac{\partial}{\partial t} + 1$$

and Equation (2) re-casts to

$$\tau\frac{\partial V(t)}{\partial t} + V(t) = aP(t).$$

These expressions hold for excitatory and inhibitory synapses.

The synaptic receptors are major targets of anesthetic agents. The present work considers the action of propofol on inhibitory synaptic and extra-synaptic GABA$_A$-receptors. The former receptor is supposed to be a major anesthetic target (Franks and Lieb, 1994) and there is growing evidence that extra-synaptic inhibitory receptors may play an important role in anesthesia as well (Orser, 2006; Hutt, 2012). The subsequent sections consider effects on synaptic receptors due to the well-established experimental evidence. Hence, the synaptic parameters of inhibitory synaptic receptors depend on the anesthetic concentration and are parameterized by the factor $p \geq 1$ (Steyn-Ross et al., 2001), i.e., the decay time of inhibitory synapses $\tau_2 = \tau_2(p)$ and the corresponding synaptic efficacy $a_i = a_i(p)$ depend on p.

The input in Equation (1) fluctuates randomly in space and time with $\xi(x, t)$ about a constant value $I_0 = $ const, i.e., $I(x, t) = I_0 + \xi(x, t)$. The random fluctuations are independent in space and time and thus obey $\langle\xi(x, t)\rangle = 0$, $\langle\xi(x, t)\xi(y, T)\rangle = 2D\delta(t - T)\delta(x - y)$, where $\langle\cdot\rangle$ denotes the ensemble average.

Considering the latter definitions of synaptic properties, anesthetic action and external input, the final model equations read

$$\begin{aligned}\tau_1\frac{\partial V_e(x,t)}{\partial t} &= -V_e(x,t) + a_e\int_{\mathcal{D}} K_e(x-y)S_e[V_e(y,t) \\ &\quad - V_i(y,t)]dy + I_0 + \xi(x,t) \\ \tau_2(p)\frac{\partial V_i(x,t)}{\partial t} &= -V_i(x,t) + a_i(p)\int_{\mathcal{D}} K_i(x-y)S_i[V_e(y,t) \\ &\quad - V_i(y,t)]dy \end{aligned} \quad (3)$$

with the decay time of excitatory synapses τ_1.

Assuming that the random fluctuations are small and do not affect the stationary state [in contrast to recent results gained from non-linear systems (Hutt et al., 2007; Hutt, 2008)], the stationary state $V_e(x, t) = V_e^0 = $ const, $V_i(x, t) = V_i^0 = $ const obeys $V_e^0 = a_e S_e[V_-] + I_0$, $V_i^0 = a_i(p)S_i[V_-]$ with $V_- = V_e^0 - V_i^0 = a_e S_e[V_-] - a_i(p)S_i[V_-] + I_0$ (Hutt and Longtin, 2009).

2.2. THEORETICAL POWER SPECTRUM

To compute the power spectrum, we employ the method of Greens function. Let us assume the activity variable vector $\mathbf{x}(t) \in \mathcal{R}^N$, the matrix $\mathbf{A}$, the external input vector $\xi(t) \in \mathcal{R}^N$, the Greens function matrix $\mathbf{G}(t) \in \mathcal{R}^{N\times N}$ and

$$\dot{\mathbf{x}}(t) = \mathbf{A}\mathbf{x} + \xi(t).$$

Then, for $t \to \infty$, the solution of the system is

$$\mathbf{x}(t) = \int_{-\infty}^{\infty} \mathbf{G}(t-\tau)\xi(\tau)d\tau. \quad (4)$$

and the Greens function obeys

$$\dot{\mathbf{G}} - \mathbf{A}\mathbf{G}(t) = \mathbf{1}\delta(t)$$

with te unitary matrix $\mathbf{1} \in \mathcal{R}^{N\times N}$. Applying the Fourier transform

$$\mathbf{G}(t) = \frac{1}{\sqrt{2\pi}}\int_{-\infty}^{\infty} \tilde{\mathbf{G}}(\omega)e^{i\omega t}d\omega. \quad (5)$$

yields

$$\tilde{\mathbf{G}}(\omega) = \frac{1}{\sqrt{2\pi}}(i\omega\mathbf{1} - \mathbf{A})^{-1} \quad (6)$$

$$= \frac{1}{\sqrt{2\pi}} \frac{\mathbf{F}(i\omega)}{P(i\omega)} \quad (7)$$

with the matrix $\mathbf{F}(i\omega)$ and the characteristic polynom $P(i\omega)$. The matrix $\mathbf{F}$ in Equation (7) includes the matrix elements of the inverse of $i\omega\mathbf{1} - \mathbf{A}$ and the characteristic polynom P represents the corresponding matrix determinant.

Inserting Equation (6) into (5) allows to compute $\mathbf{G}(t)$ by the residue theorem in functional analysis

$$\mathbf{G}(t) = 2\pi i \sum_{n=1}^{r} \mathbf{Res}(z_n, t)\Theta(t) \quad (8)$$

with the Heaviside function $\Theta(t)$ and the residues matrix $\mathbf{Res}(z_n, t)$ of $\mathbf{F}(z)/P(z)$ at the roots z_n of the characteristic equation $P(z) = 0$. The condition $t > 0$ considered by the Heaviside function is the mathematical condition for the validity of Equation (8) while it also guarantees the causality of the system response. Equation (8) together with Equation (4) determines the time dependence of the solution x and is computed explicitly in section 3.4.

Finally, the power spectral density matrix $\mathbf{S}(\omega)$ of $\mathbf{x}$ is the Fourier transform of the auto-correlation function matrix $\langle \mathbf{x}^t(t)\mathbf{x}(t-T)\rangle$ (Wiener-Khinchine Theorem) leading to

$$\mathbf{S}(\omega) = 2D\sqrt{2\pi}\tilde{\mathbf{G}}(\omega)\tilde{\mathbf{G}}^t(-\omega),$$

where the high index t denotes the transposed vector or matrix.

3. RESULTS

3.1. EFFECT OF PROPOFOL

The effect of the anesthetic propofol on neural properties is manifold (Alkire et al., 2008). It affects properties of membrane ion channels, synaptic receptors and extra-synaptic receptors, see Franks and Lieb (1994) for a review. Kitamura et al. (2002) have revealed in an experimental study how propofol affects post-synaptic phasic responses of inhibitory synapses to spontaneous neurotransmitter release. They have found that the decay time constant decreases with increasing anesthetic blood concentration, the charge transfer increases while the amplitude of the responses remains constant. Some previous studies (Hutt and Longtin, 2009; Hindriks and van Putten, 2012) have implemented these effects for a bi-exponential synaptic response function. The present work considers an exponential decay phase due to its mathematical simplicity, which nevertheless reflects the major anesthetic impact. To this end, the phasic response at inhibitory synapses is determined by the decay time constant and the response amplitude. Introducing the parameter $p = \tau_2(p)/\tau_2(1)$, $p = 1$ reflects the absence of anesthetic agents and increases of the anesthetic concentration yields an increase of p. In addition Kitamura et al. (2002) have shown that the amplitude in cortical neurons remains constant or changes slightly only, i.e., $h(0) = a/\tau_2(p) \approx$ const and the charge transfer $\rho(p) = a$ increase with increasing anesthetic concentration. In the case of constant the model

$$\tau_2(p) = \tau_2(1)p, \quad a_i(p) = H_0 p. \quad (9)$$

with the constant $H_0 > 0$. These choices of anesthetic actions reflect different synaptic mechanism. The first relation reflects the increase of the time constant with increasing anesthetic concentration, and the second one both the constant amplitude and the resulting increasing charge transfer. However, synapses may have different properties in different brain areas, e.g., synapses in cortico-thalamic connections increase their amplitude with increasing propofol concentrations (Ying and Goldstein, 2005). Hence the relations (Equation 9) are specific properties of inhibitory synapses on cortical neurons only.

3.2. THE LINEAR MODEL

The following investigation considers the stability of stationary states and spectral properties of small deviations about them. These small deviations represent fluctuating currents on the dendritic trees of the neurons in the population generating an electric field on the scalp. They originate from fluctuations in the neuron membranes or from spontaneous neurotransmitter emission at synapses. The generated electric field is measured in terms of voltage differences between two spatial locations on the scalp which is the electroencephalogram (EEG) (Nunez and Srinivasan, 2006).

The small fluctuations about the stationary states $u_e(x, t) = V_e(x, t) - V_e^0$, $u_i(x, t) = V_i(x, t) - V_i^0$ obey

$$\tau_1 \frac{du_e(x, t)}{dt} = -u_e(x, t) + a_e S_e' \int_{\mathcal{D}} K_e(x - y)\left(u_e(y, t) - u_i(y, t)\right) dy + \xi(x, t)$$

$$\tau_2(p) \frac{du_i(x, t)}{dt} = -u_i(x, t) + a_i(p) S_i' \int_{\mathcal{D}} K_i(x - y)\left(u_e(y, t) - u_i(y, t)\right) dy$$

with the somatic non-linear gain $S'_{e,i} = dS_{e,i}(x)/dx$ at $x = \{V_e^0, V_i^0\}$. By virtue of the finite spatial domain, the small deviations about the stationary state may be expanded into a discrete infinite Fourier series. The major contribution of neuronal activity to encephalographic activity on the scalp is modeled successfully by a spatially constant Fourier mode $u_e(x, t) = x(t)$, $u_i(x, t) = y(t)$ (Nunez and Srinivasan, 2006). Then $x(t)$, $y(t)$ obey

$$\tau_1 \frac{dx(t)}{dt} = (-1 + N_1)x(t) - N_1 y(t) + \gamma(t)$$

$$\tau_2(p) \frac{dy(t)}{dt} = N_2 x(t) + (-1 - N_2)y(t) \quad (10)$$

with the synaptic non-linear gains $N_1 = a_e S_e' \tilde{K}_e(0)\sqrt{L}$, $N_2 = N_2(p) = a_i(p) S_i' \tilde{K}_i(0)\sqrt{L}$, the spatial Fourier transform of the kernels $\tilde{K}_e(k)$, $\tilde{K}_i(k)$ and the spatial Fourier transform of the external noise at zero wavenumber $\gamma(t)$. We point out that $\langle\gamma(t)\rangle = 0$, $\langle\gamma(t)\gamma(T)\rangle = 2D\delta(t - T)$.

3.3. STABILITY ANALYSIS

To study the dynamics about the stationary state, at first let us neglect the external input $\xi(t)$ since in a first approximation the stability of the linear system does not depend on the external input. Then the stationary state is asymptotically stable if the characteristic equation of Equation (10)

$$\lambda^2 - \lambda Tr + det = 0 \tag{11}$$

with $\lambda \in \mathbb{C}$ and

$$Tr = \frac{N_1 - 1}{\tau_1} - \frac{N_2 + 1}{\tau_2} \tag{12}$$

$$det = \frac{N_1 N_2}{\tau_1 \tau_2} - \frac{N_1 - 1}{\tau_1}\frac{N_2 + 1}{\tau_2}. \tag{13}$$

has solutions $Re(\lambda) < 0$. Here Tr and det are the trace and determinant of the linear matrix in Equation (10), respectively. In addition, the stationary state is a stable focus if $Im(\lambda) = \Omega \neq 0$, $\Omega \in \mathbb{R}$ and

$$\Omega^2 = \frac{N_1 N_2}{\tau_1 \tau_2} - \frac{1}{4}\left(\frac{N_1 - 1}{\tau_1} + \frac{N_2 + 1}{\tau_2}\right)^2.$$

We observe immediately from Equation (12), that the stable focus is asymptotically stable if $Tr < 0$ or $N_1 < 1$ for all other parameters and the system may lose stability only if $N_1 > 1$. Since the present work aims to give conditions for certain oscillation frequencies in the population, the subsequent part of the work considers stable foci only. In addition the inhibitory synaptic time scale $\tau_2 = \tau_2(p)$ depends on the anesthetic concentration, but not τ_1. Thus τ_1 is treated as a constant.

The new variables $a = (N_1 - 1)^2$, $b = N_1 N_2 - N_1 + N_2 + 1$ and $c = (N_2 + 1)^2$ depend solely on N_1, N_2, and simplify the notation in the following analysis. Then for $N_1 > 1$, stable foci stipulate

$$Tr = \frac{\sqrt{a}}{\tau_1} - \frac{\sqrt{c}}{\tau_2} < 0 \quad \text{or} \quad \frac{\tau_2}{\tau_1} < \sqrt{\frac{c}{a}}, \tag{14}$$

$$\Omega = \frac{1}{2}\sqrt{\frac{1}{\tau_1}\left(\frac{2b}{\tau_2} - \frac{a}{\tau_1} - \frac{c\tau_1}{\tau_2^2}\right)} \in \mathbb{R}. \tag{15}$$

The last equation implies that the determinant is positive definite, i.e.,

$$d(\tau_2) = a\tau_2^2 - 2b\tau_1\tau_2 + c\tau_1^2 < 0.$$

A comparison to Equation (15) reveals that $d(\tau_2) = 0$ leads to $\Omega = 0$ which permits to compute the range of τ_2 for which the system exhibits stable foci:

$$\frac{\tau_2^-}{\tau_1} \leq \frac{\tau_2}{\tau_1} \leq \frac{\tau_2^+}{\tau_1} \tag{16}$$

$$\frac{\tau_2^-}{\tau_1} = \frac{b}{a}\left(1 + \sqrt{1 - \frac{ac}{b^2}}\right), \; \frac{\tau_2^+}{\tau_1} = \frac{b}{a}\left(1 - \sqrt{1 - \frac{ac}{b^2}}\right)$$

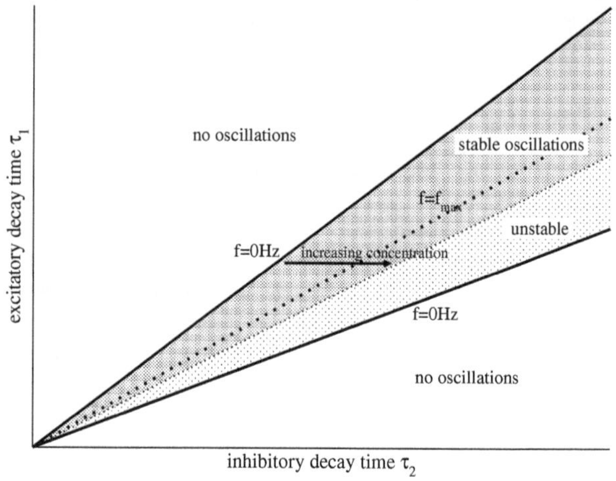

FIGURE 1 | Illustration of the parameter areas which exhibit stable, unstable, and no oscillations. The upper and lower solid lines denote τ_2^-/τ_1 and τ_2^+/τ_1, respectively. The dotted line denotes the maximum frequency $f_{\max} = 2\pi\omega_m$ with $\tau_2/\tau_1 = b/c$, cf. Equation (20), and the stability threshold is given by $\tau_2/\tau_1 = \sqrt{c/a}$, see Equation (14).

implying $(b/a)^2 > c/a$. Condition (16) constrains the relation of both synaptic time scales τ_2/τ_1 by N_1 and N_2, see **Figure 1** for the corresponding parameter space.

To learn more about the dynamics of the model, we consider parameters yielding strong oscillations with a predefined frequency, such as $f = 4$ Hz (δ-band), $f = 10$ Hz (α-band), or $f = 15$ Hz (β-band) as observed in experiments (Cimenser et al., 2011). To this end, we fix the frequency $\Omega = 2\pi f$ in Equation (15). Then inserting the threshold condition $\tau_2/\tau_1 = \sqrt{c/a}$ given in Equation (14) into (15) for a fixed τ_1 yields a relation between N_1 and N_2, see **Figure 2A**. Similarly the condition $\Omega = 0$ given by Equation (16) determines the values of N_1 and N_2 at the threshold of oscillations. **Figures 2B–E** plot the parameter space $\tau_2/\tau_1 - N_2$ where the system exhibits stable oscillations. The figure also shows how the values change when increasing p (arrows in panels), i.e., increasing the propofol concentration, and it turns out that the system always approaches the stability threshold.

3.4. THE SPECTRAL POWER

To compute the power spectrum, we employ the method of Greens function. Equations (10) show that the solutions of the system obey

$$x(t) = \int_{-\infty}^{\infty} G_{11}(t - \tau)\gamma(\tau)d\tau, \quad y(t) = \int_{-\infty}^{\infty} G_{21}(t - \tau)\gamma(\tau)d\tau$$

with the Greens functions

$$G_{11}(t) = \frac{1}{2\pi}\int_{-\infty}^{\infty} \frac{i\omega + (N_2 + 1)/\tau_2}{P(i\omega)} e^{i\omega t} d\omega \tag{17}$$

$$G_{21}(t) = -\frac{1}{2\pi}\int_{-\infty}^{\infty} \frac{N_2/\tau_2}{P(i\omega)} e^{i\omega t} d\omega \tag{18}$$

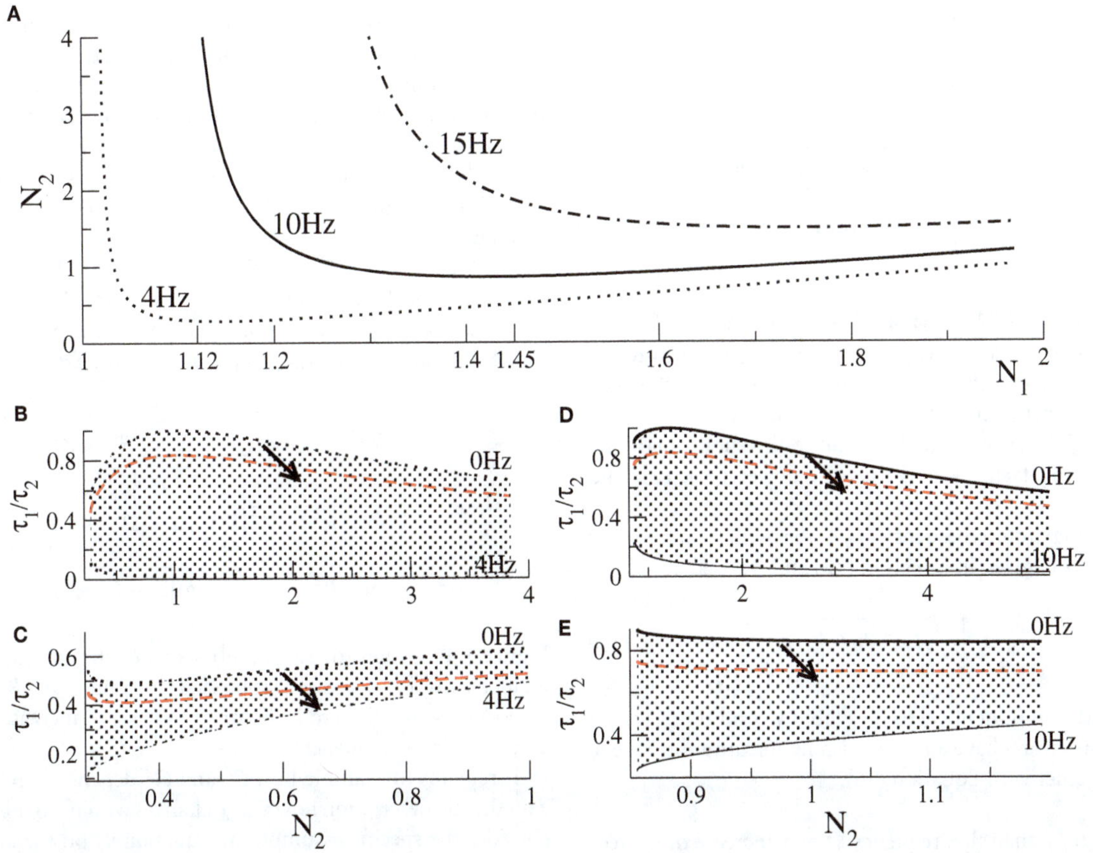

FIGURE 2 | Conditions for Hopf-instabilities and the effect of propofol action. (A) threshold of Hopf-instability at 4, 10, and 15 Hz dependent on N_1, N_2. Panels **(B,C)** show parameters for Hopf-instabilities at 4 Hz dependent on N_2 for which the corresponding values of N_1 obey $N_1 < N_{1,\min} = 1.12$ and **(C)** $N_1 \geq 1.12$, respectively. Panels **(D,E)** show parameters for Hopf-instabilities at 10 Hz for $N_1 < N_{1,\min} = 1.45$ and $N_1 \geq 1.45$, respectively. In each panel **(B–E)** the top line reflects no oscillations, i.e., $f = 0$ Hz, and the bottom line denotes the corresponding stability threshold. Hence the shaded areas include parameters for which the system exhibits stable oscillations. The black solid and dotted lines reflect the situation of no anesthetic action, i.e., $p = 1.0$. The red-dashed line denotes the values of $\tau_1/\tau_2 \times p$ with $p = 1.3$. The arrows illustrate how the parameters change when anesthetic action is increased, i.e., when p is increased.

and $P(i\omega) = -\omega^2 - i\omega Tr + det$ using the definitions of Tr and det in Equations (12) and (13). In fact, $P(i\omega)$ in Equations (17) and (18) is the characteristic polynom in Equation (11) for $\lambda = i\omega$.

In the following in a good approximation (Nunez and Srinivasan, 2006) we assume that the experimental encephalographic data that we want to model originates from the excitatory synapses, i.e., $x(t)$. This assumption is reasonable since the encephalographic activity is observed due to aligned apical dendritic branches and more excitatory synapses than inhibitory synapses are located on the apical branches of dendrites on cortical neurons. However, it is also possible to derive the power spectral density for the difference of excitatory and inhibitory potentials $x(t) - y(t)$ (Hutt and Longtin, 2009). Now the application of the residue theorem allows to compute the integrals in Equation (17) by

$$G_{11}(t) = \frac{1}{2\pi i}\sum_{n=1}^{2} \mathrm{Res}(z_n)\Theta(t)$$

with the residues

$$\mathrm{Res}(z_1) = \frac{1}{2\pi i}\frac{\lambda_1 + (N_2+1)/\tau_2}{\lambda_1 - \lambda_2}e^{\lambda_1 t},$$

$$\mathrm{Res}(z_2) = \frac{1}{2\pi i}\frac{\lambda_2 + (N_2+1)/\tau_2}{\lambda_2 - \lambda_1}e^{\lambda_2 t}$$

and the roots $\lambda_1 = \lambda_2^* = R + i\Omega$ of the characteristic polynom $P(\lambda) = 0$ in Equation (11). This solution is valid if and only if $\mathrm{Res}(\lambda_n) = R < 0$. These yields

$$G_{11}(t) = e^{Rt}\left(\frac{R+Z}{\Omega}\sin(\Omega t) + \cos(\Omega t)\right)\Theta(t)$$

with $Z = -(N_2+1)/\tau_2$, i.e., the Greens function of x, and hence $x(t)$ itself oscillates with frequency Ω and is damped with the factor $|R|$. In other words, the solution x oscillates with the imaginary part of the root of the characteristic equation, and this frequency is already determined in the stability analysis.

Finally, the power spectral density $S(\omega)$ of x is the Fourier transform of the auto-correlation function $\langle x(t)x(t-T)\rangle$:

$$S(\omega) = 2D\sqrt{2\pi}|\tilde{G}_{11}(\omega)|^2$$
$$= 2D\sqrt{2\pi}\frac{Z^2+\omega^2}{(R^2+\Omega^2-\omega^2)^2+4R^2\omega^2} \quad (19)$$

where $\tilde{G}_{11}(\omega)$ is the Fourier transform of the Greens function $G_{11}(t)$.

3.5. THE FREQUENCY OF MAXIMUM POWER SPECTRAL DENSITY

According to the reversed-engineering approach motivated in the previous section, this section aims to derive further conditions on model constants for certain oscillations close to instabilities. This vicinity to the stability threshold guarantees a small damping factor R and thus the power peak is located close to Ω.

There is a maximum frequency ω_m of the oscillation frequency with respect to τ_2 given in Equation (15) and reached at

$$\frac{\tau_2}{\tau_1} = \frac{b}{c} \rightarrow \omega_m = \frac{1}{2}\sqrt{c/\tau_2^2 - a/\tau_1^2} \quad \text{if} \quad \frac{\tau_2}{\tau_1} < \sqrt{c/a}. \quad (20)$$

The last condition is identical to the stability condition (14), i.e., stable systems always have a non-vanishing maximum frequency $\omega_m > 0$. Together with Equation (16):

- If $b/c < \sqrt{c/a}$, then the frequency Ω may increase or decrease while increasing τ_2 with

$$\frac{d\Omega}{d\tau_2} > 0 \quad \text{for} \quad \frac{\tau_2^-}{\tau_1} \leq \frac{\tau_2}{\tau_2} < \frac{b}{c}, \quad (21)$$

$$\frac{d\Omega}{d\tau_2} \leq 0 \quad \text{for} \quad \frac{b}{c} \leq \frac{\tau_2}{\tau_2} \leq \sqrt{\frac{c}{a}}. \quad (22)$$

- If $b/c \geq \sqrt{c/a}$, then the frequency Ω increases only while increasing τ_2 with

$$\frac{d\Omega}{d\tau_2} > 0 \quad \text{for} \quad \frac{\tau_2^-}{\tau_1} \leq \frac{\tau_2}{\tau_2} \leq \sqrt{\frac{c}{a}}. \quad (23)$$

Figure 1 shows the case $b/c < \sqrt{c/a}$. There increasing τ_2 by increasing p from small frequencies on the left border for constant τ_1 increases the oscillation frequency until reaching the dotted line, i.e., $d\Omega/d\tau_2 > 0$. Then a further increase of p decreases the frequency of the oscillations again, $d\Omega/d\tau_2 < 0$. Although this reasoning assumes that $N_2(p)$ does not change with p, it gives a first insight into the dependence of the systems oscillation frequencies on p.

Now considering the power spectral density (Equation 19), for $R^4 + R^2(2\Omega^2 - 3Z^2) + \Omega^2(\Omega^2 + Z^2) > 0$ $S(\omega)$ has a global maximum at

$$\Omega_{\text{peak}} = \sqrt{\Omega^2 + R^2\left(1 - 4\frac{Z^2}{R^2+\Omega^2+Z^2}\right)}.$$

We learn that a vanishing real part of the characteristic root $|R|$ yields a global maximum of the power spectral density at the imaginary part of the characteristic root Ω. From a reversed-engineer point of view, one could say that a strong peak in the experimental power spectral density reflects a characteristic root in the underlying linear system with a small real part. This way to interpret the spectral results allows to find analytical conditions for physiological parameters, as will be seen below.

If $R^4 + R^2(2\Omega^2 - 3Z^2) + \Omega^2(\Omega^2 + Z^2) < 0$, then the system exhibits a global maximum at $\Omega_{\text{peak}} = 0$. Since R and Ω depend on the anesthetic concentration, i.e., the parameter p, it is interesting to examine how Ω_{peak} depends on R and Ω:

$$\frac{d\Omega_{\text{peak}}}{dR} > 0 \quad \text{for} \quad R^2 > Z^2(p) - \Omega^2 \text{ or } R^2 < Z^2(p) - \Omega^2 \quad (24)$$

$$\frac{d\Omega_{\text{peak}}}{d\Omega} > 0 \quad \text{for} \quad R^2 > \sqrt{2}|Z(p)|\Omega - \Omega^2 + Z^2(p)$$
$$\text{or} \quad R^2 < -\sqrt{2}|Z(p)|\Omega - \Omega^2 + Z^2(p) \quad (25)$$

Figure 3 illustrates these conditions and shows that Ω_{peak} is increased or decreased subjected to values of R and Ω. Importantly, we observe in **Figure 3** that Ω_{peak} increases with R and Ω for large frequencies Ω.

It remains to examine how R^2 and Ω^2 depend on p to finally gain the full description how Ω_{peak} changes with p. To this end, we consider the specific assumption (Equation 9) on the anesthetic action yielding the specific dependence of Ω^2 and R^2 to p

$$\frac{d^2R}{dp} = -2\frac{R}{\tau_2(1)}\frac{1}{p^2} > 0$$

$$\frac{d\Omega^2}{dp} = -\frac{2}{\tau_2(1)p^2}\left(A - \frac{1}{\tau_2(1)p}\right)$$

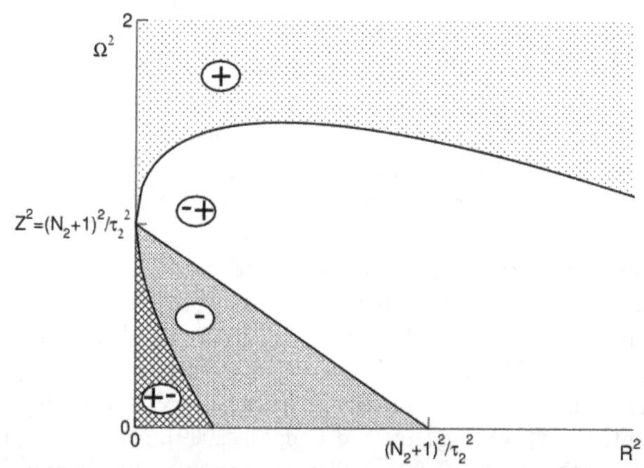

FIGURE 3 | Illustration of the conditions (24) and (25). The regions are marked as follows: (+): $d\Omega_{\text{peak}}/d\Omega > 0$, $d\Omega_{\text{peak}}/dR > 0$; (∓): $d\Omega_{\text{peak}}/d\Omega < 0$, $d\Omega_{\text{peak}}/dR > 0$; (−): $d\Omega_{\text{peak}}/d\Omega < 0$, $d\Omega_{\text{peak}}/dR < 0$; (±): $d\Omega_{\text{peak}}/d\Omega > 0$, $d\Omega_{\text{peak}}/dR < 0$.

with $A = (1 - N_1)/\tau_1 - N_2(1)/\tau_2(1)$, $N_2(p) = N_2(1)p$, and $\tau_2 = \tau_2(1)p$. Defining $p_0 = (N_2(1) + \tau_2(1)(N_1 - 1)/\tau_1)^{-1}$ and re-calling $p \geq 1$, then there exist two distinct cases:

- If $p_0 < 1$, then $d\Omega^2/dp > 0$ for all p. Specifically, this stipulates
$$N_2(1) > 1 + \frac{\tau_2(1)}{\tau_1} - \frac{\tau_2(1)}{\tau_1}N_1.$$
- If $p_0 \geq 1$, then there is a small interval $1 \leq p \leq p_0$ for which $d\Omega^2/dp \leq 0$. For larger p, $d\Omega/dp > 0$. For instance, for $p_0 = 1.3$, i.e.,
$$N_2(1) = 1/1.3 + \frac{\tau_2(1)}{\tau_1} - \frac{\tau_2(1)}{\tau_1}N_1,$$
the frequency decreases with increasing p for clinically reasonable concentrations, i.e., $1 \leq p \leq 1.3$ (Hutt and Longtin, 2009).

Figure 4 illustrates the parameter space where $d\Omega^2/dp$ has different signs and we observe that the system may exhibit either increasing or decreasing frequencies while increasing p.

To elucidate the systems behavior at the stability threshold, we set $\tau_2(1)/\tau_1 = (N_2(1) + 1)/(N_1 - 1)$ according to Equation (14) and find $p_0 = 1/(2N_2(1) + 1) < 1$. Consequently, oscillations close to the stability threshold always increase their frequencies with increasing p. In contrast, for $1 < \tau_2(1)/\tau_1 \ll (N_2(1) + 1)/(N_1 - 1)$, i.e., systems far from the stability threshold, may exhibit values $p_0 > 1$.

Finally, **Figure 5** illustrates the temporal dynamics in two different frequency bands close to the corresponding Hopf-instabilities and shows the effect of increased propofol concentration. The power increases and the peak of maximum power moves to larger frequencies as predicted by the theory and as observed in experiments (Hindriks and van Putten, 2012).

4. DISCUSSION

The introduced model considers first-order synaptic responses and take into account experimental findings on the propofol effect in synaptic $GABA_A$-receptors in cortical neurons. It describes the evolution of neural populations on a mesoscopic level involving major properties of underlying neurons and synapses on the microscopic description level.

The analytical study reveals that the frequency of maximum power may increase or decrease with increasing anesthetic concentration subjected to the physiological constants, cf. **Figure 3**. In detail, close to the oscillatory instability the frequency of maximum power always increases with increasing p as observed in EEG (Gugino et al., 2001; Feshchenko et al., 2004; Hindriks and van Putten, 2012), whereas far from the stability threshold the maximum power frequency may also decrease as observed recently in EEG (Ching et al., 2010; Cimenser et al., 2011), cf. **Figures 3, 4**. The analytical treatment shows clearly that these two findings depend strongly on the physiological parameters, which are derived analytically in section 3.5, i.e., the phenomena depend on the brain area in which they are generated.

Moreover, the analytically predicted increase of the power at higher frequencies explains the power enhancement in the α- and β-band in anesthesia (Gugino et al., 2001; McCarthy et al., 2008) by a dynamic oscillatory instability. In fact, the analytical treatment in the present work suggests that power enhancement always starts from oscillatory activity at lower frequencies

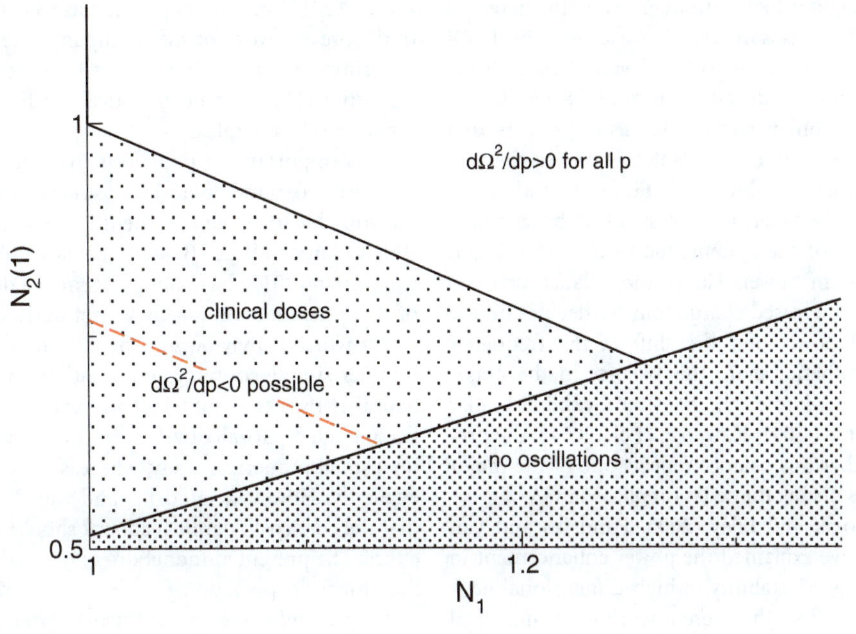

FIGURE 4 | Parameter space for different signs of $d\Omega^2/dp$. The red line denotes $p_0 = 1.3$ and the parameter space of clinical doses (red) implies $d\Omega^2/dp < 0$ for clinically reasonable drug doses, i.e., $p \leq 1.3$. An additional parameter is $r = \tau_2(1)/\tau_1 = 1.11$.

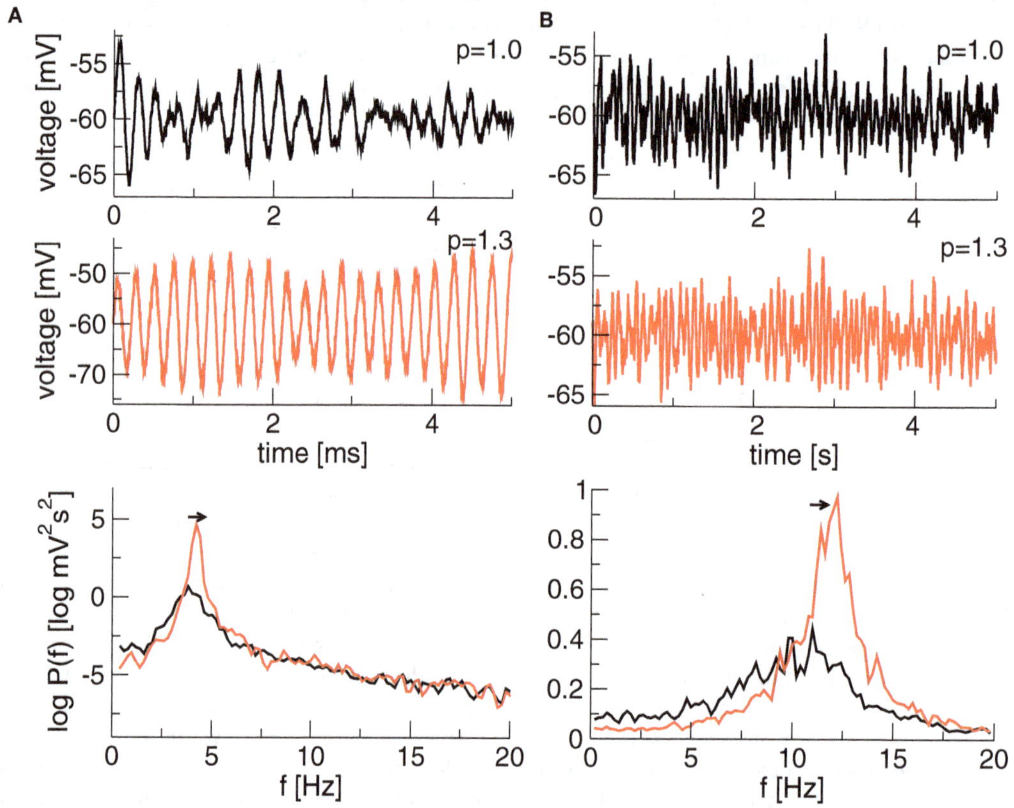

FIGURE 5 | Simulated time series of $x(t) + V_e^0$ and the corresponding power spectrum of $x(t)$. (A) $N_1 = 1.1$, $N_2 = p \times 0.25128$, $\tau_2 = \tau_1 \times p/0.10$ generating a maximum power in the δ-band. **(B)** $N_1 = 1.1$, $N_2 = 0.2236 \times p$, $\tau_2 = \tau_1 \times p/0.10$ generating a maximum in the α-band. Other parameters are $\tau_1 = 2\,\text{ms}$, the noise strength $\kappa = 0.01\,\text{mV}$ and $V_e^0 = -60\,\text{mV}$. The Equation (10) is simulated with a Euler–Maryuama method for 200 s, time step was $\Delta t = 0.05\,\text{ms}$.

and are generated at slightly higher frequencies with increased concentration (**Figure 5**). This is in accordance to previous EEG-studies (Gugino et al., 2001; Hindriks and van Putten, 2012) showing power enhancement induced in the α- and β-band.

The analytical discussion in section 3.3 also predicts that decreasing the inhibitory time constant always moves the system toward an oscillatory instability, cf. **Figure 1**, and hence increases the spectral power, whereas increasing the charge transfer yields a stabilization of the system due to $dR/dP < 0$ and consequently a decrease of power. Hence the balance between decay prolongation and increased charge transfer decides on the change of the spectral power and the shift of the frequency peaks. Since many anesthetics share this balance in the major target $GABA_A$-receptor (Alkire et al., 2008) and exhibit similar EEG-change (Gugino et al., 2001; Kuizenga et al., 2001), the presented work suggests that this balance reflects one of the major underlying mechanisms during the sedation phase in GA.

Previous studies (Bojak and Liley, 2005; Hindriks and van Putten, 2012) already have explained the power enhancement in anesthesia by an oscillatory instability in high-dimensional neural models. As one of the first, the present work gives analytical conditions on physiological parameters for this effect, while Bojak and Liley (2005) and Hindriks and van Putten (2012) mainly performed numerical studies. The recent work of Hindriks and van Putten (2012) resembles in some aspects the analytical approach of the present work by discussing in some detail the dynamics of superimposed oscillation modes subjected to the propofol concentration. However, no analytical conditions are given due to the higher model complexity.

It is important to point out that the current model is low-dimensional, physiologically reasonable and analytically treatable but still able to explain the neural phenomenon of the frequency shift to larger values. Bojak and Liley (2005) and Hindriks and van Putten (2012) have not performed a detailed analytical study of this phenomenon and have not derived analytical conditions under which it may occur. The current work shows that already a rather simple coupling of excitation and inhibition in cortical neural networks is sufficient to explain this phenomenon. This is concluded partially by Hindriks and van Putten (2012) based on a small numerical study, whereas the present work shows this explicitly. However, Hindriks and van Putten (2012) also argue that the cortico-thalamic feedback should be negative to gain this effect. The presented model does not need the thalamic feedback loop for the explanation.

In principle, the present work extends the work of Bojak and Liley (2005) studying just numerically a rather complicated model with tens of unknown parameters, while the current model allows to achieve some insights into the effect of few parameters.

For instance, the maximum of spectral power and the corresponding frequency are highly sensitive to modification of the relation between excitatory and inhibitory synaptic time scales. This confirms the general observation that many different anesthetics share effects on the activity spectrum.

The work both supports the hypothesis of cortical generation of α-activity and predicts the presence of oscillating neural circuits where each circuit generates a certain oscillation observed experimentally. This can be observed in **Figure 5** showing emerging δ- and α-activity for different parameters. Hence two neural circuits with different properties may explain the occurrence of both δ- and α-activity observed in experimental data. This interpretation of the results complements the findings of Hindriks and van Putten (2012) showing implicitly a linear decomposition into eigenmodes with corresponding eigenvalues and manifests the notion of interacting oscillation modes generated by interacting networks as observed experimentally (Fries, 2009; Spaak et al., 2012).

Of course the present model is limited since it cannot explain the increase of activity in the δ-band as observed in experiments and modeled by the previous studies. In the present work, we observe clearly that this synchronous modeling of two rhythms is not possible since the model is too low-dimensional and just can describe a single rhythm such as the α- or the δ-rhythm. Consequently further neural elements should be considered to gain this additional rhythm such as the thalamic loop. This may be possible due to the linear superposition of oscillatory activity originating from different networks. This linear superposition proposes the interaction of different sub-networks each oscillating in a certain frequency band. Future work will consider such entangled neural networks on the basis of the presented neural field to explain the spontaneous emergence or diminution of spectral peaks in experimentally observed data such as the δ-rhythms or transient phenomena such as paradoxical excitation.

ACKNOWLEDGMENTS

The author thanks Meysam Hashemi for fruitful discussions and acknowledges funding from the European Research Council for support under the European Union's Seventh Framework Programme (FP7/2007-2013)/ERC grant agreement No. 257253. The author thanks the referees for valuable comments.

REFERENCES

Alkire, M., Hudetz, A., and Tononi, G. (2008). Consciousness and anesthesia. *Science* 322, 876–880.

Amari, S. (1977). Dynamics of pattern formation in lateral-inhibition type neural fields. *Biol. Cybern.* 27, 77–87.

Angelucci, A., and Bressloff, P. (2006). The contribution of feedforward, lateral and feedback connections to the classical receptive field center and extra-classical receptive field surround of primate v1 neurons. *Prog. Brain Res.* 154, 93–121.

Bojak, I., and Liley, D. (2005). Modeling the effects of anesthesia on the electroencephalogram. *Phys. Rev. E* 71:041902. doi: 10.1103/PhysRevE.71.041902

Boly, M., Moran, R., Murphy, M., Boveroux, P., Bruno, M. A., Noirhomme, Q., et al. (2012). Connectivity changes underlying spectral eeg changes during propofol-induced loss of consciousness. *J. Neurosci.* 32, 7082–7090.

Ching, S., Cimenser, A., Purdon, P. L., Brown, E. N., and Kopell, N. J. (2010). Thalamocortical model for a propofol-induced-rhythm associated with loss of consciousness. *Proc. Natl. Acad. Sci. U.S.A.* 107, 22665–22670.

Cimenser, A., Purdon, P. L., Pierce, E. T., Walsh, J. L., Salazar-Gomez, A. F., Harrell, P. G., et al. (2011). Tracking brain states under general anesthesia by using global coherence analysis. *Proc. Natl. Acad. Sci. U.S.A.* 108, 8832–8837.

Coombes, S., Venkov, N., Shiau, L., Bojak, I., Liley, D., and Laing, C. (2007). Modeling electrocortical activity through improved local approximations of integral neural field equations. *Phys. Rev. E* 76, 051901–051908.

Ermentrout, G. (1998). Neural networks as spatio-temporal pattern-forming systems. *Rep. Progr. Phys.* 61, 353–430.

Ermentrout, G., and Cowan, J. (1979). A mathematical theory of visual hallucination patterns. *Biol. Cybern.* 34, 137–150.

Feshchenko, V. A., Veselis, R. A., and Reinsel, R. A. (2004). Propofol-induced alpha rhythm. *Neuropsychobiology* 50, 257–266.

Franks, N., and Lieb, W. (1994). Molecular and cellular mechanisms of general anesthesia. *Nature* 367, 607–614.

Fries, P. (2009). Neuronal gamma-band synchronization as a fundamental process in cortical computation. *Annu. Rev. Neurosci.* 32, 209–224.

Gugino, L. D., Chabot, R. J., Prichep, L. S., John, E. R., Formanek, V., and Aglio, L. S. (2001). Quantitative eeg changes associated with loss and return of conscious- ness in healthy adult volunteers anaesthetized with propofol or sevoflurane. *Br. J. Anaesth.* 87, 421–428.

Hindriks, R., and van Putten, M. J. A. M. (2012). Meanfield modeling of propofol-induced changes in spontaneous eeg rhythms. *Neuroimage* 60, 2323–2344.

Huang, X., Troy, W., Schiff, S., Yang, Q., Ma, H., Laing, C., et al. (2004). Spiral waves in disinhibited mammalian neocortex. *J. Neurosci.* 24, 9897–9902.

Hutt, A. (2008). Additive noise may change the stability of nonlinear systems. *Europhys. Lett.* 84:34003. doi: 10.1209/0295-5075/84/34003

Hutt, A. (ed.). (2011). *Sleep and Anesthesia: Neural Correlates in Theory and Experiment.* Springer Series in Computational Neuroscience, Vol. 15. New York, NY: Springer.

Hutt, A. (2012). The population firing rate in the presence of gabaergic tonic inhibition in single neurons and application to general anaesthesia. *Cogn. Neurodyn.* 6, 227–237.

Hutt, A., and Longtin, A. (2009). Effects of the anesthetic agent propofol on neural populations. *Cogn. Neurodyn.* 4, 37–59.

Hutt, A., Longtin, A., and Schimansky-Geier, L. (2007). Additive global noise delays turing bifurcations. *Phys. Rev. Lett.* 98:230601. doi: 10.1103/PhysRevLett.98.230601

Kitamura, A., Marszalec, W., Yeh, J., and Narahashi, T. (2002). Effects of halothane and propofol on excitatory and inhibitory synaptic transmission in rat cortical neurons. *J. Pharmacol.* 304, 162–171.

Koch, C. (1999). *Biophysics of Computation.* Oxford: Oxford University Press.

Kuizenga, K., Wierda, J., and Kalkman, C. (2001). Biphasic eeg changes in relation to loss of consciousness during induction with thiopental, propofol, etomidate, midazolam or sevoflurane. *Br. J. Anaesth.* 86, 354–360.

Liley, D., and Bojak, I. (2005). Understanding the transition to seizure by modeling the epileptiform activity of general anaesthetic agents. *J. Clin. Neurophysiol.* 22, 300–313.

McCarthy, M. M., Brown, E. N., and Kopell, N. (2008). Potential network mechanisms mediating electroencephalographic beta rhythm changes during propofol-induced paradoxical excitation. *J. Neurosci.* 28, 13488–13504.

Murphy, M., Bruno, M.-A., Riedner, B. A., Boveroux, P., Noirhomme, Q., Landsness, E. C., et al. (2011). Propofol anesthesia and sleep: a high-density eeg study. *Sleep* 34, 283–291.

Nunez, P., and Srinivasan, R. (2006). *Electric Fields of the Brain: The Neurophysics of EEG.* Oxford, NY: Oxford University Press.

Orser, B. (2006). Extrasynaptic gabaa receptors are critical targets for sedative-hypnotic drugs. *J. Clin. Sleep Med.* 2, S12–S18.

Schwabe, L., Obermayer, K., Angelucci, A., and Bressloff, P. (2006). The role of feedback in shaping the extra-classical receptive field of cortical neurons: a recurrent network model. *J. Neurosci.* 26, 9117–9126.

Spaak, E., Bonnefond, M., Maier, A., Leopold, D. A., and Jensen, O. (2012). Layer-specific entrainment of gamma-band neural activity by the alpha rhythm in monkey visual cortex. *Curr. Biol.* 22, 2313–2318.

Steyn-Ross, M., Steyn-Ross, D., and Sleigh, J. (2004). Modelling general anaesthesia as a first-order phase transition in the cortex. *Prog. Biophys. Molec. Biol.* 85, 369–385.

Steyn-Ross, M., Steyn-Ross, D., Sleigh, J., and Wilcocks, L. (2001). Toward a theory of the general-anesthetic-induced phase transition of the cerebral cortex: I. a thermodynamic analogy. *Phys. Rev. E* 64:011917. doi: 10.1103/PhysRevE.64.011917

Steyn-Ross, M., Steyn-Ross, D., and Sleigh, J. W. (2012). Gap junctions modulate seizures in a mean-field model of general anesthesia for the cortex. *Cogn. Neurodyn.* 6, 215–225.

Steyn-Ross, M., Steyn-Ross, D., Sleigh, J. W., and Liley, D. T. J. (1999). Theoretical electroencephalogram stationary spectrum for a white-noise-driven cortex: evidence for a general anesthetic-induced phase transition. *Phys. Rev. E* 60, 7299–7311.

Wilson, H., and Cowan, J. (1972). Excitatory and inhibitory interactions in localized populations of model neurons. *Biophys. J.* 12, 1–24.

Ying, S., and Goldstein, P. (2005). Propofol suppresses synaptic responsiveness of somatosensory relay neurons to excitatory input by potentiating gabaa receptor chloride channels. *Mol. Pain* 1:2. doi: 10.1186/1744-8069-1-2

2

Neural masses and fields in dynamic causal modeling

Rosalyn Moran [1,2,3*†], Dimitris A. Pinotsis [1†] and Karl Friston [1]

[1] Wellcome Trust Centre for Neuroimaging, Institute of Neurology, University College London, London, UK
[2] Virginia Tech Carilion Research Institute, Virginia Tech, Roanoke, VA, USA
[3] Bradley Department of Electrical and Computer Engineering, Virginia Tech, Blacksburg, VA, USA

Correspondence:
Rosalyn Moran, Virginia Tech Carilion Research Institute, Virginia Tech, 2 Riverside Drive, Roanoke, 24016 VA, USA
e-mail: rosalynj@vtc.vt.edu

† These authors have contributed equally to this work.

Dynamic causal modeling (DCM) provides a framework for the analysis of effective connectivity among neuronal subpopulations that subtend invasive (electrocorticograms and local field potentials) and non-invasive (electroencephalography and magnetoencephalography) electrophysiological responses. This paper reviews the suite of neuronal population models including neural masses, fields and conductance-based models that are used in DCM. These models are expressed in terms of sets of differential equations that allow one to model the synaptic underpinnings of connectivity. We describe early developments using neural mass models, where convolution-based dynamics are used to generate responses in laminar-specific populations of excitatory and inhibitory cells. We show that these models, though resting on only two simple transforms, can recapitulate the characteristics of both evoked and spectral responses observed empirically. Using an identical neuronal architecture, we show that a set of conductance based models—that consider the dynamics of specific ion-channels—present a richer space of responses; owing to non-linear interactions between conductances and membrane potentials. We propose that conductance-based models may be more appropriate when spectra present with multiple resonances. Finally, we outline a third class of models, where each neuronal subpopulation is treated as a field; in other words, as a manifold on the cortical surface. By explicitly accounting for the spatial propagation of cortical activity through partial differential equations (PDEs), we show that the topology of connectivity—through local lateral interactions among cortical layers—may be inferred, even in the absence of spatially resolved data. We also show that these models allow for a detailed analysis of structure–function relationships in the cortex. Our review highlights the relationship among these models and how the hypothesis asked of empirical data suggests an appropriate model class.

Keywords: dynamic causal modeling, electroencephalography, magnetoencephalography (MEG), local field potential (LFP), neural mass models

INTRODUCTION

Over the past two decades, BOLD neuroimaging techniques have been successfully applied in human studies to identify regions of functional specialization, to within a scale of a few millimeters (Ashburner, 2012). Electrophysiological recordings including magneto- and electro-encephalography (M/EEG) offer an aggregate measure of neuronal activity (in the order of hundreds of thousands of neurons) but at a millisecond timescale (Baillet et al., 2001; Nunez and Srinivasan, 2006). Though localizing activity is mathematically ill-posed in these electromagnetic modalities, the wealth of spatial information from fMRI studies can now support M/EEG as a powerful modality for the analysis of functional integration in the human brain.

Dynamic causal modeling (DCM) is designed to probe the mechanisms of effective connectivity (the influence of one brain region on another) that underlie multi-region network responses in neuroimaging (fMRI, M/EEG) data. The approach uses a neurobiologically motivated model which is inverted or fitted to empirical observations using Bayesian techniques (Daunizeau et al., 2011). These comprise separate generative processes at the neuronal level and at the observation level. For M/EEG, neural mass and neural field models in particular are used, to support this analysis by quantifying the temporal and spatiotemporal evolution of macroscopic brain activity, using physiologically plausible dynamics. In DCM; as implemented in the SPM software (Litvak et al., 2011), neural mass and field models are used as generative models to infer the synaptic parameters and effective connectivity that constitute active brain networks. More recently, these models have been applied in (single-region) DCMs as a "mathematical microscope"—to test synaptic hypotheses at the level of specific laminae and receptors (Moran et al., 2011b), and disambiguate between structural and functional hypotheses; for example, explaining intersubject variations in gamma oscillations (Pinotsis et al., 2013b). In this review, we summarize the state-of-the-art in modeling such population-based activity and demonstrate their use in the context of DCM. The development of these modeling approaches has been underpinned by pioneering developments several decades ago that produced generative models of EEG data characteristics based on neural masses (Wilson and Cowan, 1972; Nunez, 1974; Freeman, 1975, 1987;

Jansen and Rit, 1995; Valdes et al., 1999; Wendling et al., 2000). These models have since been refined and extended (Wright and Liley, 1996; Rennie et al., 2000) to examine a myriad of neurobiological processes including anesthesia (Steyn-Ross et al., 1999), epilepsy (Breakspear et al., 2006; Marten et al., 2009; Nevado-Holgado et al., 2012), "resting state" brain dynamics (Deco and Jirsa, 2012), and so on. The types of models we will review here have played a direct implementational role in DCM and do not represent an exhaustive overview—a non DCM-centric treatment is provided in Deco et al. (2008). Here we consider, in particular, how DCM treats ensemble neuronal activity as a point process (neural mass models) or explicitly incorporate a spatial dimension (neural field models). Both types describe so-called "mesoscopic" properties of neural activity, employing statistical mechanics to transform single unit activity into population activity—where appropriate composites can be used to generate macroscopic data. Since this mesoscale is hidden from direct observation, we demonstrate how these models rely upon and exploit knowledge about synaptic and cell physiology, as well as neuroanatomy.

Two distinct biological perspectives have informed the development of neural models, leading to a taxonomy of "convolution" or "conductance-based" models. These distinctions arose from the consideration of cortical mesocolumns—convolution models (Freeman, 1975); and separately from the consideration of a single cell's electrophysiological properties—conductance models (Hodgkin and Huxley, 1952). Early work by Wilson and Cowan (1973) derived a sigmoidal relationship for transforming population membrane potential to an average population firing rate. These models consisted of sigmoidal and convolution-based operators and were refined on the basis of empirical observations by Freeman, Wendling and others (Freeman, 1987; Jansen and Rit, 1995; Wendling et al., 2000). In contrast, conductance based models were formulated as an equivalent circuit model of an excitable cell membrane: Hodgkin–Huxley's original description of the giant squid axon is the classical example of this sort of model—and was reduced to a two dimensional form by Morris and Lecar (1981). Their reduced circuit has been scaled up for M/EEG analysis in DCM using the Fokker-Planck formalism (Breakspear et al., 2010) to describe the evolution of population densities (Marreiros et al., 2009). In this setting, when only the first order statistics (e.g., mean) of the population density are considered, the model describes a neural mass (where the population density can be regarded as a point of mass). When higher order statistics are considered, we obtain a "mean-field" model (where the full density of one population depends on the mean of another). We note that the terminology here is rather specific to DCM; the focus of this review. In other settings, and in other treatments of neuronal activity (Coombes, 2010; Buice and Chow, 2013), mean-field models often refer to population dynamics with interacting means only. However, here we use the term *neural-mass* to refer to an interaction in population means and *mean-field* to higher-order interactions to remain consistent with the DCM literature and to acknowledge the early neural-mass nomenclature developed by Valdez-Sosa and other pioneering work in this field (Valdes et al., 1999). Both neural mass and mean field formulations can be applied to convolution and conductance based models: The choice of either convolution or conductance based model depends on the type of inference required (when applying the model to real data), with the latter offering a richer and biologically more realistic parameterization of synaptic currents.

The deployment of neural mass (or mean field) models of populations in DCM entails further neurobiological plausibility, through a laminar specification of cell types and their interconnectivity. For neocortical studies, a laminar architecture is populated with neuronal ensembles, so that forward (e.g., thalamo-cortical), backward or lateral (e.g., inter-hemispheric) extrinsic connections impinge upon pyramidal, spiny stellate or inhibitory interneurons (David et al., 2006). This construction is motivated by tracing studies in the macaque (Felleman and Van Essen, 1991) and demonstrates the first constraint under which these models were developed for DCM. Namely; that they conform to known physiological and anatomical principles. A second constraint is that they must be able to generate stereotypical features of empirical macroscopic measurements; for example, dominant alpha rhythms (David and Friston, 2003) or late potentials in evoked transients (Garrido et al., 2007a). In this sense, none of the models are "right" or "wrong"—but can be usefully compared to test a particular hypothesis (Box, 1976).

In addition to the distinction between neural mass and mean field formulations of either convolution or conductance based models, we also have to consider the distinction between models based upon ordinary differential equations and partial differential equations (PDEs) that endow neuronal populations with spatial attributes: incorporating the spatial domain into DCM was motivated by the advent of spatially resolved population recording modalities (Pinotsis et al., 2012). This use of neural fields, was proposed as a semi-quantitative treatment of electromagnetic brain activity by Jirsa and Haken (1996, 1997) and Robinson (2006). Crucially neural fields enable local axonal arborization to be modeled directly and can generate topological data features. These may be particularly resolved in high-density subdural grid electrodes (electrocorticography) and optical imaging techniques and also contribute to the topographical distribution of sensor/scalp space measurements in M/EEG.

In this review, we hope to provide a didactic treatment of the neural mass and neural field models available in DCM and highlight application studies that exemplify their use. This complements more general treatments of neural population modeling (Deco et al., 2008). The first section considers convolution-based neural mass models. We will demonstrate their use in inferring causal interactions among multiple brain regions and highlight the minimal assumptions needed to form—and test—competing hypotheses. In this section, we will also introduce the important distinction between different models and different data features; noting that the same models can be used for (and indeed should be capable of generating) different data features. We will focus on the distinction between time and frequency domain responses—highlighting the use of identical neural mass models when modeling evoked and steady state responses. In the second section, we examine conductance-based models and how new currents can be added to enhance physiological detail at the synaptic level. We also examine the impact of second-order interactions among neuronal ensembles in mean field models, particularly in the spectral domain. The third section introduces the spatial parameterization in the form of partial differential or neural field equations—and how these have been applied to test alternative explanations for gamma activity in the visual cortex. In this example, we reconsider lateral connections and the role of distinct pyramidal cell populations. This final model recapitulates "a canonical microcircuit" and provides a framework for investigating differences in directed oscillations. This development was motivated by theoretical considerations about message passing in the brain; namely predictive coding and implications for spectral asymmetries in laminar specific communication (Friston, 2005, 2009). Important asymmetries of the sort are evident in several recent empirical observations (Maier et al., 2010; Buffalo et al., 2011; Bastos et al., 2012) on the laminar specificity of oscillation frequencies. In principle, these sorts of observations can be used with DCM, to address key questions about reciprocal message passing in the brain and its hierarchical architecture.

CONVOLUTION BASED NEURAL MASS MODEL

GENERATIVE MODELS OF EVOKED RESPONSES: THE ERP MODEL

In DCM, event related potentials are modeled as the response of a dynamic input–output system to exogenous (experimental) inputs (David et al., 2006; Kiebel et al., 2006; Garrido et al., 2007b). The DCM generates a predicted ERP as the response of a network of coupled sources to sensory (thalamic) input—with the form of a narrow (16 ms) Gaussian impulse function that accounts for some temporal smoothing in thalamic volleys. Each source is modeled as a point source (c.f., equivalent current dipole) comprising three subpopulations, each assigned to a particular cortical layer. For simplicity, we place an inhibitory subpopulation in the supragranular layer. This receives inputs from excitatory deep pyramidal cells in an infra-granular layer which are, in turn, driven by excitatory spiny cells in the granular layer; layer IV. These three subpopulations are connected with intrinsic coupling parameters as shown in **Figure 1**. Though these models operate as a point process, by specifying different layers we can call on anatomical rules of extrinsic (region to region) connectivity (Felleman and Van Essen, 1991). Specifically,

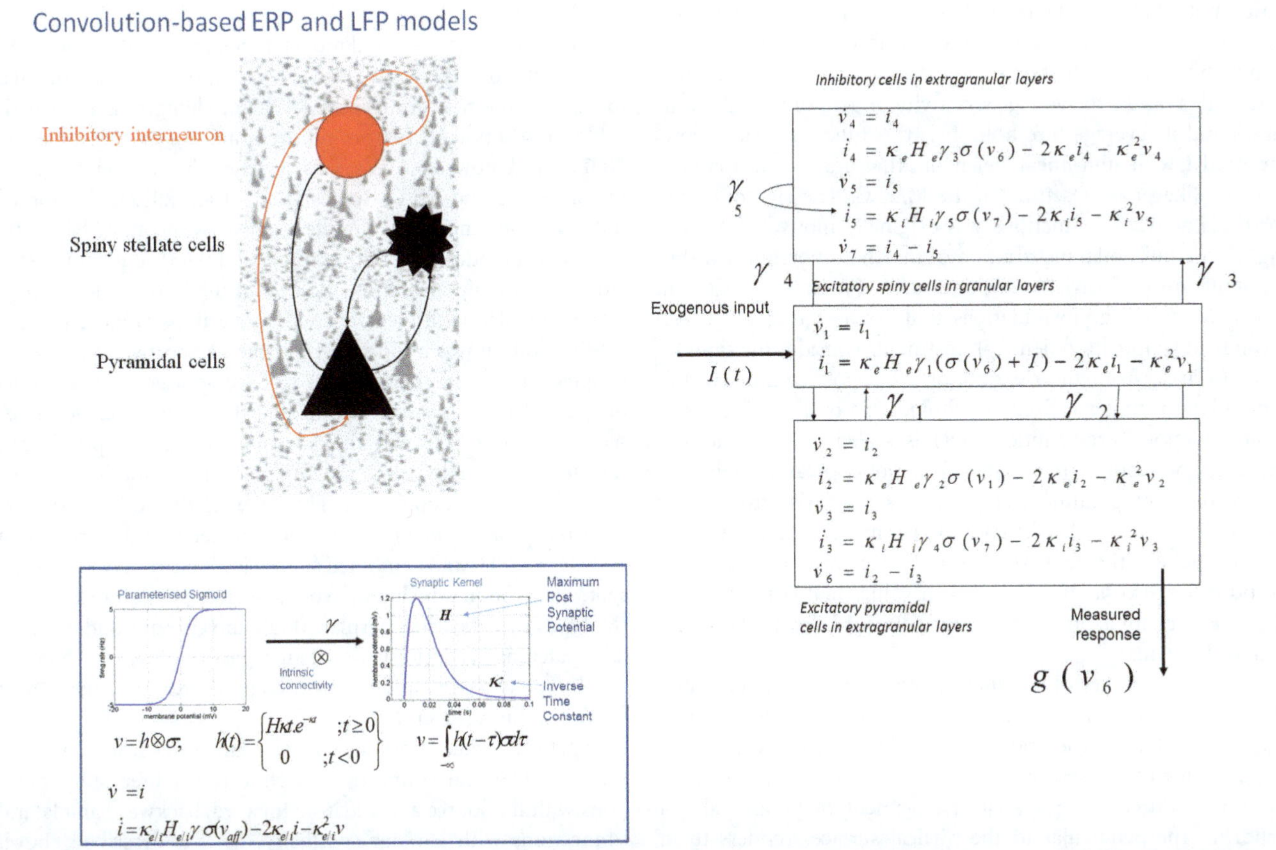

FIGURE 1 | Convolution-based neural mass models: "ERP" and "LFP". Neural mass model used to represent a cortical source. Three cell subpopulations contribute to the ongoing dynamics. These include spiny stellate cells in granular layer IV, pyramidal cells and inhibitory interneurons in extra granular layers (II and III; V and VI). Intrinsic connections, $\gamma_{1,2,3,4,5}$ link subpopulations in each source. Neuronal states include currents, i, and membrane potentials v. Extrinsic connections enter at specific cortical layers (see main text). Right: The functions controlling ongoing dynamics and their parameterization are summarized by synaptic kernels, which are used to convolve presynaptic (firing) input [a sigmoidal function of presynaptic membrane depolarization $\sigma(v)$] to produce postsynaptic depolarization (v), dependent on membrane time constants ($1/\kappa_{e/i}$) and average post-synaptic depolarizations ($H_{e/i}$) at excitatory (e) and inhibitory (i) synapses.

the "ERP" and "LFP" convolution based models can be assembled within a generative network using three distinct types of connections. Forward connections correspond to afferent pyramidal axons and synapse on layer IV stellate cells, while backward afferents impinge upon pyramidal and inhibitory interneurons outside of layer IV. Lateral, inter-hemispheric connections are modeled with a postsynaptic response that is elicited in all layers.

The evolution of neuronal activity in this anatomical architecture is controlled by two simple operations following Jansen and Rit (1995). The first is a convolution operation (**Figure 1**) that lends the model its name and models the average membrane depolarization response as a low-pass impulse response. This transforms the average density of pre-synaptic firing arriving at the population into the average postsynaptic membrane potential (PSP). This response is specified by two biologically informed parameters; one tunes the maximum amplitude of PSPs and represents the receptor density and the second is a lumped representation of the sum of synaptic rate constants (of passive membrane and other spatially distributed delays in the dendritic tree). The output operator (**Figure 1**) then transforms this average membrane potential into the average rate of action potentials fired by the population. This transformation is assumed to be instantaneous and is described by a sigmoid function with parameters that determine its shape and location. These parameters model the voltage sensitivity or gain of the subpopulation and its average threshold. It is this function that endows the model with non-linear behaviors that are crucial for phenomena like phase-resetting of the M/EEG. The sigmoid form for these activation functions was originally motivated as arising from a unimodal distribution of threshold potentials within a population of Heaviside response units (Wilson and Cowan, 1973). More recent formulations that connect directly to full mean field (population density) treatments consider the sigmoid form to arise from the distribution of depolarizations within a population, under a fixed threshold. This output of this sigmoid function (presynaptic input) is scaled by intrinsic and extrinsic connectivity parameters from subpopulations within a source or from pyramidal cell afferents that arise from other sources in the network. Thus activity promulgates and reverberates throughout the network (**Figure 1**). Delays along these connections are also parameterized with values that correspond to the time taken for axonal propagation between layers (~2 ms) and regions (~16 ms).

A pair of ordinary differential equations completely describes the dynamics of each subpopulation within a source (**Figure 1**). These are deterministic and—for a DCM of ERPs—a thalamic impulse timed to correspond to some experimental stimulus perturbs the sources. The spatial arrangement of pyramidal cell dendrites (perpendicular to the cortical surface) renders them the prominent sources of measurable electromagnetic signals and are thus harvested from each source in the network and passed through a lead field, to produce the spatiotemporal patterns observed in M/EEG sensors.

Early applications of this model led to a series of EEG-based investigations into oddball effects by Garrido et al. (2007a, 2008, 2009). The mismatch negativity (MMN) is a negative change in the auditory evoked potential that occurs after an unpredictable change in the acoustic stream. It is elicited, for example, when deviant frequency tones are embedded in a stream of repeated tones. The MMN has a fronto-temporal topology and is thought to reflect the updating of an internal model of the sensorium, where by a sensory prediction error is registered and a new prediction formed (Näätänen et al., 2005). Competing "ERP" neural mass models were compared (in terms of their model evidence, using standard Bayesian techniques) to probe the type of extrinsic connection changes that mediate the MMN. Indicating both a bottom-up sensory prediction error and a top-down change in predictions, a stimulus specific modulation of both forward and backward connections among hierarchically deployed sources exhibited trial specific (deviant compared to standard) modulation (Garrido et al., 2007b). This network and paradigm has since been investigated in pathological settings. A striking example by Boly et al. (2011) used the same model comparison procedure to distinguish between top-down and bottom-up extrinsic connections and their changes with levels of consciousness.

GENERATIVE MODELS OF EVOKED AND SPECTRAL RESPONSES: THE LFP MODEL

A second convolution-based model, named the "LFP" model was developed from the "ERP" model. The model was augmented to address the neurotransmitter basis of changes in intracortical local field potentials from rat prefrontal cortex (Moran et al., 2007)—and now also serves as a generative model for non-invasive EEG and MEG studies (Boly et al., 2012). The model differed from the "ERP" model in two ways: first, based on biophysical models by Whittington et al. (1995) of gamma oscillations in the hippocampus, the role of inhibitory interneurons was augmented with recurrent self-connections (**Figure 1**). This subtle addition was important from the perspective of a new set of questions. Here our goal was to develop a generative model of spectral responses can exhibit high-frequency oscillations. A second extension refined the neurophysiological input-output transforms; whereby spike-rate adaptation was modeled at the input stellate cell population. This involves the addition of currents based on the phenomenological model described by Benda and Herz (2003) and combined several ionic currents modulating spike generation—including voltage-gated potassium currents (M-type currents), the interplay of calcium currents and intracellular calcium dynamics with calcium-gated potassium channels (AHP-type currents) and the slow recovery from inactivation of the fast sodium current.

Practically these additions lead to a larger dynamic repertoire using an identical connectivity architecture (three subpopulations within a source and extrinsic forward, backward and lateral connections with laminar specificity) as that described above. The focus of the LFP model was the reproduction of fast synchronous activity as summarized with the steady-state spectral density (Fourier transform) of time series data. In order to generate steady-state spectral responses, we linearized the model's differential equations around an equilibrium point. This equilibrium or operating point is obtained by integrating the system over a protracted time window. The linearity assumption will accommodate parameter spaces in the region of fixed points and local bifurcations (Friston et al., 2012), known to emerge from this sort of model (Grimbert and Faugeras, 2006). In DCM, the neural masses are treated as a system that is perturbed by white and pink noise; which is explicitly parameterized. This provides a compact summary of the system, where the system's spectral responses can be obtained from its transfer functions, which depend on the physiological parameters of the model (and neural noise) (Nunez, 1974; Steyn-Ross et al., 1999; Robinson et al., 2001; Moran et al., 2007). In other words, the transfer function links unobserved physiological processes to measured spectral responses and is an essential part of forward or generative models of spectral measures. This "LFP" neural mass model was first used in a single-region DCM analysis to demonstrate how one can make inferences about synaptic function at the neuronal level, using macroscopic electrophysiological measurements. This proof of principle used microdialysis measures of extracellular neurotransmitter for validation (Moran et al., 2008) and extended the breadth of applications of DCM—in this case by inferring condition specific modulations of synaptic parameters.

CONDUCTANCE BASED NEURAL MASS MODELS

THE NMM AND MFM

In DCM, the first biophysical model of ensemble activity to receive the three-letter acronym "NMM" was described in Marreiros et al. (2008, 2009). These models parameterize neuronal dynamics at the level of a single neuron and employ density-based flow (the time derivative of neural activity) mechanics to represent the dynamics of a population of neurons. In coupling multiple subpopulations with different characteristics within and between regions, the framework used a mean-field reduction (assumption); where each type of population comprises a probability density and is only affected by the main activity of other neuronal populations or ensembles in the model. This formal population treatment was applied in the context of a conductance-based model predicated on the Morris–Lecar equivalent RC-circuit description of oscillatory membrane properties in barnacle muscle fiber (Morris and Lecar, 1981). These models equate capacitive current (according to Kirchhoff's current law) with the summed active and passive currents across the membrane. Morris–Lecar models can be thought of as reductions of Hodgkin and Huxley's model of the squid axon. They include active currents that describe ligand-gated excitatory (Na^+) and inhibitory (Cl^-) ion flow, mediated through fast glutamatergic and GABAergic receptors, with a potassium leak current used to account for all passive ionic currents (Gutkin et al., 2003); where the conductance of the active channels display first order dynamics that depend on the time constant of the channel and their current state (**Figure 2**).

It may seem that we are conflating the introduction of mean field (versus neural mass) formulations with the introduction of conductance-based models. However, there is a fundamental reason for doing this: in full mean field treatments, the ordinary differential equations describe the dynamics of first and higher-order statistics of population densities—such as the covariance among neuronal states within a population. Crucially, the covariance depends upon the mean of the neuronal states when, and only when, the equations are non-linear in the states (i.e., where the states interact multiplicatively). In other words, the weakly non-linear (sigmoidal) equations of motion of convolution-based models mean that the covariances are not functions of the population averages and therefore do not change with time. This is why one only has to consider first-order statistics in neural mass models based upon (linear) synaptic convolution operators. However, when we move to conductance-based models, there is a necessary interaction between conductance and depolarization, which renders the models intrinsically non-linear. This means that the covariances depend upon the means (and vice versa). It therefore only makes sense to consider mean field treatments of conductance-based models.

Mean field treatments start with a description of a single neuronal response in terms of stochastic differential equations (presented in **Figure 2**) that accommodate noise or fluctuations in neuronal states (Note: In physics generally a mean-field reduction refers to any statistical summary i.e., to first or higher order, to describe population responses. In the context of neuronal population models of brain function, the literature has a adopted a standard where a neural-mass refers to first order and a mean-field; first and higher order interactions (Deco et al., 2008). Marreiros et al. (2009) used these stochastic differential equations to form a set of non-linear ordinary differential equations by applying the Fokker-Planck formalism using the Laplace assumption (or method of moments). This meant that ensemble activity could be modeled without the need to simulate individual unit activity with noisy fluctuations—the neuronal fluctuations are implicit in the population density dynamics. Heuristically, the population density approach is important because it provides a unique prediction or generative model of an empirical response. Mean field formulations of conductance-based models are therefore invertible (can be fitted to data) in the setting of DCM. The resulting expression for the population dynamics; the evolution of the population's mean and variance, decomposes into deterministic flow and diffusion. In turn, these reduce to simple forms under Gaussian (Laplace) assumptions about the population density—where first order population dynamics are a function of flow and the curvature of the flow, and the second order statistics a function of the gradients of flow. However, a DCM of a single source typically comprises three coupled populations (David and Friston, 2003).

For conductance based models in DCM, we employed a similar structure to the "ERP" and "LFP" mass models—with interacting populations of excitatory spiny stellate cells, pyramidal cells and inhibitory interneurons, coupled through intrinsic connections (**Figure 2**). The mean field partition means that these operations can be applied to each population in turn, and lead to simple expressions; given that the gradient and curvature of the equations of motion are only non-zero within a particular ensemble. These equations describe a mean-field model; the "MFM," in which the first and second order sufficient statistics interact, influencing each other when the curvature (derivative of the flow) is non-zero. The formally reduced model, where only first order interactions are considered is termed the "NMM". This point mass interaction is identical to the ERP and LFP

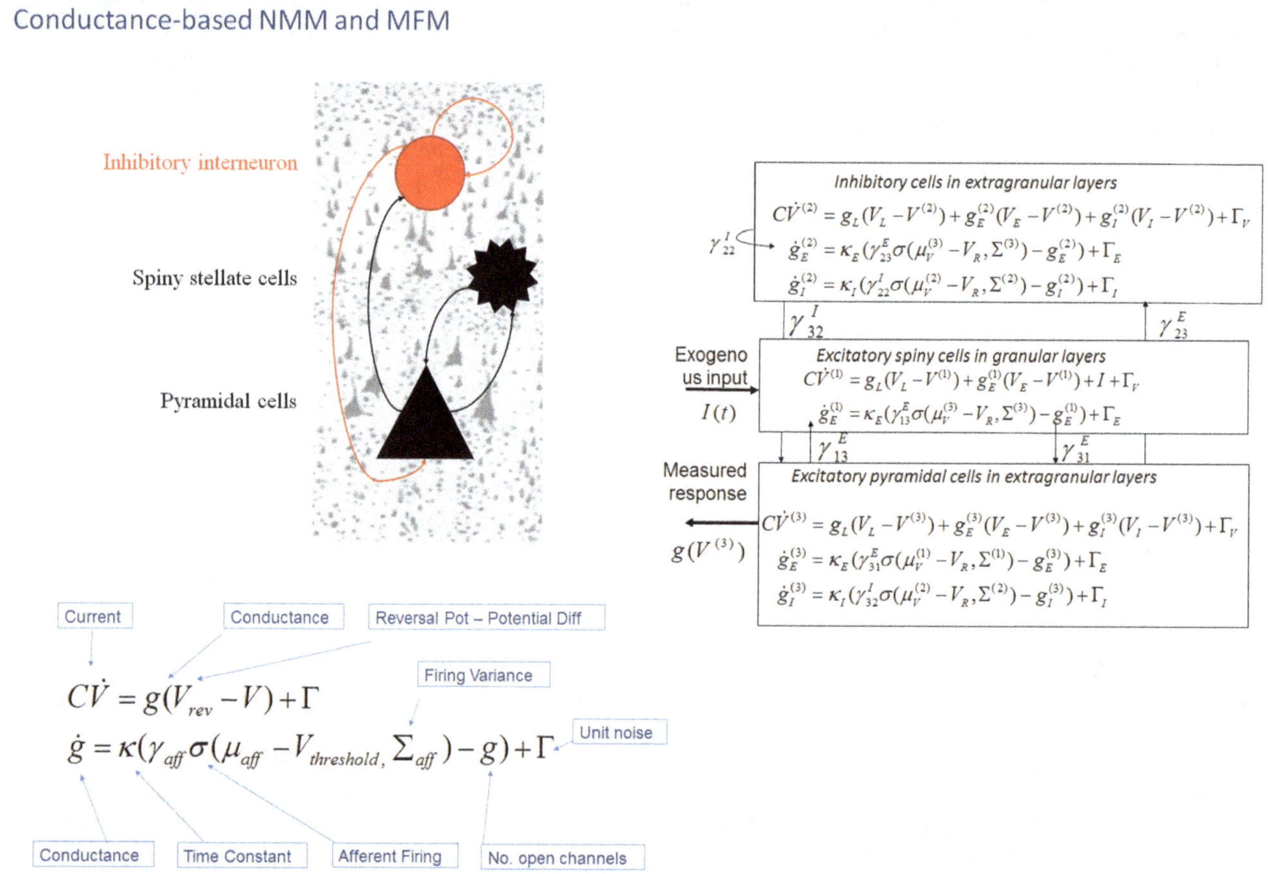

FIGURE 2 | Conductance-based neural mass models: "NMM" and "MFM". This figure shows Morris–Lecar-type differential equations describing the time evolution of a single cell current (capacitance × change of membrane potential: $C\dot{V}$) and conductance (g) at inhibitory interneurons (extra granular layers), spiny stellate cells (granular layers) and pyramidal cells (extra granular layers). In this model, all cell types possess AMPA receptors, $GABA_A$; with ion-channel time constants ($1/\kappa_{e/i}$). Layers are connected with strengths parameterized by γ V_L, V_E, and V_I are reversal potentials for leak potassium channels, sodium, and chloride channels, respectively, at V_T is the threshold potential. NMDA receptors at pyramidal cells and inhibitory interneurons can be added using a conductance equation of similar form, weighted by a voltage dependent switch (Moran et al., 2011a,b). For a full population Fokker-Planck characterization see Marreiros et al. (2008).

models in terms of the effects different subpopulations exert on others, but have a different dynamic form through the equivalent RC circuit description. Unlike the NMM, the MFM allows for expansion (dynamic increase in the variance of the state's associated probability distribution) and contraction (dynamic reduction in the variance of the state's associated probability distribution) of dispersed neuronal states to influence the average flow.

Marreiros et al. (2010) compared DCM using mean-field models (MFM) with dynamically coupled means and variances to a model where the variance was fixed (NMM). In the time domain, a simulated evoked potential elegantly demonstrated the effect of this coupling with the variance of the pyramidal cell population's depolarization contracting to close to zero when the mean approaches its maximum. Within the spectral domain, they similarly showed qualitative differences in the dynamic repertoire—with the MFM displaying limit-cycle attractors after bifurcation from a fixed-point (Marreiros et al., 2009). In this setting, the mean-field model is inherently more non-linear, because it entails non-linear interactions between the first and second order statistics of the hidden states (i.e., dynamic processes that affect the observations, but cannot be directly measured. the activity in interneurons affect signal propagation within regions but due to the random pattern of their dendrites do not directly contribute to the measured field). This speaks to many similar investigations of non-linearity in neural systems (Lopes Da Silva et al., 1989; Destexhe and Babloyantz, 1991; Daffertshofer et al., 2000; Breakspear, 2002; Breakspear and Terry, 2002; Stam, 2005), where the emergence of quasiperiodic, chaotic and itinerant attractors belies a rich set of dynamic phenomena with physiologically plausible interpretations.

THE NMM AND MFM WITH VOLTAGE GATED NMDA RECEPTORS

An extension to the NMM and MFM was presented in Moran et al. (2011a) through the inclusion of a third ligand-gated ion channel to model conductances controlled by the NMDA receptor. NMDA receptor controlled ion channels were considered in a separate treatment since they are both ligand- and voltage-gated. For an NMDA channel to open, following the binding of glutamate, there must first be a large transmembrane potential to remove a magnesium ion blocking the channel. Hence, the dynamics for this particular current are given by an extended equation, which includes the magnesium component using a voltage gated function (**Figure 2**). By introducing NMDA ion channels to pyramidal cells and inhibitory interneurons (Brunel and Wang, 2001), we further constrained and distinguished laminar specific responses. This type of channel afforded another source of non-linearity due to its voltage dependency (Jahr and Stevens, 1990), and required an extension of the steady-state linearization, for both the NMM and MFM case.

To characterize the dynamic repertoire of these models, we examined steady-state responses in the frequency domain to identify regimes where the system settles to a fixed point (i.e., the average activity reaches steady-state) or a limit cycle. In the first regime the spectrum observed is generated by noise, where neuronal populations act as a filter—shaping the noise spectrum to produce a profile of output frequencies. In the second dynamic regime, the average neuronal states themselves may oscillate. In this situation, the system exhibits what is known as a quasiperiodic attractor and the frequency response to noise changes with different points on the attractor (Moran et al., 2011a). This means one has to take the average frequency response over the attractor manifold (i.e., over the limit cycle). Crucially, the frequencies that are preferentially passed by the system are also the frequency of the oscillation (limit cycle). This means the predicted spectral responses to noise under steady state can be seen (and treated mathematically) as a special case that obtains when the attractor collapses to a fixed point. This second regime was particularly evident in the MFM case, where attractor subspaces characteristic of heteroclinic channels were observed—and produced bimodal spectral peaks from local and global state space trajectories.

This richly parameterized neural mass model was then used to examine distinctions among the type of receptors underlying empirical neural activations in EEG and MEG. In Moran et al. (2011b), we tried to recover pharmacologically induced changes in receptor processing using MEG, during a visuo-spatial working memory task. Specifically, parameter estimates from the spectral response in superior frontal gyrus, disclosed an effect of L-Dopa on delay period activity—in terms of how L-dopa changed specific synaptic (connectivity) parameters (**Figure 2**). These effects were exactly commensurate with predictions from the animal and computational literature (Goldman-Rakic, 1996; Durstewitz et al., 2000; Gorelova and Yang, 2000; Gonzalez-Islas and Hablitz, 2003; Durstewitz and Seamans, 2008) and revealed the dual mechanisms of dopaminergic modulation of glutamatergic processing; where L-Dopa increased the non-linearity of post-synaptic responses mediated by NMDA receptors, and decreased AMPA coupling between pyramidal cells and stellate cells. In this study, we also found an L-Dopa-dependent change in exogenous input into the frontal region, which effectively suppresses this region during delay-related reverberatory processing. Moreover, individual parameter estimates from the DCM correlated with individual performance indices (Moran et al., 2011b), a crucial finding that is often used to show that parameter estimates from an NMM reflect real neuronal processes.

SPATIAL HARMONICS AND THE NEURAL FIELD

THE NFM

Pinotsis et al. (Pinotsis and Friston, 2011; Pinotsis et al., 2012) introduced the spatial domain into DCM with neural field models. Neural fields model current fluxes as continuous processes on the cortical sheet, using PDEs. The key advance that neural field models offer, over conventional neural mass models, is that they embody spatial parameters (like the density and extent of lateral connections). This means that, in principle, one can infer the spatial parameters of cortical infrastructures generating electrophysiological signals (and infer changes in those parameters over different levels of an experimental factor) from empirical data. This rests on modeling responses not just in time but also over space. This sort of model should be ideally suited to exploit the temporal dynamics of observed cortical responses with a high spatial resolution; for example, with high-density recordings, at the epidural or intracortical level. However, as demonstrated in early DCM-NFM, the impact of spatially extensive dynamics is not restricted to expression over space but can also have profound effects on temporal (e.g., spectral) responses at one point (or averaged locally over the cortical surface) (Pinotsis et al., 2012). This means that neural field models may also play a key role in the modeling of non-invasive electrophysiological data that does not resolve spatial activity directly. Although, neural mass models can describe patterns in sensor space, the spatial attributes of these patterns result from the coupling among states at different points in source space and not from hidden states that are functions space (i.e., they are described by equations that are time dependent but not spatially dependent).

In terms of anatomical and physiological constraints, functional specialization demands that cells with common functional properties are grouped together. This architectural constraint necessitates both convergence and divergence of cortical connections (Zeki, 1990), of the sort that can be modeled with a neural field model. To model these spatial aspects of connectivity one needs partial differential or integro differential equations that accommodate lateral interactions over spatially extended cortical manifolds. In Pinotsis and Friston (2011), the repertoire of steady state regimes engendered by sparse (patches of) intrinsic connections was examined. Specifically, we considered a bimodal, non-centric distribution and showed (through a Turing instability analysis) that the dispersion relation from this particular arrangement of spatial delays leads to infinite branches of complex spectra. These branches undergo similar conformational changes, under both increased propagation velocity and decreased spatial separation (range) of lateral connections. The resulting fall in the amplitude of high frequency oscillations was also apparent in the spectral summaries of these responses, in terms of cross spectral densities. For example, as the separation of coupled neuronal populations increases, the total spectral power decreases and falls faster for higher frequencies in a manner similar to local coherence functions based on primate recordings (see Leopold et al., 2003) In brief, both the spatial deployment and the speed of lateral connections can have a profound effect on the behavior of spatial harmonics over different scales. Interestingly, it turned out that only synaptic gain was capable of producing phase-transitions: when increasing gain, the system was driven to an unstable regime and oscillations appeared as a result of a Hopf bifurcation.

This neural field model was later extended to a three layered architecture comprising pyramidal cells, inhibitory interneurons and spiny stellate cells (**Figure 3**), where spatial delays result from signals propagating with finite conduction speeds along axonal arbors (Pinotsis et al., 2012). These arbors were arranged with a central distribution of synaptic densities, which decayed exponentially in space. Spatial delays operated along the same intrinsic connections used in ERP neural mass models: the cortical micro circuitry in the "ERP" and "NFM" models. This means that the neural mass and field models are essentially the same; describing the same neurobiological dynamics over time, but where the "NFM" is equipped with spatially extended hidden states that characterize presynaptic input as a spatially-extended process that is propagated along axonal arbors. In contrast the hidden states in a neural mass model are a function of time only. As with the "ERP" and "LFP" models, this model ("NFM") uses a convolution operator to characterize post synaptic filtering and a sigmoid function to accommodate the dispersion of the hidden states of the afferent population (**Figure 3**).

The advantage of neural field models is that they can accommodate spatially extended activity on cortical manifold or patches that endows the predicted responses with a complicated frequency dependency. This allows one to distinguish between spatial effects and other factors (such as intrinsic cell properties) on

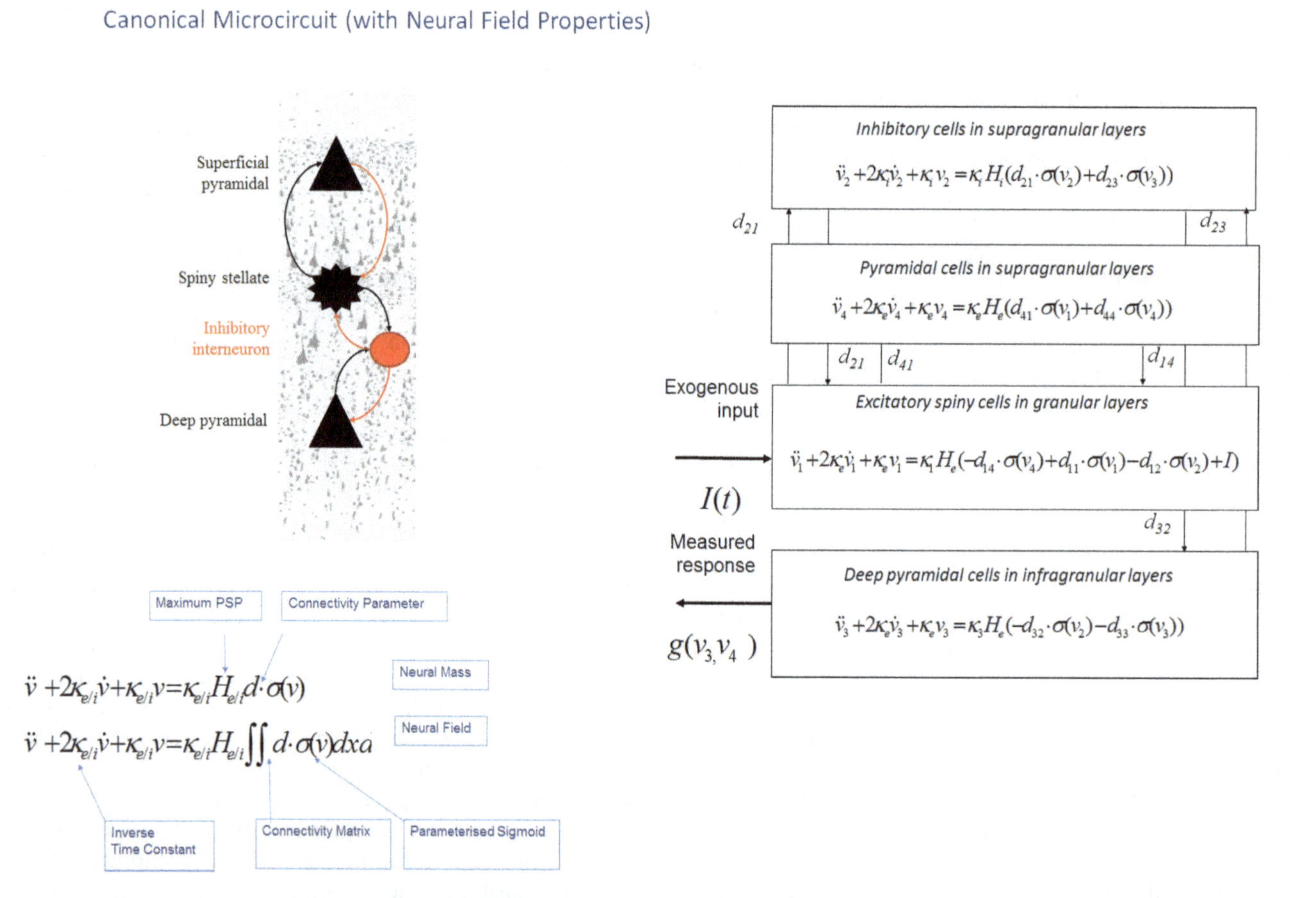

FIGURE 3 | Canonical microcircuit neural field model: "CMC". This figure shows the evolution equations that specify a canonical microcircuit (CMC) neural mass model of a single source. This model contains four populations occupying different cortical layers: the pyramidal cell population of the Jansen and Rit model is effectively split into two subpopulations allowing a separation of the neuronal populations that elaborate forward and backward connections in cortical hierarchies. As with the ERP and LFP models, second-order differential equations (shown earlier in **Figure 1** decomposed into two first order ODEs), mediate a linear convolution of presynaptic activity [a sigmoidal function of presynaptic membrane depolarization $\sigma(v)$] to produce postsynaptic depolarization (v), dependent on membrane time constants ($1/\kappa_{e/i}$) and average post-synaptic depolarizations ($H_{e/i}$) at excitatory (e) and inhibitory (i) synapses. This depolarization gives rise to firing rates within each sub-population that provide inputs to other populations. Replacing connectivity parameters d, with a connectivity matrix over space and time $D(x,t)$ enables one to generalize the neural mass model to a neural field model. This effectively converts the ordinary differential equations in this figure into partial differential equations or neural field equations.

the basis of observed (empirical) responses. The incorporation of neural field models in the DCM framework allowed spatial parameters of the sources—like the spatial decay rate of synaptic connections and intrinsic conduction speed—to be optimized even using spatially unresolved data, like a time series from a single LFP channel. For example, Bayesian model selection (BMS) correctly distinguished between mass and field models. This type of comparison was formalized using DCM and Bayesian model evidence in the context of invasive local field potentials from rat auditory cortex. With these invasive data, the neural-field model had a much greater evidence than the equivalent neural mass variant; this could be attributed to the increased repertoire of predictions that these models afford and indicates a key role for—and parameterization of—spatial as well as temporal dynamics on the cortical manifold.

STRUCTURE, FUNCTION, AND THE CANONICAL MICROCIRCUIT (CMC)

Pinotsis et al. (2013b) showed that DCM with neural fields can provide a detailed analysis of correlations between cortical structure and function. This analysis was motivated by previous results suggesting two hypotheses regarding the biophysical basis of inter-individual differences in peak gamma frequencies—one based on functional differences and one based on structural differences: Muthukumaraswamy et al. (2009) suggested that peak gamma frequency is determined by the level of inhibition in V1, as described by resting GABA concentration measured with MR spectroscopy. Later, Schwarzkopf et al. (2012) found a correlation between peak gamma frequency and the surface area of primary visual cortex as measured with retinotopic mapping. These authors suggested that the size of V1 and associated differences in structural microanatomy could be true determinants of peak gamma frequency. The above two hypotheses suggest that both GABA concentration and V1 size can influence gamma frequency; however, these factors may or may not be causally linked. In other words, a larger V1 may have a higher GABA concentration that may or may not be due to a higher local GABA density.

DCM with neural fields incorporate parameters pertaining to both microanatomy and the density of GABA receptors (that determine inhibitory intrinsic connection strengths) and allow one to investigate alternative explanations for differences in gamma peak frequency. These differences could be mediated by either a kinetic (functional) parameter, summarizing the level of cortical inhibition or the (structural) macrocolumn width or both of these parameters. Pinotsis et al. (2013b) looked at the correlations over subjects between peak gamma frequency, V1 surface area and the Bayesian estimates of these structural and functional parameters and found that both hypotheses were confirmed. In brief, they found correlations between columnar width, gamma peak and V1 size and also between the GABAergic parameter and the gamma peak. This correlation remained significant when controlling for V1 size and width. This suggests that the correlation between gamma peak and V1 inhibition cannot be accounted for completely by the spatial parameters (at the microscopic or macroscopic level). Structural equation modeling was used to characterize the causal dependencies among observed quantities and the model parameters: in the winning structure equation model, peak gamma frequency was mediated proximately by excitatory drive to inhibitory (GABAergic) interneurons and the strength of this drive was determined, in part, by the size of macrocolumns. In turn, the size of the macrocolumn was constrained by the macroscopic (retinotopic) size of V1 (under the assumption that V1 size is determined genetically or epigenetically). These results suggested that both cortical microstructure and excitability may be important for visual perception and are in accord with empirical studies showing that the size of V1 is negatively correlated with the strength of visual illusions (Schwarzkopf et al., 2010)—and that GABA concentration correlates with orientation discrimination ability (Edden et al., 2009).

This work also introduced an expanded neuronal architecture based upon the canonical microcircuit. These models comprise four subpopulations (as opposed to three subpopulations in mass and field models above, see **Figure 3**). The canonical microcircuit or "CMC" models a refinement of the Jansen and Rit convolution models that explicitly accommodates the neuronal sources of forward and backward connections in cortical hierarchies (Bastos et al., 2012). These are distinct superficial and deep pyramidal cell populations, respectively that, crucially, may exhibit different spectral outputs. Specifically gamma responses have been recorded in superficial layers, while slower dynamics (in the alpha and beta range) arise concurrently in infra granular populations (Maier et al., 2010; Buffalo et al., 2011; Bastos et al., 2012). The CMC proposes an intrinsic connectivity architecture to account for this non-linear transformation though dendritic and population effects (Bastos et al., 2012). The canonical microcircuit model is based upon intracellular recordings in cat visual cortex by Douglas and Martin (1991) who investigated the laminar propagation of afferent signals and produced pathways that are thought to reflect canonical input–output processing streams for forward and backward signals throughout the cortex. These models are currently being used to test hypotheses about asymmetries in forward and backward message passing that may shed light on the distributed neural processing that underlies perceptual synthesis and inference.

SUMMARY

The basic idea behind DCM is that neural activity propagates through brain networks in a way that can be modeled as an input-state-output-system, where causal interactions within the system are mediated by unobservable (hidden) dynamics. The resulting multi-input-multi-output (MIMO) neuronal model is then supplemented with a observation model (e.g., classical electromagnetic forward model) that describes the mapping from neural activity to observed responses (Daunizeau et al., 2011). It is the dynamics of the hidden states that are prescribed by the neural mass and neural field models outlined above. The type of data and data features determine the combination of neuronal and observation models. For example, EEG and MEG data require a different observation model than LFP data, while evoked responses necessitate a parameterized Gaussian pulse input—in contrast with spectral density data features that require parameterized neuronal noise spectra. In all of these different applications, the underlying "LFP," "ERP,"

"NMM," "MFM," "NFM," and "CMC" models are, in principle, interchangeable.

The choice of the appropriate neuronal model should reflect the research question at hand: for example, whether the focus is on topographic as opposed to intrinsic neurotransmitter properties or drug effects etc. This choice may also be informed by previous applications, where a particular model has already proven useful within a DCM context (for example, fast oscillations in the gamma band for the "CMC" model). One generally designs a DCM study to assess the effects of task manipulation, group, pathology or drug on a particular parameter or set of parameters of interest. In other words, the choice of model should be evident at the outset and often conforms to the "minimal model approach" necessary to access that parameter—this is because, in general, a simpler model has more constraints and can use the degrees of freedom in the data to estimate model parameters and evidence more efficiently. For example, where differences in effective extrinsic connectivity are of interest, a convolution based model—that is agnostic to specific intrinsic ion channel mediators—will suffice to address the hypothesis (Campo et al., 2012). The direction of empirical research using DCM as a "mathematical microscope" of synaptic processes—where particular receptor and neurotransmitter changes are important—may call for the finer grained physiological details of the NMM or MFM (Moran et al., 2011b). In other cases the form of the dynamics, for example whether field (or propagation) effects should be considered, may itself embody the central hypothesis. In this case, as demonstrated in Pinotsis et al. (2013b), BMS may be sufficient to disambiguate among competing hypotheses about neuronal architecture (Penny et al., 2004). In effect, BMS usurps all other arguments as the best method to test which model should be applied to which data; though computational and time constraints, particularly as the suite of options in DCM is expanded, may determine the extensiveness and overall feasibility of such a search. In principle, researchers may employ their own neuronal model (or feature extraction process) by compositing a parameterized state space and utilizing the modularity of SPM's source code. Wrapper routines which specify parameter priors, integration schemes and variational expectation maximization can be applied to a function of neuronal activity that is user-specified (In SPM's DCM toolbox: http://www.fil.ion.ucl.ac.uk/spm/, The current routines are described in files "spm_fx_nmm") (Kiebel et al., 2009; Litvak et al., 2011). Construct validity would then need to be tested by simulating data from different regions of parameter space and investigating parameter identify ability i.e., whether the framework can recover the simulated parameters given different initializations. These tests are particularly important in the case of highly nonlinear state space models, given the potential of the gradient ascent to converge to local maxima (Friston et al., 2012).

The models we have reviewed in this paper may also be useful beyond the DCM inference framework. For example, in the study of large scale generative processes underlying resting-state networks in fMRI, neural mass (Deco and Jirsa, 2012) and neural field models (Pinotsis et al., 2013a) have been embedded in anatomical graphs to study emergent behaviors and dynamic properties (Gray et al., 2009; Robinson et al., 2009). This suggests that these models may have some utility as neural state equations in DCM for fMRI, though currently we deploy coarser models with far less physiological detail (Daunizeau et al., 2011). The field of inquiry using these types of models is varied and rich, with DCM applications including the locus of consciousness and unconsciousness in vegetative state patients (Boly et al., 2011), diaschisis in temporal lobe epilepsy (Campo et al., 2012) and the effects of ketamine on synaptic plasticity (Schmidt et al., 2012). The set of distinct dynamics within which these types of effects can be parameterized will no doubt grow beyond the current suite of models available. Indeed their exchangeability within the DCM framework allows researchers to define their own favorite or interesting model and proceed in the usual Bayesian way (Friston et al., 2003).

ACKNOWLEDGMENTS

This work was supported by the Wellcome Trust and Virginia Tech Carilion Research Institute.

REFERENCES

Ashburner, J. (2012). SPM: a history. *Neuroimage* 62, 791–800.

Baillet, S., Mosher, J. C., and Leahy, R. M. (2001). Electromagnetic brain mapping. *Signal Process. Mag. IEEE* 18, 14–30.

Bastos, A. M., Usrey, W. M., Adams, R. A., Mangun, G. R., Fries, P., and Friston, K. J. (2012). Canonical microcircuits for predictive coding. *Neuron* 76, 695–711.

Benda, J., and Herz, A. V. M. (2003). A universal model for spike-frequency adaptation. *Neural Comput.* 15, 2523–2564.

Boly, M., Garrido, M. I., Gosseries, O., Bruno, M. A., Boveroux, P., Schnakers, C., et al. (2011). Preserved feedforward but impaired top-down processes in the vegetative state. *Science* 332, 858–862.

Boly, M., Moran, R., Murphy, M., Boveroux, P., Bruno, M. A., Noirhomme, Q., et al. (2012). Connectivity changes underlying spectral EEG changes during propofol-induced loss of consciousness. *J. Neurosci.* 32, 7082–7090.

Box, G. E. P. (1976). Science and statistics. *J. Am. Stat. Assoc.* 71, 791–799.

Breakspear, M. (2002). Nonlinear phase desynchronization in human electroencephalographic data. *Hum. Brain Mapp.* 15, 175–198.

Breakspear, M., Heitmann, S., and Daffertshofer, A. (2010). Generative models of cortical oscillations: neurobiological implications of the Kuramoto model. *Front. Hum. Neurosci.* 4:190. doi: 10.3389/fnhum.2010.00190

Breakspear, M., Roberts, J., Terry, J. R., Rodrigues, S., Mahant, N., and Robinson, P. (2006). A unifying explanation of primary generalized seizures through nonlinear brain modeling and bifurcation analysis. *Cereb. Cortex* 16, 1296–1313.

Breakspear, M., and Terry, J. (2002). Topographic organization of nonlinear interdependence in multichannel human EEG. *Neuroimage* 16, 822–835.

Brunel, N., and Wang, X. (2001). Effects of neuromodulation in a cortical network model of object working memory dominated by recurrent inhibition. *J. Comput. Neurosci.* 11, 63–85.

Buffalo, E. A., Fries, P., Landman, R., Buschman, T. J., and Desimone, R. (2011). Laminar differences in gamma and alpha coherence in the ventral stream. *Proc. Natl. Acad. Sci. U.S.A.* 108, 11262–11267.

Buice, M. A., and Chow, C. C. (2013). Dynamic finite size effects in spiking neural networks. *PLoS Comput. Biol* 9:e1002872. doi: 10.1371/journal.pcbi.1002872

Campo, P., Garrido, M. I., Moran, R. J., Maestú, F., García-Morales, I., Gil-Nagel, A., et al. (2012). Remote effects of hippocampal sclerosis on effective connectivity during working memory encoding: a case of connectional diaschisis? *Cereb. Cortex* 22, 1225–1236.

Coombes, S. (2010). Large-scale neural dynamics: simple and complex. *Neuroimage* 52, 731–739.

Daffertshofer, A., Peper, C., Frank, T., and Beek, P. (2000).

Spatio-temporal patterns of encephalographic signals during polyrhythmic tapping. *Hum. Mov. Sci.* 19, 475–498.

Daunizeau, J., David, O., and Stephan, K. E. (2011). Dynamic causal modelling: a critical review of the biophysical and statistical foundations. *Neuroimage* 58, 312–322.

David, O., and Friston, K. J. (2003). A neural mass model for MEG/EEG:-coupling and neuronal dynamics. *Neuroimage* 20, 1743–1755.

David, O., Kiebel, S., Harrison, L., Mattout, J., Kilner, J., and Friston, K. (2006). Dynamic causal modeling of evoked responses in EEG and MEG. *Neuroimage* 30, 1255–1272.

Deco, G., and Jirsa, V. K. (2012). Ongoing cortical activity at rest: criticality, multistability, and ghost attractors. *J. Neurosci.* 32, 3366–3375.

Deco, G., Jirsa, V. K., Robinson, P. A., Breakspear, M., and Friston, K. (2008). The dynamic brain: from spiking neurons to neural masses and cortical fields. *PLoS Comput. Biol.* 4:e1000092. doi: 10.1371/journal.pcbi.1000092

Destexhe, A., and Babloyantz, A. (1991). Pacemaker-induced coherence in cortical networks. *Neural Comput.* 3, 145–154.

Douglas, R. J., and Martin, K. (1991). A functional microcircuit for cat visual cortex. *J. Physiol.* 440, 735–769.

Durstewitz, D., Seamans, J., and Sejnowski, T. (2000). Dopamine-mediated stabilization of delay-period activity in a network model of prefrontal cortex. *J. Neurophysiol.* 83, 1733.

Durstewitz, D., and Seamans, J. K. (2008). The dual-state theory of prefrontal cortex dopamine function with relevance to catechol-o-methyltransferase genotypes and schizophrenia. *Biol. Psychiatry* 64, 739–749.

Edden, R. A., Muthukumaraswamy, S. D., Freeman, T. C., and Singh, K. D. (2009). Orientation discrimination performance is predicted by GABA concentration and gamma oscillation frequency in human primary visual cortex. *J. Neurosci.* 29, 15721–15726.

Felleman, D. J., and Van Essen, D. C. (1991). Distributed hierarchical processing in the primate cerebral cortex. *Cereb. Cortex* 1, 1.

Freeman, W. J. (1975). *Mass Action in the Nervous System.* New York, NY: Academic Press.

Freeman, W. J. (1987). Simulation of chaotic EEG patterns with a dynamic model of the olfactory system. *Biol. Cybern.* 56, 139–150.

Friston, K. (2005). A theory of cortical responses. *Philos. Trans. R. Soc. B Biol. Sci.* 360, 815–836.

Friston, K. (2009). The free-energy principle: a rough guide to the brain? *Trends Cogn. Sci.* 13, 293–301.

Friston, K., Bastos, A., Litvak, V., Stephan, K., Fries, P., and Moran, R. (2012). DCM for complex-valued data: cross-spectra, coherence and phase-delays. *Neuroimage* 59, 439–455.

Friston, K., Harrison, L., and Penny, W. (2003). Dynamic causal modelling. *Neuroimage* 19, 1273–1302.

Garrido, M., Friston, K., Kiebel, S., Stephan, K., Baldeweg, T., and Kilner, J. (2008). The functional anatomy of the MMN: a DCM study of the roving paradigm. *Neuroimage* 42, 936–944.

Garrido, M., Kilner, J., Kiebel, S., and Friston, K. (2007a). Evoked brain responses are generated by feedback loops. *Proc. Natl. Acad. Sci. U.S.A.* 104, 20961.

Garrido, M. I., Kilner, J. M., Kiebel, S. J., Stephan, K. E., and Friston, K. J. (2007b). Dynamic causal modelling of evoked potentials: a reproducibility study. *Neuroimage* 36, 571–580.

Garrido, M., Kilner, J., Stephan, K., and Friston, K. (2009). The mismatch negativity: a review of underlying mechanisms. *Clin. Neurophysiol.* 120, 453–463.

Goldman-Rakic, P. (1996). Regional and cellular fractionation of working memory. *Proc. Natl. Acad. Sci. U.S.A.* 93, 13473.

Gonzalez-Islas, C., and Hablitz, J. (2003). Dopamine enhances EPSCs in layer II-III pyramidal neurons in rat prefrontal cortex. *J. Neurosci.* 23, 867.

Gorelova, N., and Yang, C. (2000). Dopamine D1/D5 receptor activation modulates a persistent sodium current in rat prefrontal cortical neurons *in vitro*. *J. Neurophysiol.* 84, 75.

Gray, R., Fung, C., and Robinson, P. (2009). Stability of small-world networks of neural populations. *Neurocomputing* 72, 1565–1574.

Grimbert, F., and Faugeras, O. (2006). Bifurcation analysis of Jansen's neural mass model. *Neural Comput.* 18, 3052–3068.

Gutkin, B., Pinto, D., and Ermentrout, B. (2003). Mathematical neuroscience: from neurons to circuits to systems. *J. Physiol. Paris* 97, 209–219.

Hodgkin, A., and Huxley, A. (1952). Propagation of electrical signals along giant nerve fibres. *Proc. R. Soc. Lond. B Biol. Sci.* 140, 177–183.

Jahr, C. E., and Stevens, C. F. (1990). A quantitative description of NMDA receptor-channel kinetic behavior. *J. Neurosci.* 10, 1830–1837.

Jansen, B. H., and Rit, V. G. (1995). Electroencephalogram and visual evoked potential generation in a mathematical model of coupled cortical columns. *Biol. Cybern.* 73, 357–366.

Jirsa, V., and Haken, H. (1996). Field theory of electromagnetic brain activity. *Phys. Rev. Lett.* 77, 960–963.

Jirsa, V., and Haken, H. (1997). A derivation of a macroscopic field theory of the brain from the quasi-microscopic neural dynamics. *Physica D.* 99, 503–526.

Kiebel, S., David, O., and Friston, K. (2006). Dynamic causal modelling of evoked responses in EEG/MEG with lead field parameterization. *Neuroimage* 30, 1273–1284.

Kiebel, S. J., Garrido, M. I., Moran, R., Chen, C. C., and Friston, K. J. (2009). Dynamic causal modeling for EEG and MEG. *Hum. Brain Mapp.* 30, 1866–1876.

Leopold, D. A., Murayama, Y., and Logothetis, N. K. (2003). Very slow activity fluctuations in monkey visual cortex: implications for functional brain imaging. *Cereb. Cortex* 13, 422–433.

Litvak, V., Mattout, J., Kiebel, S., Phillips, C., Henson, R., Kilner, J., et al. (2011). EEG and MEG data analysis in SPM8. *Comput. Intell. Neurosci.* 2011:852961. doi: 10.1155/2011/852961

Lopes Da Silva, F., Pijn, J. P., and Boeijinga, P. (1989). Interdependence of EEG signals: linear vs. nonlinear associations and the significance of time delays and phase shifts. *Brain Topogr.* 2, 9–18.

Maier, A., Adams, G. K., Aura, C., Leopold, D. A., Maier, A., Adams, G., et al. (2010). Distinct superficial and deep laminar domains of activity in the visual cortex during rest and stimulation. *Front. Syst. Neurosci.* 4:31. doi: 10.3389/fnsys.2010.00031

Marreiros, A., Kiebel, S., Daunizeau, J., Harrison, L., and Friston, K. (2009). Population dynamics under the Laplace assumption. *Neuroimage* 44, 701–714.

Marreiros, A. C., Daunizeau, J., Kiebel, S. J., and Friston, K. J. (2008). Population dynamics: variance and the sigmoid activation function. *Neuroimage* 42, 147–157.

Marreiros, A. C., Kiebel, S. J., and Friston, K. J. (2010). A dynamic causal model study of neuronal population dynamics. *Neuroimage* 51, 91–101.

Marten, F., Rodrigues, S., Suffczynski, P., Richardson, M. P., and Terry, J. R. (2009). Derivation and analysis of an ordinary differential equation mean-field model for studying clinically recorded epilepsy dynamics. *Phys. Rev. E* 79:021911. doi: 10.1103/PhysRevE.79.021911

Moran, R., Kiebel, S., Stephan, K., Reilly, R., Daunizeau, J., and Friston, K. (2007). A neural mass model of spectral responses in electrophysiology. *Neuroimage* 37, 706–720.

Moran, R., Stephan, K., Kiebel, S., Rombach, N., O'connor, W., Murphy, K., et al. (2008). Bayesian estimation of synaptic physiology from the spectral responses of neural masses. *Neuroimage* 42, 272–284.

Moran, R. J., Stephan, K. E., Dolan, R. J., and Friston, K. J. (2011a). Consistent spectral predictors for dynamic causal models of steady state responses. *Neuroimage* 55, 1694–1708.

Moran, R. J., Symmonds, M., Stephan, K. E., Friston, K. J., and Dolan, R. J. (2011b). An *in vivo* assay of synaptic function mediating human cognition. *Curr. Biol.* 21, 1320–1325.

Morris, C., and Lecar, H. (1981). Voltage oscillations in the barnacle giant muscle fiber. *Biophys. J.* 35, 193–213.

Muthukumaraswamy, S. D., Edden, R. A., Jones, D. K., Swettenham, J. B., and Singh, K. D. (2009). Resting GABA concentration predicts peak gamma frequency and fMRI amplitude in response to visual stimulation in humans. *Proc. Natl. Acad. Sci. U.S.A.* 106, 8356–8361.

Näätänen, R., Jacobsen, T., and Winkler, I. (2005). Memory-based or afferent processes in mismatch negativity (MMN): a review of the evidence. *Psychophysiology* 42, 25–32.

Nevado-Holgado, A. J., Marten, F., Richardson, M. P., and Terry, J. R. (2012). Characterising the dynamics of EEG waveforms as the path through parameter space of a neural mass model: application to epilepsy seizure evolution. *Neuroimage* 59, 2374–2392.

Nunez, P. L. (1974). The brain wave equation: a model for the EEG. *Math. Biosci.* 21, 279–297.

Nunez, P. L., and Srinivasan, R. (2006). *Electric Fields of the Brain: The Neurophysics of EEG.* New York, NY: Oxford University Press.

Penny, W., Stephan, K., Mechelli, A., and Friston, K. (2004). Comparing dynamic causal models. *Neuroimage* 22, 1157–1172.

Pinotsis, D., and Friston, K. (2011). Neural fields, spectral responses and lateral connections. *Neuroimage* 55, 39–48.

Pinotsis, D., Hansen, E., Friston, K., and Jirsa, V. (2013a). Anatomical connectivity and the resting state activity of large cortical networks. *Neuroimage* 65, 127–138.

Pinotsis, D., Schwarzkopf, S., Litvak, V., Rees, G., Barnes, G., and Friston, K. (2013b). Dynamic causal modelling of lateral interactions in the visual cortex. *Neuroimage* 66, 563–576.

Pinotsis, D., Moran, R., and Friston, K. (2012). Dynamic causal modeling with neural fields. *Neuroimage* 59, 1261–1274.

Rennie, C. J., Wright, J. J., and Robinson, P. A. (2000). Mechanisms of cortical electrical activity and emergence of gamma rhythm. *J. Theor. Biol.* 205, 17–35.

Robinson, P. (2006). Patchy propagators, brain dynamics, and the generation of spatially structured gamma oscillations. *Phys. Rev. E* 73:041904. doi: 10.1103/PhysRevE.73.041904

Robinson, P., Henderson, J., Matar, E., Riley, P., and Gray, R. (2009). Dynamical reconnection and stability constraints on cortical network architecture. *Phys. Rev. Lett.* 103:108104. doi: 10.1103/PhysRevLett.103.108104

Robinson, P., Rennie, C., Wright, J., Bahramali, H., Gordon, E., and Rowe, D. (2001). Prediction of electroencephalographic spectra from neurophysiology. *Phys. Rev. E* 63:021903. doi: 10.1103/PhysRevE.63.021903

Schmidt, A., Diaconescu, A. O., Kometer, M., Friston, K. J., Stephan, K. E., and Vollenweider, F. X. (2012). Modeling ketamine effects on synaptic plasticity during the mismatch negativity. *Cereb. Cortex.* doi: 10.1093/cercor/bhs238. [Epub ahead of print].

Schwarzkopf, D. S., Robertson, D. J., Song, C., Barnes, G. R., and Rees, G. (2012). The frequency of visually induced gamma-band oscillations depends on the size of early human visual cortex. *J. Neurosci.* 32, 1507–1512.

Schwarzkopf, D. S., Song, C., and Rees, G. (2010). The surface area of human V1 predicts the subjective experience of object size. *Nat. Neurosci.* 14, 28–30.

Stam, C. (2005). Nonlinear dynamical analysis of EEG and MEG: review of an emerging field. *Clin. Neurophysiol.* 116, 2266–2301.

Steyn-Ross, M. L., Steyn-Ross, D. A., Sleigh, J. W., and Liley, D. (1999). Theoretical electroencephalogram stationary spectrum for a white-noise-driven cortex: evidence for a general anesthetic-induced phase transition. *Phys. Rev. E* 60, 7299.

Valdes, P., Jimenez, J., Riera, J., Biscay, R., and Ozaki, T. (1999). Nonlinear EEG analysis based on a neural mass model. *Biol. Cybern.* 81, 415–424.

Wendling, F., Bellanger, J., Bartolomei, F., and Chauvel, P. (2000). Relevance of nonlinear lumped-parameter models in the analysis of depth-EEG epileptic signals. *Biol. Cybern.* 83, 367–378.

Whittington, M. A., Traub, R. D., and Jefferys, J. G. R. (1995). Synchronized oscillations in interneuron networks driven by metabotropic glutamate receptor activation. *Nature* 373, 612–615.

Wilson, H. R., and Cowan, J. D. (1972). Excitatory and inhibitory interactions in localized populations of model neurons. *Biophys. J.* 12, 1–24.

Wilson, H. R., and Cowan, J. D. (1973). A mathematical theory of the functional dynamics of cortical and thalamic nervous tissue. *Biol. Cybern.* 13, 55–80.

Wright, J., and Liley, D. (1996). Dynamics of the brain at global and microscopic scales: neural networks and the EEG. *Behav. Brain Sci.* 19, 285–294.

Zeki, S. (1990). Parallelism and functional specialization in human visual cortex. *Cold. Spring Harb. Symp. Q. Biol.* 55, 651–661.

3

On the dynamics of cortical development: Synchrony and synaptic self-organization

James Joseph Wright*[1,2] ***and Paul David Bourke*[3]**

[1] *Department of Psychological Medicine, Faculty of Medicine, The University of Auckland, Auckland, New Zealand*
[2] *Liggins Institute, The University of Auckland, Auckland, New Zealand*
[3] *iVEC@UWA, University of Western Australia, Perth, WA, Australia*

***Correspondence:**
James Joseph Wright, Department of Psychological Medicine, Faculty of Medical and Health Sciences, School of Medicine, The University of Auckland, PB 92019, Auckland, New Zealand.
e-mail: james.wright@auckland.ac.nz

We describe a model for cortical development that resolves long-standing difficulties of earlier models. It is proposed that, during embryonic development, synchronous firing of neurons and their competition for limited metabolic resources leads to selection of an array of neurons with ultra-small-world characteristics. Consequently, in the visual cortex, macrocolumns linked by superficial patchy connections emerge in anatomically realistic patterns, with an ante-natal arrangement which projects signals from the surrounding cortex onto each macrocolumn in a form analogous to the projection of a Euclidean plane onto a Möbius strip. This configuration reproduces typical cortical response maps, and simulations of signal flow explain cortical responses to moving lines as functions of stimulus velocity, length, and orientation. With the introduction of direct visual inputs, under the operation of Hebbian learning, development of mature selective response "tuning" to stimuli of given orientation, spatial frequency, and temporal frequency would then take place, overwriting the earlier ante-natal configuration. The model is provisionally extended to hierarchical interactions of the visual cortex with higher centers, and a general principle for cortical processing of spatio-temporal images is sketched.

Keywords: synchronous oscillation, cortical development, synaptic organization, cortical response properties, cortical information flow

INTRODUCTION

During its embryological development the mammalian brain differentiates from a group of stem cells into an organized form ready to begin a life-long adaptive interaction with signals from the sensory environment. At the beginning of extra-uterine life, despite exposure to a limited milieu, it is somehow already organized to begin this engagement, as tho a matrix of connections has formed in which signal flows are pre-adapted to learn specific recurring patterns of the experiential world. A large body of work, following the pioneering work of Hubel and Wiesel (1959), has addressed just this issue, taking as the main target for research the primary visual cortex (V1). The majority of this work has sought to understand the emerging connections in terms of stimulus "features"—that is, elementary properties of sensory stimuli—rather than as a process independent of sensation until the post-natal stage. Our approach depends on alternative assumptions. Here we summarize and extend our earlier work (Wright et al., 2006; Wright and Bourke, 2008, 2013; Wright, 2009, 2010) relating the basic dynamics of neuron firing and competition among developing neurons for the resources needed for their growth, to the emergent connections at birth.

Our model draws on two recent experimental observations. Firstly, neurons in neonatal cerebral cortical slices show increased apoptosis when their capacity to enter into synchronous firing is disrupted by pharmacological means (Heck et al., 2008). Secondly, embryonic neurons developing *in vitro* develop synchronous firing, and as their growth proceeds, show self-organization into "small world" networks (Downes et al., 2012). We propose that the synchronous firing and protection from apoptosis are directly causally related, because during cortical embryogenesis there is competition among developing neurons and synapses, which, although mediated by trophic factors (Harris et al., 1997; van Ooyen and Willshaw, 1999; van Ooyen, 2001) is ultimately a competition for available metabolic energy and/or some other scarce resource needed to promote metabolism (Montague, 1996; Thomaidou et al., 1997). We suppose that pre-synaptic pulse synchrony increases uptake of critical metabolic resources by some action not presently specified, and we argue that the assembly of cells that maximizes synchronous firing, and thus energy uptake, is also that which has the minimum metabolic cost per neuron in the length of axonal connections—the combination optimum for their survival.

Synchronous oscillation of pulses and local field potentials is a ubiquitous aspect of cortical activity (Eckhorn et al., 1988, 1990; Gray et al., 1989; Bressler et al., 1993; Singer, 1999) and has been proposed as a mechanism solving the "binding problem" of perceptual grouping and cognitive processing (Eckhorn et al., 1990; Singer, 1999; Crick and Koch, 2003). "Synchrony" refers to the broadband cross-correlation of neuron firing and field potentials at zero time-lag. The mechanism of origin of synchrony itself is controversial. In this paper we rely on an explanation that appears best applicable to the synchrony seen in neuron cultures, brain slices, or the early embryonic brain, and depends on a universal property of networks with summing junctions, including dendrites (Robinson et al., 1998; Wright et al., 2000; Chapman et al.,

2002). This type of synchrony appears in simulations that also accurately reproduce spectra, cross-correlations, and excitatory/inhibitory timings characteristic of activated cortex (Wright, 2009, 2010).

GEOMETRY OF RESPONSE ORGANIZATION IN THE DEVELOPED BRAIN

Since the discovery that individual cells in the primary visual cortex (V1) respond with an orientation preference (OP) to visual lines of differing orientation (Hubel and Wiesel, 1959), analysis of the response organization and its relationship to cortical function has remained both conceptually influential and controversial (von der Malsburg, 1973; Willshaw and von der Malsburg, 1976; Swindale, 1996). The surface organization of OP in V1 has recently been compared with appropriate random surrogates, and shown to exhibit significant hexagonal rotational periodicity, in which each roughly delineated macrocolumnar unit exhibits all values of OP arrayed around a pinwheel (Paik and Ringach, 2011; Muir et al., 2011). Varying chirality and orientation of the pinwheels achieves continuity of OP at the columnar margins, thus producing zones of irregular but continuously varying OP, known as linear zones and saddles.

Some species exhibit little or no sign of this hexagonal and continuous ordering, and because of the marked interspecies variation, serious doubt has been expressed that the pattern is of functional significance at all, since species showing little such organization have no apparent deficit in vision (Horton and Adams, 2005). Interspecies variation seems, in part, to be related to both variation in size of V1 between species, and a relative constancy of the size of macrocolumns, independently of species. Measurements of the average distance of separation of OP singularities (the singularity taken as demarcating the center of a macrocolumn) show this distance to be relatively constant over a 40-fold variation of body size, and related size of V1 (Kaschube et al., 2010; Keil et al., 2012). Models using symmetry arguments indicate that macrocolumns must undergo divisions during cortical development to maintain uniform surface density of singularities (Wolf and Geisel, 1998; Oster and Bressloff, 2006). Kaschube and colleagues conclude that self-organization has canalized the evolution of the underlying OP maps into a single common design—subject to the proviso that, from further symmetry arguments, this can only be the case where long-range interactions between developing macrocolumns, suppressing some possible connections, can take place. Thus, in animals with very small V1, this organization breaks down, creating a "pepper and salt" OP map pattern (Meng et al., 2012).

THE SUPERFICIAL PATCH SYSTEM

A related puzzle of V1 organization is posed by the superficial patch system. This system, composed of relatively long-range, largely excitatory (Hirsch and Gilbert, 1991; McGuire et al., 1991) patchy connections (Gilbert and Wiesel, 1979; Rockland and Lund, 1983) is ubiquitous in cortex (Muir and Douglas, 2011) and has a functional relationship to OP. Patchy connections develop before sensory afferents reach the cortex (Price, 1986; Callaway and Katz, 1990; Durack and Katz, 1996; Ruthazer and Stryker, 1996) but do not arise or terminate in the vicinity of OP singularities. Instead, near singularities, connections are apparently diffuse and local (Sharma et al., 1995; Yousef et al., 2001; Mariño et al., 2005; Buzás et al., 2006; Muir and Douglas, 2011). Patchy connections link areas of common OP ("like-to-like") over distances several times the diameter of a macrocolumn (Gilbert and Wiesel, 1989; Buzás et al., 2006; Muir et al., 2011), are periodic on roughly the same interval as OP, and are largely patch-reciprocal (Rockland and Lund, 1983; Angelucci et al., 2002). It has been shown that development of patchy connections must depend on the supply of organizing information from the neural field, and is not explicable from considerations of local neural growth *per se* (Muir and Douglas, 2011). Just as for maps of response properties, there is variation of patchy connection orderliness between species. Muir et al. (2011) have pointed out that those species with less orderliness have smaller visual cortices and/or less defined organization of "like-to-like" connections—an argument congruent with the findings on brain size, orderliness of response maps, and surface density of OP singularities cited above (viz. Kaschube et al., 2010; Keil et al., 2012, etc.).

PROBLEMS OF STANDARD MODELS OF FEATURE RESPONSES

Explanation of organization of OP has been undertaken in a group of now-classical theories, which we will refer to as "standard models," following the comparative description of Swindale (Swindale, 1996). Descriptive dimension reduction methods (Kohonen, 1982; Durbin and Willshaw, 1987; Durbin and Mitchison, 1990) show that the response maps of OP, eye preference (OC), direction preference (DP), and spatial frequency preference (SF) are consequences of requiring continuity and completeness of representation of each response property, in a two-dimensional representation in which every type of response property occurs within any small area on the surface of V1 (Swindale, 1996; Carriera-Perpiñán et al., 2005). The same ordering is also explained as a consequence of competitive Hebbian learning among small neighborhood assemblies of excitatory neurons, driven by spatially filtered cortical noise. Separate spatial filters each distinguish a type of response, and total synaptic gain is conserved during the training (Grossberg and Olson, 1994).

Classical standard models depend on seeding with oriented lines, in one way or another (von der Malsburg, 1973; Swindale, 1982, 1992; Durbin and Mitchison, 1990; Obermayer et al., 1990, 1992; Tanaka, 1990; Miyashita and Tanaka, 1992; Grossberg and Olson, 1994) and recently, initial belief that primary response to static oriented lines in the visual field forms the basis of OP maps has been undermined in two ways:

Firstly, in large species particularly, maps of OP appear in the cortex prior to visual experience (Wiesel and Hubel, 1974; Blakemore and Van Sluyters, 1975; Sherk and Stryker, 1976). This problem has been addressed by arguments for the normal occurrence of line-like structure in ante-natal retinal input (Albert et al., 2008; Ringach, 2007; Paik and Ringach, 2011). In contrast to all the above models, Kang et al. (2003) have proposed a model which breaks with the traditional dependence on the primacy of lines, and depends instead on time-invariant correlations in cortical "Mexican Hat" inhibitory surrounds. This model accounts successfully for the apparent isotropy of local intracortical connections and the observed uniformity of sharpness of definition of OP independent of proximity to singularities, and provides a mechanism which might plausibly operate before eye-opening. It requires instead, that LGM inputs to cortex become tuned according to orientation. A further model avoiding the problem of ascription of OP as a primary, stimulus dependent property, explains the conjoint development of OP and ocular dominance columns as a consequence of Hebbian connection formation driven by correlation of visual inputs as a declining function of retinotopic distance of separation at short distances, and reversed correlation of activity in ON and OFF V1 simple cells at greater distances (Erwin and Miller, 1998). All these models however, result in the emergence of OP as a property of line orientation alone, rather than as one attribute of some more complex mechanism of feature response.

Secondly, and more recently, Basole and colleagues, who tested OP using stimulus lines moving at different speeds, and oriented at differing angles to the line of movement of the stimulus, found OP to be a function of these variables to such a degree that for lines oriented non-orthogonally to the direction of movement, OP could vary progressively with increments of speed to an asymptotic limit of 90° (Basole et al., 2003, 2006). Longer lines showed less variation of OP with increasing speed. This finding challenged all models which depended on OP being a fixed "feature" of cortical response, whether or not direct visual stimuli was required to prime the process of self-organization. Basole and colleagues at first concluded that the primal stimulus characteristics are not isolated features such as orientation, direction and speed, but a single characteristic—the "spatio-temporal energy"—that is, the combined spatial and temporal Fourier components of the moving visual stimulus' projection to V1. Subsequent workers explained these results by retaining OP as a primary characteristic, and adding separate consideration of the temporal and spatial frequencies associated with the moving stimuli (Baker and Issa, 2005; Mante and Carandini, 2005; Basole et al., 2006). This analysis was consistent with earlier single unit results, in which tuning of V1 neurons to spatial and temporal frequencies was demonstrated (DeAngelis et al., 1993). Issa and colleagues (Baker and Issa, 2005; Issa et al., 2008) reported that a total of six parameters are required to explain response maps—OP, SF preference, and temporal frequency preference, and the tuning bandwidths of all three. This account is referred to as the spatio-temporal filter model. How these response characteristics arise during cortical development and how neurons become tuned to just those features is the subject of continuing research (Rosenberg et al., 2010), and of this paper.

In common with the model of Erwin and Miller (1998) and that of Kang et al. (2003) the model reviewed here depends upon time-average correlations—that is, the common occurrence of synchronous oscillation in the cortex—although it does not share their other assumptions or conclusions. It seeks to avoid the ascription of "features" as primary characteristics, and to explain both the findings of Basole et al. (2003) and the empirical reduction to alternative feature attributes used in the spatio-temporal model, as well as explaining the emergence of the anatomical features described above.

DESCRIPTION OF MODEL

NEURAL FIELD EQUATIONS

As alternatives to neural network models, lumped neural models and neural field equations have been expressed in many forms (e.g., Wilson and Cowan, 1973; Freeman, 1975; Haken, 1996; Amari, 1977; Nunez, 1981; van Rotterdam et al., 1982; Jirsa and Haken, 1996; Robinson et al., 2001; Wright et al., 2003; beim Graben, 2008; Bressloff, 2012). These offer means of approximating the properties of ensembles of cells on a larger scale then neural networks *per se*. Here we have used a generic form of neural field equations to represent an idealized, isotropic, neural field, representing the developing cortex as if it were not subject to apoptosis—a potentiality from which connections are selected during development. The scale of the field is that of a cortical area such as V1, representing intracortical connections rather than cortico-cortical. Thus, the density of connection between neurons declines with increasing separation of their cell bodies (Braitenberg and Schüz, 1991). The high non-linearity of synapto-dendritic summations are linearized at the field level, and axonal conduction speed is considered single-valued. Subject to these strictures, the following equations include features relevant to the present context:

$$\varphi_p^{\mathbf{qr}'}(t) = f_p^{\mathbf{qr}'} \times Q_p\left(\mathbf{r}', t - \frac{|\mathbf{q}-\mathbf{r}'|}{\nu}\right) \quad (1)$$

$$\psi_p^{\mathbf{qr}'}(t) = M_p^{\mathbf{qr}'} * \varphi_p^{\mathbf{qr}'}(t) \quad (2)$$

$$\Psi_p(\mathbf{q}, t) = \int_{\mathbf{r}'} \psi_p^{\mathbf{qr}'}(t)d\mathbf{r}' \quad (3)$$

$$V_p(\mathbf{q}, t) = \sum_{p=e \wedge p=i} G_p * \Psi_p(\mathbf{q}, t) \quad (4)$$

$$Q_p(\mathbf{q}, t) = f_\Sigma(V_p(\mathbf{q}, t)) + E_p(\mathbf{q}, t) \quad (5)$$

Subscript $p = e, i$ refers to excitatory or inhibitory neurons; superscript $\mathbf{qr}'$ refers to synaptic connection from $\mathbf{r}'$ to $\mathbf{q}$ where $\mathbf{q}$, $\mathbf{r}'$ are cortical positions occupied by single neurons.

$\varphi_p^{\mathbf{qr}'}(t)$ is the flux of pulses reaching pre-synapses at the neuron at $\mathbf{q}$, from the neuron at $\mathbf{r}'$.

$\psi_p^{\mathbf{qr}'}(t)$is the synaptic current generated by $\varphi_p^{\mathbf{qr}'}(t)$.

$\Psi_p(\mathbf{q}, t)$ is the aggregate synaptic current of type p generated at $\mathbf{q}$.

$V_p(\mathbf{q}, t)$ is the soma membrane potential (relative to the resting potential) generated at $\mathbf{q}$.

$Q_p(\mathbf{q}, t)$ is the pulse emission rate at $\mathbf{q}$.

$f_p^{\mathbf{qr}'}$ is the probability density of occurrence of pre-synapses generated by axons of the neuron at $\mathbf{r}'$ terminating at $\mathbf{q}$.

ν is axonal conduction speed.

$M_p^{\mathbf{qr}'}$ is the steady-state term in a convolution transforming pre-synaptic flux to synaptic current.

G_p is the steady-state term in a convolution transforming pre-synaptic flux into dendritic potentials.

$f_\Sigma(V_q(\mathbf{q}, t))$ is a sigmoid function describing the local conversion of dendritic potentials into the rate of generation of action potentials.

$E_p(\mathbf{q}, t)$ is a driving signal noise, arising from intrinsic random cell action potentials.

Restriction of the field to the scale of a cortical area carries several implications important for the model, all because the probability of connections between any two neurons declines with distance of separation. Firstly, descriptively we can consider "reciprocal couplings" as an idealization/representation of field coupling symmetry, and in many instances reciprocal couplings will in fact exist. Secondly because of more generally dense connections among near neighbors, smoothing at dendritic summation requires that $Q_p(\mathbf{q}, t)$ is spatially and temporally "brown"—i.e., has high correlation at short distances and times of separation. Thirdly, the average "degree" of separation—i.e., the average number of neighboring cells traversed by synaptic connections linking one cell to another—will also increase in proportion to physical distance of separation.

Experimental observations (Freeman, 1975, 1991; Hassenstaub et al., 2005) show intrinsic cortical oscillation arises from alternating excitatory cell and inhibitory cell firing at lags ¼ of the period of oscillation. Simulations of the oscillations (Wright, 2009, 2010) show that traveling waves are thus generated, the intersection of which produces broadband synchrony. In conditions of uniform cortical excitation without strong perturbation from external inputs the exchange of pulses between all cells reaches an equilibrium—that is, a steady-state of symmetrical exchange of signals between excitatory cells at any two positions on the cortex, so that over sufficient intervals, T,

$$\frac{1}{T}\int_T \left(\varphi_{p1}(\mathbf{q}) - \bar{\varphi}_{p1}\right)dt = \frac{1}{T}\int_T \left(\varphi_{p2}(\mathbf{r}') - \bar{\varphi}_{p2}\right)dt \tag{6}$$

where $\bar{\varphi}_p$ is the time-average presynaptic flux, uniform throughout the cortical field. The equilibrium reached implies differences in timing between the firing of excitatory and inhibitory cells. The interaction of excitatory and inhibitory cells ($p1 \vee p2 = e$, and $p1 \vee p2 = i$,) leads to closely correlated firing of both cells if they are very closely situated, as a consequence the similar local values of $E(\mathbf{q}, t)$ equation (5), while ¼-cycle-out-of-phase oscillation develops between more separated excitatory and inhibitory cells. Inhibitory/inhibitory or excitatory/excitatory interactions ($p1 \wedge p2 = e$, or $p1 \wedge p2 = i$,) between reciprocally connected neurons lead to zero-lag synchrony, and since conduction delays are short compared to the period of oscillation, the equality of equation (6) is generally approached even when T is smaller than the period of oscillation (Chapman et al., 2002). As there are equal time-lags in both directions of conduction excitatory pulse trains throughout the cortex have maximum correlation at zero lag—i.e., where $\overline{Q}_e$ is the time-average firing rate—also uniform throughout the cortical field -

$$(Q_e - \overline{Q}_e)(\mathbf{r}', t) \approx (Q_e - \overline{Q}_e)(\mathbf{q}, t) \tag{7}$$

Figures 1 and **2** show these properties generated in a simulation of cortical dynamics with physiologically realistic parameters (Wright, 2009, 2010). In conditions of strong cortical excitation local oscillation is autonomous and corresponds to cortical gamma rhythm, while in conditions of lower cortical excitation, damped gamma oscillation, and a predominance of background $1/f^2$ is seen.

MAGNITUDE OF PRE-SYNAPTIC PULSE SYNCHRONY

Zero-lag synchronous oscillation thus entails presynaptic pulse synchrony, with a magnitude of presynaptic flux variation which can be defined respectively for individual synapses, individual cells, and in aggregate, as

$$J^{\mathbf{qr}'} = \left[\frac{1}{T}\int_T (\varphi_e^{\mathbf{qr}'} - \bar{\varphi}_e)^2 dt\right]^{1/2} \tag{8}$$

$$J^{\mathbf{q}} = \left[\frac{1}{T}\int_T \int_{\mathbf{r}'} (\varphi_e^{\mathbf{qr}'} - \bar{\varphi}_e)^2 dt d\mathbf{r}'\right]^{1/2} \tag{9}$$

$$J = \left[\frac{1}{T}\int_T \int_{\mathbf{r}'} \int_{\mathbf{q}} (\varphi_e^{\mathbf{qr}'} - \bar{\varphi}_e)^2 dt d\mathbf{r}' d\mathbf{q}\right]^{1/2} \tag{10}$$

$J^{\mathbf{qr}'}$ is RMS presynaptic flux variation between $\mathbf{q}$ and $\mathbf{r}'$, $J^{\mathbf{q}}$ is the sum of $J^{\mathbf{qr}'}$ at a single excitatory neuron, and J is the aggregate of $J^{\mathbf{q}}$ over the cortex.

SELECTION OF SCALE-FREE SMALL-WORLD CONFIGURATIONS OF NEURONS

For any given level of cortical excitation, J is greatest for that ensemble of C connected neurons, in which excitatory pulses arrive at dendrites, from all sources at differing distances of separation, as closely in-phase as possible, so as to maximize their summation. Axonal delays, small compared to the period of gamma oscillation, contribute a phase difference between cell firing at $\mathbf{r}'$ and the arrival of presynaptic pulses at $\mathbf{q}$, of

$$\Delta\Phi^{\mathbf{qr}'} = 2\pi \frac{|\mathbf{q} - \mathbf{r}'|}{P\nu} \tag{11}$$

where P is the period of oscillation. Therefore that ensemble selected by its capacity to maximize presynaptic synchrony must approach minimal total axonal length, $L = \int_{\mathbf{r}'} \int_{\mathbf{q}} |\mathbf{q} - \mathbf{r}'|\, d\mathbf{q}d\mathbf{r}'$, and minimization of this length minimizes the metabolic requirements of the axons.

It has been shown generally (Cohen and Havlin, 2003) for all systems of connected elements, the path length in a topological sense is at a minimum where degree distribution follows a power law. As was pointed out in conjunction with equations (1–5), in our idealized neural field, average degree of separation, in the topological sense, increases linearly as metric distance of separation of the cell bodies, so that if L, their total length of axonal connections, is minimal, then the path length in the topological sense is also minimal, and the degree distribution is that of a scale-free, or ultra-small world. Therefore, the connection density between cells vs. their metric distance of separation should also be approximated by a power-law distribution. Further, according to Cohen and Havlin

$$L \sim \log\log C \tag{12}$$

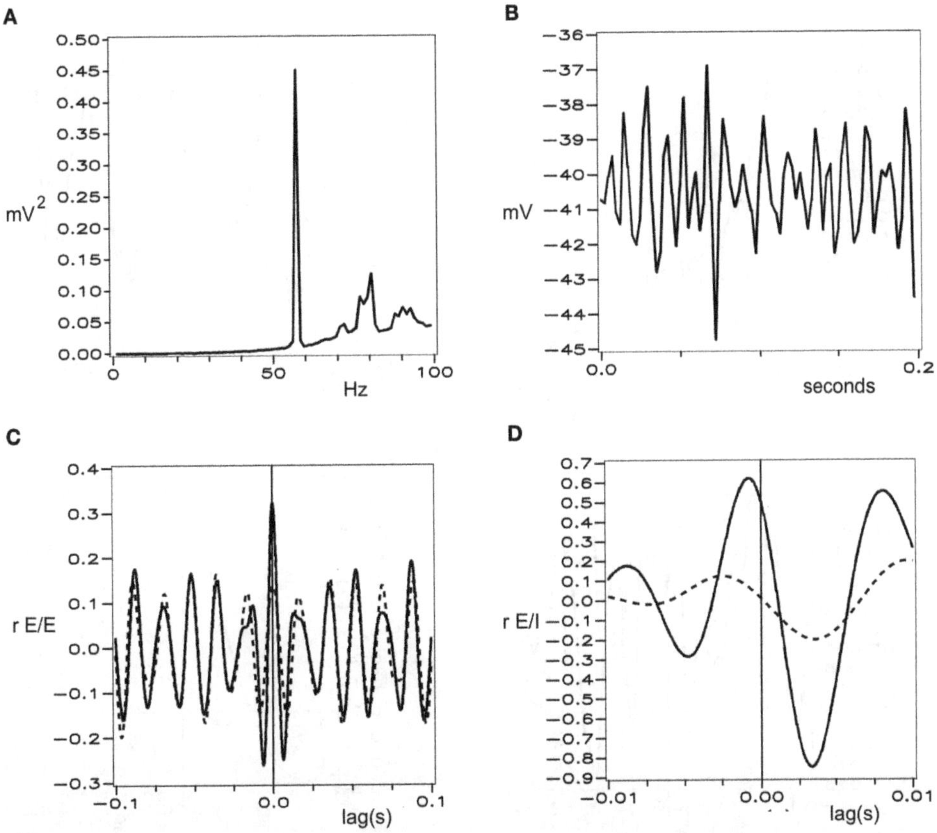

FIGURE 1 | Simulated electrocortical activity in the excited cortex, from Wright (2010). (A) Power spectrum of a local field potential time-series, shown in **(B)**. **(C)** and **(D)** Cell firing correlations, vs. time-lag. Dashed line—cells remote from each other. Solid lines—cells adjacent to each other. **(C)** Between excitatory cells. **(D)** Between excitatory and inhibitory cells.

so the metabolic efficiency of the connection system is further enhanced if the surviving cells are linked into a continuum, as opposed to separate pools of neurons.

In accord with equation (1), the number of neighboring excitatory cells connected to a given excitatory neuron, as a function of distance of separation, is proportional to $2\pi \times f_e^{\mathbf{qr}'}(|\mathbf{q}-\mathbf{r}'|)$—so the ensemble of neurons selected by greatest synchrony must have a connection density function of the form:

$$f_e^{\mathbf{qr}'} \sim \left(2\pi\left|\mathbf{q}-\mathbf{r}'\right|\right)^{-A} \qquad A > 0 \tag{13}$$

Intracortical axonal trees have approximately exponential density/range relations (Scholl, 1956; Braitenberg and Schüz, 1991) and a power function is fitted exactly by an infinite sum of exponential functions—i.e.:

$$\left(2\pi\left|\mathbf{q}-\mathbf{r}'\right|\right)^{-A} = \frac{1}{\Gamma(A)}\int_0^\infty u^{A-1}\mathbf{exp}\left[-u2\pi\left|\mathbf{q}-\mathbf{r}'\right|\right]du \tag{14}$$

so an ultra-small-world connectivity can be achieved by sets of populations of cells with differing axonal characteristic lengths. During embryogenesis primal cells divide sequentially by layer (Rakic, 1988; Shi et al., 2012) with differences in growth pattern and characteristic axonal length programmed in sequential cell divisions. For simplicity, we consider only two populations of excitatory cells, with cell bodies partially separated by layer, but with intermingled axonal and dendritic trees, and axonal tree connection probabilities described by:

$$f_\alpha^{\mathbf{qr}'} = \frac{N_\alpha}{N}2\pi\lambda_\alpha \exp\left[-\lambda_\alpha 2\pi\left|\mathbf{q}-\mathbf{R}\right|\right] \tag{15}$$

$$f_\beta^{\mathbf{qr}'} = \frac{N_\beta}{N}2\pi\lambda_\beta \exp\left[-\lambda_\beta 2\pi\left|\mathbf{q}-\mathbf{r}\right|\right] \tag{16}$$

$$f_e^{\mathbf{qr}'} = f_\alpha^{\mathbf{qR}} + f_\beta^{\mathbf{qr}}$$

$f_\alpha^{\mathbf{qR}}$ refers to the axonal trees with longest axonal extensions, and $f_\beta^{\mathbf{qr}}$ refers to the axonal trees with short axonal extension, thus $\lambda_\alpha < \lambda_\beta$. $N = N_\alpha + N_\beta$ is the number of synapses received/generated by each cell. Distances from $\mathbf{r}'$ to $\mathbf{q}$ are substituted as $\mathbf{r}, \mathbf{R}$ to indicate equal distances, $|\mathbf{q}-\mathbf{r}|$ and $|\mathbf{q}-\mathbf{R}|$, measured along the axonal trees of the respective populations.

The further defining characteristic of small-world connectivity—the occurrence of connection nodes—emerges as a consequence of the formation of the superficial patch system, as follows.

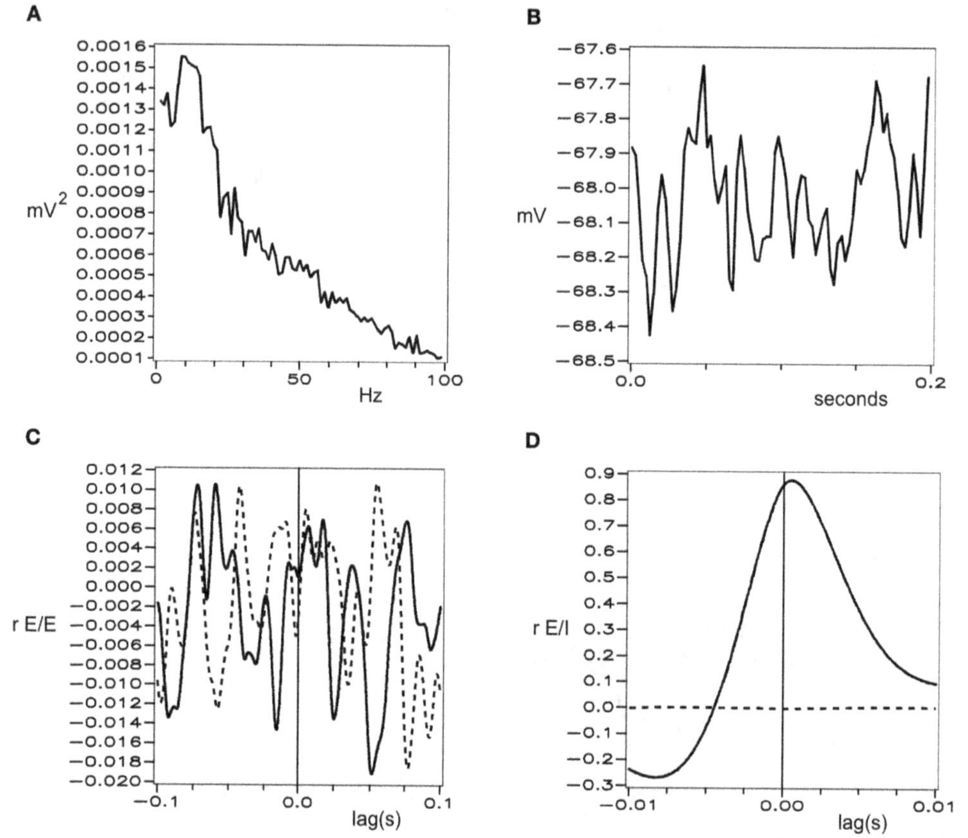

FIGURE 2 | Simulated background electrocortical activity, in conditions of low cortical excitation. Graphical format is the same as in **Figure 1**.

THE ORIGIN OF THE SUPERFICIAL PATCH SYSTEM

The two populations of cells described by equations (15) and (16), and the synapses they give rise to can be referred to as α-cells and synapses, and β-cells and synapses. We first make a provisional assumption (later justified on a species-specific basis) that $N_\beta >>> N_\alpha$, so that α-cells with long-range axons are embedded among much more numerous β-cells, all with sparse connectivity. Equation (10) can be written by separately summing contributions from α-cells at positions $\{\mathbf{q}\alpha\}$ and β-cells at positions $\{\mathbf{q}\beta\}$, to give:

$$J = \int_{q\alpha}\int_{\mathbf{R}} J^{\mathbf{qR}} d\mathbf{q}\alpha d\mathbf{R} + \int_{q\beta}\int_{\mathbf{r}} J^{\mathbf{qr}} d\mathbf{q}\beta d\mathbf{r} \quad (17)$$

so J is at a maximum if $\int_{q\alpha}\int_{\mathbf{R}} J^{\mathbf{qR}} d\mathbf{q}\alpha d\mathbf{R}$ and $\int_{q\beta}\int_{\mathbf{r}} J^{\mathbf{qr}} d\mathbf{q}\beta d\mathbf{r}$ are individually at maxima. Applying equations (15) and (16) via equation (1) to find values of $J^{\mathbf{qr}'}$ in equation (8) as functions of $|\mathbf{q}-\mathbf{r}, \mathbf{R}|$, shows that:

$$\begin{aligned} J^{\mathbf{qr}} &= J^{\mathbf{qR}} \quad \text{if} \quad |\mathbf{q}-\mathbf{r}, \mathbf{R}| = x \\ J^{\mathbf{qr}} &> J^{\mathbf{qR}} \quad \text{if} \quad |\mathbf{q}-\mathbf{r}, \mathbf{R}| < x \\ J^{\mathbf{qr}} &< J^{\mathbf{qR}} \quad \text{if} \quad |\mathbf{q}-\mathbf{r}, \mathbf{R}| > x \end{aligned} \quad (18)$$

where $x = -\ln\left(\frac{N_\alpha \lambda_\alpha}{N_\beta \lambda_\beta}\right)/2\pi(\lambda_\beta - \lambda_\alpha)$

Consequently $\int_{q\beta}\int_{\mathbf{r}} J^{\mathbf{qr}} d\mathbf{q}\beta d\mathbf{r}$ is at a maximum if β-cells are clustered so they make reciprocal connections at minimum distance and maximum density (β-clusters). β-cells at the center of β-clusters, for which $J^{\mathbf{qr}}$ attains the maximum possible value, must give and receive all their connections as β-connections to a radial distance of x.

Since β-cells are clustered, α-cells necessarily are also clustered (α-clusters), and since maximization of reciprocal β-connections excludes formation of short-range reciprocal α- connections, α-cells must form reciprocal synaptic connections at distances greater than x, to maximize $\int_{q\alpha}\int_{\mathbf{R}} J^{\mathbf{qR}} d\mathbf{q}\alpha d\mathbf{R}$. Similarly, reciprocal connections between α- and β-cells must occur at cluster margins, over distances approximate to x. Since we made the provisional assumption that $N_\beta >>> N_\alpha$, then fitting the sum of equations (15) and (16) to a power function requires $\lambda_\alpha <<< \lambda_\beta$. Consequently α-cells may form multiple patches of synaptic connections, skipping from α-cluster to α-cluster.

Since β-clusters have radius x and α-clusters are separated by distance x, α-clusters are necessarily placed at the vertices of hexagons tiling the cortical surface, with each hexagon embracing a β-cluster. Analogy to the superficial patch system in some species is apparent.

As noted earlier, hexagonal symmetry of OP and the superficial patch system is an idealization that is roughly approached in some species, while in others it is effectively absent (Horton and Adams, 2005). Since approximation of a power law distribution by two populations of neurons requires $N_\alpha <<< N_\beta$ if $\lambda_\alpha <<< \lambda_\beta$, this case is more closely approached for larger cortical sizes, and the patchy connection system will have higher orderliness and hexagonal rotational symmetry. If $\lambda_\alpha < \lambda_\beta$ by only a small amount, as in animals with small cortical size, then N_β is not necessarily greater than N_α, and an ordered hexagonal structure need not be apparent. Such reduction of the apparent orderliness does not imply the absence of "small world" connectivity, nor imply impairment of function. The comparative invariance of distance between OP singularities across species reported by Kaschube et al. (2010) and Keil et al. (2012) implies that $x = -\ln\left(\frac{N_\alpha \lambda_\alpha}{N_\beta \lambda_\beta}\right)/2\pi(\lambda_\beta - \lambda_\alpha)$ [equation (18)] is also relatively constant over species in the middle to large range of V1 size. Since the ratios N_β/N_α, and $\lambda_\alpha/\lambda_\beta$ must vary inversely in value in different species, according to cortical size, as required if the sum of the two synaptic distributions maintains a power law distribution, then comparative invariance of OP singularity density is to be expected.

LOCAL SYNAPTIC COMPETITION FOR METABOLIC SUPPLY

Turning from optimization of energy demand of axons, to that of dendrites, we can modify equation (2) to a form representing complex distinct processes of synaptic adaptation, impulse decay, and pre-synaptic synergy, including the limiting rate of metabolic energy supplied to excitatory synapses—viz:

$$\psi_e^{qr'}(t) = \Gamma^{qr'} M_e^{qr'} * \varphi_e^{qr'}(t) \tag{19}$$

$$M_e^{qr'} = D \times S \tag{20}$$

$\Gamma^{qr'}$ is the available fraction of the metabolic supply rate needed to attain maximum current flow. Since we have assumed increasing synaptic current in synchronously activated synapses increases the available metabolic supply, the value of $\Gamma^{qr'}$ must follow that of $\psi_e^{qr'}$.

$$D = \frac{1}{B}\exp[-Bt] \quad B > 0 \tag{21}$$

represents impulse decay following delivery of an afferent action potential, with time-integral of 1 (after Rennie et al., 2000).

$$S = 1/(1 + \exp[-g(J^q(t))] \tag{22}$$

is a sigmoid function with range 0–1, representing synaptic adaptation to the afferent pulse rate, and including the effect of pre-synaptic co-operation (Tsukada and Fukushima, 2010) upon individual synaptic current flow as $g(J^q)$—a suitable ascending function in J^q, such that if $J^q = 0$, there is no current flow at the synapse.

As well as inter-cellular competition between assemblies of neurons, we assume competition takes place between adjacent individual synapses arising from the same neuron. Therefore those neurons that survive apoptosis must have found an efficient deployment of resource to the synapses best positioned to maximize the magnitude of synchrony. Any two adjacent synapses arising from the same pre-synaptic neuron may terminate on the same, or different, post-synaptic neurons. If they terminate on the same neuron their conditions are essentially identical in terms of equations (19–22). If they terminate on different neurons, then the relevant values of J^q need not identical—and their competition for resources would lead, via the feedback between $\psi_e^{qr'}$ and $\Gamma^{qr'}$, to low synaptic current at one synapse, and high current at the other. Just what the physiological corollary of these opposite high and low-activity states is, and the critical metabolic component for which the synapses compete, we do not specify. A likely, but by no means unique contributing factor is the supply of extracellular calcium (Montague, 1996). Whatever the critical component(s), the important consequence is that, at synchronous equilibrium, closely situated neurons have either high, or low, pulse correlations with each other.

ORGANIZATION OF PRE-VISION RESPONSE PROPERTIES

We can now term those synapses that are transmitting impulses more strongly near equilibrium "saturated" synapses, and those which are more quiescent, but potentially able to be activated, "sensitive" synapses, and can consider what spatial patterns of saturated connections would best meet the requirement to maximize synchrony. Here a further property of the neural field commented on in relation to equations (1–5)—higher spatial cross-correlation of pulses and field potentials at shorter range—has a decisive impact on the equilibrium pattern of synaptic saturations. These emergent patterns, diagrammed in **Figure 3**, arise for the following reasons:

(a) Maximum synchrony generation with highest cross-correlation among near-neighbors in each β-cluster requires saturated couplings link near-neighbor cells—but sensitive connections must also form between closely adjacent β-cells. Both requirements are met when saturated connections within each β-cluster form a re-entrant network analogous to a Möbius strip. A similar argument regarding connections formed within macrocolumns has been advanced earlier (Wright et al., 2006; Wright and Bourke, 2008).
(b) The α-cluster system and each of the β-clusters must enter into maximum joint resonance. This requires the formation of a homeomorphic projection between scales. The projection must be homeomorphic, since spatial cross-correlation is constrained to decline with distance at both scales, and so if resonance is at a maximum, the projection map must be one preserving topological identity between scales. This is possible because a disk can be mapped to a Möbius strip. Thus saturated α-cell to β-cell synapses must systematically map limited angular ranges of the surrounding α-system onto limited angular ranges on the margins of each β-cluster, and receive reciprocal saturated β-cell to α-cell synapses. Such a mapping requires specification of an orientation and chirality for each β-cluster, and requires a reciprocal distribution of saturated and sensitive synapses from opposite sides of the α-system to neurons in a limited angular range within each β-cluster.
(c) Maximum synchrony generation with high cross-correlation among near-neighbors in the α-system requires α-cells be

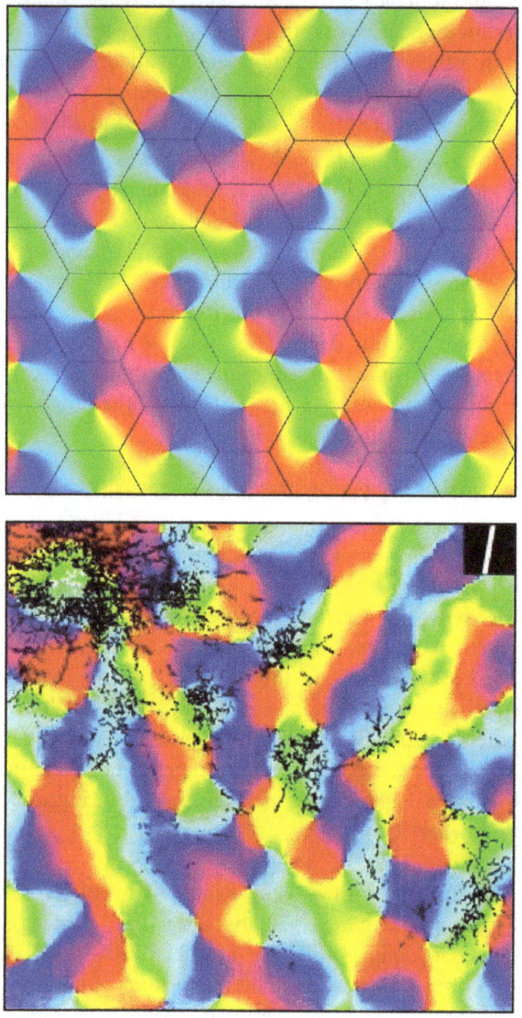

FIGURE 3 | Simulated and real maps of orientation preference in V1, from Wright et al. (2006). Top: Simulation. Colors of the spectrum, from red to violet, represent average OP of V1 neurons for slow-moving visual lines of orientation $0 - \pi$. Adjacent macrocolumns, of diameter $\sim 300\,\mu m$ are set within a hexagonal frame (the patch system) with OP forming color wheels about OP singularities. Orientations and chiralities of the color wheels are arranged to approach a minimum total of angular disparity from mirror reflection of OP between each macrocolumn and its neighbors. **Bottom:** Real OP. Visualized in the tree shrew by Bosking et al. (1997). Superficial patchy connections are demarcated in black by a selective stain. Scale of macrocolumns is approximate to that of the simulation.

linked by saturated synapses. This requirement is concordant with deployment of the excess sensitive α-connections to neurons in β-clusters at positions outside the homeomorphic projection.

(d) Saturated and sensitive $\beta - \beta$ connections between adjacent β-clusters must also be arranged to maximize resonance. Therefore β-clusters must project to each of their six neighbors as closely as possible to mirror symmetry, with both saturated and sensitive synapses linking homologous points—that is to say, points with similar OP as classically measured with low object speeds—within each cluster. Perfect mirror symmetry is not possible between all adjacent clusters within a hexagonal array, so mirror-symmetry can be only approximate and irregular and the necessarily broken symmetry permits the particular pattern generated to be one of a large set of possible combinations.

Further analogy between the hypothetical α- and β-systems and real anatomical structures can now be drawn. As well as the α-system's congruence with the superficial patch system, the β-systems, each with a dense system of local connections that are centrally spared from patchy connections, are analogous to macrocolumns each centred about an OP singularity. The distribution of OP for lines of orientation $0 - \pi$ to angles $0 - 2\pi$ in pinwheels about a singularity finds analogy in the wrapping of a Euclidean plane onto a Möbius strip. It has also been earlier shown that arrangements of adjacent pinwheels in broken mirror symmetry match classical OP maps (Wright et al., 2006).

The structure of real patchy connections and classical OP response maps, contrasted with the results of simulating the arrangement of adjacent macrocolumnar structures in accord with the description above, are shown in **Figure 3**, while **Figure 4** shows diagrammatically the proposed arrangement of saturated and sensitive synapses, and foreshadows the effect of structured visual stimuli, once the post-natal phase of development begins—to be described in the next section.

Figure 5 shows a further impact upon response map organization—the emergence of OD columns.

Just as OP organization in some species is apparent before eye opening, so too is the organization into OD columns (Blakemore and Van Sluyters, 1975; Erwin and Miller, 1998). Explanation of this can be included in the present model by an argument similar to that of Erwin and Miller, who suppose the correlation of cell firing at short distances of separation of V1 cells to be greater than the correlation of visual inputs over a similar distance. This forces a columnar OD organization because of instability—in the present model's terms, the resulting disruption of the synchronous field at equilibrium produced by binocular inputs to the same cells—resolved by formation of columns in Turing patterns. A corollary of this effect is impact on the hexagonal arrangement, with broken mirror symmetry of OP organization, predicted in (d) above. The required alternation of OD columns would imposes a frustration on the approach to hexagonal tiling of the cortical surface—forcing approach closer to a square tiling. The occurrence of mirror symmetry within a square tiling accounts for the way that lines of OP cross orthogonally between OP columns. (Obermayer and Blasdel, 1993). Following eyeopening inputs from the two eyes transmit images which are necessarily cross-correlated at a small spatial lag, because of angular disparity in their line of focus. Spatial lag correlation in their inputs at V1 level could then help maintain the columnar organization (Wright and Bourke, 2008).

WAVE TRANSMISSION OF VISUAL INFORMATION, FOLLOWING EYE-OPENING

We compactly express the emergent map by which the patchy connections over a part of V1 link to positions within each

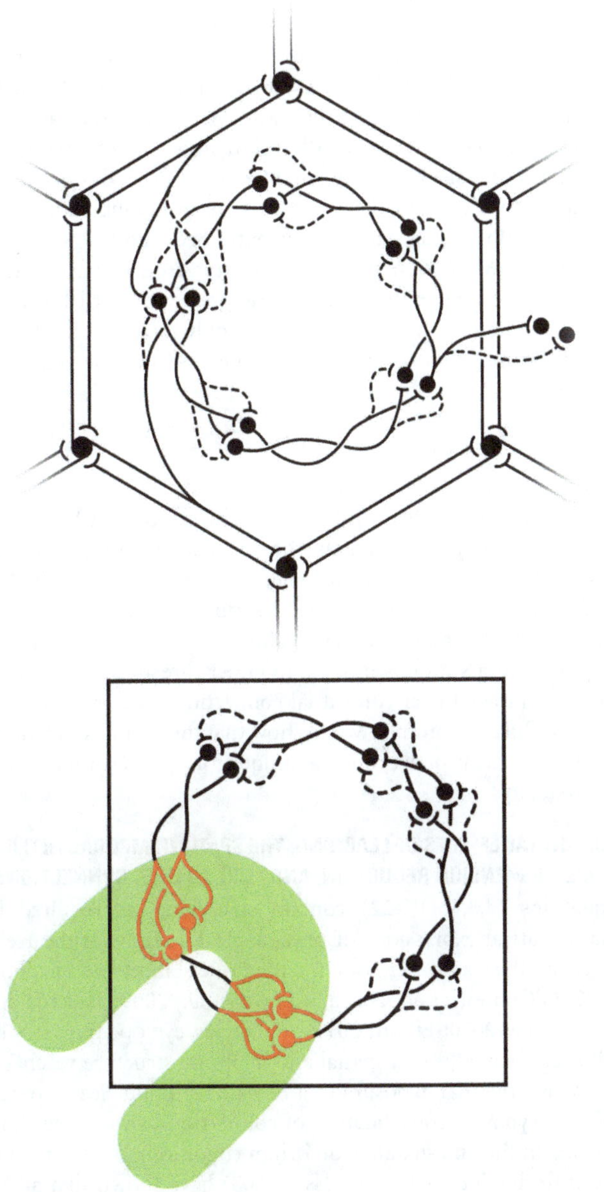

FIGURE 4 | Equilibrium distribution of synaptic activity, and the impact of visual inputs disrupting equilibrium from Wright and Bourke (2013). Top: equilibrium disposition of saturated and sensitive synapses. Black circles represent cell bodies and dendrites. Synapses are indicated as saturated (solid) or sensitive (dashed) terminations of axons. Reciprocal connections between α-patches (patchy connections) form the hexagonal array. (Other connections, although shown as unidirectional, are also reciprocal.) A representative pair of connections from α-cells to the β-patch is displayed in the upper-and lower-aspects of the figure. At the center of the figure, saturated and sensitive synapses show the network's analogy to a Möbius-strip within a β-patch (macrocolumn). To the right, representative links from the central macrocolumn to cells at homologous positions in neighboring macrocolumns. **Bottom**: exposed to strong transient signals conveyed over the superficial patch system, summing with direct visual inputs conveyed to the cRF, the equilibrium configuration breaks down. The green bar represents the field of excitation of cells by the contextual signals, within which cells also directly excited in the cRF, fire at high rates.

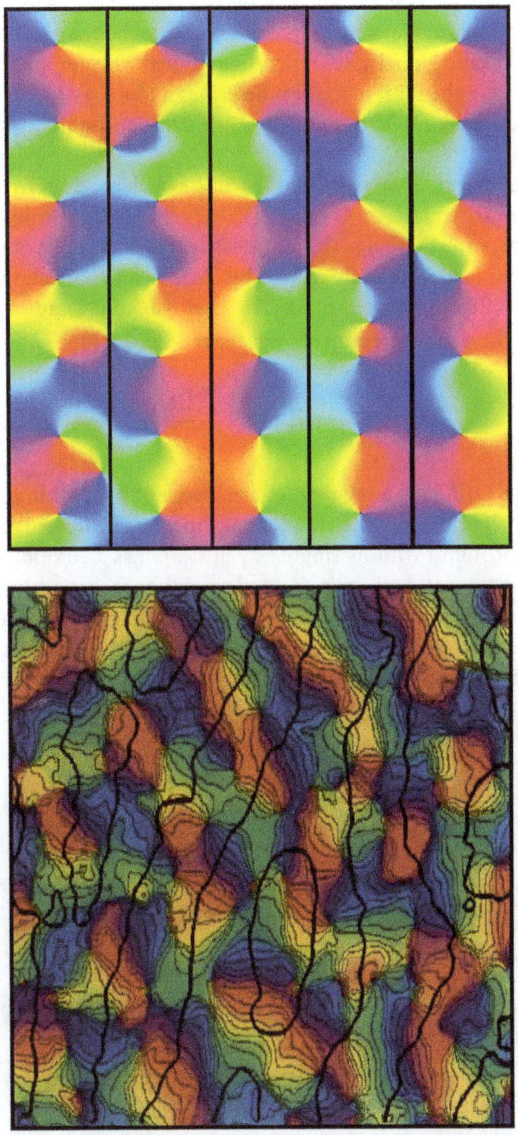

FIGURE 5 | Top: Simulation of OD columns in accord with Wright and Bourke (2008). **Bottom:** Real OD columns, visualized by Obermayer and Blasdel (1993). Color coding of OP and scale as for **Figure 3**. Black lines demarcate alternation of OD between columns. Fine black lines in the lower figure trace the way OP is aligned so it matches orthogonally across OD column boundary.

macrocolumn, as an homeomorphic projection from a disk on a Euclidean plane, **P**, to a Möbius strip, $\mathbf{p}^{[2]}$ - the square brackets [2] indicating the map's resemblance, if viewed from a third dimension, to a 2:1 map formed by squaring a complex vector. Defined in polar co-ordinates,

$$\mathbf{P}\left(\left|\mathbf{R}-\mathbf{C}_j\right|,\boldsymbol{\vartheta}\right)\rightarrow\mathbf{p}^{[2]}\left(\left|\mathbf{r}-\mathbf{C}_j\right|,\pm\boldsymbol{\vartheta}+\varphi\right) \tag{23}$$

where $\mathbf{C}_j$ is the origin of both **P** and $\mathbf{p}^{[2]}$ for the $j-th$ local map, and corresponds to the position of the OP singularity in that macrocolumn. ϑ is the polar angle of **R**, chirality of the local map is indicated by $\pm\vartheta$, and φ is the orientation of the local map relative to the global map. $\vartheta + \varphi$ is defined on the range $0 - 2\pi$ in both local and global maps, but is represented with apparent angle doubling in the local map. This describes a topology for "contextual" connections (Li et al., 2000; Angelucci and Bullier, 2003) to each macrocolumn.

Visual input after eye opening will cause departures from the equilibrium condition. Let $O(\mathbf{P}, t)$ be a visual image projected to V1 by the direct visual pathway. Laterally traveling waves of pulses and local field potentials relayed by the patchy connections can transmit that image to each local map with a point to point delay, $\frac{|\mathbf{R}-\mathbf{r}|}{\upsilon}$, where υ now represents wave speed, so that

$$O(\mathbf{P}, t) \to O\left(\mathbf{p}^{[2]}, t + \frac{|\mathbf{R} - \mathbf{r}|}{\boldsymbol{\nu}}\right) \tag{24}$$

Suppose $O(\mathbf{P}, t)$ is a segment of the image of a visual line, traveling with uniform velocity, $\mathbf{V}_x$, along an $x-$axis directed toward a macrocolumn with its singularity at $\mathbf{C}_j$. O has a component of its extension on the $x-$axis, O_x, and an orthogonal component of extension, on the $y-$axis, O_y. K_x is the dominant spatial frequency of O_x, and K_y is the dominant spatial frequency of O_y. Then the local map projection of O has a transformed spatial frequency in the $x-$axis but not in the $y-$axis—i.e.:

$$k_x \propto \frac{\nu}{\boldsymbol{\nu} \pm \mathbf{V}_x} K_x \tag{25}$$

$$k_y \propto K_y \tag{26}$$

where k_x, k_y are the spatial frequencies in the local map projection of O, and the sign $\pm$ in equation (25) depends on whether O is approaching or departing from $\mathbf{C}_j$. That is, O's orientation in the global map is transformed to its projection to corresponding areas in the local map, by Doppler shift, with a difference in orientation, $\delta\vartheta$;

$$\delta\boldsymbol{\vartheta} = \left|\mathbf{tan}^{-1}[K_y/K_x] - \mathbf{tan}^{-1}[k_y/k_x]\right| \tag{27}$$

INTERACTION OF CONTEXTUAL SIGNALS AND THE CLASSIC RECEPTIVE FIELD

Laterally transmitted contextual signals generally do not trigger cell firing, until the classic receptive field (cRF) is directly stimulated (Li et al., 2000; Angelucci and Bullier, 2003) via the visual pathway. Those cells that then fire within a macrocolumn are those that reflect the supra-threshold summations of sub-threshold signals conveyed over the contextual, patchy, connections, and the direct pathway. We next assume that the summation of contextual and direct cRF inputs acts as an impulse causing a transient breakdown of equilibrium, during which synapses that were in the sensitive state in equilibrium briefly generate substantial synaptic currents [See **Figure 4** (Bottom) and **Figure 6**]. Action potentials are triggered in surrounding cells, and subsequently there is a restoration toward the equilibrium state on withdrawal of the stimulus. During the breakdown the mapping of activity from the global to the local map becomes:

$$O(\mathbf{P}, t) \to O\left(\mathbf{p}^{2}, t + \frac{|\mathbf{R} - \mathbf{r}|}{\nu}\right) \tag{28}$$

The change from equation (24) made by removal of the square brackets from $p^{[2]}$ represents the breakdown's form, as itself a map from global to local scale, resembling a 2:1 complex-multiplication map, as initially described by Alexander et al. (2004). The 2:1 map implies that single cells would show similar responses to a stimulus moving in either direction, but because firing is initiated over contextual connections in a 1:1 mapping, multi-cellular recordings would show that the spatial and temporal order of firing of neurons was unique for a given stimulus form and velocity.

POST-NATAL EFFECTS OF LEARNING, THE SPATIO-TEMPORAL FILTER MODEL, DIMENSION REDUCTION, AND "LIKE TO LIKE" CONNECTIONS

Equations (2,3,4, 19–22) contain state-variables required by mathematical expressions of physiological versions of the Hebb rule, and the spatio-temporal learning rule (Elliott and Shadbolt, 2002; O'Connor et al., 2005a,b; Enoki et al., 2009; Tsukada and Fukushima, 2010; Elliott, 2011). Following eye opening, stimuli with regularly repeated spatial and temporal structure reach V1, so we assume that exposure to a repeated stimulus leads to permanent synaptic consolidation of connections, overlaying those formed in the ante-natal, equilibrium condition. As remarked in the Introduction, Baker and Issa (2005) have shown that all V1 response features can be described in terms of six variables—optimal values of OP, spatial frequency preference, and temporal

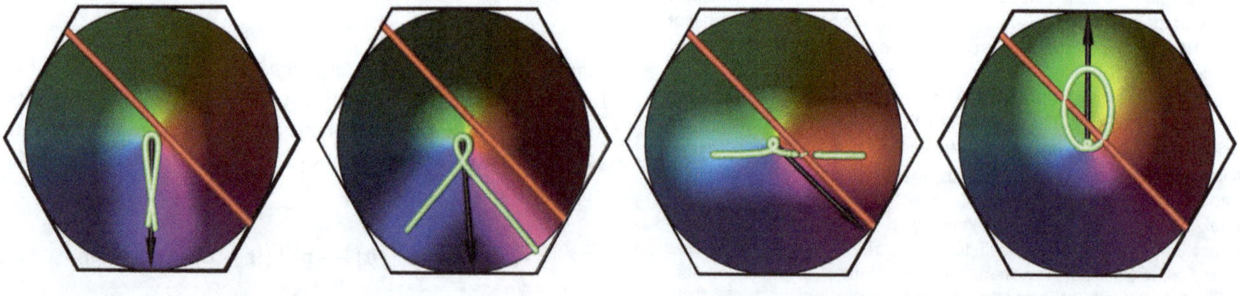

FIGURE 6 | The effect of increasing stimulus speed on apparent OP, for a bar of length 6 units, oriented at 45° to its direction of motion, and traveling left to right. Examples shown are freeze-frames, from separate simulation movies, at similar positions in the visual stimulus' transit across the macrocolumn. From left to right, in each example, the bar speed/wave speed is 0.1, 0.5, 1.0, 1.5, respectively.

frequency preference, each associated with a Gaussian bandwidth of tuning of the cortical response to these features. These define three hypothetical filter proceeses. However, stimulus variables in the present model have equivalents to those used in the spatio-temporal filter model. These are:

Spatio-temporal model	Present model
Object orientation	Orientation relative to the y-axis defined for equations (25, 26)
Object velocity	$\mathbf{V}_x$
Object drift angle	$\tan^{-1}[K_y/K_x]$
Object spatial frequency	$K_x/\lvert\cos(\tan^{-1}[K_y/K_x])\rvert$
Object temporal frequency	$\mathbf{V}_x K_x$

Repeated stimulation with a particular stimulus will therefore lead, under Hebbian learning, to maximization of the response to that stimulus, thus creating an apparent "tuning" of particular neurons to that particular combination of stimulus features. Thus, the spatio-temporal model can be regarded as a consequence of the present model. Optimization by learning of the parameters for each of the three filters must be competitive between adjacent cells, providing the necessary condition for fitting response maps with continuity and completeness, by dimension-reduction methods (Kohonen, 1982; Durbin and Willshaw, 1987; Durbin and Mitchison, 1990).

Finally, the consolidation of saturated long-range patchy connections by Hebbian learning would result in mature "like to like" connections.

SIMULATIONS—A CRITICAL TEST

A critical test of our model, then, is whether we can reproduce in simulation the results of Basole et al. (2003), without *a priori* feature-specific responses to orientation, spatial frequency, or temporal frequency. Our simulations assume the steady-state presence of the Mobius synaptic configuration and its perturbation by visual signals, intended to reflect the state of the visual cortex shortly after birth, when first exposed to visual stimuli.

Equation (28) was applied in simulations of an hexagonal array of seven adjacent macrocolumns. Results reported here are for the central macrocolumn of the array of 7. Examples are shown in **Figure 6**, which shows the orthogonal transformation of apparent OP from the lowest to the highest bar speed for a moving line stimulus oriented at 45° to its line of passage.

Diameter for each macrocolumn is 300 microns, and wave speed for transcortical polysynaptic propagation 0.1 m/s (Bringuier et al., 1999). Units of length subsequently referred to, are multiples of the radius of a macrocolumn—150 microns. Simulation time-step was 0.1 ms.

A moving line in the visual field, relayed by the direct visual pathway to the cRF of each macrocolumn is represented as a red bar. In a single simulation the red bar traveled across the entire hexagonal array from left to right, with constant speed, direction and orientation. The orientation of the red bar to the line of passage is measured as *bar angle* from 0°, where the bar is oriented orthogonally to the direction of travel, to ±90°, where the bar is oriented in the direction of travel.

The lag-transmitted image of the red bar, relayed as subthreshold activation to each macrocolumn via the superficial patch system, is shown in green, with illumination about the zone of subthreshold activation, to indicate that input to the cRF from the direct visual pathway and contextual signals caused triggering of action potentials. The average angle from the macrocolumn singularity to the centers of action potential generation (i.e., all points on the green line with illumination) was calculated at each time-step, and shown as a black arrow, thus indicating the part of the macrocolumn with a response preference (*apparent OP*) for the particular bar movement. (A change in the sector of the macrocolumn that is maximally stimulated is equivalent to an equal change in the angle of approach of the bar needed to maintain stimulation of the same sector). The black arrow angle was averaged over a window beginning after the red bar had passed the center of the macrocolumn by a distance equal to 10% of macrocolumn radius, and extending from the 10th percentile to the 20th percentile of that radius, thus obtaining an estimate of the apparent OP during the cRF activation time. The standard error (SE) of the black arrow angles was calculated from 11 equally spaced time steps through the averaging window.

Combinations of bar-length, orientation of the bar to the direction of movement, and bar speed, were then systematically varied in separate simulations, results of which are supplied as supplementary animated movies. Their effects on OP, measured at the central local map of the hexagonal group, were obtained as *OP difference,* $\Delta\phi$—a measure of the change in OP as a function of these variables—calculated as

$$\Delta\phi = \begin{cases} \phi_1 - \phi_0 - \pi & \text{when} \quad \pi/2 < \phi_1 - \phi_0 \\ \phi_1 - \phi_0 & \text{when} \quad -\pi/2 \le \phi_1 - \phi_0 \le \pi/2 \\ \phi_1 - \phi_0 + \pi & \text{when} \quad \phi_1 - \phi_0 < -\pi/2 \end{cases} \quad (29)$$

The *reference OP,* $\phi_0 \in [0, \pi)$, was the OP found at the lowest bar speed applied (bar speed/wave speed = 0.1) and the *apparent OP,* $\phi_1 \in [0, \pi)$, was the OP found at higher speeds.

Systematic results are shown in **Figure 7**, which graphs OP difference vs. bar speed/wave speed, for bar angles 0 to ±90°, calculated for a bar length of 6 units. Variation of bar length showed progressive lessening of the effect of velocity on OP for greater bar lengths.

For the case of bar-angle zero degrees (a line oriented orthogonally to its direction of passage, as in classical measurements of OP) no OP difference is seen until, as bar speed approaches wave speed, a 90° change in apparent OP takes place at a single increment in speed. This corresponds to transition to a "motion streak," as object movement blurs resolution in the direction of motion. Increasing OP difference with bar speed at other bar angles is a more gradual development of the same effect—that is, mixing of responses to object speed and to object orientation. The illuminated field of supra-threshold excitation generated is not that expected to accompany a Gaussian-shaped tuning

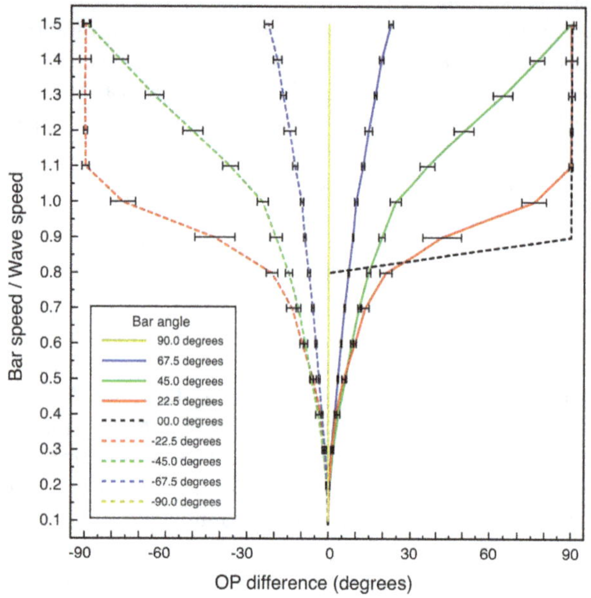

FIGURE 7 | Change in apparent OP, and standard error of the estimate, as a function of bar speed to wave speed, for lines at different orientations to their directions of motion. Bar length 6 units.

curve, but is roughly bimodal at medium speeds—e.g., bar-speed/wave-speed = 0.5. The form of the field of excitation is a combination of the classical preferred OP and the orthogonal orientation, expected as a consequence of Doppler shifts in the laterally-transmitted cortical signals generated by the moving visual input.

Variation of the window over which the apparent OP was estimated did not affect the qualitative results so long as averaging was conducted over a window beginning after the center point of the macrocolumn was crossed by the red bar. Variation of the estimate of wave speed was also without effect, so long as results were expressed in terms of bar speed/wave speed.

For comparative purposes similar simulations were performed in which contextual (green bar) responses were constrained to occur only with a limited angular response within a macrocolumn. That is, a restricted response to the line, according only to its orientation was imposed, in analogy to conventional models of OP, but with conduction delays of "like to like" fibers included. Then, systematic variation of OP with bar velocity did not occur.

These results match the findings of Basole et al. (2003) with respect to variation of OP peak responses as a function of line velocity and length. They do not reproduce the form of the experimentally observed Gaussian tuning curves, but as argued in the prior section, subsequent post-natal Hebbian learning progressively over-writing the Mobius configuration, and strengthening the peak response to the optimal visual signal, would concurrently strengthen responses to signals which are close to the optimum, resulting in Gaussian tuning curves in the more mature animals studied by Basole et al. (2003) and Issa et al. (2008).

INTER-AREAL INTERACTIONS OF V1 AND HIGHER VISUAL AREAS

The principle underlying the development of connections between macrocolumns and the superficial patch system may be generalized to the emergence of inter-areal connections. To recap, taking V1 as an example we have argued above that, because co-variance of activity declines with metric distance at both the scale of the patchy connections and within a macrocolumn, a homeotypic mapping between scales can emerge. This requires that relative distances on the maps at each scale must be in the ratio of correlation lengths of synchronous oscillation at the two scales, and adjacent maps must themselves have a correlated structure over a distance approximate to the correlation length of the patch system. It then follows that superposition of adjacent local maps, with appropriate rotation and correction to a common chirality, would result in a further map with co-variance of activity declining with metric distance, over the correlation length of the patch system.

Inter-areal connections, made by cortico-cortical axonal projections, could permit maps of this type to arise during ante-natal development, with the composite map at the higher cortical-area level itself folded into the Möbius configuration. The selection of saturated connections, projecting between areas with normalization of rotations and chiralities, would be possible by selection from the larger set of possible connections made by branches of cortico-cortical axons, diverging from their cells of origin to their cells of termination, overlapping as they terminate, and generally reciprocal between areas (Braitenberg and Schüz, 1991; Boucsein et al., 2011). Thus, antenatally, sets of macrocolumns at both the lower, V1, level and higher levels, could resonate with, and form preferential connections with, superimposed and overlapping groups at the other level, in accord with the developmental selection requirement to maximize joint synchrony. With the occurrence of eye-opening, Hebbian learning would then begin to overwrite the equilibrium resonance configuration between areas, in analogy to the process at intra-areal level—with the added property of associating concurrent patterns of activity in the V1 macrocolumns.

Illustrating this effect, **Figure 8** shows, at the bottom, a system of seven macrocolumns at V1 level, driven via the direct visual pathway by a pair of intersecting lines in the visual field.

The top part of the figure shows a projection of activity in conjointly activated macocolumns in V1, to a higher visual area, in which responses in the seven macrocolumns in V1 have been superimposed, with disparities in their orientation and chirality eliminated. Summations of points stimulated by both lines, shown by highlighted white points, occur frequently in the forward projection—much more so than at the level of V1 itself. These indicate response to angles of intersection of the lines at the lower level, and, commonly at the higher level, summating responses to time-lagged correlations between disparate positions of the moving visual stimulus. This effect is consistent with the preferential responses to angular and complex stimuli, characteristic of higher cortical levels (Merigan and Maunsell, 1993).

Conversely, since connections between higher and lower levels are generally reciprocal, a possible mechanism permitting control of attention (Rao and Ballard, 1997; Kveraga et al., 2007;

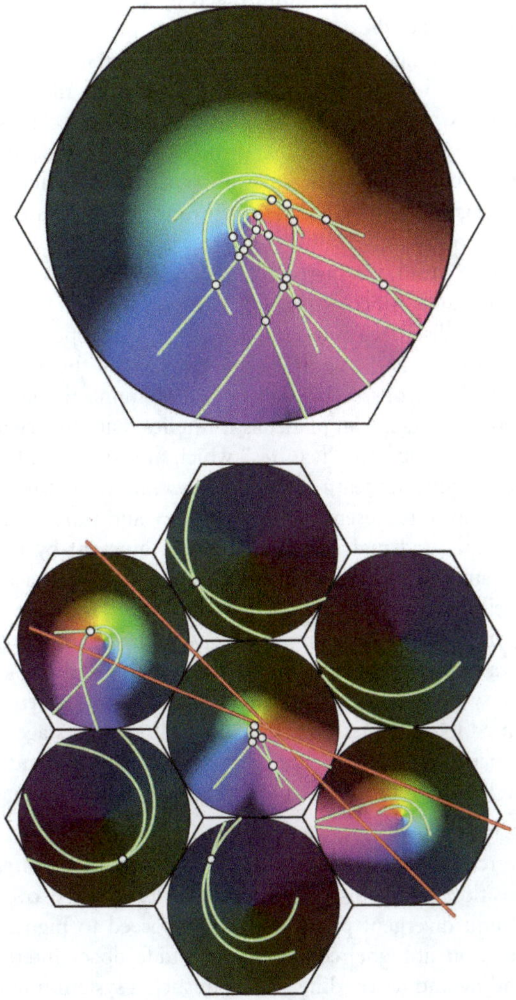

FIGURE 8 | Projection of a complex object (a double bar) from V1 (bottom) to a large macrocolumn in, e.g., V2 (top). Brightened dots show the intersections of lines, producing more frequent enhanced responses to stimulus angles in V2 than V1.

Swindale, 2008; Naci et al., 2012) is suggested, since the backward flow would continuously modify the forward flow of sensory information.

CONCLUSION

The model of cortical development we have outlined above is efficient from both energetic and information-processing perspectives, and has considerable anatomical and physiological explanatory power. It leads to an explanation of the spatial organization of signal flow in the cortex that differs from any other model. The proposed antenatal self-organization of cortical synapses leads to the creation of a *tabula rasa* on which homeomorphic maps, in a form disguised by the Möbius-strip-like folding of connections, occur in lateral connections at the millimetric scale, embedding the statistics of spatial organization of the sensory world to first approximation, before any detailed sensory inputs are received. The assumptions and findings of the model overlap with, and although not necessarily contradictory to, are not identical to, those of other models (Erwin and Miller, 1998; Wolf and Geisel, 1998; Kang et al., 2003; Oster and Bressloff, 2006). Distinguishing features include the explanation of the relationship of superficial patch connections to macrocolumn centers, and their hexagonal rotational symmetry, and crucially, the findings of Basole et al. (2003), which cannot be explained by any model dependent on "like-to-like" connections between feature-specific neurons. Nor can any model with otherwise similar assumptions about the self-organizing effect of synchrony be formulated without introducing a Möbius configuration to the connections, since an equivalent model utilizing only Euclidian conformations would represent a given OP twice, rather than once, around a singularity.

In review, the assumptions and conclusions reached, were as follows. By assuming that cells surviving apoptosis are selected by competition for metabolic substrates, and that synchronous oscillation mediates the uptake of metabolic substrates, we showed the outcome was a neural system with ultra-small world axonal configuration. Further assuming the small world connections were necessarily constructed from neuron populations characterized by respective axonal length, we showed that long range patchy connections and regular macro-column-like areas with central sparing of patchy connections emerge, with some degree of hexagonal rotational symmetry, with species variation in orderliness according to cortical size, and were able to show that this result was consistent with anatomical observations of limited interspecies variation of singularity density. A crucial further assumption made, was that metabolic competition between synapses from the same neuron leads to particular configuration of synaptic current flows at equilibrium, in which active connection networks within each macrocolumn are arranged in a Möbius-strip-like conformation. Then, with the introduction of visual inputs, signals conveyed by contextual fibers transfer a visual image from the global map to each local map, determining the pattern of neuron firing induced by activation of the cRF, and synaptic consolidation on Hebbian principles begins—thus storing information based on visual experience—explaining how response maps for OP, SF, and TF become organized in accord with the spatio-temporal filter model (Baker and Issa, 2005; Issa et al., 2008), and how "like to like" anatomical connections emerge, as well as providing conditions for dimension-reduction description of response features. The model is also compatible with explanation of ocular columns and direction preference fractures, as proposed in our earlier work (Wright et al., 2006).

The resulting synaptic storage of learned information in local topological maps of Möbius configuration offers a further compression of format, adding to the efficiency of the "small world" arrangement, by minimizing the distance which need be spanned by connections between positions on the local map representing positions widely separated on the global map. The development of cross-links also offers large potential information storage, since the regular spatial organization of links in the Möbius configuration implies the synaptic connections have low joint entropy in their ante-natal state. With visual experience, and the storage of image information in cross-links, joint entropy could, in principle, increase to a limit where all synaptic states are independent, and equally distributed about some mean connection strength, as implied by Montague's (1996) resource consumption principle. In effect, before eye-opening, the cortex has "learnt" the underlying statistical structure of visual space—that of cross-correlation declining with metric distance—and subsequently stores information about departures from this "first component" of structure in the visual world.

The antenatal development of response maps (Wiesel and Hubel, 1974; Blakemore and Van Sluyters, 1975; Sherk and Stryker, 1976) presents no paradox in this model, since emergence of organized response properties within the Möbius configuration does not depend upon structured visual stimuli. EEG activity progressively matures toward alternating alert and sleeping states in the later antenatal period (Marks et al., 1995; Mirmiran, 1995) providing the widespread co-ordination of pre-synaptic activity required for initial synaptic self-organization. Conversely, overwriting by learning in the immediate and later post-natal periods explains why representation in adult response maps of stimuli to which the subject as has not been exposed would not be present—as also seen experimentally (e.g., Blakemore and Van Sluyters, 1975).

No direct evidence yet exists of Möbius-like patterns of connections in cortex, yet this is scarcely surprising if transient dynamic couplings, present only in the equilibrium state, are overwritten by post-natal learning-related changes. However, relaxation toward the equilibrium condition is still to be expected in the mature state, so it is important whether or not some anatomical substrate exists in which the dynamic state of synapses may be capable of transient assembly into Möbius patterns. Markram and colleagues (Perin et al., 2011) found that pyramidal neuron networks cluster into multiple groups of a few dozen neurons each, with the neurons composing each group typically more than 100 μm apart, allowing for multiple groups to be interlaced in the same space. Connections within groups were largely reciprocal, and those between groups relatively sparse. Transient interlinkages between such interwoven linked groups could form Möbius-like networks. The temporal plasticity of synaptic connections near singularities (Dragoi et al., 2001) is also consistent with this interpretation. As well as plasticity of responses near OP singularities, Dragoi and colleagues found lack of plasticity in linear zones—the areas of strong patchy connection termination. This is to be expected if the patch system is composed of well consolidated connections suitable for consistent transmission with delay from fixed points in V1, while of the other hand, more complex, continually modified, information processing goes on in the areas around singularities. Consequently, an anatomical test of the model may be possible, in regard to the terminations of patchy connections in the periphery of the patch-free areas about singularities. As indicated in **Figure 3**, two populations of synaptic connections should be demonstrable in principle, by double injection/staining methods, near the singularity/patch edge. If some Hebbian consolidation occurs both antenatally and postnatally, then, in principle it should be possible to observe Möbius-like connections within macrocolumns antenatally, and the overwriting of these connections during post-natal learning.

If later testing supports this model, current conceptions of cortical information processing will require modification. Synchronous oscillation has been regarded as a mechanism for feature-binding—requiring that groups of cells in synchrony stand out in some way against a non-synchronized background. Instead, this model emphasizes synchrony as the organizer of a matrix of connections within which each macrocolumn gathers information from its surround, and organizes these connections systematically according to spatial position and time-lag, as functions of distance from each singularity. The topology of signal organization is markedly different to that of the association of "feature" neurons embedded in neural connections that are deployed on a Euclidean plane, as it implies that sensory images are not broken up into "features" which are subsequently associated in an abstract feature space, but retain, in modified form, an organization representing sensory space and time. Upon this more complicated matrix of connections, moment-by-moment states of autonomous local firing could interact with each other via traveling waves, generating internal images adding to those arising from sensation—all selectively strengthening preferred pathways by Hebbian learning, under the supervision of motivational systems. This gives a modified basis to Sherrington's "enchanted loom" (Sherrington, 1906, 1940), and a stage for the kind of neuro-dynamic events progressively observed and envisaged by Freeman for many years (Freeman, 1975; Freeman and Quiroga, 2013).

Hierarchical interaction of V1 with higher visual areas, by superposition of spatio-temporal images transmitted over convergent and divergent pathways might proceed to higher levels of abstraction, at higher cortical levels, and feedback interactions of ascending and descending signals in such a system might permit very complex image manipulation. Analogous processes may apply to other modalities throughout the cortex in general, since all sensory input systems are analogous to the visual system, in as much as they encode the sensory world by imposing a topological order to inputs as they arrive at the sensory cortices. Again, the ubiquitous distribution of patchy connections throughout the cortex, and the basic modular similarity of the paleo- and neocortex throughout, supports the notion that a single schema of information flow may be characteristic of all. The principle of organization might even extend to the motor cortex, with the efferent pyramidal motor neurons simply reversing the role of neurons in the direct visual pathway.

ACKNOWLEDGMENTS

A special debt of gratitude is owed to Adrienne Edith Wright.

This work was supported by the Frank P. Hixon Fund of the California Institute of Technology and the Oakley Foundation of New Zealand, and by iVEC, through the use of advanced computing resources located at the University of Western Australia.

REFERENCES

Albert, M. V., Schnabel, A., and Field, D. J. (2008). Innate visual learning through spontaneous activity patterns. *PLoS Comput. Biol.* 4:e1000137. doi: 10.1371/journal.pcbi.1000137

Alexander, D. M., Bourke, P. D., Sheridan, P., Konstandatos, O., and Wright, J. J. (2004). Intrinsic connections in tree shrew V1 imply a global to local mapping. *Vision Res.* 44, 857–876.

Amari, S.-I. (1977). Dynamics of pattern formation in lateral-inhibition type neural fields. *Biol. Cybern.* 27, 77–87.

Angelucci, A., and Bullier, J. (2003). Reaching beyond the classical receptive field of V1 neurons; horizontal or feedback axons? *J. Physiol.* 97, 141–154.

Angelucci, A., Levitt, J. B., and Lund, J. S. (2002). Anatomical origins of the classic receptive field and modulatory surround field of single neurons in macaque visual cortical area V1. *Prog. Brain Res.* 136, 373–388.

Baker, T. I., and Issa, N. P. (2005). Cortical maps of separable tuning properties predict population responses of complex visual stimuli. *J. Neurophysiol.* 94, 775–787.

Basole, A., Kreft-Kerekes, V., White, L. E., and Fitzpatrick, D. (2006). Cortical cartography revisited: a frequency perspective on the functional architecture of visual cortex. *Prog. Brain Res.* 154, 121–134.

Basole, A., White, L. E., and Fitzpatrick, D. (2003). Mapping of multiple features in the population response of visual cortex. *Nature* 423, 986–990.

beim Graben, P. (2008). "Foundations of neurophysics," in *Lectures in Supercomputational Neuroscience: Dynamics in Complex Brain Networks*, eds P. Graben, C. Zhou, M. Thiel, and J. Kurths (Berlin: Springer), 3–48.

Blakemore, C., and Van Sluyters, R. C. (1975). Innate and environmental factors in the development of the kitten's visual cortex. *J. Physiol.* 248, 663–716.

Bosking, W. H., Zhang, Y., Schofield, B., and Fitzpatrick, D. (1997). Orientation selectivity and the arrangement of horizontal connections in tree shrew striate cortex. *J. Neurosci.* 17, 2112–2127.

Boucsein, C., Nawrot, M., Schnepel, P., and Aertsen, A. (2011). Beyond the cortical column: abundance and physiology of horizontal connections imply a strong role for inputs from the surround. *Front. Neurosci.* 5:32. doi: 10.3389/fnins.2011.00032

Braitenberg, V., and Schüz, A. (1991). *Anatomy of the Cortex: Statistics and Geometry*. Berlin, New York: Springer.

Bressler, S. L., Coppola, R., and Nakamura, R. (1993). Episodic multiregional cortical coherence at multiple frequencies during visual task performance. *Nature* 366, 153–156.

Bressloff, P. (2012). Spatiotemporal dynamics of continuum neural fields. *J. Phys. A Math. Theor.* 45:033001. doi: 10.1088/1751-8113/45/3/033001

Bringuier, V., Chavane, F., Glaeser, L., and Frégnac, Y. (1999). Horizontal propagation of visual activity in the synaptic integration field of area 17 neurons. *Science* 283, 695–699.

Buzás, P., Kovács, K., Ferecskó, A. S., Budd, J. M. L., Eysel, U. T., and Kisvárday, Z. F. (2006). Model-based analysis of excitatory lateral connections in the visual cortex. *J. Comp. Neurol.* 499, 861–881.

Callaway, E. M., and Katz, L. C. (1990). Emergence and refinement of clustered horizontal connections in cat striate cortex. *J. Neurosci.* 10, 1134–1153.

Carriera-Perpiñán, M. Á., Lister, R. J., and Goodhill, G. J. (2005). A computational model for development of multiple maps in primary visual cortex. *Cereb. Cortex* 15, 1222–1233.

Chapman, C. L., Bourke, P. D., and Wright, J. J. (2002). Spatial eigenmodes and synchronous oscillation: coincidence detection in simulated cerebral cortex. *J. Math. Biol.* 45, 57–78.

Cohen, R., and Havlin, S. (2003). Scale-free networks are ultra-small. *Phys. Rev. Lett.* 90:058701. doi: 10.1103/PhysRevLett.90.058701

Crick, F. C., and Koch, C. (2003). A framework for consciousness. *Nat. Neurosci.* 6, 119–126.

DeAngelis, G. C., Ohzawa, I., and Freeman, R. D. (1993). Spatiotemporal organization of simple-cell receptive fields in the cat's striate cortex. I. General character-istics and postnatal development. *J. Neurophysiol.* 69, 1091–1117.

Downes, J. H., Hammond, M. W., Xydas, D., Spencer, M., Becerra, V. M., Warwick, K., et al. (2012). Emergence of a small-world functional network in cultured neurons. *PLoS Comput. Biol.* 8:e1002522. doi: 10.1371/journal.pcbi.1002522

Dragoi, V., Rivadulla, C., and Sur, M. (2001). Foci of orientation plasticity in visual cortex. *Nature* 411, 80–86.

Durack, J. C., and Katz, L. C. (1996). Development of horizontal projections in layer 2/3 of ferret visual cortex. *Cereb. Cortex* 6, 178–183.

Durbin, R., and Mitchison, G. (1990). A dimension reduction framework for understanding cortical maps. *Nature* 343, 644–647.

Durbin, R., and Willshaw, D. J. (1987). An analogue approach to the travelling salesman problem using an elastic net method. *Nature* 326, 689–691.

Eckhorn, R., Bauer, R., Jordon, W., Brosch, M., Kruse, W., Monk, M., et al. (1988). Coherent oscillations: a mechanism of feature linking in the in the visual cortex? *Biol. Cybern.* 60, 121–130.

Eckhorn, R., Reitboeck, H. J., Arndt, M., and Dicke, P. (1990). Feature linking via synchronization among distributed assemblies: simulations of results from cat visual cortex. *Neural Comput.* 2, 293–307.

Elliott, T. (2011). Stability against fluctuations: scaling, bifurcations, and spontaneous symmetry breaking in stochastic models of synaptic plasticity. *Neural Comput.* 23, 674–734.

Elliott, T., and Shadbolt, N. R. (2002). Multiplicative synaptic normalization and a nonlinear Hebb rule underlie a neurotrophic model of competitive synaptic plasticity. *Neural Comput.* 14, 1311–1322.

Enoki, R., Hu, Y.-L., Hamilton, D., and Fine, A. (2009). Expression of long-term plasticity at individual synapses in hippocampus is graded, bi-directional, and mainly pre-synaptic: optic quantal analysis. *Neuron* 62, 242–253.

Erwin, E., and Miller, K. D. (1998). Correlation-based development of ocular matched orientation and ocular dominance maps: determination of required input activities. *J. Neurosci.* 18, 9870–9895.

Freeman, W. J. (1975). *Mass Action in the Nervous System*. New York, NY: Academic Press.

Freeman, W. J. (1991). "Predictions on neocortical dynamics derived from studies in paleocortex," in *Induced Rhythms of the Brain*, eds E. Basar and T. H. Bullock (Boston, MA: Berkhäuser), 183–195.

Freeman, W. J., and Quiroga, R. Q. (2013). *Imaging Brain Function*. New York, Heidelberg, Dordrecht, London: Springer.

Gilbert, C. D., and Wiesel, T. N. (1979). Morphology and intracortical projections of functionally characteristic neurons in cat visual cortex. *Nature* 280, 120–125.

Gilbert, C. D., and Wiesel, T. N. (1989). Columnar specificity of intrinsic horizontal and corticocortical connections in cat visual cortex. *J. Neurosci.* 9, 2432–2442.

Gray, C. M., Konig, P., Engel, A. K., and Singer, W. (1989). Oscillatory responses in cat visual cortex exhibit intercolumnar synchronisation which reflects global stimulus properties. *Nature* 388, 334–337.

Grossberg, S., and Olson, S. J. (1994). Rules for the cortical map of ocular dominance and orientation columns. *Neural Netw.* 7, 883–894.

Haken, H. (1996). *Principles of Brain Functioning*. Berlin: Springer.

Harris, A. E., Ermentrout, G. B., and Small, S. L. (1997). A model of ocular column development by competition for trophic factor. *Proc. Natl. Acad. Sci. U.S.A.* 94, 9944–9949.

Hassenstaub, A., Shu, Y., Haider, B., Krauschaar, U., Duque, A., and McCormick, D. A. (2005). Inhibitory postsynaptic potentials carry synchronized frequency information in active cortical networks. *Neuron* 47, 423–435.

Heck, N., Golbs, A., Riedemann, T., Sun, J.-J., Lessmann, V., and Luhmann, H. J. (2008). Activity dependent regulation of neuronal apoptosis in neonatal mouse cerebral cortex. *Cereb. Cortex* 18, 1335–1349.

Hirsch, J. A., and Gilbert, C. D. (1991). Synaptic physiology of horizontal connections in the cat's visual cortex. *J. Neurosci.* 11, 1800–1809.

Horton, C. H., and Adams, D. L. (2005). The cortical column: a structure without a function. *Philos. Trans. R. Soc. Lond. B Biol. Sci.* 360, 837–862.

Hubel, D. H., and Wiesel, T. N. (1959). Receptive fields of single neurones in the cat's striate cortex. *J. Physiol.* 148, 574–591.

Issa, P., Rosenberg, A., and Husson, T. R. (2008). Models and measurements of functional maps in V1. *J. Neurophysiol.* 99, 2745–2754.

Jirsa, V. K., and Haken, H. (1996). Field theory of electromagnetic brain activity. *Phys. Rev. Lett.* 77, 960–963.

Kang, K., Shelley, M., and Sompolinsky, H. (2003). Mexican hats and pinwheels in visual cortex. *Proc. Natl. Acad. Sci. U.S.A.* 100, 2848–2853.

Kaschube, M., Schnabel, M., Löwel, S., Coppola, D. M., White, L. E., and Wolf, F. (2010). Universality in the evolution of orientation columns in the visual cortex. *Science* 330, 1113.

Keil, W., Kaschube, M., Schnabel, M., Kisvarday, Z. F., Löwel, S., Coppola,

D. M., et al. (2012). Response to comment on "Universality in the evolution of orientation columns in the visual cortex". *Science* 336, 413.

Kohonen, T. (1982). Self-organized formation of topologically correct feature maps. *Biol. Cybern.* 43, 59–69.

Kveraga, K., Ghuman, A. S., and Bar, M. (2007). Top-down predictions in the cognitive brain. *Brain Cogn.* 65, 145–168.

Li, W., Their, P., and Wehrhahn, C. (2000). Contextual influence on orientation discrimination of humans and responses of neurons in V1 of alert monkeys. *J. Neurophysiol.* 83, 941–954.

Mariño, J., Schummers, J., Lyon, D. C., Schwabe, L., Beck, O., Wiesing, P., et al. (2005). Invariant computations in local cortical networks with balanced excitation and inhibition. *Nat. Neurosci.* 8, 194–201.

Marks, G. A., Shaffery, J. P., Okensberg, A., Speciale, S. G., and Roffwarg, H. P. (1995). A functional role for REM sleep in brain maturation. *Behav. Brain Res.* 69, 1–11.

McGuire, B. A., Gilbert, C. D., Rivlin, P. K., and Wiesel, T. N. (1991). Targets of horizontal connections in macaque primary visual cortex. *J. Comp. Neurol.* 305, 370–392.

Mante, V., and Carandini, M. (2005). Mapping of stimulus energy in primary visual cortex. *J. Neurophysiol.* 94, 788–798.

Meng, Y., Tanaka, S., and Poon, C.-S. (2012). Comment on "Universality in the evolution of orientation columns in the visual cortex". *Science* 336, 413. Available online at: www.sciencemag.org/cgi/content/full/336/6080/413-d

Merigan, W. H., and Maunsell, J. H. R. (1993). How parallel are the primate visual pathways? *Annu. Rev. Neurosci.* 16, 369–402.

Mirmiran, M. (1995). The function of fetal/neonatal rapid eye movement sleep. *Behav. Brain Res.* 69, 13–22.

Miyashita, M., and Tanaka, S. (1992). A mathematical model for the self-organization of orientation columns in visual cortex. *Neuroreport* 3, 69–72.

Montague, P. R. (1996). The resource consumption principle: attention and memory in volumes of neural tissue. *Proc. Natl. Acad. Sci. U.S.A.* 93, 3619–3623.

Muir, D. R., Da Costa, N. M. A., Girardin, C. C., Naaman, S., Omer, D. B., Ruesch, E., et al. (2011). Embedding of cortical representations by the superficial patch system. *Cereb. Cortex* 21, 2244–2260.

Muir, D. R., and Douglas, R. J. (2011). From neural arbours to daisies. *Cereb. Cortex* 21, 1118–1133.

Naci, L., Taylor, K. I., Cusak, R., and Tyler, L. K. (2012). Are the senses enough for sense? Early high-level feedback shapes our comprehension of multisensory objects. *Front. Integr. Neurosci.* 6:82. doi: 10.3389/fnint.2012.00082

Nunez, P. L. (1981). *Electric Fields of the Brain*. London: Oxford University Press.

Obermayer, K., and Blasdel, G. G. (1993). Geometry of orientation and ocular dominance columns in monkey striate cortex. *J. Neurosci.* 13, 4114–4129.

Obermayer, K., Ritter, H., and Schulten, K. (1990). A principle for the formation of the spatial structure of cortical feature maps. *Proc. Natl. Acad. Sci. U.S.A.* 87, 8345–8349.

Obermayer, K., Ritter, H., and Schulten, K. (1992). A model for the development of the spatial structure of retinotopic maps and orientation columns. *IEICE Trans. Fundamentals* E75A, 537–545.

O'Connor, D. H., Wittenberg, G. M., and Wang, S. S.-H. (2005a). Dissection of bidirectional synaptic plasticity into saturable unidirectional processes. *J. Neurophysiol.* 94, 1565–1573.

O'Connor, D. H., Wittenberg, G. M., and Wang, S. S.-H. (2005b). Graded bidirectional synaptic plasticity is composed of switch-like unitary events. *Proc. Natl. Acad. Sci. U.S.A.* 102, 9679–9684.

Oster, A. M., and Bressloff, P. C. (2006). A developmental model of ocular dominance column formation on a growing cortex. *Bull. Math. Biol.* 68, 73–98.

Paik, S.-B., and Ringach, D. L. (2011). Retinal origin of orientation maps in visual cortex. *Nat. Neurosci.* 14, 919–925.

Perin, R., Berger, T. K., and Markram, H. (2011). A synaptic organizing principle for cortical neuronal groups. *Proc. Natl. Acad. Sci. U.S.A.* 108, 5419–5424.

Price, D. J. (1986). The postnatal development of clustered intrinsic connections in area 18 of the visual cortex in kittens. *Dev. Brain Res.* 24, 31–38.

Rakic, P. (1988). Specification of cerebral cortical areas. *Science* 241, 170–176.

Rao, R. P. N., and Ballard, D. H. (1997). Dynamic model of visual recognition predicts neural response properties in the visual cortex. *Neural Comput.* 9, 721–763.

Rennie, C. J., Wright, J. J., and Robinson, P. A. (2000). Mechanisms of cortical electrical activity and the emergence of gamma rhythm. *J. Theor. Biol.* 205, 17–35.

Ringach, D. L. (2007). On the origin of the functional architecture of the cortex. *PLoS ONE* 2:e251. doi: 10.1371/journal.pone.0000251

Robinson, P. A., Rennie, C. J., and Wright, J. J. (1998). Synchronous oscillations in the cerebral cortex. *Phys. Rev. E* 57, 4578–4588.

Robinson, P. A., Rennie, C. J., Wright, J. J., Bahramali, H., Gordon, E., and Rowe, D. L. (2001). Prediction of electroencephalographic spectra from neurophysiology. *Phys. Rev. E* 63, 701–702.

Rockland, K. S., and Lund, J. S. (1983). Intrinsic laminar lattice connections in primate visual cortex. *J. Comp. Neurol.* 216, 303–318.

Rosenberg, A., Husson, T. R., and Issa, N. P. (2010). Subcortical representation of non-Fourier image features. *J. Neurosci.* 30, 1985–1993.

Ruthazer, E. S., and Stryker, M. P. (1996). The role of activity in the development of long-range horizontal connections in area 17 of the ferret. *J. Neurosci.* 16, 7253–7269.

Scholl, D. A. (1956). *The Organization of the Cerebral Cortex*. New York, NY: Wiley.

Sharma, J., Angelucci, A., Rao, S. C., and Sur, M. (1995). *Relationship of Intrinsic Connections to Orientation Maps in Ferret Primary Visual Cortex: Iso-Orientation Domains and Singularities*. San Diego, CA: Presented at Society for Neuroscience.

Sherk, H., and Stryker, M. P. (1976). Quantitative study of orientation selectivity in visually inexperienced kittens. *J. Neurophysiol.* 39, 63–70.

Sherrington, C. S. (1906). *The Integrative Action of the Nervous System*. New Haven, CT: Yale University Press.

Sherrington, C. S. (1940). *Man on His Nature. Gifford Lecture, Edinburgh, 1937–1938*. Cambridge, UK: Cambridge University Press.

Shi, Y., Kirwan, P., Smith, J., Robinson, H. P. C., and Livesey, F. J. (2012). Human cerebral cortex development from pluripotent stem cells to functional cortical synapses. *Nat. Neurosci.* 15, 477–486.

Singer, W. (1999). Neuronal synchrony: a versatile code for the definition of relations? *Neuron* 24, 49–65.

Swindale, N. V. (1982). A model for the formation of orientation columns. *Proc. R. Soc. Lond. B Biol. Sci.* 215, 211–230.

Swindale, N. V. (1992). A model for the coordinated development of columnar systems in primate striate cortex. *Biol. Cybern.* 66, 217–230.

Swindale, N. V. (1996). The development of topography in the visual cortex: a review of models. *Network* 7, 161–247.

Swindale, N. V. (2008). Feedback decoding of spatially structured population activity in cortical maps. *Neural Comput.* 20, 176–204.

Tanaka, S. (1990). Theory of self-organization of cortical maps: mathematical framework. *Neural Netw.* 3, 625–640.

Thomaidou, D., Mione, M. C., Cavanagh, J. F. R., and Parnavelas, J. G. (1997). Apoptosis and its relation to the cell cycle in the developing cerebral cortex. *J. Neurosci.* 17, 1075–1085.

Tsukada, M., and Fukushima, Y. (2010). A context dependent mechanism in hippocampal CA1 networks. *Bull. Math. Biol.* 73, 417–435.

van Ooyen, A. (2001). Competition in the development of nerve connections: a review of models. *Network* 12, R1–R47.

van Ooyen, A., and Willshaw, D. J. (1999). Competition for neurotrophic factor in the development of nerve connections. *Proc. Biol. Sci.* 266, 883–892.

van Rotterdam, A., Lopes da Silva, F. H., van den Ende, J., Viergever, M. A., and Hermans, A. J. (1982). A model of the spatio-temporal characteristics of the alpha rhythm. *Bull. Math. Biol.* 44, 283–305.

von der Malsburg, C. (1973). Self organization of orientation sensitive cells in the striate cortex. *Kybernetic* 14, 85–100.

Wiesel, T. N., and Hubel, D. H. (1974). Ordered arrangement of orientation columns in monkeys lacking visual experience. *J. Comp. Neurol.* 158, 307–318.

Willshaw, D. J., and von der Malsburg, C. (1976). How patterned neural connections can be be set up by self-organization. *Proc. R. Soc. Lond. B Biol. Sci.* 194, 431–435.

Wilson, H. R., and Cowan, J. D. (1973). A mathematical theory of the functional dynamics of cortical and thalamic nervous tissue. *Kybernetik* 13, 55–80.

Wolf, F., and Geisel, T. (1998). Spontaneous pinwheel annihilation during visual development. *Nature* 395, 73–78.

Wright, J. J. (2009). Generation and control of cortical gamma: findings from simulation at two scales. *Neural Netw.* 22, 373–384.

Wright, J. J. (2010). Attractor dynamics and thermodynamic analogies in the cerebral cortex: synchronous oscillation, the background EEG, and the regulation of attention. *Bull. Math. Biol.* 73, 436–457.

Wright, J. J., Alexander, D. M., and Bourke, P. D. (2006). Contribution of lateral interactions in V1 to organization of response properties. *Vision Res.* 46, 2703–2720.

Wright, J. J., and Bourke, P. D. (2008). An outline of functional self-organization in V1: synchrony, STLR and Hebb rules. *Cogn. Neurodyn.* 2, 147–157.

Wright, J. J., and Bourke, P. D. (2013). A model for embryogenesis of cortical macrocolumns and superficial patchy connections: consequent neuronal responses at maturity. *Cereb. Cortex* (in press).

Wright, J. J., Bourke, P. D., and Chapman, C. L. (2000). Synchronous oscillation in the cerebral cortex and object coherence: simulation of basic electrophysiological findings. *Biol. Cybern.* 83, 341–353.

Wright, J. J., Rennie, C. J., Lees, G. J., Robinson, P. A., Bourke, P. D., Chapman, C. L., et al. (2003). Simulated electrocortical activity at microscopic, mesoscopic and global scales. *Neuropsychopharmacology* 28, S80–S93.

Yousef, T., Tóth, É., Rausch, M., Eysel, U. T., and Kisvárday, Z. F. (2001). Topography of orientation centre connections in the primary visual cortex of the cat. *Neuroreport* 12, 1693–1699.

4

Traveling pulses in a stochastic neural field model of direction selectivity

Paul C. Bressloff* and Jeremy Wilkerson

Department of Mathematics, University of Utah, Salt Lake City, UT, USA

Correspondence:
Paul C. Bressloff, Department of Mathematics, University of Utah, 155 South 1400 East, Salt Lake City, UT 84112, USA.
e-mail: bressloff@math.utah.edu

We analyze the effects of extrinsic noise on traveling pulses in a neural field model of direction selectivity. The model consists of a one-dimensional scalar neural field with an asymmetric weight distribution consisting of an offset Mexican hat function. We first show how, in the absence of any noise, the system supports spontaneously propagating traveling pulses that can lock to externally moving stimuli. Using a separation of time-scales and perturbation methods previously developed for stochastic reaction-diffusion equations, we then show how extrinsic noise in the activity variables leads to a diffusive-like displacement (wandering) of the wave from its uniformly translating position at long time-scales, and fluctuations in the wave profile around its instantaneous position at short time-scales. In the case of freely propagating pulses, the wandering is characterized by pure Brownian motion, whereas in the case of stimulus-locked pulses, it is given by an Ornstein–Uhlenbeck process. This establishes that stimulus-locked pulses are more robust to noise.

Keywords: stochastic processes, traveling waves, neural field theory, direction selectivity, stimulus-driven

INTRODUCTION

Continuum neural field models represent the large-scale dynamics of spatially structured networks of neurons in terms of non-linear integro-differential equations, whose associated integral kernels represent the spatial distribution of neuronal synaptic connections (Wilson and Cowan, 1972, 1973; Amari, 1977). As in the case of non-linear partial differential equation (PDE) models of diffusively coupled excitable systems (Keener, 1981; Kuramoto, 1984), non-local neural fields can exhibit a diverse range of spatiotemporal dynamics, including solitary traveling fronts and pulses, stationary pulses, and spatially localized oscillations (breathers), spiral waves, and Turing-like patterns. See, for example, the reviews Ermentrout (1998), Coombes (2005), and Bressloff (2012). In recent years, neural fields have been used to model a wide range of neurobiological phenomena, including wave propagation in cortical slices (Pinto and Ermentrout, 2001; Richardson et al., 2005) and *in vivo* (Huang et al., 2004), geometric visual hallucinations (Ermentrout and Cowan, 1979; Bressloff et al., 2001), EEG rhythms (Nunez, 1995; Robinson et al., 2001; Liley et al., 2002; Steyn-Ross et al., 2003), orientation tuning in primary visual cortex (V1) (Ben-Yishai et al., 1995; Somers et al., 1995), short term working memory (Camperi and Wang, 1998; Laing and Chow, 2002), control of head direction (Zhang, 1996), direction selectivity (Xie and Giese, 2002), motion perception (Giese, 1999), and binocular rivalry waves (Bressloff and Webber, 2012a). One particularly useful feature of neural fields is that analytical techniques for solving these integro-differential equations can be adapted from previous studies of non-linear PDEs. These include regular and singular perturbation methods, weakly non-linear analysis and pattern formation, symmetric bifurcation theory, Evans functions and wave stability, and homogenization theory (Bressloff, 2012). In particular, we have recently shown how perturbation methods for studying fluctuating fronts in reaction-diffusion PDEs (Schimansky-Geier et al., 1983; de Pasquale et al., 1992; Armero et al., 1998; Sagues et al., 2007) can be extended to the problem of front propagation in stochastic neural fields (Bressloff and Webber, 2012b), and have used this to investigate the effects of noise on binocular rivalry waves (Webber and Bressloff, submitted). Such methods exploit a separation of time-scales in which there is a diffusive-like displacement (wandering) of the front from its uniformly translating position at long time-scales, and fluctuations in the front profile around its instantaneous position at short time-scales.

In this paper, we extend our theory of wave propagation in stochastic neural fields to the case of a neural field that supports traveling pulses rather than fronts. A typical mechanism for generating traveling pulses in an excitatory network is to include some form of slow adaptation, such as spike frequency adaptation (Pinto and Ermentrout, 2001; Coombes and Owen, 2005) or synaptic depression (Kilpatrick and Bressloff, 2010a,b), which suppresses the trailing edge of the wave. One of the motivations for considering excitatory neural fields is that traveling pulses are observed in *in vitro* cortical slices that have been disinhibited. Here we consider an alternative mechanism for generating pulses, based on asymmetric excitatory/inhibitory synaptic connections. Such a network architecture supports freely propagating pulses without any adaptation, and has been proposed as a simple recurrent mechanism for generating direction selectivity in a network driven by moving stimuli (Mineiro and Zipser, 1998; Xie and Giese, 2002). Most classical models for the direction selectivity of cortical neurons are based on feedforward mechanisms, namely, the linear or non-linear spatiotemporal filtering of afferent thalamo-cortical inputs (Reichardt, 1961; Adelson and Bergen, 1985; Koch and Poggio, 1985; van Santen and Sperling, 1985). Some of these models also involve a combination of lagged (time-delayed) and non-lagged inputs (Saul and Humphrey, 1990; Baker and Bair, 2012). However, there is now considerable experimental data demonstrating that the response of cortical cells is strongly influenced by intracortical circuitry. This has motivated a number of modeling studies that show how direction selectivity can be reproduced by recurrent neural network models with asymmetric lateral excitatory or inhibitory connections and non-direction-selective inputs (Suarez et al., 1995; Maex and Urban, 1996; Mineiro and Zipser, 1998; Xie and Giese, 2002). In this paper, we base our investigation of stochastic traveling pulses on the particular version introduced by Xie and Giese (2002).

The main results of the paper are as follows. We first analyze freely propagating pulses and stimulus-locked pulses in the deterministic case, expanding the analysis of Xie and Giese (2002). In particular, we construct a stability diagram showing the existence and stability of stimulus-locked pulses as a function of stimulus velocity and amplitude. We then turn to a corresponding stochastic version of the model. We show how extrinsic noise in the activity variable leads to a diffusive-like displacement (wandering) of the wave from its uniformly translating position at long time-scales, and fluctuations in the wave profile around its instantaneous position at short time-scales. In the case of freely propagating pulses, the wandering is characterized by pure Brownian motion, whereas in the case of stimulus-locked pulses, it is given by an Ornstein–Uhlenbeck process. This establishes that stimulus-locked pulses are more robust to noise. One major difference between pulses and fronts is that, in principle, noise could significantly affect both the location (center-of-mass) and width of the pulse. We find that fluctuations in the width can be neglected in the case of freely propagating pulses, whereas the saturation of the mean-square displacement of the center-of-mass of the pulse for stimulus-locked pulses means that fluctuations in pulse width can no longer be ignored.

MATERIALS AND METHODS

NEURAL FIELD MODEL OF DIRECTION SELECTIVITY

In this paper we consider a scalar neural field equation of the form

$$\tau \frac{\partial u(x,t)}{\partial t} = -u(x,t) + \int_{-\infty}^{\infty} w(x-x')F(u(x',t))dx' + h(x,t) \tag{1}$$

Here $u(x, t)$ is a measure of activity (current or voltage) within a local population of excitatory and inhibitory neurons at position $x \in \mathbb{R}$ and time t, τ is a membrane time constant (of order 10 msec), $w(x)$ denotes the spatial distribution of synaptic connections between local populations, $F(u)$ is a non-linear firing rate function and $h(x, t)$ is an external input. (We fix the time-scale by setting $\tau = 1$). F is usually taken to be a sigmoid function

$$F(u) = \frac{1}{1 + e^{-\gamma(u-\kappa)}} \tag{2}$$

with gain γ and threshold κ. In the high-gain limit $\gamma \to \infty$, this reduces to the Heaviside function

$$F(u) \to H(u-\kappa) = \begin{cases} 1 & \text{if } u > \kappa \\ 0 & \text{if } u \le \kappa. \end{cases} \tag{3}$$

The function $w(x - x')$ represents the distribution of synaptic weights from the local population at x' to the population at x. Usually, w is taken to be a symmetric or even function such that $w(x) = w(-x)$. A common choice for the weight distribution is a "Mexican hat" function, with a center excitatory region surrounded by flanking inhibitory regions. As originally shown by Amari (1977), symmetric Mexican hat functions tend to support stationary activity "bumps." Following Xie and Giese (2002), however, we will use an asymmetric Mexican hat function whose maximum is offset by an amount x_0, that is $w(x - x_0) = w(-[x - x_0])$; the resulting neural field then supports freely propagating pulses that depend on the degree of offset. Note that such a choice should be contrasted with a symmetric function w with peaks offset from zero see e.g., (Hutt and Atay, 2005). In the case of exponential functions, w takes the form (see **Figure 1**)

$$w(x) = a_e e^{-\sigma_e|x-x_0|} - a_i e^{-\sigma_i|x-x_0|}, \tag{4}$$

where $a_e > a_i$ and $\sigma_e > \sigma_i$. Setting $x_0 = 0$ recovers the standard Mexican hat function. Note that one could equally use other functions such as a difference-of-Gaussians without changing the main results of the paper; the advantage of exponentials is that one can carry out explicit calculations.

Finally, the external input $h(x, t)$ consists of two components:

$$h(x,t) = I(x - vt) + \sqrt{\epsilon} g(u(x,t))\xi(x,t). \tag{5}$$

Here $I(x - vt)$ represents an external pulse-like stimulus moving with constant speed v and amplitude I_0, whereas the second term represents an extrinsic, multiplicative noise source. In particular, $\xi(x, t)$ is a Gaussian process with zero mean and two-point correlations

$$\langle \eta(x,t)\eta(x',t')\rangle = 2C(|x-x'|/\lambda)\delta(t-t'). \tag{6}$$

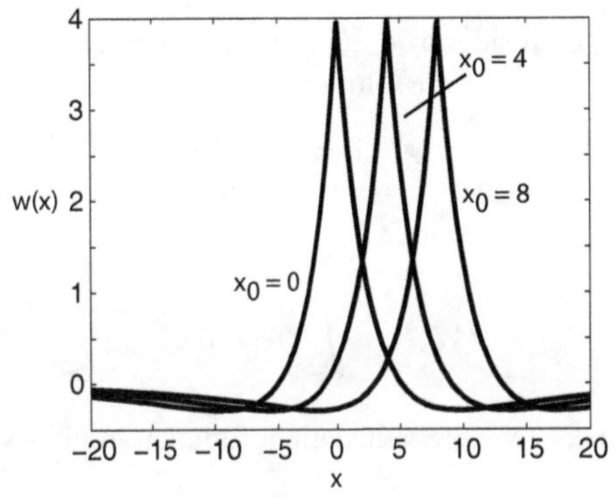

FIGURE 1 | Plot of weight distribution for various values of the shift x_0. Here $a_e = 5$, $a_i = 1$, $\sigma_e = 0.42$, and $\sigma_i = 0.1$.

Thus the noise is white in time and colored in space with correlation length λ. Formally speaking, $\eta(x,t)dt = dW(x,t)$ where $dW(x,t)$ is a corresponding Wiener process.The amplitude of the noise is determined by the parameter ϵ, and the function $g(u)$ incorporates any activity-dependence. Note that (Xie and Giese, 2002) only considered the deterministic case ($\epsilon = 0$). They showed how the deterministic neural field supports freely propagating pulses of fixed speed c when $I_0 = 0$. This then provides a mechanism for direction selectivity, since these pulses can lock to a moving stimulus of speed v provided that $|c - v|$ is sufficiently small; the range of locking depends on the amplitude I_0. In this paper, we develop a more systematic analysis of stimulus-locking in the absence of noise, and then investigate the effects of noise on both freely propagating and stimulus-locked pulses.

RESULTS

DETERMINSTIC NEURAL FIELD

We begin by analyzing traveling pulse solutions of the neural field Equation (1) in the absence of noise ($\epsilon = 0$). Following the original formulation of Amari (1977), we investigate the existence and stability of traveling pulses by setting the firing rate function to be the Heaviside (Equation 3).

Freely propagating pulses

For the moment, suppose that there are no external inputs so that $h(x,t) = 0$ in Equation (1). A traveling pulse of velocity c is then defined according to $u(x,t) = U(\xi)$, with $\xi = x - ct$ a traveling wave coordinate such that $\lim_{\xi\to\pm\infty} U(\xi) = 0$. Moreover, the wave profile is restricted to be super threshold in a connected interval of width d. Since the neural field is equivariant with respect to uniform translations (in the absence of external stimuli), we choose the two threshold crossing points to be

$$U(0) = \kappa, \quad U(d) = \kappa. \tag{7}$$

Thus, $U(\xi) > \kappa$ for $0 < \xi < d$, $U(\xi) < \kappa$ for $\xi < 0$, and $\xi > d$. It turns out the wave travels in the same direction as the offset so we restrict ourselves to the case $x_0 > 0$ and $c > 0$. Substituting the traveling pulse solution into Equation (1) gives

$$-c\frac{\partial U(\xi)}{\partial \xi} = -U(\xi) + \int_0^d w(\xi - \xi')d\xi' \tag{8}$$

Multiplying both sides by $e^{-\xi/c}$ and integrating gives the following equation for the wave solution:

$$U(\xi) = \frac{e^{\xi/c}}{c}\int_\xi^\infty W(\xi')e^{-\xi'/c}\,d\xi', \tag{9}$$

where

$$W(\xi) \equiv \int_{\xi-d}^{\xi} w(x)\,dx.$$

It is convenient to express the weight function in piecewise form as follows:

$$w(x) = \begin{cases} a_e e^{-\sigma_e(x-x_0)} - a_i e^{-\sigma_i(x-x_0)} \equiv w_1(x), & \text{if } x \geq x_0 \\ a_e e^{\sigma_e(x-x_0)} - a_i e^{\sigma_i(x-x_0)} \equiv w_2(x), & \text{if } x \leq x_0 \end{cases} \tag{10}$$

We then obtain a piecewise expression for $W(\xi)$ of the form

$$W(\xi) = \begin{cases} W_3(\xi) \equiv \int_{\xi-d}^{\xi} w_2(x)\,dx, & \text{if } \xi \leq x_0 \\ W_2(\xi) \equiv \int_{\xi-d}^{x_0} w_2(x)\,dx \\ \qquad + \int_{x_0}^{\xi} w_1(x)\,dx, & \text{if } x_0 \leq \xi \leq x_0 + d \\ W_1(\xi) \equiv \int_{\xi-d}^{\xi} w_1(x)\,dx, & \text{if } \xi \geq x_0 + d \end{cases} \tag{11}$$

We then have

$$U(\xi) = \begin{cases} \frac{1}{c}e^{\xi/c}(M_3(\xi) + M_1(x_0+d) \\ \qquad + M_2(x_0)), & \text{if } \xi \leq x_0 \\ \frac{1}{c}e^{\xi/c}(M_2(\xi) + M_1(x_0+d)), & \text{if } x_0 \leq \xi \leq x_0 + d \\ \frac{1}{c}e^{\xi/c}M_1(\xi), & \text{if } \xi \geq x_0 + d \end{cases}.$$

where

$$M_n(\xi) = \int_\xi^{\xi_n} W_n(\xi')e^{-\xi'/c}d\xi' \tag{12}$$

with $\xi_1 = \infty$, $\xi_2 = x_0 + d$ and $\xi_3 = x_0$.

Having obtained the piecewise wave profile $U(\xi)$, the threshold conditions (Equation 7) can now be used to determine the pulse speed c and width d; the resulting transcendental equations have to be solved numerically. **Figure 2** shows solutions for the pulse speed and width as functions of the threshold. It turns out that the solution with slower speed (and larger width)

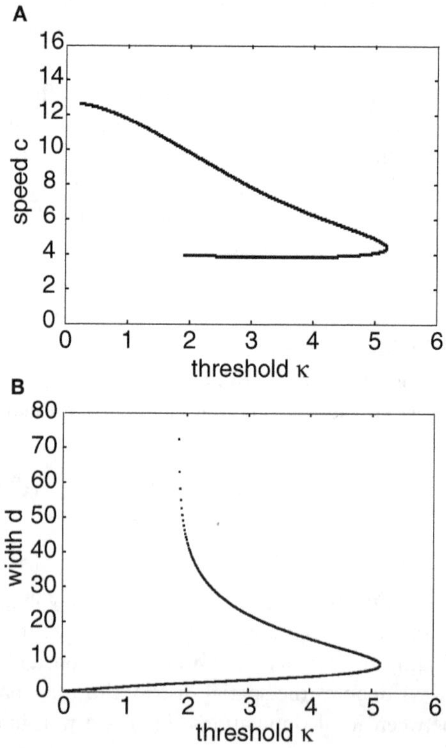

FIGURE 2 | (A) Plots of pulse speed ***c*** and **(B)** pulse width ***d*** as a function of the threshold **κ**. Weight parameters are as in **Figure 1** with offset $x_0 = 3$. Stable (unstable) branches are indicated by black (gray) curves.

is stable (see below). This differs from traveling pulse solutions found in adaptive neural fields, where the faster wave (with larger width) tends to be stable (Pinto and Ermentrout, 2001; Kilpatrick and Bressloff, 2010a). **Figure 3A** shows a typical pulse waveform and **Figure 3B** shows a numerical simulation of the neural field Equation (1) using the wave solution as the initial condition. The pulse propagates at the predicted speed without changing shape significantly. This occurs because the parameters were chosen to make the pulse solution linearly stable.

Stability

In order to determine the linear stability of a traveling pulse solution $U(\xi)$ in the moving frame, we linearize Equation (1) with $h(x, t) = 0$ by setting

$$U(\xi, t) = U(\xi) + \varphi(\xi, t),$$

and Taylor expanding to first order in φ. This gives

$$\frac{\partial \varphi(\xi, t)}{\partial t} = c\frac{\partial \varphi(\xi, t)}{\partial \xi} - \varphi(\xi, t) + \int_{-\infty}^{\infty} w(\xi - y) \times F'(U(y))\varphi(y, t)\, dy. \tag{13}$$

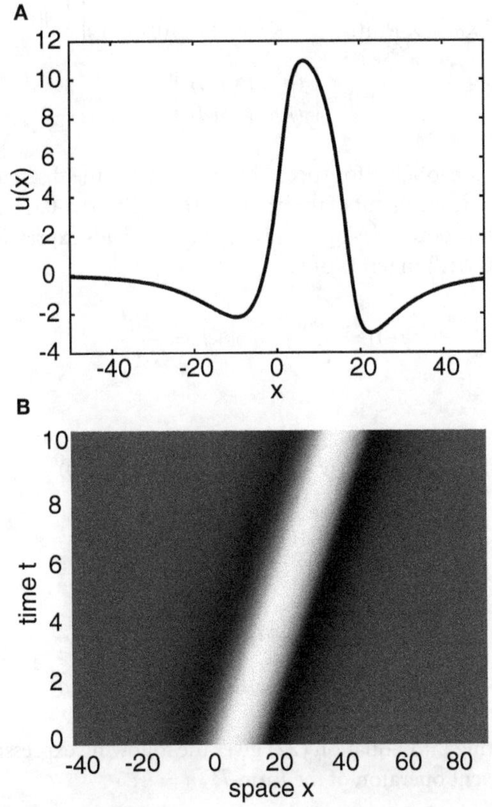

FIGURE 3 | (A) Plot of traveling wave profile $U(\xi)$ obtained analytically. Same parameters as **Figure 2** for threshold $\kappa = 4$. **(B)** Spacetime plot of a traveling pulse using the profile of **(A)** as the initial condition. High (low) activity indicated by light (gray).

In the case of the Heaviside rate function (Equation 3), we have

$$F'(U(\xi)) = \frac{\delta(\xi)}{|U'(0)|} + \frac{\delta(\xi - d)}{|U'(d)|}. \tag{14}$$

Moreover, differentiating Equation (9) with respect to ξ shows that

$$U'(\xi) = \frac{1}{c}(U(\xi) - W(\xi)).$$

Substituting the previous two results into Equation (13) gives

$$\begin{aligned} \frac{\partial \varphi(\xi, t)}{\partial t} &= \mathcal{L}\varphi(\xi, t) \\ &\equiv c\frac{\partial \varphi(\xi, t)}{\partial \xi} - \varphi(\xi, t) + \frac{c\varphi(0, t)}{|\kappa - W(0)|}w(\xi) \\ &\quad + \frac{c\varphi(d, t)}{|\kappa - W(d)|}w(\xi - d). \end{aligned} \tag{15}$$

where κ is the threshold. Looking for solutions of the form

$$\varphi(\xi, t) = e^{\lambda t}\varphi(\xi). \tag{16}$$

then leads to the spectral problem

$$\mathcal{L}\varphi(\xi, t) = \lambda\varphi(\xi, t). \tag{17}$$

We take the linear operator $\mathcal{L}$ to act on a Banach space $\mathcal{B}$ of continuous, bounded functions $\psi(\xi)$ that are defined for $\xi \in \mathbb{R}$, and that decay exponentially as $\xi \to \pm\infty$. Let $\sigma(\mathcal{L})$ denote the spectrum of the linear operator $\mathcal{L}$, and define the associated resolvent operator according to $\mathcal{R}_\lambda \equiv (\mathcal{L} - \lambda I)^{-1}$, where I is the identity operator. The spectrum can be defined as those values of λ for which $\mathcal{T}_\lambda \equiv \mathcal{L} - \lambda I$ is not bijective. The spectrum is composed of three disjoint sets, the point or discrete spectrum, the residual spectrum, and the continuous spectrum. The point spectrum is defined as the values of λ (eigenvalues) for which the resolvent does not exist. The residual spectrum are the spectral values for which the resolvent exists but is not defined on a dense subset of $\mathcal{B}$. The continuous spectrum are the spectral values for which the resolvent exists and is densely defined but is unbounded (Kreyszig, 1978). Given these definitions, the traveling pulse is said to be linearly stable if (1) $\mathrm{Re}(\lambda) < 0$ for all $\lambda \in \sigma(\mathcal{L})$, $\lambda \neq 0$ and (2) the zero eigenvalue is simple. The existence of a zero eigenvalue with corresponding eigenfunction $\varphi(\xi, t) = U'(\xi)$ reflects translation invariance, and immediately follows from differentiating (Equation 9) with respect to ξ.

We first consider the discrete spectrum by solving the eigenvalue equation

$$\frac{d\psi(\xi)}{d\xi} - \frac{\lambda + 1}{c}\psi(\xi) + K_0\psi(0)w(\xi) + K_d\psi(d)w(\xi - d) = 0,$$

where we have introduced the constants

$$K_0 = \frac{1}{|\kappa - W(0)|} \text{ and } K_d = \frac{1}{|\kappa - W(d)|}.$$

Multiplying both sides by $e^{-(\lambda+1)\xi/c}$ and integrating gives

$$\psi(\xi) = K_0\psi(0)\int_{\xi}^{\infty} w(y)e^{(\lambda+1)(\xi-y)/c}\,dy + K_d\psi(d)\int_{\xi-d}^{\infty} w(y)e^{(\lambda+1)(\xi-d-y)/c}\,dy,$$

which can be rewritten in the more compact form

$$\psi(\xi) = K_0\psi(0)(w\times P_\lambda)(\xi) + K_d\psi(d)(w\times P_\lambda)(\xi-d) \quad (18)$$

with

$$(w\times P_\lambda)(\xi) = \int_{-\infty}^{\infty} w(y)P_\lambda(\xi-y)\,dy,\ P_\lambda(\xi) = H(-\xi)e^{(\lambda+1)\xi/c} \quad (19)$$

The eigenvalues are now determined by imposing self-consistency at $\xi = 0$ and $\xi = d$. Setting $\xi = 0$ and $\xi = d$ in Equation (18) leads to the vector equation

$$\begin{bmatrix} K_0(w\times P_\lambda)(0)-1 & K_d(w\times P_\lambda)(-d) \\ K_0(w\times P_\lambda)(d) & K_d(w\times P_\lambda)(0)-1 \end{bmatrix}\begin{bmatrix}\psi(0)\\ \psi(d)\end{bmatrix} = \mathbf{0} \quad (20)$$

This has a non-trivial solution if and only if the determinant of the matrix is zero. The determinant expressed as a function of λ, $\mathcal{E}(\lambda)$, is a complex analytic function known as the Evans function:

$$\mathcal{E}(\lambda) = [K_0(w\times P_\lambda)(0)-1]\,[K_d(w\times P_\lambda)(0)-1] - K_0K_d(w\times P_\lambda)(d)(w\times P_\lambda)(-d). \quad (21)$$

Thus, the zeros of the Evans function determine the discrete spectrum of the linear operator formed by linearizing the neural field equation about the pulse solution. Evans functions were originally introduced within the context of the stability of solitary pulses in diffusive Hodgkin–Huxley type equations describing action potential propagation in nerve axons (Evans, 1975). Since then the Evans function construction has been extended to a wide range of PDEs, see the review (Sandstede, 2002). It has also recently been applied to neural field equations (Zhang, 2003; Coombes and Owen, 2004; Rubin, 2004; Folias and Bressloff, 2005; Pinto et al., 2005; Sandstede, 2007) and more general non-local problems (Kapitula et al., 2004). An example plot of the real and imaginary parts of $\mathcal{E}(\lambda) = 0$ on the complex plane is shown in **Figure 4**. It can be seen that there is a zero eigenvalue and one negative real eigenvalue, indicating that the corresponding traveling pulse is linearly stable.

To find the essential spectrum, which is the union of the residual and continuous spectra, we will derive an explicit expression for the resolvent $\mathcal{R}_\lambda$. We start by writing an inhomogeneous equation of the form $\mathcal{T}_\lambda\psi(\xi) = h(\xi)$, where $h(\xi)$ represents a general function from the Banach space $\mathcal{B}$. This can be manipulated as before to give

$$\psi(\xi) = -(h\times P_\lambda)(\xi) + K_0\psi(0)(w\times P_\lambda)(\xi) + K_d\psi(d)(w\times P_\lambda)(\xi-d) \quad (22)$$

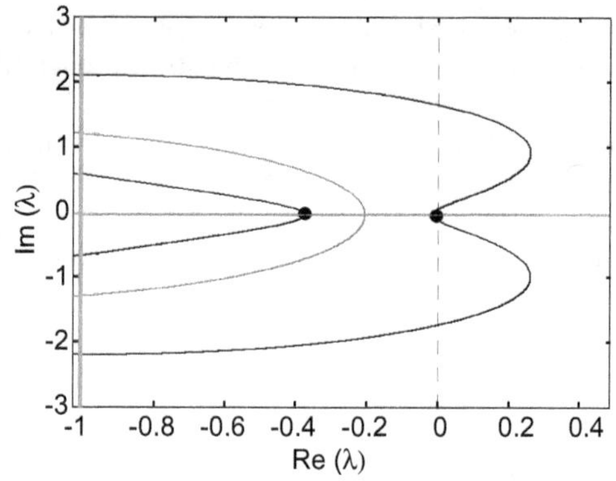

FIGURE 4 | Graphs of the zero sets of the real (*dark curves*) and imaginary (*light curves*) parts of the Evans function determining the stability of a freely propagating pulse; intersection points (filled circles) indicate eigenvalues. The line $\operatorname{Im}\lambda = -1$ indicates the essential spectrum. Same parameter values as **Figure 3**.

By evaluating at $\xi = 0$ and $\xi = d$ as before, we arrive at the following vector equation, which differs from (Equation 20) only on the right-hand side:

$$\begin{bmatrix} K_0(w\times P_\lambda)(0)-1 & K_d(w\times P_\lambda)(-d) \\ K_0(w\times P_\lambda)(d) & K_d(w\times P_\lambda)(0)-1 \end{bmatrix}\begin{bmatrix}\psi(0)\\ \psi(d)\end{bmatrix} = \begin{bmatrix}(h\times P_\lambda)(0)\\ (h\times P_\lambda)(d)\end{bmatrix}.$$

Since we are looking for spectral values outside the discrete spectrum, the determinant of the matrix satisfies $\mathcal{E}(\lambda) \neq 0$. Therefore, multiplying both sides by the inverse matrix yields expressions for $\psi(0)$ and $\psi(d)$ in terms of h:

$$\psi(0) = \frac{S_0h}{\mathcal{E}(\lambda)},\quad \psi(d) = \frac{S_dh}{\mathcal{E}(\lambda)}$$

where

$$S_0h = (K_d(w\times P_\lambda)(0)-1)\,(h\times P_\lambda)(0) - K_d(w\times P_\lambda)(-d)(h\times P_\lambda)(d)$$

and

$$S_dh = -K_0(w\times P_\lambda)(d)(h\times P_\lambda)(0) + (K_0(w\times P_\lambda)(0)-1)\,(h\times P_\lambda)(d).$$

Substituting into Equation (22) gives the following expression for the resolvent operator, of the form $\mathcal{R}_\lambda h = \varphi$:

$$-(h\times P_\lambda)(\xi) + \frac{K_0S_0h}{\mathcal{E}(\lambda)}(w\times P_\lambda)(\xi) + \frac{K_dS_dh}{\mathcal{E}(\lambda)}(w\times P_\lambda)(\xi-d) = \psi(\xi) \quad (23)$$

The resolvent is well-defined for all h in $\mathcal{B}$, so the residual spectrum of $\mathcal{L}$ is empty. To find the continuous spectrum, we Fourier transform Equation (23):

$$-\hat{h}(k)\hat{P}_\lambda(k) + \frac{K_0 S_0 h}{\varepsilon(\lambda)}\hat{w}(k)\hat{P}_\lambda(k) + \frac{K_d S_d h}{\varepsilon(\lambda)}\hat{w}(k)\hat{P}_\lambda(k)e^{-2\pi i d k} = \hat{\psi}(k) \tag{24}$$

It follows that the resolvent operator is unbounded when $\hat{P}_\lambda$ is unbounded. Equation (19) implies that

$$\hat{P}_\lambda(k) = \int_{-\infty}^{\infty} P_\lambda(\xi)e^{2\pi i k\xi}\, d\xi = \frac{1}{\dfrac{\lambda+1}{c} + 2\pi i k}. \tag{25}$$

Hence, $\hat{P}_\lambda$ is unbounded for $\lambda = -1 - 2\pi i k c$ so that the continuous spectrum of $\mathcal{L}$ is a vertical line in the complex plane at $\mathrm{Re}(\lambda) = -1$. Since $\mathrm{Re}(\lambda) < 0$, the continuous spectrum will not make any pulse solution of our model unstable.

Stimulus-locked pulses

Now suppose that the neural field is driven by a moving external pulse stimulus of speed v so that Equation (1) becomes

$$\frac{\partial u(x,t)}{\partial t} = -u(x,t) + \int_{-\infty}^{\infty} w(x-y)\, H\left(u(y,t) - \kappa\right) dy + I(x - vt). \tag{26}$$

In order to study the existence of stimulus-locked pulses, we will define a "stimulus coordinate" $\xi = x - vt$ and look for pulse solutions that move at the same speed as the stimulus, that is, $u(x,t) = U(\xi)$ with

$$-v\frac{\partial U(\xi)}{\partial \xi} = -U(\xi) + \int_{-\infty}^{\infty} w(\xi - y)H(U(y) - \kappa)\, dy + I(\xi). \tag{27}$$

For concreteness, the stimulus will be represented by a rectangular wave of amplitude I_0 and width d, defined formally as

$$I(\xi) = \begin{cases} I_0, & \text{if } 0 \le \xi \le d \\ 0, & \text{if } \xi < 0 \text{ or } \xi > d. \end{cases}$$

Since translation invariance no longer holds, it is necessary to determine both threshold crossing points, which we denote by $\xi = d_1$ and $\xi = d_2$. Proceeding in a similar fashion to the case of freely propagating pulses, we find that

$$U(\xi) = \frac{e^{\xi/v}}{v}\int_{\xi}^{z_0} e^{-y/v}W(y)\, dy + \frac{e^{\xi/v}}{v}\int_{\xi}^{z_0} e^{-y/v}I(y)\, dy,$$

where $z_0 = \infty$ if $v > 0$, $z_0 = -\infty$ if $v < 0$, and

$$W(\xi) \equiv \int_{\xi-d_2}^{\xi-d_1} w(x)\, dx.$$

The latter can be expressed in the piecewise form

$$W(\xi) = \begin{cases} W_3(\xi) \equiv \int_{\xi-d_2}^{\xi-d_1} w_2(x)\, dx, & \text{if } \xi \le x_0 + d_1 \\ W_2(\xi) \equiv \int_{\xi-d_2}^{x_0} w_2(x)\, dx + \int_{x_0}^{\xi-d_1} w_1(x)\, dx, & \text{if } x_0 + d_1 \le \xi \le x_0 + d_2 \\ W_1(\xi) = \int_{\xi-d_2}^{\xi-d_1} w_1(x)\, dx, & \text{if } \xi \ge x_0 + d_2 \end{cases} \tag{28}$$

where w_1 and w_2 are defined as in Equation (10). After evaluating the integrals along similar lines to section "Neural Field Model of Direction Selectivity," we obtain the following expressions for the pulse solution, defined independently for positive and negative stimulus directions:

$\underline{v > 0:}$

$$U(\xi) = \begin{cases} U_3(\xi), & \text{if } \xi \le x_0 + d_1 \\ U_2(\xi), & \text{if } x_0 + d_1 \le \xi \le x_0 + d_2, \\ U_1(\xi), & \text{if } \xi \ge x_0 + d_2, \end{cases}$$

with

$$U_3(\xi) = \frac{1}{v}e^{\xi/v}\left(M_3(\xi) + M_1(x_0 + d_2) + M_2(x_0 + d_1)\right) + Z(\xi)$$

$$U_2(\xi) = \frac{1}{v}e^{\xi/v}\left(M_2(\xi) + M_1(x_0 + d_2)\right) + Z(\xi)$$

$$U_1(\xi) = \frac{1}{v}e^{\xi/v}M_1(\xi) + Z(\xi),$$

$$M_n(\xi) = \int_{\xi}^{\xi_n} W_n(\xi')e^{-\xi'/v}d\xi'$$

for $\xi_1 = \infty$, $\xi_2 = x_0 + d_2$, $\xi_3 = x_0 + d_1$, and

$$Z(\xi) = \begin{cases} \left(e^{\xi/v} - e^{(\xi-d)/v}\right) I_0, & \text{if } \xi < 0 \\ \left(1 - e^{(\xi-d)/v}\right) I_0, & \text{if } 0 \le \xi \le d. \\ 0, & \text{if } \xi > d \end{cases}$$

$\underline{v < 0:}$

$$U(\xi) = \begin{cases} U_3(\xi), & \text{if } \xi \le x_0 + d_1 \\ U_2(\xi), & \text{if } x_0 + d_1 \le \xi \le x_0 + d_2, \\ U_1(\xi), & \text{if } \xi \ge x_0 + d_2 \end{cases}$$

with

$$U_3(\xi) = -\frac{1}{v}e^{\xi/v}N_3(\xi) + Z(\xi)$$

$$U_2(\xi) = -\frac{1}{v}e^{\xi/v}\left(N_2(\xi) + N_3(x_0 + d_1)\right) + Z(\xi)$$

$$U_1(\xi) = -\frac{1}{v}e^{\xi/v}\left(N_1(\xi) + N_2(x_0 + d_1) + N_3(x_0 + d_1)\right) + Z(\xi)$$

$$N_n(\xi) = \int_{\xi_n}^{\xi} W_n(\xi')e^{-\xi'/v}d\xi'$$

for $\xi_3 = -\infty, \xi_2 = x_0 + d_1, \xi_1 = x_0 + d_2$, and

$$Z(\xi) = \begin{cases} 0, & \text{if } \xi < 0 \\ \left(1 - e^{\xi/v}\right) I_0, & \text{if } 0 \le \xi \le d. \\ \left(e^{(\xi-d)/v} - e^{\xi/v}\right) I_0, & \text{if } \xi > d \end{cases}$$

The threshold crossing points (d_1 and d_2) are determined in the same way the pulse speed and width were determined in the no-stimulus case, which is by numerically solving a system of two transcendental equations. The first equation is given by $U_3(d_1) = \kappa$. The second equation is $U_3(d_2) = \kappa$ if $d_2 < x_0 + d_1$, else it is given by $U_2(d_2) = \kappa$. **Figure 5** shows a plot of d_1 (black curves) and d_2 (gray curves) vs. the threshold κ. It can be seen that for a certain range of thresholds there exists more than one stable/unstable pair of pulses. **Figure 6** shows the linear stability and the number of solutions for different combinations of stimulus speed (v) and strength (I_0). The offset $x_0 = 3$ and the corresponding spontaneous wave speed is $c = 4$. (Note that for smaller offsets x_0 and thus smaller wave speeds c, one finds stimulus-locked waves for negative values of v). The stability of solutions in the presence of a stimulus is determined in much the same way as without a stimulus. We again define $u(x, t) = U(\xi) + \varphi(\xi, t)$ and look at the behavior of the perturbations described by $\varphi(\xi, t)$. Substituting into Equation (26), the stimulus term drops out when we perform the linearization, so that

$$\frac{\partial\varphi(\xi, t)}{\partial t} = v\frac{\partial\varphi(\xi, t)}{\partial\xi} - \varphi(\xi, t) + \int_{-\infty}^{\infty} w(\xi - y) \times F'(U(y))\varphi(y, t)\,dy.$$

Setting $\varphi(\xi, t) = e^{\lambda t}\varphi$ ultimately yields the spectral problem

$$\lambda\varphi(\xi) \equiv \mathcal{L}\varphi(\xi) = v\frac{\partial\varphi(\xi, t)}{\partial\xi} - \varphi(\xi, t) + \frac{|v|\varphi(d_1)}{|\kappa - W(d_1) - I(d_1)|}w(\xi - d_1) + \frac{|v|\varphi(d_2)}{|\kappa - W(d_2) - I(d_2)|}w(\xi - d_2). \quad (29)$$

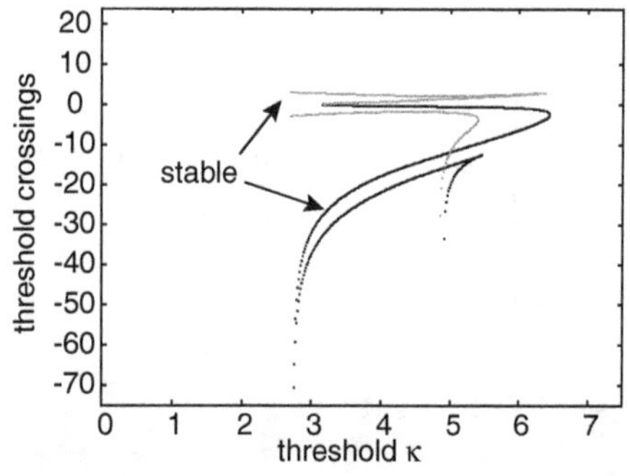

FIGURE 5 | Plot of leading threshold crossing position d_2 (gray curves) and trailing threshold crossing position d_1 (black curves) of stimulus-locked pulses as a function of threshold κ. There exists at most one stable pulse (indicated by arrows) and up to three unstable pulses. Weight parameters as in **Figure 2** and $\kappa = 4$. Stimulus parameters are $d = 5$, $I_0 = 5$, and $v = 5$.

The corresponding Evans function is now

$$\mathcal{E}(\lambda) = [K_1(w \times P_\lambda)(0) - 1]\,[K_2(w \times P_\lambda)(0) - 1] - K_1K_2(w \times P_\lambda)(d_2 - d_1)(w \times P_\lambda)(d_1 - d_2), \quad (30)$$

where

$$K_n = \frac{\text{sgn}(v)}{|\kappa - W(d_n) - I(d_n)|}, \quad n = 1, 2,$$

and

$$P_\lambda(\xi) = H(-\text{sgn}(v)\xi)e^{(\lambda+1)\xi/v}.$$

It is easy to establish as before that the residual spectrum is empty and that the continuous spectrum consists of a vertical line in the complex plane at $\text{Re}(\lambda) = -1$. So the stability is again determined only by the discrete spectrum, which consists of the zeros of the Evans function. **Figure 7A** shows an example of a numerical simulation of a stable stimulus-locked pulse solution of Equation (26) with the analytical pulse solution $U(x)$ as an initial condition. **Figure 7B** shows the same simulation except with the zero initial condition $u(x, 0) = 0$. It can be seen from **Figure 7C** that both initial conditions converge to the same pulse profile.

STOCHASTIC NEURAL FIELD

Several recent studies have considered stochastic versions of neural field equations that are based on a corresponding Langevin

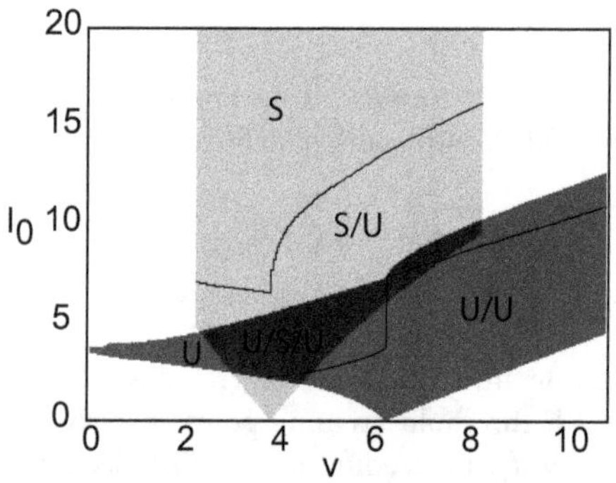

FIGURE 6 | Stability diagram for stimulus-locked pulses in (v, I_0)-parameter space. Weight parameters as in **Figure 2**, $\kappa = 4$, and $d = 5$. Emerging from the stable pulse solution when $I_0 = 0$ is a tongue consisting of a stable/unstable pair of pulses (light gray). Similarly, emerging from the unstable solution when $I_0 = 0$ is a tongue consisting of two unstable pulses (medium gray). As I_0 increases within a tongue an unstable pulse can disappear due to the development of multiple super-threshold regions (indicated by solid curves). All solutions coexist when tongues overlap (dark gray).

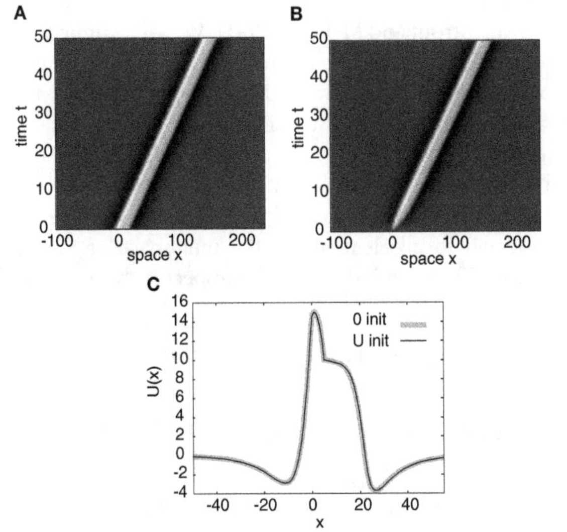

FIGURE 7 | Space-time plots of a stimulus-locked pulse for (A) $u(x,\ 0) = U(x)$ and (B) $u(x,\ 0) = 0$. Both initial conditions converge to the same wave profile in the large t limit as indicated in **(C)** for $t = 50$. Weight parameters as in **Figure 2** and $\kappa = 4$. Stimulus parameters are $d = 5,\ I_0 = 8,$ and $v = 3$.

equation formulation (Brackley and Turner, 2007; Hutt et al., 2008; Faugeras et al., 2009; Bressloff and Webber, 2012b). Motivated by these examples, we consider the following Langevin equation (or stochastic PDE) for the stochastic activity variable $U(x, t)$, which is a rewriting of Equation (1) with $h(x, t)$ given by Equation (5) for $I_0 = 0$ and $\epsilon > 0$:

$$dU(x,t) = \left[-U(x,t) + \int_{-\infty}^{\infty} w(x-y)F(U(y,t))dy\right]dt + \epsilon^{1/2} g(U(x,t))dW(x,t), \tag{31}$$

where $dW(x, t)$ is an independent Wiener process with zero mean and correlation given by

$$\langle dW(x,t)dW(x',t')\rangle = 2C(|x-x'|/\lambda)\delta(t-t')dtdt'. \tag{32}$$

Here λ is the spatial correlation length of the noise such that $C(x/\lambda) \to \delta(x)$ in the limit $\lambda \to 0$, and ϵ determines the strength of the noise, which is assumed to be weak. For the sake of generality, we take the noise to be multiplicative rather than additive; however, the main results of the paper hold for both. Following standard formulations of Langevin equations (Gardiner, 2009), the multiplicative noise term is taken to be of Stratonovich form in the case of extrinsic noise. Note, however, that an alternative formulation of stochastic neural field theory has been developed in terms of a neural master equation (Buice and Cowan, 2007; Bressloff, 2009, 2010; Buice et al., 2010), in which the underlying deterministic equations are recovered in the thermodynamic limit $N \to \infty$, where N is a measure of the system size of each local population. In the case of large but finite N, a Kramers-Moyal expansion of the master equation yields a Langevin neural field equation with multiplicative noise of the Ito form Bressloff (2009, 2010). Multiplicative noise in the Stratonovich sense causes a shift in the speed and width of the pulse. This happens because $\langle g(U)dW\rangle \neq 0$, even though $\langle dW\rangle = 0$. We can use Novikov's theorem (Novikov, 1965) to calculate the former average:

$$\epsilon^{1/2}\langle g(U)dW\rangle = \epsilon C(0)\langle g'(U)g(U)\rangle dt.$$

The average can also be calculated by Fourier transforming Equation (31) and taking averages using the corresponding Fokker–Planck equation (Armero et al., 1998; Bressloff and Webber, 2012b). In the limit that λ approaches 0, we set $C(0) \to 1/\Delta x$, where Δx is a lattice cut-off that can be identified with the spatial discretization step size in numerical simulations (Bressloff and Webber, 2012b). Following Ref. Armero et al. (1998), we rewrite Equation (31) so the fluctuating term has zero mean:

$$dU(x,t) = \left[h(U(x,t)) + \int_{-\infty}^{\infty} w(x-y)F(U(y,t))dy\right]dt + \epsilon^{1/2} dR(U,x,t), \tag{33}$$

where

$$h(U) = -U + \epsilon C(0)g'(U)g(U) \tag{34}$$

and

$$dR(U,x,t) = g(U)dW(x,t) - \epsilon^{1/2}C(0)g'(U)g(U)dt. \tag{35}$$

The stochastic process R has zero mean and correlation

$$\langle dR(U,x,t)dR(U,x',t')\rangle = \langle g(U(x,t))dW(x,t)g(U(x',t'))dW(x',t')\rangle + \mathcal{O}(\epsilon^{1/2}). \tag{36}$$

Separation of time-scales

The effects of additive or multiplicative extrinsic noise on traveling waves can be analyzed using multiple time-scale methods originally developed for reaction-diffusion equations (Schimansky-Geier et al., 1983; de Pasquale et al., 1992; Armero et al., 1998; Sagues et al., 2007), which were recently extended to neural field equations in Ref. Bressloff and Webber (2012b). The main idea is to assume that the fluctuating term generates two distinct phenomena that occur on different time-scales: a diffusive-like displacement of the traveling wave from its uniformly translating position at long time-scales, and fluctuations in the wave profile around its instantaneous position at short time-scales. It is important to point out that, in contrast to traveling front solutions of scalar neural field equations (Bressloff and Webber, 2012b), we are now considering traveling pulse solutions. Thus in addition to the center-of-mass of the traveling pulse wave, which moves with speed c in the absence of noise, there is an additional degree of freedom corresponding to the "width" of the pulse. (In the case of a Heaviside rate function, the width Δ is determined by the threshold crossing points). For simplicity, we assume that the width of the wave is only weakly affected by the noise; this is consistent with what is found numerically. We now express the solution U of Equation (33) as a combination of a fixed wave profile U_0 that is displaced by an amount $\Delta(t)$ from its uniformly translating position $\xi = x - c_\epsilon t$, where c_ϵ is a noise-dependent speed, and a time-dependent fluctuation Φ in the wave shape about its instantaneous position:

$$U(x,t) = U_0(\xi - \Delta(t)) + \epsilon^{1/2}\Phi(\xi - \Delta(t), t). \tag{37}$$

The wave profile U_0 and associated wave speed/width c_ϵ, Δ_ϵ are obtained by solving the modified deterministic equation

$$-c_\epsilon \frac{dU_0(\xi)}{d\xi} - h(U_0(\xi)) = \int_{\infty}^{\infty} w(\xi - \xi')F(U_0(\xi'))d\xi'. \tag{38}$$

The results depend on ϵ due to the ϵ-dependence of h. Equation (38) is chosen so that that to leading order, the stochastic variable $\Delta(t)$ undergoes unbiased Brownian motion with a diffusion coefficient $D(\epsilon) = \mathcal{O}(\epsilon)$ (see below). The next step is to substitute the decomposition Equation (37) into (33) and expand to first order in $\mathcal{O}(\varepsilon^{1/2})$:

$$\begin{aligned}
-[c_\varepsilon + \dot{\Delta}]U_0'(\xi_\Delta)dt &+ \epsilon^{1/2}\left[d\Phi(\xi_\Delta, t) - [c_\epsilon + \dot{\Delta}]\Phi'(\xi_\Delta, t)dt\right] \\
&= h(U_0(\xi_\Delta))dt + \epsilon^{1/2}h'(U_0(\xi_\Delta))\Phi(\xi_\Delta, t)dt \\
&+ \int_{-\infty}^{\infty} w(\xi - \xi')F(U_0(\xi'_\Delta))d\xi' dt \\
&+ \epsilon^{1/2}\int_{-\infty}^{\infty} w(\xi - \xi')F'(U_0(\xi'_\Delta))\Phi(\xi'_\Delta, t)d\xi' dt \\
&+ \epsilon^{1/2} dR(U_0(\xi_\Delta), \xi, t) + \mathcal{O}(\epsilon).
\end{aligned}$$

where we have set $\xi_\Delta = \xi - \Delta(t)$ and $\xi'_\Delta = \xi' - \Delta(t)$. We now use Equation (38) for U_0, after shifting $\xi \to \xi - \Delta(t)$, to eliminate terms and then divide through by $\sqrt{\epsilon}$. This gives the inhomogeneous equation to $\mathcal{O}(\epsilon^{1/2})$

$$\begin{aligned}
d\Phi(\xi_\Delta, t) - \widehat{L}\Phi(\xi_\Delta, t)dt &= \epsilon^{-\frac{1}{2}}U_0'(\xi_\Delta)d\Delta(t) \\
&+ dR(U_0(\xi_\Delta), \xi, t)
\end{aligned} \tag{39}$$

where the non-self-adjoint linear operator

$$\begin{aligned}
\widehat{L}A(\xi) \equiv c_\epsilon \frac{dA(\xi)}{d\xi} &+ h'(U_0(\xi))A(\xi) \\
&+ \int_{-\infty}^{\infty} w(\xi - \xi')F'(U_0(\xi'))A(\xi')d\xi'
\end{aligned} \tag{40}$$

is defined for all functions $A(\xi)$ in $\mathcal{L}_2(\mathbb{R})$. Note that for all terms in Equation (40) to be of the same order we have taken $\Delta(t) = \mathcal{O}(\varepsilon^{1/2})$. It then follows that $U_0(\xi - \Delta(t)) = U_0(\xi) + \mathcal{O}(\varepsilon^{1/2})$ etc., and Equation (39) reduces to

$$d\Phi(\xi, t) - \widehat{L}\Phi(\xi, t)dt = \epsilon^{-\frac{1}{2}}U_0'(\xi)d\Delta(t) + dR_u(U_0(\xi), \xi, t) \tag{41}$$

If $U_0(\xi)$ were a traveling front solution of a neural field model with a symmetric, excitatory weight distribution w, then it could be proven that the operator $\widehat{L}$ has a 1D null space spanned by $U_0'(\xi)$ (Ermentrout and McLeod, 1993). We will assume that such a result carries over to traveling pulse solutions of a neural field with w given by an asymmetric Mexican hat function; the fact that $U_0'(\xi)$ belongs to the null space follows immediately from differentiating Equation (38) with respect to ξ. We then have the solvability condition for the existence of a non-trivial bounded solution of Equation (41), namely, that the inhomogeneous part is orthogonal to all elements of the null space of the adjoint operator $\widehat{L}^*$. The latter is defined with respect to the inner product

$$\int_{-\infty}^{\infty} B(\xi)\widehat{L}A(\xi)\, d\xi = \int_{-\infty}^{\infty} \left[\widehat{L}^* B(\xi)\right] A(\xi)\, d\xi.$$

Integrating by parts and using (Equation 14) leads to

$$\begin{aligned}
\widehat{L}^* B(\xi) = -c_\epsilon \frac{dB(\xi)}{d\xi} &+ h'(U_0(\xi))B(\xi) \\
&+ F'(U_0(\xi))\int_{-\infty}^{\infty} w(\xi' - \xi)B(\xi')d\xi'.
\end{aligned} \tag{42}$$

We will assume that the null space of the adjoint operator $\widehat{L}^*$ is also one-dimensional and is spanned by some yet to be determined function $\mathcal{V}(\xi)$. (In the case of a Heaviside firing function, we will determine the null space explicitly). Hence, we can write the solvability condition as

$$\int_{-\infty}^{\infty} \mathcal{V}(\xi)\left[U_0'(\xi)d\Delta(t) + \epsilon^{1/2}dR(U_0(\xi), \xi, t)\right]\, d\xi = 0.$$

which leads directly to the stochastic differential equation

$$d\Delta(t) = -\epsilon^{1/2}\frac{\int_{-\infty}^{\infty} \mathcal{V}(\xi)dR(U_0, \xi, t)\, d\xi}{\int_{-\infty}^{\infty} \mathcal{V}(\xi)U_0'(\xi)d\xi}.$$

Using the lowest order approximations $dR(U_0, \xi, t) = g(U_0(\xi))dW(\xi, t)$, we deduce that [for $\Delta(0) = 0$]

$$\langle \Delta(t)\rangle = 0, \quad \langle \Delta(t)^2\rangle = 2D(\varepsilon)t, \tag{43}$$

where $D(\epsilon)$ is the effective diffusivity

$$D(\epsilon) = \epsilon \frac{\int_{-\infty}^{\infty} \mathcal{V}^2(\xi)g(U_0(\xi))^2\, d\xi}{\left[\int_{-\infty}^{\infty} \mathcal{V}(\xi)U_0'(\xi)\, d\xi\right]^2}. \tag{44}$$

Explicit results for Heaviside rate function

In order to illustrate the above analysis, we consider a particular example where the mean speed c_ϵ and diffusion coefficient $D(\epsilon)$ can be calculated explicitly. That is, set $g(U) = g_0 U$ for the multiplicative noise term and take $F(U) = H(u - \kappa)$. (The constant g_0 has units of $\sqrt{\text{length/time}}$). Note that the choice for $g(U)$ can be interpreted physiologically in terms of an effective modification in the membrane time constant of neurons due to stochastic background synaptic activity (Bernander et al., 1991; Rapp et al., 1992; Bressloff, 1994). The deterministic Equation (38) for U_0

then reduces to

$$-\frac{dU_0(\xi)}{d\xi}+\Gamma(\epsilon)U_0(\xi)=\frac{1}{c_\epsilon}\int_{\infty}^{\infty}w(\xi-\xi')H(U_0(\xi')-\kappa)d\xi', \tag{45}$$

where $\Gamma(\epsilon)=(1-\epsilon C(0)g_0^2)/c_\epsilon$. Hence,

$$U(\xi)=\frac{e^{\Gamma\xi}}{c_\epsilon}\int_{\xi}^{\infty}W(\xi')e^{-\Gamma\xi'}\,d\xi'. \tag{46}$$

The deterministic pulse profile can be evaluated along identical lines to section "Neural Field Model of Direction Selectivity." In order to calculate the diffusion coefficient, it is first necessary to determine the null vector $\mathcal{V}(\epsilon)$ of the adjoint linear operator $\widehat{L}^*$. Substituting $F(U)=H(U-\kappa)$ and $g(U)=g_0U$ into Equation (42) shows that

$$\frac{d\mathcal{V}(\xi)}{d\xi}+\Gamma(\epsilon)\mathcal{V}(\xi)=\frac{\delta(\xi)}{c|U_0'(0)|}\int_{-\infty}^{\infty}w(z)\mathcal{V}(z)dz+\frac{\delta(\xi-\Delta)}{c|U_0'(\Delta)|}\int_{-\infty}^{\infty}w(z-\Delta)\mathcal{V}(z)dz. \tag{47}$$

Proceeding along similar lines to Bressloff (2001) and Kilpatrick et al. (2008), we make the ansatz that

$$\mathcal{V}(\xi)=AH(\xi)e^{-\Gamma\xi}+BH(\xi-\Delta)e^{-\Gamma(\xi-\Delta)}. \tag{48}$$

Substituting into Equation (47) shows that

$$A=\frac{1}{|U_0'(0)|}[Ab(0)+Bb(\Delta)],\quad B=\frac{1}{|U_0'(\Delta)|}[Ab(-\Delta)+Bb(0)]$$

where

$$b(z)\equiv\frac{1}{c}\int_{z}^{\infty}e^{-\Gamma(\xi'-z)}w(\xi')\,d\xi'. \tag{49}$$

Differentiating Equation (46) shows that $U'(\xi)=b(\xi)-b(\xi-\Delta)$, so that we obtain the vector equation

$$\begin{bmatrix}\frac{b(0)}{b(0)-b(-\Delta)}-1 & \frac{b(\Delta)}{b(0)-b(-\Delta)}\\ \frac{b(-\Delta)}{b(0)-b(\Delta)} & \frac{b(0)}{b(0)-b(\Delta)}-1\end{bmatrix}\begin{bmatrix}A\\B\end{bmatrix}=0$$

The matrix has rank 1, confirming that the linear operator $\widehat{L}^*$ has a 1D null-space. The latter is spanned by the function

$$\mathcal{V}(\xi)=b(\Delta)H(\xi)e^{-\Gamma\xi}-b(-\Delta)H(\xi-\Delta)e^{-\Gamma(\xi-\Delta)}. \tag{50}$$

In **Figure 8** we show the temporal evolution of a freely propagating stochastic traveling pulse, which is obtained by numerically solving the Langevin Equation (31) for $F(U)=H(U-\kappa)$, $g(U)=U$ and the asymmetric difference-of-exponentials (Equation 4). Note that the location of the stochastic wave appears to coincide with the underlying mean solution. However, over longer time-scales the wandering of the pulse about its mean position would be seen. In **Figure 9** we plot the mean position $\overline{X}(t)$ and variance $\sigma_X^2(t)$ of the leading and trailing edges of the pulse as a function of t. It can be seen that they all vary linearly with t, consistent with the assumption that there is a diffusive-like displacement of the center-of-mass of the pulse from its uniformly translating position at long time-scales. The slopes of these curves then determine the effective wave speed and diffusion coefficient according to $\overline{X}(t)\sim c_\varepsilon t$ and $\sigma_X^2(t)\sim 2D(\varepsilon)t$. Both the leading and trailing edges exhibit the same speeds and diffusivities (after a transient phase). The transients are caused by fluctuations in the mean width of the pulse which can be neglected for large t, where the difference in the size of fluctuations of the leading and trailing edges can be neglected.

In order to find the mean location of the leading or trailing edge of the pulse as a function of time, we numerically carry out

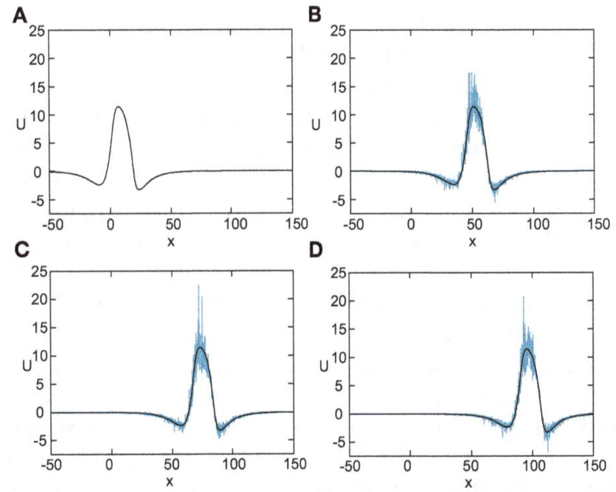

FIGURE 8 | Numerical simulation of freely propagating pulse solution of the stochastic neural field Equation (31) for a Heaviside rate function $F(U)=H(U-\kappa)$ with $\kappa=4$, and weight function (Equation 4) with $a_e=5$, $a_i=1$, $\sigma_e=0.42$, $\sigma_i=0.1$, and $x_0=3$. The multiplicative noise is taken to be $g(U)=U$, the noise strength is $\epsilon=0.005$, and $C(0)=10$. The wave profile is shown at successive times **(A)** $t=0$ **(B)** $t=12$ **(C)** $t=18$, and **(D)** $t=24$, with the initial profile at $t=0$ given by equation U_0. In numerical simulations we take the discrete space and time steps $\Delta x=0.1$, $\Delta t=0.01$. The deterministic part U_0 of the stochastic wave is shown by the black curves.

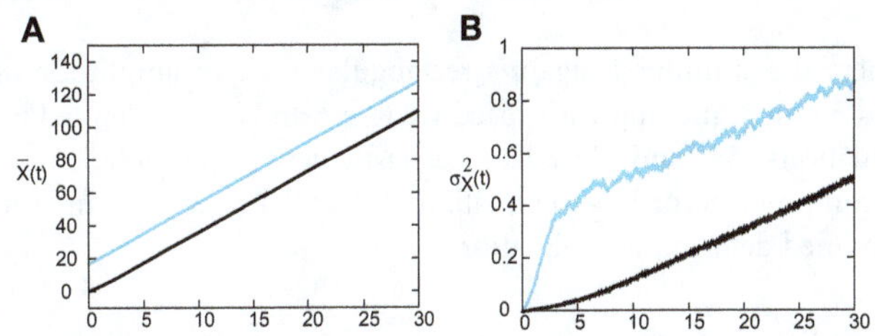

FIGURE 9 | (A) Plot of mean position $\overline{X}(t)$ of leading (blue) and trailing (black) edges of pulse as a function of time t averaged over $N=4096$ trials. **(B)** Corresponding plots of the variance $\sigma_X^2(t)$. Same parameter values as **Figure 8**.

a large number of level set position measurements. That is, we determine the positions $X_a(t)$ such that $U(X_a(t), t) = a$, for various level set values a and then define the mean location to be $\overline{X}(t) = \mathbb{E}[X_a(t)]$, where the expectation is first taken with respect to the sampled values a and then averaged over N trials. The corresponding variance is given by $\sigma_X^2(t) = \mathbb{E}[(X_a(t) - \bar{X}(t))^2]$. In order to compare the numerical results with our theoretical analysis, we assume that $X_a(t) = \Delta(t) + c_\epsilon t + X_a(0)$ for each a on either the leading or trailing edge. It then follows that $\bar{X}(t) = c_\epsilon t + X_a(0)$ and $\sigma_X^2(t) = \langle \Delta(t)^2 \rangle$. In **Figure 10** we plot the numerically estimated diffusion coefficient for various values of the threshold κ and compare these to the corresponding theoretical curves obtained using the above analysis. It can be seen that there is excellent agreement with our theoretical predictions. Finally, note that we can also use the level set data to estimate fluctuations in the width of the pulse. Suppose that $X_d(t)$ and $Y_d(t)$ denote the threshold crossing points of the leading and trailing edges of the pulse at time t. Then the stochastic width of the pulse can be defined according to $D(t) = X_d(t) - Y_d(t)$. We find that after a transient phase, $\langle D(t)^2 \rangle - \langle D(t) \rangle^2 \ll \sigma_X^2(t)$.

Stimulus-locked pulses

We now add a stimulus term I to the stochastic neural field Equation (33), that is

$$dU(x, t) = \left[h(U(x, t)) + \int_{-\infty}^{\infty} w(x - y) F(U(y, t))\, dy \right] dt$$
$$+ I(x - vt)dt + \epsilon^{1/2} dR(U, x, t), \tag{51}$$

where the stimulus is again a rectangular wave of amplitude I_0 and width d, moving with speed v. Here h and dR are defined by Equations (34) and (35). The stochastic activity variable is now decomposed according to Equation (37), with $\xi = x - vt$, and the modified deterministic equation

$$-v\frac{dU_0}{d\xi} - h(U_0(\xi)) - I(\xi) = \int_{\infty}^{\infty} w(\xi - \xi') F(U_0(\xi'))\, d\xi'. \tag{52}$$

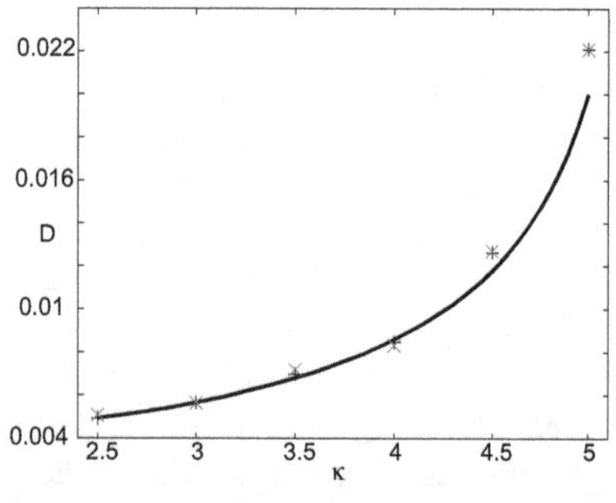

FIGURE 10 | Plot of diffusion coefficient $D(\epsilon)$ as a function of threshold κ. Numerical results ("+" for leading edge,"X" for trailing edge) are obtained by averaging over $N = 4096$ trials starting from the initial condition given by U_0. Corresponding theoretical predictions (solid curves) for $D(\epsilon)$ are based on Equation (44). Other parameters as in **Figure 8**.

Through a similar process as in the previous section, we expand to $\mathcal{O}(\epsilon^{1/2})$ to obtain the inhomogeneous equation

$$d\Phi(\xi, t) - \widehat{L}\Phi(\xi, t)dt = -\epsilon^{-1/2} \left[U_0'(\xi) - I'(\xi) \right] d\Delta(t)$$
$$- dR(U_0(\xi), \xi, t) + \mathcal{O}(\epsilon^{1/2}), \tag{53}$$

where $\widehat{L}$ is defined as in Equation (40) but with $c_\epsilon \to v$. The solvability condition is now

$$\int_{-\infty}^{\infty} \mathcal{V}(\xi) \left[U_0'(\xi) d\Delta(t) + I'(\xi) d\Delta(t) \right.$$
$$\left. + \epsilon^{1/2} dR(U_0(\xi), \xi, t) \right] d\xi = 0. \tag{54}$$

This can be manipulated to give, to leading order, the Ornstein–Uhlenbeck equation (Gardiner, 2009):

$$d\Delta(t) + A\Delta(t)dt = d\widehat{W}(t), \tag{55}$$

where

$$A = \frac{\int_{-\infty}^{\infty} \mathcal{V}(\xi) I'(\xi) d\xi}{\int_{-\infty}^{\infty} \mathcal{V}(\xi) U_0'(\xi) d\xi},$$

and

$$d\widehat{W}(t) = -\epsilon^{1/2} g_0 \frac{\int_{-\infty}^{\infty} \mathcal{V}(\xi) U_0(\xi) dW(\xi, t)\, d\xi}{\int_{-\infty}^{\infty} \mathcal{V}(\xi) U_0'(\xi) d\xi}.$$

Solving the stochastic differential equation in Equation (55) and taking averages shows that $\langle \Delta(t) \rangle = \Delta(0) e^{-At}$ and

$$\langle \Delta(t)^2 \rangle - \langle \Delta(t) \rangle^2 \approx \frac{D(\epsilon)}{A} \left[1 - e^{-2At} \right], \tag{56}$$

where $D(\epsilon)$ is given by Equation (44) except for a modified null vector $\mathcal{V}(\xi)$. Thus the variance of $\Delta(t)$ approaches $D(\epsilon)/A$ in the large t limit.

As in the case of freely propagating pulses, we can explicitly solve for $\mathcal{V}(\epsilon)$ and thus calculate the diffusion coefficient $D(\epsilon)$ when $F(U) = H(U - \kappa)$ and $g(U) = U$. Since the steps are similar to the previous case, we simply present our results here. In **Figure 11** we show the temporal evolution of a single stimulus-locked front, which is obtained by numerically solving the Langevin Equation (51) for $F(U) = H(U - \kappa)$, $g(U) = U$ and the weight distribution (Equation 4). The external input is taken to be a square pulse of amplitude $I_0 = 5$, width $d = 5$, and speed $v = 5$. Next we determine the mean $\overline{X}(t)$ and variance $\sigma_X^2(t)$ of the position of the leading and trailing edges by averaging over level sets along identical lines to the freely-propagating case. The results are shown in **Figure 12**. It can be seen that, as predicted by the analysis, $\overline{X}(t)$ varies linearly with t with a slope equal to the stimulus speed $v = 5$. Moreover, the variance $\sigma_X^2(t)$ approaches a constant value as $t \to \infty$ for both the trailing and leading edges. Thus, we find that stimulus-locked pulses are much more robust to noise than freely propagating pulses, since the variance of the mean position of the leading and

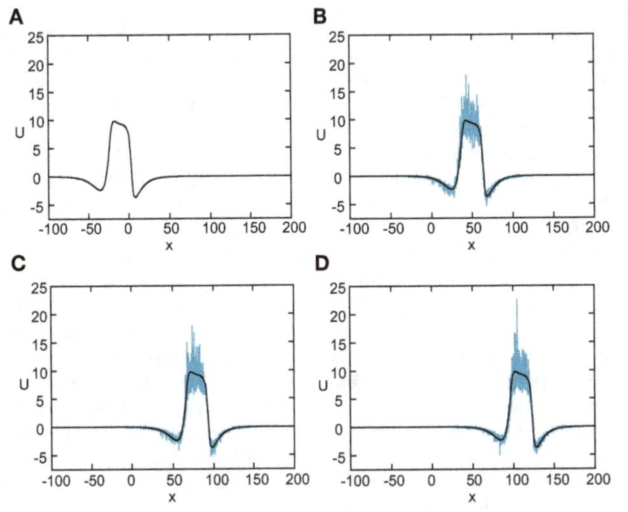

FIGURE 11 | Numerical simulation showing the propagation of a stimulus-locked pulse solution of the stochastic neural field Equation (51). The external input is taken to be a square pulse with amplitude $I_0 = 5$, width $d = 5$, and speed $v = 5$. All other parameters are as in **Figure 8**. The wave profile is shown at successive times **(A)** $t = 0$ **(B)** $t = 6$ **(C)** $t = 12$, and **(D)** $t = 24$, with the initial profile at $t = 0$ given by the solution U_0. In numerical simulations we take the discrete space and time steps $\Delta x = 0.1$, $\Delta t = 0.01$.

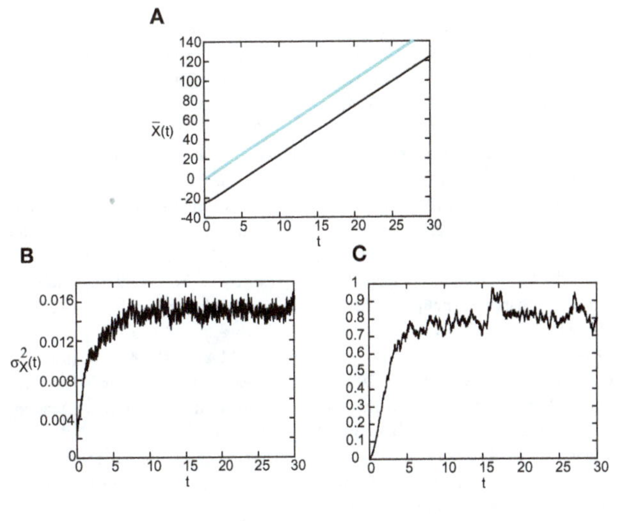

FIGURE 12 | (A) Plot of mean position $\overline{X}(t)$ of leading (blue) and trailing (black) edges of stimulus-locked pulse as a function of time t averaged over $N = 1000$ trials. **(B,C)** Corresponding plots of the variance $\sigma_X^2(t)$ of the leading and trailing edges. Same parameter values as **Figure 11**.

trailing edges saturate as $t \to \infty$. Consequently, stimulus locking persists in the presence of noise over most of the parameter range for which stimulus locking is predicted to occur. However, the trailing edge has an asymptotic variance that is at least an order of magnitude larger than the leading edge, which implies that fluctuations in the width of the pulse can no longer be neglected.

DISCUSSION

In this paper we have explored the effects of extrinsic noise on propagating pulses in a one-dimensional scalar neural field with asymmetric weights. Such a network has previously been proposed as a continuum model of direction selectivity. We have shown that the effects of noise on the wandering of the mean front position depends on properties of the underlying deterministic pulse. In the case of a freely propagating pulse, we find diffusive wandering with the mean square displacement growing linearly with time t. Moreover, in the large time limit, fluctuations in the width of the pulse can be neglected. On the other hand, if the pulse is locked to a moving pulse-like stimulus, then the wandering is described by an Ornstein–Uhlenbeck process and the mean square displacement saturates in the long time limit. However, we find that fluctuations in the pulse width can no longer be ignored.

In summary, this paper further illustrates how methods developed for studying wave propagation in stochastic PDEs can be adapted to study wave propagation in stochastic neural fields. As we have previously found for fronts, stimulus-locked waves are more robust to noise, which is a desirable property of a network performing some form of stimulus-processing such as direction selectivity.

REFERENCES

Adelson, E. H., and Bergen, J. R. (1985). Spatiotemporal energy models for the perception of motion. *J. Opt. Soc. Am.* 2, 284–299.

Amari, S. (1977). Dynamics of pattern formation in lateral inhibition type neural fields. *Biol. Cybern.* 27, 77–87.

Armero, J., Casademunt, J., Ramirez-Piscina, L., and Sancho, J. M. (1998). Ballistic and diffusive corrections to front propagation in the presence of multiplicative noise. *Phys. Rev. E* 58, 5494–5500.

Baker, P. M., and Bair, W. (2012). Inter-neuronal correlation distinguishes mechanisms of direction selectivity in cortical circuit models. *J. Neurosci.* 32, 8800–8816.

Ben-Yishai, R., Bar-Or, R. L., and Sompolinsky, H. (1995). Theory of orientation tuning in visual cortex. *Proc. Natl. Acad. Sci. U.S.A.* 92, 3844–3848.

Bernander, O., Douglas, R. J., Martin, K. A. C., and Koch, C. (1991). Synaptic background activity influences spatiotemporal integration in single pyramidal cells. *Proc. Natl. Acad. Sci. U.S.A.* 88, 11569–11573.

Brackley, C. A., and Turner, M. S. (2007). Random fluctuations of the firing rate function in a continuum neural field model. *Phys. Rev. E* 75, 041913.

Bressloff, P. C. (1994). A green's function approach to analysing the effects of random synaptic background activity in a model neural network. *J. Phys. A* 27, 4097–4113.

Bressloff, P. C. (2001). Traveling fronts and wave propagation failure in an inhomogeneous neural network. *Physica D* 155, 83–100.

Bressloff, P. C. (2009). Stochastic neural field theory and the system-size expansion. *SIAM J. Appl. Math* 70, 1488–1521.

Bressloff, P. C. (2010). Metastable states and quasicycles in a stochastic Wilson-Cowan model of neuronal population dynamics. *Phys. Rev. E* 85, 051903.

Bressloff, P. C. (2012). Spatiotemporal dynamics of continuum neural fields. *J. Phys. A* 45, 033001.

Bressloff, P. C., Cowan, J. D., Golubitsky, M., Thomas, P. J., and Wiener, M. (2001). Geometric visual hallucinations, Euclidean symmetry and the functional architecture of striate cortex. *Phil. Trans. R. Soc. Lond. B* 356, 299–330.

Bressloff, P. C., and Webber, M. A. (2012a). Neural field model of binocular rivalry waves. *J. Comput. Neurosci.* 32, 233–252.

Bressloff, P. C., and Webber, M. A. (2012b). Front propagation in stochastic neural fields. *SIAM J. Appl. Dyn. Syst.* 11, 708–740.

Buice, M., and Cowan, J. D. (2007). Field-theoretic approach to fluctuation effects in neural networks. *Phys. Rev. E* 75, 051919.

Buice, M., Cowan, J. D., and Chow, C. C. (2010). Systematic fluctuation expansion for neural network activity equations. *Neural Comput.* 22, 377–426.

Camperi, M., and Wang, X.-J. (1998). A model of visuospatial short-term memory in prefrontal cortex: recurrent network and cellular bistability. *J. Comput. Neurosci.* 5, 383–405.

Coombes, S. (2005). Waves, bumps and patterns in neural field theories. *Biol. Cybern.* 93, 91–108.

Coombes, S., and Owen, M. R. (2004). Evans functions for integral neural field equations with Heaviside firing rate function. *SIAM J. Appl. Dyn. Syst.* 4, 574–600.

Coombes, S., and Owen, M. R. (2005). Bumps, breathers, and waves in a neural network with spike frequency adaptation. *Phys. Rev. Lett.* 94, 148102.

de Pasquale, F., Gorecki, J., and Poielawski., J. (1992). On the stochastic correlations in a randomly perturbed chemical front. *J. Phys. A* 25, 433.

Ermentrout, G. B. (1998). Neural networks as spatio-temporal pattern-forming systems. *Rep. Prog. Phys.* 61, 353–430.

Ermentrout, G. B., and Cowan, J. (1979). A mathematical theory of visual hallucination patterns. *Bio. Cybern.* 34, 137–150.

Ermentrout, G. B., and McLeod, J. B. (1993). Existence and uniqueness of travelling waves for a neural network. *Proc. R. Soc. Edinburgh A* 123, 461–478.

Evans, J. (1975). Nerve axon equations iv: the stable and unstable impulse. *Indiana Univ. Math. J.* 24, 1169–1190.

Faugeras, O., Touboul, J., and Cessac, B. (2009). A constructive mean–field analysis of multi–population neural networks with random synaptic weights and stochastic inputs. *Front. Compt. Neurosci.* 3:1. doi: 10.3389/neuro.10.001. 2009

Folias, S. E., and Bressloff, P. C. (2005). Stimulus–locked traveling pulses and breathers in an excitatory neural network. *SIAM J. Appl. Math.* 65, 2067–2092.

Gardiner, C. W. (2009). *Handbook of Stochastic Methods, 4th Edn*. Berlin: Springer.

Giese, M. A. (1999). *Neural Field Theory for Motion Perception*. Dordrecht: Kluwer Academic Publishers.

Huang, X., Troy, W. C., Yang, Q., Ma, H., Laing, C. R., Schiff, S. J., et al. (2004). Spiral waves in disinhibited mammalian neocortex. *J. Neurosci.* 24, 9897–9902.

Hutt, A., and Atay, F. (2005). Analysis of nonlocal neural fields for both general and gamma-distributed connectivities. *Physica D* 203, 30–54.

Hutt, A., Longtin, A., and Schimansky-Geier, L. (2008). Additive noise-induces turing transitions in spatial systems with application to neural fields and the swift-hohenberg equation. *Physica D* 237, 755–773.

Kapitula, T., Kutz, N., and Sandstede, B. (2004). The Evans function for nonlocal equations. *Indiana Univ. Math. J.* 53, 1095–1126.

Keener, J. P. (1981). Waves in excitable media. *SIAM J. Appl. Math.* 39, 528–548.

Kilpatrick, Z. P., and Bressloff, P. C. (2010a). Effects of synaptic depression and adaptation on spatiotemporal dynamics of an excitatory neuronal network. *Physica D* 239, 547–560.

Kilpatrick, Z. P., and Bressloff, P. C. (2010b). Spatially structured oscillations in a two-dimensional neuronal network with synaptic depression. *J. Comput. Neurosci.* 28, 193–209.

Kilpatrick, Z. P., Folias, S. E., and Bressloff, P. C. (2008). Traveling pulses and wave propagation failure in inhomogeneous neural media. *SIAM J. Appl. Dyn. Syst.* 7, 161–185.

Koch, C., and Poggio, T. (1985). "Orientation selectivity in the visual cortex?" in *Models of the Visual Cortex*, eds D. Rose and V. G. Dobson (New York, NY: Wiley), 408–419.

Kreyszig, E. (1978). *Introductory Functional Analysis with Applications*. New York, NY: Wiley.

Kuramoto, Y. (1984). *Chemical Oscillations, Waves and Turbulence*. New York, NY: Springer-Verlag.

Laing, C. R., and Chow, C. C. (2002). A spiking neuron model for binocular rivalry. *J. Comput. Neurosci.* 12, 39–53.

Liley, D. J. T., Cadusch, P. J., and Dafilis, M. P. (2002). A spatially continuous mean field theory of electrocortical activity. *Network* 13, 67–113.

Maex, R., and Urban, G. A. (1996). Model circuit of spiking neurons generating directional selectivity in simple cells. *J. Neurophysiol.* 75, 1515–1545.

Mineiro, P., and Zipser, D. (1998). Analysis of direction selectivity arising from recurrent cortical interactions. *Neural Comput.* 10, 353–371.

Novikov, E. A. (1965). Functionals and the random-force method in turbulence theory. *Sov. Phys. JETP* 20, 1290.

Nunez, P. I. (1995). *Neocortical Dynamics and Human EEG Rhythms*. New York, NY: Oxford University Press.

Pinto, D., and Ermentrout, G. B. (2001). Spatially structured activity in synaptically coupled neuronal networks: I. Traveling fronts and pulses. *SIAM J. Appl. Math* 62, 206–225.

Pinto, D., Jackson, R. K., and Wayne, C. E. (2005). Existence and stability of traveling pulses in a continuous neuronal network. *SIAM J. Appl. Dyn. Syst.* 4, 954–984.

Rapp, M., Yarom, Y., and Segev, I. (1992). The impact of parallel fiber background activity on the cable properties of cerebellar purkinje cells. *Neural Comput.* 4, 518–533.

Reichardt, W. (1961). "Autocorrelation, a principle for the evaluation of sensory information by the central nervous system," in *Sensory Communication*, ed A. Rosenblith (Cambridge, MA: MIT Press), 303–317.

Richardson, K. A., Schiff, S. J., and Gluckman, B. J. (2005). Control of traveling waves in the mammalian cortex. *Phys. Rev. Lett.* 94, 028103.

Robinson, P. A., Rennie, C. J., Wright, J. J., Bahramali, H., Gordon, E., and Rowe, D. I. (2001). Prediction of electroencephalographic spectra from neurophysiology. *Phys. Rev. E* 63, 021903.

Rubin, J. E. (2004). A nonlocal eigenvalue problem for the stability of a traveling wave in a neuronal medium. *Discrete Contin. Dyn. Syst.* 10, 925–940.

Sagues, F., Sancho, J. M., and Garcia-Ojalvo, J. (2007). Spatiotemporal order out of noise. *Rev. Mod. Phys.* 79, 829–882.

Sandstede, B. (2002). "Stability of travelling waves," in *Handbook of Dynamical Systems, Vol. 2*, ed B. Fiedler (Amsterdam: North-Holland), 983–1055.

Sandstede, B. (2007). Evans functions and nonlinear stability of traveling waves in neuronal network models. *Int. J. Bifurcation Chaos Appl. Sci. Eng.* 17, 2693–2704.

Saul, A. B., and Humphrey, A. L. (1990). Spatial and temporal response properties of lagged and nonlagged cellscells in cat lateral geniculate nucleus. *J. Neurophysiol.* 64, 206–224.

Schimansky-Geier, L., Mikhailov, A. S., and Ebeling., W. (1983). Effects of fluctuations on plane front propagation in bistable nonequilibrium systems. *Ann. Phys.* 40, 277.

Somers, D. C., Nelson, S., and Sur, M. (1995). An emergent model of orientation selectivity in cat visual cortical simple cells. *J. Neurosci.* 15, 5448–5465.

Steyn-Ross, M. L., Steyn-Ross, D. A., Sleigh, J. W., and Whiting, D. R. (2003). Theoretical predictions for spatial covariance of the electroencephalographic signal during the anesthetic-induced phase transition: increased correlation length and emergence of spatial self-organization. *Phys. Rev. E* 68, 021902.

Suarez, H., Koch, C., and Douglas, R. J. (1995). Modeling direction selectivity of simple cells in striate visual cortex using the canonical microcircuit. *J. Neurosci.* 15, 6700–6719.

van Santen, J. P., and Sperling, G. (1985). Elaborated reichardt detectors. *J. Opt. Soc. Am. A* 256, 300–320.

Wilson, H. R., and Cowan, J. D. (1972). Excitatory and inhibitory interactions in localized populations of model neurons. *Biophys. J.* 12, 1–23.

Wilson, H. R., and Cowan, J. D. (1973). A mathematical theory of the functional dynamics of cortical and thalamic nervous tissue. *Kybernetik* 13, 55–80.

Xie, X., and Giese, M. A. (2002). Nonlinear dynamics of direction-selective recurrent neural media. *Phys. Rev. E* 65, 051904.

Zhang, K. (1996). Representation of spatial orientation by the intrinsic dynamics of the head-direction cell ensemble: a theory. *J. Neurosci.* 16, 2112–2126.

Zhang, L. (2003). On the stability of traveling wave solutions in synaptically coupled neuronal networks. *Diff. Integral Equat.* 16, 513–536.

5

The mesoscopic modeling of burst suppression during anesthesia

David T. J. Liley * and Matthew Walsh

Brain and Psychological Sciences Research Centre, Faculty of Life and Social Sciences, Swinburne University of Technology, Hawthorn, VIC, Australia

Correspondence:
David T. J. Liley, Brain and Psychological Sciences Research Centre, Faculty of Life and Social Sciences, Swinburne University of Technology, P.O. Box 218, Hawthorn, VIC 3122, Australia.
e-mail: dliley@swin.edu.au

The burst-suppression pattern is well recognized as a distinct feature of the mammalian electroencephalogram (EEG) waveform. Consisting of alternating periods of high amplitude oscillatory and isoelectric activity, it can be induced in health by deep anesthesia as well as being evoked by a range of pathophysiological processes that include coma and anoxia. While the electroencephalographic phenomenon and clinical implications of burst suppression have been studied extensively, the physiological mechanisms underlying its emergence remain unresolved and obscure. Because electroencephalographic bursting phenomenologically resembles the bursting observed in single neurons, it would be reasonable to assume that the theoretical insights developed to understand bursting at the cellular ("microscopic") level would enable insights into the dynamical genesis of bursting at the level of the whole brain ("macroscopic"). In general action potential bursting is the result of the interplay of two time scales: a fast time scale responsible for spiking, and a slow time scale that modulates such activity. We therefore hypothesize that such fast-slow systems dynamically underpin electroencephalographic bursting. Here we show that a well-known mean field dynamical model of the electroencephalogram, the Liley model, while unable to produce burst suppression unmodified, is able to give rise to a wide variety of burst-like activity by the addition of one or more slow systems modulating model parameters speculated to be major "targets" for anesthetic action. The development of a physiologically plausible theoretical framework to account for burst suppression will lead to a more complete physiological understanding of the EEG and the mechanisms that serve to modify ongoing brain activity necessary for purposeful behavior and consciousness.

Keywords: burst suppression, anesthesia, electroencephalogram, mean field model, neuronal hyperexcitability

1. INTRODUCTION

Prior to the development of the modern intensive care unit in the early 1960s, that featured intubation, artificial respiration, and comprehensive physiological monitoring, reports of the electroencephalographic pattern of burst suppression (BS) were confined to animal studies involving deep anesthesia and the occasional case of psychosurgery (Niedermeyer, 2009). Since then the burst-suppression pattern has become well recognized as a major diagnostic feature of the EEG waveform that is encountered in a range of encephalopathic conditions, in addition to its appearance in health during deep anesthesia. Typically the BS pattern consists of bursts of high amplitude slow, sharp, or spiking electroencephalographic activity separated by periods of electroencephalographic suppression (isoelectricity). The oscillatory features of the bursts, together with their duration and the duration of suppressed periods show a high degree of variability (see **Figure 1** for examples) that presumably reflects its myriad of initiating causes. First identified during deep anesthesia with tribromoethanol in cats (Derbyshire et al., 1936), labeled burst-suppression pattern by Swank and Watson (1949) during barbiturate and ether anesthesia in dogs, it is now associated with cortical deafferentation (Henry and Scoville, 1952), cerebral anoxia and hypoxia, various types of intracortical lesions (Fischer-Williams and Cooper, 1963), deep coma, various infantile encephalopathies, the final stages of deteriorated status epilepticus (Treiman et al., 1990), hypothermia, and high levels of many sedative and anesthetic agents (Schwartz et al., 1989; Akrawi et al., 1996).

Burst suppression in the absence of anesthesia is in general associated with a very poor prognosis. For example in neonates (Grigg-Damberger et al., 1989) the appearance of BS, even if transient, is a portent of death or severe neurodevelopmental disability. In contrast, in adult populations while an anoxic/hypoxic BS pattern signals a serious pathophysiological event the outcome is not necessarily fatal and recovery with or without severe neurological damage is possible (Niedermeyer, 2009). Consistent with this are results of experimental work with EEG monitoring in rats revealing that animals with greater rates of high amplitude bursts have a better survival and neurological outcome compared to those with lower rates of low amplitude bursts (Geocadin et al., 2002).

While the electroencephalographic phenomenon and clinical implications of BS have been studied extensively (Brenner, 1985; Niedermeyer, 2009) the physiological mechanisms underlying its emergence remain in general unresolved and obscure.

Burst suppression is typically thought to be spatially homogeneous with burst onset and termination reported to occur near simultaneously across the entire scalp (Brenner, 1985; An et al.,

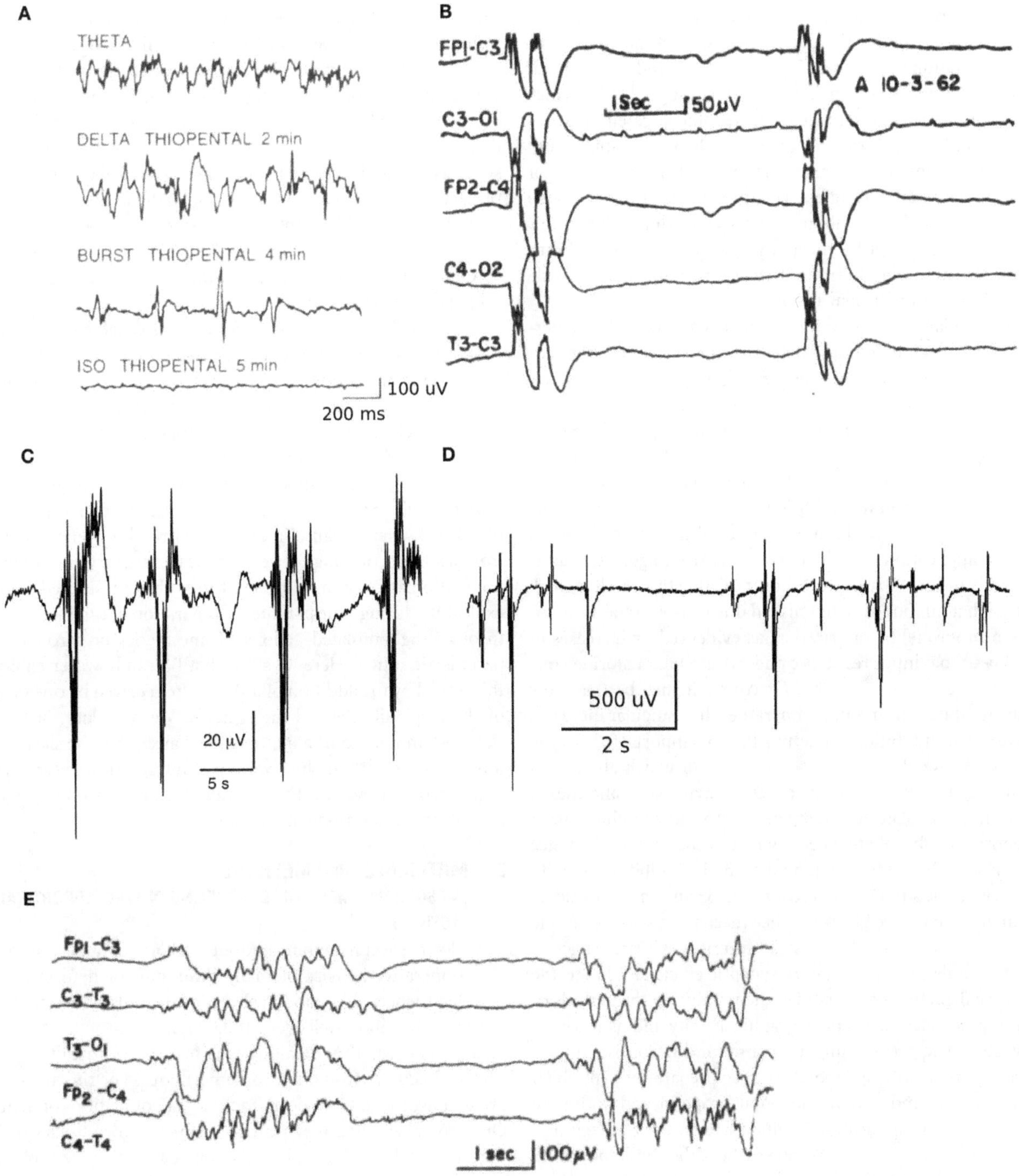

FIGURE 1 | Example traces of electroencephalogram and electrocorticogram illustrating the heterogeneity of BS patterns. **(A)** Changes in neocortical electroencephalogram in the rat, recorded using dural surface electrodes, in response to a 5 mg/kg/min thiopental infusion [figure reproduced with permission from Lukatch and MacIver (1996)]. **(B)** Electroencephalogram recorded in acute anoxia showing a clear burst-suppression pattern with grouped spikes [figure reproduced with permission from Hockaday et al. (1965)]. **(C)** BS pattern during closed loop target controlled propofol infusion at a target level of approximately 15 μg/ml (data courtesy of Professor Michel Struys, Groningen). Note the bursts consist of fast activity (>10 Hz) on a slow wave background. **(D)** Electrocorticogram obtained from an adult merino sheep during deep enflurane anesthesia, demonstrating high amplitude spikes interspersed with isoelectric periods of variable length [figure reproduced with permission from Voss et al. (2006)]. **(E)** Electroencephalogram recorded from a 3-month-old infant suffering from infantile myoclonic encephalopathy [reproduced with permission from Niedermeyer (2005)].

1996; Ching et al., 2012), indicating that low level subcortical mechanisms may be playing a decisive role. However arguing against this is the fact that this pattern persists subsequent to cortical deafferentation (Lukatch and MacIver, 1996), indicating that it probably represents an intrinsic, though physiologically abnormal, dynamical mode of cortex. Indeed the phenomenal resemblance of the patterns of BS to disorders of neuronal hyperexcitability suggests the involvement of similar physiological mechanisms. For example the bursting during burst suppression is often associated with myoclonic jerks resembling those seen during epileptic fits. Like generalized epileptiform activity, bursts are recorded simultaneously at multiple electrode derivations, implying the wide synchronization of neuronal activity.

At the cellular level a commonly reported finding is that hyperpolarization of the membrane potential of cortical neurons reliably precedes any overt electroencephalographic activity of BS (Steriade et al., 1994). Such hyperpolarization, which has been attributed to an increase in neuronal membrane potassium conductance (Steriade et al., 1994), has been hypothesized to play a major role in the induction of BS. This implied importance of inhibition in the genesis of BS is further supported by results involving rat neocortical brain slice micro-EEG preparations in which the application of a direct acting $GABA_A$ agonist, muscimol, readily induces BS. However contradicting this result is work reporting that inhibition is diminished during isoflurane-induced BS, in an *in vivo* feline preparation, as evidenced by increases in cortical neuronal input resistance and extracellular chloride concentration (Ferron et al., 2009). Of course it may be that slow periodic modulations in inhibition, rather than singular increases or decreases in inhibition, underpin BS. In support of this view is the recent model of Ching et al. (2012), in which alterations in brain metabolism, due to the effects of hypoxia or anesthesia, parametrically regulate an activity dependent slow modulation of an adenosine triphosphate-gated potassium channel conductance to give rise to BS. However modulations in inhibitory activity alone may not be sufficient to account for BS and more consideration might need to be given to other mechanisms. For example Kroeger and Amzica (2007) present empirical evidence suggesting that modulations in excitatory synaptic efficiency, due to the progressive depletion of interstitial calcium during the periods of high amplitude electroencephalographic activity and its recovery during isoelectric periods, might account for BS. Consistent with this are reports involving laboratory slice preparations in which burst suppression induced by thiopental, propofol, and isoflurane is abolished by the application of glutamate receptor antagonists (Lukatch and MacIver, 1996). Whatever the pathophysiology of BS is it is reasonably clear that it is unlikely to be accounted for by a unitary physiological perturbation. That the physiological factors identified to date in BS all lead to a single well defined state suggests the possibility of an unifying dynamical mechanism. Thus the best hope for progress in understanding the phenomena of BS may be theoretical.

How might we theoretically approach BS? The well studied dynamical mechanisms of action potential bursting (Izhikevich, 2007) may be able to provide vital insights into the mechanisms of bursting in the EEG. In general the dynamical mechanisms underlying bursting can be divided into two broad classes (i) fast-slow bursters in which there is a clear separation of the underlying time scales, with a fast system responsible for the fast spiking, and a slow system its slow modulation, and (ii) "hedgehog" bursters (Izhikevich, 2000) in which there is no clear separation of time scales. In terms of developing a theory of BS the former might represent the preferable starting point as the little empirical evidence that is available (Ching et al., 2012), at least in humans, suggests that alphoid activity, indicative of normal resting EEG, is preserved during the bursts of BS. Thus a theoretical starting point to understanding BS might be to consider the slow modulation of a dynamical system developed to describe the resting EEG.

One such dynamical system is the mesoscopic electrocortical model of Liley et al. (Liley et al., 1999, 2002, 2011; Bojak and Liley, 2005; Frascoli et al., 2011). This model is capable of accounting for a range of resting electroencephalographic phenomena that includes the alpha rhythm (Liley et al., 2002), the modulation of resting activity by sedative and anesthetic action (Bojak and Liley, 2005) as well as the proconvulsant properties of the latter (Liley and Bojak, 2005), all within a physiologically plausible/admissible parameter space. This model is therefore well suited as a foundation from which to explore the physiological and dynamical genesis of BS. However, because in this model rhythmogenesis emerges from a strong coupling between cortical excitatory and inhibitory population activity, in its present form it has a restricted ability to exhibit BS through the parametric separation of time scales, either through the simulated actions of anesthetics or through other parametric routes. Here we show that BS can however emerge in this model by the addition of a slow system driven by one or more of the originally defined mean fields. We speculate that such a slow system represents a mathematical ansatz for the slow neuromodulation of activity by a variety of intracortical, inter-cortical, and subcortical systems that include thalamus and the ascending neurotransmitter modulatory systems.

2. MATERIALS AND METHODS

2.1. MESOSCOPIC MEAN FIELD MODELING OF ELECTROCORTICAL ACTIVITY

The electroencephalogram and electrocorticogram arise out of the cooperative activity of many thousands of neurons. A single electroencephalographic electrode records the synaptically induced currents of well over a 100,000 neurons (Nunez and Srinivasan, 2005) and thus detailing each neurons contribution to this summed activity would appear superfluous. For this reason it is preferable instead to model the activity of populations of neurons. One general way of achieving this, in which known stochastic fluctuations can be included, is to dynamically evolve the probability distributions associated with the states of the neuronal ensemble. While in principle providing a rigorous way forward the formulation of such stochastic equations of motion entails a great deal of physiological uncertainty. For this and other reasons (Deco et al., 2008) a more resolute path is to dynamically evolve some average quantity such as the mean soma membrane potential or the mean firing rate of some suitably defined neuronal ensemble. In this manner a mesoscopic level model can be developed which acts as a bridge between cellular (or microscopic) level activity and whole brain (or macroscopic) level behavior. While the current mathematical approach for formulating the equations of motion for the activity of neuronal populations or masses, stems principally from the works of Wilson and Cowan (1972, 1973), Nunez (1974), Freeman (1975), and Amari (1975), they are not particularly successful in articulating the genesis of rhythmic activity in the EEG and its modulation by pharmacological agents, due to a range of mathematical simplifications that cannot be justified by an appeal to physiology. For this reason a range of biologically more refined neuronal populations models have been developed (Deco et al., 2008) that form a more appropriate basis from which to model the physiological genesis of the electroencephalogram. The model of Liley et al. (Liley et al., 1999, 2002, 2011; Bojak and Liley, 2005; Frascoli et al., 2011) is one such model and will be the focus of our attempts to account for the phenomenon of BS.

The model of Liley et al. is able to account for the major features of the mammalian electroencephalogram in the context of a parameterization that accords with physiological measurement and experiment. Because it aims to provide a dynamical description of the electroencephalogram the model is spatially coarse-grained over the approximate extent of a cortical macrocolumn, reflecting the general physiological wisdom that such columniation signifies populations of neurons having similar functional behavior and anatomical connectivity. The multiple interactions between individual neurons are replaced by effective feed-forward and feedback interactions between the mean activity (or mean fields) of excitatory and inhibitory populations of neurons over the spatial extent of the column. In this way mammalian neocortex is conceived as consisting of localized populations of excitatory and inhibitory neurons interacting by all possible combinations of feed-forward and feed-back connectivity interacting globally via long-range excitatory connections (**Figure 2**).

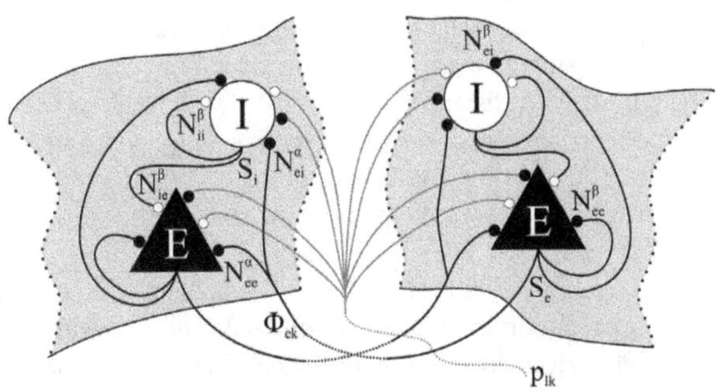

FIGURE 2 | Schematic overview of the essential intracortical and cortico-cortical interactions between excitatory and inhibitory neuronal populations in the model of Liley et al. (Liley et al., 1999, 2002, 2011; Bojak and Liley, 2005; Frascoli et al., 2011). Following conductance based approaches typically used to model networks of synaptically interacting networks of individual model neurons, excitatory and inhibitory neuronal populations are modeled as single passive resistive-capacitive compartments into which all synaptically induced postsynaptic currents flow. Functionally these populations are equivalent to the excitatory and inhibitory KO sets of Freemans K-set hierarchy (Freeman, 1975). Cortical activity is then described by the mean soma membrane potentials of the spatially distributed excitatory (h_e) and inhibitory (h_i) neuronal populations. The connection with physiological measurement is obtained through h_e, which is assumed to be linearly related to the surface recorded electroencephalogram (Freeman, 1975; Nunez and Srinivasan, 2005). Figure reproduced with permission from Frascoli et al. (2011).

Thus the response of the mean soma membrane potential h_k ($k = e, i$) at position r on a two-dimensional cortical sheet, in response to induced post synaptic activity I_{lk} ($l =$ source, $k =$ target population) is given by

$$\tau_k \frac{\partial h_k(r,t)}{\partial t} = h_k^r - h_k(r,t) + \sum_{l=e,i} \frac{h_{lk}^{eq} - h_k(r,t)}{|h_{lk}^{eq} - h_k^r|} I_{lk}(r,t) \quad (1)$$

The postsynaptic response to a single pre-synaptic action potential (at $t = 0$) is modeled by the well-known synaptic alpha function of cable theory as $\Gamma_{lk}\gamma_{lk}t \exp(1 - \gamma_{lk}t)\Theta(t)$ where Γ_{lk} is peak amplitude (occurring at $t = t_{\text{peak}} = 1/\gamma_{lk}$) of the respective excitatory ($l = e$) or inhibitory ($l = i$) postsynaptic potential (PSP), and $\Theta(t)$ is the Heaviside step function. Thus we assume that the time course of the synaptically induced excitatory and inhibitory currents is described by a critically damped oscillator driven respectively by the mean rate of incoming excitatory and inhibitory axonal pulses:

$$\left(\frac{\partial}{\partial t} + \gamma_{lk}\right)^2 I_{lk}(r,t) = \exp(1)\Gamma_{lk}\gamma_{lk}A_{lk}(r,t), \quad (2)$$

with

$$A_{ek}(r,t) = N_{ek}^{\beta} S_e[h_e(r,t)] + \phi_{ek} + p_{ek}(r,t), \quad (3)$$

and

$$A_{ik}(r,t) = N_{ik}^{\beta} S_i[h_i(r,t)] + p_{ik}(r,t), \quad (4)$$

where A_{lk} comprises the different sources of pre-synaptic spikes: $N_{lk}^{\beta} S_i$ (input from local cortical neuronal populations), ϕ_{ek} (input from long-range excitatory cortico-cortical fibers), and p_{lk} (extra-cortical sources). While the present consensus is that extra-cortical sources (thalamo-cortical afferents) are purely excitatory in nature and thus $p_{ik} = 0$, we choose to retain these terms as when time independent they can be utilized to include the effects of tonic inhibition that are known to be induced by anesthetic action. The time courses of the synaptically induced currents, $1/\gamma_{lk}$ are taken to describe the time course of "fast" excitatory [$l = e$: α-amino-3-hydroxl-5-methyl-4-isoxazole-propionate (AMPA) and kainate] and inhibitory [$l = i$: γ-amino-butyric-acid type A ($GABA_A$)] neurotransmitter kinetics. Thus each type of PSP (excitatory, inhibitory) is described by two parameters Γ_{lk}, γ_{lk}. However, as we will describe later, a parametrically more flexible description of the PSP is required to meaningfully model the effects of anesthetics in which we can independently vary peak amplitude, rise (t_{peak}) and decay times. Mean neuronal population firing rates, S_l, are assumed to instantaneous sigmoid functions of the mean soma membrane potential i.e.,

$$S_l[h_l(r,t)] = S_l^{\max}/\{1 + \exp[\sqrt{2}(h_l(r,t) - \bar{\mu}_l/\sigma_l)]\} \quad (5)$$

The axonal pulses ϕ_{ek} propagated by the exclusively excitatory long-range cortico-cortical fiber system is in the simplest case described by the following two-dimensional telegraph equation,

$$\left(\frac{\partial}{\partial t} + v_{ek}\Lambda_{ek}\right)^2 \phi_{ek}(r,t) - \frac{3}{2}v_{ek}^2\nabla^2\phi_{ek}(r,t) = v_{ek}^2\Lambda_{ek}^2 N_{ek}^{\alpha} S_e[h_e(r,t)] \quad (6)$$

where N_{ek}^{α} is the total number of excitatory connections formed by long-range cortico-cortical axons on long on local population k, and assumes a single axonal conduction velocity v_{ek} and an exponential fall off with distance (characteristic scale $= 1/\Lambda_{ek}$) of the strength of cortico-cortical connectivity. For simplicity, and given the fact that at least in anesthesia BS appears to have a degree of spatial uniformity, we chose to only study the spatially homogeneous case, i.e., $\nabla^2 = 0$.

Equations (1)–(4) and (6) represent a system of 8 coupled non-linear partial differential equations that typically defines the Liley model of electrocortical rhythmogenesis, which is capable of reproducing the main features of spontaneous human electroencephalogram (alpha resonance, "$1/f$" activity). **Table 1** summarizes all model parameters, their definitions, and approximate ranges.

2.2. MODEL PARAMETERIZATION: GENERATION OF NORMATIVE PARAMETER SETS

Because BS activity (at least that induced by anesthetic and sedative action) is assumed to ultimately arise out of a background of normal electroencephalographic activity it is important to define parametrically normative states in order to study how they may be perturbed during health and disease. We therefore chose to utilize previously defined parameter sets (Bojak and Liley, 2005) that have the following properties: (i) are confined to the physiologically admissible parameter space (see **Table 1**), (ii) give rise to electroencephalographically and physiologically plausible activity ("$1/f$" decay at low frequencies plus a relatively sharp peak at alpha frequencies, 8–13 Hz; mean excitatory/inhibitory neuronal firing rates $<20\,\mathrm{s}^{-1}$) and (iii) that exhibit transient increases in total power and monotonic reductions in mean frequency with respect to modeled anesthetic action (see below). In general such sets can be found by randomly searching the high dimensional physiologically admissible (and plausible) parameter space. For further details see Bojak and Liley (2005).

Table 1 | List of spatially averaged parameters for different types $k, l \in \{e, i\}$ of neuronal target populations in the electrocortical model of Liley et al. (Liley et al., 1999, 2002, 2011; Bojak and Liley, 2005; Frascoli et al., 2011), with typical ranges that are assumed to be physiologically admissible.

	Definition	Min	Max	Units
h_k^r	Resting membrane potential	−80	−60	mV
τ_k	Passive membrane decay time	5	150	ms
h_{ek}^{eq}	Excitatory reversal potential	−20	10	mV
h_{ik}^{eq}	Inhibitory reversal potential	−90	$h_k^r - 5$	mV
Γ_{ek}	EPSP peak amplitude	0.1	2.0	mV
Γ_{ik}	IPSP peak amplitude	0.1	2.0	mV
$1/\gamma_{ek}$	EPSP rise time to peak	1	10	ms
$1/\gamma_{ik}$	IPSP rise time to peak	2	100	ms
N_{ek}^{α}	Number of excitatory cortico-cortical synapses	1000	5000	-
N_{ek}^{β}	Number of excitatory intracortical synapses	2000	5000	-
N_{ik}^{β}	Number of inhibitory intracortical synapses	100	1000	-
v_{ek}	Axonal conduction velocity	0.1	1	mm ms^{-1}
$1/\Lambda_{ek}$	Decay scale cortico-cortical connectivity	10	100	mm
S_k^{max}	Maximum firing rate	0.05	0.5	ms^{-1}
$\bar{\mu}_k$	Mean firing threshold	−55	−40	mV
σ_k	Firing threshold standard deviation	2	7	mV
p_{lk}	Extra-cortical synaptic input rate	0	10	ms^{-1}

Table adapted from Liley et al. (2011). EPSP, excitatory PSP; IPSP, inhibitory PSP.

2.3. MODELING ANESTHETIC ACTION

The range of molecular and cellular targets identified to date as sites of anesthetic action is so varied that a unitary biological mechanism for anesthetic effect seems unlikely. Nevertheless, at least functionally, at the level of cortex anesthetics seem to act principally by enhancing the actions of inhibitory activity (Liley et al., 2011). Indeed from the perspective of the mean field model we have described many of its parameters can be related in a fairly straightforward way to these alterations in inhibitory activity and other identified sites of anesthetic action in cortex (see **Table 2**). However a parametrically more flexible description of the PSP, than is presently incorporated, is required to meaningfully model the effects of anesthetics in which we can independently vary peak amplitude, rise (t_{peak}) and decay times. For example isoflurane, a volatile halogenated anesthetic, has been shown to prolong the decay time of the unitary IPSP without altering its time to peak. Fortunately a simple modification of the equation describing the dynamics of the PSP enables independent adjustment of the peak amplitude, rise (t_{peak}) and decay times. By defining I_{lk} to satisfy

$$\left[\frac{\partial}{\partial t} + \gamma_{lk}(\varepsilon_{lk})\right]\left[\frac{\partial}{\partial t} + \tilde{\gamma}_{lk}(\varepsilon_{lk})\right] I_{lk}(r,t) = \tilde{\gamma}_{lk}(\varepsilon_{lk}) \exp[\gamma_{lk}(\varepsilon_{lk})/\gamma_{lk}^{0}]\Gamma_{lk} A_{lk}(r,t), \tag{7}$$

$$\gamma_{lk}(\varepsilon_{lk}) = \varepsilon_{lk}\gamma_{lk}^{0}/(e^{\varepsilon_{lk}} - 1), \quad \tilde{\gamma}_{lk} = \gamma_{lk}(\varepsilon)e^{\varepsilon_{lk}} \tag{8}$$

Table 2 | Relationship between major experimentally identified sites of cortical anesthetic action and parameters of the electrocortical model of Liley et al. (Liley et al., 1999, 2002; Bojak and Liley, 2005).

Site of action	Main anesthetic effect	Parameters
2PK channels and extrasynaptic GABA$_A$	Increase in tonic inhibition	p_{ik}, h_k^r
nACh receptors	Reduction in tonic excitation	p_{ek}, h_k^r
Synaptic GABA$_A$	Increase of IPSPs	γ_{ik}, Γ_{ik}
AMPA/kainate receptors and NMDA receptors*	Reduction of EPSPs	γ_{ek}, Γ_{ek}
Myelinated axons	Slowdown of conduction†	v_{ek}
Na channels	Alteration of neuronal firing	S_k^{max}, $\bar{\mu}_k$, σ_k

**Parameters will depend on membrane potential in this case.*

†Effect demonstrated in periphery, speculative in cortex (Swindale, 2003).

where $1/\gamma^0_{lk}$ defines the time to peak, we can control the decay of the unitary PSP by altering $\varepsilon_{lk} > 0$. Increasing ε_{lk} will monotonically increase the decay time of the tail of the unitary PSP (see lower left panel, **Figure 6**). Empirically it is found that increasing the aqueous concentration of a range of GABAergic anesthetic agents leads to a progressive increase in the decay time of the unitary inhibitory PSP (e.g., Banks and Pearce, 1999) and thus ε_{ik} will be a monotonic function of anesthetic concentration c, i.e., $\varepsilon_{ik}(c)$. Liley et al. (2011), based on a range of empirical evidence, have numerically estimated $\varepsilon_{ik}(c)$ for the volatile anesthetic agent isoflurane. However because $\varepsilon_{ik}(c)$ is not currently known for other GABAergic anesthetic agents we will assume that in general $\varepsilon_{ik} \propto c$.

It is worth noting that equation (7) reduces to equation (2) as $\varepsilon_{lk} \rightarrow 0$. Further details regarding this formulation can be found in Bojak and Liley (2005).

2.4. DEFINING A THEORETICAL BASIS FOR BURSTING

We call a bursting system *fast-slow* if it can be written in the following form

$$\dot{x} = f(x, y) \quad \textit{(fast oscillatory system)} \tag{9}$$

$$\dot{y} = \mu g(x, y) \quad \textit{(slow modulatory system)} \tag{10}$$

where $x \in \mathbb{R}^m$ describes the m-dimensional system responsible for the fast oscillatory (spiking in single neuron models) dynamics and $y \in \mathbb{R}^n$ the n-dimensional slow system that modulates the fast oscillations (or spiking behavior). The parameter μ represents the ratio of the time scales between the slow and fast system. It is typically assumed that $\mu \ll 1$. Because μ can be made as small as we like equations (9) and (10) represent a singularly perturbed system.

We will assume that equations (1)–(4) and (6), which putatively describe the genesis of the "fast oscillatory" resting EEG, correspond to the m-dimensional fast system. To motivate the slow n-dimensional slow modulatory system we will make a plausible appeal to the biophysics of synaptic resource depletion and recovery during periods of sustained neuronal population activity. During periods of high firing neural activity a variety of factors come into play to diminish synaptic efficiency. The most important of these are receptor desensitization and synaptic vesicle depletion. Tsodyks and Markram (1997) developed a model to account for the biophysics of such activity dependent short term synaptic depression estimating that its onset is rapid, of the order of milliseconds, but that its recovery is quite slow, of the order of 800 ms. Given that such a time scale is approximately at least an order of magnitude greater than the characteristic time scales associated with resting EEG activity, this may represent a candidate slow EEG modulatory system. On this basis we choose to include this activity dependent short term synaptic depression using the following two different formulations, referred respectively to as SS1 and SS2,

$$\dot{\Gamma}_{lk} = \mu_l[\theta_l - k_l S_l(h_l)], \quad (SS1) \tag{11}$$

$$\dot{\Gamma}_{lk} = \mu_l[\Gamma^0_{lk}/(1 + \exp[\kappa_l(h_l - \xi_l)]) - \Gamma_{lk}], \quad (SS2) \tag{12}$$

where $1/\mu_l$ is the characteristic time scale of the respective slow modulatory system. Based on Tsodyks and Markram (1997) we will fix $1/\mu_l$ to 1000 ms. The advantage of the first formulation is that the rates of synaptic recovery ($\mu_l\theta_l$) and depletion ($\mu_l k_l$) can be separately specified. The advantage of the second formulation is that Γ_{lk} remains bounded between Γ^0_{lk} (the resting value) and zero decreasing monotonically with increasing mean soma membrane potential h_l, with Γ^0_{lk} remaining as a free parameter. For low levels of the respective neuronal activity (h_l) there is very little decrease in Γ_{lk} until a threshold ξ_l is reached, with the parameter κ_l controlling the sensitivity of the change at this threshold to variations in neuronal activity. This formulation has previously been used by Tabak and Rinzel (2005) in their mean field model for spontaneous electrical bursting activity in embryonic chick spinal cord.

2.5. COMPUTATIONAL METHODS

All numerical integrations and one-dimensional dynamical continuations were performed using the XPPAUT package (Ermentrout, 2002). A 4-th order Runge-Kutta scheme with a time step of 0.1 ms was used to numerically integrate the differential equations. Because of the multiple time scales our differential system may suffer from stiffness and numerical solutions may not converge. In these cases we have used the recommended "stiff" integrator CVODE (Cohen and Hindmarsh, 1994) as implemented in XPPAUT.

3. RESULTS

All numerical simulations were performed using a single model parameter set having a physiologically plausible white noise fluctuation spectrum (see top left panel **Figure 3**) and a single stable fixed point. This parameter set was found using the methods described in section 2.2. The parameters used, all within the physiologically admissible domain, can be found in the **Table 3**.

Figure 3 shows the effects of the activity dependent modulation of Γ_{ii} on simulated mean field EEG activity using SS1 [equation (11)]. Bursts emerge periodically, with intervening near isoelectric intervals, apparently driven by slow variations in Γ_{ii} (red line, top right panel). A spectrogram of a sufficiently long simulated time series reveals that the frequency of the model EEG activity decreases from low beta ($\cong$ 15 Hz) to high alpha ($\cong$ 12 Hz) over the period of the bursts. Such intra-burst "chirping" is a common feature of many of the topologically identified single neuronal bursters (Izhikevich, 2007). Of interest are the multiple harmonics of this dominant oscillatory activity.

Figure 4 illustrates how we might dynamically account for the transition to, and cessation from, bursting and follows the now standard method of the dissection of neural bursting pioneered by Rinzel (1985). Here we have set $\mu_i = 0$ and consider how the "fast" EEG system responds. **Figure 4** shows a one-dimensional bifurcation diagram of this "fast" EEG system with Γ_{ii} as the bifurcation parameter. Thick black lines show the fixed points as a function of Γ_{ii}. For small values of Γ_{ii} there is a single stable fixed point. As Γ_{ii} is increased this fixed point loses stability by a super-critical Hopf bifurcation, thus signaling the onset of limit cycle activity. Periodic continuations of this low amplitude activity reveals that it, and a stable fixed point, co-exist with a higher amplitude limit

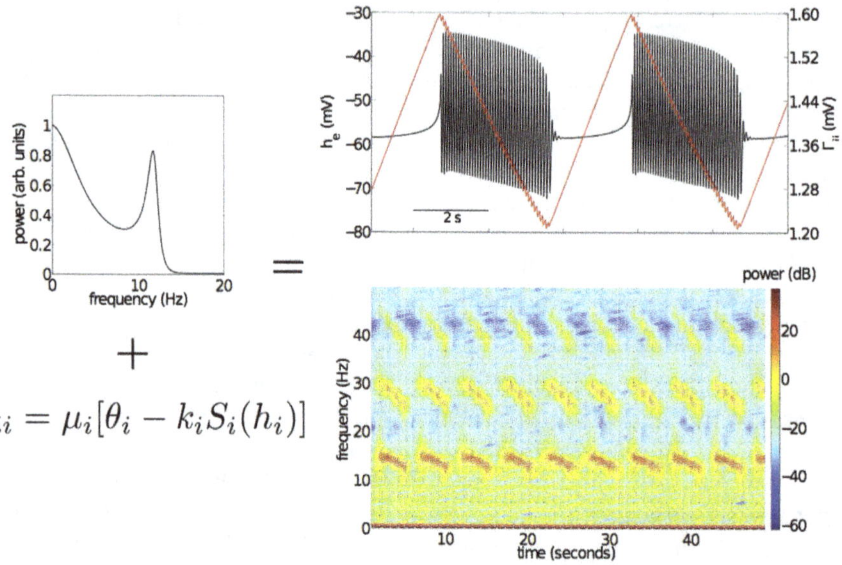

FIGURE 3 | Effects of the slow, activity dependent modulation of IPSPs on the inhibitory neuronal population, Γ_{ik} using the SS1 model of equation (11). The top left panel shows the fluctuation spectrum of the unmodulated "fast" EEG system (Bojak and Liley, 2005). When Γ_{ik} of this system is slowly modulated ($\mu_i = 0.001$ ms^{-1}, $\theta_i = 0.1818$ mV, $k_i = 10$ mV s) bursting emerges (top right panel). Bursting is associated with the periodic modulation of Γ_{ii} (red line, top right panel) on a much longer time scale than that of intra-burst oscillatory activity. Time-frequency analysis (bottom right panel) reveals that intra-burst activity sweeps down through a range of frequencies from low beta (13–30 Hz) to high alpha (8–12 Hz). Parameter values used for the "fast" EEG system can be found in **Table 3**.

cycle, thus suggesting that an activity dependent hysteresis drives the system between a fixed point and a high amplitude oscillation, thus giving rise to the bursting activity observed. This can be better seen by superimposing on this diagram the trajectory of a single burst (thin solid black line). Here we can see that the burst terminates through a fold-limit cycle bifurcation. At this stage it is not clear what bifurcation accounts for the emergence of the burst.

A well described feature of anesthetic action is the reduction in cerebral blood flow and metabolism (Kaisti et al., 2003). Therefore during anesthetic action it would be reasonable to assume that the recovery of pre-synaptic neurotransmitter levels will be impaired. In particular as the anesthetic level increases then the rate of synaptic recovery should decrease. **Figure 5** shows the effects of systematic reductions in the synaptic recovery rate for the SS1 model. As θ_i (synaptic recovery) is decreased the burst duration decreases and the period of non-oscillatory isoelectric activity increases until the model EEG becomes fully isoelectric. This trend is also observed clinically during anesthesia.

Short term synaptic depression would be expected to affect all synapses, though the depression would not be expected to be uniform. So far we have assumed that the synaptic depression would principally affect inhibitory synapses between inhibitory neurons. Will such bursting survive when all types of "fast" synaptic activity is subject to the biological forces of short term synaptic depression? **Figure 6** reveals that bursting does occur when both excitatory and inhibitory synaptic activity undergoes activity dependent short term synaptic depression. Further, the bursting that emerges is strongly modulated by parameters of the "fast"

Table 3 | Model parameter set used in simulations of Figures 3–8.

Parameter	Value	Parameter	Value
h_e^{rest} (mV)	−68.1355	N_{ee}^{α}	4994.4860
h_i^{rest} (mV)	−77.2602	N_{ei}^{α}	2222.9060
h_{ee}^{eq} (mV)	−15.8527	N_{ee}^{β}	4582.0661
h_{ei}^{eq} (mV)	7.4228	N_{ei}^{β}	4198.1829
h_{ie}^{eq} (mV)	−85.9896	N_{ie}^{β}	989.5281
h_{ii}^{eq} (mV)	−84.5363	N_{ii}^{β}	531.9419
τ_e (ms)	138.3660	v_{ek} (cm ms^{-1})	0.1714
τ_i (ms)	89.3207	Λ_{ek} (cm^{-1})	0.2433
Γ_{ee} (mV)	0.3127	S_e^{max} (ms−^{1})	0.2801
Γ_{ei} (mV)	0.9426	S_i^{max} (ms−^{1})	0.1228
Γ_{ie} (mV)	0.4947	μ_e (mV)	−47.1364
Γ_{ii} (mV)	1.4122	μ_i (mV)	−45.3751
γ_{ee} (ms^{-1})	0.4393	σ_e (mV)	2.6120
γ_{ei} (ms^{-1})	0.2350	σ_i (mV)	2.8294
γ_{ie} (ms^{-1})	0.0791	p_{ee} (ms^{-1})	3.6032
γ_{ii} (ms^{-1})	0.0782	p_{ei} (ms^{-1})	0.3639

Parameter set taken from Bojak and Liley (2005). Because parameters were obtained as part of a numerical search their full precision had been detailed, however their sensitivity to perturbation is much less than the precision reported (Bojak and Liley, 2005).

EEG system (see **Table 2**) that have been identified as targets for the action of anesthetic agents. Prolonging the decay of the unitary IPSP and reducing subcortical input are both found to significantly modulate modeled EEG bursting. In particular it is found that reducing excitatory extra-cortical input (p_{ee}), which

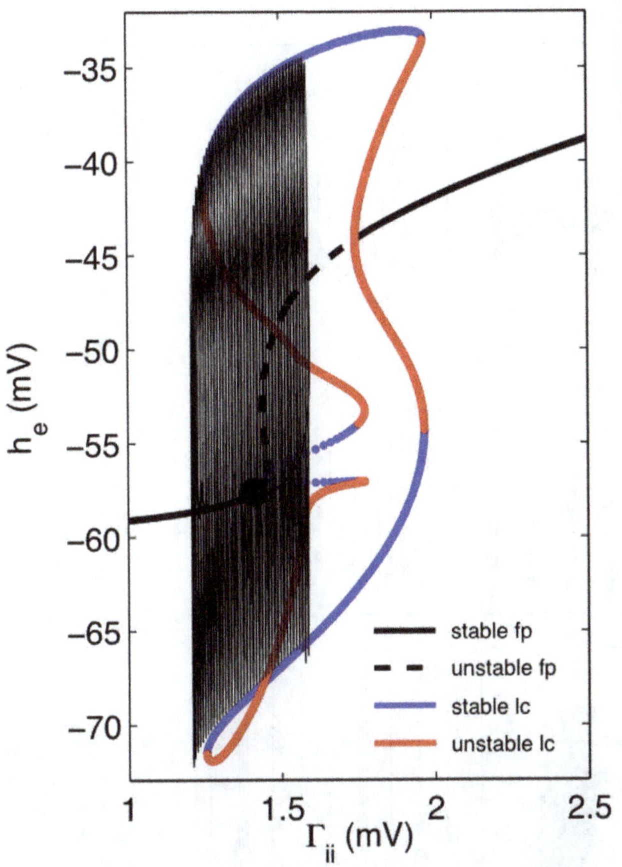

FIGURE 4 | One-dimensional continuation of the "fast" EEG system in h_e suggests how we might account for the dynamics of bursting. Thick black lines (solid = stable, dashed = unstable) shows the fixed points (fp) as a function of Γ_{ii}. Solid black circle indicates fixed point for the default parameter values for "fast" EEG system (parameters as for **Figure 3**). Solid blue lines indicate the locus of maximum and minimum amplitudes respectively of stable limit cycle (lc) activity, whereas solid red lines correspond similarly to locus of unstable limit activity. Transitions between stable and unstable lc activity is predominantly through fold-limit cycle bifurcations, except for middle limit cycle branch where transition is through a torus bifurcation. Superimposed on this one-dimensional bifurcation diagram is the trajectory of a single burst.

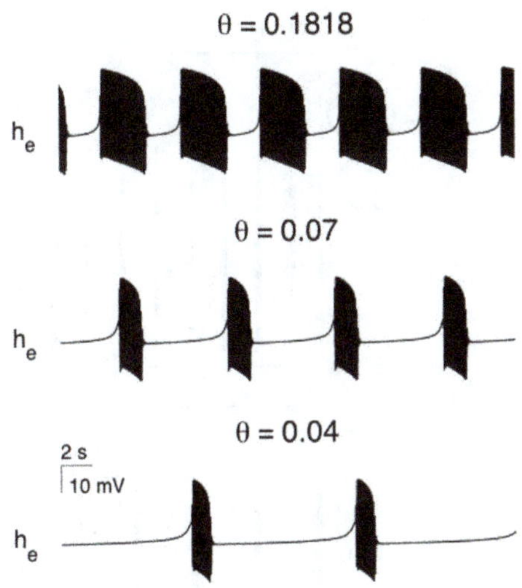

FIGURE 5 | The effect of parametrically varying the rate of recovery of synaptic efficacy in modulating the modeled burst duration and the quiescent (isoelectric) period. If θ_i is made small enough the bursting solutions will undergo a bifurcation to a non-oscillatory state. All parameters as per **Figure 4**.

presumably dominantly arises from thalamus, leads to very long quiescent (isoelectric) periods.

One of the limitations in using SS1 is that the PSPs are, in principle, free to take any value whereas physiology would dictate that they should remain bounded. To explore the effects of this restriction we chose to define an alternative slow modulating system [SS2, equation (12)]. **Figure 7** shows the effect of utilizing this system to provide a slow activity dependent modulation of excitatory and inhibitory synaptic efficacy of our "fast" EEG system. In the left panel of this figure we have plotted $c_e \equiv \Gamma_{el}/\Gamma^0_{el}$ as a function of time. The interesting thing to note is that in contrast to **Figure 3** excitatory synaptic efficacy decreases during the quiescent inter-burst period and increases during the burst. The left hand panel however shows that there is a significant phase difference between the normalized excitatory synaptic efficacy $c_e \equiv \Gamma_{el}/\Gamma^0_{el}$ and the normalized inhibitory synaptic efficacy $c_i \equiv \Gamma_{il}/\Gamma^0_{il}$. This suggests that there is an important dynamical interplay between excitatory and inhibitory synaptic efficacy to regulate neuronal population excitability such that bursting occurs. This may explain why there is confusion in the empirical literature regarding the role alterations in synaptic efficiency have in the genesis of BS.

An important difference between SS2 and SS1 is that parameters hypothesized to be important targets of anesthetic action p_{ee} and ε_{il} are able not only to parametrically regulate bursting but appear also able to switch bursting on (presumably through a bifurcation from a stable fixed point). **Figure 8** illustrates this. If the inhibitory neuronal IPSP decay time is not long enough then a single fixed point dominates which has an associated white noise fluctuation spectrum. But as the IPSP decay time increases (beyond $\varepsilon_{ii} > 1.8$ for the parameter set chosen) then bursting emerges. However if p_{ee} is decreased, as we would expect during anesthesia, then the isoelectric period is prolonged until at some critical value of p_{ee} bursting is extinguished to be replaced by an infinitely long quiescent/isoelectric period.

4. DISCUSSION

We have described here how a well-known model of the "fast" dynamics of the EEG can be modulated by a number of slow systems to produce bursting activity that bears some resemblance to BS seen clinically. The slow systems that we used were all based on some form of activity dependent short term plasticity that has been empirically observed, and used successfully in other models of macroscopic level bursting (Tabak and Rinzel, 2005). While we were able to clearly show the existence of bursting, because we did not include any additive or multiplicative noise sources, we were unable to account for the quasi-periodicity of BS. Thus all our busting arises from purely deterministic processes, presumably involving a range of well described bifurcations (Izhikevich,

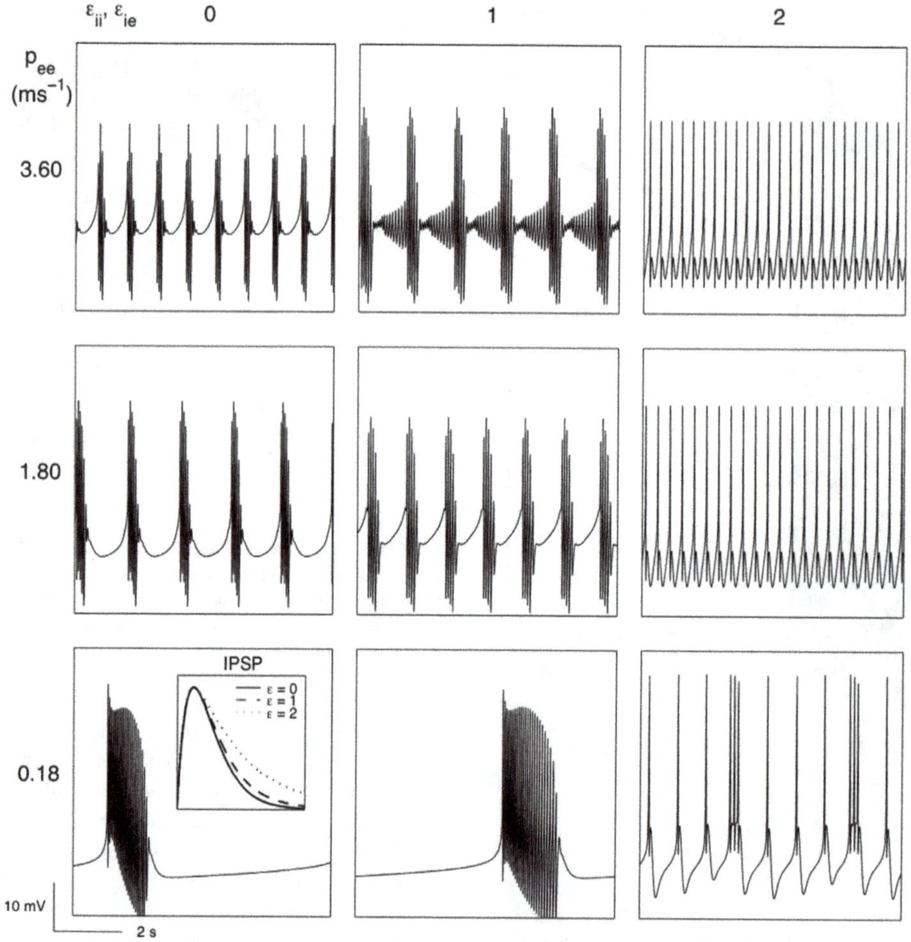

FIGURE 6 | The effects of short term synaptic depression of both excitatory and inhibitory cortical synapses in the genesis of burst suppression and its modulation by variations in extra-cortical input (p_{ee}) and the IPSP decay time (ε_{ii}, ε_{ie}) (see section 2.3 for further details). Parameters: $\theta_e = 0.1818$ mV, $\theta_i = 0.07$ mV, $k_e = 14$ mV s. All other parameters as for **Figure 3**.

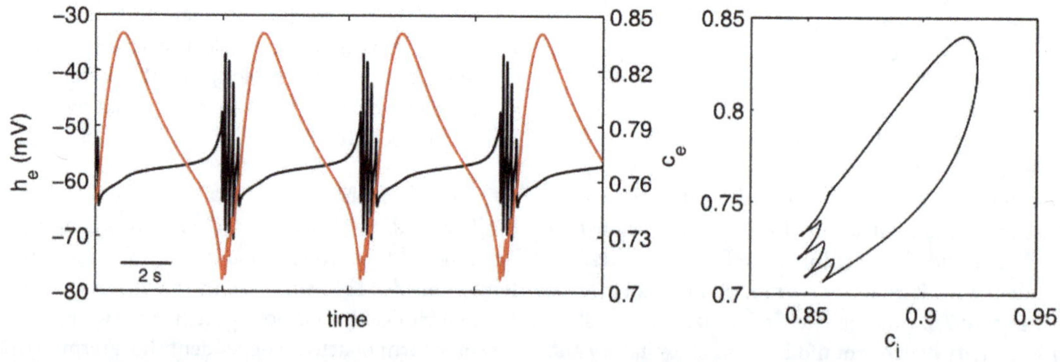

FIGURE 7 | Bursting produced by the activity dependent slow modulation of excitatory and inhibitory synaptic efficacy according to SS2 [equation (12)]. Left panel shows h_e (solid black line) and normalized excitatory synaptic efficacy $c_e \equiv \Gamma_{el}/\Gamma^0_{el}$ (solid red line) as a function of time. The left hand panel shows the phase relationship between normalized excitatory and inhibitory ($c_i \equiv \Gamma_{il}/\Gamma^0_{il}$) synaptic efficacies. Parameters: $\kappa_e = 0.2\ \mathrm{mV}^{-1}$, $\kappa_i = 0.1\ \mathrm{mV}^{-1}$, $\varepsilon_{ii} = 1.8$, $\varepsilon_{ie} = 1.5$.

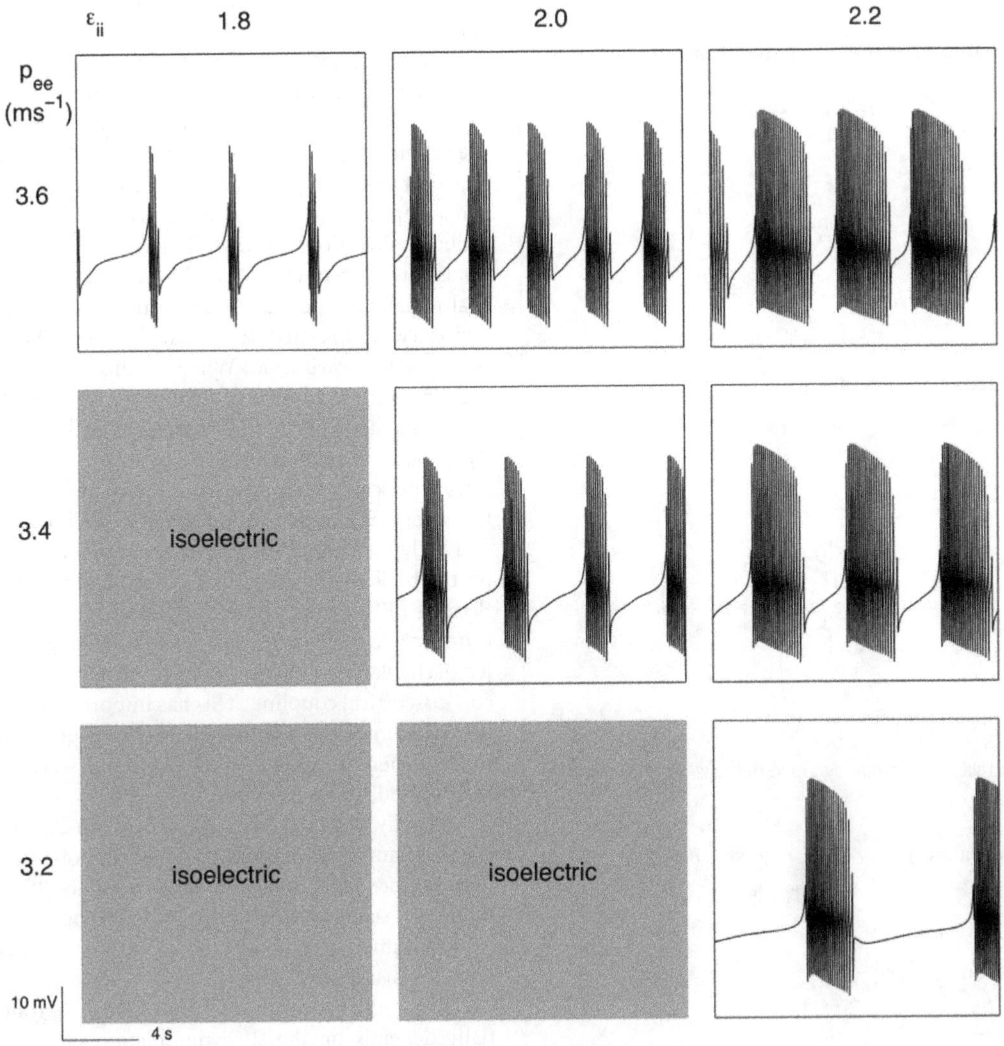

FIGURE 8 | Parametric variability of bursting produced by the activity dependent slow modulation of excitatory and inhibitory synaptic efficacy according to SS2 [equation (12)]. For $\varepsilon_{ii} < 1.8$ simulated EEG was isoelectric as was the case for labeled combinations of ε_{ii} and p_{ee}. Parameters as for **Figure 7**.

2007). However because our system clearly exhibited bistability (see **Figure 4**) it is almost certain that our system will be able to exhibit some form of burst excitability in response to stochastic forcing. Such burst excitability has been described experimentally. For example during BS induced by various halogenated anesthetic agents, bursts can be readily evoked by auditory, visual, or somatosensory stimuli (Hartikainen et al., 1995). Nevertheless while burst onset and duration may be random variables it would seem that the bursts themselves should reveal a high degree of determinism (weak non-linearity) when compared to EEG in which bursting or epileptiform activity is not evident.

Because the parameter space of the underlying "fast" EEG model is potentially extremely large it is not possible to systematically explore its dynamical repertoire and it may be possible that this system, not augmented with one of the slow systems described, is able to burst. Nevertheless, on the basis of our results, and what is known regarding the dynamical mechanisms of bursting, it would seem likely that multiple pathways to BS exist through a variety of activity dependent slow modulatory systems.

Further we might hypothesize that such slow modulatory systems might span a number of functional scales in the brain. **Figure 9** diagrammatically illustrates some possible candidate systems. An obvious activity driven slow modulatory system would be that associated with thalamus and the corresponding thalamo-cortical feed-back. Mean field models of the EEG that incorporate thalamo-cortical feed-back have been developed (Rennie et al., 2002) and it will be interesting to see if they are structurally configured to support BS. In addition to synaptic fatigue another obvious cortical system that might be marshaled to provide slow activity dependent modulation is the cortico-cortical conduction system. Although at this stage there is currently little evidence to suggest anesthetics slow conduction velocities, it is widely documented that axonal conduction velocities are significantly decreased in

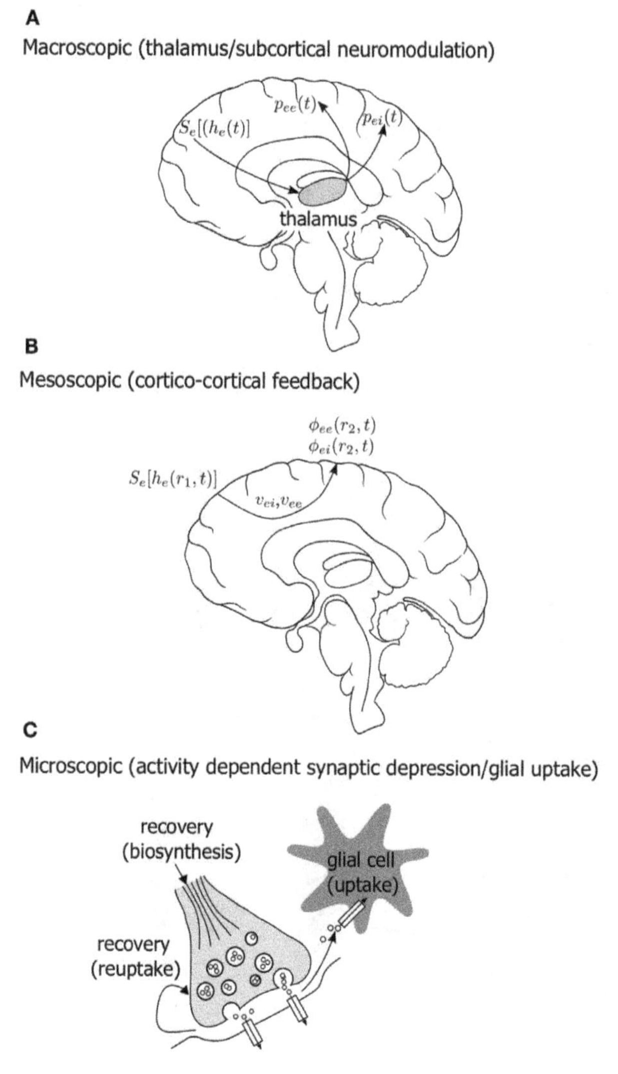

FIGURE 9 | Diagram illustrating a number of hypothesized, physiologically plausible, multiple scale slow modulatory systems that could be important in the genesis of electroencephalographic bursting in the context mean field model of Liley et al. (A) Thalamo-cortical feed-back **(B)** changes in the conduction properties of the long-range cortico-cortical fiber system **(C)** slow changes in the efficacy of synaptic function due to activity dependent resource depletion and restitution. See accompanying text for symbol definitions.

hypothermia. Decreases of up to 5% per °C for conduction velocity have been reported (Waxman, 1980). As BS has been observed to occur in hypothermia (Schwartz et al., 1989; Akrawi et al., 1996) we can conclude that a slow system emerging in the long-range coupling via a slowing of axonal conduction velocity is a possible route to BS.

Our attempts to account for the dynamical pathogenesis of burst suppression differ from other approaches, most notably Ching et al. (2012). Ching et al. described the scalp EEG in terms of the activity of a small scale, biophysically detailed, computational model of interacting populations of cortical and thalamic neurons. Burst suppression was modeled as arising from metabolically induced alterations in an ATP-gated slow neuronal membrane potassium current ($I_{K_{ATP}}$) on the basis that the reduction in cerebral metabolic rate (CMRO2) induced by anesthetic agents and hypoxia was associated with the depletion of ATP, and hence membrane hyperpolarization. While on this basis they claim to have accounted for a number of defining features of BS that included (i) the spatial synchrony of burst onset (ii) the parametric variability of burst duration/isoelectricity and (iii) the characteristically long time scales associated with bursting/isoelectricity compared to resting EEG, some caution needs to be exercised.

Firstly their model of resting/spontaneous EEG is constructed on the basis of the activity of no more than 20 model neurons. Because EEG is a distributed large scale phenomena such a model is unlikely to meaningfully account for resting/spontaneous activity particularly given the absence of any long-range excitatory cortico-cortical coupling. This has important implications for the propagation of burst activity particularly given that the onset of bursts, when examined at fine temporal scales, is probably not truly spatially homogeneous.

Secondly while the relationship between CMRO2 and ATP production cannot be reasonably disputed, not all anesthetic agents that produce reductions in CMRO2 produce BS. For example the noble gas xenon has been reported to reduce CMRO2 by up to 33% in human participants (Rex et al., 2006) yet is not associated with any discernable BS.

Thirdly the approach they have taken to producing BS essentially depends on the slow modulation of a faster system, the approach we have adopted here. The modeled time scales of $I_{K_{ATP}}$ variability are very long, of the order of tens of seconds.

For clarity and tractability the current investigations have focused on the spatially homogeneous case for the model of Liley et al. [i.e., $\nabla^2 = 0$ in equation (6)]. Clearly the emergence of BS in the spatially extended case will need to be investigated through the appropriate numerical solution of the defining partial differential equations. Because the cortical phase synchrony (Hartikainen et al., 1995) of burst suppression has not, as far as we are aware, been explicitly investigated it will be crucial to empirically determine the spatiotemporal emergence of bursts in order to assess the importance of excitatory cortico-cortical connectivity in the emergence and modulation of BS as implied by the model and as we have suggested. This will require recording high density EEG during anesthesia in which BS is present.

REFERENCES

Akrawi, W. P., Drummond, J. C., Kalkman, C. J., and Patel, P. M. (1996). A comparison of the electrophysiologic characteristics of eeg burst-suppression as produced by isoflurane, thiopental, etomidate, and propofol. *J. Neurosurg. Anesthesiol.* 8, 40–46.

Amari, S.-I. (1975). Homogeneous nets of neuron-like elements. *Biol. Cybern.* 17, 211–220.

An, D. S., Straumann, D., and Wieser, H. G. (1996). 'One-way asynchrony' of burst-suppression activity. *Neurophysiol. Clin.* 26, 329–334.

Banks, M. I., and Pearce, R. A. (1999). Dual actions of volatile anesthetics on GABA(A) IPSCs: dissociation of blocking and prolonging effects. *Anesthesiology* 90, 120–134.

Bojak, I., and Liley, D. T. J. (2005). Modeling the effects of anesthesia on the electroencephalogram. *Phys. Rev. E Stat. Nonlin. Soft Matter Phys.* 71, 041902.

Brenner, R. P. (1985). The electroencephalogram in altered states of consciousness. *Neurol. Clin.* 3, 615–631.

Ching, S., Purdon, P. L., Vijayan, S., Kopell, N. J., and Brown, E. N. (2012). A neurophysiological-metabolic model for burst suppression. *Proc. Natl. Acad. Sci. U.S.A.* 109, 3095–3100.

Cohen, S. D., and Hindmarsh, A. C. (1994). *CVODE User Guide.* Technical Report. Livermore: Lawrence Livermore National Laboratory.

Deco, G. R., Jirsa, V. K., Robinson, P. A., Breakspear, M., and Friston, K. J. (2008). The dynamic brain: from spiking neurons to neural masses and cortical fields. *PLoS Comput. Biol.* 4:e1000092. doi:10.1371/journal.pcbi.1000092

Derbyshire, A. J., Rempel, B., Forbes, A., and Lambert, E. F. (1936). The effects of anesthetics on action potentials in the cerebral cortex of the cat. *Am. J. Physiol.* 116, 577–596.

Ermentrout, B. (2002). *Simulating, Analyzing and Animating Dynamical Systems: A Guide to XPPAUT for Researchers and Students.* Philadelphia: SIAM.

Ferron, J. F., Kroeger, D., Chever, O., and Amzica, F. (2009). Cortical inhibition during burst suppression induced with isoflurane anesthesia. *J. Neurosci.* 29, 9850–9860.

Fischer-Williams, M., and Cooper, R. A. (1963). Depth recording from the human brain in epilepsy. *Electroencephalogr. Clin. Neurophysiol.* 15, 568–587.

Frascoli, F., van Veen, L., Bojak, I., and Liley, D. T. J. (2011). Metabifurcation analysis of a mean field model of the cortex. *Physica D* 240, 949–962.

Freeman, W. J. (1975). *Mass Action in the Nervous System: Examination of the Neurophysiological Basis of Adaptive Behavior Through the EEG,* 1st Edn. New York: Academic Press.

Geocadin, R. G., Sherman, D. L., Hansen, H. C., Kimura, T., Niedermeyer, E., Thakor, N. V., et al. (2002). Neurological recovery by eeg bursting after resuscitation from cardiac arrest in rats. *Resuscitation* 55, 193–200.

Grigg-Damberger, M. M., Coker, S. B., Halsey, C. L., and Anderson, C. L. (1989). Neonatal burst suppression: its developmental significance. *Pediatr. Neurol.* 5, 84–92.

Hartikainen, K. M., Rorarius, M., Perakyla, J. J., Laippala, P. J., and Jantti, V. (1995). Cortical reactivity during isoflurane burst-suppression anesthesia. *Anesth. Analg.* 81, 1223–1228.

Henry, C. E., and Scoville, W. B. (1952). Suppression-burst activity from isolated cerebral cortex in man. *Electroencephalogr. Clin. Neurophysiol.* 4, 1–22.

Hockaday, J. M., Potts, F., Epstein, E., Bonazzi, A., and Schwab, R. S. (1965). Electroencephalographic changes in acute cerebral anoxia from cardiac or respiratory arrest. *Electroencephalogr. Clin. Neurophysiol.* 18, 575–586.

Izhikevich, E. M. (2000). Neural excitability, spiking, and bursting. *Int. J. Bifurcat. Chaos* 10, 1171–1266.

Izhikevich, E. M. (2007). *Dynamical Systems in Neuroscience: The Geometry of Excitability and Bursting.* Cambridge, MA: The MIT Press.

Kaisti, K. K., Langsjo, J. W., Aalto, S., Oikonen, V., Sipila, H., Teras, M., et al. (2003). Effects of sevoflurane, propofol, and adjunct nitrous oxide on regional cerebral blood flow, oxygen consumption, and blood volume in humans. *Anesthesiology* 99, 603–613.

Kroeger, D., and Amzica, F. (2007). Hypersensitivity of the anesthesia-induced comatose brain. *J. Neurosci.* 27, 10597–10607.

Liley, D. T. J., and Bojak, I. (2005). Understanding the transition to seizure by modeling the epileptiform activity of general anesthetic agents. *J. Clin. Neurophysiol.* 22, 300–313.

Liley, D. T. J., Cadusch, P. J., and Dafilis, M. P. (2002). A spatially continuous mean field theory of electrocortical activity. *Network* 13, 67–113.

Liley, D. T. J., Cadusch, P. J., and Wright, J. J. (1999). A continuum theory of electro-cortical activity. *Neurocomputing* 26–27, 795–800.

Liley, D. T. J., Foster, B. L., and Bojak, I. (2011). "A mesoscopic modelling approach to characterising anaesthetic action on brain electrical activity," in *Sleep and Anesthesia: Neural Correlates in Theory and Experiment, Springer Series in Computational Neuroscience,* ed. A. Hutt (New York: Springer), 139–166.

Lukatch, H. S., and MacIver, M. B. (1996). Synaptic mechanisms of thiopental-induced alterations in synchronized cortical activity. *Anesthesiology* 84, 1425–1434.

Niedermeyer, E. (2005). "Epileptic seizure disorders," in *Electroencephalography: Basic Principles, Clinical Applications, and Related Fields,* 5th Edn, eds E. Niedermeyer and F. H. Lopes da Silva (Philadelphia: Lippincott), 505–619.

Niedermeyer, E. (2009). The burst-suppression electroencephalogram. *Am. J. Electroneurodiagnostic Technol.* 49, 333–341.

Nunez, P. L. (1974). The brain wave equation: a model for the EEG. *Math. Biosci.* 21, 279–297.

Nunez, P. L., and Srinivasan, R. (2005). *Electric Fields of the Brain: The Neurophysics of EEG,* 2nd Edn. New York: Oxford University Press.

Rennie, C. J., Robinson, P. A., and Wright, J. J. (2002). Unified neurophysical model of EEG spectra and evoked potentials. *Biol. Cybern.* 86, 457–471.

Rex, S., Schaefer, W., Meyer, P. H., Rossaint, R., Boy, C., Setani, K., et al. (2006). Positron emission tomography study of regional cerebral metabolism during general anesthesia with xenon in humans. *Anesthesiology* 105, 936–943.

Rinzel, J. (1985). "Bursting oscillations in an excitable membrane model," in *Ordinary and Partial Differential Equations: Proceedings of the 8th Dundee Conference, Number 1151 in Lecture Notes in Mathematics,* eds B. D. Sleeman and R. J. Jarvis (Berlin: Springer), 304–316.

Schwartz, A. E., Tuttle, R. H., and Poppers, P. J. (1989). Electroencephalographic burst suppression in elderly and young patients anesthetized with isoflurane. *Anesth. Analg.* 68, 9–12.

Steriade, M., Amzica, F., and Contreras, D. (1994). Cortical and thalamic cellular correlates of electroencephalographic burst-suppression. *Electroencephalogr. Clin. Neurophysiol.* 90, 1–16.

Swank, R. L., and Watson, C. W. (1949). Effects of barbiturates and ether on spontaneous electrical activity of dog brain. *J. Neurophysiol.* 12, 137–160.

Swindale, N. V. (2003). Neural synchrony, axonal path lengths and general anesthesia: a hypothesis. *Neuroscientist* 9, 440–445.

Tabak, J., and Rinzel, J. (2005). "Bursting in excitatory neural networks," in *Bursting: The Genesis of Rhythm in the Nervous System,* eds S. Coombes and P. C. Bressloff (Singapore: World Scientific), 273–301.

Treiman, D. M., Walton, N. Y., and Kendrick, C. (1990). A progressive sequence of electroencephalographic changes during generalized convulsive status epilepticus. *Epilepsy Res.* 5, 49–60.

Tsodyks, M. V., and Markram, H. (1997). The neural code between neocortical pyramidal neurons depends on neurotransmitter release probability. *Proc. Natl. Acad. Sci. U.S.A.* 94, 719–723.

Voss, L. J., Ludbrook, G., Grant, C., Sleigh, J. W., and Barnard, J. P. (2006). Cerebral cortical effects of desflurane in sheep: comparison with isoflurane, sevoflurane and enflurane. *Acta Anaesthesiol. Scand.* 50, 313–319.

Waxman, S. G. (1980). Determinants of conduction velocity in myelinated nerve fibers. *Muscle Nerve* 3, 141–150.

Wilson, H. R., and Cowan, J. D. (1972). Excitatory and inhibitory interactions in localized populations of model neuron. *Biophys. J.* 12, 1–24.

Wilson, H. R., and Cowan, J. D. (1973). A mathematical theory of the functional dynamics of cortical and thalamic nervous tissue. *Kybernetik* 13, 55–80.

6

A biophysical observation model for field potentials of networks of leaky integrate-and-fire neurons

Peter beim Graben[1,2]* and Serafim Rodrigues[3]

[1] Bernstein Center for Computational Neuroscience Berlin, Berlin, Germany
[2] Department of German Language and Linguistics, Humboldt-Universität zu Berlin, Berlin, Germany
[3] Centre for Robotics and Neural Systems, School of Computing and Mathematics, University of Plymouth, Plymouth, UK

We present a biophysical approach for the coupling of neural network activity as resulting from proper dipole currents of cortical pyramidal neurons to the electric field in extracellular fluid. Starting from a reduced three-compartment model of a single pyramidal neuron, we derive an observation model for dendritic dipole currents in extracellular space and thereby for the dendritic field potential (DFP) that contributes to the local field potential (LFP) of a neural population. This work aligns and satisfies the widespread dipole assumption that is motivated by the "open-field" configuration of the DFP around cortical pyramidal cells. Our reduced three-compartment scheme allows to derive networks of leaky integrate-and-fire (LIF) models, which facilitates comparison with existing neural network and observation models. In particular, by means of numerical simulations we compare our approach with an *ad hoc* model by Mazzoni et al. (2008), and conclude that our biophysically motivated approach yields substantial improvement.

Correspondence:
Peter beim Graben, Department of German Language and Linguistics, Humboldt-Universität zu Berlin, Unter den Linden 6, D–10099, Berlin, Germany.
e-mail: peter.beim.graben@hu-berlin.de

Keywords: biophysics, neural networks, leaky integrate-and-fire neuron, current dipoles, extracellular medium, field potentials

1. INTRODUCTION

Since Hans Berger's 1924 discovery of the human *electroencephalogram (EEG)* (Berger, 1929), neuroscientists achieved much progress in clarifying its neural generators (Creutzfeldt et al., 1966a,b; Nunez and Srinivasan, 2006; Schomer and Lopes da Silva, 2011). These are the cortical pyramidal neurons, as sketched in **Figure 1**, that possess a long dendritic trunk separating mainly excitatory synapses at the apical dendritic tree from mainly inhibitory synapses at the soma and at the perisomatic basal dendritic tree (Creutzfeldt et al., 1966a; Spruston, 2008). In addition, they exhibit an axial symmetry and are aligned in parallel to each other, perpendicular to the cortex' surface, thus forming a palisade of cell bodies and dendritic trunks. When both kinds of synapses are simultaneously active, inhibitory synapses generate current sources and excitatory synapses current sinks in extracellular space, hence causing the pyramidal cell to behave as a microscopic dipole surrounded by its characteristic electrical field, the *dendritic field potential (DFP)*. The densely packed pyramidal cells form then a dipole layer whose superimposed currents give rise to the *local field potential (LFP)* of neural masses and eventually to the EEG (Nunez and Srinivasan, 2006; Lindén et al., 2010; Lindén et al., 2011; Schomer and Lopes da Silva, 2011).

Despite of the progress from experimental neuroscience, theoretically understanding the coupling of complex neural network dynamics to the electromagnetic field in the extracellular space poses challenging problems; some of them have been addressed to some extent by Bédard et al. (2004); Bédard and Destexhe (2009), and Bédard and Destexhe (2012).

In computer simulation studies, neural mass potentials, such as LFP and EEG are most realistically simulated by means of multicompartmental models (Protopapas et al., 1998; Sargsyan et al., 2001; Lindén et al., 2010; Lindén et al., 2011). Lindén et al. (2010) calculated the current dipole momentum of the DFP for single pyramidal and stellate cells, based on several hundreds compartments of the dendritic trees. Their results were in compliance with the standard dipole approximation of the electrostatic multipole expansion in the far-field (more than 1 mm remote from the dendritic trunk), but they found rather poor agreement with that approximation in the vicinity of the cell body. For comparison they also computed a "two-monopole" model of one synaptic current and its counterpart, the somatic return current, estimated from the current dipole momentum of the whole dendritic tree. This "two-monopole" model, which corresponds to an electrically equivalent single dipole model, obtained from the decomposition of the dendrite into two compartments, better approximates the true current dipole momentum in the vicinity of the pyramidal neuron. By superimposing the DFPs of pyramidal cells to the ensemble LFP, Lindén et al. (2011) found that LFP properties cannot be attributed to the far-field dipole approximation.

However, realistic multicompartmental models are computationally too expensive for large-scale neural network simulations. Therefore, various techniques have been proposed and employed to overcome computational complexity. These include networks of point models (i.e., devoid from any spatial representation), based on conductance models (Hodgkin and Huxley, 1952; Mazzoni et al., 2008), population density models

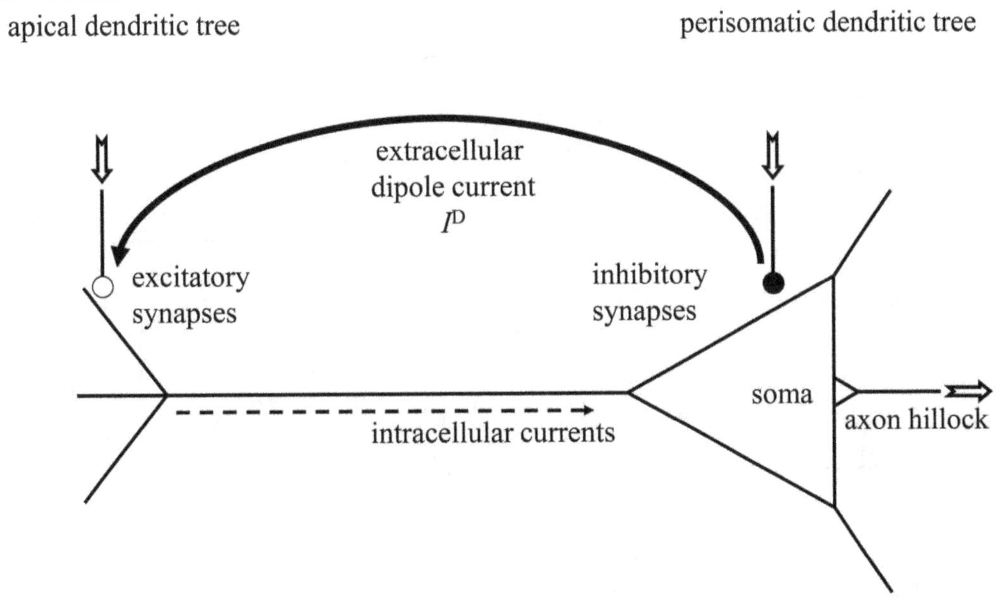

FIGURE 1 | Sketch of a cortical pyramidal neuron with extracellular current dipole between spatially separated excitatory (open bullet) and inhibitory synapses (filled bullet). Neural in- and outputs are indicated by the jagged arrows. Dendritic current I^D causes dendritic field potential (DFP).

(Omurtag et al., 2000), or firing rate models (Wilson and Cowan, 1972), which can be seen as a sub class of population density models, with uniform density distribution (Chizhov et al., 2007). In these kinds of models, mass potentials such as LFP or EEG are conventionally described as averaged membrane potential. A different class of models are neural mass models (Jansen and Rit, 1995; Wendling et al., 2000; David and Friston, 2003; Rodrigues et al., 2010), where mass potentials are estimated either through sums (or actually differences) of excitatory postsynaptic potentials (EPSP) (David and Friston, 2003) or of excitatory postsynaptic currents (EPSC) (Mazzoni et al., 2008).

In particular, the model of Mazzoni et al. (2008) which is based on Brunel and Wang (2003), recently led to a series of follow-up studies (Mazzoni et al., 2010, 2011) addressing the correlations between numerically simulated and experimentally measured LFP/EEG with spike rates by means of statistical modeling and information theoretic measures. In all of the above point models and their extension to population models, it is assumed that the extracellular space is iso-potential and the majority of studies thereby neglect the effect of extracellular resistance. That is, the extracellular space constitutes a different and isolated domain with no effect on neuronal dynamics.

In this article we extend the *ad hoc* model of Mazzoni et al. (2008) toward a biophysically better justified approach, taking the dipole character of extracellular currents and fields into account. Basically, our model corresponds to the "two-monopole," or, equivalent dipole model of Lindén et al. (2010) which gave a good fit of the DFP close to the cell body of a cortical pyramidal neuron. However, we aim to keep the simplicity of the Mazzoni et al. (2008) model in terms of computational complexity, by endowing the extracellular space with resistance and by keeping point-like neuronal circuits. That is, in our case we do not quite consider point neurons, nor spatially extended models with detailed compartmental morphology, yet an intermediate level of description is achieved. To this end we propose a *reduced three-compartmental model* of a single pyramidal neuron (Destexhe, 2001; Wang et al., 2004; beim Graben, 2008), and derive an observation model for the dendritic dipole currents in the extracellular space and thereby for the DFP that contributes to the LFP of a neural population. Interestingly, our reduced three-compartmental model enables us to derive a leaky integrate-and-fire (LIF) mechanism [as for a point model (Mazzoni et al., 2008)], with additional observation equations for the DFP, which all together allows to study the relationship between spike rates and LFP. Our derivations also nicely map realistic electrotonic parameters to phenomenological parameters considered in Mazzoni et al. (2008).

2. MATERIALS AND METHODS

Mazzoni et al. (2008) consider three populations of neurons, namely excitatory cortical pyramidal cells (population 1), inhibitory cortical interneurons (population 2), and excitatory thalamic relay neurons (population 3), passing sensory input to the cortex that is simulated by a random (Erdős–Rényi) graph of $K = 4000$ pyramidal and $L = 1000$ interneurons with connection probability $P = 0.2$.

2.1. THEORY

We describe the ith cortical pyramidal neuron (**Figure 1**) from population 1 via the electronic equivalent (reduced) three-compartment model (**Figure 2**) (Destexhe, 2001; Wang et al., 2004; beim Graben, 2008), which is parsimonious to derive our observation model: one compartment for the apical dendritic

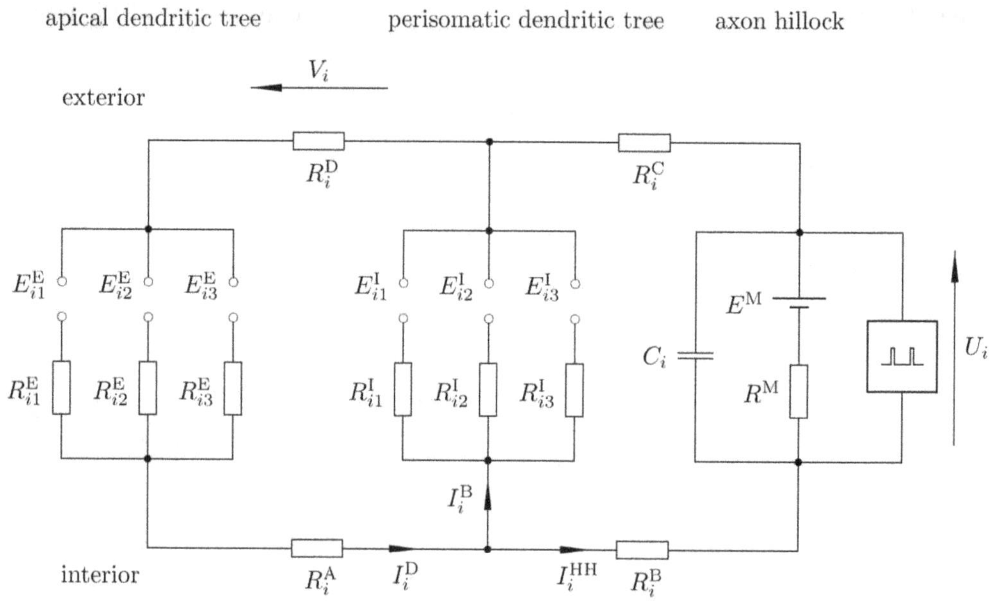

FIGURE 2 | Proposed electronic equivalent circuit for a pyramidal neuron (reduced three-compartmental model). Note that the apical and basal dendrites are not true compartments since capacitors are not explicitly represented, rather, these are implicitly taken into account via EPSP and IPSP static functions, thus keeping computational complexity low.

tree, another one for soma and perisomatic basal dendritic tree (Lindén et al., 2010), and the third—actually a LIF unit—for the axon hillock where membrane potential is converted into spike trains by means of an integrate-and-fire mechanism.

Excitatory synapses are represented by the left-most branch, where EPSP at a synapse between a neuron j from population 1 or 3 and neuron i act as electromotoric forces E_{ij}^{E}. These potentials drive EPSC I_{ij}^{E}, essentially consisting of sodium ions, through the cell plasma with resistance R_{ij}^{E} from the synapse toward the axon hillock.

The middle branch describes the inhibitory synapses between a neuron k from population 2 and neuron i. Here, inhibitory postsynaptic potentials (IPSP) E_{ik}^{I} provide a shortcut between the excitatory branch and the trigger zone, where inhibitory postsynaptic currents (IPSC) I_{ik}^{I} (essentially chloride ions) close the loop between the apical and perisomatic dendritic trees. The resistivity of the current paths along the cell plasma is given by R_{ik}^{I}.

The cell membrane at the axon hillock itself is represented by the branch at the right hand side. Here, a capacitor C_i reflects the temporary storage capacity of the membrane. The serial circuit consisting of a battery E^{M} and a resistor R^{M} denotes the Nernst resting potential and the leakage conductance of the membrane, respectively (Johnston and Wu, 1997). Finally, a spike generator (Hodgkin and Huxley, 1952; Mazzoni et al., 2008) (indicated by a "black box") is regarded of having infinite input impedance. Both, EPSP and IPSP result from the interaction of postsynaptic receptor kinetics with dendritic low-pass filtering in compartments one and two, respectively (Destexhe et al., 1998; Lindén et al., 2010). Hence the required capacitances, omitted in **Figure 2**, are already taken into account by E_{ij}^{E}, E_{ik}^{I}. Therefore, we refer to our model as to a "reduced compartment model" here.

The three compartments are coupled through longitudinal resistors, R_i^{A}, R_i^{B}, R_i^{C}, and R_i^{D} where R_i^{A}, R_i^{B} denote the resistivity of the cell plasma and R_i^{C}, R_i^{D} that of extracellular space (Holt and Koch, 1999).

Finally, the membrane voltage at the axon hillock U_i (the dynamical state variable) and the DFP V_i, which measures the drop in electrical potential along the extracellular resistor R_i^{D} are indicated. For the aim of calculation, the mesh currents I_i^{D} (the dendritic current), I_i^{B} (the basal current), and I_i^{IF} (the integrate-and-fire current) are indicated.

The circuit in **Figure 2** obeys the following equations:

$$I_i^{\mathrm{D}} = \sum_{j=1}^{p} I_{ij}^{\mathrm{E}} \tag{1}$$

$$I_i^{\mathrm{B}} = \sum_{k=1}^{q} I_{ik}^{\mathrm{I}} \tag{2}$$

$$I_i^{\mathrm{IF}} = I_i^{\mathrm{D}} - I_i^{\mathrm{B}} \tag{3}$$

$$I_i^{\mathrm{IF}} = C_i \frac{\mathrm{d}U_i}{\mathrm{d}t} + \frac{U_i - E^{\mathrm{M}}}{R^{\mathrm{M}}} \tag{4}$$

$$E_{ij}^{\mathrm{E}} = R_{ij}^{\mathrm{E}} I_{ij}^{\mathrm{E}} + \left(R_i^{\mathrm{A}} + R_i^{\mathrm{D}}\right) I_i^{\mathrm{D}} + \left(R_i^{\mathrm{B}} + R_i^{\mathrm{C}}\right) I_i^{\mathrm{IF}} + U_i,\ 1 \le j \le p \tag{5}$$

$$E_{ik}^{\mathrm{I}} = R_{ik}^{\mathrm{I}} I_{ik}^{\mathrm{I}} + \left(R_i^{\mathrm{B}} + R_i^{\mathrm{C}}\right) I_i^{\mathrm{IF}} + U_i,\ 1 \le k \le q \tag{6}$$

$$V_i = R_i^{\mathrm{D}} I_i^{\mathrm{D}}. \tag{7}$$

Here, p is the number of excitatory and q is the number of inhibitory synapses connected to neuron i.

The circuit described by Equations (1–7) shows that the neuron i is likely to fire when the excitatory synapses are activated. Then, the integrate-and-fire current I_i^{IF} equals the dendritic current I_i^{D}. If, by contrast, also the inhibitory synapses are active, the dendritic current I_i^{D} is shunted between the apical and perisomatic basal dendritic trees and only a portion could evoke spikes at the trigger zone (Equation 4). On the other hand, the large dendritic current I_i^{D} flowing through the extracellular space of resistance R_i^{D}, gives rise to a large DFP V_i.

In order to simplify the following derivations, we gauge the resting potential (Equation 4) to $E^{\mathrm{M}} = 0$, yielding

$$I_i^{\mathrm{IF}} = C_i \frac{\mathrm{d}U_i}{\mathrm{d}t} + \frac{U_i}{R^{\mathrm{M}}}. \tag{8}$$

From Equation (5) we obtain the individual EPSC's as

$$I_{ij}^{\mathrm{E}} = \frac{1}{R_{ij}^{\mathrm{E}}} \left[E_{ij}^{\mathrm{E}} - \left(R_i^{\mathrm{A}} + R_i^{\mathrm{D}}\right) I_i^{\mathrm{D}} - \left(R_i^{\mathrm{B}} + R_i^{\mathrm{C}}\right) I_i^{\mathrm{IF}} - U_i \right]. \tag{9}$$

And accordingly, the individual IPSC's from Equation (6)

$$I_{ik}^{\mathrm{I}} = \frac{1}{R_{ik}^{\mathrm{I}}} \left[E_{ik}^{\mathrm{I}} - \left(R_i^{\mathrm{B}} + R_i^{\mathrm{C}}\right) I_i^{\mathrm{IF}} - U_i \right]. \tag{10}$$

Inserting Equation (9) into Equation (1) yields the excitatory dendritic current

$$I_i^{\mathrm{D}} = \sum_{j=1}^{p} \frac{1}{R_{ij}^{\mathrm{E}}} E_{ij}^{\mathrm{E}} - g_i^{\mathrm{E}} \left[\left(R_i^{\mathrm{A}} + R_i^{\mathrm{D}}\right) I_i^{\mathrm{D}} + \left(R_i^{\mathrm{B}} + R_i^{\mathrm{C}}\right) I_i^{\mathrm{IF}} + U_i \right], \tag{11}$$

where we have introduced the excitatory dendritic conductivity

$$g_i^{\mathrm{E}} = \sum_{j=1}^{p} \frac{1}{R_{ij}^{\mathrm{E}}}. \tag{12}$$

Likewise we obtain the inhibitory dendritic currents from Equations (2) and (10) as

$$I_i^{\mathrm{B}} = \sum_{k=1}^{q} \frac{1}{R_{ik}^{\mathrm{I}}} E_{ik}^{\mathrm{I}} - g_i^{\mathrm{I}} \left[\left(R_i^{\mathrm{B}} + R_i^{\mathrm{C}}\right) I_i^{\mathrm{IF}} + U_i \right], \tag{13}$$

with the inhibitory dendritic conductivity

$$g_i^{\mathrm{I}} = \sum_{k=1}^{q} \frac{1}{R_{ik}^{\mathrm{I}}}. \tag{14}$$

With these results, we obtain an interface equation for an observation model as follows. Rearranging Equation (11) yields

$$I_i^{\mathrm{D}} \left[1 + g_i^{\mathrm{E}} \left(R_i^{\mathrm{A}} + R_i^{\mathrm{D}}\right) \right] = \sum_{j=1}^{p} \frac{1}{R_{ij}^{\mathrm{E}}} E_{ij}^{\mathrm{E}} - g_i^{\mathrm{E}} \left[\left(R_i^{\mathrm{B}} + R_i^{\mathrm{C}}\right) I_i^{\mathrm{IF}} + U_i \right] \tag{15}$$

Next, we eliminate I_i^{IF} through Equation (8):

$$I_i^{\mathrm{D}} \left[1 + g_i^{\mathrm{E}} \left(R_i^{\mathrm{A}} + R_i^{\mathrm{D}}\right) \right] = \sum_{j=1}^{p} \frac{1}{R_{ij}^{\mathrm{E}}} E_{ij}^{\mathrm{E}} - g_i^{\mathrm{E}} \times \left[C_i \left(R_i^{\mathrm{B}} + R_i^{\mathrm{C}}\right) \frac{\mathrm{d}U_i}{\mathrm{d}t} + U_i \left(1 + \frac{R_i^{\mathrm{B}} + R_i^{\mathrm{C}}}{R^{\mathrm{M}}} \right) \right].$$

Division by $1 + g_i^{\mathrm{E}} \left(R_i^{\mathrm{A}} + R_i^{\mathrm{D}}\right)$ gives the desired expression for the extracellular dendritic dipole current:

$$I_i^{\mathrm{D}} = \sum_{j=1}^{p} \alpha_{ij} E_{ij}^{\mathrm{E}} - \beta_i \frac{\mathrm{d}U_i}{\mathrm{d}t} - \gamma_i U_i, \tag{16}$$

with the following electrotonic parameters

$$\alpha_{ij} = \frac{1}{R_{ij}^{\mathrm{E}} \left[1 + g_i^{\mathrm{E}} \left(R_i^{\mathrm{A}} + R_i^{\mathrm{D}}\right) \right]} \tag{17}$$

$$\beta_i = \frac{C_i g_i^{\mathrm{E}} \left(R_i^{\mathrm{B}} + R_i^{\mathrm{C}}\right)}{1 + g_i^{\mathrm{E}} \left(R_i^{\mathrm{A}} + R_i^{\mathrm{D}}\right)} \tag{18}$$

$$\gamma_i = \frac{g_i^{\mathrm{E}} \left(R^{\mathrm{M}} + R_i^{\mathrm{B}} + R_i^{\mathrm{C}}\right)}{R^{\mathrm{M}} \left[1 + g_i^{\mathrm{E}} \left(R_i^{\mathrm{A}} + R_i^{\mathrm{D}}\right) \right]}. \tag{19}$$

In order to derive the evolution equation we consider the integrate-and-fire current I_i^{IF} that is given through Equation (3). The individual EPSCs and IPSCs have already been obtained in Equations (9) and (10), respectively. Inserting Equation (13) into Equation (3) yields

$$I_i^{\mathrm{IF}} \left[1 - g_i^{\mathrm{I}} \left(R_i^{\mathrm{B}} + R_i^{\mathrm{C}}\right) \right] - g_i^{\mathrm{I}} U_i = I_i^{\mathrm{D}} - \sum_{k=1}^{q} \frac{1}{R_{ik}^{\mathrm{I}}} E_{ik}^{\mathrm{I}}.$$

Next we insert our interface equation Equation (16) and also Equation (8):

$$\left[C_i \frac{\mathrm{d}U_i}{\mathrm{d}t} + \frac{U_i}{R^{\mathrm{M}}} \right] \left[1 - g_i^{\mathrm{I}} \left(R_i^{\mathrm{B}} + R_i^{\mathrm{C}}\right) \right] - g_i^{\mathrm{I}} U_i = \sum_{j=1}^{p} \alpha_{ij} E_{ij}^{\mathrm{E}} - \beta_i \frac{\mathrm{d}U_i}{\mathrm{d}t} - \gamma_i U_i - \sum_{k=1}^{q} \frac{1}{R_{ik}^{\mathrm{I}}} E_{ik}^{\mathrm{I}}$$

and obtain after some rearrangements

$$\left\{ C_i \left[1 - g_i^{\mathrm{I}} \left(R_i^{\mathrm{B}} + R_i^{\mathrm{C}}\right) \right] + \beta_i \right\} \frac{\mathrm{d}U_i}{\mathrm{d}t} + \frac{1 - g_i^{\mathrm{I}} \left(R_i^{\mathrm{B}} + R_i^{\mathrm{C}} + R^{\mathrm{M}}\right) + R^{\mathrm{M}} \gamma_i}{R^{\mathrm{M}}} U_i = \sum_{j=1}^{p} \alpha_{ij} E_{ij}^{\mathrm{E}} - \sum_{k=1}^{q} \frac{1}{R_{ik}^{\mathrm{I}}} E_{ik}^{\mathrm{I}}$$

and after multiplication with

$$r_i = \frac{R^{\mathrm{M}}}{1 - g_i^{\mathrm{I}} \left(R_i^{\mathrm{B}} + R_i^{\mathrm{C}} + R^{\mathrm{M}}\right) + R^{\mathrm{M}} \gamma_i}$$

the dynamical law for the membrane potential at axon hillock:

$$\tau_i \frac{dU_i}{dt} + U_i = \sum_{j=1}^{p} w_{ij}^{E} E_{ij}^{E} - \sum_{k=1}^{q} w_{ik}^{I} E_{ik}^{I}, \tag{20}$$

where we have introduced the following parameters:

- *time constants*

$$\tau_i = r_i \left\{ C_i \left[1 - g_i^{I} \left(R_i^{B} + R_i^{C} \right) \right] + \beta_i \right\} \tag{21}$$

- *excitatory synaptic weights*

$$w_{ij}^{E} = r_i \alpha_{ij} \tag{22}$$

- *inhibitory synaptic weights*

$$w_{ik}^{I} = \frac{r_i}{R_{ik}^{I}}. \tag{23}$$

Using the result Equation (20), we can also eliminate the temporal derivative in the interface equation Equation (16) through

$$\frac{dU_i}{dt} = \frac{1}{\tau_i} \left[\sum_{j=1}^{p} w_{ij}^{E} E_{ij}^{E} - \sum_{k=1}^{q} w_{ik}^{I} E_{ik}^{I} - U_i \right] \tag{24}$$

which yields

$$I_i^{D} = \sum_{j=1}^{p} \left(\alpha_{ij} - \frac{\beta_i}{\tau_i} w_{ij}^{E} \right) E_{ij}^{E} + \sum_{k=1}^{q} \frac{\beta_i}{\tau_i} w_{ik}^{I} E_{ik}^{I} + \left(\frac{\beta_i}{\tau_i} - \gamma_i \right) U_i.$$

And eventually, by virtue of Equation (7) after multiplication with R_i^{D} the DFP

$$V_i = \sum_{j=1}^{p} \tilde{w}_{ij}^{E} E_{ij}^{E} + \sum_{k=1}^{q} \tilde{w}_{ik}^{I} E_{ik}^{I} + \xi_i U_i, \tag{25}$$

with parameters

$$\tilde{w}_{ij}^{E} = R_i^{D} w_{ij}^{E} \left(\frac{1}{r_i} - \frac{\beta_i}{\tau_i} \right) \tag{26}$$

$$\tilde{w}_{ik}^{I} = R_i^{D} w_{ik}^{I} \frac{\beta_i}{\tau_i} \tag{27}$$

$$\xi_i = R_i^{D} \left(\frac{\beta_i}{\tau_i} - \gamma_i \right). \tag{28}$$

The change in sign of the inhibitory contribution from Equation (20) to Equation (25) has an obvious physical interpretation: In Equation (20), the change of membrane potential U_i and therefore the spike rate is enhanced by EPSPs but diminished by IPSPs. On the other hand, the dendritic shunting current I_i^{D} in Equation (25) is large for both, large EPSPs and large IPSPs.

From Equation (20) we eventually obtain the neural network's dynamics by taking into account that postsynaptic potentials are obtained from presynaptic spike trains through temporal convolution with postsynaptic impulse response functions, i.e.,

$$E_{ij}^{E|I}(t) = \int_{-\infty}^{t} s_i^{E|I}(t - t') R_j(t') \, dt' \tag{29}$$

where $s_i^{E|I}(t)$ are excitatory and inhibitory synaptic impulse response functions, respectively, and R_j is the spike train

$$R_j(t) = \sum_{t_\nu} \delta \left(t - t_\nu - \tau_L \right) \tag{30}$$

coming from presynaptic neuron j, when spikes were emitted at times t_ν. The additional time constant τ_L is attributed to synaptic transmission delay (Mazzoni et al., 2008). These events are obtained by integrating Equation (20) with initial condition

$$U_i \left(t_\nu \right) = E. \tag{31}$$

where E is some steady-state potential (Mazzoni et al., 2008). If at time $t = t_\nu$ the membrane reaches a threshold

$$U_i(t) \geq \theta_i(t) \tag{32}$$

[with possibly a time-dependent activation threshold $\theta_i(t)$] from below $\frac{dU_i(t)}{dt} > 0$ then an output spike $\delta(t - t_\nu)$ is generated, which is then followed by a potential resetting as follows

$$U_i(t_{\nu+1}) \leftarrow E. \tag{33}$$

Additionally, the integration of the dynamical law is restarted at time $t = t_{\nu+1} + \tau_{rp}$ after interrupting the dynamics for a refractory period τ_{rp}.

Inserting Equation (29) into Equation (20) entails the evolution equation of the neural network

$$\tau_i \frac{dU_i}{dt} + U_i = \sum_{j=1}^{p} w_{ij}^{E} s_i^{E}(t) * R_j(t) + \sum_{k=1}^{q} w_{ik}^{I} s_i^{I}(t) * R_k(t), \tag{34}$$

where the signs had been absorbed by the synaptic weights, such that $w_{ij}^{E} > 0$ for excitatory synapses and $w_{ik}^{I} < 0$ for inhibitory synapses, respectively.

Following Mazzoni et al. (2008) an individual postsynaptic current $I_{ij}^{E|I}$ at a synapse between neurons i and j obeys

$$\tau_d^{E|I} \frac{dI_{ij}^{E|I}}{dt} + I_{ij}^{E|I} = x_{ij}^{E|I} \tag{35}$$

$$\tau_r^{E|I} \frac{dx_{ij}^{E|I}}{dt} + x_{ij}^{E|I} = F_{ij}^{E|I}, \tag{36}$$

where $\tau_d^{E|I}$ are decay time constants and $\tau_r^{E|I}$ are rise time constants of EPSC and IPSC, respectively. Auxiliary variables are denoted by

$x_{ij}^{\mathrm{E|I}}$, while $F_{ij}^{\mathrm{E|I}}$ prescribes presynaptic forcing

$$F_{ij}^{\mathrm{E|I}} = \tau_i J_{ij} R_j(t) \quad (37)$$

with spike train Equation (30). Here, $J_{ij} = v w_{ij}^{\mathrm{E|I}}$ denotes synaptic gain with $v = 1$ mV as voltage unit.

Note that Equation (37) is essentially a weighted sum of delta functions, such that a single spike can be assumed as particular forcing

$$F = F_0 \delta(t), \quad (38)$$

with some constant F_0.

Derivating Equation (35) and eliminating $x_{ij}^{\mathrm{E|I}}$ transforms Equations (35, 36) into a linear second-order differential equation with constant coefficients

$$\tau_d^{\mathrm{E|I}} \tau_r^{\mathrm{E|I}} \frac{\mathrm{d}^2 I_{ij}^{\mathrm{E|I}}}{\mathrm{d}t^2} + \left(\tau_d^{\mathrm{E|I}} + \tau_r^{\mathrm{E|I}}\right) \frac{\mathrm{d}I_{ij}^{\mathrm{E|I}}}{\mathrm{d}t} + I_{ij}^{\mathrm{E|I}} = F_{ij}^{\mathrm{E|I}}. \quad (39)$$

Equation (39) with the particular forcing Equation (38) is solved by a Green's function $s_i^{\mathrm{E|I}}(t)$ such that the general solution of Equation (39) is obtained as the temporal convolution

$$I_{ij}^{\mathrm{E|I}}(t) = \int_{-\infty}^{t} s_i^{\mathrm{E|I}}(t - t') F_{ij}^{\mathrm{E|I}}(t)\, \mathrm{d}t'. \quad (40)$$

For $t \neq 0$, Equation (39) assumes its homogeneous form and is easily solved by means of the associated characteristic polynomial

$$\tau_d^{\mathrm{E|I}} \tau_r^{\mathrm{E|I}} \lambda^2 + \left(\tau_d^{\mathrm{E|I}} + \tau_r^{\mathrm{E|I}}\right) \lambda + 1 = 0 \quad (41)$$

with roots $\lambda_1 = -1/\tau_d^{\mathrm{E|I}}$ and $\lambda_2 = -1/\tau_r^{\mathrm{E|I}}$, entailing the Green's functions

$$s_i^{\mathrm{E|I}}(t) = \left(A^{\mathrm{E|I}} \mathrm{e}^{t/\tau_r^{\mathrm{E|I}}} - B^{\mathrm{E|I}} \mathrm{e}^{t/\tau_d^{\mathrm{E|I}}}\right) \Theta(t) \quad (42)$$

with the Heaviside step function $\Theta(t)$.

The constants $A^{\mathrm{E|I}}, B^{\mathrm{E|I}} > 0$ are obtained from the initial conditions $s_i^{\mathrm{E|I}}(t) = 0$, reflecting causality, and a suitable normalization

$$\int_0^{\infty} s_i^{\mathrm{E|I}}(t)\mathrm{d}t = 1.$$

The initial condition yields $A^{\mathrm{E|I}} = B^{\mathrm{E|I}} \equiv S^{\mathrm{E|I}}$, while the remaining constant

$$S^{\mathrm{E|I}} = \frac{1}{\tau_d^{\mathrm{E|I}} - \tau_r^{\mathrm{E|I}}},$$

due to normalization. Therefore, the normalized Green's functions are those of Brunel and Wang (2003)

$$s_i^{\mathrm{E|I}}(t) = v \frac{\tau_i}{\tau_d^{\mathrm{E|I}} - \tau_r^{\mathrm{E|I}}} \left(\mathrm{e}^{t/\tau_r^{\mathrm{E|I}}} - \mathrm{e}^{t/\tau_d^{\mathrm{E|I}}}\right) \Theta(t). \quad (43)$$

Now, we are able to compare our DFP V_i (Equation 25) with the estimate of Mazzoni et al. (2008) which is given (in our notation) as the sums of the moduli of excitatory and inhibitory synaptic currents, i.e.,

$$V_i^{\mathrm{MPLB}} = \sum_j |I_{ij}^{\mathrm{E}}| + \sum_k |I_{ik}^{\mathrm{I}}| \quad (44)$$

where "MPLB" refers to the authors Mazzoni et al. (2008).

From Equations (25) and (44), respectively, we compute two models of the LFP. First, by summing DFP across all pyramidal neurons (beim Graben and Kurths, 2008; Mazzoni et al., 2008), and, second by taking the DFP average (Nunez and Srinivasan, 2006), which yields

$$L_1 = \sum_i V_i^{\mathrm{MPLB}} \quad (45)$$

$$L_2 = \frac{1}{K} \sum_i V_i^{\mathrm{MPLB}} \quad (46)$$

$$L_3 = \sum_i V_i \quad (47)$$

$$L_4 = \frac{1}{K} \sum_i V_i, \quad (48)$$

where K is number of pyramidal neurons.

2.2. PARAMETER ESTIMATION

Next, we relate the electrotonic parameters of our model to the phenomenological parameters of Mazzoni et al. (2008). To this end, we first report their synaptic efficacies in **Table 1**.

From these, we compute the synaptic weights through

$$w_{ij}^{\mathrm{E}} = J_{ij}^{\mathrm{E}}/v = \begin{cases} 0.42 & \text{if } j \text{ "cortical"} \\ 0.55 & \text{if } j \text{ "thalamic"} \end{cases} \quad (49)$$

and

$$w_{ik}^{\mathrm{I}} = J_{ik}^{\mathrm{I}}/v = 1.7$$

Next, we determine the factors r_i by virtue of Equation (23) through

$$r_i = \frac{w_{ik}^{\mathrm{I}}}{\bar{g}_{\mathrm{GABA}}} = \frac{1.7}{1\,\mathrm{nS}} = 1.7\,\mathrm{G}\Omega$$

using the inhibitory synaptic conductivity $\bar{g}_{\mathrm{GABA}} = 1$ nS, correspondingly, Equation (22) allows us to express α_{ij} in terms of the

Table 1 | Parameters laid as in Mazzoni et al. (2008).

Synaptic efficacies/mV	On interneurons	On pyramidal neurons
GABA	2.7	1.7
Recurrent cortical AMPA	0.7	0.42
External thalamic AMPA	0.95	0.55

excitatory synaptic weights through

$$\alpha_{ij} = \frac{w_{ij}^{\mathrm{E}}}{r_i} = \begin{cases} 0.25\,\mathrm{nS} & \text{if } j\text{ "cortical"} \\ 0.32\,\mathrm{nS} & \text{if } j\text{ "thalamic"} \end{cases}$$

From α_{ij} we can determine the total excitatory synaptic conductivities g_i^{E} according to Equation (17) through

$$\alpha_{ij} = \frac{1}{R_{ij}^{\mathrm{E}}\left[1 + g_i^{\mathrm{E}}\left(R_i^{\mathrm{A}} + R_i^{\mathrm{D}}\right)\right]}$$

$$g_i^{\mathrm{E}}\left[1 - \left(R_i^{\mathrm{A}} + R_i^{\mathrm{D}}\right)\sum_{j=1}^{p}\alpha_{ij}\right] = \sum_{j=1}^{p}\alpha_{ij}$$

$$g_i^{\mathrm{E}} = \frac{\sum_{j=1}^{p}\alpha_{ij}}{1 - \left(R_i^{\mathrm{A}} + R_i^{\mathrm{D}}\right)\sum_{j=1}^{p}\alpha_{ij}} \tag{50}$$

and hence

$$R_{ij}^{\mathrm{E}} = \frac{1}{\alpha_{ij}\left[1 + g_i^{\mathrm{E}}\left(R_i^{\mathrm{A}} + R_i^{\mathrm{D}}\right)\right]} \tag{51}$$

Inserting next Equation (18) into Equation (21) yields

$$\tau_i = r_i C_i \frac{1 + g_i^{\mathrm{E}}\left(R_i^{\mathrm{A}} + R_i^{\mathrm{D}}\right) + \left(R_i^{\mathrm{B}} + R_i^{\mathrm{C}}\right)\left\{g_i^{\mathrm{E}} - g_i^{\mathrm{I}}\left[1 + g_i^{\mathrm{E}}\left(R_i^{\mathrm{A}} + R_i^{\mathrm{D}}\right)\right]\right\}}{1 + g_i^{\mathrm{E}}\left(R_i^{\mathrm{A}} + R_i^{\mathrm{D}}\right)}. \tag{52}$$

Equation (52) could constraint the choice of the membrane capacitance C_i by choosing $\tau_i = 20$ ms (Mazzoni et al., 2008).

In order to also determine the DFP parameters Equations (26–28), we finally compute the ratios

$$\frac{\beta_i}{\tau_i} = \frac{g_i^{\mathrm{E}}\left(R_i^{\mathrm{B}} + R_i^{\mathrm{C}}\right)}{r_i\left\{1 + g_i^{\mathrm{E}}\left(R_i^{\mathrm{A}} + R_i^{\mathrm{D}}\right) + \left(R_i^{\mathrm{B}} + R_i^{\mathrm{C}}\right)\left\{g_i^{\mathrm{E}} - g_i^{\mathrm{I}}\left[1 + g_i^{\mathrm{E}}\left(R_i^{\mathrm{A}} + R_i^{\mathrm{D}}\right)\right]\right\}\right\}}.$$

The remaining electrotonic parameters R_i^{M}, R_i^{A}, R_i^{B}, R_i^{C}, and R_i^{D} are estimated from cell geometries as follows. The resistance R of a volume conductor is proportional to its length ℓ and reciprocally proportional to its cross-section A, i.e.,

$$R = \rho\frac{\ell}{A} \tag{53}$$

where ρ is the (specific) resistivity of the medium. **Table 2** shows the resistivities of the three kinds of interest which then allows to evaluate the various volume conductor resistances according to Equation (53).

We consider a total dendritic length of $2\ell = 20\,\mu$m and a dendritic radius of $a = 7\,\mu$m, that are generally subjected to variation. Equally, parameters that were allowed to vary are the length and radius of the axon hillock, yet herein we consider a length of $2\ell = 20\,\mu$m and radius of $a = 0.5\,\mu$m (Mainen et al., 1995; Destexhe, 2001; Kole and Stuart, 2012). To evaluate the intracellular (R_A, R_B) and extracellular (R_D, R_C) resistances, respectively, according to Equation (53), we consider a simple implementation

Table 2 | Resistivities of cell membrane, cell plasma and extracellular space.

Medium	ρ/Ωcm
Cell membrane (at axon hillock)	5×10^7
Cell plasma (cytoplasm)	200
Extracellular space	333

Parameters from Rall (1977); Mainen et al. (1995); Kole and Stuart (2012), and Gold et al. (2007). Note that the resistivity of the cell membrane has to be related to the constant membrane thickness (≈10 nm).

where the length ℓ is half of the dendritic length (i.e., basal and apical length are symmetrical, but this can be broken). However, the cross sectional area for the cytoplasm is simply $A = \pi a^2$. Finally, the area of the axon hillock is simply the surface area of a cylinder.

In order to also determine the cross-section of extracellular space between dendritic trunks we make the following approximations. We assume that dendritic trunks are parallel aligned cylinders of radius a and length ℓ that are hexagonally dense packed. Then the centers of three adjacent trunks form an equilateral triangle with side length $2a$ and hence area $2\sqrt{3}a^2$. The enclosed space is then given by the difference of the triangle area and the area of three sixth circle sectors, therefore

$$A_{\mathrm{space}} = 2\sqrt{3}a^2 - \frac{3}{6}\pi a^2 = \left(2\sqrt{3} - \frac{1}{2}\pi\right)a^2.$$

Hence, the cross-section of extracellular space surrounding one trunk is

$$A = 6A_{\mathrm{space}} = \left(12\sqrt{3} - 3\pi\right)a^2. \tag{54}$$

2.3. SIMULATIONS

Subsequently, we implement an identical network to the one considered by Mazzoni et al. (2008) with *Brian Simulator*, that is a Python-based environment (Goodman and Brette, 2009). However, the derivations from the previous section enables the possibility of setting a dipole observable that measures the local DFP on each pyramidal neurons, given by Equation (25). This allows then to define a mesoscopic LFP observable, which can be equated either as averaged DFP or simply given as the sum of DFP, given by Equations (45–48). Primarily, we compare our LFP measure L_4, proposed as the average of DFP, with the Mazzoni et al. LFP L_1 which is defined as the sum of absolute values of GABA and AMPA currents (Equation 44). Additionally, we also compare all possible measures, namely, mean membrane potential $\frac{1}{K}\sum_i U_i$, Mazzoni et al. LFP L_1, average of Mazzoni et al. DFP L_2, sum of DFP L_3, and the average of DFP L_4.

For completeness, we briefly summarize the description of the network [we refer the reader to Mazzoni et al. (2008) for details]. The network models a cortical tissue with LIF neurons, composed of 1000 inhibitory interneurons and 4000 pyramidal neurons, which are described by the evolution Equation (34). The threshold crossings given by Equation (32) is considered static with

$\theta_i = 18\,\text{mV}$ and the reset potential $E = 11\,\text{mV}$. The refractory period for excitatory neurons is $\tau_{rp} = 2\,\text{ms}$ while for inhibitory neurons it is $\tau_{rp} = 1\,\text{ms}$. The network connectivity is random and sparse with a 0.2 probability of directed connection between any pair of neurons. The evolution of synaptic currents, fast GABA (inhibitory) and AMPA (excitatory) are described via the second order evolution Equations (35, 36), which are activated by incoming presynaptic spikes represented by Equation (30). The latency of the postsynaptic currents is set to $\tau_L = 1\,\text{ms}$ and the rise and decay times are given by **Table 3**.

Moreover, synaptic efficacies, $J_{ij}^{E|I}$, for simulation were presented in **Table 1**. Note that Relation (49) then allows to determine the synaptic weights. Additionally, all neurons receive external thalamic excitatory inputs, that is, via AMPA-type synapses, which are activated by random Poisson spike trains, with a time varying rate that is identical for all neurons. Specifically, the thalamic inputs are the only source of noise, which attempts to account for both cortical heterogeneity and spontaneous activity. This is achieved by modeling a two level noise, where the first level is an Ornstein–Uhlenbeck process superimposed with a constant signal and the second level is a time varying inhomogeneous Poisson process. Thus, we have the following time varying rate, $\lambda(t)$, that feeds into inhomogeneous Poisson process:

$$\tau_n \frac{dn(t)}{dt} = -n(t) + \sigma_n \sqrt{\frac{2}{\tau_n}}\, \eta(t) \quad (55)$$

$$\lambda(t) = [c_0 + n(t)]_+ \quad (56)$$

where $\eta(t)$ represents Gaussian white noise, c_0 represents a constant signal (but equally could be periodic or other), and the operation $[\cdot]$ is the threshold-linear function, $[x]_+ = x$ if $x > 0$, $[x]_+ = 0$ otherwise, which circumvents negative rates. The constant signal c_0 can range between 1.2 and 2.6 spikes/ms. The parameters of the Ornstein–Uhlenbeck process are $\tau_n = 16\,\text{ms}$ and the standard deviation $\sigma_n = 0.4$ spikes/ms.

For complete exposition, we note that from an implementation viewpoint (within the Brian simulator), a copy of the postsynaptic impulse response function (Equation 29) has to be evaluated to calculate the DFP (Equation 25) with weights $\tilde{w}_{ij}^{E|I}$. This implies evaluating the second order process (Equations 35, 36) with a different forcing term. Specifically, starting from $I_{ij}^{E|I}(t) \equiv w_{ij}^{E|I} E_{ij}^{E|I}(t) = s_i^{E|I}(t) * F_{ij}^{E|I}$ and pre-multiplying both sides with $\tilde{w}_{ij}^{E|I}$ and subsequently re-arranging we obtain the desired forcing term $\tilde{F}_{ij}^{E|I} = \tilde{w}_{ij}^{E|I} F_{ij}^{E|I} / w_{ij}^{E|I}$. Note further that by expanding the term $F_{ij}^{E|I}$ with Equation (37) and using Relation (49) we finally obtain $\tilde{F}_{ij}^{E|I} = \tilde{w}_{ij}^{E|I} \tau_i \nu R_j(t)$.

Table 3 | Synaptic rise (τ_r) and decay times (τ_d).

Synaptic times	τ_r/ms	τ_d/ms
GABA	0.25	5
AMPA on interneurons	0.2	1
AMPA on pyramidal neurons	0.4	2

Parameters laid as in Mazzoni et al. (2008).

3. RESULTS

Following Mazzoni et al. (2008), the network simulations are run for 2 s with three different noise levels, specifically, receiving a constant signal with three different rates 1.2, 1.6, and 2.4 spikes/ms as depicted in **Figure 3**. Note that these input rates do not mean that a single neuron fires at these high rates. Rather, it can be obtained from multiple neurons that jointly fire with slower, yet desynchronized, rates converging at the same postsynaptic cell. The Poisson process ensures that this is well represented.

The focus is to compare our proposed measure L_4, defined as mean of the DFP (Equation 48), with the Mazzoni et al. LFP L_1 from Equation (45). In **Figure 3** one sees two main striking differences between the two measures, namely in frequency and in amplitude. Specifically, L_1 responds instantaneously to the spiking network activity by means of high frequency oscillations. Moreover, L_1 also exhibits a large amplitude. In contrast, our mean DFP L_4 measures comparably to experimental LFP, that is, in the order of millivolts, and although it responds to population activity, it has a relatively smoother response. Actually one can realize that our LFP estimate represents low-pass filtered thalamic input.

The physiological relevance of this is not yet clear in our work. However, recent work (Poulet et al., 2012) shows that desynchronized cortical state during active behavior is driven by a centrally generated increase in thalamic action potential firing (i.e., thalamic firing controls cortical states). Thus, it seems that cortical synchronous activity is suppressed when thalamic input increases, thereby suggesting that cortical desynchronized states to be related to sensory processing. This work further quantifies these observations by applying Fast Fourier Transform (FFT) to cortical EEG and subsequently comparing with thalamic firing rate by means of Pearson correlation coefficient. Unfortunately they do not quantify the amount of thalamic oscillations contained within the cortical EEG.

Yet, to keep a comparable comparison between measures, we also compute the average of the Mazzoni et al. DFP L_2 (Equation 48) and additionally the mean membrane potential (the standard considered in the neuroscientific literature). These are shown in **Figure 4**.

Clearly, in terms of time profile, the summed and averaged observables are similar within the same class of LFP measures. However, in all cases the Mazzoni et al. LFP L_1 exhibits a significantly larger order of magnitude, which diverges substantially from experimental LFP amplitudes, typically varying between 0.5 and 2 mV (Lakatos et al., 2005; Niedermeyer, 2005). In contrast, although the mean DFP is not contained within the interval from 0.5 to 2 mV it arguably performs better. However, we do concede further work is required. Some gains in improving the different LFP measures can be achieved by applying for example a weighted average, which would mimic the distance of an electrode to a particular neuron by means of a lead field kernel (Nunez and Srinivasan, 2006). For example, a convolution of either L_1

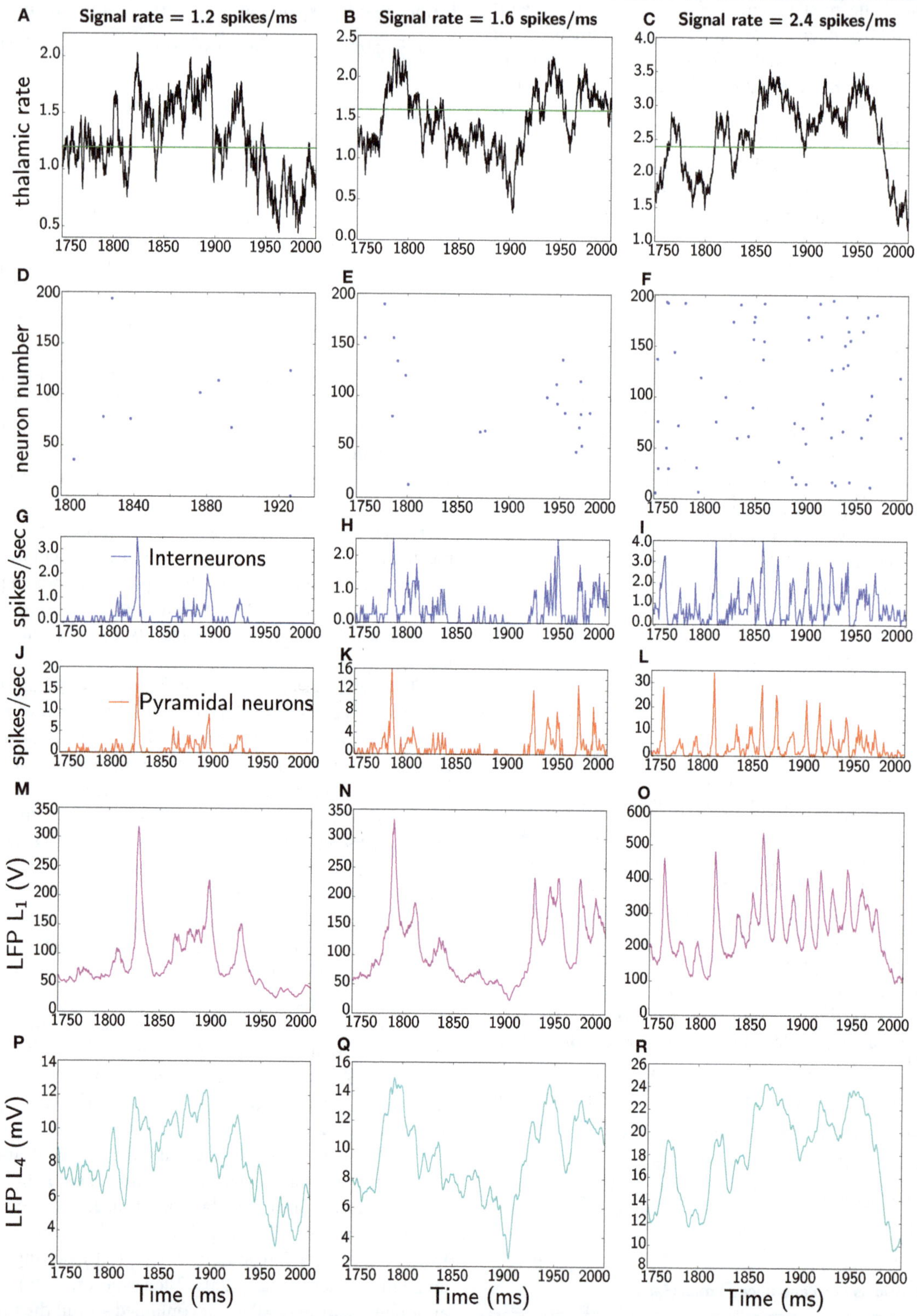

FIGURE 3 | Dynamics of the network and LFP comparisons: the three columns represent different runs of the network for three different rates, 1.2, 1.6, and 2.4 spikes/ms. In each column, all panels show the same 250 ms (extracted from 2 s simulations). The first panels **(A–C)** represent thalamic inputs with the different rates. The second panels **(D–F)** corresponds to a raster plot of the activity of 200 pyramidal neurons. The third panels **(G–I)** depict average instantaneous firing rate (computed on a 1 ms bin) of interneurons (blue) and fourth panels **(J–L)** correspond to average instantaneous firing rate of pyramidal neurons. The fifth panels **(M–O)** show the Mazzoni et al. LFP L_1 from Equation (45). Finally, the last panels **(P–R)** depict our proposed LFP measure L_4, which is the average of dendritic field potential (DFP) (Equation 48).

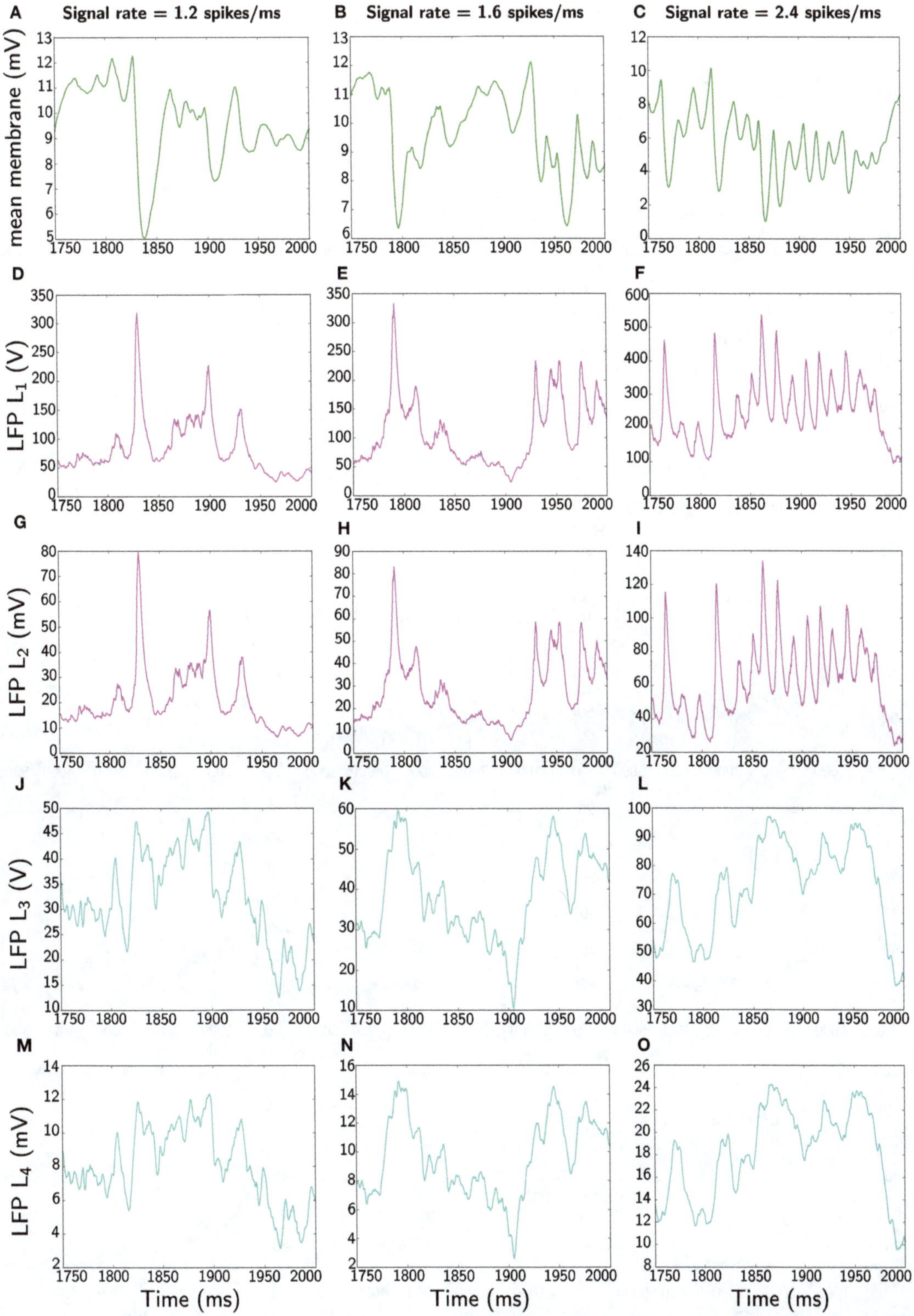

FIGURE 4 | Comparison of different LFP measures when the network receives constant signal with three different rates (1.2, 1.6, and 2.4 spikes/ms). Again, only 250 ms is represented (extracted from 2 s simulation). The first panels **(A–C)** corresponding to the different rates shows the most widespread LFP measure used in the literature, namely average membrane potential $\frac{1}{K}\sum_i U_i$. The second panels **(D–F)** shows the Mazzoni et al. LFP L_1 from Equation (45). The third panels **(G–I)** displays the average of the Mazzoni et al. DFP L_2 (Equation 46). Similarly, the fourth panels **(J–L)** shows the total, L_3, (Equation 47) and the last panels **(M–O)** depicts the averaged, L_4, (Equation 48) LFP measure. Note the different amplitude scales between measures.

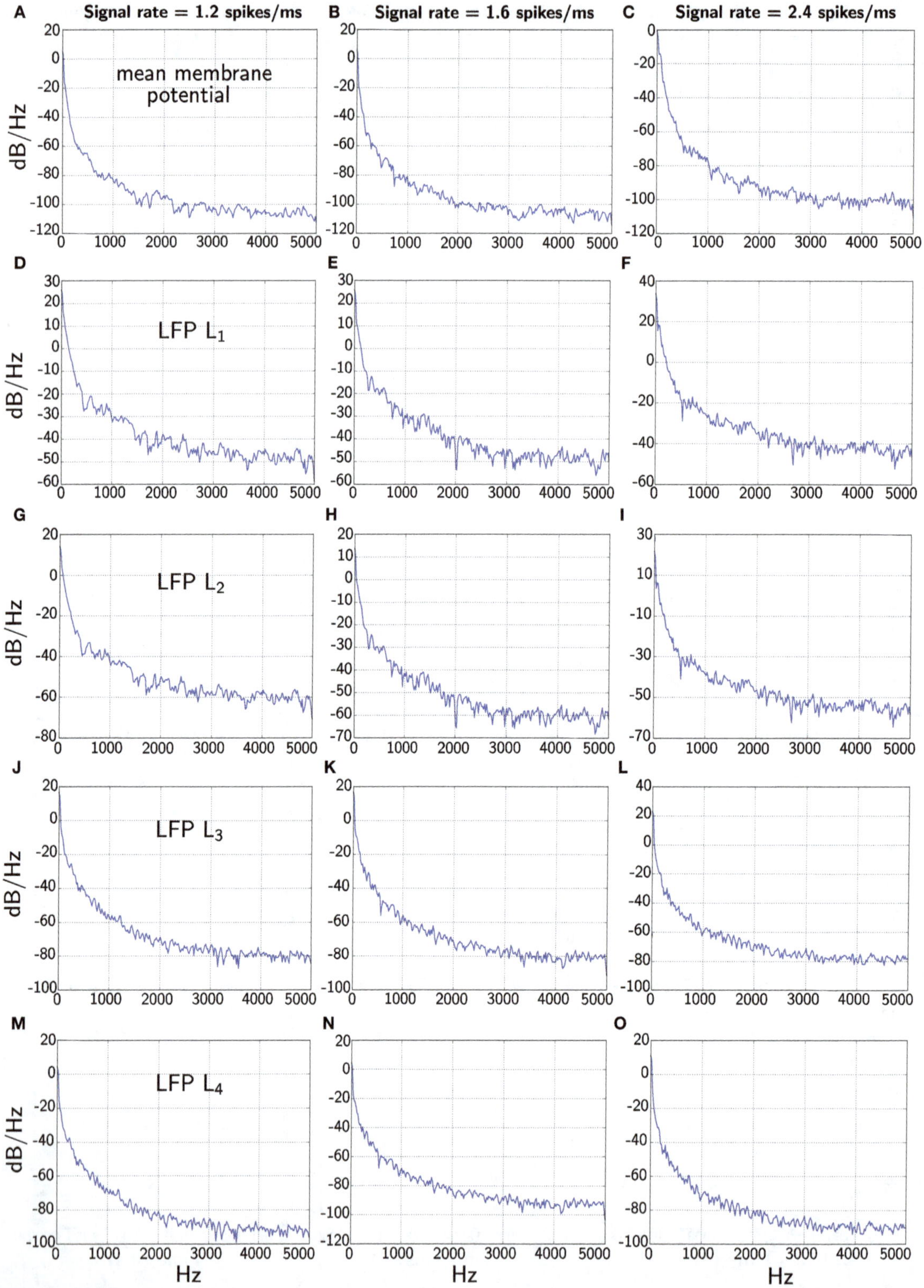

FIGURE 5 | Comparison of power spectra of the various LFP measures when the network receives constant signal with three different rates (1.2, 1.6, and 2.4 spikes/ms). The first panels **(A–C)** corresponding to the different rates shows the power spectrum of the average membrane potential $\frac{1}{K}\sum_i U_i$. The second panels **(D–F)** and third panels **(G–I)** show power spectra of the total and average of L_1 and L_2 corresponding to Mazzoni et al. (2008), respectively. The fourth panels **(J–L)** and the last panels **(M–O)** display power spectra of the L_3 and L_4 measures from our model, respectively. Note we show the full spectrum up to 5 kHz only for convenience due to the fine sample rate.

or L_2 with a Gaussian kernel (representing the distance to a neuron), would yield a measure that captures better the LFP or better the DFP of the nearest neurons. However, further work will be required to properly quantify the gain when space is taken into account.

In **Figure 5** we finally contrast the power spectra of the different LFP measures.

One interesting feature is that the power spectrum of the Mazzoni et al. LFP measures decays much more slowly that the average membrane potential for higher frequencies. This observation is true for both, L_1 and L_2. In contrast, our LFP measures L_3 and L_4 fare better, and in particular, L_4 decays at an approximately similar rate as the average membrane potential.

4. DISCUSSION

In this article we derived a model for cortical dipole fields, such as DFP/LFP from biophysical principles. To that aim we decomposed a cortical pyramidal cell, the putative generator of those potentials, into three compartments: the apical dendritic tree as the place of mainly excitatory (AMPA) synapses, the soma and the perisomatic dendritic tree as the place of mainly inhibitory (GABA) synapses, and the axon hillock as the place of wave-to-spike conversion by means of an integrate-and-fire mechanism. From Kirchhoff's laws governing an electronic equivalent circuit of our model, we were then able to derive the evolution equation for neural network activity (Equation 34) and, in addition, an observation equation (25) for the dendritic dipole potential contributing to the LFP of a cortical population.

In order to compare our approach with another model discussed in the recent literature (Mazzoni et al., 2008, 2010, 2011) we aligned the parameters of our model with the model of Mazzoni et al. (2008) who approximated DFP as the sum of moduli of excitatory and inhibitory synaptic currents (Equation 44). From both approaches, we computed four different LFP estimates: L_1, the sum of Mazzoni et al. DFP, L_2, the population average of Mazzoni et al. DFP, L_3 the sum of our dipole DFP, and L_4 the population average of our dipole DFP (Equations 45–48).

Our results indicate two main effects between our dipole LFP measures and those of Mazzoni et al. Firstly, the measures based on Mazzoni et al. (2008) systematically overestimate LFP amplitude by almost one order of magnitude. One reason for that could be attributed to the direct conversion of synaptic current into voltage without taking extracellular conductivity into account, as properly done in our approach. Yet, another, even more crucial reason is disclosed by our equivalent circuit (**Figure 2**). In our approach there is just *one* extracellular current I^D flowing from the perisomatic to the apical dendritic tree. In the model of Mazzoni et al. (2008), however, two synaptic currents that might be of the same order of magnitude are superimposed to the DFP. Secondly, the measures based on Mazzoni et al. (2008) also systematically overestimate LFP frequencies. This could probably be attributed partly to spurious higher harmonics introduced by computing absolute values. Moreover, taking the power spectrum shows that the Mazzoni et al. (2008) measure decays much more slowly than the average membrane potential, which is at variance with experimental data.

However, at the current stage, both models, that of Mazzoni et al. (2008) and our own, agree with respect to the polarity of DFP and LFP. The measures based on Mazzoni et al. (2008) have positive polarity simply due to the moduli. On the other hand, also the direction of current dipoles in our model is constrained by the construction of the equivalent circuit (**Figure 2**) where current sources are situated at the perisomatic and current sinks are situated at apical dendritic tree. Taking this polarity as positive also entails positive DFP and LFP that could only change in strength. However, it is well known from brain anatomy that pyramidal cells appear in at least two layers, III and VI, of neocortex. This is reflected in experiments when an electrode traverses different layers by LFP polarity reversals, and, of course, by the fact that LFP and EEG oscillate between positive and negative polarity. Adapting our model to this situation could be straightforwardly accomplished in the framework of neural field theory by fully representing space and simulating layered neural fields (Amari, 1977; Jirsa and Haken, 1996; beim Graben, 2008). By contrast such a generalization is impossible at all with the model of Mazzoni et al. (2008) due to the presence of absolute values.

On theses grounds we have good indication that our measure is an improvement to the Mazzoni et al. LFP measures, and, quite importantly, it is biophysically better motivated than the *ad hoc* model of Mazzoni et al. (2008). However, much considerable effort is still required to underpin all the relevant LFP mechanisms and to better represent experimental LFP/EEG dynamics.

Finally, our work provides a new framework where DFPs and the relationship between firing rates and local fields can be explored without the extreme demand on computational complexity involved in multicompartmental modeling (Protopapas et al., 1998; Sargsyan et al., 2001; Lindén et al., 2010; Lindén et al., 2011) by adopting reduced compartment circuits. For example, we envisage to extend our recent work which maps firing rate model (derived from LIF models) to population density models (Chizhov et al., 2007), but now incorporating our observational DFP model. In addition, our framework is analytically amenable and thus can be applied to any linear differential equation, for instance, GIF (Gif-sur-Yvette Integrate Fire) models, which are improvements to the LIF models and compute more accurately spike activations (Rudolph-Lilith et al., 2012). Also resonant membranes (mediated by Ca^{2+} and a Ca^{2+}-activated K^+ ionic currents) that describe sub-threshold oscillations and which can be easily expressed by linear equations (Mauro et al., 1970) can be incorporated in our derivations. We note, however, that our framework can be applied to non-linear equations, with Hodgkin and Huxley (1952) type activation, but it will fall short from explicit and analytical observation equations.

ACKNOWLEDGMENTS

We thank Michelle Lilith, Claude Bédard, Alain Destexhe, and Jürgen Kurths for fruitful discussion. In addition, we would like to thank Samantha Adams for providing help with Brian Simulator installations and initial discussions of Brian usage. This research was supported by a DFG Heisenberg grant awarded to PbG (GR 3711/1-1).

REFERENCES

Amari, S.-I. (1977). Dynamics of pattern formation in lateral-inhibition type neural fields. *Biol. Cybern.* 27, 77–87.

Bédard, C., and Destexhe, A. (2009). Macroscopic models of local field potentials and the apparent 1/*f* noise in brain activity. *Biophys. J.* 96, 2589–2603.

Bédard, C., and Destexhe, A. (2012). "Modeling local field potentials and their interaction with the extracellular medium," in *Handbook of Neural Activity Measurement*, eds R. Brette and A. Destexhe (Cambridge, MA: Cambridge University Press), 136–191.

Bédard, C., Kröger, H., and Destexhe, A. (2004). Modeling extracellular field potentials and the frequency-filtering properties of extracellular space. *Biophys. J.* 86, 1829–1842.

beim Graben, P. (2008). "Foundations of neurophysics," in *Lectures in Supercomputational Neuroscience: Dynamics in Complex Brain Networks*, Springer Complexity Series, eds P. b. Graben, C. Zhou, M. Thiel, and J. Kurths (Berlin: Springer), 3–48.

beim Graben, P., and Kurths, J. (2008). Simulating global properties of electroencephalograms with minimal random neural networks. *Neurocomputing* 71, 999–1007.

Berger, H. (1929). Über das Elektroenkephalogramm des Menschen. *Archiv für Psychiatrie* 87, 527–570.

Brunel, N., and Wang, X.-J. (2003). What determines the frequency of fast network oscillations with irregular neural discharges? I. synaptic dynamics and excitation-inhibition balance. *J. Neurophysiol.* 90, 415–430.

Chizhov, A. V., Rodriguesb, S., and Terryb, J. R. (2007). A comparative analysis of a firing-rate model and conductance-based neural population model. *Phys. Lett. A* 369, 31–36.

Creutzfeldt, O. D., Watanabe, S., and Lux, H. D. (1966a). Relations between EEG phenomena and potentials of single cortical cells. I. evoked responses after thalamic and epicortical stimulation. *Electroencephalogr. Clin. Neurophysiol.* 20, 1–18.

Creutzfeldt, O. D., Watanabe, S., and Lux, H. D. (1966b). Relations between EEG phenomena and potentials of single cortical cells. II. spontaneous and convulsoid activity. *Electroencephalogr. Clin. Neurophysiol.* 20, 19–37.

David, O., and Friston, K. J. (2003). A neural mass model for MEG/EEG: coupling and neuronal dynamics. *Neuroimage* 20, 1743–1755.

Destexhe, A. (2001). Simplified models of neocortical pyramidal cells preserving somatodendritic voltage attenuation. *Neurocomputing* 38–40, 167–173.

Destexhe, A., Mainen, F., and Sejnowski, T. J. (1998). "Kinetic models of synaptic transmission," in *Methods in Neuronal Modelling. From Ions to Networks*, eds C. Koch and I. Segev (Cambridge, MA: MIT Press), 1–25.

Gold, C., Henze, D., and Koch, C. (2007). Using extracellular action potential recordings to constrain compartmental models. *J. Comput. Neurosci.* 23, 39–58.

Goodman, D., and Brette, R. (2009). The Brian simulator. *Front. Neurosci.* 3, 192–197: doi: 10.3389/neuro.01.026.2009

Hodgkin, A. L., and Huxley, A. F. (1952). A quantitative description of membrane current and its application to conduction and excitation in nerve. *J. Physiol.* 117, 500–544.

Holt, G. R., and Koch, C. (1999). Electrical interactions via the extracellular potential near cell bodies. *J. Comput. Neurosci.* 6, 169–184.

Jansen, B. H., and Rit, V. G. (1995). Electroencephalogram and visual evoked potential generation in a mathematical model of coupled cortical columns. *Biol. Cybern.* 73 357–366.

Jirsa, V. K., and Haken, H. (1996). Field theory of electromagnetic brain activity. *Phys. Rev. Lett.* 77, 960–963.

Johnston, D., and Wu, S. M.-S. (1997). *Foundations of Cellular Neurophysiology*. Cambridge, MA: MIT Press.

Koch, C., and Segev, I. (eds.). (1998). *Methods in Neuronal Modelling. From Ions to Networks*, 2nd Edn., Computational Neuroscience. Cambridge, MA: MIT Press.

Kole, M., and Stuart, G. (2012). Signal processing in the axon initial segment. *Neuron* 73, 235–247.

Lakatos, P., Shah, A., Knuth, K., Ulbert, I., Karmos, G., and Schroeder, C. (2005). An oscillatory hierarchy controlling neuronal excitability and stimulus processing in the auditory cortex. *J. Neurophysiol.* 94, 1904–1911.

Lindén, H., Pettersen, K., and Einevoll, G. (2010). Intrinsic dendritic filtering gives low-pass power spectra of local field potentials. *J. Comput. Neurosci.* 29, 423–444.

Lindén, H., Tetzlaff, T., Potjans, T. C., Pettersen, K. H., Grün, S., Diesmann, M., et al. (2011). Modeling the spatial reach of the LFP. *Neuron* 72, 859–872.

Mainen, Z., Joerges, J., Huguenard, J., and Sejnowski, T. (1995). A model of spike initiation in neocortical pyramidal neurons. *Neuron* 15, 1427–1439.

Mauro, A., Conti, F., Dodge, F., and Schor, R. (1970). Subthreshold behavior and phenomenological impedance of the squid giant axon. *J. Gen. Physiol.* 55, 497–532.

Mazzoni, A., Brunel, N., Cavallari, S., Logothetis, N. K., and Panzeri, S. (2011). Cortical dynamics during naturalistic sensory stimulations: experiments and models. *J. Physiol.* 105, 2–15.

Mazzoni, A., Panzeri, S., Logothetis, N. K., and Brunel, N. (2008). Encoding of naturalistic stimuli by local field potential spectra in networks of excitatory and inhibitory neurons. *PLoS Comput. Biol.* 4:e1000239. doi: 10.1371/journal.pcbi.1000239

Mazzoni, A., Whittingstall, K., Brunel, N., Logothetis, N. K., and Panzeri, S. (2010). Understanding the relationships between spike rate and delta/gamma frequency bands of LFPs and EEGs using a local cortical network model. *Neuroimage* 52, 956–972.

Niedermeyer, E. (2005). "The normal EEG of the waking adult," in *Electroencephalography: Basic Principles, Clinical Applications, and Related Fields, 5th Edn*, eds E. Niedermeyer and F. L. D. Silva (Philadelphia, PA: Lippincott Williams & Wilkins), 167–192.

Nunez, P. L., and Srinivasan, R. (2006). *Electric Fields of the Brain: The Neurophysics of EEG*. 2nd Edn. New York, NY: Oxford University Press.

Omurtag, A., Knight, B., and Sirovich, L. (2000). On the simulation of large populations of neurons. *J. Comput. Neurosci.* 8, 51–63.

Poulet, J. F., Fernandez, L. M., Crochet, S., and Petersen, C. C. (2012). Thalamic control of cortical states. *Nat. Neurosci.* 15, 370–372.

Protopapas, A., Vanier, M., and Bower, J. M. (1998). "Simulating large networks of neurons," in *Methods in Neuronal Modelling. From Ions to Networks*, eds C. Koch and I. Segev (Cambridge, MA: MIT Press), 461–498.

Rall, W. (1977). "Core conductor theory and cable properties of neurons," in *Handbook of Physiology – The Nervous System, Cellular Biology of Neurons*, Vol. 1, ed E. R. Kandel (Bethesda, MD: American Physiological Society), 39–97.

Rodrigues, S., Chizhov, A., Marten, F., and Terry, J. (2010). Mappings between a macroscopic neural-mass model and a reduced conductance-based model. *Biol. Cybern.* 102, 361–371.

Rudolph-Lilith, M., Dubois, M., and Destexhe, A. (2012). Analytical integrate-and-fire neuron models with conductance-based dynamics and realistic postsynaptic potential time course for event-driven simulation strategies. *Neural Comput.* 34, 1426–1461.

Sargsyan, A. R., Papatheodoropoulos, C., and Kostopoulos, G. K. (2001). Modeling of evoked field potentials in hippocampal CA1 area describes their dependence on NMDA and GABA receptors. *J. Neurosci. Methods* 104, 143–153.

Schomer, D. L., and Lopes da Silva, F. H. (eds.). (2011). *Niedermayer's Electroencephalography. Basic Principles, Clinical Applications, and Related Fields.* 6th Edn. Philadelphia, PA: Lippincott Williams & Wilkins.

Spruston, N. (2008). Pyramidal neurons: dendritic structure and synaptic integration. *Nat. Rev. Neurosci.* 9, 206–221.

Wang, X.-J., Tegnér, J., Constantinidis, C., and Goldman-Rakic, P. S. (2004). Division of labor among distinct subtypes of inhibitory neurons in a cortical microcircuit of working memory. *Proc. Natl. Acad. Sci. U.S.A.* 101, 1368–1373.

Wendling, F., Bellanger, J. J., Bartolomei, F., and Chauvel, P. (2000). Relevance of nonlinear lumped-parameter models in the analysis of depth-EEG epileptic signals. *Biol. Cybern.* 83, 367–378.

Wilson, H. R., and Cowan, J. D. (1972). Excitatory and inhibitory interactions in localized populations of model neurons. *Biophys. J.* 12, 1–24.

7

Ketamine, propofol and the EEG: A neural field analysis of HCN1-mediated interactions

Ingo Bojak[1,2]*, Harry C. Day[1] and David T. J. Liley[3,4]

[1] *Centre for Computational Neuroscience and Cognitive Robotics, School of Psychology, University of Birmingham, Birmingham, UK*
[2] *Donders Centre for Neuroscience, Donders Institute for Brain, Cognition and Behaviour, Radboud University Nijmegen Medical Centre, Nijmegen, Netherlands*
[3] *Brain and Psychological Sciences Research Centre, Faculty of Life and Social Sciences, Swinburne University of Technology, Hawthorn, VIC, Australia*
[4] *Cortical Dynamics Ltd., Hawthorn, VIC, Australia*

***Correspondence:**
Ingo Bojak, Centre for Computational Neuroscience and Cognitive Robotics, School of Psychology, University of Birmingham, Birmingham West Midlands B15 2TT, UK.
e-mail: i.bojak@bham.ac.uk

Ketamine and propofol are two well-known, powerful anesthetic agents, yet at first sight this appears to be their only commonality. Ketamine is a dissociative anesthetic agent, whose main mechanism of action is considered to be *N*-methyl-d-aspartate (NMDA) antagonism; whereas propofol is a general anesthetic agent, which is assumed to primarily potentiate currents gated by γ-aminobutyric acid type A ($GABA_A$) receptors. However, several experimental observations suggest a closer relationship. First, the effect of ketamine on the electroencephalogram (EEG) is markedly changed in the presence of propofol: on its own ketamine increases θ (4–8 Hz) and decreases α (8–13 Hz) oscillations, whereas ketamine induces a significant shift to beta band frequencies (13–30 Hz) in the presence of propofol. Second, both ketamine and propofol cause inhibition of the inward pacemaker current I_h, by binding to the corresponding hyperpolarization-activated cyclic nucleotide-gated potassium channel 1 (HCN1) subunit. The resulting effect is a hyperpolarization of the neuron's resting membrane potential. Third, the ability of both ketamine and propofol to induce hypnosis is reduced in HCN1-knockout mice. Here we show that one can theoretically understand the observed spectral changes of the EEG based on HCN1-mediated hyperpolarizations alone, without involving the supposed main mechanisms of action of these drugs through NMDA and $GABA_A$, respectively. On the basis of our successful EEG model we conclude that ketamine and propofol should be antagonistic to each other in their interaction at HCN1 subunits. Such a prediction is in accord with the results of clinical experiment in which it is found that ketamine and propofol interact in an infra-additive manner with respect to the endpoints of hypnosis and immobility.

Keywords: ketamine, propofol, EEG, HCN1, neural field theory, drug interaction, anesthesia, infra-additivity

INTRODUCTION

Ketamine, a phenylcyclohexylpiperidine (PCP) derivative, is a powerful psychoactive drug that is predominantly used as a sedative and general anesthetic agent in humans and animals (Sinner and Graf, 2008). Ketamine occurs as two stereoisomers, R(−) and S(+), in which the latter is found to be some three to four times more potent (White et al., 1985), but despite such differences in potency the drug is generally made available clinically as a racemate (racemic mixture) that contains both stereoisomers in equal proportion. Ketamine is classified as a dissociative agent due to its ability to induce hallucinations and perceptual/environmental detachment (Wolff and Winstock, 2006). Because of these properties it has become popular recreationally. At sufficiently high doses it has been reported to induce a state of dissociation comparable to that of schizophrenia, and as a consequence has found use as a pharmacological model for psychosis (Bubenikova-Valesova et al., 2008; Corlett et al., 2011). More recently its therapeutic use has been re-evaluated in light of evidence suggesting that sub-anesthetic doses may aid in the treatment of bipolar affective disorder and major depression (Mathew et al., 2012; Murrough, 2012; Murrough et al., 2012).

While ketamine is widely believed to act principally through the non-competitive antagonism of *N*-methyl-D-aspartate (NMDA) receptor mediated glutamatergic activity (Irifune et al., 1992; Oye et al., 1992), two significant pieces of empirical evidence have emerged that challenge such a unitary view. Firstly, dizocilpine (also known as MK801), an even more potent non-competitive NMDA antagonist, produces no significant hypnotic effect (Kelland et al., 1993; Irifune et al., 2007). Secondly, ketamine's effect on spontaneous electroencephalogram (EEG) activity is qualitatively altered when administered in the presence of propofol, a widely used intravenous general anesthetic agent that, at clinically meaningful concentrations, has little or no effect on NMDA mediated currents. Ketamine alone has been shown to reduce spectral edge frequencies, an effect that is driven predominately by increases in absolute θ band (4–8 Hz) power at the expense of α band (8–13 Hz) power (Schuttler et al., 1987; Kochs et al., 1996), see **Figure 1A**. In contrast, ketamine administered in the presence of steady state propofol levels is associated with a definite acceleration of α band activity; increasing its peak frequency by up to 4.7 Hz (Hayashi et al., 2007; Tsuda et al., 2007), see **Figure 1C**. Propofol on its own roughly maintains the α peak frequency with an

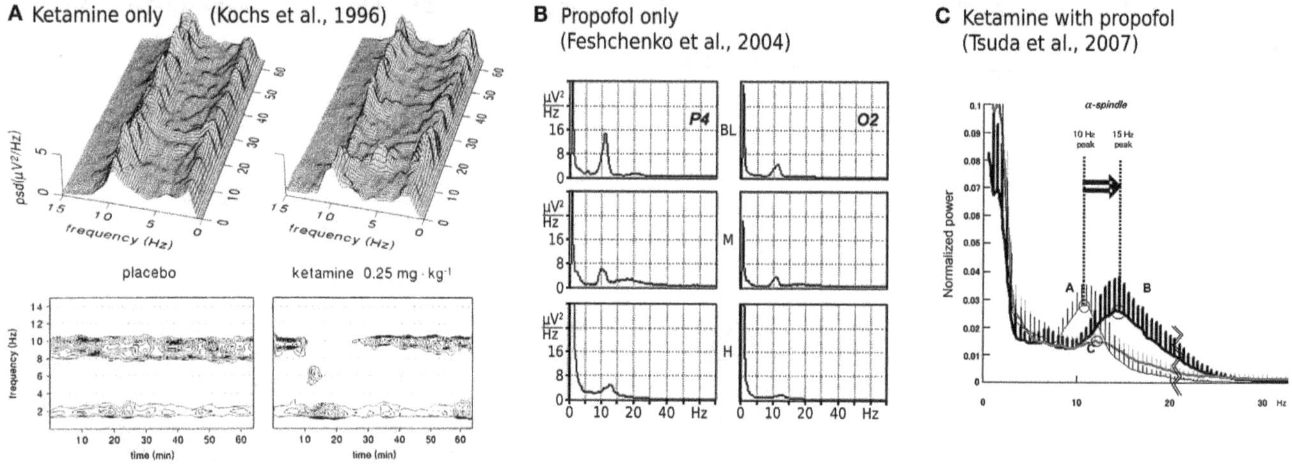

FIGURE 1 | Experimentally described EEG power spectral changes induced by ketamine and propofol. (A) A single bolus dose of ketamine (0.25 mg/kg) is associated with resting α activity being transiently replaced by θ band activity. Data shown is the mean power spectral density (PSD) of EEG recorded in three subjects from a Cz-A1/A2 (vertex-linked ears) montage. Figure adapted and used with permission from Kochs et al. (1996). **(B)** Average spectra of EEG recorded during two sequential target concentrations of propofol in a single subject. BL = baseline, M = 1.25 μg/ml propofol, H = 2.5 μg/ml propofol. α band EEG recorded from parietal (P4) and occipital (O2) electrodes reveals minimal changes in peak frequency with increasing propofol concentration. At medium propofol concentrations (M) the α rhythm shifts to central and frontal areas (figure not shown) without any significant change in frequency. Figure adapted and used with permission from Feshchenko et al. (2004). **(C)** Fifteen minutes after the administration of a ketamine bolus (1 mg/kg; bold line labeled B), in the presence of a steady state target controlled propofol level (3.5 μg/ml; thin line labeled A), peak α band EEG activity is markedly shifted to higher frequencies. Data shown is mean PSD recorded at Fp1-A1, with an Fpz reference, from nine subjects undergoing elective abdominal surgery. Figure used with permission from Tsuda et al. (2007).

anteriorization of power (decrease occipital, increase frontal), see **Figure 1B**; though an additional broadband "beta buzz" just above α frequencies, "biphasic" response dynamics and smooth transitions to lower frequencies can confound the picture (Schwender et al., 1996; Kuizenga et al., 1998, 2001; Feshchenko et al., 2004; Breshears et al., 2010; Cimenser et al., 2011). We assume here from previous theoretical studies (Liley et al., 2003; Hutt and Schimansky-Geier, 2008; Hutt and Longtin, 2010; Hindriks and van Putten, 2012) that these complications can be accounted for by mechanisms not considered in this work, in particular the prominent γ-aminobutyric acid type A ($GABA_A$) agonism of propofol that affects dominantly inhibitory postsynaptic currents (Kitamura et al., 2003). Furthermore, the acceleration due to ketamine observed by Hayashi et al. (2007) and Tsuda et al. (2007) that we wish to describe occurred on top of a clear α rhythm at steady propofol concentration, see **Figure 1C**. Thus we assume in the following that the action of propofol is largely neutral concerning the α peak frequency (while unspecified concerning total α band spectral power).

Recently a number of alternative, behaviorally relevant, molecular targets for ketamine action have been identified (Schnoebel et al., 2005; Hevers et al., 2008; Chen et al., 2009). Of particular significance is the identification of hyperpolarization-activated cyclic nucleotide-gated (HCN) potassium channel subunits as a target for ketamine action (Chen et al., 2009). HCN subunits, of which there are four isoforms (HCN1–4), assemble to form a tetrameric ion channel that mediates an inward (i.e., depolarizing) hyperpolarization-activated pacemaker current I_h implicated in neuronal rhythmogenesis (Biel, 2009; Biel et al., 2009). In particular the HCN1 isoform has been identified as a molecular substrate for the actions of ketamine (Chen et al., 2009): ketamine causes inhibition of HCN1-mediated I_h currents, and hence membrane hyperpolarization, in pyramidal neurons from wild-type but not HCN1-knockout mice. The potency of ketamine to provoke a loss of the righting reflex (the ability to regain footing from a back position), which is a behavioral correlate of hypnosis, is also strongly reduced in HCN1-knockout mice. Hence a causal relationship between ketamine-induced membrane hyperpolarization and its clinical effects can be made. The existence of such a causal relationship is made more likely by evidence indicating that the hypnotic potency of propofol is also reduced in HCN1-knockout mice, in approximate proportion to its ability to inhibit HCN1-mediated membrane depolarization (Chen et al., 2009).

It should be noted though that the hypnotic response was not abolished entirely in HCN1-knockout mice by either ketamine or propofol (Chen et al., 2009), thus other effects like the mentioned $GABA_A$ agonism will be required to fully understand the hypnotic action of these agents. However, etomidate, which has no effect on HCN1 channels, showed no loss of hypnotic effect in HCN1-knockout mice (Chen et al., 2009), suggesting the specific involvement of HCN1-mediated I_h currents for ketamine and propofol. The identification of a shared molecular target for ketamine and propofol action could offer a new possibility to account for the qualitatively disparate electroencephalographic effects of ketamine alone and in the presence of propofol. On this basis we hypothesized that by modeling the differential effects of ketamine and propofol on neuronal membrane hyperpolarization, in the context of an established theory of resting EEG (Liley et al., 2002, 2010, 2011; Bojak and Liley, 2005), we would be able to describe the observed effects on the EEG at least qualitatively. Because current depth of anesthesia monitoring approaches are either insensitive (Faraoni et al., 2009; Nonaka et al., 2012), or respond anomalously (Hans et al., 2005; Sengupta et al., 2011), to the hypnotic effects of ketamine, understanding the mechanism by which ketamine and propofol interact electroencephalographically will ultimately assist in the development of improved approaches to clinically monitor the hypnotic effects of combinations of these drugs. The combination of propofol and ketamine (often referred to as *ketofol*) is becoming increasingly important in the procedural sedation setting where rapid and effective sedation and analgesia, with minimal cardiorespiratory/hemodynamic compromise, is required (Hui et al., 1995; Frizelle et al., 1997; Sakai et al., 1999; Phillips et al., 2010).

MATERIALS AND METHODS

MODELING DRUG RESPONSE AND INTERACTIONS

The simplest pharmacodynamic model of drug effect involving two or more agonists is that of competitive ligand-receptor binding. It is easily shown for two full agonists competing for the same receptor binding site, that the fractional receptor occupancy θ, as a function of the respective drug concentrations (D_1, D_2) is (Shafer et al., 2008)

$$\theta = \frac{k_2 D_1 + k_1 D_2}{k_2 D_1 + k_1 D_2 + k_1 k_2}, \text{ or} \tag{1}$$

$$\frac{\theta}{1-\theta} = \frac{D_1}{k_1} + \frac{D_2}{k_2}. \tag{2}$$

For $D_1 \to \infty$ and/or $D_2 \to \infty$, one then finds $\theta \to 1$, i.e., full receptor occupancy. k_1, $k_2 > 0$ are the respective drug-receptor dissociation constants, which are equivalent to single drug concentrations that produce 50% receptor occupancy, i.e., $\theta = 1/2$. In general a pharmacodynamic effect E is assumed to be some monotonic function of θ, i.e., $E = f(\theta) \equiv g(D_1, D_2)$. For a fixed effect E the locus of points (D_1, D_2) defines a *response isobole* and $E = g(D_1, D_2)$ a *response surface.* Now consider the case of competitive binding and drug interaction (Greco et al., 1995)

$$\frac{\theta}{1-\theta} = \frac{D_1}{k_1} + \frac{D_2}{k_2} + \frac{\eta D_1 D_2}{k_1 k_2}, \tag{3}$$

where η defines an interaction term. It can be easily demonstrated that

$$\begin{aligned} \tfrac{\theta-1}{\theta} < \eta < 0 &\Rightarrow \text{infra-additivity / antagonism,} \\ \eta = 0 &\Rightarrow \text{additivity,} \\ \eta > 0 &\Rightarrow \text{synergy.} \end{aligned} \tag{4}$$

Inspired by these considerations, we chose here to describe the general pharmacodynamic effect of our two ligands by the following bilinear form

$$E = c_1 D_1 + c_2 D_2 + c_{12} D_1 D_2. \tag{5}$$

This ansatz represents the simplest extension beyond the purely additive; and the sign of c_{12} then has the same interpretation as the sign of η in Eq. 4. We will use this bilinear form below to parameterize the dependence of the induced hyperpolarizations on normalized concentrations of propofol and ketamine, respectively.

One can however relate Eqs 3 and 5 more directly. Assume first that the pharmacodynamic effect is directly proportional to receptor occupancy, i.e., $E \propto \theta$. Then k_1 and k_2 become the respective "half maximum effective concentrations" (EC50s) at which 50% of the maximum response is observed for each drug applied alone. Furthermore, assume that the receptor occupancy remains relatively small $\theta \approx \theta/(1-\theta) = D_1/k_1 + D_2/k_2 + \eta D_1 D_2/(k_1 k_2) < 1/2$, so that the effect $E < E_{max}/2$. The half-maximal inhibition of HCN1 subunit-mediated ionic currents by racemic ketamine occurs at a concentration of approximately 16 μM (Chen et al., 2009), which is significantly greater than the estimated minimum free plasma concentrations of 2.9 μM required to produce surgical anesthesia in humans (Grant et al., 1983). Data for the half-maximal inhibition of HCN1-mediated ionic currents by propofol is to our knowledge not available. However, because HCN1-knockout mice are significantly less sensitive to the effects of propofol than wild-type ones, we can speculate that the ED50 (the "half maximum effective dose") for unresponsiveness with propofol in wild-type mice corresponds roughly to the half maximum of the neuronal changes (EC50). Chen et al. (2009) found this to be approximately 7 mg/kg. Using the volume of distribution of 1.38 l/kg (Cox et al., 1998) in the rat (murine values not available), EC50 is then about 5.1 mg/l or 29 μM, which is significantly greater than the minimum free plasma concentration ~8.5 μM for surgical anesthesia. Thus $D_{ketamine}/k_{ketamine} + D_{propofol}/k_{propofol} + \eta D_{ketamine} D_{propofol}/(k_{propofol} k_{ketamine}) < 1/2$ is approximately satisfied as long as $\eta < \frac{1}{2}$. While the E_{max} for ketamine-induced membrane hyperpolarization in murine pyramidal neurons is of the order of -4 mV, the actual value of E_{max} will depend on the species and the recording conditions/preparation. In the absence of any information to the contrary one can assume that $E < E_{max}/2$. Thus our ansatz Eq. 5 can be considered as following from Eq. 3 under a range of reasonable assumptions.

LILEY MODEL AND EIGENSPECTRUM CALCULATION

We base our investigation in this paper on the Liley et al. (2002) model, which is a typical neural field model (Deco et al., 2008; Coombes, 2010; Bressloff, 2012; Liley et al., 2012). In Bojak and Liley (2005) 73,454 different parameter sets, which produce biologically plausible resting state activity, were found for this model. We use here also the "eigenspectrum" approach introduced in Bojak and Liley (2005) to directly predict EEG power spectral densities (PSDs) from a given parameter set. In the following we will briefly review a few key features of the Liley et al. (2002) model and of the eigenspectrum approach that will play a role for the analysis in this paper, and refer the reader to the original reference for more detail. The Liley et al. (2002) model can be written concisely as follows:

$$\tau_k \frac{\partial}{\partial t} h_k(\mathbf{x},t) = h_k^r - h_k(\mathbf{x},t) + \sum_{l=e,i} \frac{h_{lk}^{eq} - h_k(\mathbf{x},t)}{\left|h_{lk}^{eq} - h_k^r\right|} I_{lk}(\mathbf{x},t), \tag{6}$$

$$\left(\frac{1}{\gamma_{lk}}\frac{\partial}{\partial t} + 1\right)^2 I_{lk}(\mathbf{x},t) = \frac{\Gamma_{lk} e}{\gamma_{lk}} \left\{ \frac{N_{lk}^{\beta} S_l^{\max}}{1 + e^{-\sqrt{2}[h_l(\mathbf{x},t) - \mu_l]/\sigma_l}} + \Phi_{lk}(\mathbf{x},t) + p_{lk}(\mathbf{x},t) \right\}, \tag{7}$$

$$\left[\left(\frac{1}{\nu_{lk}\Lambda_{lk}}\frac{\partial}{\partial t} + 1\right)^2 - \frac{3}{2}\frac{1}{\Lambda_{lk}^2}\nabla^2\right] \Phi_{lk}(\mathbf{x},t) = \frac{N_{lk}^{\alpha} S_l^{\max}}{1 + e^{-\sqrt{2}[h_l(\mathbf{x},t) - \mu_l]/\sigma_l}}. \tag{8}$$

In all these equations $l, k = e, i$ serve as indices for excitatory and inhibitory neural populations, respectively, and $\mathbf{x}$ gives their position on a two-dimensional cortical sheet. The mean excitatory soma membrane potential $h_e(\mathbf{x}, t)$ of Eq. 6 is taken to predict the EEG. In the absence of postsynaptic inputs these potentials $h_k(\mathbf{x}, t)$ decay to their resting values h_k^r. The inputs $I_{lk}(\mathbf{x}, t)$ correspond to postsynaptic potentials and are weighted by ionic driving forces $h_{lk}^{\text{eq}} - h_k(\mathbf{x}, t)$, where the h_{lk}^{eq} are the respective Nernst potentials. These weights are normalized at rest to +1 (excitatory) and −1 (inhibitory), respectively. A postsynaptic input in Eq. 7 uses double indices to indicate source and target (for example, $I_{ei}(\mathbf{x}, t)$ is excitatory input to an inhibitory neural population). Γ_{lk} is the mean peak amplitude induced by a single presynaptic pulse $\delta(t - t_p)$, and $1/\gamma_{lk}$ the corresponding rise time to this peak of a postsynaptic "α form" response $I(\mathbf{x}, t) \propto \gamma^2 t e^{-\gamma t}\Theta(t - t_p)$, where Θ is the Heaviside step function and δ the Dirac delta function. Extra-cortical input is given by $p_{lk}(\mathbf{x}, t)$, and is here assumed to be shaped noise (p_{ee}), static (p_{ei}), or absent (p_{ik}). The noise represents the average of uncorrelated input to the many neurons in the neural mass. For simplicity it is imposed only on the excitatory extra-cortical input to excitatory neurons, which is sufficient to generate the full dynamical range of the model. Finally, activity is propagated cortico-cortically via Eq. 8 with a standard damped wave equation (Jirsa and Haken, 1996; Robinson et al., 1997). The activity propagation through $\Phi_{lk}(\mathbf{x}, t)$ represents a synaptic footprint which falls off exponentially with characteristic distance scale Λ_{lk}, and fibers having conduction velocity ν_{lk}. Since there are no long-range inhibitory fibers, we can set $\Phi_{ik} \equiv 0$ in the following. Short range connectivity is both excitatory and inhibitory, and is represented by the first term in the curly brackets of Eq. 7. Note that Eq. 8 can be improved upon (Bojak and Liley, 2010), but its main role is in this case to include a larger variety of EEG wavelengths as will become apparent. Our main conclusions are not affected even for the radical choice of an entirely homogeneous cortex, i.e., upon removing all spatial dependence.

The eigenspectrum approach (Bojak and Liley, 2005) assumes that Eqs 6–8 have a "fixed point" solution for a homogeneous cortex with static p_{ee}. All variables are then linearly expanded around this solution, and auxiliary variables $\tilde{I}_{lk} = \partial I_{lk}/\partial t$ and $\tilde{\Phi}_{ek} = \partial\Phi_{ek}/\partial t$ are used to turn Eqs 6–8 into 14 first order ODEs. One can then Fourier-transform in space and time, and obtains an equation for the 14-dimensional state vector $\mathbf{s}$ in the form

$$i\omega\mathbf{s}(\omega,\mathbf{k}) = \mathbf{J}\left(\mathbf{k}^2\right)\cdot\mathbf{s}(\omega,\mathbf{k}) + \mathbf{P}(\omega,\mathbf{k}), \tag{9}$$

where $\mathbf{J}$ is the Jacobian matrix and $\mathbf{P}(\omega, \mathbf{k})$ contains the remainder of the extra-cortical input, i.e., the variation of p_{ee} with subtracted mean. Note that the only spatial derivative here is the Laplacian in Eq. 8, hence the Fourier-transformed Jacobian is a function of the square of wavenumber $\mathbf{k}$. One can then show (Bojak and Liley, 2005) that

$$|h_e(\omega,k)|^2 = \left|\sum_{n=1}^{14} \frac{c_n(k)}{i\omega - \lambda_n(k)}\right|^2, \tag{10}$$

where both the coefficients c_n and the eigenvalues λ_n can be obtained from a decomposition of the Jacobian in both left and right eigenmatrices, and $k \equiv |\mathbf{k}|$.

Furthermore, if one makes the simplifying assumption that an EEG electrode aggregates the contributions of a disk-shaped part of the cortical sheet with radius R, then one can compute a prediction of the PSD as follows (Bojak and Liley, 2005)

$$PSD(f) = 2\pi R^2 \int_0^{\infty} \frac{dk}{k} J_1^2(kR)\left|h_e(\omega \equiv 2\pi f, k)\right|^2, \tag{11}$$

where J_1 is a Bessel function of the first kind. In practice we evaluate the integral Eq. 11 numerically using a 64 point $0 < k_i < 14.14$/cm Gauss–Legendre quadrature, and hence need to evaluate Eq. 10 for all these $k = k_i$. PSDs calculated in this manner from 10 parameter sets selected out of the 73,454 in Bojak and Liley (2005) are shown in **Figure 2.** We call a solution *stable* if for all 64 $k = k_i$, as well as for homogeneous cortex $k = 0$ cm, the eigenvalues are such that $\forall n$: $\Re\lambda_n(k) < 0$. Only for stable cases do all the approximations leading up to Eq. 11 make sense. The largest contributions to Eq. 10 arise when $\omega = \Im\lambda_n(k)$; and if one disregards the $c_n(k)$, then the "least stable" eigenvalue with largest $\Re\lambda_n(k) < 0$ will contribute most.

Consider now only those λ_m that have non-zero frequencies $f_m \equiv \Im\lambda_m(k = 0/\text{cm})/(2\pi) \neq 0$: due to the selection process (Bojak and Liley, 2005), the "least stable" $\lambda_{\max}$ of these λ_m will have 8 Hz $\leq f_{\max} \leq$ 13 Hz, i.e., a frequency in the α rhythm range. If we change from parameter set $\{\mathbf{P}_1\}$ to $\{\mathbf{P}_2\}$, we can compute the resulting frequency shift $\Delta f \equiv f_{\max}^{\{P_2\}} - f_{\max}^{\{P_1\}}$ of this eigenvalue α frequency. We find that for the parameter changes considered below, this "theoretical" α frequency shift Δf estimated directly from the eigenvalues provides a reasonable approximation for a more "experiment-like" calculation of the α peak shift. In an experiment one would typically seek the maxima of the measured PSDs in the 8–13 Hz range, and then compute their difference in frequency in order to determine an α frequency shift, cf. **Figure 1C** (Hayashi et al., 2007; Tsuda et al., 2007). We can do something similar here by evaluating the full PSDs with Eq. 11 for $\{\mathbf{P}_1\}$ and $\{\mathbf{P}_2\}$, respectively, and then compute the difference of the maxima of these theoretical predictions. However, we use the "theoretical" Δf

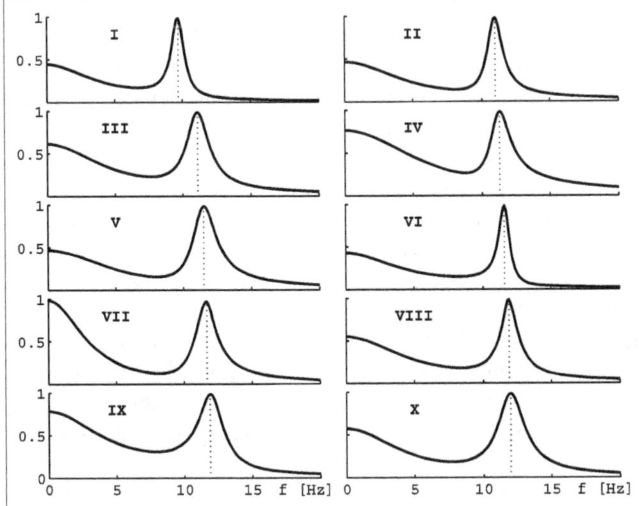

FIGURE 2 | Eigenspectra of 10 parameter sets. The panels show eigenspectra estimated with Eq. 11 from 10 different parameter sets in Bojak and Liley (2005). These 10 sets are selected for the behavior of their α peak frequency under hyperpolarization, see text and **Figures 3B,D**.

Table 1 | α peak frequency shifts predicted from the leading eigenvalue (Δf) and the full PSD, respectively, for the parameter sets of Figure 2.

	Propofol only $P=1.2, K=0$		Ketamine only $P=0, K=1.4$		Both $P=1.2, K=1.4$	
	Δf (Hz)	**PSD (Hz)**	**Δf (Hz)**	**PSD (Hz)**	**Δf (Hz)**	**PSD (Hz)**
I	0.25	0.07	−1.42	−1.70	1.84	1.85
II	0.40	0.29	−1.60	−1.69	2.70	2.61
III	0.24	0.13	−1.37	−1.69	1.91	2.27
IV	0.45	0.37	−1.10	−0.96	2.55	2.54
V	−0.20	−0.21	−1.39	−1.30	1.51	1.40
VI	0.12	−0.18	−1.00	−1.44	1.47	1.44
VII	0.10	0.16	−2.12	−2.11	2.72	2.81
VIII	0.02	−0.15	−1.33	−1.50	1.45	1.59
IX	0.20	−1.46	−1.89	−3.02	2.09	2.05
X	0.15	0.15	−1.38	−1.66	1.86	2.14

P and K are normalized propofol and ketamine concentrations, respectively.

in the following. It is much easier to compute, since it involves only one eigendecomposition for $k=0$/cm compared to 64 for $k=k_i$ needed in the numerical PSD integration Eq. 11. Furthermore, the "theoretical" Δf separates the change of the α peak frequency from other changes to the spectrum. "Experiment-like" calculations of shifts directly from local maxima in the full spectrum can be confounded easily by other spectral changes, and a prior subtraction of the spectral "background" around these maxima would closely match our "theoretical" procedure. For the parameter sets shown in **Figure 2**, a comparison between "theoretical" and "experiment-like" frequency shifts is provided by **Table 1**. How these shifts are generated will be discussed in the following, but note for now that most results are quite similar. The big discrepancies for parameter set IX are caused precisely by a rise of the spectral "background," as discussed.

DRUG EFFECT PARAMETERIZATION AND SELECTION OF SETS

The effect of the action of both ketamine and propofol on HCN1 channels is to hyperpolarize the resting membrane potentials of pyramidal (excitatory) cells (Chen et al., 2009). Consider Eq. 6 in the absence of synaptic inputs $I_{lk}(\mathbf{x},t)\equiv 0$, then $\lim_{t\to\infty} h_k(\mathbf{x},t) = h_k^r$. Thus h_e^r and h_i^r parameterize the excitatory and inhibitory resting membrane potentials, respectively. In the spirit of Eq. 5 we hence use the following ansatz:

$$\Delta h_e^r \equiv h_e^r\big|_{P,K} - h_e^r\big|_{P=K=0} = -\left(a_1 P + a_2 K + a_{12} PK\right) = -\Delta h \cos\theta, \quad (12)$$

$$\Delta h_i^r \equiv h_i^r\big|_{P,K} - h_i^r\big|_{P=K=0} = -\left(b_1 P + b_2 K + b_{12} PK\right) = -\Delta h \sin\theta, \quad (13)$$

where P, K are normalized (dimensionless) concentrations of propofol and ketamine, respectively; and $\Delta h_e^r, \Delta h_i^r$ are changes of the excitatory and inhibitory resting membrane potentials, respectively, due to these drugs. For convenience we have factored out the sign corresponding to hyperpolarization, and we have assumed that inhibitory neurons would react qualitatively like the pyramidal cells, i.e., $\Delta h_e^r, \Delta h_i^r \le 0$ mV in the considered ranges $0 \le P \le P_{\max}$ and $0 \le K \le K_{\max}$, while quantitative differences are expressed by potentially different coefficients. Since the drugs applied individually lead to hyperpolarization, we must have coefficients $a_1, a_2, b_1, b_2 > 0$, whereas the sign of the interaction coefficients a_{12}, b_{12} carries the same meaning as that of η in Eq. 4. In the following it often will be useful to express the "Cartesian" $\Delta h_e^r, \Delta h_i^r \le 0$ mV in the corresponding "polar coordinate" form as $\Delta h \equiv \sqrt{\left(\Delta h_e^r\right)^2 + \left(\Delta h_i^r\right)^2} \ge 0$ mV and $\theta \equiv \arctan \frac{\Delta h_i^r}{\Delta h_e^r} \in [0°, 90°]$.

As a first step, we have investigated which of the 73,454 human α rhythm sets from Bojak and Liley (2005) can be extended viably via Eq. 12 and Eq. 13. Chen et al. (2009) found for rat pyramidal neurons that $\Delta h_e^r = -4.0$ mV for ketamine at 20 μM concentration and $\Delta h_e^r = -3.7$ mV for propofol at 5 μM concentration. Assuming that in humans (and in inhibitory neurons) hyperpolarizations of similar sizes occur, we varied both h_e^r and h_i^r away from their original values in steps of -0.05 mV up to a hyperpolarization of -6 mV, while the remaining parameters were left unchanged. This leads to a grid of 121×121 hyperpolarization combinations $\left(\Delta h_e^r, \Delta h_i^r\right)$, for which we tested whether the changed parameter sets remain stable, i.e., we computed eigendecompositions for $64+1$ values of k and made sure that all eigenvalues had negative real parts. We also calculated the resulting shift in the α peak frequency as compared to the original parameter set in the "theoretical" manner discussed above: $\Delta f(\Delta h_e^r, \Delta h_i^r) \equiv f_{\max}^{\{P(\Delta h_e^r, \Delta h_i^r)\}} - f_{\max}^{\{P(0,0)\}}$.

We find that of the 73,454 parameter sets only 1,627 remain stable for all 121×121 combinations of hyperpolarizations up to -6 mV. This does not mean that the other parameter sets are thereby rejected on biological or physiological grounds;

rather their PSDs cannot be calculated with the eigenspectrum approximation used here, but would have to be estimated from explicit simulations with the fully non-linear Eqs 6–8. This ordinary numerical procedure is several orders of magnitude slower and hence not employed here. **Figure 3A** displays the average $\langle\Delta f(\Delta h_e^r, \Delta h_i^r)\rangle$ over the 1,627 stable sets. The color bar indicates the corresponding frequency values. We can see that in this average there is little effect of Δh_i^r, whereas decreasing Δh_e^r (increasing the hyperpolarization of the pyramidal neurons) leads to an increasingly negative $\langle\Delta f\rangle$. The lowest average value for the 1,627 sets in **Figure 3A** is $\langle\Delta f(-6\,\text{mV}, -6\,\text{mV})\rangle = -2.03$ Hz, whereas the highest is $\langle\Delta f(0\,\text{mV}, -6\,\text{mV})\rangle = 0.336$ Hz.

Since more substantial increases in frequency are expected for the interaction of ketamine and propofol (Hayashi et al., 2007; Tsuda et al., 2007), we introduce the following cut: a set will be kept only if for at least one of the 121 × 121 hyperpolarization combinations $(\Delta h_e^r, \Delta h_i^r)$ we find $\Delta f > 1.6$ Hz. Similarly, since ketamine on its own should introduce a decrease in Δf (Schuttler et al., 1987; Kochs et al., 1996), we require that for at least one other hyperpolarization combination $\Delta f < -0.8$ Hz. Finally, propofol on its own is assumed here to not change the α frequency significantly $\Delta f \approx 0$ Hz (Schwender et al., 1996; Kuizenga et al., 1998, 2001; Feshchenko et al., 2004; Bresheärs et al., 2010; Cimenser et al., 2011), at least not by a HCN1-mediated mechanism, as was discussed in the Introduction. It is more difficult to introduce a simple cut for this property, since for small hyperpolarizations by definition one finds $\Delta f \approx 0$ Hz. We orient ourselves here to $\Delta h_e^r = -3.7$ mV for propofol from Chen et al. (2009), and require that at least for one combination with $\Delta h_i^r \leq -4.3$ mV one has $|\Delta f(-3.7\,\text{mV}, \leq 4.3\,\text{mV})| < 0.4$ Hz. Considered individually, the low frequency cut for ketamine eliminates only 80 parameter sets, whereas the high frequency cut for the interaction of ketamine and propofol leaves only 66 parameter sets. Combining these two cuts then leaves 64 parameter sets in total. Individually, the cut for propofol limiting the frequency shift leaves 149 parameter sets. Combined with the other two cuts, we arrive at 10 parameter sets. Their original PSDs are the ones that were displayed previously in **Figure 2**, and we display their parameter values in **Table A1** in the Appendix. We show the resulting $\langle\Delta f\rangle$, now averaging over only the 10 selected sets, in **Figure 3B**. It is immediately apparent that there are now three zones: for small Δh_e^r but large (negative) Δh_i^r one sees large increases in frequency, for large (negative) Δh_e^r but small Δh_i^r large decreases in frequency, and in between there is a corridor with little change in frequency. This same basic structure is found in all 10 selected sets individually.

Now we can use this structure to determine the coefficients in Eq. 12 and Eq. 13. Starting with the case of giving ketamine only, we can write

$$P = 0 : \tan\theta_K = \frac{b_2}{a_2}. \tag{14}$$

Thus the effect of increasing ketamine concentration in the plane of hyperpolarizations is to move out along a line through the origin with angle θ_K. Ketamine on its own is supposed to deliver shifts to low frequencies, for which we have set a cut $\Delta f < -0.8$ Hz above. We now determine for every hyperpolarization combination how many of the 10 selected parameter sets have $\Delta f\left(\Delta h_e^r, \Delta h_i^r\right) < -0.8$ Hz. This leads to a 121 × 121 grid of values between 0 and 10. In **Figure 3C** this is shown by blue contour lines for 4, 7, and 10 sets fulfilling this cut. We choose the mean of all $\left(\Delta h_e^r, \Delta h_i^r\right)$ in the "maximal fulfillment" (10 sets) region (tip of blue arrow) to determine $\tan\theta_K = 0.315$. Given that we do not know the dependence of hyperpolarizations on ketamine concentrations in humans, we choose $\Delta h_e^r \equiv -4$ mV at $K = 1$ and thus consequently $a_2 \equiv 4$ mV. This implies an unknown normalization $K \equiv c_K/c_K^*$, so that at a ketamine concentration c_K^* one finds $\Delta h_e^r = -4$ mV in humans. Given this choice, we have $b_2 \equiv 1.26$ mV from the ketamine angle $\tan\theta_K = 0.315$. Since $a_2 > b_2$, we can now also find $K_{\max} = (6\,\text{mV})/a_2 = 1.5$ as the largest value for the normalized ketamine concentration for which both hyperpolarizations remain below −6 mV.

In a similar manner we can deal with the case of propofol as the sole drug. Then we find the angular dependence:

$$K = 0 : \tan\theta_P = \frac{b_1}{a_1}. \tag{15}$$

Figure 3C shows contour lines for 4, 7, and 10 parameter sets fulfilling the cut for an α frequency shift $\left|\Delta f\left(\Delta h_e^r, \Delta h_i^r\right)\right| < 0.4$ Hz, this time in green color. Since the cut was evaluated for $\Delta h_e^r = -3.7$ mV only to find these sets, we determine the mean of combinations $\left(\Delta h_e^r \equiv -3.7\,\text{mV}, \Delta h_i^r\right)$ that have "maximal fulfillment" (10 sets) in order to obtain $\tan\theta_P = 1.297$, indicated by the tip of the green arrow. We choose $\Delta h_e^r \equiv -3.7$mV at $P \equiv c_P/c_P^* = 1$, so that $a_1 \equiv 3.7$ mV and at an unknown propofol concentration c_P^* one finds $\Delta h_e^r = -3.7$ mV in humans. Then $b_1 \equiv 4.8$ mV, and since $b_1 > a_1$ it follows that $P_{\max} = (6\,\text{mV})/b_1 = 1.25$.

Finally, **Figure 3C** shows red contour lines for 4, 7, and 10 parameter sets fulfilling $\Delta f(\Delta h_e^r, \Delta h_i^r) > 1.6$ Hz. Again we find the mean of "maximal fulfillment" (10 parameter sets), as indicated by the tip of the red arrow. These mean values are $\Delta\overline{h}_e^r \equiv -0.177$ mV and $\Delta\overline{h}_i^r \equiv -5.903$ mV in this case. We now extend to the −6 mV hyperpolarization limit by setting $\Delta\overline{h}_i^{\max} \equiv -6$ mV and $\Delta\overline{h}_e^{\max} \equiv (-6\,\text{mV})(-0.177\,\text{mV})/(-5.903\,\text{mV}) = -0.180$ mV. We can now solve the following two equations

$$\Delta\overline{h}_e^{\max} = -\left(a_1 P_{\max} + a_2 K_{\max} + a_{12} P_{\max} K_{\max}\right), \tag{16}$$

$$\Delta\overline{h}_i^{\max} = -\left(b_1 P_{\max} + b_2 K_{\max} + b_{12} P_{\max} K_{\max}\right). \tag{17}$$

This will then mean that our entire hyperpolarization grid $-6\,\text{mV} \leq \Delta h_e^r, \Delta h_i^r \leq 0$ mV will be projected onto a rectangular area bounded by $0 \leq P \leq P_{\max}$ and $0 \leq K \leq K_{\max}$, respectively. Solving Eq. 16 and Eq. 17 with our previous results yields $a_{12} = -5.57$ mV and $b_{12} = -1.01$ mV. **Figure 3D** shows the projected $\langle\Delta f(P, K)\rangle$. Clearly the intended α frequency shifts are now achieved: negative ones for only ketamine, none for only propofol, and positives ones for propofol and ketamine together.

RESULTS

We have parameterized the HCN1-mediated hyperpolarizations of neuron membrane potentials in order to reproduce

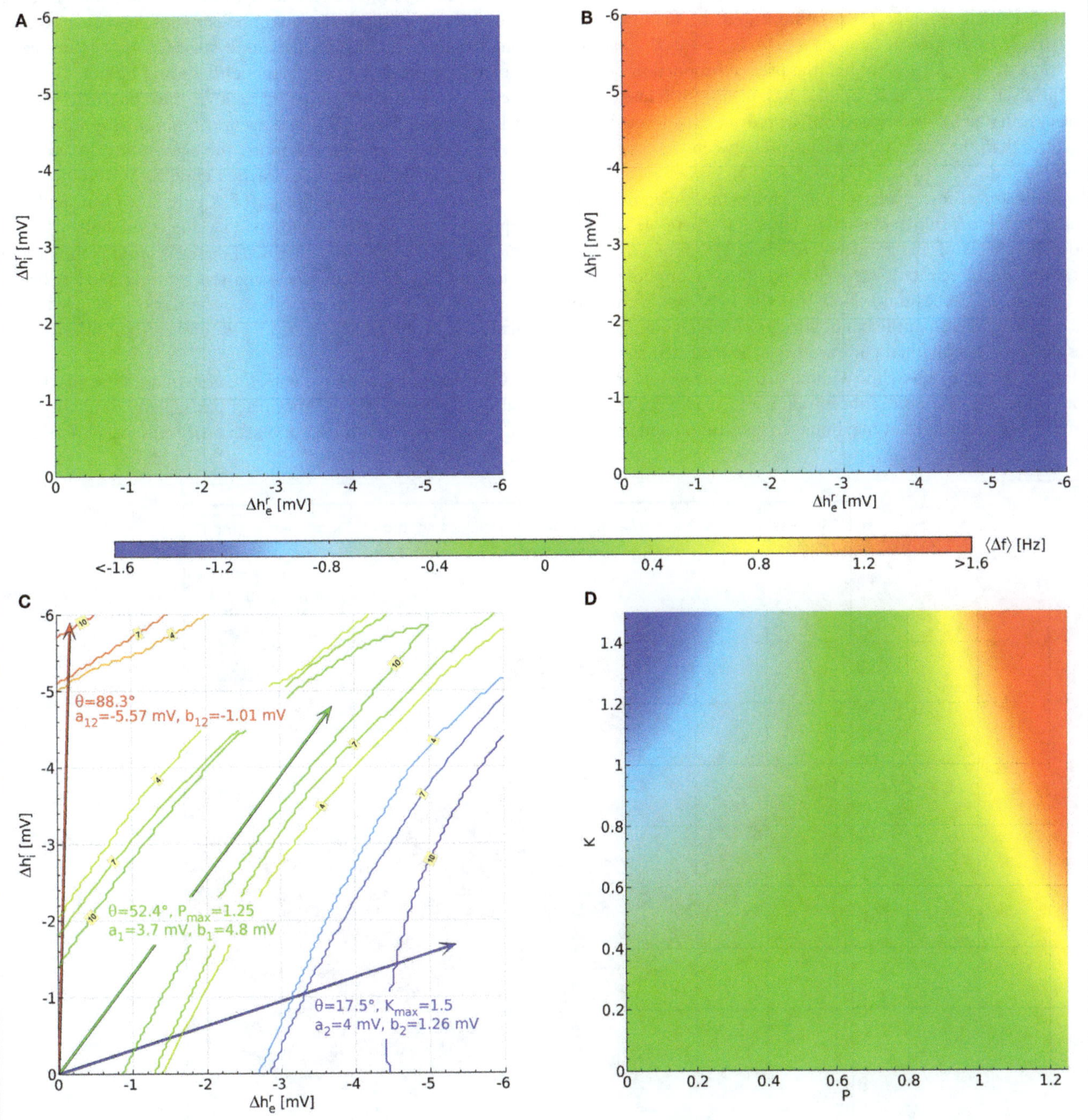

FIGURE 3 | Parameterization of the hyperpolarization effects of propofol and ketamine. (A) Shift of the α peak frequency, average over all 1,627 sets estimated as described below Eq. 11. **(B)** Likewise, but averaged over the 10 sets shown in **Figure 2**, which were selected for having large up ($\Delta f > 1.6$ Hz) and down ($\Delta f < -0.8$ Hz) shifts of α peak frequency, as well as a lack of shift for some large hyperpolarizations ($|\Delta f(-3.7\text{ mV}, \leq 4.3\text{ mV})| < 0.4$ Hz). **(C)** Blue contours indicate areas where 4, 7, or 10 sets have the required down-shift. A blue arrow points to the midpoint of this area, and drug effect parameters for Eq. 12 and Eq. 13 derived from this are listed in blue text. Likewise, parameters are derived for up-shift in red and a lack of shift in green. **(D)** These are the same results as in **(B)**, but now plotted against normalized propofol P and ketamine K concentrations using the drug effect parameters found in **(C)**.

the observed EEG effects of ketamine and propofol, and in particular of their interaction when concurrent. The coefficients that we have obtained for Eqs 12–13 afford the following interpretation: pyramidal neurons react similarly to ketamine and propofol ($a_1 = 0.925 \times a_2$), whereas inhibitory neurons react much more strongly to propofol than to ketamine ($b_1 = 3.81 \times b_2$). Furthermore, and perhaps most interestingly, there is an antagonism of ketamine and propofol (a_{12},

$b_{12} < 0$), which leads to infra-additivity in the investigated effect of HCN1-mediated hyperpolarization, cf. Eq. 4. This antagonism is stronger in pyramidal neurons $a_{12}/(a_1 P_{\max} + a_2 K_{\max}) = 4.10$ $b_{12}/(b_1 P_{\max} + b_2 K_{\max})$, though the precise proportion depends on the given concentrations of the drugs. Intuitively it makes sense however that in inhibitory neurons, where one drug is much more effective than the other, the antagonism between the drugs is less pronounced.

To illustrate these results we look again at the "theoretical" estimates of the α peak frequency in **Figure 4**, where we compare now the effects of changing propofol and ketamine concentration on the 10 selected sets (red) with those computed for all the valid 1,627 sets (gray). Note that the 1,627 sets include the 10 selected ones. Quantile bands are computed to summarize the results for the individual parameter sets, as indicated by the legend. Starting from a baseline without drugs, four phases are being considered: first, propofol concentration is increased linearly; then propofol is maintained at maximum concentration and ketamine concentration is increased linearly; next propofol concentration is decreased linearly while ketamine is maintained at maximum concentration, and finally ketamine concentration is decreased linearly for a return to the baseline. It should be noted that no attempt at modeling the pharmacodynamics/pharmacokinetics of ketamine and propofol drug action beyond drug interaction has been made here. Furthermore, the eigenspectrum approach assumes that the system has reached equilibrium for the given parameters. Thus every single $f_{\max}(P, K)$ predicted here, and consequently every single quantile band value, represents a "steady state" result for that particular drug concentration combination. Hence one can for example view **Figure 4** from right to left, beginning with an increase in ketamine concentration, followed by an increase in ketamine at maximum propofol concentration, and so forth.

Comparing now the red with the gray quantile bands, we see that our cuts selected sets that react particularly dramatically to the concurrence of propofol and ketamine (phases 2 and 3), while

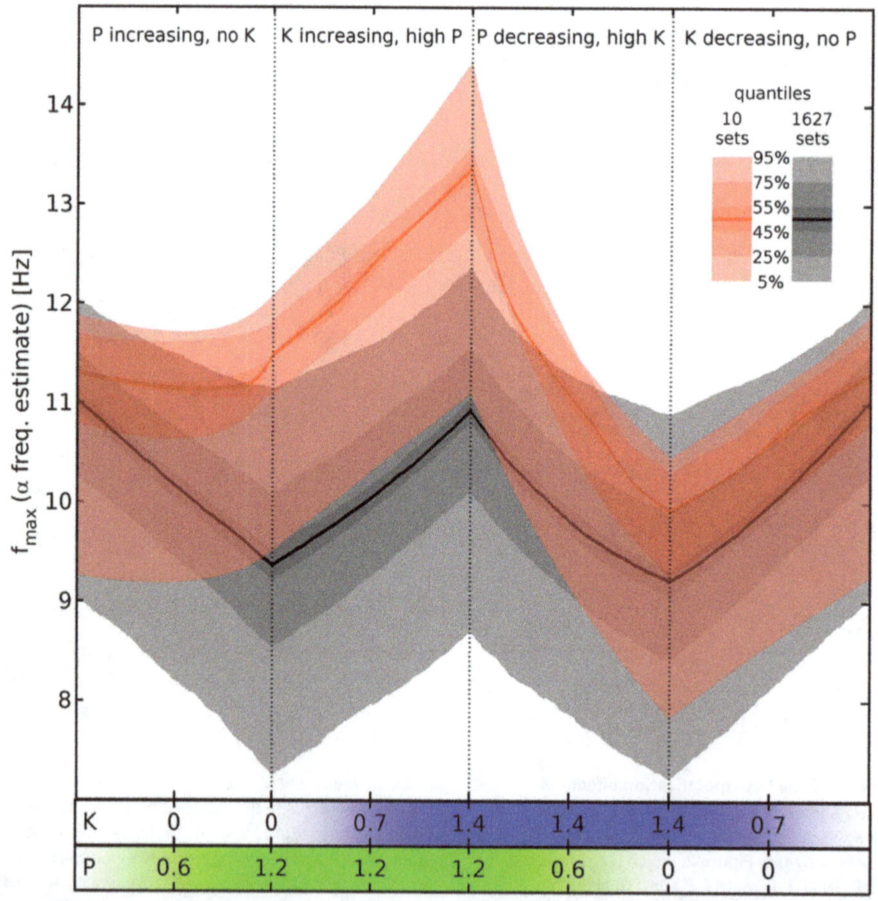

FIGURE 4 | Estimated α peak frequency shifts. Shifts of the α peak frequency for normalized propofol P and ketamine K concentrations estimated as described below Eq. 11, using the hyperpolarizations in Eq. 12 and Eq. 13. Either all 1,627 (gray) or the 10 selected sets (red) are used to compute quantile bands, as indicated by the legend. The median value is shown by a thick black or red line, respectively. There are four phases of drug variation, as indicated by the titles and dotted lines, quantified by bars below the main panel: first, $P = 0 \rightarrow 1.2$ linearly, while $K = 0$. Then $K = 0 \rightarrow 1.4$ linearly, while $P = 1.2$. Next $P = 1.2 \rightarrow 0$, while $K = 1.4$. Finally, $K = 1.4 \rightarrow 0$, while $P = 0$. No pharmacodynamics has been modeled here, so every (P, K) combination yields an independent "steady state" result. Hence for example an increase of P at high K is shown by the third phase viewed from right to left.

being unresponsive to propofol alone (phase 1). Nevertheless, it is not the case that the results for the 1,627 sets show a totally divergent response pattern. In fact, the median rise of estimated α peak frequency in phase 2 (upon introducing ketamine at maximum propofol concentration) is comparable: 1.88 Hz for the selected sets (from 11.48 to 13.36 Hz) vs. 1.56 Hz for all sets (from 9.37 to 10.93 Hz). Thus the predicted boost of α peak frequencies due to the interaction between ketamine and propofol is a robust result for all sets given our drug effect parameterization, which is infra-additive concerning HCN1-mediated hyperpolarization. The main difference appears to be rather that the α peak frequencies of the selected sets do not react significantly to propofol, whereas they are similar to all other sets in the reaction to ketamine and the interaction between these drugs.

Turning to results for full PSDs from Eq. 11, we will consider the 10 selected sets only due to the higher computational demands. **Figure 5** shows results for one individual set (Set III of **Figure 2**) under three variations of drug concentration. In **Figure 5A** we see that as desired and estimated, the α peak frequency stays roughly the same during propofol anesthesia (Schwender et al., 1996; Kuizenga et al., 1998, 2001; Feshchenko et al., 2004; Breshears et al., 2010; Cimenser et al., 2011). The damping seen here would be more characteristic of occipital than frontal regions, though other processes in particular related to the $GABA_A$ agonism could modify these results. The "theoretical" $\Delta f = 0.24$ Hz at $P = 1.2$ is larger than the "experiment-like" shift of 0.13 Hz. In **Figure 5B** we can see the reaction to increasing ketamine concentration. As expected, the α peak gets shifted to lower frequencies. The "theoretical" $\Delta f = -1.37$ Hz estimate at $K = 1.4$ is somewhat lower than the "experiment-like" shift of the local maxima of the PSDs of -1.69 Hz. While the α oscillations get dampened, they contribute to a net increase in the θ frequency range (Schuttler et al., 1987; Kochs et al., 1996) thanks to their downward frequency shift. But one sees also a general rise in power at lower frequencies. **Figure 5C** shows that adding ketamine in the presence of high doses of propofol leads to a shift of the α peak into the beta band, as observed by Hayashi et al. (2007) and Tsuda et al. (2007). The "theoretical" $\Delta f = 1.91$ Hz at $P = 1.2$ and $K = 1.4$ is smaller than the "experiment-like" shift of 2.27 Hz. We predict here an increase in power, unlike the experiment, which observed a small but significant reduction, and our frequency shift of 2.27 Hz is less than half the observed 4.7 Hz. But this could be explained easily by the missing $GABA_A$ and NMDA mechanisms, or the precise circumstances of the experiment. A bolus of ketamine was given by intravenous injection in the experiment, whereas here we calculate "steady state" results. Furthermore, while the frequency shifts from our "theoretical" Δf method are largely in agreement with those obtained from the local α maxima of the PSDs, they do not

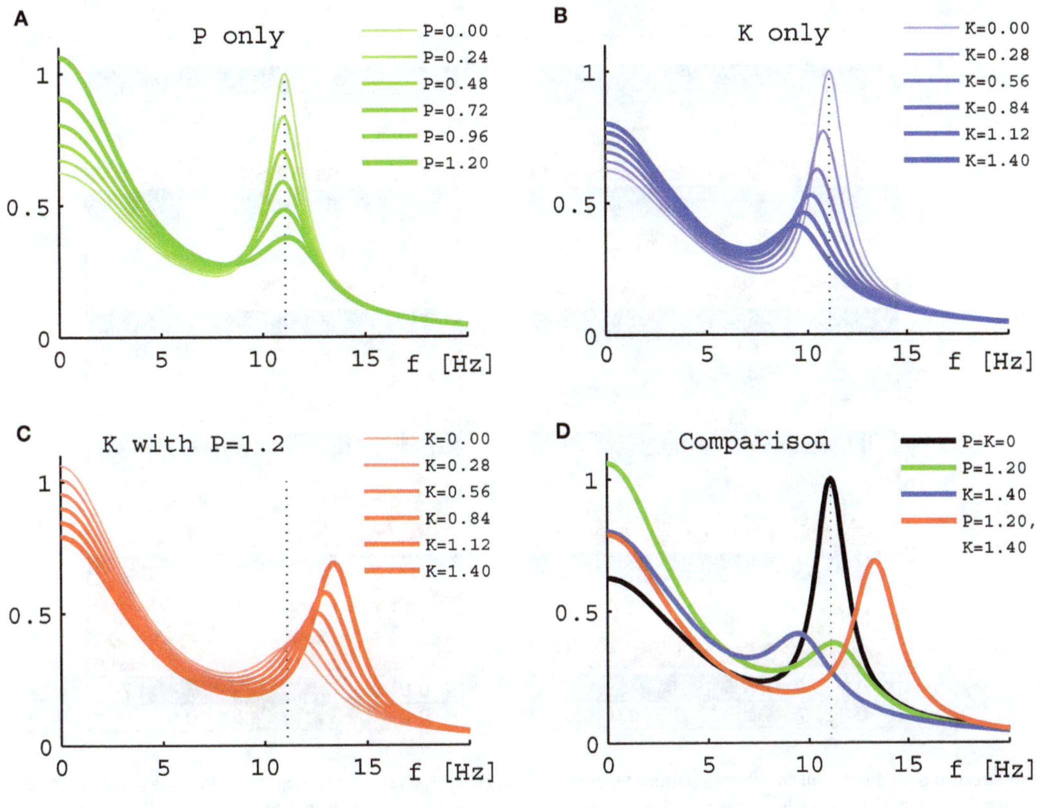

FIGURE 5 | Power spectral densities for Set III under drug variations. **(A)** PSDs for increasing normalized propofol concentration from none (thinnest green line) to 1.2 (thickest green line). **(B)** PSDs for increasing normalized ketamine concentration from none (thinnest blue line) to 1.4 (thickest blue line). **(C)** PSDs for increasing normalized ketamine concentration from none (thinnest red line) to 1.4 (thickest red line), while normalized propofol concentration is held constant at 1.2. **(D)** Comparison of the PSDs representing the highest normalized concentrations from **(A)** in green, **(B)** in blue, and **(C)** in red. The black curve is the PSD without drugs. In all four panels the dotted line represents the position of the α peak of this curve.

agree perfectly – in spite of both being derived using the same eigenspectrum technique. The difference is that by looking at the maxima the results are influenced by changes to the overall spectrum, which provide the "background" on which the α resonance sits. **Table 1** gives Δf and "experiment-like" α peak frequency shifts for the 10 sets at the three highlighted drug concentrations.

Finally, in **Figure 6** we show similar results for all the 10 selected sets. We follow here the same scheme of changing drug concentrations as in **Figure 4**. We see that the α peaks of the full PSDs (here shown in decibels by color) of the individual sets indeed follow the "zigzag" shape we saw in the quantile bands of **Figure 4**. Panel III in **Figure 6** can be directly compared to **Figure 5**, which we have just discussed. For example, **Figure 5A** corresponds to the first phase in panel III here. Overall we see that while the sets clearly change in a similar way, they all have individual features that set them apart from the others. For example, parameter set IV shows particularly strong changes in the low frequency range, whereas parameter set VII reacts with a particularly strong lowering of the α peak frequency in the presence of ketamine. These variations can be considered as representing the variations that one can also observe in humans.

DISCUSSION

We have shown that observed changes of the EEG α peak frequency induced by the presence of the anesthetic agents propofol and ketamine, but in particular also by their interaction when given concurrently, can be explained based on the modeling of HCN1-mediated hyperpolarizations alone, at least qualitatively. This is surprising, since the main mechanism of action of these drugs is supposed to be through NMDA antagonism (ketamine) and $GABA_A$ agonism (propofol), respectively. However, since HCN1-knockout mice are indeed less sensitive to the hypnotic effects of both drugs (Chen et al., 2009), this would indicate that the EEG remains useful as an indicator of anesthetic action. It is perhaps interesting to note that while ketamine is famous for its hallucinatory action (Wolff and Winstock, 2006), and hence is considered a dissociative anesthetic agent, propofol as a classic general anesthetic agent is also capable of inducing a range of hallucinatory phenomena (Balasubramaniam and Park, 2003). Hence it is possible that psychotropic HCN1-mediated effects are simply masked behaviorally more by propofol's $GABA_A$ agonism than by ketamine's NMDA antagonism, but that the EEG is particularly sensitive to these underlying changes.

Only a fraction of all considered parameter sets (1,627 of the 73,454 parameter sets from Bojak and Liley (2005) proved "stable" under the HCN1-mediated hyperpolarization changes up to −6 mV on both excitatory and inhibitory neurons. However, this is at least partly due to the computational methods used here: the eigenspectrum method (Bojak and Liley, 2005) can only be used for "fixed point" dynamics. Rejected sets could follow the

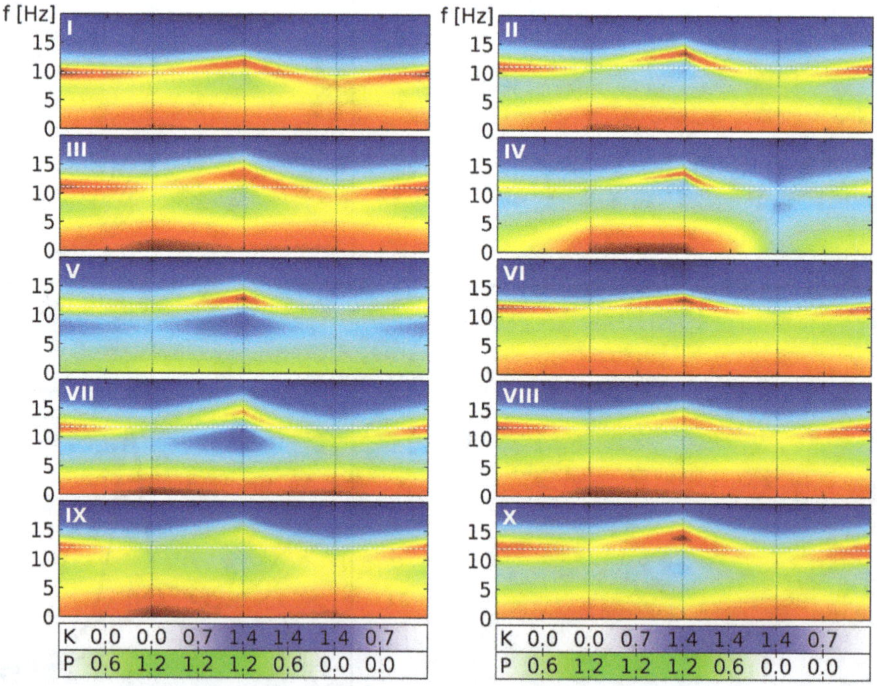

FIGURE 6 | Power spectral densities for all 10 selected parameter sets under drug variation. We use here the same four phases of drug variation as in **Figure 4**, as indicated by the dotted lines and quantified by bars below the main panels: first, $P = 0 \rightarrow 1.2$ linearly, while $K = 0$. Then $K = 0 \rightarrow 1.4$ linearly, while $P = 1.2$. Next $P = 1.2 \rightarrow 0$, while $K = 1.4$. Finally, $K = 1.4 \rightarrow 0$, while $P = 0$. Every panel corresponds to 1 of the 10 selected parameter sets, as indicated by a white roman numeral. The PSD for one specific (P, K) combination is indicated in the panel by a colored vertical line corresponding to frequencies from 0 to 20 Hz. Colors here indicate decibels of the PSD, with dark red corresponding to large, green to medium and dark blue to small values. (The "jet" colormap of Matlab has been mapped for each panel individually, to the full range of PSD decibel values shown in the panel.) A white dashed line indicates the α peak frequency in the absence of drugs.

same kind of drug-induced changes, but be inaccessible with our method chosen for its computational speed. In principle it would be desirable to carry out fully non-linear calculations instead, but under extra-cortical noise input it takes about a minute to estimate a sufficiently detailed and accurate power spectrum on a regular PC. For the 121 × 121 hyperpolarization changes of **Figure 3** that would lead to about 10 days of calculations even for a single parameter set – but we investigate here 73,454 different ones. The eigenspectrum method is several orders of magnitude faster even for a single neural mass. Yet we include here also effects due to the spatial distribution of neural masses, see Eq. 11. The computational load scales roughly linearly with the number of integration points for the eigenspectrum method, but roughly as a square for an equivalent fully non-linear simulation based on spatial grids. This increases the difference in computation speed even further. Thus for the investigations carried out here only the eigenspectrum method proves practicable. In addition, limit cycle or chaotic dynamics are often more representative of seizures or other pathological brain states, which in clinical practice would lead to the termination of the pharmacological intervention that we intend to describe here. Other than by numerical simulation in every single case, we do not know how to determine the characteristics of the dynamics past the point of instability.

Furthermore, our current investigation does not include the NMDA and $GABA_A$ actions commonly assumed to be dominant in these drugs. We speculate that a more complete simulation could allow the use of a larger fraction of the 73,454 parameter sets, since these omitted actions can affect the required stability. A prolongation of the inhibitory postsynaptic potentials due to $GABA_A$, for example, could suppress excessive excitation and thus stabilize a parameter set. These neglected stabilizing effects would increase also in due proportion to the agent concentration, just as the potentially destabilizing hyperpolarizations we have modeled here do. In order to obtain spectral changes that demonstrate clearly the expected frequency shifts, we introduced three further selection cuts, leaving us with only 10 parameter sets out of the 1,627. Again we speculate that NMDA and $GABA_A$ actions may ameliorate this reduction. If this is not the case, then this may point to underlying correlations between neural parameters or functional properties that were not considered in Bojak and Liley (2005), but which now prove crucial for a realistic description. Note that in terms of the hyperpolarizations, cf. **Figures 3B,C**, the non-reactivity to propofol means that for the 10 selected parameter sets an increase in the hyperpolarization of excitatory neurons can be compensated by an increase in the hyperpolarization of inhibitory neurons. This could suggest a particular intrinsic balance of excitation and inhibition maintaining functional stability against extrinsic disturbances.

As is apparent from **Figure 2**, most of our 10 selected sets have relatively high α peak frequencies. However, this simply reflects an underlying bias in the original 73,454 parameter sets, cf. Figure 8 in Bojak and Liley (2005); and we were able to lower base α frequencies through the adjustment of a few parameters (e.g., cortico-cortical connectivity N^{β}_{lk}) within physiological limits, without thereby qualitatively changing the relative frequency shifts due to propofol and ketamine. Other spectral features that could be selected for are also unlikely to affect the α frequency shifts here qualitatively. The constraints used by Bojak and Liley (2005) leave plenty of room for such adjustments: effectively only four out of 14 system eigenvalues were used to establish the "$1/f$" background and the α resonance. Adding a weak beta frequency resonance to enhance realism, for example, would only require the adjustment of two further system eigenvalues. Thus we expect that our results here would hold true if one were to redo the parameter space search of Bojak and Liley (2005) first with additional constraints on the base power spectra. Finally, for concurrent application of propofol and ketamine we predict increases of the α peak frequency of around 2 Hz, falling short of the 4.7 Hz seen experimentally (Hayashi et al., 2007; Tsuda et al., 2007). Yet our calculations were for "steady state" concentrations, and for rapid increases in dosage, as in the experimental injection of a single ketamine bolus here, one often finds a more complex response due the pharmacodynamics and transient neural responses. The so-called biphasic responses to anesthetic agents (Kuizenga et al., 1998, 2001) has received theoretical attention from several groups (Bojak and Liley, 2005; Wilson et al., 2006; Molaee-Ardekani et al., 2007; Hutt and Longtin, 2010; Steyn-Ross and Steyn-Ross, 2010), see also the review in Foster et al. (2008). Hints of such a biphasic response could be visible in **Figure 5** of Tsuda et al. (2007), which shows a significant drop of the α peak shift with time from the initial 4.7 Hz to values around 2 Hz. However, this would have to be disentangled from the decrease in ketamine concentration due to natural clearance after the bolus. We intend to investigate all the mentioned issues in future work.

We found that we could account for the heterogeneous effects of ketamine on the EEG if we assumed that propofol and ketamine interacted in an *infra-additive or antagonistic* manner in their inhibition of HCN1-mediated neuronal membrane hyperpolarization. While most anesthetic and sedative agents are reported to interact synergistically ketamine is well-known to be a major exception (Hendrickx et al., 2008). The interaction between ketamine and $GABA_A$ agonists (most sedative/anesthetic agents) to produce hypnosis is reported to range from additivity to infra-additivity/antagonism (Hendrickx et al., 2008). On the basis of the limited clinical data available it appears that the $GABA_A$ agonist propofol can interact infra-additively to produce a given hypnotic endpoint. For instance Hui et al. (1995), in a study involving 180 female patients presenting for minor gynecological surgery, calculated quantal dose-response curves for propofol and ketamine administered alone and in combination. On the basis of logarithmic regression of a response surface model, it was first suggested that the dose-response for the combination was best explained by additivity, but on reanalysis (Hendrickx et al., 2008), by infra-additivity (significantly so for immobility, as trend for hypnosis). In apparent contradiction, Sakai et al. (1999) claim a significantly additive interaction between propofol and ketamine for the endpoints of unresponsiveness to vocal command and the loss of eyelash reflex. However, the former study determined the probability of a given hypnotic endpoint in response to *single doses* of fixed proportions of ketamine and propofol, whereas the latter gave *continuous infusions* of ketamine and propofol until a given hypnotic endpoint was reached. Another study by Frizelle et al. (1997) used smaller doses of ketamine and targeted a lower level of sedation (rousable to verbal stimuli) with a bolus of propofol and ketamine followed by concomitant infusion. They found no statistical evidence that the addition of ketamine reduced the required amount of propofol to reach their intended sedation level, suggesting once more infra-additivity. Clearly, additional work regarding the pharmacodynamic interactions of ketamine and propofol are required, as it is difficult to reconcile the results of these studies.

The use of neural field/mass approaches to modeling drug action on the EEG is emerging as a powerful explanatory framework (Liley and Bojak, 2005; Foster et al., 2008; Hutt, 2011), which is able to retain meaningful connections to the brain's physiology despite its mesoscopic scale of description. Because neural field/mass models generally have much smaller parameter and state spaces than biophysically plausible neural network models, they are not only much easier to parameterize and simulate, but offer a simpler framework from which to make predictions and derive hypotheses that can be empirically tested. Our ability to account qualitatively for the effects that propofol and ketamine have on the EEG adds to a growing list of phenomena that are amenable to neural field/mass description (Deco et al., 2008; Coombes, 2010; Bressloff, 2012; Liley et al., 2012). Ultimately it is hoped that by accounting for large scale phenomena using neural field/mass models, genuine and enduring insights into brain function and physiology will emerge.

ACKNOWLEDGMENTS

Harry C. Day is supported by a scholarship from the College of Life and Environmental Sciences at the University of Birmingham.

REFERENCES

Balasubramaniam, B., and Park, G. R. (2003). Sexual hallucinations during and after sedation and anaesthesia. *Anaesthesia* 58, 549–553.

Biel, M. (2009). Cyclic nucleotide-regulated cation channels. *J. Biol. Chem.* 284, 9017–9021.

Biel, M., Wahl-Schott, C., Michalakis, S., and Zong, X. (2009). Hyperpolarization-activated cation channels: from genes to function. *Physiol. Rev.* 89, 847–885.

Bojak, I., and Liley, D. T. J. (2005). Modeling the effects of anesthesia on the electroencephalogram. *Phys. Rev. E Stat. Nonlin. Soft Matter Phys.* 71, 041902.

Bojak, I., and Liley, D. T. J. (2010). Axonal velocity distributions in neural field equations. *PLoS Comput. Biol.* 6:e1000653. doi:10.1371/journal.pcbi.1000653

Breshears, J. D., Roland, J. L., Sharma, M., Gaona, C. M., Freudenburg, Z. V., Tempelhoff, R., et al. (2010). Stable and dynamic cortical electrophysiology of induction and emergence with propofol anesthesia. *Proc. Natl. Acad. Sci. U.S.A.* 107, 21170–21175.

Bressloff, P. C. (2012). Spatiotemporal dynamics of continuum neural fields. *J. Phys. A* 45, 033001.

Bubenikova-Valesova, V., Horacek, J., Vrajova, M., and Hoschl, C. (2008). Models of schizophrenia in humans and animals based on inhibition of NMDA receptors. *Neurosci. Biobehav. Rev.* 32, 1014–1023.

Chen, X., Shu, S., and Bayliss, D. A. (2009). HCN1 channel subunits are a molecular substrate for hypnotic actions of ketamine. *J. Neurosci.* 29, 600–609.

Cimenser, A., Purdon, P. L., Pierce, E. T., Walsh, J. L., Salazar-Gomez, A. F., Harrell, P. G., et al. (2011). Tracking brain states under general anesthesia by using global coherence analysis. *Proc. Natl. Acad. Sci. U.S.A.* 108, 8832–8837.

Coombes, S. (2010). Large-scale neural dynamics: simple and complex. *Neuroimage* 52, 731–739.

Corlett, P. R., Honey, G. D., Krystal, J. H., and Fletcher, P. C. (2011). Glutamatergic model psychoses: prediction error, learning, and inference. *Neuropsychopharmacology* 36, 294–315.

Cox, E. H., Knibbe, C. A., Koster, V. S., Langemeijer, M. W., Tukker, E. E., Lange, R., et al. (1998). Influence of different fat emulsion-based intravenous formulations on the pharmacokinetics and pharmacodynamics of propofol. *Pharm. Res.* 15, 442–448.

Deco, G., Jirsa, V. K., Robinson, P. A., Breakspear, M., and Friston, K. J. (2008). The dynamic brain: from spiking neurons to neural masses and cortical fields. *PLoS Comput. Biol.* 4:e1000092. doi:10.1371/journal.pcbi.1000092

Faraoni, D., Salengros, J. C., Engelman, E., Ickx, B., and Barvais, L. (2009). Ketamine has no effect on bispectral index during stable propofol-remifentanil anaesthesia. *Br. J. Anaesth.* 102, 336–339.

Feshchenko, V. A., Veselis, R. A., and Reinsel, R. A. (2004). Propofol-induced alpha rhythm. *Neuropsychobiology* 50, 257–266.

Foster, B. L., Bojak, I., and Liley, D. T. J. (2008). Population based models of cortical drug response: insights from anaesthesia. *Cogn. Neurodyn.* 2, 283–296.

Frizelle, H. P., Duranteau, J., and Samii, K. (1997). A comparison of propofol with a propofol-ketamine combination for sedation during spinal anesthesia. *Anesth. Analg.* 84, 1318–1322.

Grant, I. S., Nimmo, W. S., Mcnicol, L. R., and Clements, J. A. (1983). Ketamine disposition in children and adults. *Br. J. Anaesth.* 55, 1107–1111.

Greco, W. R., Bravo, G., and Parsons, J. C. (1995). The search for synergy: a critical review from a response surface perspective. *Pharmacol. Rev.* 47, 331–385.

Hans, P., Dewandre, P. Y., Brichant, J. F., and Bonhomme, V. (2005). Comparative effects of ketamine on bispectral index and spectral entropy of the electroencephalogram under sevoflurane anaesthesia. *Br. J. Anaesth.* 94, 336–340.

Hayashi, K., Tsuda, N., Sawa, T., and Hagihira, S. (2007). Ketamine increases the frequency of electroencephalographic bicoherence peak on the alpha spindle area induced with propofol. *Br. J. Anaesth.* 99, 389–395.

Hendrickx, J. F., Eger, E. I. II, Sonner, J. M., and Shafer, S. L. (2008). Is synergy the rule? *Anesth. Analg.* 107, 494–506.

Hevers, W., Hadley, S. H., Luddens, H., and Amin, J. (2008). Ketamine, but not phencyclidine, selectively modulates cerebellar GABA(A) receptors containing alpha6 and delta subunits. *J. Neurosci.* 28, 5383–5393.

Hindriks, R., and van Putten, M. J. (2012). Meanfield modeling of propofol-induced changes in spontaneous EEG rhythms. *Neuroimage* 60, 2323–2334.

Hui, T. W., Short, T. G., Hong, W., Suen, T., Gin, T., and Plummer, J. (1995). Additive interactions between propofol and ketamine when used for anesthesia induction in female patients. *Anesthesiology* 82, 641–648.

Hutt, A. (2011). *Sleep and Anesthesia: Neural Correlates in Theory and Experiment.* New York: Springer.

Hutt, A., and Longtin, A. (2010). Effects of the anesthetic agent propofol on neural populations. *Cogn. Neurodyn.* 4, 37–59.

Hutt, A., and Schimansky-Geier, L. (2008). Anesthetic-induced transitions by propofol modeled by non-local neural populations involving two neuron types. *J. Biol. Phys.* 34, 433–440.

Irifune, M., Katayama, S., Takarada, T., Shimizu, Y., Endo, C., Takata, T., et al. (2007). MK-801 enhances gabaculine-induced loss of the righting reflex in mice, but not immobility. *Can. J. Anaesth.* 54, 998–1005.

Irifune, M., Shimizu, T., Nomoto, M., and Fukuda, T. (1992). Ketamine-induced anesthesia involves the N-methyl-D-aspartate receptor-channel complex in mice. *Brain Res.* 596, 1–9.

Jirsa, V. K., and Haken, H. (1996). Field theory of electromagnetic brain activity. *Phys. Rev. Lett.* 77, 960–963.

Kelland, M. D., Soltis, R. P., Boldry, R. C., and Walters, J. R. (1993). Behavioral and electrophysiological comparison of ketamine with dizocilpine in the rat. *Physiol. Behav.* 54, 547–554.

Kitamura, A., Marszalec, W., Yeh, J. Z., and Narahashi, T. (2003). Effects of halothane and propofol on excitatory and inhibitory synaptic transmission in rat cortical neurons. *J. Pharmacol. Exp. Ther.* 304, 162–171.

Kochs, E., Scharein, E., Mollenberg, O., Bromm, B., and Schulte Am Esch, J. (1996). Analgesic efficacy of low-dose ketamine. *Anesthesiology* 85, 304–314.

Kuizenga, K., Kalkman, C. J., and Hennis, P. J. (1998). Quantitative electroencephalographic analysis of the biphasic concentration-effect relationship of propofol in surgical patients during extradural analgesia. *Br. J. Anaesth.* 80, 725–732.

Kuizenga, K., Wierda, J. M., and Kalkman, C. J. (2001). Biphasic EEG changes in relation to loss of consciousness during induction with thiopental, propofol, etomidate, midazolam or sevoflurane. *Br. J. Anaesth.* 86, 354–360.

Liley, D. T., and Bojak, I. (2005). Understanding the transition to seizure by modeling the epileptiform activity of general anesthetic agents. *J. Clin. Neurophysiol.* 22, 300–313.

Liley, D. T., Cadusch, P. J., Gray, M., and Nathan, P. J. (2003). Drug-induced modification of the system properties associated with spontaneous human electroencephalographic activity. *Phys. Rev. E Stat. Nonlin. Soft Matter Phys.* 68, 051906.

Liley, D. T. J., Bojak, I., Dafilis, M. P., Veen, L., Frascoli, F., and Foster, B. L. (2010). "Bifurcations and state changes in the human alpha rhythm: theory and experiment," in *Modeling Phase Transitions in the Brain*, eds D. A. Steyn-Ross, and M. Steyn-Ross (New York: Springer), 117–145.

Liley, D. T. J., Cadusch, P. J., and Dafilis, M. P. (2002). A spatially continuous mean field theory of electrocortical activity. *Network* 13, 67–113.

Liley, D. T. J., Foster, B. L., and Bojak, I. (2011). "A mesoscopic modelling approach to anaesthetic action on brain electrical activity," in *Sleep and Anesthesia: Neural Correlates in Theory and Experiment*, ed. A. Hutt (New York: Springer), 139–166.

Liley, D. T. J., Foster, B. L., and Bojak, I. (2012). "Co-operative populations of neurons: mean field models of mesoscopic brain activity," in *Computational Systems Neurobiology*, ed. N. Le Novère (Dordrecht: Springer), 315–362.

Mathew, S. J., Shah, A., Lapidus, K., Clark, C., Jarun, N., Ostermeyer, B., et al. (2012). Ketamine for treatment-resistant unipolar depression: current evidence. *CNS Drugs* 26, 189–204.

Molaee-Ardekani, B., Senhadji, L., Shamsollahi, M. B., Vosoughi-Vahdat, B., and Wodey, E. (2007). Brain activity modeling in general anesthesia: enhancing local mean-field models using a slow adaptive firing rate. *Phys. Rev. E Stat. Nonlin. Soft Matter Phys.* 76, 041911.

Murrough, J. W. (2012). Ketamine as a novel antidepressant: from synapse to behavior. *Clin. Pharmacol. Ther.* 91, 303–309.

Murrough, J. W., Perez, A. M., Pillemer, S., Stern, J., Parides, M. K., Aan Het Rot, M., et al. (2012). Rapid and longer-term antidepressant effects of repeated ketamine infusions in treatment-resistant major depression. *Biol. Psychiatry.* doi:10.1016/j.biopsych.2012.06.022

Nonaka, A., Makino, K., Suzuki, S., Ikemoto, K., Furuya, A., Tamaki, F., et al. (2012). Low doses of ketamine have no effect on bispectral index during stable propofol-remifentanil anesthesia. *Masui* 61, 364–367.

Oye, I., Paulsen, O., and Maurset, A. (1992). Effects of ketamine on sensory perception: evidence for a role of N-methyl-D-aspartate receptors. *J. Pharmacol. Exp. Ther.* 260, 1209–1213.

Phillips, W., Anderson, A., Rosengreen, M., Johnson, J., and Halpin, J. (2010). Propofol versus propofol/ketamine for brief painful procedures in the emergency department: clinical and bispectral index scale comparison. *J. Pain Palliat. Care Pharmacother.* 24, 349–355.

Robinson, P. A., Rennie, C. J., and Wright, J. J. (1997). Propagation and stability of waves of electrical activity in the cerebral cortex. *Phys. Rev. E Stat. Nonlin. Soft Matter Phys.* 56, 826–840.

Sakai, T., Singh, H., Mi, W. D., Kudo, T., and Matsuki, A. (1999). The effect of ketamine on clinical endpoints of hypnosis and EEG variables during propofol infusion. *Acta Anaesthesiol. Scand.* 43, 212–216.

Schnoebel, R., Wolff, M., Peters, S. C., Brau, M. E., Scholz, A., Hempelmann, G., et al. (2005). Ketamine impairs excitability in superficial dorsal horn neurones by blocking sodium and voltage-gated potassium currents. *Br. J. Pharmacol.* 146, 826–833.

Schuttler, J., Stanski, D. R., White, P. F., Trevor, A. J., Horai, Y., Verotta, D., et al. (1987). Pharmacodynamic modeling of the EEG effects of ketamine and its enantiomers in man. *J. Pharmacokinet. Biopharm.* 15, 241–253.

Schwender, D., Daunderer, M., Mulzer, S., Klasing, S., Finsterer, U., and Peter, K. (1996). Spectral edge frequency of the electroencephalogram to monitor "depth" of anaesthesia with isoflurane or propofol. *Br. J. Anaesth.* 77, 179–184.

Sengupta, S., Ghosh, S., Rudra, A., Kumar, P., Maitra, G., and Das, T. (2011). Effect of ketamine on bispectral index during propofol – fentanyl anesthesia: a randomized controlled study. *Middle East J. Anesthesiol.* 21, 391–395.

Shafer, S. L., Hendrickx, J. F., Flood, P., Sonner, J., and Eger, E. I. II (2008). Additivity versus synergy: a theoretical analysis of implications for anesthetic mechanisms. *Anesth. Analg.* 107, 507–524.

Sinner, B., and Graf, B. M. (2008). Ketamine. *Handb Exp Pharmacol.* 182, 313–333.

Steyn-Ross, A., and Steyn-Ross, M. (2010). *Modeling Phase Transitions in the Brain.* New York: Springer.

Tsuda, N., Hayashi, K., Hagihira, S., and Sawa, T. (2007). Ketamine, an NMDA-antagonist, increases the oscillatory frequencies of alpha-peaks on the electroencephalographic power spectrum. *Acta Anaesthesiol. Scand.* 51, 472–481.

White, P. F., Schuttler, J., Shafer, A., Stanski, D. R., Horai, Y., and Trevor, A. J. (1985). Comparative pharmacology of the ketamine isomers. *Br. J. Anaesth.* 57, 197–203.

Wilson, M. T., Sleigh, J. W., Steyn-Ross, D. A., and Steyn-Ross, M. L. (2006). General anesthetic-induced seizures can be explained by a mean-field model of cortical dynamics. *Anesthesiology* 104, 588–593.

Wolff, K., and Winstock, A. R. (2006). Ketamine: from medicine to misuse. *CNS Drugs* 20, 199–218.

APPENDIX

Table A1 | The 10 selected parameter sets, whose PSDs are shown in Figure 2.

	I	II	III	IV	V	VI	VII	VIII	IX	X
h_e^r (mV)	−68.718	−70.286	−69.774	−78.169	−63.407	−60.745	−67.15	−64.128	−64.061	−60.588
h_i^r (mV)	−71.115	−78.148	−69.325	−79.978	−72.375	−70.488	−79.864	−79.399	−70.777	−69.941
τ_e (ms)	149.16	83.072	125.02	104.53	69.026	86.932	134.75	77.855	96.538	109.63
τ_i (ms)	125.78	122.72	116.58	112.75	118.65	50.200	66.766	137.77	43.662	76.350
h_{ee}^{eq} (mV)	1.8642	−16.433	3.2177	8.7034	−2.5551	1.9520	−18.571	−9.8354	8.4179	0.83573
h_{ei}^{eq} (mV)	−13.716	5.2227	8.2845	−14.231	−17.725	−15.828	−19.572	−4.4417	4.0220	2.4429
h_{ie}^{eq} (mV)	−86.369	−85.969	−86.775	−86.941	−85.466	−83.939	−86.449	−87.012	−82.833	−87.292
h_{ii}^{eq} (mV)	−80.439	−85.348	−77.200	−86.445	−83.047	−79.708	−87.791	−87.906	−78.523	−78.755
Γ_{ee} (mV)	0.22666	0.15856	0.17189	0.11073	0.25964	0.18606	0.31401	0.11187	0.10671	0.15192
Γ_{ei} (mV)	0.72933	1.8661	1.7385	1.8429	1.7030	0.91706	1.7073	1.2797	0.60619	1.7838
Γ_{ie} (mV)	1.9579	1.6800	1.5436	1.6612	1.8285	1.1699	0.53775	1.2751	0.31684	1.2942
Γ_{ii} (mV)	1.0898	0.68575	0.61488	0.53105	0.87001	0.38026	0.10299	0.59535	0.38033	1.2539
γ_{ee} (s^{-1})	768.09	979.20	626.91	494.19	399.13	848.11	964.40	795.80	689.20	355.38
γ_{ei} (s^{-1})	128.26	399.71	357.24	170.95	246.39	219.24	238.50	191.63	224.39	258.87
γ_{ie} (s^{-1})	192.29	178.41	135.36	411.10	251.74	82.043	468.53	221.95	133.21	203.10
γ_{ii} (s^{-1})	57.060	58.091	52.773	53.437	49.217	50.113	43.132	57.302	59.581	49.348
N_{ee}^{β}	3393.0	2552.5	2337.7	4557.9	3571.9	2945.1	2002.9	3941.9	2061.2	2718.0
N_{ei}^{β}	4520.7	4183.2	4168.8	4922.0	4290.5	2771.2	3297.8	4833.0	4357.1	4964.4
N_{ie}^{β}	270.31	674.75	566.64	934.52	927.91	520.26	703.66	838.55	835.88	607.11
N_{ii}^{β}	125.69	453.59	594.80	141.53	472.96	658.36	294.98	890.80	314.72	147.19
N_{ee}^{α}	4223.4	2234.3	4974.3	2517.6	2871.9	2230.2	2678.3	2874.7	4781.7	4128.1
N_{ei}^{α}	2892.3	1559.1	2837.9	2412.1	2952.9	1441.3	1693.6	2896.0	2095.3	2078.7
Λ (cm^{-1})	0.69280	0.27742	0.2529	0.76041	0.16148	0.22388	0.84812	0.56276	0.83448	0.51625
ν (cm^{-1})	116.05	137.60	483.12	158.20	156.22	283.76	483.97	504.36	790.03	325.52
S_e^{max} (s^{-1})	311.08	201.57	474.21	126.59	88.686	103.54	280.25	422.80	190.77	246.41
S_i^{max} (s^{-1})	249.73	280.48	287.93	171.23	227.44	238.74	473.82	294.99	485.67	411.64
$\bar{\mu}_e$(mV)	−45.365	−49.195	−53.432	−54.004	−44.616	−46.851	−46.811	−43.850	−47.622	−51.391
$\bar{\mu}_i$ (mV)	−49.046	−45.093	−51.480	−44.165	−48.954	−47.996	−51.395	−50.619	−42.285	−44.831
$\hat{\sigma}_e$(mV)	6.5908	6.7284	5.2051	6.8209	6.9030	5.9824	5.9045	6.6268	5.6959	5.0919
$\hat{\sigma}_i$ (mV)	4.3224	4.7270	4.4501	4.1542	5.4314	3.0605	5.4229	5.8536	5.6195	6.6326
$\bar{p}_{ee}$ (s^{-1})	7795.9	7344.6	7966.7	5876.2	4496.4	3882.5	6781.8	2649.9	9342.5	2833.6
p_{ei} (s^{-1})	329.39	2554.0	999.87	2120.3	2188.8	2337.9	1196.8	2063.5	914.37	1339.4

8

Modulation of epileptic activity by deep brain stimulation: A model-based study of frequency-dependent effects

Faten Mina[1,2], **Pascal Benquet**[1,2], **Anca Pasnicu**[3], **Arnaud Biraben**[1,2,3] **and Fabrice Wendling**[1,2]*

[1] INSERM, U1099, Universite de Rennes 1, Rennes, France
[2] Laboratoire Traitement du Signal et de L'Image, Université de Rennes 1, Rennes, France
[3] Unité d'Épileptologie, Service de Neurologie, CHU, Rennes, France

Correspondence:
Fabrice Wendling, Laboratoire Traitement du Signal et de L'Image, INSERM, Université de Rennes 1, Campus de Beaulieu, Bat. 22 - 35042 Rennes Cedex, France
e-mail: fabrice.wendling@univ-rennes1.fr

A number of studies showed that deep brain stimulation (DBS) can modulate the activity in the epileptic brain and that a decrease of seizures can be achieved in "responding" patients. In most of these studies, the choice of stimulation parameters is critical to obtain desired clinical effects. In particular, the stimulation frequency is a key parameter that is difficult to tune. A reason is that our knowledge about the frequency-dependant mechanisms according to which DBS indirectly impacts the dynamics of pathological neuronal systems located in the neocortex is still limited. We address this issue using both computational modeling and intracerebral EEG (iEEG) data. We developed a macroscopic (neural mass) model of the thalamocortical network. In line with already-existing models, it includes interconnected neocortical pyramidal cells and interneurons, thalamocortical cells and reticular neurons. The novelty was to introduce, in the thalamic compartment, the biophysical effects of direct stimulation. Regarding clinical data, we used a quite unique data set recorded in a patient (drug-resistant epilepsy) with a focal cortical dysplasia (FCD). In this patient, DBS strongly reduced the sustained epileptic activity of the FCD for low-frequency (LFS, < 2 Hz) and high-frequency stimulation (HFS, > 70 Hz) while intermediate-frequency stimulation (IFS, around 50 Hz) had no effect. Signal processing, clustering, and optimization techniques allowed us to identify the necessary conditions for reproducing, in the model, the observed frequency-dependent stimulation effects. Key elements which explain the suppression of epileptic activity in the FCD include: (a) feed-forward inhibition and synaptic short-term depression of thalamocortical connections at LFS, and (b) inhibition of the thalamic output at HFS. Conversely, modeling results indicate that IFS favors thalamic oscillations and entrains epileptic dynamics.

Keywords: DBS, thalamocortical model, computational, centromedian nucleus, FCD, premotor cortex, epilepsy

INTRODUCTION

Deep brain stimulation (DBS) for Parkinson's disease (PD) and other movement and psychiatric disorders—including dystonia, tremor, and depression—is clinically used today as a conventional therapeutic procedure for the alleviation of symptoms (Sillay and Starr, 2009). Since the early 90s, neurologists also attempted to apply DBS to other neurological disorders, typically to intractable epilepsies in order to suppress—or at least dramatically reduce—the occurrence of seizures [see recent review in Boon et al. (2009)]. These studies followed early scientific evidence showing potentially beneficial effects of DBS on epileptic neural dynamics in animal models (Reimer et al., 1967; Hablitz, 1976) as well as in patients (Cooper et al., 1973; Davis et al., 1982; Wright and Weller, 1983). However, contrary to PD, the optimal "antiepileptic parameters" of DBS for reducing the frequency of seizures are much more variable among patients and the number of non-responders to stimulation still perplexes scientists. Moreover, in responding patients, the fine tuning of stimulation parameters in a patient-specific manner remains indispensable for maximizing antiepileptic effects. On that account, many fundamental questions are frequently raised: where and when to stimulate, at which frequency, at which current intensity, and with which current waveform?

The answers to these questions remain bound to our current, and still limited, understanding of the mechanisms by which DBS modulates neuronal dynamics, whether normal or pathological. Today, the precise mechanisms of neuronal modulation by DBS remain elusive. In addition, these mechanisms are controversial as observed effects are sometimes opposite (McIntyre et al., 2004b). Among the many studies reported over the last decade, identified mechanisms regarding HFS include: local depolarization blockade by HFS (Beurrier et al., 2001), synaptic depression due to neurotransmitter depletion (Shen et al., 2003; Kim et al., 2012), synaptic inhibition (Filali et al., 2004), disruption of

Abbreviations: CMN, Centromedian Nucleus; DBS, Deep Brain Stimulation; EPSP, Excitatory Postsynaptic Potentials; FCD, Focal Cortical Dysplasia; FFI, Feed-Forward Inhibition; GPi, Globus Pallidus; HFS, High Frequency Stimulation; iEEG, Intracerebral EEG (depth electrodes); IFS, Intermediate Frequency Stimulation; IPSP, Inhibitory Postsynaptic Potentials; LFP, Local Field Potential; $LFPs_{FCD}$, Local Field Potentials recorded in the FCD; LFS, Low Frequency Stimulation; NS, No Stimulation; PMC, Premotor cortex; RtN, Reticular thalamic Nucleus, STD, Short-Term Depression; STN, Subthalamic Nucleus.

the thalamocortical network's dysrhythmia (McIntyre and Hahn, 2010; Kendall et al., 2011). As far as LFS is concerned, some studies described a transient synaptic depression that alters synaptic transmission (Jiang et al., 2003; Speechley et al., 2007). Finally, IFS is routinely used in the context of presurgical evaluation of patients with drug resistant epilepsy to map epileptogenic and functional brain areas. It has long been observed that this type of stimulation is prone to trigger epileptic afterdischarges (Goddard, 1967). This brief overview shows that the spectrum of involved mechanisms is very large and that distinct stimulation frequencies trigger distinct cellular/network processes. More precise insights into these processes will come with increased knowledge about both biophysical and neurophysiological effects of stimulation currents on underlying neuronal systems.

However, the access to cellular and network mechanisms induced by DBS is rather difficult in animal models of epilepsy and (almost) impossible in patients especially in large-scale systems like the thalamocortical loop. An alternative approach is the use of computational models based on physiological data to first reproduce and then explain changes in cerebral activity as a function of stimulation conditions (stimulation site, intensity, and frequency). This is precisely the objective of this study, with a special focus on the distinct effects of DBS frequency on cortical epileptic dynamics.

Our investigation combines computational modeling and clinical data. We explored stimulation effects in a lumped-parameter mesoscopic neural mass model of the thalamacortical loop, inspired from previously published models (Suffczynski et al., 2004; Lopes Da Silva, 2006; Roberts and Robinson, 2008; Crunelli et al., 2011).

Although these models are lumped representations of underlying neuronal systems, they offer a number of advantages in the context of this study. First, neural mass models include subpopulations of principal excitatory cells and inhibitory interneurons. Second, these models were shown to produce realistic activity as observed in LFPs or EEG under normal (Freeman, 1973; Lopes Da Silva et al., 1974) or epileptic conditions [review in Lytton (2008); Wendling (2008)]. Third, main parameters (mean membrane potential and firing rate) provide access to the investigation of several stimulation-induced (patho)physiological mechanisms. For instance, a neural mass model was successfully used in the context of direct low-intensity pulse stimulation in the hippocampus to explain the behavior of evoked responses during the transition to seizures (Suffczynski et al., 2008).

In particular, using this model, we analyzed the neurophysiological effects induced by direct thalamic stimulation on epileptic cortical dynamics at low frequency (LF, < 20 Hz), intermediate frequency (IF, 20–70 Hz) and high frequency (HF, 70–130 Hz). Model parameters were tuned to reproduce a typical pathological oscillatory activity observed in a neocortical lesion (focal cortical dysplasia, or FCD) in a patient with drug-resistant epilepsy. Intracerebral EEG (iEEG) signals observed during thalamic stimulation (centromedian nucleus) of this patient revealed particularly pronounced frequency-dependent modulation of the FCD pathological activity. Therefore, this data set offered the unique opportunity to identify key model parameters for which such a frequency-dependent modulation could be reproduced and, subsequently to get insights regarding the mechanisms underlying the modulatory effects, in the FCD, of thalamic stimulation. Results revealed that LFS favors feed-forward inhibition and short-term depression at the cortical level and that HFS inhibits the thalamic activity, while IFS reinforces reticulothalamic oscillations thus entraining cortical pathological epileptic dynamics.

MATERIALS AND METHODS

In this section, we present (1) the neurophysiologically-relevant computational model that we developed to study thalamic DBS, (2) the real depth-EEG dataset used for model tuning and, (3) the signal processing methods used for characterizing real and simulated EEG signals.

MODEL OF THE THALAMOCORTICAL LOOP

In order to study the effects of thalamic DBS on cortical dynamics, we implemented a physiologically-plausible mesoscopic model of the thalamocortical loop. This model accounts for the average activity of both cortical and thalamic compartments which include various types of neuronal populations interacting via synaptic transmission. This modeling approach was first proposed in the early 70s (Wilson and Cowan, 1972) and further enriched in order to interpret electrophysiological recordings and study brain dynamics, in the olfactory (Freeman, 1973) and the thalamocortical (Lopes Da Silva et al., 1974) system, for instance, as well as the dynamics of cortical oscillations (Nunez, 1974). This approach was then developed by other research groups in the context of state changes in brain dynamics (Wright et al., 1985), visual evoked potentials (Jansen et al., 1993), dynamics of the human alpha rhythm (Stam et al., 1999) or pathophysiological mechanisms of ictal transitions in epilepsy (Wendling et al., 2000, 2002; Suffczynski et al., 2001; Robinson et al., 2002; Liley and Bojak, 2005; Breakspear et al., 2006). Later, neural mass models were also used in studies dealing with the connectivity among cortical regions and the impact of model parameters on the power spectrum of EEG or MEG signals (Robinson et al., 1997; David and Friston, 2003; Zavaglia et al., 2006).

Model architecture

The model architecture was inspired from previously published models of the thalamocortical loop (Suffczynski et al., 2004; Lopes Da Silva, 2006; Roberts and Robinson, 2008; Crunelli et al., 2011). In a global view, the model was built of three interconnected compartments: a cortical compartment, a thalamic compartment, and a reticular compartment, in accordance with previously published models (**Figure 1A**) and with anatomical data (**Figure 1B**). Each compartment includes one or several subpopulation(s) of neurons, either excitatory or inhibitory. Generally speaking, the input/output functions of a considered subpopulation are represented by two mathematical equations that were respectively named "pulse-to-wave" (input) and "wave-to-pulse" (output) by Walter Freeman (Freeman, 1992). The former is a linear transfer function that converts the presynaptic average density of afferent action potentials into an average postsynaptic membrane potential (PSP), either excitatory (EPSP) or inhibitory (IPSP). The output function is a static nonlinear function (sigmoid) that

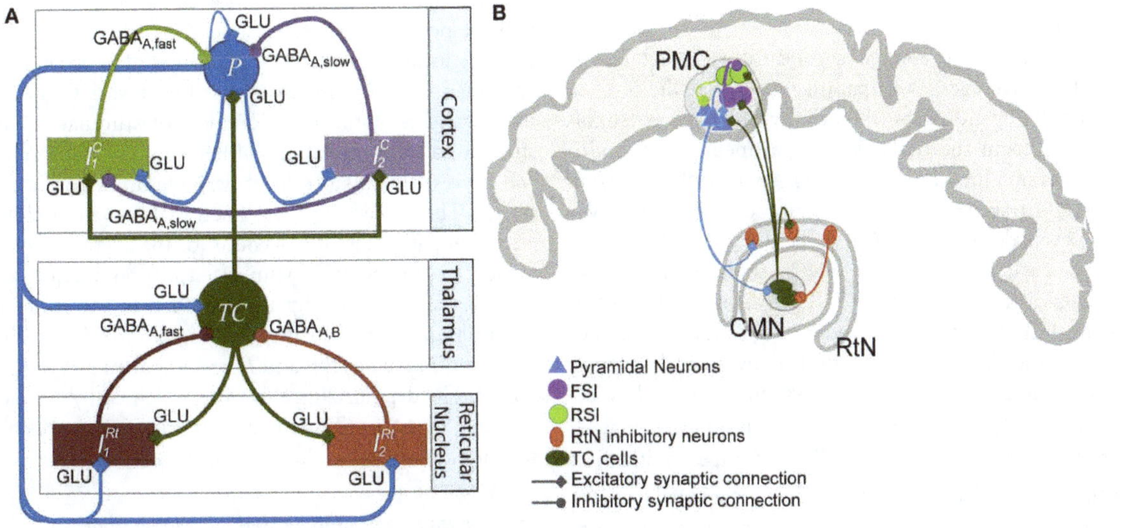

FIGURE 1 | Model of the thalamocortical loop. (A) The model architecture comprises three main compartments: cortical, thalamic, and reticular. The cortical compartment includes three subpopulations: P (pyramidal principal neurons), I_1^C (soma- and proximal-dendrite targeting interneurons mediating $GABA_{A,\ fast}$ currents), and I_2^C, (dendrite-targeting interneurons mediating $GABA_{A,\ slow}$ currents). The thalamic compartment represents a generic thalamic nucleus including a subpopulation of excitatory thalamocortical (*TC*) cells. The reticular nucleus (RtN) compartment is made up of two GABAergic neuronal populations (I_1^{Rt}, $GABA_{A,\ fast}$ currents and I_2^{Rt}, $GABA_{A,\ slow}$). Excitatory synaptic transmission among the considered subpopulations is glutamatergic (GLU). **(B)** *Anatomical connectivity of the CMN, PMC, and RtN.* This diagram represents the anatomy of a particular thalamocortical loop interconnecting the CM thalamic nucleus, the PMC, and the RtN. Connectivity patterns were inferred from the literature. It is compatible with the thalamocortical model diagram presented in **(A)**.

provides the average pulse density of action potentials fired by neurons depending on the sum of EPSPs and IPSPs at the input. This non-linear function accounts for threshold and saturation effects that take place at the somas and initial axonal segments of considered cells.

Formally, the input function is represented by a second order low-pass filter $H(s) = W/(s+1/\tau_w)^2$ (where s is the Laplace variable). The impulse response of this filter is given by

$$h(t) = \frac{W}{\tau_w} \cdot t \cdot e^{-t/\tau_w} \tag{1}$$

Parameters W and τ_w are tuned such that $h(t)$ approximates the shape of real excitatory (glutamatergic) or inhibitory (GABAergic) postsynaptic potentials (Lopes Da Silva et al., 1976). The quantity $W.\tau_w^2$ is the static gain of filter h. Lumped parameter τ_w (expressed in s) is linked to the kinetics of synaptic currents. It determines both the rise time ($t_{rise} = \tau_w$) and the decay time ($t_{decay} = 3.146\tau_w$) of the second order filter impulse response h and it is usually adjusted with respect to the physiological rise and decay times of actual PSPs (Molaee-Ardekani et al., 2010). Given the time constantτ_w, parameter W can be used to adjust the sensitivity of synapses (the maximal PSP amplitude is $W.e^{-1}$). An alternative implementation of the h function was introduced in Bojak and Liley (2005) and is described in detail in Molaee-Ardekani et al. (2013). It is based on a bi-exponential pulse-to-wave function with two time constant parameters. This implementation allows for the separate adjustment of the rise and decay times of PSPs, and therefore a better approximation of actual PSPs in some circumstances. Besides, the output function is represented by $S(v) = \frac{2e_0}{1+e^{r(v_0-v)}}$, where $2e_0$ is the maximum firing rate, v_0 is the postsynaptic potential corresponding to a firing rate of e_0 and r is the steepness of the sigmoid.

The cortical compartment

The cortical compartment was inspired from an existing model of the neocortex which proved its capability of generating both normal and epileptiform activity. Readers may refer to Molaee-Ardekani et al. (2010) for details. In brief, the cortical compartment integrates a subpopulation of pyramidal cells (P, $W = A_C$, $\tau_w = \tau_{ac}$ in Equation 1) and two inhibitory neuronal populations (I_1^c and I_2^c, **Figure 1A**) representing soma- and proximal-dendrite targeting interneurons ($GABA_{A,\ fast}$ currents, $W = G_C$, $\tau_w = \tau_{gc}$ in Equation 1) and dendrite-targeting interneurons ($GABA_{A,\ slow}$ currents, $W = B_C$, $\tau_w = \tau_{bc}$ in Equation 1), respectively. Pyramidal collateral excitation was implemented as in Jansen et al. (1993).

In addition, these three cortical subpopulations receive excitatory input from the thalamic compartment. Therefore, feed-forward inhibition (FFI) is represented in the model as the two subpopulations of interneurons project to the pyramidal subpopulation (see *The Thalamic and Reticular Compartments* paragraph below).

Short-term synaptic depression (STD)

STD is present in the neocortex (Boudreau and Ferster, 2005). It can be potentially involved in the context of direct stimulation of the thalamus as TC cells directly project to cortical pyramidal cells. Consequently, this mechanism was implemented at the interface of thalamic/cortical compartments. To our knowledge, an implementation of STD in neural mass models has not been proposed before.

In our model, we represented a modulatory effect of the amplitude of the average EPSP (parameter A_C') at the level of subpopulation P depending on the density of action potentials $[d_{AP}(t)]$ coming from the thalamic compartment. This modulatory effect was obtained by multiplying A_C' by a time-varying coefficient $\kappa(t) \in [0.6, 1]$ where the function describing the evolution of $\kappa(t)$ was derived from Chung et al. (2002). This study shows that: (i) cortical EPSPs drop by 40% under periodic low-frequency intense thalamocortical (*TC*) cell firing and, (ii) this drop in cortical EPSP is directly linked to transient depression of thalamocortical monosynaptic projections to pyramidal neurons.

In line with these observations, STD was implemented as follows. First, signal $d_{AP}^{(t)}$ is low-pass filtered (cutoff frequency = 10 Hz) to restrict the STD effect to LFS. Then, from each time t_η at which the filtered signal $d^f_{AP}(t)$ exceeds a firing rate equal to η, the $\kappa(t)$ coefficient undertakes an exponential decay given by $\kappa(t) = \kappa_\eta \cdot e^{-t/\tau}$ where $\kappa_\eta = \kappa(t_\eta^-)$ and where t_η^- is the time instant that just precedes t_η. The decrease of $\kappa(t)$ is limited to the time interval $[t_\eta + 0.45\text{ s}]$ and cannot exceed 40%, total. Parameters η and τ were set to 0.8 and 8 s, respectively.

The thalamic and reticular compartments

The thalamic compartment was limited to one population of excitatory neurons (known as glutamatergic thalamocortical - *TC* - cells) receiving glutamatergic EPSPs ($W = A_{Th}$, $\tau_w = \tau_{aTh}$ in Equation 1) from cortical pyramidal cells (*P*) and GABAergic IPSPs with slow ($W = B_{Th}$, $\tau_w = \tau_{bTh}$ in Equation 1) and fast ($W = G_{Th}$, $\tau_w = \tau_{gTh}$ in Equation 1) kinetics from the reticular compartment (RtN). Here, we increased the time constant (τ_{bTh}) with respect to τ_{bc} to account for both $GABA_{A,\ slow}$- and $GABA_B$-receptor mediated currents in a single variable. *TC* cells directly target both cortical pyramidal cells and interneurons. The activation of these GABAergic interneurons subsequently promotes inhibition of pyramidal cells after a di-synaptic delay. Therefore, *TC* cells activation induces first an EPSP followed later on by an IPSP on cortical pyramidal cells, resulting in feed-forward inhibition (FFI). The *RtN* compartment comprised two inhibitory subpopulations, namely I_1^{RT} and I_2^{RT} which both receive excitatory input from the cortical ($W = A_{Rt}$, $\tau_w = \tau_{aRt}$ in Equation 1) and the thalamic ($W = A_{Rt}$, $\tau_w = \tau_{aRt}$ in Equation 1) compartments.

Simulation of stimulation effects

Stimulation currents induce a perturbation of the membrane potential of neurons. At cellular level, this effect can be accounted for by the "λE model", which is well grounded in the biophysics of compartment models (Rattay, 1998; McIntyre et al., 2004a; Manola et al., 2005, 2007) (see Miranda et al., 2009 for a review) and supported by *in vitro* experiments (Bikson et al., 2004; Frohlich and McCormick, 2010). This model $\Delta V \approx \vec{\lambda}.\vec{E}$ approximates the membrane potential variation ΔV as a linear function of the electrical field $\vec{E}$ induced by stimulation ($\vec{\lambda}$ representing the membrane space constant). In our neural mass model, the situation is less straightforward as space is not explicitly represented, conversely to detailed or mean-field models. However, within a certain range of intensity values, it has been shown that the membrane potential variation ΔV is modified in a linear way with respect to the electrical field which is itself proportional to the stimulation intensity (Bikson et al., 2004). These considerations led us to also assume a linear variation for the mean membrane potential as a function of stimulation intensity, in stimulated sub-populations of neurons. In addition, stimulation was represented by a train of periodic monophasic depolarizing pulses. The pulse width was fixed to 1 ms (as in clinics). Pulses were low-pass filtered to account for the average time of repolarization (set to 4.8 ms) in stimulated sub-populations of cells. The resulting stimulation signal was added to the mean membrane potential of neuronal sub-populations included in the thalamic (*TC*) and reticular (I_1^{RT} and I_2^{RT}) compartments of the proposed model. The depolarizing effect was weighted by three coefficients S_{TC}, S_{Rt1} and S_{Rt2} (**Table 1**) accounting for the possibly different stimulation impact at the thalamic and reticular level.

Model parameters, outputs, and implementation

Parameter values as well as physiological interpretation are provided in **Table 1**. Note that each synaptic connection in the model is weighted by a connectivity constant denoted by $C_{SP1-SP2}$ where *SP1* and *SP2*, respectively, denote the source and target subpopulations. In addition, two Gaussian noise inputs $p_P(t) \sim N(\mu_P, \sigma_P)$ and $p_{TC}(t) \sim N(\mu_{TC}, \sigma_{TC})$ were used to represent nonspecific inputs on pyramidal and thalamocortical cell subpopulations. Finally, signals simulated at the level of pyramidal cells in the cortical compartment and at the level of *TC* cells in the thalamic compartment were chosen as model outputs. They correspond to the sum of PSPs at each compartment respectively. The temporal dynamics of these signals provide a good approximation of actual LFPs. The model was implemented in Simulink®, and all other complementary scripts were implemented in MATLAB®.

REAL DATA FOR MODEL TUNING

We used real clinical data to tune the model into a functioning mode which simulates pathological activity. The clinical data set was limited to a unique patient who underwent thalamic DBS during the presurgical intracerebral EEG exploration (iEEG performed with depth electrodes implanted under stereotaxic conditions) at the Epilepsy Surgery Unit, Rennes University Hospital. This particular patient was chosen for two main reasons: (1) the pronounced frequency-dependent stimulation effects observed during his preoperative diagnostic iEEG exploration at LF, IF and HF in addition to (2) the existence of an epileptogenic zone in a limited area of the premotor cortex (PMC).

In brief, this patient suffered from partial drug-resistant epilepsy since the age of two. MRI scans and EEG recordings pointed out the existence of a neuronal malformation known as FCD in the PMC at the origin of seizures. This type of cortical malformation is known for its epileptogenic features like neuronal hyperexcitability and hypersynchronization and its characteristic epileptiform discharges (continuous, rhythmic or semirhythmic spikes, and polyspikes) (Avoli et al., 2003; Palmini, 2010) as shown in **Figure 2C**. Based on various clinical studies reporting the modulation of epileptic cortical activity by the

Table 1 | Model parameters, values and interpretation.

Parameter	Value	Interpretation
A_C	6 (optimized, pathological) 3 (normal) mV	Amplitude of the cortical average EPSP
A_C'	$\kappa(t).A_C$ mV	Amplitude of the cortical average EPSP in response to thalamic input (only on subpopulation P)
B_C	14 (optimized, pathological) 50 (normal) mV	Amplitude of the cortical average IPSP ($GABA_{A,slow}$ mediated currents)
G_C	16.5 (optimized, pathological) 22 (normal) mV	Amplitude of the cortical average IPSP ($GABA_{A,fast}$ mediated currents)
A_{Th}	3.5 mV	Amplitude of the thalamic average EPSP
B_{Th}	30 mV	Amplitude of the thalamic average IPSP ($GABA_{A,slow}$ and $GABA_B$ receptors)
G_{Th}	22 mV	Amplitude of the thalamic average IPSP ($GABA_{A,fast}$ receptors)
A_{Rt}	3.5 mV	Amplitude of the reticular average EPSP
τ_{ac}	1/80 s	Time constant of cortical glutamate-mediated synaptic transmission.
τ_{bc}	1/35 s	Time constant of cortical GABA-mediated synaptic transmission ($GABA_{A,\ slow}$ receptors)
τ_{gc}	1/180 s	Time constant of cortical GABA-mediated synaptic transmission ($GABA_{A,\ fast}$ receptors)
τ_{aTh}	1/100 s	Time constant of thalamic glutamate-mediated synaptic transmission
τ_{bTh}	1/20 s	Time constant of thalamic GABA-mediated synaptic transmission ($GABA_{A,\ slow}$ and $GABA_B$ receptors)
τ_{gTh}	1/150 s	Time constant of thalamic GABA-mediated synaptic transmission ($GABA_{A,\ fast}$ receptors)
τ_{aRt}	1/100 s	Time constant of reticular glutamate-mediated synaptic transmission
$\nu_0,\ e_0,\ r$	$\nu_0 = 6$mV, $e_0 = 2.5\ s^{-1}$ $r = 0.56$mV^{-1}	Parameters of the nonlinear sigmoid function (transforming the average membrane potential to an average density of action potentials)
$C_{P-P'}$	135	Collateral excitation connectivity constant
$C_{P'-P}$	108	Collateral excitation connectivity constant
$C_{P-I_2^C}$	33.75	P to I_2^C connectivity constant
$C_{I_2^C-P}$	33.75	I_2^C to P connectivity constant
$C_{P-I_1^C}$	40.5	P to I_1^C connectivity constant
$C_{I_2^C-I_1^C}$	13.5	I_1^C to I_2^C connectivity constant
$C_{I_1^C-P}$	91.125	I_1^C to P connectivity constant
C_{TC-P}	120	TC to P connectivity constant
$C_{TC-I_1^C}$	30	TC to I_1^C connectivity constant
$C_{TC-I_2^C}$	45	TC to I_2^C connectivity constant
$C_{TC-I_1^{Rt}}$	20	TC to I_1^{Rt} connectivity constant
$C_{TC-I_2^{Rt}}$	20	TC to I_2^{Rt} connectivity constant
$C_{P-I_1^{Rt}}$	30	P to I_1^{Rt} connectivity constant
$C_{P-I_2^{Rt}}$	30	P to I_2^{Rt} connectivity constant
C_{P-TC}	20	P to TC connectivity constant
$C_{I_1^{Rt}-TC}$	35	I_1^{Rt} to TC connectivity constant
$C_{I_2^{Rt}-TC}$	5	I_2^{Rt} to TC connectivity constant
μ_{P1}	0	Mean of nonspecific cortical input
μ_{P2}	70	Mean of nonspecific subcortical input
σ_{P1}	20.v6	Standard deviation of nonspecific cortical input
σ_{P2}	35.v6	Standard deviation of nonspecific subcortical input
S_{TC}	5	Stimulation impact on subpopulation TC
S_{Rt1}	4	Stimulation impact on subpopulation I_1^{Rt}
S_{Rt2}	4	Stimulation impact on subpopulation I_2^{Rt}
f_s	1 Hz – 150Hz	Frequency of the stimulation signal (pulse train)
A_{fs}	1	Stimulation signal amplitude

Model parameters used to reproduce $LFPs_{FCD}$. Stimulation impact parameters S_{TC}, S_{Rt1} and S_{Rt2} are set to zero during the simulation of the NS scenario. These parameters are held constant for all other stimulation scenarios.

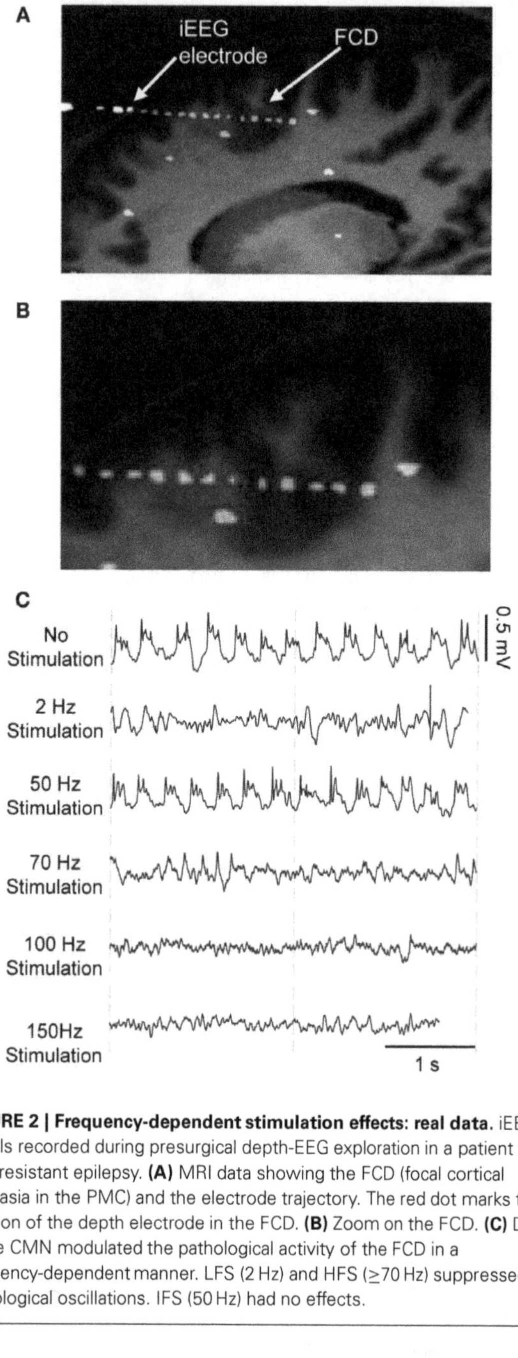

FIGURE 2 | Frequency-dependent stimulation effects: real data. iEEG signals recorded during presurgical depth-EEG exploration in a patient with drug-resistant epilepsy. **(A)** MRI data showing the FCD (focal cortical dysplasia in the PMC) and the electrode trajectory. The red dot marks the position of the depth electrode in the FCD. **(B)** Zoom on the FCD. **(C)** DBS of the CMN modulated the pathological activity of the FCD in a frequency-dependent manner. LFS (2 Hz) and HFS (≥70 Hz) suppressed pathological oscillations. IFS (50 Hz) had no effects.

stimulation of the CM nucleus (Velasco et al., 1995, 1997, 2000, 2001, 2007), it was decided by neurologists and neursosurgeons to implant a depth electrode in this nucleus, as potentially beneficial for the patient who gave his informed consent.

During the presurgical exploration, the stimulation of the thalamic CM nucleus (CMN) induced frequency-dependent modulation of the pathologic activity of the FCD (**Figure 2**). Readers may refer to (Pasnicu et al., 2013) for detailed information. Interestingly, LFS (2 Hz, 4 mA) and HFS (70, 100, and 150 Hz, 0.8 mA) desynchronized the pathological activity of the FCD, while IFS (50 Hz, 0.8 mA) barely affected it. These segments of signals corresponding to either typical pathological activity or modulated activity (depending on stimulation conditions) were used to optimize the model parameters.

PROCESSING OF REAL AND SIMULATED SIGNALS

The use of signal processing techniques was necessary (i) to quantify the above-described effects of stimulation in real iEEG signals, and (ii) to define a feature-vector-based cost function for model parameter optimization. **Figure 3A** illustrates the feature extraction methodology. iEEG signals recorded in the FCD in absence of stimulation ($LFPs_{FCD}$) and under different stimulation conditions were decomposed using an orthogonal matching pursuit algorithm [matching pursuit toolkit—MPTK—(Krstulovic and Gribonval, 2006)]. First introduced in 1993 (Mallat and Zhifeng, 1993), matching pursuit is signal processing algorithm used to decompose any time series into a linear sum of waveforms selected from a predefined dictionary based on a mother wavelet. To proceed, a proper multi-scalar dictionary of Gabor, Fourier, and Dirac atoms was first defined to account for real iEEG signal components (time-frequency atoms are waveforms well localized in both the time and the frequency domains). In line with (Krstulovic and Gribonval, 2006), the multi-scalar dictionary was formed by translation in time and amplitude/frequency modulation of atoms (defined as Gabor and Fourier functions in our case), over ten different user-defined time scales (i.e. the atom durations, ranging from 0.125 to 5 s). Then, the algorithm provided a table of time-frequency parameters associated to the detected atoms (atom type, central frequency, phase, scale, amplitude, position). Identified atoms were reconstructed using the extracted parameter table and their analytical expression. They were then associated to a given frequency band depending on their central frequency. These frequency bands corresponded to the classical EEG bands as defined in normal adults (δ_1 [0 – 1.9Hz], δ_2 [1.9 – 3.4 Hz], θ_1 [3.4 – 5.4 Hz], θ_2 [5.4 – 7.4 Hz], α_1 [7.4 – 10 Hz], α_2 [10 – 12 Hz], β_1 [12 –18 Hz], β_2 [18 – 24 Hz], γ [24 – 128 Hz]) (**Figure 3A**, blue). Finally, a 9D feature vector V_F was defined from the normalized energy distribution in these frequency bands, itself computed as the sum of averaged (over time) atom energies relative to the total signal energy (**Figure 3A**, green).

MODEL OPTIMIZATION UNDER THE "NO STIMULATION" CONDITION

In order to simulate $LFPs_{FCD}$, we optimized the excitation/inhibition ratio of the cortical compartment. Thus, the average EPSP/IPSP amplitude parameters of the cortical compartment $\{A_C, B_C, G_C\}$ were considered as free parameters while all other model parameters were set to fixed values (**Table 1**). The optimization method is illustrated in **Figure 3B**. For each triplet $\{A_C, B_C, G_C\}$, the feature vector $V_{F,\,model}$ of the model's output signal (cortical compartment's LFP) was calculated and compared to $V_{F,\,real}$, i.e., the feature vector computed from the average of the 20 feature vectors, each computed on a 5 s signal segment of real $LFPs_{FCD}$. Feature vectors $V_{F,\,model}$ and $V_{F,\,real}$ were computed as described in section Processing of Real and Simulated Signals. The optimization procedure aimed at finding the triplet $\left\{\widehat{A_C}, \widehat{B_C}, \widehat{G_C}\right\}$ that minimizes a cost function simply corresponding to the Euclidean

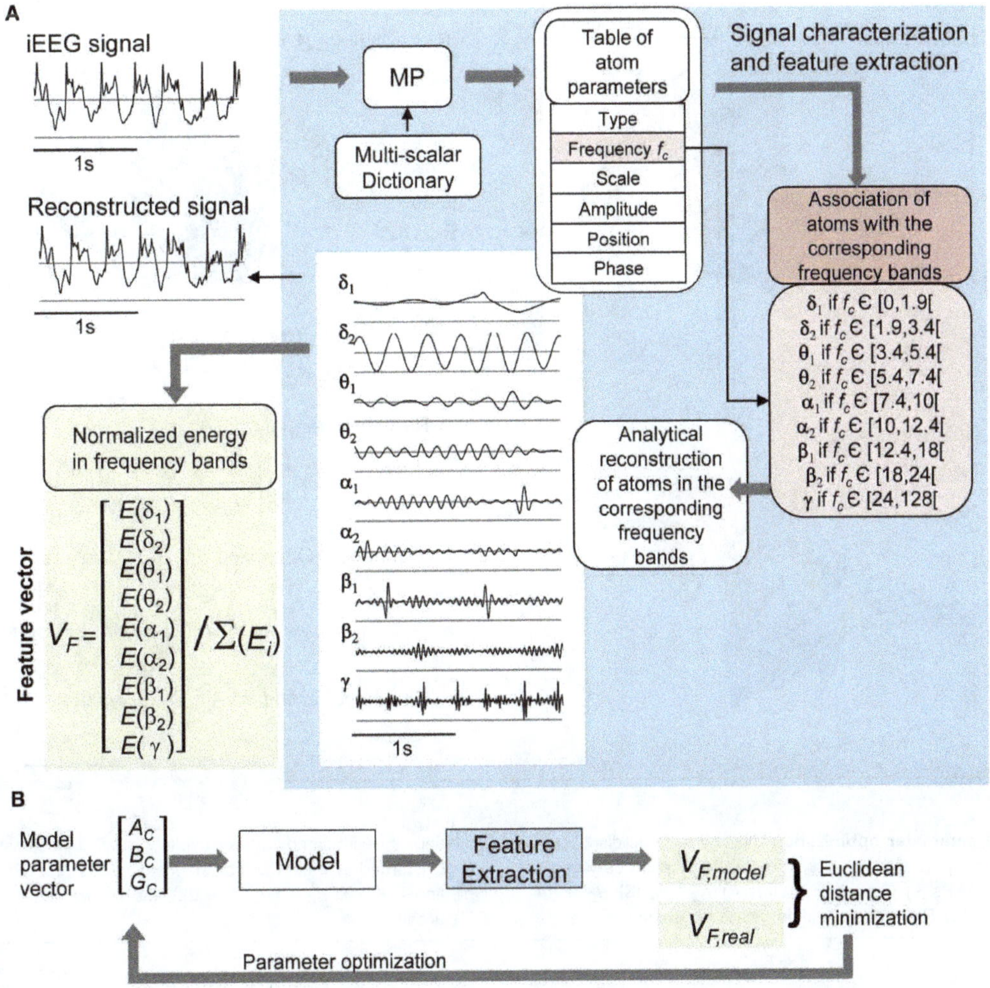

FIGURE 3 | iEEG signal processing. (A) *Feature vector extraction.* Input signals were characterized using the matching pursuit (MP) method (dictionary of Gabor, Fourier, and Dirac atoms). Parameters of detected atoms (atom type, central frequency f_C, scale, phase, amplitude, and position) are extracted by MP from input signals. Detected atoms are then associated with frequency bands (δ_1 to γ) depending on their proper central frequency. Sub-band (δ_1 to γ) signals were reconstructed from the sum of corresponding atoms, themselves obtained by fitting parameters into their analytic expression (see top left: input and reconstructed signals). The normalized energy vector $[E(\delta_1) \ldots E(\gamma)]/(E(\delta_1) + \ldots + E(\gamma))$ was chosen as the feature vector for further *optimization of model parameters.* **(B)** The model's free parameters A_C, B_C, and G_C were optimized by minimizing the distance between the feature vector $V_{F,\ model}$ of the simulated cortical LFP and the average of real feature vectors $V_{F,\ real}$ of $LFPs_{FCD}$.

distance $d(V_{F,\ real}, V_{F,\ model})$ when parameters A_C, B_C, and G_C span pre-defined ranges of values according to a Brute-Force procedure.

RESULTS

In this section, results regarding the identification of cellular mechanisms underlying the modulation of cortical activity by thalamic DBS are reported. First, the model capability to reproduce signals similar to those recorded from the FCD in the patient was assessed, under two conditions (no stimulation and during stimulation). Three mechanisms contributing to frequency-dependant stimulation effects could be identified. Then, simulations were performed to analyze the marginal or joint contribution of these mechanisms at low, intermediate or high frequency stimulation.

SIMULATION OF $LFPs_{FCD}$ UNDER NO STIMULATION CONDITION

As a first step, we verified the ability of the model to generate signals that resemble those recorded from the FCD in the considered patient ($LFPs_{FCD}$). This procedure, described in sections Processing of Real and Simulated Signals and Model Optimization Under the "No Stimulation" Condition, led us to identify a minimal distance (**Figures 4A–C**) and thus an optimal parameter vector $\{\widehat{A_C}, \widehat{B_C}, \widehat{G_C}\} = \{6, 14, 16.5\}$ for which simulated signals under the no stimulation condition have similar features as compared with those of real signals (**Figure 4D**).

SIMULATION OF $LFPs_{FCD}$ UNDER STIMULATION CONDITIONS

Actual $LFPs_{FCD}$ recorded at various stimulation frequencies (2, 50, 70, 100, and 150 Hz) were first characterized using the matching pursuit method described in section Processing of

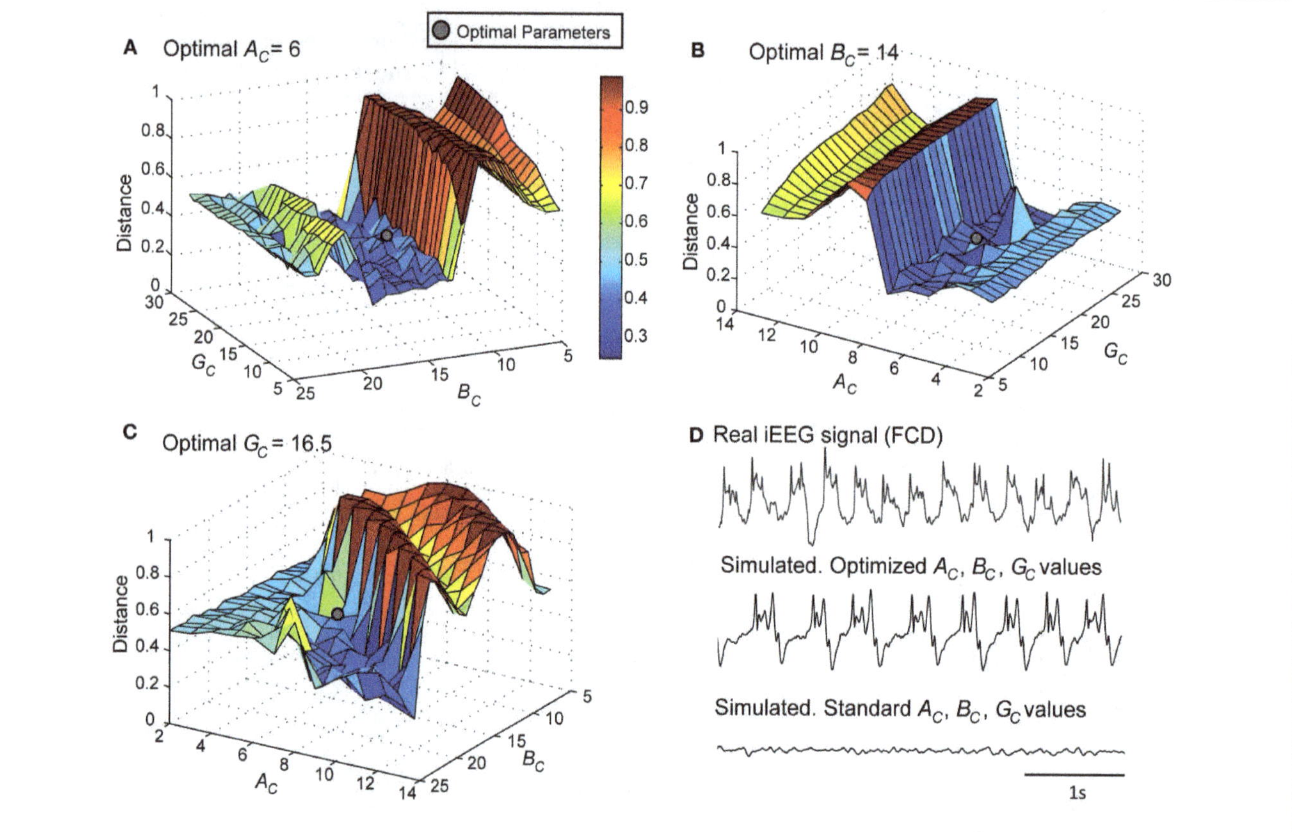

FIGURE 4 | Model parameter optimization. Normalized Euclidian distance between $V_{E,\ real}$ and $V_{E,\ model}$. Best fit (gray disk) between simulated and real LFPs$_{FCD}$ was obtained for **(A)** $A_C = 6$, **(B)** $B_C = 14$, and **(C)** $G_C = 16.5$. **(D)** For these modified values of excitation and inhibition, the simulated signal exhibits similar characteristics as the iEEG signal recorded in the FCD. For standard values of excitation and inhibition ($A_C = 3$, $B_C = 50$, $G_C = 22$), the model generates background EEG activity.

Real and Simulated Signals (**Figure 3A**). Results are shown in **Figure 5A** where feature vectors of segments of LFPs$_{FCD}$ are represented in a 3D space where axes correspond to merged typical EEG frequency bands (δ_2 to θ_1, θ_2 to β_1, β_2 to γ). Results show that the distribution of points in the 3D frequency space is not random but clustered, indicating that the frequency content of LFPs$_{FCD}$ segments depends on the stimulation frequency. In addition, some clusters are very close. This is typically the case for i) the no stimulation (yellow) and the 50 Hz stimulation conditions (red) on the one hand, and ii) the 70 Hz (violet) and 150 Hz (cyan) stimulation conditions on the other hand. To go beyond the qualitative clustering performed by visual inspection of 3D plots, a K-means clustering algorithm implemented in MATLAB and using a Mahalanobis distance was used to automatically detect the three types of stimulation effects. Initial centroids were randomly chosen. The optimal clustering that globally minimizes intra-cluster inertia is presented in **Figure 5B**. LFPs$_{FCD}$ segments were automatically classified into three subgroups. The first subgroup contains LFPs$_{FCD}$ segments obtained for low-frequency stimulation (LFS). The second subgroup gathers all segments recorded for high frequency stimulations (HFS, > 70 Hz). And finally, in the third subgroup, segments obtained under the no stimulation and the intermediate stimulation frequency (IFS, 50 Hz) conditions are merged together, suggesting that this stimulation frequency does not reduce the "epileptiform aspect" of the activity reflected in the LFP.

Based on this characterization of local field potentials recorded in the FCD (LFPs$_{FCD}$), parameters S_{TC}, S_{Rt1} and S_{Rt2} were manually tuned to lead the model to generate simulated signals which have spectral characteristics similar to those of actual LFPs$_{FCD}$. Such a manual procedure was sufficient to reproduce stimulation effects observed in one patient. However, extending the study to a larger group of patients would have made imperative an automated parameter fitting procedure based on the spectral characteristics of real EEG signals as in Rowe et al. (2004). **Figure 5B** shows the projection of representative simulated LFPs$_{FCD}$ in the 3D frequency space ("M" triangles). As depicted, simulated signals obtained for LFS, IFS and HFS were close to corresponding clusters obtained from real signals for the exact same computation of feature vectors. Shown in **Figure 5C**, these representatives simulated LFPs$_{FCD}$ do not perfectly match actual signals. However, qualitatively similar bifurcations were observed in the model when the stimulation conditions are changed. Indeed, under the no stimulation (NS) and the IFS condition the model generates rhythmic slow oscillations (δ) with superimposed faster activity (β, γ), as observed in real data. For LFS and HFS conditions, strong modulation of this activity was also obtained in the model.

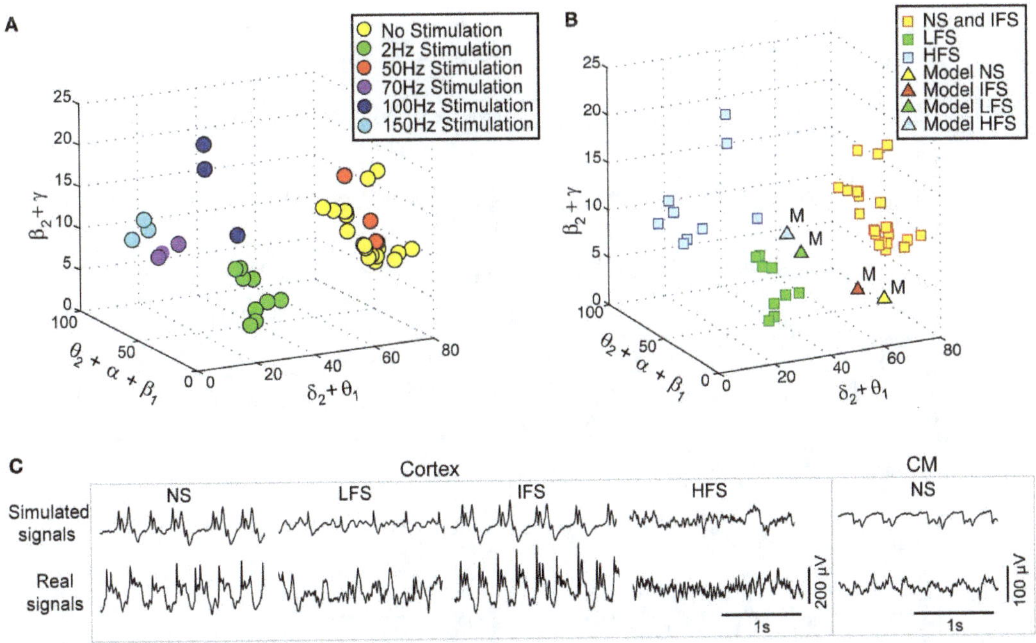

FIGURE 5 | Characterization and classification of real and simulated data. (A) 3-dimensional (3D) projection of feature vectors ($V_{F,\ real}$) corresponding to different stimulation conditions. This projection was obtained by summing some coordinates of initial 9D feature vectors to get 3D vectors $[E(\delta_2)+E(\theta_1),\ E(\theta_2)+E(\alpha_1)+E(\alpha_2)+E(\beta_1),\ E(\beta_2)+E(\gamma)]/[E(\delta_1)+\cdots+E(\gamma)]$. Each vector was then represented by a point in the 3D space $(\delta_2+\theta_1,\ \theta_2+\alpha_1+\alpha_2+\beta_1,\ \beta_2+\gamma)$.Three main classes can be visually identified. **(B)** Clusters obtained using the k-means algorithm (Mahalanobis distance). The three clusters correspond to (i) low-frequency stimulation (LFS) effects (green squares), (ii) no stimulation (NS) and intermediate-frequency stimulation (IFS) effects (yellow squares), and (iii) high-frequency stimulation (HFS) effects (blue squares). Simulated signals corresponding to the four types of scenarios (NS, LFS, IFS, and HFS) were also projected in the same space (triangles). **(C)** Two-second segments of real and simulated signal during NS, LFS, IFS, and HFS.

At LFS, in the model, the slow wave activity was strongly reduced but spike events occurred in the signals at the instant times of stimulation, mimicking, to some extent, comparable events also present in actual LFPs_{FCD}. Finally, at HFS, slow oscillations (δ) were abolished in the model which generates quasi-normal background activity. This simulated activity was also comparable to real activity observed for HFS stimulation but disclosed less γ activity. Note that these are the effects which were quantified in **Figure 5B**. The qualitative optimization procedure of parameters S_{TC}, S_{Rt1}, and S_{Rt2} was then complemented by an evaluation of parameter sensitivity aimed at studying the impact of random changes affecting the parameter vector $\Theta = \{A_C, B_C, G_C, A_{Th}, B_{Th}, G_{Th}, A_{Rt}\}$ on simulated signals. Parameter vector Θ determines the excitability properties in the three model compartments. As shown in **Figure 6**, results show that the simulated signals obtained under the four stimulation conditions (NS, LFS, IFS, HFS) stay "quite robust" (in the sense that waveforms are conserved) when parameters stay in the range $[\widehat{\Theta} \pm \zeta.\ \widehat{\Theta}]$ with $0 \leq \zeta \leq 0.2$.

MECHANISMS UNDERLYING FREQUENCY-DEPENDANT STIMULATION EFFECTS

Three main mechanisms implemented in the model are required to mimic actually observed effects of the CM nucleus stimulation. These mechanisms are the following: (i) the presence of feed-forward inhibition (FFI) at the level of thalamic projections to the FCD, (ii) the presence of short-term depression (STD) at the level of the thalamocortical glutamatergic synapses and, (iii) the depolarization of RtN inhibitory interneurons targeting *TC* cells.

This result raises an additional question: to what extent the joint effect of these mechanisms is necessary to reproduce frequency-dependant stimulation effects (LFS, IFS, and HFS). In order to assess their individual contribution, we performed simulations where each mechanism was either present in—or removed from—the model (the model parameters remaining unchanged). Results are displayed in **Figure 7**. First, they confirmed that both FFI and STD mechanisms are jointly necessary in the model to suppress the epileptic activity in the FCD when LFS is being used since the withdrawal of either STD or FFI leads the model to generate epileptic activity at LFS. Second, results indicated that the RtN inhibitory interneurons targeting *TC* cells (both I_1^{RT} and I_2^{RT} subpopulations) must be affected (i.e., depolarized) by the stimulation to obtain a suppression of epileptic activity when HFS is being used, as observed in the patient. Third, and interestingly, an unexpected effect was observed at IFS when the depolarization of I_2^{RT} interneurons was removed from the model. Indeed, epileptic activity was abolished in this case, which is really unlikely to occur during actual stimulation as both subtypes of neurons are expected to be affected by the direct stimulation of the CM nucleus.

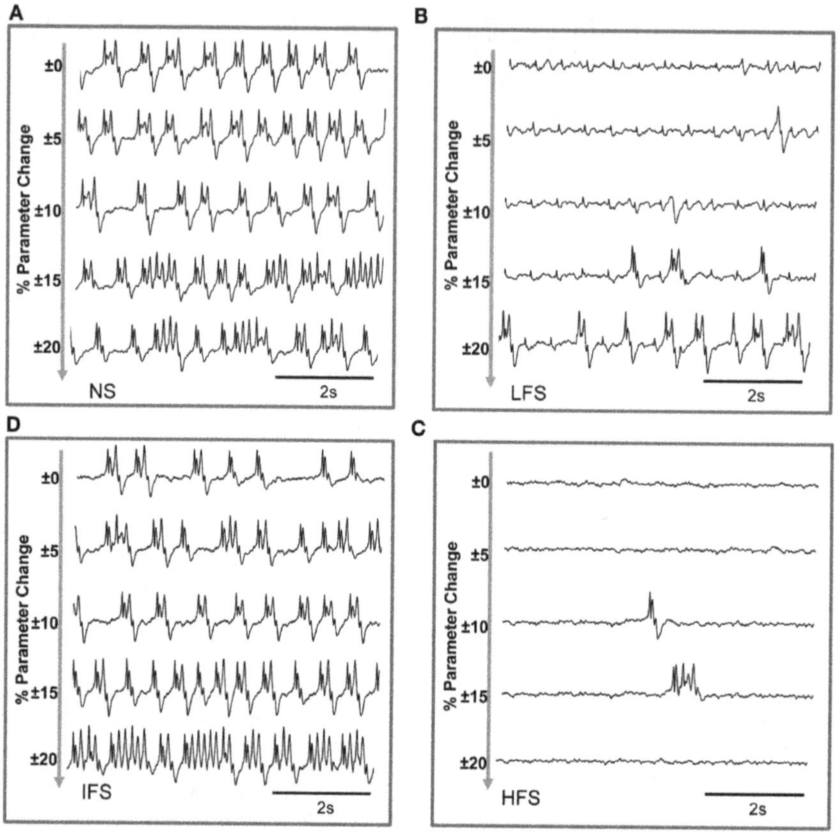

FIGURE 6 | Evaluation of parameter sensitivity. Model output sensitivity to variations of excitatory and inhibitory key parameters. Realizations of parameter vector $\Theta = \{A_C, B_C, G_C, A_{Th}, B_{Th}, G_{Th}, A_{Rt}\}$ were randomly (uniform law) generated around the optimal parameter vector Θ_0 over a variation domain defined by $(1 \pm \varsigma).\ \Theta_0$. For $\varsigma \leq 0.2$ (±20% variation), stimulation effects are preserved in the model for **(A)** no stimulation, **(B)** low-frequency stimulation, **(C)** intermediate-frequency stimulation, and **(D)** high-frequency stimulation.

These results were complemented by a deeper analysis of the thalamic output (i.e., the firing rate of *TC* cells) in response to stimulation at low, intermediate and high frequency. Results are provided in **Figure 8**. First, they showed that the thalamic output dramatically differs depending on the stimulation frequency (**Figure 8A**). Under the no stimulation condition, the firing rate continuously oscillates around a certain value (referred to as Λ, **Figure 8A**). At LFS, the firing rate was found to be lower, except at the stimulation times where it abruptly and transiently increased. At IFS, a balance was observed between time intervals for which the *TC* firing is above and below Λ. Finally, at HFS, the output of *TC* cells was found to be very low, i.e., systematically under the threshold Λ. From these observations, we could define (i) two time intervals, Δ1 and Δ2, for which the *TC* cells firing rate is either below Λ(Δ1) or above Λ (Δ2) and (ii) a "high to low firing" ratio (*HtoLR*) which provides an indication on the amount of time the *TC* cells spend firing (up state) relatively to the amount of time they do not fire (down state). **Figure 8B** provides the evolution of the *HtoLR* when the stimulation frequency is progressively changing from 0 to 150 Hz in the model. As depicted, these simulations indicated that three stimulation frequency ranges have dramatic effects on the firing of *TC* cells. First, from 0 to 20 Hz, the down state is predominant. Then, an abrupt jump was observed around 22 Hz indicating that beyond this value, the firing rate dramatically increased. Interestingly, from 55 to 65 Hz, a progressive decrease of the *HtoLR* was observed. Then, after 70 Hz, the ratio is equal to zero indicating that *TC* cells did not fire anymore. Finally, in order to relate the thalamic activity with the cortical activity, we plotted the phase portraits (*TC* cell firing vs. cortical LFP) as illustrated in **Figure 8C**. Results confirmed the visual inspection of signals simulated at the two sites. For the no stimulation (NS) and for the intermediate frequency stimulation (IFS) conditions, phase portraits were found to be quite similar. They indicated the presence of mixed slow/fast oscillations in both signals. For the low frequency stimulation (LFS) condition, oscillations in the simulated LFP in the FCD were reduced. They came along with short-duration, abrupt and rhythmic augmentations of the *TC* firing corresponding to stimulation pulses. Finally, for the high frequency stimulation (HFS) condition, oscillations in both types of activity stayed confined to small amplitude values.

DISCUSSION

We modeled the thalamocortical loop in order to investigate frequency-dependent effects of electrical stimulation performed

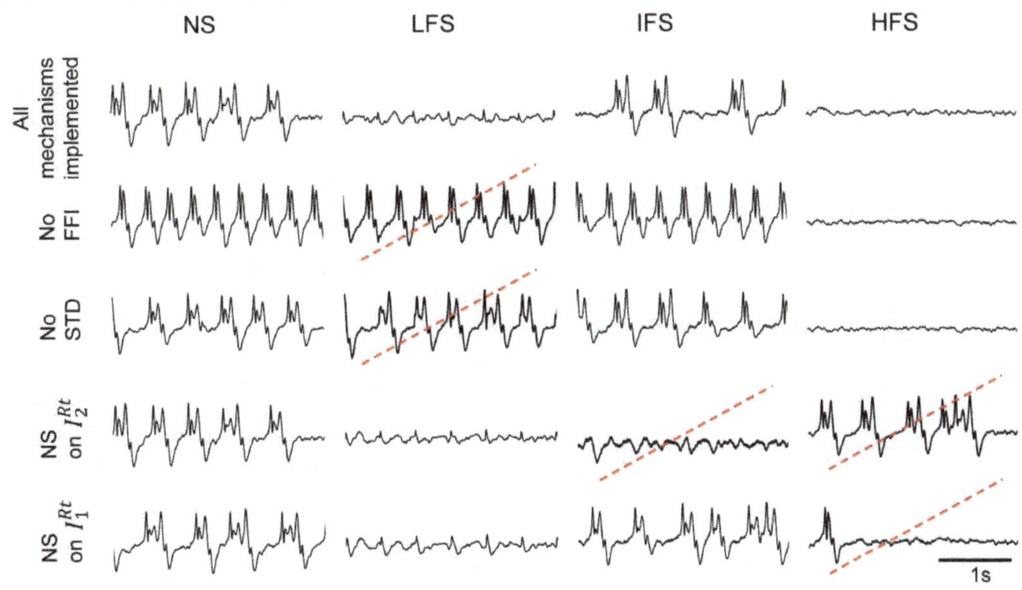

FIGURE 7 | Conditions to reproduce frequency-dependent stimulation effects. Model output in the case where one of the implemented mechanisms (FFI, STD, depolarization of I_2^{Rt}, and I_1^{Rt},, respectively) is removed at a time. LFS effects are not reproduced when the model does not account for FFI and STD. HFS effects require the depolarization of both reticular populations I_2^{Rt} and I_1^{Rt}. Suppression of epileptic activity is observed at IFS when I_2^{Rt} interneurons are removed. Red dotted lines indicate situations where simulated signals do not match real ones for given stimulation condition.

in the thalamus and aimed at modulating the neocortical activity. We chose to elaborate our model at a mesoscopic level, i.e., intermediate between microsocopic and macroscopic.

Regarding the model architecture, we followed a similar approach to that used in previously proposed models of the thalamocortical loop (Robinson et al., 2002; Suffczynski et al., 2004; Breakspear et al., 2006; Roberts and Robinson, 2008; Marten et al., 2009; Crunelli et al., 2011). Our model includes three main compartments: cerebral cortex, reticular nucleus and thalamic relay. Subpopulations of neurons and interneurons located in these three structures interact via excitatory and/or inhibitory synaptic connections. The novelty with respect to aforementioned studies is threefold. First, we modified the cortical compartment in order to better approximate the temporal dynamics of epileptic signals recorded in the FCD. This modification consisted in the use of two types of interneurons (mediating GABAergic IPSPs with slow and fast kinetics on cortical principal cells), as reported in a previous study (Molaee-Ardekani et al., 2010). Second, our model accounts for the direct effects of electrical stimulation. At this stage, we used the $\Delta V \approx \vec{\lambda}.\vec{E}$ assumption according to which the perturbation of the mean membrane potential of neurons is a linear function of the electrical field magnitude induced by bipolar stimulation. This "λE" assumption was already used in neural mass models in the context of low-intensity direct hippocampal stimulation to anticipate seizures (Suffczynski et al., 2008) as well as in the analysis of the stimulus-response relationship of DBS in healthy animals (Adhikari et al., 2009). However, it is worth mentioning that in our model, the three subtypes of neurons (*TC* cells and both subpopulations of inhibitory neurons in the RtN) are depolarized by the stimulation, as suggested in (Molaee-Ardekani et al., 2013) and conversely to (Adhikari et al., 2009) where only principal cells are impacted. And third, our model includes two well-known mechanisms at the cortical level: feed-forward inhibition (FFI) and short-term depression (STD).

As in any modeling approach, our approach has some limitations. First, the chosen modeling level does not allow for analyzing sub-cellular mechanisms involved in stimulation-evoked changes. Similarly, it does not account for direct activation of axons by stimulation versus somatic inhibition (McIntyre et al., 2004b), nor for the mechanisms of orthodromic/antidromic propagation of action potentials due to stimulation (Degos et al., 2005; Hammond et al., 2007; Dorval et al., 2008). Second, a strong assumption in the type of model we used (neural mass) is related to the intrinsic synchronization among neurons included in a given sub-population. This assumption does not allow for representing either de- or weakly-synchronized firing patterns that may be observed during epileptic activity, in particular during high frequency oscillations that can be encountered in FCDs (Brázdil et al., 2010). Nevertheless, we could accurately reproduce the abnormal rhythms generated in the FCD suggesting that main pyramidal cells have a relatively synchronized activity in this epileptogenic tissue. Third, regarding plasticity-related mechanisms, we only implemented short-term effects (i.e., STD) and neglected long-term plastic changes that may be induced by DBS (Shukla et al., 2013).

Despite these limitations, we could identify a number of mesoscopic factors which could explain the frequency-dependent mechanisms of thalamic stimulation. The model was tuned using electrophysiological data recorded in a patient in whom the centromedian nucleus (CMN) stimulation was particularly efficient

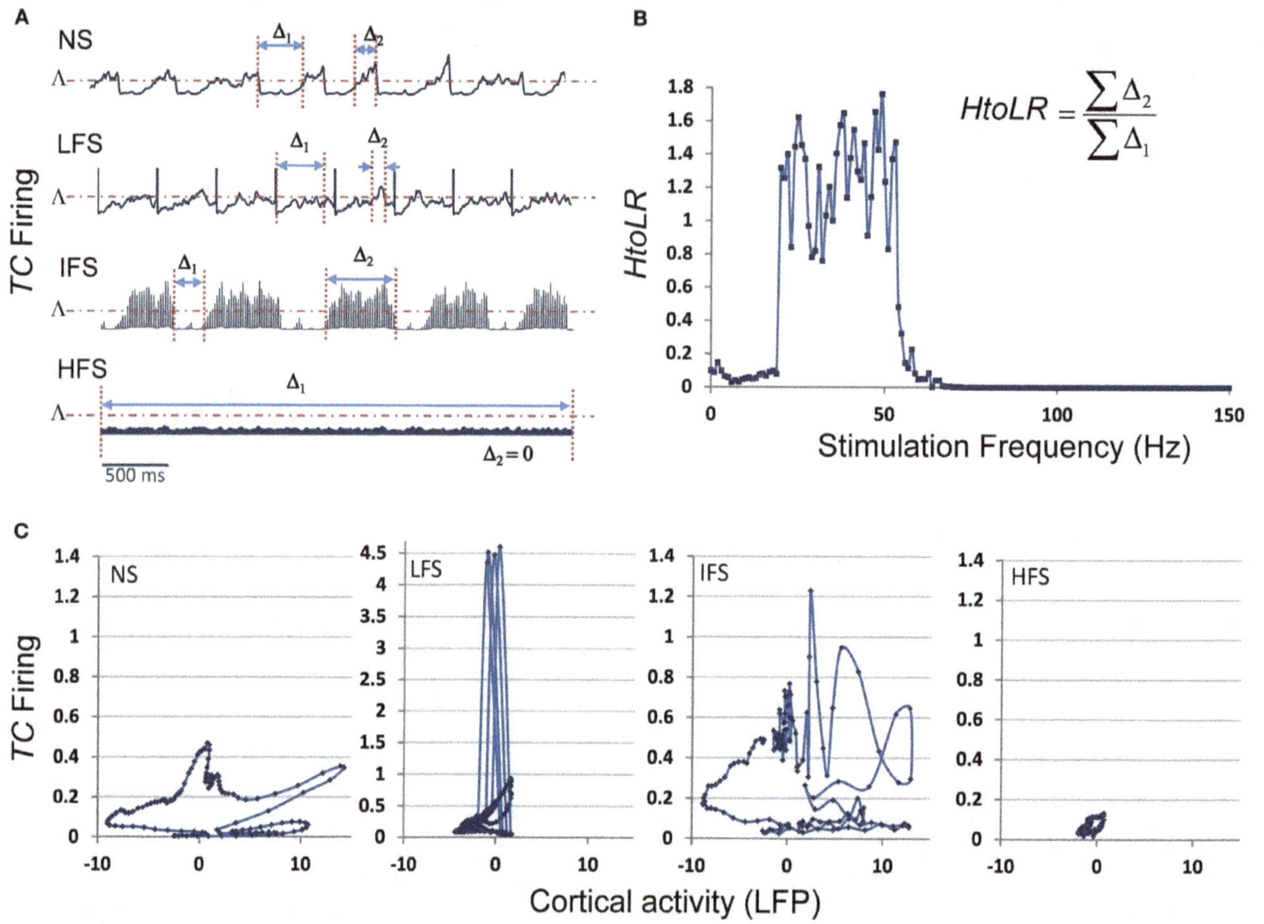

FIGURE 8 | Model behavior as a function of the stimulation frequency. (A) The firing rate of TC cells depends on the stimulation frequency (Δ_1: time interval for which this firing is lower than a threshold Λ, Δ_2: time interval for which this firing is higher than Λ). **(B)** Evolution of the "High to Low firing Ratio" (*HtoLR*) as a function of stimulation frequency. **(C)** Phase portraits (FCD activity vs. CM firing) for the four stimulation conditions (NS, LFS, IFS, and HFS).

to reduce the epileptic activity of a FCD located in the premotor cortex, in a frequency-specific manner. The main findings are summarized in **Figure 9**.

"NO STIMULATION" (NS) CONDITION

In the model, under the NS condition, excitation among pyramidal cells had to be increased and inhibition had to be reduced in the cortical compartment for producing "pathological" oscillatory rhythms, as observed in the FCD. The thalamocortical loop was found to be responsible for these pathological dynamics, characteristic of FCDs. These findings are in line with histological studies showing that these typical oscillations are generated in altered brain tissue, where inhibition is partially deteriorated or dysfunctioning (Calcagnotto et al., 2005), and where excitation is heavily increased (Avoli et al., 2003). In addition to neuron alterations in the dysplastic tissue (Sisodiya et al., 2009), FCD keeps sufficient projections to—and input from—other brain structures to propagate pathological dynamics (Avoli et al., 2003). As mentioned, the presence of connections with subcortical structures was a necessary condition in the model for producing pathological oscillations resembling those actually recorded in the FCD (**Figure 9A**).

LOW-FREQUENCY STIMULATION (LFS) CONDITION

For the low-frequency stimulation (LFS, $f < 20$ Hz) condition, two mechanisms were found to play a major role for the abortion of epileptic activity in the FCD: short-term depression (STD, i.e., decreased excitatory synaptic efficacy in thalamus-to-cortex connections) and feed-forward inhibition (FFI, i.e., excitation of inhibitory cortical interneurons by *TC* cells) (**Figure 9B**).

STD was reported in previous studies concerning cortical adaptation to thalamic stimulation, and suggesting that electrical LFS of *TC* cell axons *in vivo* resulted in a 40% reduction in cortical EPSPs (Chung et al., 2002). In the same context, LFS trains in adult anaesthetized rats provoked transient long-term depression of thalamocortical synapses; this was measured by up to 40% drop in cortical EPSPs after LFS trains and under the effect of GABA antagonist (Speechley et al., 2007).

As mentioned above, the LFS effects could not be reproduced by the model without incorporating also FFI. Actually,

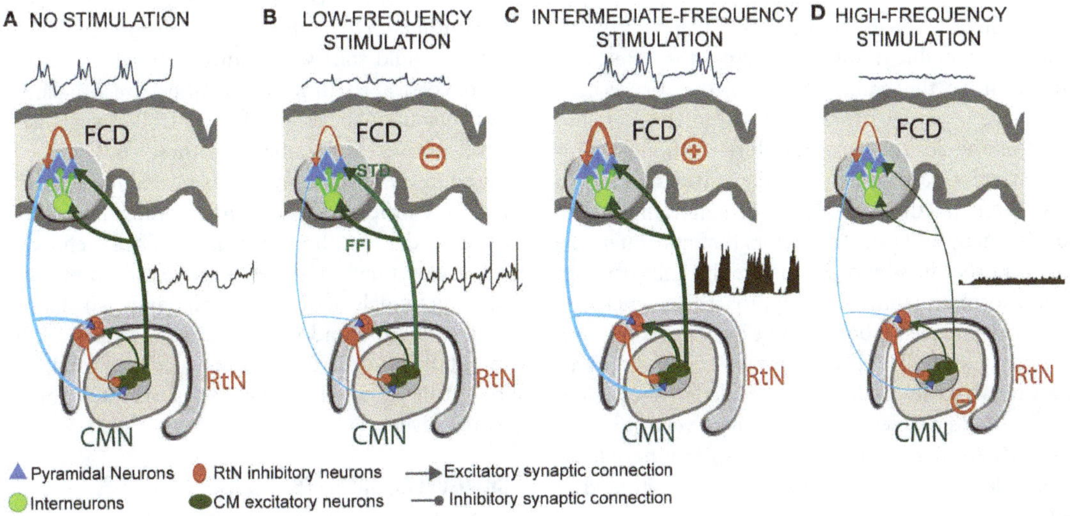

FIGURE 9 | Frequency-dependent mechanisms underlying DBS. (A) Under the no stimulation (NS) condition, the thalamocortical loop is responsible for pathological oscillatory rhythms observed in the FCD. **(B)** For low-frequency stimulation (LFS), feed-forward inhibition (FFI, i.e., excitation of inhibitory cortical interneurons by *TC* cells) and short-term depression (STD, i.e., decreased excitatory synaptic efficacy in thalamus-to-cortex connections) was found to play a major role for the abortion of epileptic activity in the FCD. **(C)** For the intermediate-frequency stimulation (IFS) condition, thalamic output is reinforced (increase of *TC* cells firing) leading to an increase of the average excitatory post-synaptic potential (EPSP) on cortical pyramidal cells and to no "anti-epileptic" effect. **(D)** For high-frequency stimulation (HFS), the direct and sustained excitation of reticular nucleus (RtN) interneurons leads to dramatic decrease of *TC* cells firing rate and to a suppression of epileptic activity.

thalamocortical ascending fibers directly target pyramidal neurons as well as cortical GABAergic interneurons inducing EPSPs in both cell types (Pouille and Scanziani, 2001). In the model, while less efficient (STD) thalamic EPSPs arrive directly onto pyramidal neurons, IPSPs induced by thalamic stimulation also arrive on pyramidal neurons (FFI) lagging by 1–2 ms. This short latency between the onset of thalamocortical excitation and the onset of feed-forward inhibition presents a temporal "window of opportunity" for pyramidal cells to integrate excitatory and inhibitory inputs, thus keeping the transmembrane potential below firing threshold. In the literature, neuroanatomical and neurophysiological studies (Isaacson and Scanziani, 2011) showed the functional importance of FFI in regulating cortical dynamics by controlling cortical excitability (Gabernet et al., 2005). Our study suggests that LFS regulates cortical excitability by a dual mechanism of FFI and STD (**Figure 9B**).

INTERMEDIATE-FREQUENCY STIMULATION (IFS) CONDITION

For the intermediate-frequency stimulation (IFS, $20 < f < 70$ Hz) condition, results indicated that the thalamic output is reinforced (increase of *TC* cells firing) and leads to an increase of the average excitatory post-synaptic potential (EPSP) on cortical pyramidal cells (**Figure 9C**). This effect corresponds to an increase of the spatiotemporal summation of unitary EPSPs. In this case, both the cortical excitability and the gain in the excitatory thalamocortical loop is increased, leading to "no anti-epileptic" effect. We did not find much studies using DBS stimulation in the intermediate frequency range of (20–60 Hz) in the context of epilepsy. Nevertheless, it is noteworthy that 50 Hz stimulation frequency is classically used during the presurgical evaluation of patient with intractable partial epilepsy in order to trigger seizures and delineate the epileptogenic zone (Talairach et al., 1974; Jayakar et al., 1992). The same frequency range is also known to provoke afterdischarges and was actually used in the kindling model of epilepsy (Goddard, 1967; Racine, 1972).

HIGH-FREQUENCY STIMULATION (HFS) CONDITION

Finally, for the high-frequency stimulation (HFS, $f > 70$ Hz) condition, the direct and sustained excitation of reticular nucleus (RtN) interneurons leads to strong inhibition of *TC* cells and thus to dramatic decrease of their firing rate. Despite the fact that *TC* neurons are also affected by stimulation, the response of reticular GABAergic neurons to stimulation and the higher efficiency of GABA-mediated currents ensure that IPSPs override EPSPs on *TC* cells. In this case, the reduced excitatory input to cortical pyramidal cells also leads to a suppression of epileptic activity (**Figure 9D**). This result corroborates reported stimulation studies where HFS (>100 Hz) was associated with significant decrease in epileptiform discharges *in vitro*, and reduction in seizure frequency in responding patients (Velasco et al., 2006; Fisher et al., 2010). This hypothesis is in line with recent findings suggesting that HFS of the globus pallidus (GPi) in dystonia patients decreased its firing by stimulation-evoked GABA release from afferent fibers and thereby the enhancement of inhibitory synaptic transmission by HFS (Liu et al., 2012). Similarly, HFS (100 Hz–130 Hz) of the STN neurons in vitro showed a suppression of the activity of the majority of neurons by the reinforcement of inhibitory responses (Filali et al., 2004). Other HFS studies also provided evidence on the inhibition of GPi output during HFS in human patients (Dostrovsky et al., 2000) as well as the disruption thalamocortical network's dysrhythmia (McIntyre and Hahn, 2010; Kendall et al., 2011).

CONCLUSION

In epilepsy research, it is well-admitted that there is, unfortunately, a lack of tangible results regarding the effects of electrical stimulation in the brain. Therefore, the very crucial issue of choosing the "optimal" stimulation parameters remains unsolved, whatever the stimulation procedure. Although computational models are always based on a number of simplifying assumptions, we think that they provide an efficient framework to (i) account for the many and essential factors that may intervene during stimulation procedures and (ii) analyze the links between these factors in a formal manner. This approach is particularly fruitful when models are well grounded in experimental/clinical data (Wendling et al., 2012). This is somehow a weak point of this study since we could make use of data sets recorded in one patient only. However, it should be mentioned that these very informative data sets stay relatively rare since many conditions have to be met (patient candidate to surgery, FCD, electrodes positioned in appropriate structures).

At this stage, the face value of the model is satisfactory. The next step is obviously to test the model predictions using animal models. Experiments can be undertaken in rodents with electrodes implanted in the cerebral cortex and in the thalamus. First, we could start with control animals to assess the modulation of cortical rhythms during/after direct thalamic stimulation at various frequencies and for controlled vigilance states (sleep, awake, resting, exploratory). In these controls, some drugs can be used to alter some parameters related to synaptic transmission (in a more or less specific manner) which have a correspondence in the model, on the other hand. Then, refined experimental models could be introduced to get closer to the epilepsy context including models of developmental dysplastic lesions [see review in Schwartzkroin and Wenzel (2012)]. Hopefully, this combined computational/experimental approach will help us to disclose some of the highly intricate effects of DBS either at local or at network level.

ACKNOWLEDGMENTS

This study was supported by Region Bretagne, France. The first author benefits from a research allocation (ARED) in the context of the project entitled "STIMULE."

REFERENCES

Adhikari, M. H., Heeroma, J. H., Di Bernardo, M., Krauskopf, B., Richardson, M. P., Walker, M. C., et al. (2009). Characterisation of cortical activity in response to deep brain stimulation of ventral-lateral nucleus: modelling and experiment. *J. Neurosci. Methods* 183, 77–85. doi: 10.1016/j.jneumeth.2009.06.044

Avoli, M., Louvel, J., Mattia, D., Olivier, A., Esposito, V., Pumain, R., et al. (2003). Epileptiform synchronization in the human dysplastic cortex. *Epileptic Disord.* 5(Suppl. 2), S45–S50.

Beurrier, C., Bioulac, B., Audin, J., and Hammond, C. (2001). High-frequency stimulation produces a transient blockade of voltage-gated currents in subthalamic neurons. *J. Neurophysiol.* 85, 1351–1356.

Bikson, M., Inoue, M., Akiyama, H., Deans, J. K., Fox, J. E., Miyakawa, H., et al. (2004). Effects of uniform extracellular DC electric fields on excitability in rat hippocampal slices *in vitro*. *J. Physiol.* 557, 175–190. doi: 10.1113/jphysiol.2003.055772

Bojak, I., and Liley, D. T. (2005). Modeling the effects of anesthesia on the electroencephalogram. *Phys. Rev. E Stat. Nonlin. Soft Matter Phys.* 71:041902. doi: 10.1103/PhysRevE.71.041902

Boon, P., Raedt, R., De Herdt, V., Wyckhuys, T., and Vonck, K. (2009). Electrical stimulation for the treatment of epilepsy. *Neurotherapeutics* 6, 218–227. doi: 10.1016/j.nurt.2008.12.003

Boudreau, C. E., and Ferster, D. (2005). Short-term depression in thalamocortical synapses of cat primary visual cortex. *J. Neurosci.* 25, 7179–7190. doi: 10.1523/JNEUROSCI.1445-05.2005

Brázdil, M., Halámek, J., Jurák, P., Daniel, P., Kuba, R., Chrastina, J., et al. (2010). Interictal high-frequency oscillations indicate seizure onset zone in patients with focal cortical dysplasia. *Epilepsy Res.* 90, 28–32. doi: 10.1016/j.eplepsyres.2010.03.003

Breakspear, M., Roberts, J. A., Terry, J. R., Rodrigues, S., Mahant, N., and Robinson, P. A. (2006). A unifying explanation of primary generalized seizures through nonlinear brain modeling and bifurcation analysis. *Cereb. Cortex* 16, 1296–1313. doi: 10.1093/cercor/bhj072

Calcagnotto, M. E., Paredes, M. F., Tihan, T., Barbaro, N. M., and Baraban, S. C. (2005). Dysfunction of synaptic inhibition in epilepsy associated with focal cortical dysplasia. *J. Neurosci.* 25, 9649–9657. doi: 10.1523/JNEUROSCI.2687-05.2005

Chung, S., Li, X., and Nelson, S. B. (2002). Short-term depression at thalamocortical synapses contributes to rapid adaptation of cortical sensory responses *in vivo*. *Neuron* 34, 437–446. doi: 10.1016/S0896-6273(02)00659-1

Cooper, I. S., Amin, I., and Gilman, S. (1973). The effect of chronic cerebellar stimulation upon epilepsy in man. *Trans. Am. Neurol. Assoc.* 98, 192–196.

Crunelli, V., Cope, D. W., and Terry, J. R. (2011). Transition to absence seizures and the role of GABA(A) receptors. *Epilepsy Res.* 97, 283–289.

David, O., and Friston, K. J. (2003). A neural mass model for MEG/EEG: coupling and neuronal dynamics. *Neuroimage* 20, 1743–1755. doi: 10.1016/j.neuroimage.2003.07.015

Davis, R., Engle, H., Kudzma, J., Gray, E., Ryan, T., and Dusnak, A. (1982). Update of chronic cerebellar stimulation for spasticity and epilepsy. *Appl. Neurophysiol.* 45, 44–50.

Degos, B., Deniau, J. M., Thierry, A. M., Glowinski, J., Pezard, L., and Maurice, N. (2005). Neuroleptic-induced catalepsy: electrophysiological mechanisms of functional recovery induced by high-frequency stimulation of the subthalamic nucleus. *J. Neurosci.* 25, 7687–7696. doi: 10.1523/JNEUROSCI.1056-05.2005

Dorval, A. D., Russo, G. S., Hashimoto, T., Xu, W., Grill, W. M., and Vitek, J. L. (2008). Deep brain stimulation reduces neuronal entropy in the MPTP-primate model of Parkinson's disease. *J. Neurophysiol.* 100, 2807–2818. doi: 10.1152/jn.90763.2008

Dostrovsky, J. O., Levy, R., Wu, J. P., Hutchison, W. D., Tasker, R. R., and Lozano, A. M. (2000). Microstimulation-induced inhibition of neuronal firing in human globus pallidus. *J. Neurophysiol.* 84, 570–574.

Filali, M., Hutchison, W. D., Palter, V. N., Lozano, A. M., and Dostrovsky, J. O. (2004). Stimulation-induced inhibition of neuronal firing in human subthalamic nucleus. *Exp. Brain Res.* 156, 274–281. doi: 10.1007/s00221-003-1784-y

Fisher, R., Salanova, V., Witt, T., Worth, R., Henry, T., Gross, R., et al. (2010). Electrical stimulation of the anterior nucleus of thalamus for treatment of refractory epilepsy. *Epilepsia* 51, 899–908. doi: 10.1111/j.1528-1167.2010.02536.x

Freeman, W. J. (1973). "A model of the olfactory system," in, *Neural Modeling*, eds M. A. B. Brazier, D. O. Walter, and D. Schneider (Los Angeles, CA: University. of California), 41–62.

Freeman, W. J. (1992). Tutorial on neurobiology: from single neurons to brain chaos. *Int. J. Bifurcat. Chaos* 2, 451–482. doi: 10.1142/S0218127492000653

Frohlich, F., and McCormick, D. A. (2010). Endogenous electric fields may guide neocortical network activity. *Neuron* 67, 129–143. doi: 10.1016/j.neuron.2010.06.005

Gabernet, L., Jadhav, S. P., Feldman, D. E., Carandini, M., and Scanziani, M. (2005). Somatosensory integration controlled by dynamic thalamocortical feed-forward inhibition. *Neuron* 48, 315–327. doi: 10.1016/j.neuron.2005.09.022

Goddard, G. V. (1967). Development of epileptic seizures through brain stimulation at low intensity. *Nature* 214, 1020–1021. doi: 10.1038/2141020a0

Hablitz, J. J. (1976). Intramuscular penicillin epilepsy in the cat: effects of chronic cerebellar stimulation. *Exp. Neurol.* 50, 505–514. doi: 10.1016/0014-4886(76)90022-4

Hammond, C., Bergman, H., and Brown, P. (2007). Pathological synchronization in Parkinson's disease:

networks, models and treatments. *Trends Neurosci.* 30, 357–364. doi: 10.1016/j.tins.2007.05.004

Isaacson, J. S., and Scanziani, M. (2011). How inhibition shapes cortical activity. *Neuron* 72, 231–243. doi: 10.1016/j.neuron.2011.09.027

Jansen, B. H., Zouridakis, G., and Brandt, M. E. (1993). A neurophysiologically-based mathematical model of flash visual evoked potentials. *Biol. Cybern.* 68, 275–283. doi: 10.1007/BF00224863

Jayakar, P., Alvarez, L. A., Duchowny, M. S., and Resnick, T. J. (1992). A safe and effective paradigm to functionally map the cortex in childhood. *J. Clin. Neurophysiol.* 9, 288–293. doi: 10.1097/00004691-199204010-00009

Jiang, B., Akaneya, Y., Hata, Y., and Tsumoto, T. (2003). Long-term depression is not induced by low-frequency stimulation in rat visual cortex *in vivo*: a possible preventing role of endogenous brain-derived neurotrophic factor. *J. Neurosci.* 23, 3761–3770.

Kendall, H. L., Frederick, L. H., Su-Youne, C., Dongchul, C. L., David, W. R., Cameron, C. M., et al. (2011). High frequency stimulation abolishes thalamic network oscillations: an electrophysiological and computational analysis. *J. Neural Eng.* 8:046001. doi: 10.1088/1741-2560/8/4/046001

Kim, E., Owen, B., Holmes, W. R., and Grover, L. M. (2012). Decreased afferent excitability contributes to synaptic depression during high frequency stimulation in hippocampal area CA1. *J. Neurophysiol.* 108, 1965–1976. doi: 10.1152/jn.00276.2011

Krstulovic, S., and Gribonval, R. (2006). "Mptk: Matching Pursuit Made Tractable," in: *IEEE International Conference on Acoustics, Speech and Signal Processing*, (Toulouse), 496–499.

Liley, D. T., and Bojak, I. (2005). Understanding the transition to seizure by modeling the epileptiform activity of general anesthetic agents. *J. Clin. Neurophysiol.* 22, 300–313.

Liu, L. D., Prescott, I. A., Dostrovsky, J. O., Hodaie, M., Lozano, A. M., and Hutchison, W. D. (2012). Frequency-dependent effects of electrical stimulation in the globus pallidus of dystonia patients. *J. Neurophysiol.* 108, 5–17. doi: 10.1152/jn.00527.2011

Lopes Da Silva, F. H. (2006). Event-related neural activities: what about phase? *Prog. Brain Res.* 159, 3–17. doi: 10.1016/S0079-6123(06)59001-6

Lopes Da Silva, F. H., Hoeks, A., Smits, H., and Zetterberg, L. H. (1974). Model of brain rhythmic activity. The alpha-rhythm of the thalamus. *Kybernetik* 15, 27–37. doi: 10.1007/BF00270757

Lopes Da Silva, F. H., van Rotterdam, A., Barts, P., van Heusden, E., and Burr, W. (1976). Models of neuronal populations: the basic mechanisms of rhythmicity. *Prog. Brain Res.* 45, 281–308. doi: 10.1016/S0079-6123(08)60995-4

Lytton, W. W. (2008). Computer modelling of epilepsy. *Nat. Rev. Neurosci.* 9, 626–637. doi: 10.1038/nrn2416

Mallat, S. G., and Zhifeng, Z. (1993). Matching pursuits with time-frequency dictionaries. *Signal Processing, IEEE Transactions* 41, 3397–3415. doi: 10.1109/78.258082

Manola, L., Holsheimer, J., Veltink, P., and Buiteweg, J. R. (2007). Anodal vs cathodal stimulation of motor cortex: a modeling study. *Clin. Neurophysiol.* 118, 464–474. doi: 10.1016/j.clinph.2006.09.012

Manola, L., Roelofsen, B. H., Holsheimer, J., Marani, E., and Geelen, J. (2005). Modelling motor cortex stimulation for chronic pain control: electrical potential field, activating functions and responses of simple nerve fibre models. *Med. Biol. Eng. Comput.* 43, 335–343. doi: 10.1007/BF02345810

Marten, F., Rodrigues, S., Benjamin, O., Richardson, M. P., and Terry, J. R. (2009). Onset of polyspike complexes in a mean-field model of human electroencephalography and its application to absence epilepsy. *Philos. Trans. A Math. Phys. Eng. Sci.* 367, 1145–1161. doi: 10.1098/rsta.2008.0255

McIntyre, C. C., Grill, W. M., Sherman, D. L., and Thakor, N. V. (2004a). Cellular effects of deep brain stimulation: model-based analysis of activation and inhibition. *J. Neurophysiol.* 91, 1457–1469.

McIntyre, C. C., and Hahn, P. J. (2010). Network perspectives on the mechanisms of deep brain stimulation. *Neurobiol. Dis.* 38, 329–337. doi: 10.1016/j.nbd.2009.09.022

McIntyre, C. C., Savasta, M., Kerkerian-Le Goff, L., and Vitek, J. L. (2004b). Uncovering the mechanism(s) of action of deep brain stimulation: activation, inhibition, or both. *J. Clin. Neurophysiol.* 115, 1239–1248.

Miranda, P. C., Wendling, F., Ruffini, G., Merlet, I., Molaee-Ardekani, B., Dunne, S., et al. (2009). *Brain Stimulation: Models, Experiments and Open Questions, Deliverable D1.1: Review of the State of the Art in Currents Distribution and Effects* HIVE (FET Open FP7 EU project), Available online at: http://hive-eu.org

Molaee-Ardekani, B., Benquet, P., Bartolomei, F., and Wendling, F. (2010). Computational modeling of high-frequency oscillations at the onset of neocortical partial seizures: from 'altered structure' to 'dysfunction'. *Neuroimage* 52, 1109–1122. doi: 10.1016/j.neuroimage.2009.12.049

Molaee-Ardekani, B., Marquez-Ruiz, J., Merlet, I., Leal-Campanario, R., Gruart, A., Sanchez-Campusano, R., et al. (2013). Effects of transcranial Direct Current Stimulation (tDCS) on cortical activity: a computational modeling study. *Brain Stimul.* 6, 25–39. doi: 10.1016/j.brs.2011.12.006

Nunez, P. L. (1974). The brain wave equation: a model for the EEG. *Math. Biosci.* 21, 279–297. doi: 10.1016/0025-5564(74)90020-0

Palmini, A. (2010). Electrophysiology of the focal cortical dysplasias. *Epilepsia* 51(Suppl. 1), 23–26. doi: 10.1111/j.1528-1167.2009.02437.x

Pasnicu, A., Denoyer, Y., Haegelen, C., Pasqualini, E., and Biraben, A. (2013). Modulation of paroxysmal activity in focal cortical dysplasia by centromedian thalamic nucleus stimulation. *Epilepsy Res.* 104, 264–268. doi: 10.1016/j.eplepsyres.2012.10.012

Pouille, F., and Scanziani, M. (2001). Enforcement of temporal fidelity in pyramidal cells by somatic feed-forward inhibition. *Science* 293, 1159–1163. doi: 10.1126/science.1060342

Racine, R. J. (1972). Modification of seizure activity by electrical stimulation. II. Motor seizure. *Electroencephalogr. Clin. Neurophysiol.* 32, 281–294. doi: 10.1016/0013-4694(72)90177-0

Rattay, F. (1998). Analysis of the electrical excitation of CNS neurons. *IEEE Trans. Biomed. Eng.* 45, 766–772. doi: 10.1109/10.678611

Reimer, G. R., Grimm, R. J., and Dow, R. S. (1967). Effects of cerebellar stimulation on cobalt-induced epilepsy in the cat. *Electroencephalogr. Clin. Neurophysiol.* 23, 456–462. doi: 10.1016/0013-4694(67)90188-5

Roberts, J. A., and Robinson, P. A. (2008). Modeling absence seizure dynamics: implications for basic mechanisms and measurement of thalamocortical and corticothalamic latencies. *J. Theor. Biol.* 253, 189–201. doi: 10.1016/j.jtbi.2008.03.005

Robinson, P. A., Rennie, C. J., and Rowe, D. L. (2002). Dynamics of large-scale brain activity in normal arousal states and epileptic seizures. *Phys. Rev. E Stat. Nonlin. Soft Matter Phys.* 65:041924. doi: 10.1103/PhysRevE.65.041924

Robinson, P. A., Rennie, C. J., and Wright, J. J. (1997). Propagation and stability of waves of electrical activity in the cerebral cortex. *Phys. Rev. E Stat. Nonlin. Soft Matter Phys.* 56, 826–840. doi: 10.1103/PhysRevE.56.826

Rowe, D. L., Robinson, P. A., and Rennie, C. J. (2004). Estimation of neurophysiological parameters from the waking EEG using a biophysical model of brain dynamics. *J. Theor. Biol.* 231, 413–433. doi: 10.1016/j.jtbi.2004.07.004

Schwartzkroin, P. A., and Wenzel, H. J. (2012). Are developmental dysplastic lesions epileptogenic? *Epilepsia* 53(Suppl. 1), 35–44. doi: 10.1111/j.1528-1167.2012.03473.x

Shen, K. Z., Zhu, Z. T., Munhall, A., and Johnson, S. W. (2003). Synaptic plasticity in rat subthalamic nucleus induced by high-frequency stimulation. *Synapse* 50, 314–319. doi: 10.1002/syn.10274

Shukla, A. W., Moro, E., Gunraj, C., Lozano, A., Hodaie, M., Lang, A., et al. (2013). Long-term subthalamic nucleus stimulation improves sensorimotor integration and proprioception. *J. Neurol. Neurosurg. Psychiatry*. doi:10.1136/jnnp-2012-304102. [Epub ahead of print].

Sillay, K., and Starr, P. (2009). "Chapter 42 - deep brain stimulation in Parkinson's Disease," in *Neuromodulation*, eds E. S. Krames, P. H. Peckham, and A. R. Rezai (San Diego, CA: Academic Press), 539–548.

Sisodiya, S. M., Fauser, S., Cross, J. H., and Thom, M. (2009). Focal cortical dysplasia type II: biological features and clinical perspectives. *Lancet Neurol.* 8, 830–843. doi: 10.1016/S1474-4422(09)70201-7

Speechley, W. J., Hogsden, J. L., and Dringenberg, H. C. (2007). Continuous white noise exposure during and after auditory critical period differentially alters bidirectional thalamocortical plasticity in rat auditory cortex *in vivo*. *Eur. J. Neurosci.* 26, 2576–2584. doi: 10.1111/j.1460-9568.2007.05857.x

Stam, C. J., Pijn, J. P., Suffczynski, P., and Lopes Da Silva, F. H. (1999). Dynamics of the human alpha rhythm: evidence for non-linearity? *Clin. Neurophysiol.* 110, 1801–1813.

Suffczynski, P., Kalitzin, S., Da Silva, F. L., Parra, J., Velis, D., and Wendling, F. (2008). Active paradigms of seizure anticipation: computer model evidence for necessity of stimulation. *Phys. Rev. E Stat. Nonlin. Soft Matter Phys.* 78:051917. doi: 10.1103/PhysRevE.78.051917

Suffczynski, P., Kalitzin, S., and Lopes Da Silva, F. H. (2004). Dynamics of non-convulsive epileptic phenomena modeled by a bistable neuronal network. *Neuroscience* 126, 467–484. doi: 10.1016/j.neuroscience.2004.03.014

Suffczynski, P., Kalitzin, S., Pfurtscheller, G., and Lopes Da Silva, F. H. (2001). Computational model of thalamo-cortical networks: dynamical control of alpha rhythms in relation to focal attention. *Int. J. Psychophysiol.* 43, 25–40. doi: 10.1016/S0167-8760(01)00177-5

Talairach, J., Bancaud, J., Szikla, G., Bonis, A., Geier, S., and Vedrenne, C. (1974). [New approach to the neurosurgery of epilepsy. Stereotaxic methodology and therapeutic results. 1. Introduction and history]. *Neurochirurgie* 20(Suppl. 1), 1–240.

Velasco, A. L., Velasco, F., Jiménez, F., Velasco, M., Castro, G., Carrillo-Ruiz, J. D., et al. (2006). Neuromodulation of the centromedian thalamic nuclei in the treatment of generalized seizures and the improvement of the quality of life in patients with Lennox–Gastaut syndrome. *Epilepsia* 47, 1203–1212. doi: 10.1111/j.1528-1167.2006.00593.x

Velasco, F., Velasco, A. L., Velasco, M., Jimenez, F., Carrillo-Ruiz, J. D., and Castro, G. (2007). Deep brain stimulation for treatment of the epilepsies: the centromedian thalamic target. *Acta Neurochir. Suppl.* 97, 337–342. doi: 10.1007/978-3-211-33081-4_38

Velasco, F., Velasco, M., Velasco, A. L., Jimenez, F., Marquez, I., and Rise, M. (1995). Electrical stimulation of the centromedian thalamic nucleus in control of seizures: long-term studies. *Epilepsia* 36, 63–71. doi: 10.1111/j.1528-1157.1995.tb01667.x

Velasco, M., Velasco, F., and Velasco, A. L. (2001). Centromedian-thalamic and hippocampal electrical stimulation for the control of intractable epileptic seizures. *J. Clin. Neurophysiol.* 18, 495–513. doi: 10.1097/00004691-200111000-00001

Velasco, M., Velasco, F., Velasco, A. L., Brito, F., Jimenez, F., Marquez, I., et al. (1997). Electrocortical and behavioral responses produced by acute electrical stimulation of the human centromedian thalamic nucleus. *Electroencephalogr. Clin. Neurophysiol.* 102, 461–471. doi: 10.1016/S0013-4694(96)95203-0

Velasco, M., Velasco, F., Velasco, A. L., Jimenez, F., Brito, F., and Marquez, I. (2000). Acute and chronic electrical stimulation of the centromedian thalamic nucleus: modulation of reticulo-cortical systems and predictor factors for generalized seizure control. *Arch. Med. Res.* 31, 304–315. doi: 10.1016/S0188-4409(00)00085-0

Wendling, F. (2008). Computational models of epileptic activity: a bridge between observation and pathophysiological interpretation. *Expert Rev. Neurother.* 8, 889–896. doi: 10.1586/14737175.8.6.889

Wendling, F., Bartolomei, F., Bellanger, J. J., and Chauvel, P. (2002). Epileptic fast activity can be explained by a model of impaired GABAergic dendritic inhibition. *Eur. J. Neurosci.* 15, 1499–1508. doi: 10.1046/j.1460-9568.2002.01985.x

Wendling, F., Bartolomei, F., Mina, F., Huneau, C., and Benquet, P. (2012). Interictal spikes, fast ripples and seizures in partial epilepsies - combining multi-level computational models with experimental data. *Eur. J. Neurosci.* 36, 2164–2177. doi: 10.1111/j.1460-9568.2012.08039.x

Wendling, F., Bellanger, J. J., Bartolomei, F., and Chauvel, P. (2000). Relevance of nonlinear lumped-parameter models in the analysis of depth-EEG epileptic signals. *Biol. Cybern.* 83, 367–378. doi: 10.1007/s004220000160

Wilson, H. R., and Cowan, J. D. (1972). Excitatory and inhibitory interactions in localized populations of model neurons. *Biophys. J.* 12, 1–24. doi: 10.1016/S0006-3495(72)86068-5

Wright, G. D., and Weller, R. O. (1983). Biopsy and post-mortem findings in a patient receiving cerebellar stimulation for epilepsy. *J. Neurol. Neurosurg. Psychiatr.* 46, 266–273. doi: 10.1136/jnnp.46.3.266

Wright, J. J., Kydd, R. R., and Lees, G. J. (1985). State-changes in the brain viewed as linear steady-states and non-linear transitions between steady-states. *Biol. Cybern.* 53, 11–17. doi: 10.1007/BF00355686

Zavaglia, M., Astolfi, L., Babiloni, F., and Ursino, M. (2006). A neural mass model for the simulation of cortical activity estimated from high resolution EEG during cognitive or motor tasks. *J. Neurosci. Methods* 157, 317–329. doi: 10.1016/j.jneumeth.2006.04.022

9

Stability constraints on large-scale structural brain networks

Richard T. Gray[1]* and Peter A. Robinson[2,3]

[1] The Kirby Institute, The University of New South Wales, Sydney, NSW, Australia
[2] School of Physics, University of Sydney, Sydney, NSW, Australia
[3] Brain Dynamics Center, Sydney Medical School – Western, University of Sydney, Westmead, NSW, Australia

***Correspondence:**
*Richard T. Gray, The Kirby Institute, The University of New South Wales, Sydney, NSW 2052, Australia.
e-mail: rgray@kirby.unsw.edu.au*

Stability is an important dynamical property of complex systems and underpins a broad range of coherent self-organized behavior. Based on evidence that some neurological disorders correspond to linear instabilities, we hypothesize that stability constrains the brain's electrical activity and influences its structure and physiology. Using a physiologically-based model of brain electrical activity, we investigated the stability and dispersion solutions of networks of neuronal populations with propagation time delays and dendritic time constants. We find that stability is determined by the spectrum of the network's matrix of connection strengths and is independent of the temporal damping rate of axonal propagation with stability restricting the spectrum to a region in the complex plane. Time delays and dendritic time constants modify the shape of this region but it always contains the unit disk. Instabilities resulting from changes in connection strength initially have frequencies less than a critical frequency. For physiologically plausible parameter values based on the corticothalamic system, this critical frequency is approximately 10 Hz. For excitatory networks and networks with randomly distributed excitatory and inhibitory connections, time delays and non-zero dendritic time constants have no impact on network stability but do effect dispersion frequencies. Random networks with both excitatory and inhibitory connections can have multiple marginally stable modes at low delta frequencies.

Keywords: brain networks, stability, network spectra, random matrices, mean-field modeling

INTRODUCTION

The brain is possibly the most complicated example of a system of interacting dynamical units whose activity self-organizes to produce complex global behavior. The human brain performs cognitive functions through the transmission of action potentials within a vast structurally dynamic network consisting of approximately 10^{11} neurons and up to 10^{15} synaptic interconnections (Kandel et al., 2000; Koch, 2004; Sporns et al., 2005). The aggregate of all neural firings within this network results in large-scale coherent electrical activity and the performance of high-level cognitive functions. Understanding the structure and physiology of the brain thus gives insight into its overall behavior.

At large scales the excitatory and inhibitory neurons in the brain are organized into a complex large-scale network of distinct anatomical and functional structures (Sporns et al., 2004, 2005; Bullmore and Sporns, 2009; van den Heuvel and Sporns, 2011) We can represent this structure as a complex network—the structure of which has been studied extensively in recent times with a number of experimental cortical connection networks determined for the cat and the macaque monkey (Felleman and van Essen, 1991; Scannell et al., 1995; Jouve et al., 1998; Hilgetag et al., 2000a,b; Sporns, 2011). These networks have a modular hierarchical structure with the small-world properties of high local clustering and short path length between structures (Hilgetag et al., 2000a,b; Sporns et al., 2000, 2004, 2005; Young, 2000; Sporns and Zwi, 2004; Bassett and Bullmore, 2006; Bullmore and Sporns, 2009, 2012).

Reasons for why the brain has evolved this particular large-scale structure are currently unknown. A number of investigations have concentrated on the effect of physical constraints on brain structure. Such constraints include brain volume, wiring length, and energy consumption or metabolic demands (Laughlin et al., 1998; Attwell and Laughlin, 2001; Lennie, 2003). Other studies have looked at functional constraints such as minimizing the conduction delay or processing steps for a signal to travel from one neuron to another (Wen and Chklovskii, 2005). Alternatively, the dynamics of the brain's electrical activity may constrain the brain's structure. If the physiology and structural characteristics of the brain produce adverse electrical activity resulting in seizures, tremors, or other neurological disorders then it is likely the structural characteristics of the brain will be constrained to limit these disorders.

One of the most important dynamical properties of complex systems such as the brain is stability. It has been associated with pattern formation (Turing, 1952; Murray, 2002), synchronized activity (Kuramoto, 1984; Pecora and Carroll, 1998; Jirsa and Ding, 2004; Acebrón et al., 2005; Feng et al., 2006), the complexity and diversity of ecosystems (May, 1972, 1974; Hogg et al., 1989; McCann, 2000; Allesina and Tang, 2012), the functioning of biological systems (Murray, 2002; Taverna and

Goldstein, 2002; Steuer, 2007), and the generation of coherent self-organized behavior. Stability is also an important aspect of the design and control of advanced technological systems (Bechhoefer, 2005).

A common approach to studying the large-scale dynamics of the brain's electrical activity is to use a continuum mean-field approximation for neural activity. This approach has been extensively studied over the past 30 years producing numerous models for the electrical activity within the brain (Wilson and Cowan, 1973; da Silva et al., 1974; Nunez, 1974, 1995; Freeman, 1975; Steriade et al., 1990; Jirsa and Haken, 1996; Wright and Liley, 1996; Robinson et al., 1997, 2003a; Wright et al., 2001; Robinson, 2005). This work has been reviewed recently (Deco et al., 2008; Bressloff, 2011). These models have been used extensively to perform stability analysis and understand pattern formation, oscillations and waves in the brain's electrical activity (Deco et al., 2008; Bressloff, 2011).

Measurements of brain activity suggest that the brain operates close to marginal stability, permitting a wide range of flexible, adaptable, and complex behavior (Stam et al., 1999; Robinson et al., 2001b; Breakspear, 2002; Breakspear et al., 2003). Physiological modeling also suggests that linear instabilities in the brain's electrical activity correspond to neurological disorders, such as epilepsy (Robinson et al., 1998, 2002; Breakspear et al., 2006; Kim and Robinson, 2007; Deco et al., 2008). It is therefore possible that stability is a dynamical property that imposes constraints on the brain's physiology and structure.

In previous work we have used a simplified version of the Robinson, Rennie, Wright (RRW) physiologically-based continuum (mean-field) model (Robinson et al., 1997, 1998, 2003a; Wright et al., 2001; Rennie et al., 2002; Robinson, 2003, 2005) to study the dynamics of the electrical activity in large-scale structural brain networks. Based on the hypothesis that stability is a dynamical constraint on the structure and physiology of structural brain networks we have investigated the effect of stability of large-scale structural brain networks (Gray and Robinson, 2006, 2008, 2009b,a; Robinson et al., 2009).

Our previous work ignored the dendritic time constants of neurons and the propagation time delays for signals to travel between neural populations. However, time delays due to axonal propagation affect stability and the possible physiology of neuronal networks (Atay and Hutt, 2004; Jirsa and Ding, 2004; Coombes, 2005; Coombes et al., 2007; Qubbaj and Jirsa, 2007, 2009; Venkov et al., 2007; Jirsa, 2009). This previous work has generally used integro-differential neural field equations with connectivity within a neural mass described by homogeneous or heterogeneous kernels. Our approach here is to focus on the temporal dynamics of the overall electrical activity of arbitrarily connected large-scale structural brain networks, ignoring the spatial spread and propagation of electrical activity within individual neuronal populations.

In this study, we increase the physiological realism of our structural brain network model by allowing propagation time delays and non-zero dendritic time constants. After reviewing the stability of structural brain networks, we aim to investigate how these physiological features might affect the dynamics and stability of networks of neuronal populations where the connection patterns between populations are arbitrary—ignoring the spatial and geometric placement of the populations and simply focusing on which populations are inter-connected.

We also investigate the dispersion frequencies of marginally stable modes of electrical activity using plausible physiological parameters. The incorporation of non-zero dendritic time constants generalizes the work in (Jirsa and Ding, 2004) which, by including time delays, extended May's original analysis on the stability of complex systems (May, 1972, 1974).

METHODS

A structural brain network of n neural populations is represented by a directed graph N whose vertices and edges represent specific neural populations and inter-population connections, respectively. Neural populations within a network are collections of neurons with an assumed effective range and of sufficient number for a mean-field approximation to be valid. For example, a neural population can represent all the neurons in a distinct region or nuclei of the brain (e.g., cortical area, thalamus), a particular neuron type (e.g., interneuron, pyramidal cell), or a particular neurotransmitter type (e.g., glutamate, GABA, dopamine). Neurons in one population do not have to be separated geometrically or physically within the brain and can be intermixed with the neurons of another population (e.g., excitatory and inhibitory neurons in the cortex).

The structure of N is represented by a connection matrix $\mathbf{C}(N) = [C_{ab}]$; where $C_{ab} = 1$ if there is a connection from population b to population a, $C_{ab} = 0$ otherwise. If $C_{ab} = C_{ba}$ for all a and b, the network is symmetric; otherwise it is asymmetric. Self-connections in structural brain networks correspond to non-zero diagonal entries in $\mathbf{C}(N)$. The connection matrix simply records whether one neuronal population sends neural signals to another neuronal population. Properties of connections are not included in $\mathbf{C}(N)$.

PHYSIOLOGICALLY-BASED STRUCTURAL BRAIN NETWORK DYNAMICS

In this section we outline the physiological model used to describe the dynamics of a brain network. If a neural population contains a sufficient number of neurons a continuum approximation can be used, whereby the properties of population neurons are averaged over. This approximation is valid for length scales greater than a few tenths of a millimeter and is thus suitable for investigating the dynamics of large-scale structural brain networks.

The continuum approximation allows the use of a previously developed model, the RRW model, for the brain's electrical activity (Robinson et al., 1997; Wright et al., 2001; Rennie et al., 2002; Robinson et al., 2003b, 2004; Robinson, 2005). This continuum model incorporates and describes three features of neural dynamics: (1) the synapto-dendritic dynamics resulting in the cell body potential; (2) from the mean cell body potential an average firing rate is determined via a non-linear sigmoid function; and (3) the population firing rate generates a neural pulse forming a field $\phi(t)$ that propagates along the populations outgoing connections. The field within a population is temporally described using a damped wave equation. Implicitly the neurons in each population are assumed to have an effective range which gives a rate at which spikes reach axonal terminals and cease existance.

This model has been extensively used to model the corticothalamic system with the linear version having been shown to produce excellent agreement with EEG spectra, ERP, and other neurophysical phenomena (Robinson et al., 1997, 2001a,b; Rennie et al., 2002; Robinson, 2003). To apply this continuum model to brain networks we previously used a number of simplifying assumptions. In particular, we assumed that all neural populations have instantaneous dendritic response times and there is no time delay for a signal to be sent from one population to the other (Gray and Robinson, 2006, 2008, 2009b,a; Robinson et al., 2009). For this study we relax some of these assumptions.

Firstly we assume time delays τ for a signal to be sent from one population to another are equal. Secondly, we assume each population in a network has the same dendritic decay rate α and rise rate β. The values of $1/\alpha$ and $1/\beta$ equal the dendritic decay and rise time constants, respectively; instantaneous rise and decay times imply $1/\alpha = 1/\beta = 0$. These assumptions are unrealistic for real structural brain networks but improve our previous analysis and allow us to analytically determine stability. Though for some structural brain networks these assumptions may be good approximations of the networks physiology. Another weakness of these assumptions is self-connections have the same time delay as connections between distinct populations—if $\tau \neq 0$ then self-connections in a network also involve a delay. Generally, self-connections represent interconnections within a neural population and would be expected to have zero time delay. However, for cortical networks self-connections can be used to represent feedback from underlying structures such as the thalamus. Time delayed self-connections would be appropriate for this type of feedback. We will generalize the assumption of equal time delays in future work.

The neurophysics and neurophysiology incorporated into the general RRW model and the equations for the linear perturbations of the neural field ϕ_a, for each neural population a, are described and derived in detail elsewhere (Robinson et al., 1997; Wright et al., 2001; Rennie et al., 2002; Robinson et al., 2003b, 2004; Robinson, 2005). This study uses the notation and equations derived in (Robinson, 2005). Under the assumptions used here the RRW equations describing linear perturbations of the neural field ϕ_a of population a about the assumed steady state in Fourier space reduce to

$$(1 - i\omega/\gamma)^2\,\phi_a(\omega) = \sum_b L(\omega) G_{ab} e^{i\omega\tau} \phi_b(\omega), \tag{1}$$

$$= L(\omega) e^{i\omega\tau} \sum_b G_{ab}\phi_b(\omega), \tag{2}$$

where ω is the angular frequency and

$$L(\omega) = \frac{\alpha\beta}{(\alpha - i\omega)(\beta - i\omega)} = \frac{1}{(1 - i\omega/\alpha)(1 - i\omega/\beta)}. \tag{3}$$

The gain G_{ab} is a dimensionless quantity describing the effect of changes in the firing rate of neurons in population b on the neurons of population a. Physiologically, G_{ab} is the number of extra action potentials produced in a per extra action potential incident from b. Hence, G_{ab} is a measure of how sensitive and responsive a is to changes in b's activity. In the general RRW model γ is a damping rate equal to the velocity of the ϕ's propagation within a neural population divided by the characteristic range of the axons that carry it. In the spatially uniform case used here, γ represents a temporal damping rate.

Letting $\mathbf{G} = [G_{ab}]$ be the matrix of gains and setting

$$D(\omega) = [L(\omega)]^{-1}(1 - i\omega/\gamma)^2 e^{-i\omega\tau}, \tag{4}$$

$$= (1 - i\omega/\alpha)(1 - i\omega/\beta)(1 - i\omega/\gamma)^2 e^{-i\omega\tau}, \tag{5}$$

which is a complex analytic function. Equation (1) can be written in matrix form as

$$\mathbf{\Delta}(\omega)\mathbf{\Phi}(\omega) = \mathbf{G}\mathbf{\Phi}(\omega), \tag{6}$$

where $\mathbf{\Phi}$ is a column vector of the ϕ_a and $\mathbf{\Delta}(\omega) = D(\omega)\mathbf{I}$, where $\mathbf{I}$ is the identity matrix. Setting $\mathbf{A} = \mathbf{G} - \mathbf{\Delta}$, Equation (6) can be simplified to

$$\mathbf{A}(\omega)\mathbf{\Phi}(\omega) = 0. \tag{7}$$

The linear stability of a network is then determined by the solutions ω of the dispersion relation,

$$\det[\mathbf{A}(\omega)] = 0. \tag{8}$$

The gain matrix $\mathbf{G} = [G_{ab}]$ encodes all of the information in $\mathbf{C}$, since $G_{ab} \neq 0$ implies $C_{ab} \neq 0$, as well as the strength of connections between populations. No assumptions (such as homogeneity or isotropy) are made for the characteristics of a connection and any attenuation or phase shifting of an incoming signal due to time delays are reflected in the exponential term of Equation (1). However, the model implicitly assumes an effective range for neurons within a population. If $G_{ab} > 0$ then the connection is excitatory and if $G_{ab} < 0$ the connection is inhibitory. Note that Equation (5) shows that if the values of α and β are exchanged, the brain network has the same dynamics and stability.

REALISTIC PARAMETER VALUES FOR LARGE-SCALE STRUCTURAL BRAIN NETWORKS

Physiologically plausible parameter values for γ, α, β, and τ are shown in **Table 1**. These values are based on the parameters used in the corticothalamic model (Robinson et al., 2003a, 2004), with the specific values taken from (Robinson et al., 2004). The nominal values in **Table 1** are the default model parameters used to illustrate our results under our assumptions α and β are the same value for all populations and τ is the same for all connections. The values for γ are based on the cortical excitatory neurons which form the long range connections within the cortex. Inhibitory inter-neurons in the cortex are short range (Nunez, 1995) and therefore have $\gamma \approx \infty$. Under the assumptions used here all neural populations are given the same γ value.

In real structural brain networks dendritic time constants and propagation time delays may vary. The spatial distribution and

Table 1 | Physiologically plausible ranges and nominal values of parameters.

Parameter	Range	Nominal value	Unit
γ	30–220	100	s^{-1}
α	5–200	60	s^{-1}
β	17–2500	240	s^{-1}
β/α	1–10	4	–
τ	0–50	10	ms

Based on the corticothalamic model parameters in Robinson et al. (2004). The nominal values are the default model parameters we use in this work.

physical separation of structures within the brain will lead to distinct time delays. The values of τ in **Table 1** are physiologically plausible values for the time delays based on corticothalamic modeling. The nominal value is a realistic value for the average delay between the large-scale neural populations (or areas) in the cerebral cortex.

RANDOMLY CONNECTED LARGE-SCALE STRUCTURAL BRAIN NETWORKS

To illustrate our results we investigate randomly connected structural brain networks where neural populations are connected randomly with probability p. The size n and probability of connection we use is based on experimentally determined cortical connection networks for animals. These have been analyzed with graph-theoretical methods and all of these networks have less than 100 neural populations with a connection density (percentage of existing connections out all possible connections) of 20–40% (Felleman and van Essen, 1991; Scannell et al., 1995; Hilgetag et al., 2000a; Sporns et al., 2000, 2004; Bullmore and Sporns, 2009; Rubinov and Sporns, 2010; Sporns, 2011). We use random networks with $n = 50$ and $p = 0.5$ to illustrate our results, allowing comparisons with real cortical networks. These values of p ensure the networks are strongly connected (Bollobás, 1985) and all populations have at least one input and one output with high probability; i.e., there are no sources or sinks of electrical activity.

The specific random networks we investigate are the same random networks we have previously investigated (Gray and Robinson, 2006, 2008, 2009a,b). These networks consist of excitatory and inhibitory connections. The probability that a connection is inhibitory is given by p_i and such a connection has a negative gain. Excitatory gains are given values from a normal distribution with a mean $\mu_e > 0$ and variance σ_e^2. Similarly, inhibitory connections have a gain sampled from a normal distribution with $\mu_i < 0$ and variance σ_i^2. In terms of the gain matrix **G** all positive entries are sampled from $\mathcal{N}(\mu_e, \sigma_e^2)$ and all negative entries are sampled from $\mathcal{N}(\mu_i, \sigma_i^2)$.

Based on these parameters we investigated the stability of three types of networks: random networks with fixed excitatory gains (RENs), random connection networks (RCNs) with excitatory and inhibitory connections distributed randomly within the network (Gray and Robinson, 2009b), and random population networks (RPNs) (Gray and Robinson, 2009a). RPNs represent random networks with excitatory and inhibitory populations of neurons, this implies the outgoing connections of a given populations are all excitatory or all inhibitory. The gain matrix of RPNs consists of columns with either all entries ≤ 0 or all entries ≥ 0.

We determine the dispersion solutions for these structural brain networks numerically using a FORTRAN program called CROOT (Botten et al., 1983). This program finds dispersion solutions by implementing a recursive algorithm that employs Cauchy's integral formula (Mitrinović and Kečkić, 1984) within a specified annulus or disk.

RESULTS

Our results describe the stability of structural brain networks by determining the criteria for a network to stable—starting from simple excitatory networks and then adding time delays and dendritic time constants. For our network model we show that stability is determined by the eigenvalues of the gain matrix with stability constraining the eigenvalues to a specific zone in the complex plain. The first subsections translate the results from previous work into the current context. In particular, when time delays are included we produce a similar tear-drop shaped stability zone found by others (Jirsa and Ding, 2004; Feng et al., 2006; Qubbaj and Jirsa, 2007; Jirsa, 2009; Qubbaj and Jirsa, 2009). However, we show the addition of dendritic time constants modifies the shape of the stability zone. Finally, we use our results to assess how stability constrains the physiology of randomly connected networks with excitatory and inhibitory connections.

STABILITY OF STRUCTURAL BRAIN NETWORKS

The solutions ω of the dispersion relation Equation (8) determine the linear stability of a network. Setting $\lambda = D(\omega)$, the dispersion relation is

$$\det(\mathbf{G} - \lambda\mathbf{I}) = 0. \tag{9}$$

Therefore, network stability is determined by the spectrum of **G**, which we denote Sp(**G**). All the dispersion solutions ω of the network can be obtained by solving

$$\lambda - D(\omega) = 0 \tag{10}$$

for each λ in Sp(**G**). If all the λ in Sp(**G**) have corresponding ω [given by Equation (10)] with $\mathrm{Im}\omega < 0$ then the network is stable. However, if there exists one λ which has a corresponding dispersion solution with $\mathrm{Im}\omega \geq 0$ then the network is unstable. The set of dispersion solutions of a brain network is termed the *dispersion spectrum*. Taking the complex conjugate of Equations (4, 10) show that if $\omega_1 = \mathrm{Re}\omega + i\mathrm{Im}\omega = \omega_r + i\omega_i$ is solution for λ then $\omega_2 = -\omega_r + i\omega_i$ is a solution for the complex conjugate $\bar{\lambda}$ of λ. Therefore, since both λ and $\bar{\lambda}$ are in Sp(**G**), the dispersion spectrum is symmetric about the real axis.

Solving Equation (10) for ω is equivalent to solving $\lambda - \mathcal{D}(\varpi) = 0$ for ϖ where

$$\mathcal{D}(\varpi) = D(\gamma\varpi) = (1 - i\varpi\gamma/\alpha)(1 - i\varpi\gamma/\beta)(1 - i\varpi)^2 e^{-i\varpi\gamma\tau}, \tag{11}$$

and $\varpi = \omega/\gamma$ is a dimensionless frequency parameter. From the ϖ solutions the dispersion solutions for the network are

$\omega = \gamma\varpi$. Since D and $\mathcal{D}$ are analytic, the dispersion spectrum can be obtained by numerically solving Equation (10) for each λ.

Boundary between unstable and stable states

As the stability of a network is determined by Sp(**G**) we are interested in the zone of the complex plane where the all the eigenvalues of **G** must lie for the network to be stable. If a dispersion solution has $\text{Im}\omega = 0$ (i.e., ω is real and marginally stable) then the λ corresponding to ω lies on the critical boundary between the unstable and stable zones in the complex plane. Therefore, the stability boundary is given by $D(\omega)$ for real ω ranging from $-\infty$ to ∞. To describe the stability boundary we use $\mathcal{D}(\varpi)$ with real ϖ. This function traces out a continuous curve in the complex plane as ϖ ranges from $-\infty$ to ∞. Points on this curve represent λ in Sp(**G**) with real dispersion solutions $\omega = \gamma\varpi$. The stability boundary of a network is a segment of this curve since, in general, $\mathcal{D}(\varpi)$ can intersect itself to form loops.

Since $\mathcal{D}$ is a re-parameterization of D using $\varpi = \omega/\gamma$, a brain network with model parameters $\gamma = \gamma'$, $\alpha = \alpha'$, $\beta = \beta'$, and $\tau = \tau'$ has the same stability boundary as a network with $\gamma = 1$, $\alpha = \alpha'/\gamma'$, $\beta = \beta'/\gamma'$, and $\tau = \gamma'\tau$. However, the dispersion spectra of these networks will differ. If an initially stable network becomes unstable due to changes in its connection gains, its spectrum initially lies in the stability zone before at least one eigenvalue moves across the stability boundary from the stable to unstable zones. The λ that crosses the boundary is an instability with frequency $\omega/2\pi = \gamma\varpi/2\pi$, where $\lambda = \mathcal{D}(\varpi)$ on the boundary.

We now describe some general properties of the stability boundary for structural brain networks with time delays and non-zero dendritic time constants. In the following sections we investigate particular cases. Firstly, $\mathcal{D} \neq 0$ for all real $-\infty < \varpi < \infty$, thus $\lambda = 0$ does not lie on the stability boundary. If $\lambda = 0$ is substituted into Equation (11) then

$$(1 - i\varpi)^2 = 0, (1 - i\varpi\gamma/\alpha)^2 = 0, \text{ or } (1 - i\varpi\gamma/\beta)^2 = 0, \quad (12)$$

for complex ϖ. The only solutions to Equation (12) are $\varpi = -i$, $\varpi = -i\alpha/\gamma$, or $\varpi = -i\beta/\gamma$ giving the dispersion solution $\omega = -i\gamma$, $\omega = -i\alpha$, and $\omega = -i\beta$. These solutions all lie in the lower half plane for $\alpha, \beta, \gamma > 0$ and hence $\lambda = 0$ is a stable eigenvalue. If $\omega = \varpi = 0$ then $\mathcal{D}(\varpi) = 1$, since $L(0) = 1$, and $\lambda = 1$ lies on the stability boundary. This implies that if $\lambda = 1$ is in Sp(**G**) then the network has a zero frequency marginally stable dispersion solution. Furthermore, if we consider

$$|\lambda| = |L(\varpi)|^{-1}|e^{-i\varpi\gamma\tau}||1 - i\varpi|^2, \quad (13)$$

$$= |1 - i\varpi\gamma/\alpha||1 - i\varpi\gamma/\beta||e^{-i\varpi\gamma\tau}||1 - i\varpi|^2, \quad (14)$$

then $|\lambda| < 1$ implies at least one of the factors on the right of Equation (14) is less than 1. Since α, β, γ, and τ are all positive, this condition can only be satisfied if $\text{Im}\omega < 0$. Therefore, the unit disk is always contained in the stability zone and if all the eigenvalues of a gain matrix lie in the unit disk the network is stable independent of α, β, γ, and τ.

Stability of excitatory networks

If the all the connections in a structural brain network are excitatory then $G_{ab} \geq 0$ and **G** is a non-negative matrix. The Perron–Frobenius theorem (Horn and Johnson, 1985; Cvetković et al., 1995) then implies that **G** has a real eigenvalue λ_p such that $|\lambda_i| \leq \lambda_p$ for all λ_i in Sp(**G**). Therefore, an excitatory brain network is stable if and only if $\lambda_p < 1$; i.e., all the eigenvalues are in the unit disk. This stability criteria follows from the discussion at the end of the previous section and the fact that if $\lambda_p = 1$ then $\omega = 0$ is a solution to Equation (11). Since 0 lies on the stability boundary this implies if $\lambda_p \geq 1$ then $\text{Im}\omega \geq 0$. This means the stability of an excitatory brain network is independent of α, β, γ, and τ (as described in the previous section). In general, structural brain networks have inhibitory connections and the Perron–Frobenius theorem does not apply. This implies the presence of inhibitory connections allows the stability zone to extend beyond the unit disk.

IMPACT OF TIME DELAYS AND DENDRITIC TIME CONSTANTS ON NETWORK STABILITY

Stability of networks with no time delays and instantaneous rise and decay times

For networks with no time delays and instantaneous dendritic rise and decay times (i.e., $1/\alpha = 1/\beta = \tau = 0$)

$$\mathcal{D}(\varpi) = (1 - i\varpi)^2, \quad (15)$$

and hence, for each λ in Sp(**G**) there are two dispersion solutions given by

$$\omega = \gamma\varpi = -\gamma(i \pm i\sqrt{\lambda}). \quad (16)$$

Taking the imaginary part of Equation (16) we obtain

$$\text{Im}\omega = -\gamma(1 \pm \text{Re}\sqrt{\lambda}). \quad (17)$$

The stability condition $\text{Im}\omega < 0$ implies that $-\gamma(1 \pm \text{Re}\sqrt{\lambda})$ or $\text{Re}\sqrt{\lambda} \leq 1$ since $\gamma > 0$. Thus the stability of a network with $1/\alpha = 1/\beta = \tau = 0$ is independent of γ and all λ must satisfy $\text{Re}\sqrt{\lambda} \leq 1$ or alternatively $\text{Re}\lambda + |\lambda| \leq 2$ [since $(\text{Re}\sqrt{\lambda})^2$ equals $(\text{Re}\lambda + |\lambda|)/2$, with equality corresponding to the stability boundary].

If $\lambda_r = \text{Re}\lambda$ and $\lambda_i = \text{Im}\lambda$ then the stability zone is a parabolic zone in the complex plane given by

$$\lambda_i^2 \leq 4 - 4\lambda_r \quad (18)$$

with equality giving the stability boundary. The axis of the parabolic boundary is along the real axis with a turning point at $(\lambda_r, \lambda_i) = (1, 0)$ and imaginary axis intercepts at $\lambda_i = \pm 2$. This stability zone is the light gray zone in **Figure 1** and is the stability region described previously in (Gray and Robinson, 2008, 2009a,b).

Stability of networks with equal time delays

We now consider the effect of time delays on the stability of networks with $1/\alpha = 1/\beta = 0$. In this section we determine how the addition of a time delay to structural brain networks modifies the parabolic stability zone described by Equation (18) and describe the characteristics of the stability boundary. As noted previously, under our assumptions any self-connection in a brain network has the same time delay as connections between populations.

In this case $L(\omega) = 1$, $\tau \neq 0$, and

$$\mathcal{D}(\varpi) = (1 - i\varpi)^2 e^{-i\varpi\gamma\tau}. \tag{19}$$

Due to the exponential in Equation (19), $\lambda - \mathcal{D}(\varpi) = 0$ has an infinite number of solutions for each eigenvalue of the gain matrix. If $\lambda = \mathrm{Re}\lambda + i\mathrm{Im}\lambda = \lambda_r + i\lambda_i$ then $\lambda = \mathcal{D}(\varpi)$ (for real ϖ) implies

$$\lambda_r = \mathrm{Re}\mathcal{D}(\varpi) = (1 - \varpi^2)\cos(\varpi\gamma\tau) - 2\varpi\sin(\varpi\gamma\tau), \tag{20}$$

and

$$\lambda_i = \mathrm{Im}\mathcal{D}(\varpi) = (\varpi^2 - 1)\sin(\varpi\gamma\tau) - 2\varpi\cos(\varpi\gamma\tau), \tag{21}$$

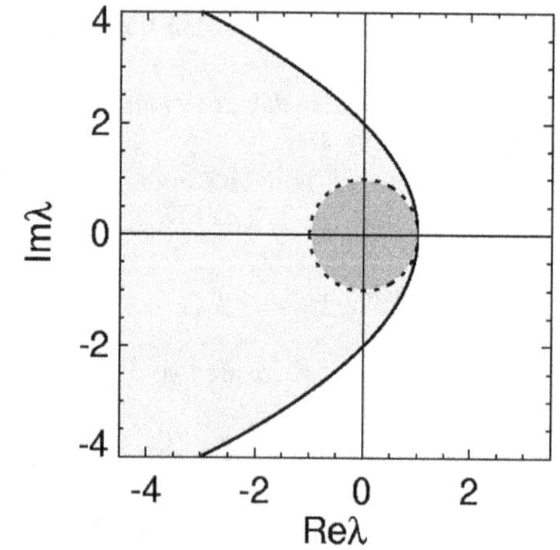

FIGURE 1 | Stability zone for a brain network with $1/\alpha = 1/\beta = \tau = 0$. The gray zone is where all the eigenvalues λ of the brain network must lie for the network to be stable. The dark region within this zone is the unit disk.

these equations can be combined giving

$$\lambda_i = -\tan(\varpi\gamma\tau)[\lambda_r + 2\varpi\mathrm{cosec}(\varpi\gamma\tau)], \tag{22}$$

which gives the stability boundary in the complex plane. For $\varpi \geq 0$, Equation (22) describes a spiral curve in the complex plane starting at the point $(\lambda_r, \lambda_i) = (1, 0)$, centered on the origin, and spiraling in a clockwise direction as ϖ increases, as seen in **Figure 2A**. For $\varpi < 0$, Equation (22) describes a similar counterclockwise spiral curve, corresponding to a reflection of the curve in **Figure 2A** about the imaginary axis.

Using Equations (20–22) we now describe the characteristics of the stability boundary and the resulting stability zone. The $\mathcal{D}(\varpi)$ curve crosses the real axis when $\lambda_i = 0$. Substituting $\lambda_i = 0$ into Equation (21) and (22) gives

$$(\varpi^2 - 1)\sin(\varpi\gamma\tau) = 2\varpi\cos(\varpi\gamma\tau), \tag{23}$$

and

$$\lambda_r = -2\varpi\mathrm{cosec}(\varpi\gamma\tau), \tag{24}$$

respectively. The values of ϖ for which $\lambda_i = 0$ can be obtained by solving Equation (23) numerically. Note that Equation (24) is only valid if $\varpi\gamma\tau \neq \pm m\pi/2$ for integers m. Due to the periodicity of the sine and cosine functions there is an infinite number of ϖ that satisfy these equations.

Thus the stability boundary consists of two spiral curves produced by bending the arms of the parabola described by Equation (18) inwards. These spiral curves intersect an infinite number of times on the real axis enclosing larger and larger regions of the complex plane as $|\varpi\gamma\tau|$ increases. The intersection of all these enclosed regions, corresponding to the innermost zone, represents the stability zone for the network. The reason eigenvalues outside this innermost zone are instabilities is because they correspond to eigenvalues outside the stability zone described by Equation (18) when transformed through multiplication by $e^{i\varpi\gamma\tau}$ (which removes the effect of the time delay).

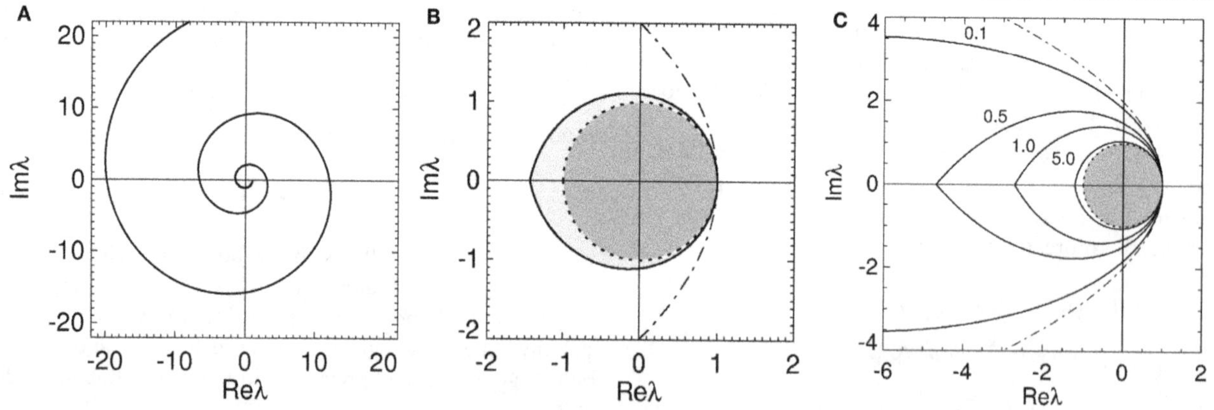

FIGURE 2 | Stability boundaries and stability zones for networks with $1/\alpha = 1/\beta = 0$. The curve $\mathcal{D}(\varpi)$ for $\varpi \geq 0$ **(A)** and corresponding stability boundary **(B)** for networks with $1/\alpha = 1/\beta = 0$ and $\gamma\tau = 3.0$. The shaded zone in **(B)** is the stability zone for a network and the dark region within this zone is the unit disk. The dot-dashed line is the boundary for $1/\alpha = 1/\beta = \tau = 0$. **(C)** Stability boundaries for brain networks with $1/\alpha = 1/\beta = 0$ and $\gamma\tau = 0.1$, 0.5, 1.0, and 5.0. The values of $\gamma\tau$ are written slightly above and to the left of the corresponding boundary. The dark gray region within this zone is the unit disk.

We define the smallest $\omega = \gamma\varpi > 0$ that gives $\lambda_i = 0$ the *critical* ω value. This critical value is denoted by ω_c with the corresponding ϖ and λ_r denoted ϖ_c and λ_r^c, respectively. The stability zone is defined by

$$|\text{Im}\lambda| < |\text{Im}[\mathcal{D}(\varpi)]|, \quad (25)$$

for $0 \leq \varpi \leq \varpi_c$. This zone has a boundary defined by Equation (19) for $-\varpi_c \leq \varpi \leq \varpi_c$. The real axis intercepts of the stability boundary are given by $\lambda_r = 1$ and $\lambda_r = \lambda_r^c = -2\varpi_c\text{cosec}(\varpi_c\gamma\tau)$. As seen in **Figure 2B** the stability zone has a teardrop shape containing the unit disc. Note that Equation (25) also defines the stability zone in **Figure 1** with $\varpi_c = \infty$. As $\gamma\tau \to 0$ then $\lambda_r \to (1 - \varpi^2)$ in Equation (20), $\lambda_i \to -2\varpi$ in Equation (21), and the stability boundary converges to the parabola $\lambda_i^2 = 4 - 4\lambda_r$, as expected.

The effect of increasing τ on the stability boundary is shown in **Figure 2C**. As $\gamma\tau$ increases, the stability boundary converges to the unit circle with the stability zone converging to the unit disk, shaded dark gray. The values of ϖ_c in **Figure 2C** for the four values of $\gamma\tau$ shown are 3.0 ($\gamma\tau = 0.1$), 1.92 ($\gamma\tau = 0.5$), 1.31 ($\gamma\tau = 1.0$), and 0.46 ($\gamma\tau = 5.0$), respectively. The corresponding λ_r^c are −9.4 (intersection not seen), −4.6, −2.7, and −1.2. For $\gamma = 100\,\text{s}^{-1}$ and $\tau = 0.01$ s (the nominal values in **Table 1**) $\omega_c/2\pi \approx 30$ Hz.

Overall, the presence of time delays bends the parabola described by Equation (18) inward, forming a teardrop-shaped stability zone containing the unit disk. As $\tau \to \infty$ the stability boundary wraps around the unit circle an infinite number of times and the stability zone converges to the unit disk, restricting the critical frequency.

Stability of networks with non-zero dendritic rise and decay time constants and no time delays

The teardrop shaped zone and the time-delay effects on stability described in the previous section produce similar results to those seen in other studies (Marcus and Westervelt, 1989; Jirsa and Ding, 2004; Feng et al., 2006). However, our model also incorporates dendritic rise and decay time constants. In the next two sections we describe the stability of structural brain networks with non-zero dendritic time constants.

We first investigate brain networks with dendritic time constants and no propagation time delays. In this case $\tau = 0$, $\alpha \neq 0$, and $\beta \neq 0$. Hence $L(\omega) \neq 1$ and

$$\mathcal{D}(\varpi) = (1 - i\varpi\gamma/\alpha)(1 - i\varpi\gamma/\beta)(1 - i\varpi)^2. \quad (26)$$

From Equation (26) the stability boundary is given by

$$\lambda_r = 1 - [1 + 2\gamma(1/\alpha + 1/\beta) + \gamma^2/(\alpha\beta)]\varpi^2 + \gamma^2/(\alpha\beta)\varpi^4, \quad (27)$$

and

$$\lambda_i = -[2 + \gamma(1/\alpha + 1/\beta)]\varpi + [\gamma(1/\alpha + 1/\beta) + 2\gamma^2/(\alpha\beta)]\varpi^3. \quad (28)$$

where $\lambda_r = \text{Re}\lambda$, $\text{Im}\lambda = \lambda_i$, and ϖ is real. In this case $\lambda - \mathcal{D}(\varpi) = 0$ only has a finite number of solutions since $\mathcal{D}(\varpi)$ is a polynomial of degree four. From Equation (28) the values of ϖ_c and ω_c are given by

$$\varpi_c^2 = \frac{2\alpha\beta + \gamma(\alpha+\beta)}{2\gamma^2 + \gamma(\alpha+\beta)}, \quad (29)$$

and

$$\omega_c = \sqrt{\frac{2\alpha\beta\gamma + \gamma^2(\alpha+\beta)}{\alpha+\beta+2\gamma}}, \quad (30)$$

respectively. An equation similar to Equation (30) was previously derived to describe gamma resonances produced by a similar mechanism (Robinson, 2005). If $\alpha\beta < \gamma^2$ then Equation (30) implies $\omega_c < \gamma$.

Unlike the case for time delays in the previous section, the $\mathcal{D}(\varpi)$ curve only crosses the real axis once for real $\varpi > 0$; an example of such a $\mathcal{D}(\varpi)$ curve is shown in **Figure 3A**. However, the region enclosed by $\mathcal{D}(\varpi)$ for $-\varpi_c \leq \varpi \leq \varpi_c$ is again the stability zone and defined by Equation (25). The corresponding stability zone for the $\mathcal{D}$ curve in **Figure 3A** is shown in **Figure 3B**.

The stability zone in **Figure 3B** contains the unit disk and has a similar teardrop shape to the zone in **Figure 2B** with the arms of the parabola given by Equation (18) bent inward. In terms of stability, this implies non-zero $1/\alpha$ and $1/\beta$ have similar effects to a propagation time delay. This is consistent with previous work on the corticothalamic model and highlights the low-pass filter effect of $L(\omega)$ (Robinson et al., 1997, 2001a,b; Rennie et al., 2002). The effective time delay resulting from γ/α and γ/β can be obtained by solving

$$e^{-i\varpi_c\gamma\tau} = (1 - i\varpi_c\gamma/\alpha)(1 - i\varpi_c\gamma/\beta), \quad (31)$$

for τ.

In the remainder of this section we explore the effect of varying γ, α, and β on the stability zone. We illustrate these effects by setting β/α to a positive constant. Firstly, for fixed β/α and large γ/α, Equations (27, 29) imply

$$\lambda_r \approx 1 + (\gamma/\alpha)^2\varpi^2(\varpi^2 - 1), \quad (32)$$

and

$$\varpi_c^2 \approx \alpha/\gamma, \quad (33)$$

respectively. From Equation (33), $\omega_c \approx 0$ for large γ/α and substituting Equation (33) into (32) shows that $\lambda_r^c \to -\infty$ as $\gamma/\alpha \to \infty$. These results are illustrated in **Figures 3C, 4**.

The change in the stability zone for fixed β/α and varying γ/α is shown in **Figure 3C**. All the stability zones contain the unit circle, and for $\gamma/\alpha = 0.1$ and 1.7 the stability zone is contained within the parabolic zone defined by Equation (18). However, the zone for $\gamma/\alpha = 100$ has expanded so that its boundary intersects the parabolic boundary at $\lambda_r \approx -11$. The ϖ_c in **Figure 3C** for $\gamma/\alpha = 100$, 0.1, and 1.7 are 0.15, 4.0, and 1.08, respectively. The corresponding λ_r^c are −66 (intersection not seen), −19, and −4.9. For $\gamma/\alpha = 1.7$, the nominal value from **Table 1**, the critical frequency is $\omega_c/2\pi \approx 17$ Hz.

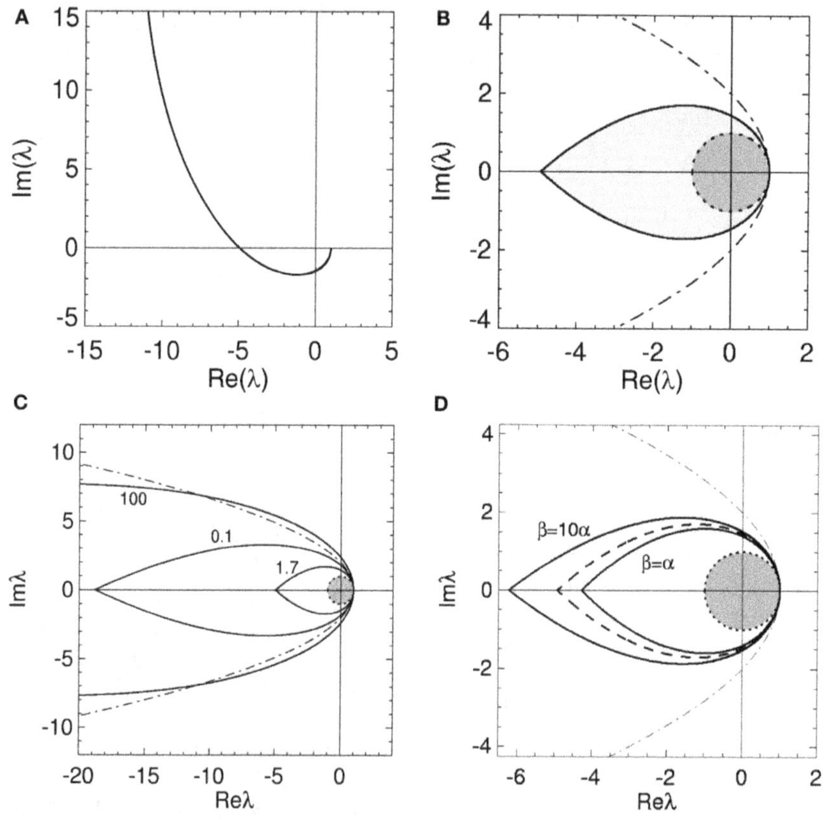

FIGURE 3 | Stability boundaries and stability zones for networks with non-zero dendritic rise and decay time constants and no time delays. The curve $\mathcal{D}(\varpi)$ for real $\varpi \geq 0$ **(A)** and corresponding stability zone and boundary **(B)** for networks with $\alpha = 60\,\mathrm{s}^{-1}$, $\beta = 240\,\mathrm{s}^{-1}$ and $\gamma = 100\,\mathrm{s}^{-1}$ and $\tau = 0\,\mathrm{s}$. The stability zone is shaded gray and the dark region within this zone is the unit disk. The dot-dashed line is the boundary for $1/\alpha = 1/\beta = \tau = 0$. **(C)** Stability boundaries for $\beta = 4\alpha$ and $\gamma/\alpha = 100$, 0.1, and 1.7. The values of γ/α are written next to their corresponding boundary. **(D)** Stability boundaries for $\gamma/\alpha = 1.7$ and $\beta/\alpha = 1$, 4 (dashed curve), and 10. The dot-dashed line in **(C,D)** is the boundary for $1/\alpha = 1/\beta = \tau = 0$ and the dark gray region in **(C,D)** is the unit disk.

The effect of changing β/α on the stability zone, while γ/α remains fixed, is shown in **Figure 3D**. The ϖ_c (λ_r^c) in **Figure 3D** for $\beta/\alpha = 1$ and $\beta/\alpha = 10$ are 0.77 ($\lambda_r^c = -4.3$) and 1.26 ($\lambda_r^c = -6.2$), respectively. Note that if $\beta/\alpha < 1$, then the values of α and β can be swapped and the results in **Figure 3** are reproduced. This is because exchanging γ/α and γ/β in Equation (4) has no effect on the dynamics and stability of a network. This implies the smallest stability zone with the minimum λ_r^c occurs when $\alpha = \beta$. Note that experimental measurements of dendritic time constants in the brain give $\beta/\alpha \approx 4$–10 (Robinson et al., 2003a, 2004), the upper range in **Table 1**, and hence, a larger stability zone for brain activity.

Figure 3 suggests that as β/α increases the stability zone expands in a similar way to decreasing τ. However, as $\tau \to 0$ the stability zone converges to the parabolic zone (Equation 18), this is not the case for $\gamma/\beta \to \infty$ and fixed γ/α. If γ/α is fixed to a positive constant and $\gamma/\beta \gg \gamma/\alpha$ then, from Equation (29), $\varpi_c^2 \lesssim 1$ and therefore

$$\lambda_r \approx 1 - \gamma\varpi^2/\beta, \tag{34}$$

and

$$\lambda_i \approx -\gamma\varpi/\beta. \tag{35}$$

When $\lambda_r = 0$, Equation (34) implies $\varpi \approx \sqrt{\beta/\gamma}$ and $\lambda_i \approx -\sqrt{\gamma/\beta}$. Therefore as $\gamma/\beta \to \infty$, the imaginary axis intercepts converge to $\pm\infty$ and the stability zone expands to cover the entire region of the complex plane defined by $\mathrm{Re}\lambda < 1$. Note that in this case, even though the eigenvalues can lie anywhere to the left of $\mathrm{Re}\lambda = 1$, the dispersion solutions have an angular frequency $\omega < \gamma$. These results explain the intersection of the stability boundary with the parabolic boundary in **Figure 3C**.

With **Figure 3C** these convergence results suggest that as γ/α increases from 0, the stability zone contracts toward the unit circle, and then expands again. **Figure 4** shows the values of λ_r^c and ω_c as a function of γ/α and β/α. As γ/α increases from 0, λ_r^c rapidly increases from $-\infty$ to a maximum value and then slowly decreases back to $-\infty$; this decrease is greatest for the $\beta/\alpha = 1$ curve which intersects the other two curves in **Figure 4A**. The maximum turning point for λ_r^c occurs when $\gamma \approx \alpha$ for each β/α, with maximum λ_r^c decreasing as β/α increases. When $\beta/\alpha = 4$ (which is the nominal value in **Table 1**), λ_r^c is approximately constant for $1 \lesssim \gamma/\alpha \lesssim 3$, with a maximum at $\gamma/\alpha \approx 1.7$, the nominal value. The corresponding ω_c curves in **Figure 4B** all show similar monotonic decreases as γ/α increases. The curves do not intersect or have a turning point as in **Figure 4A**. This decrease

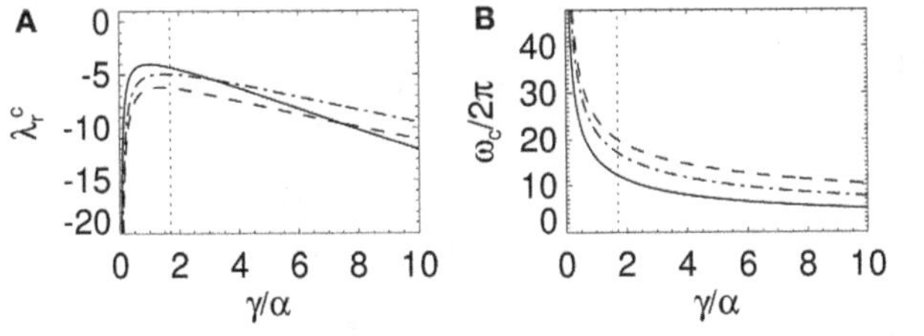

FIGURE 4 | Change in stability boundary real axis intercept and critical frequency as a function of γ/α. (A) λ_r^c and **(B)** ω_c as a function of γ/α for $\gamma\tau = 0$ and $\beta/\alpha = 1$ (solid lines), 4 (dotted lines), and 10 (dot-dashed lines). In **(B)** ω_c is determined with $\gamma = 100\,\text{s}^{-1}$. The dotted lines represent the nominal γ/α from **Table 1**.

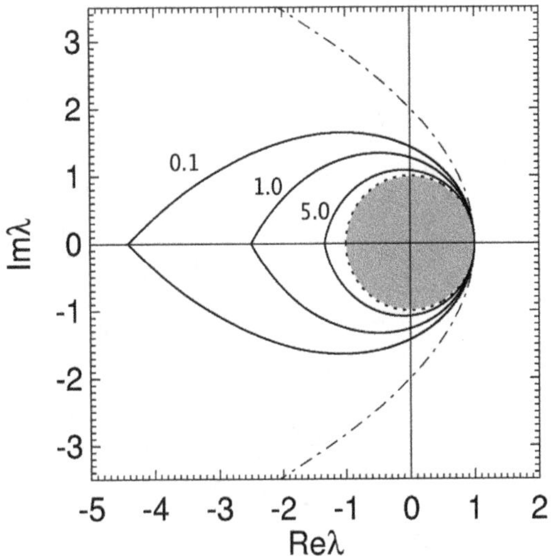

FIGURE 5 | Stability boundaries for brain networks with $\gamma/\alpha = 1.7$, $\beta/\alpha = 4$ and $\gamma\tau = 0.1, 1.0,$ and 5.0. The values of $\gamma\tau$ are written slightly to the left of their corresponding boundary. The gray region is the unit disk.

from ∞ is initially very rapid, before gradually decreasing to 0 as $\gamma/\alpha \to \infty$. This change approximately occurs at the nominal γ/α value in **Table 1**, where $\omega_c/2\pi \lesssim 20\,\text{Hz}$ for each β/α. Note that when β/α is a fixed constant, Equation (33) shows that $\omega_c \to 0$. **Figure 4B** also shows that increasing γ/α and decreasing γ/β results in a decreased value for ω_c.

In this section we have shown that physiologically realistic dendritic time constants have an effect on network stability similar to that of propagation time delays restricting, the critical frequency and the stability zone to a teardrop-shaped zone in the complex plane. However, unlike τ, for particular values of γ/α and γ/β the stability zone can expand to enclose an area outside the parabolic region described by Equation (18).

Stability of networks with time delays and non-zero dendritic time constants

The effect of having both time delays and non-zero dendritic time constants on stability is now described. In this case each of the parameters γ, $1/\alpha$, $1/\beta$, and τ are non-zero and $\mathcal{D}$ is given by Equation (11). As in the previous section, the stability boundary for these networks is defined by $\lambda_r = \text{Re}\mathcal{D}(\varpi)$ and $\lambda_i = \text{Im}\mathcal{D}(\varpi)$ for $-\infty < \varpi < \infty$. Analysis of these equations gives the properties of the stability boundary and zone. However, the effects on stability of having equal time delays and dendritic time constants are easily understood qualitatively as a combination of our previous results. Beginning with a network that has $\gamma/\alpha = \gamma/\beta = \gamma\tau = 0$ and a parabolic stability zone, given by Equation (18), adding a time delay τ contracts the stability zone toward the unit circle, by "pulling in" the parabolic boundary, forming a teardrop-shaped zone within the original parabolic region. Adding dendritic rise and decay constants then, depending on their value, expands or contracts this stability zone. In all cases the stability zone is defined by

$$|\text{Im}\lambda| < |\text{Im}[\mathcal{D}(\varpi)]|, \qquad (36)$$

for $0 \le \varpi \le \varpi_c$. Note that for large $\gamma\tau$, γ/α, and γ/β the contraction caused by $\gamma\tau$ is greater than the expansion effects due to γ/α and γ/β because of the exponential in Equation (11).

In **Figure 5** the stability zone of a brain network with plausible time delays and dendritic time constants (from **Table 1**) is shown. This shows that for realistic parameter values brain networks have a teardrop-shaped stability zone completely within the parabolic zone (Equation 18). For large realistic τ the stability zone is only slightly larger than the unit disc. The ϖ_c in **Figure 5** for increasing $\gamma\tau$ are 1.02, 0.72, and 0.35, respectively. The corresponding critical frequencies $\omega_c/2\pi$ for $\gamma = 100$ are then 16, 11.3, and 5.5 Hz, respectively.

STABILITY AND DISPERSION SOLUTIONS OF RANDOMLY CONNECTED NETWORKS

We now investigate the stability and dispersion solutions of the randomly connected structural brain networks defined in the "Methods" section. For these networks we fix the model parameters γ, α, β, and τ to their nominal values in **Table 1**. The stability and dispersion solutions of this networks are determined from Sp(**G**). If all the eigenvalues λ in Sp(**G**) satisfy Equation (25) then the network is stable. The corresponding dispersion solutions are obtained numerically by solving Equation (10) for each λ using CROOT (Botten et al., 1983) (as described in "Methods").

The spectrum of a RENs consists of one eigenvalue at $np\mu_e$ with the other $n-1$ eigenvalues uniformly distributed in a disc of radius $\mu_e\sqrt{np(1-p)} < np\mu_e$. The spectrum of RCNs and RPNs with maximum μ_e and μ_i allowed by stability is distributed within the unit disk, see (Gray and Robinson, 2009a), with multiple eigenvalues near the stability boundary. Therefore, stability constrains the spectrum of random brain networks to the unit disk and the stability of random brain networks is independent of the γ, α, β, and τ. However, the frequencies of the dispersion solutions do depend on the model parameters.

In **Figure 6** the spectrum and dispersion solutions for a REN, RCN, and RPN with the nominal model parameters are shown. The parameters of each network are set so that the networks are marginally stable and μ_e and $|\mu_i|$ are as large as possible while maintaining stability. Note the larger values of μ_e and $|\mu_i|$ for the

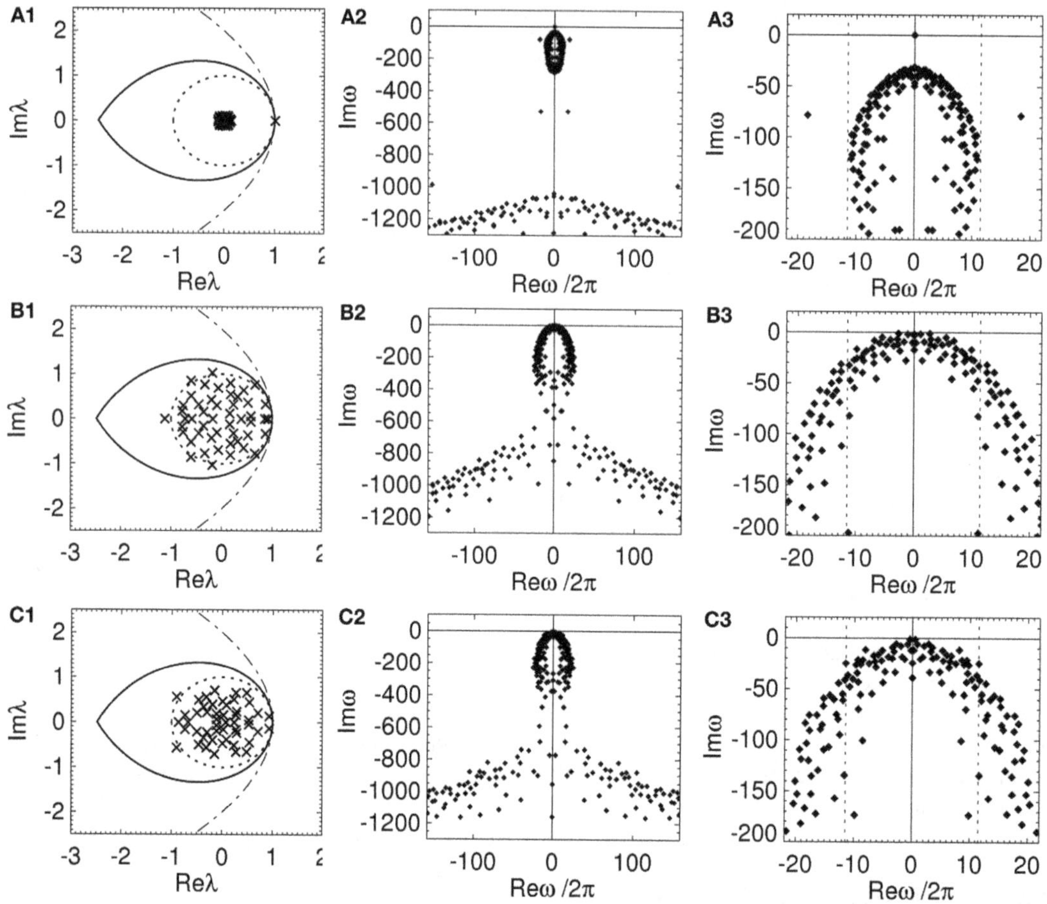

FIGURE 6 | Spectrum and dispersion solutions for a REN, a RCN, and a RPN. Each network has $n = 50$, $p = 0.5$, and the nominal parameters in **Table 1**, other parameters are set so that the network is close to marginal stability. The left column is the spectrum (crosses), the middle column shows the dispersion solutions (diamonds), and the right column shows an expanded view of the dispersion solutions near the imaginary axis with dotted lines representing the critical frequencies $\pm\ \omega_c/2\pi$. **(A)** REN with $\mu_e = 0.04$, **(B)** RCN with $p_i = 0.5$, $\mu_e = -\mu_i = 0.2$, $\sigma_e = \sigma_i = 0$, and **(C)** RPN with $p_i = 0.5$, $\mu_e = -\mu_i = 0.22$, $\sigma_e = \sigma_i = 0$.

RPN, compared to the RCN. This highlights that RPNs can have larger μ_e and $|\mu_i|$, and hence be more responsive, before becoming almost certainly unstable as shown in (Gray and Robinson, 2009a). This suggests stability may have an effect on the arrangement of inhibitory and excitatory neurons and their physiology in structural brain networks.

Each network has an infinite number of dispersion solutions because $\tau \neq 0$. The second column of **Figure 6** shows the dispersion spectrum is symmetrically placed around the real axis. Each network has a qualitatively similar dispersion spectrum, with a finite cluster of solutions near the origin and a broad "arrowhead" of solutions for $\text{Im}\omega \lesssim 800\ \text{s}^{-1}$; this arrowhead has an infinite number of solutions with $\text{Im}\omega$ decreasing as $|\text{Re}\omega|$ increases. The third column shows the dispersion solutions near the imaginary axis. In **Figure 6A3** one solution, $\omega = \omega_1$, lies on the origin, separate from the other dispersion solutions. This solution corresponds to the eigenvalue at $\lambda \approx 1$ that is separated from the rest of the spectrum in **Figure 6A1**. This implies the dynamics of an REN will be dominated by a zero-frequency mode. Since the rest of the dispersion solutions have $\text{Im}\omega \ll 0$ all other modes rapidly decay to zero amplitude. However, the RCN and RPN in **Figure 6** have a very similar dispersion spectrum with multiple dispersion solutions near the imaginary axis. The solutions closest to the imaginary axis have small frequencies $\lesssim 5$ Hz. This shows that the presence of inhibitory connections allows random networks to have multiple marginally stable low frequency modes (Gray and Robinson, 2008, 2009a,b).

DISCUSSION

We increased the physiological realism of a structural brain network model we studied previously in (Gray and Robinson, 2006, 2008, 2009a,b; Robinson et al., 2009) by allowing the network to have equal time delays τ for propagation between neuronal populations and non-zero dendritic rise $1/\beta$ and decay $1/\alpha$ time constants. Under these assumptions the stability of an arbitrarily connected network of neural populations is determined by the network's gain matrix. The addition of time delays changed the stability zone in the complex plane from a parabolic region to a teardrop-shaped zone, dependent on α, β, τ, and the temporal damping rate γ. Our results are similar to previous work investigating the effect of time delays on stability of electrical activity within spatially continuous networks of neural tissue (Marcus and Westervelt, 1989; Jirsa and Ding, 2004; Feng et al., 2006; Qubbaj and Jirsa, 2007, 2009; Jirsa, 2009). This previous work has generally used integro-differential neural field equations with connectivity within a neural mass described by homogeneous or heterogeneous kernels. While in principle this work could be applied to large-scale connection topologies of discrete neural masses, as we have investigated here, this has generally not been done as it is difficult to incorporate arbitrary connectivity patterns (Qubbaj and Jirsa, 2009). In this work we have investigated the temporal dynamics of the overall electrical activity of arbitrarily connected structural brain networks, ignoring the spatial spread and propagation of electrical activity within individual neuronal populations.

In terms of stability the effect of non-zero dendritic time constants is similar to a time delay, further suggesting that dendrites act as a low-pass filter on synaptic inputs (Robinson et al., 1997, 2001a,b; Rennie et al., 2002). However, dendritic time constants can change the shape of the stability zone even allowing it to expand and enclose areas outside the parabolic stability region for networks with zero time delays and instantaneous dendritic rise and decay times. For all values of γ, α, β, and τ the stability zone contains the unit disk. This result implies that the stability criteria originally derived by May (1972, 1974) (that a network is stable if all its eigenvalues lie in the unit disk) is a sufficient condition for the stability of structural brain networks.

We also explored the dispersion solutions and frequencies of structural brain networks. If an initially stable brain network becomes unstable through a change in its connection gains, then at least one eigenvalue moves across the stability boundary and the network has an instability at a frequency given by the eigenvalue's corresponding dispersion solution. For networks with time delays and non-zero dendritic time constants there is a maximum frequency, the critical frequency $\omega_c/2\pi$, at which initially stable networks will become unstable. For example, if all the gain matrix eigenvalues of a networks are initially inside the stability zone but then move across the stability boundary (e.g., due to changes in connection gains) then the frequency of these instabilities will be less than the critical frequency.

Measurements of brain activity (Stam et al., 1999; Robinson et al., 2001b; Breakspear, 2002; Breakspear et al., 2003) suggest the brain operates near marginal stability allowing the brain to have rich dynamics and a wide range of complex behavior. A network near marginal stability has eigenvalues near the stability boundary with corresponding modes that are the slowest to decay back to the steady state dominating the network's dynamics. These modes have a frequency less than the critical frequency. Using physiologically plausible parameter values in our structural network model (see **Table 1**) we would expect the electrical dynamics to be dominated by frequencies $\lesssim 100$ Hz. When the nominal parameter values of α, β, γ, and τ are used the critical frequency is approximately 10 Hz and decreases as $\gamma\tau$ increases (see **Figures 4, 6**).

For the randomly connected structural brain networks we investigated previously (Gray and Robinson, 2006, 2008, 2009a,b) the spectrum of the gain matrix is almost certainly contained in a disk centered on the origin with a radius dependent on the network's architecture and the average values of its excitatory and inhibitory gains. Thus, the stability zone of these networks is the unit disk and their stability is independent of time delays and dendritic time constants. Therefore, the results of that work remain valid in the more general case studied here. However, for the critical frequency is dependent on dendritic time constants, temporal damping rate, and time delays. We showed marginally stable randomly connected networks with inhibitory connections have multiple marginally stable low frequency dispersion solutions.

The primary goal of this and our previous work on structural brain networks is to understand how stability potential constrains the structure physiology of networks. For the randomly connected networks studied in (Gray and Robinson, 2006, 2008, 2009a,b), we have shown that time delays and non-zero dendritic time constants have minimal effect on their stability. One network type whose stability could be affected by these physiological properties is networks with inhibitory self-connections. The spectrum of these networks, even if they are randomly connected, is no longer restricted to a disc by stability but can have eigenvalues distributed within the teardrop-shaped region. Such networks could have marginally stable modes with frequencies (up to the critical frequency) in the alpha, beta, and gamma ranges. This will be explored in future work.

LIKELY EFFECTS OF DISTRIBUTED OR VARYING PARAMETERS ON STABILITY

Assuming structural brain networks have equal γ, α, and β for each neural population and equal τ for each connection is unrealistic. Different neuronal populations in the brain have different parameter values; for example, excitatory cortical neurons have $\gamma \approx 100\,\text{s}^{-1}$ while for inhibitory cortical neurons $\gamma \approx 10^3$–$10^4\,\text{s}^{-1}$ (Robinson et al., 2004). Also, the time delay in real cortical networks is expected to vary from $\tau = 0$ for self-connections to a large value for areas physically far apart. A realistic model of a structural brain network would therefore allow the model parameters γ, α, β, and τ to vary across neural populations. This variation could possibly be represented as a distribution.

The effect of distributed time delays on network stability has been studied using general models for network activity (Yi and Tan, 2002; Atay, 2003; Jirsa and Ding, 2004; Feng et al., 2006). In (Feng et al., 2006) and (Jirsa and Ding, 2004) networks with a distributed time delay with mean τ were shown to have a stability zone that contained the stability zone of networks with an constant delay equal to τ. These results are applicable to the brain networks studied here, since our model without dendritic time constants can be described as a specific case of the model studied in (Jirsa and Ding, 2004; Feng et al., 2006). This implies brain networks with distributed delay are more stable than networks with equal time delays; in the sense that a stable network with a distribution of delays could be unstable if its delays were replaced with a constant delay equal to the distribution mean. Hence, the equal time delay case is the least stable case and yields a bound on the stability of a structural brain network.

Here we have shown that plausible dendritic time constants have similar effects on stability as a time delay. This suggests that similar results to those found in (Jirsa and Ding, 2004; Feng et al., 2006) will likely be observed for distributed α and β. Also, we have shown that γ only affects the dispersion frequencies of a network, not its stability. A distributed γ is therefore expected to have no effect on the stability, only on the dispersion frequencies but this needs to be confirmed numerically.

Given the previous results investigating distributed parameter values we argue our results are still informative. But the exact effect of distributed γ, α, and β on structural brain network dynamics needs to be determined, particularly to understand the critical frequency and the dynamics of marginally stable modes in a networks electrical activity. To fully understand the stability and dynamics of structural brain networks with varying time delays and dendritic time constants requires a numerical approach. This will be investigated using CROOT (Botten et al., 1983) in future work.

CONCLUSIONS

We investigated the stability of discrete networks of neuronal populations using a simplified physiologically-based mean-field model of brain electrical activity. Incorporating time delays and non-zero dendritic time constants affects the stability of arbitrarily connected structural brain networks by constraining the eigenvalues of the gain matrix to a teardrop-shaped region in the complex plane. The stability of randomly connected networks of excitatory and inhibitory neuronal populations is unaffected by time delays and dendritic time constants; as stability constrains the gain matrix eigenvalues to the unit circle. However, the dispersion frequencies of instabilities are affected by network physiology. Randomly connected brain networks with the largest average excitatory and inhibitory gains allowed by stability can have multiple marginally stable low-frequency modes. Such networks would be highly responsive and adaptable to external stimuli while remaining stable, and have a wide range of flexible, adaptable, and complex behavior.

REFERENCES

Acebrón, J. A., Bonilla, L. L., Vicente, C. J. P., Ritort, F., and Spigler, R. (2005). The kuramoto model: a simple paradigm for synchronization phenomena. *Rev. Mod. Phys.* 77, 137–185.

Allesina, S., and Tang, S. (2012). Stability criteria for complex ecosystems. *Nature* 483, 205–208.

Atay, F. M. (2003). Distributed delays facilitate amplitude death of coupled oscillators. *Phys. Rev. Lett.* 91:094101. doi: 10.1103/PhysRevLett.91.094101

Atay, F. M., and Hutt, A. (2004). Stability and bifurcations in neural fields with finite propagation speed and general connectivity. *SIAM J. Appl. Math.* 65, 644–666.

Attwell, D., and Laughlin, S. B. (2001). An energy budget for signaling in the grey matter of the brain. *J. Cereb. Blood Flow Met.* 21, 1133–1145.

Bassett, D. S., and Bullmore, E. (2006). Small-world brain networks. *Neuroscientist* 12, 1–12.

Bechhoefer, J. (2005). Feedback for physicists: a tutorial essay on control. *Rev. Mod. Phys.* 77, 783–836.

Bollobás, B. (1985). *Random Graphs.* London: Academic Press.

Botten, L. C., Craig, M. S., and McPhedran, R. C. (1983). Complex zeros of analytic functions. *Comput. Phys. Commun.* 29, 245–259.

Breakspear, M. (2002). Nonlinear phase desynchronization in human electroencephalographic data. *Hum. Brain Mapp.* 15, 175–198.

Breakspear, M., Roberts, J. A., Terry, J. R., Rodrigues, S., Mahant, N., and Robinson, P. A. (2006). A unifying explanation of primary generalized seizures through nonlinear brain modeling and bifurcation analysis. *Cereb. Cortex* 16, 1296–1313.

Breakspear, M., Terry, J. R., and Friston, K. J. (2003). Modulation of excitatory synaptic coupling facilitates synchronization and complex dynamics in a nonlinear model or neuronal dynamics. *Neurocomputing* 52–54, 151–158.

Bressloff, P. (2011). Spatiotemporal dynamics of continuum neural fields. *J. Phys. A Math. Theor.* 45:033001. doi: 10.1088/1751-8113/45/3/033001

Bullmore, E., and Sporns, O. (2009). Complex brain networks: graph theoretical analysis of structural and functional systems. *Nat. Rev. Neurosci.* 10, 186–198.

Bullmore, E., and Sporns, O. (2012). The economy of brain network organization. *Nat. Rev. Neurosci.* 13, 336–349.

Coombes, S. (2005). Waves, bumps, and patterns in neural field theories. *Biol. Cybern.* 93, 91–108.

Coombes, S., Venkov, N. A., Shiau, L., Bojak, I., Liley, D. T., and Laing, C. R. (2007). Modeling electrocortical activity through improved local approximations of integral neural field equations. *Phys. Rev. E* 76:051901. doi: 10.1103/PhysRevE.76.051901

Cvetković, D., Doob, M., and Scahs, H. (1995). *Spectra of Graphs.* 3rd Edn. Heidelberg: Johann Ambrosius Barth Verlag.

da Silva, F. H. L., Hoeks, A., Smits, A., and Zetterberg, L. H. (1974). Model of brain rhythmic activity: the alpha-rhythm of the thalamus. *Kybernetik* 15, 27–37.

Deco, G., Jirsa, V., Robinson, P., Breakspear, M., and Friston, K. (2008). The dynamic brain: from spiking neurons to neural masses and cortical fields. *PLoS Comput. Biol.* 4:e1000092. doi: 10.1371/journal.pcbi.1000092

Felleman, D. J., and van Essen, D. C. (1991). Distributed hierarchical processing in the primate cerebral cortex. *Cereb. Cortex* 1, 1–47.

Feng, J., Jirsa, V. K., and Ding, M. (2006). Synchronization in networks with random interactions: theory and applications. *Chaos* 16:015109. doi: 10.1063/1.2180690

Freeman, W. J. (1975). *Mass Action in the Nervous System: Examination of the Neurophysiological Basis of Adaptive Behavior Through the EEG.* New York, NY: Academic Press.

Gray, R., and Robinson, P. (2006). Stability and spectra of randomly connected excitatory cortical networks. *Neurocomputing* 70, 1000–1012.

Gray, R., and Robinson, P. (2008). Stability and synchronization of random brain networks with a distribution of connection strengths. *Neurocomputing* 71, 1373–1387.

Gray, R. T., and Robinson, P. A. (2009a). Stability and structural constraints of random brain networks with excitatory and inhibitory neural populations. *J. Comput. Neurosci.* 27, 81–101.

Gray, R. T., and Robinson, P. A. (2009b). Stability of random brain networks with excitatory and inhibitory connections. *Neurocomputing* 72, 1849–1858.

Hilgetag, C.-C., Burns, G. A. P. C., O'Neill, M. A., Scannell, J. W., and Young, M. P. (2000a). Anatomical connectivity defines the organization of clusters of cortical areas in the macaque monkey and the cat. *Philos. Trans. R. Soc. Lond. B* 355, 91–110.

Hilgetag, C.-C., O'Neill, M. A., and Young, M. P. (2000b). Hierarchical organization of macaque and cat cortical sensory systems explored with a novel network processor. *Philos. Trans. R. Soc. Lond. B* 355, 71–89.

Hogg, T., Huberman, B. A., and McGlade, J. M. (1989). The stability of ecosystems. *Proc. R. Soc. B* 237, 43–51.

Horn, R. A., and Johnson, C. R. (1985). *Matrix Analysis.* New York, NY: Cambridge University Press.

Jirsa, V. (2009). Neural field dynamics with local and global connectivity and time delay. *Philos. Trans. R. Soc. Lond. A Math. Phys. Eng. Sci.* 367, 1131–1143.

Jirsa, V. K., and Ding, M. (2004). Will a large complex system with time delays be stable? *Phys. Rev. Lett.* 93:070602, 1–4. doi: 10.1103/PhysRevLett.93.070602

Jirsa, V. K., and Haken, H. (1996). Field theory of electromagnetic brain activity. *Phys. Rev. Lett.* 77, 960–963.

Jouve, B., Rosenstiehl, P., and Imbert, M. (1998). A mathematical approach to the connectivity between the cortical visual areas of the macaque monkey. *Cereb. Cortex* 8, 28–39.

Kandel, E. R., Schwartz, J. H., and Jessell, T. M. (2000). *Principles of Neural Science.* 4th Edn. New York, NY: McGraw-Hill.

Kim, J. W., and Robinson, P. A. (2007). Compact dynamical model of brain activity. *Phys. Rev. E* 75:031907. doi: 10.1103/PhysRevE.75.031907

Koch, C. (2004). *The Quest for Consciousness: A Neurobiological Approach*. Englewood: Roberts and Company.

Kuramoto, Y. (1984). *Chemical Oscillations, Waves, and Turbulence*. New York, NY: Dover.

Laughlin, S. B., de Ruyter van Stevenick, R. R., and Anderson, J. C. (1998). The metabolic cost of neural information. *Nat. Neurosci.* 1, 36–41.

Lennie, P. (2003). The cost of cortical computation. *Cogn. Brain Res.* 13, 493–497.

Marcus, C. M., and Westervelt, R. M. (1989). Stability of analog neural networks with delay. *Phys. Rev. A* 39, 347–359.

May, R. M. (1972). Will a large complex system be stable? *Nature* 238, 413–414.

May, R. M. (1974). *Stability and Complexity in Model Ecosystems*. 2nd Edn. Princeton, NJ: Princeton University Press.

McCann, K. S. (2000). The diversity-stability debate. *Nature* 405, 228–233.

Mitrinović, D. S., and Keckić, J. D. (1984). *The Cauchy Theory of Residues: Theory and Applications*. Dordrecht: D. Reidel Publishing Company.

Murray, J. D. (2002). *Mathematical Biology*. 3rd Edn. New York, NY: Springer.

Nunez, P. L. (1974). Wave-like properties of the alpha rhythm. *IEEE Trans. Biomed. Eng.* 21, 473–482.

Nunez, P. L. (1995). *Neocortical Dynamics and Human EEG Rhythms*. New York, NY: Oxford University Press.

Pecora, L. M., and Carroll, T. L. (1998). Master stability functions for synchronized coupled systems. *Phys. Rev. Lett.* 80, 2109–2112.

Qubbaj, M., and Jirsa, V. (2007). Neural field dynamics with heterogeneous connection topology. *Phys. Rev. Lett.* 98:238102. doi: 10.1103/PhysRevLett.98.238102

Qubbaj, M., and Jirsa, V. (2009). Neural field dynamics under variation of local and global connectivity and finite transmission speed. *Physica D* 238, 2331–2346.

Rennie, C. J., Robinson, P. A., and Wright, J. J. (2002). Unified neurophysical model of EEG spectra and evoked potentials. *Biol. Cybern.* 86, 457–471.

Robinson, P. A. (2003). Neurophysical theory of coherence and correlations of electroencephalographic and electrocorticographic signals. *J. Theor. Biol.* 222, 163–175.

Robinson, P. A. (2005). Propagator theory of brain dynamics. *Phys. Rev. E* 72:0119404. doi: 10.1103/PhysRevE.72.011904

Robinson, P. A., Henderson, J. A., Matar, E., Riley, P., and Gray, R. T. (2009). Dynamical reconnection and stability constraints on cortical network architecture. *Phys. Rev. Lett.* 103, 1–4.

Robinson, P. A., Loxley, P. N., O'Connor, S. C., and Rennie, C. J. (2001a). Modal analysis of corticothalamic dynamics, electroencephalographic spectra, and evoked potentials. *Phys. Rev. E* 63:041909. doi: 10.1103/PhysRevE.63.041909

Robinson, P. A., Rennie, C. J., Wright, J. J., Bahramali, H., Gordon, E., and Rowe, D. L. (2001b). Prediction of electroencephalographic spectra from neurophysiology. *Phys. Rev. E* 63:021903. doi: 10.1103/PhysRevE.63.021903

Robinson, P. A., Rennie, C. J., and Rowe, D. L. (2002). Dynamics of large-scale brain activity in normal arousal states and epileptic seizures. *Phys. Rev. E* 65:041924. doi: 10.1103/PhysRevE.65.041924

Robinson, P. A., Rennie, C. J., Rowe, D. L., and O'Connor, S. C. (2004). Estimation of multiscale neurophysicologic parameters by electroencephalographic means. *Hum. Brain Mapp.* 23, 53–72.

Robinson, P. A., Rennie, C. J., Rowe, D. L., O'Connor, S. C., Wright, J. J., Gordon, E., et al. (2003a). Neurophysical modeling of brain dynamics. *Neuropsychopharmacology* 28, S74–S79.

Robinson, P. A., Whitehouse, R. W., and Rennie, C. J. (2003b). Nonuniform corticothalamic continuum model of electroencephalographic spectra with application to split-alpha peaks. *Phys. Rev. E* 68:021922. doi: 10.1103/PhysRevE.68.021922

Robinson, P. A., Rennie, C. J., and Wright, J. J. (1997). Propagation and stability of waves of electrical activity in the cerebral cortex. *Phys. Rev. E* 56, 826–840.

Robinson, P. A., Rennie, C. J., Wright, J. J., and Bourke, P. D. (1998). Steady states and global dynamics of electrical activity in the cerebral cortex. *Phys. Rev. E* 58, 3557–3571.

Rubinov, M., and Sporns, O. (2010). Complex network measures of brain connectivity: uses and interpretations. *Neuroimage* 52, 1059–1069.

Scannell, J. W., Blakemore, C., and Young, M. P. (1995). Analysis of connectivity in the cat cerebral cortex. *Int. J. Neural Syst.* 15, 1463–1483.

Sporns, O. (2011). The human connectome: a complex network. *Ann. N.Y. Acad. Sci.* 1224, 109–125.

Sporns, O., Chialvo, D. R., Kaiser, M., and Hilgetag, C. C. (2004). Organization, development and function of complex brain networks. *TRENDS Neurosci.* 8, 418–425.

Sporns, O., Tononi, G., and Edelman, G. M. (2000). Theoretical neuroanatomy: relating anatomical and functional connectivity in graphs and cortical connection matrices. *Cereb. Cortex* 10, 127–141.

Sporns, O., Tononi, G., and Kötter, R. (2005). The human connectome: a structural description of the human brain. *PLoS Comput. Biol.* 1:e42. doi: 10.1371/journal.pcbi.0010042

Sporns, O., and Zwi, J. D. (2004). The small world of the cerebral cortex. *Neuroinformatics* 2, 145–161.

Stam, C., Pijn, J. P. M., Suffczynski, P., and da Silva, F. H. L. (1999). Dynamics of the human alpha rhythm: evidence for non-linearity? *Clin. Neurophysiol.* 110, 1801–1813.

Steriade, M., Gloor, P., Linas, R. P., da Silva, F. H. L., and Mesulam, M. M. (1990). Basic mechanisms of cerebral rhythmic activities. *Electroencephalogr. Clin. Neurophysiol.* 76, 481–508.

Steuer, R. (2007). Computational approaches to the topology, stability and dynamics of metabolic networks. *Phytochemistry* 68, 2139–2151.

Taverna, D. M., and Goldstein, R. A. (2002). Why are proteins marginally stable? *Proteins* 46, 105–109.

Turing, A. M. (1952). The chemical basis of morphogenesis. *Philos. Trans. R. Soc. Lond. B* 237, 37–72.

van den Heuvel, M., and Sporns, O. (2011). Rich-club organization of the human connectome. *J. Neurosci.* 31, 15775–15786.

Venkov, N. A., Coombes, S., and Matthews, P. C. (2007). Dynamic instabilities in scalar neural field equations with space-dependent delays. *Physica D* 232, 1–15.

Wen, Q., and Chklovskii, D. B. (2005). Segregation of the brain into gray and white matter: a design minimizing conduction delays. *PLoS Comput. Biol.* 1:e78. doi: 10.1371/journal.pcbi.0010078

Wilson, H. R., and Cowan, J. D. (1973). A mathematical theory of the functional dynamics of cortical and thalamic nervous tissue. *Kybernetik* 13, 55–80.

Wright, J. J., and Liley, D. T. J. (1996). Dynamics of the brain at global and microscopic scales: neural networks and the EEG. *Behav. Brain Sci.* 19, 285–320.

Wright, J. J., Robinson, P. A., Rennie, C. J., Gordon, E., Bourke, P. D., Chapman, C. L., et al. (2001). Towards an integrated continuum model of cerebral dynamics: the cerebral rhythms, synchronous oscillation and cortical stability. *Biosystems* 63, 71–88.

Yi, Z., and Tan, K. K. (2002). Dynamic stability conditions for Lotka-Volterra recurrent neural networks with delay. *Phys. Rev. E* 66:011910, 1–8. doi: 10.1103/PhysRevE.66.011910

Young, M. P. (2000). The architecture of visual cortex and inferential processes in vision. *Spat. Vis.* 13, 137–146.

10

How adaptation shapes spike rate oscillations in recurrent neuronal networks

Moritz Augustin[1,2]*†, Josef Ladenbauer[1,2]*† and Klaus Obermayer[1,2]

[1] Department of Software Engineering and Theoretical Computer Science, Technische Universität Berlin, Berlin, Germany
[2] Bernstein Center for Computational Neuroscience Berlin, Berlin, Germany

Correspondence:
Moritz Augustin and Josef Ladenbauer, Department of Software Engineering and Theoretical Computer Science, Technische Universität Berlin, Neural Information Processing Group, Marchstr. 23, MAR 5-6, 10587 Berlin, Germany.
e-mail: augustin@ni.tu-berlin.de; jl@ni.tu-berlin.de

†These authors have contributed equally to this work.

Neural mass signals from *in-vivo* recordings often show oscillations with frequencies ranging from <1 to 100 Hz. Fast rhythmic activity in the beta and gamma range can be generated by network-based mechanisms such as recurrent synaptic excitation-inhibition loops. Slower oscillations might instead depend on neuronal adaptation currents whose timescales range from tens of milliseconds to seconds. Here we investigate how the dynamics of such adaptation currents contribute to spike rate oscillations and resonance properties in recurrent networks of excitatory and inhibitory neurons. Based on a network of sparsely coupled spiking model neurons with two types of adaptation current and conductance-based synapses with heterogeneous strengths and delays we use a mean-field approach to analyze oscillatory network activity. For constant external input, we find that spike-triggered adaptation currents provide a mechanism to generate slow oscillations over a wide range of adaptation timescales as long as recurrent synaptic excitation is sufficiently strong. Faster rhythms occur when recurrent inhibition is slower than excitation and oscillation frequency increases with the strength of inhibition. Adaptation facilitates such network-based oscillations for fast synaptic inhibition and leads to decreased frequencies. For oscillatory external input, adaptation currents amplify a narrow band of frequencies and cause phase advances for low frequencies in addition to phase delays at higher frequencies. Our results therefore identify the different key roles of neuronal adaptation dynamics for rhythmogenesis and selective signal propagation in recurrent networks.

Keywords: spike frequency adaptation, adaptation, oscillations, rate models, network dynamics, Fokker–Planck, mean-field, recurrent network

INTRODUCTION

A prominent characteristic of cortical activity is its rhythmicity as shown by electroencephalography or the local field potential. Dominant oscillation frequencies in these signals range from <1 to 100 Hz and reflect synchronous activity of populations of neurons. Such oscillations are linked to behavioral states (Wang, 2010) and involved in a variety of cognitive functions (Engel et al., 2001; Fries, 2001; Melloni et al., 2007; Ghazanfar et al., 2008; Wang, 2010) as well as pathological conditions (Hammond et al., 2007; Zijlmans et al., 2009; Uhlhaas and Singer, 2010). It is therefore important to understand the mechanisms of oscillations in neuronal networks, how they are initiated and terminated, and how their frequency is determined.

Fast rhythmic activity in the beta and gamma band (>20 Hz) can be generated by network-based mechanisms, such as synaptic excitation-inhibition loops or by feedback inhibition alone (Isaacson and Scanziani, 2011). In these scenarios the oscillation frequency is largely determined by the inhibitory decay time constant (Brunel and Wang, 2003; Tiesinga and Sejnowski, 2009). Low-frequency oscillations, on the other hand, could depend on slow transmembrane outward currents (Compte et al., 2003; Gigante et al., 2007b; Destexhe, 2009), which are mediated by low-threshold voltage-dependent muscarinic (M) and high-threshold calcium-gated afterhyperpolarization (AHP) K^+ channels, respectively (Brown and Adams, 1980; Connors et al., 1982; Stocker, 2004). These currents cause spike frequency adaptation and are typically more pronounced in cortical regular spiking pyramidal (excitatory) neurons compared to fast spiking (inhibitory) interneurons (La Camera et al., 2006). Both, the M and AHP type K^+ currents, are susceptible to cholinergic modulation (McCormick, 1992). Their kinetic time constants range from milliseconds to seconds (Abel et al., 2004; Manuel et al., 2005) and can be pharmacologically manipulated (Pedarzani et al., 2001).

Here we study the interplay of the dynamics of such adaptation currents with synaptic excitation and inhibition in recurrent networks of excitatory and inhibitory neurons. Specifically, we ask (1) how adaptation can generate slow oscillations, (2) how it modulates faster rhythms based on synaptic interaction, and (3) how adaptation affects resonance properties of the network.

In-vivo recordings from behaving animals have revealed that even when the population activity oscillates, the spike trains of the constituent neurons are rather irregular and display Poisson-like characteristics (Fries, 2001; Wang, 2010). This stochasticity in neuronal responses allows us to derive a mean-field model from a recurrent network of adaptive spiking model neurons coupled through conductance-based synapses with heterogeneous strengths and delays. Our approach is based on the boosts the activity, thereby increasing the adaptation current $w_{\mathcal{E}}$ through b in a spike rate dependent way. The adaptation current in turn acts as a negative feedback which eventually outweighs the recurrent excitation. The population activity drops rapidly and the adaptation current decays slowly. Upon recovery from the adaptation current the cycle starts again.

Next, we investigate how these oscillations are affected by the external input $r^{\mathcal{E}}_{\mathrm{ext}}$, the subthreshold adaptation conductance a and the adaptation timescale τ_w, see **Figure 3**. The existence of adaptation-induced oscillations is quite sensitive to the level of $r^{\mathcal{E}}_{\mathrm{ext}}$ (**Figure 3A**). Periodic activity is stable for small values of $r^{\mathcal{E}}_{\mathrm{ext}}$ (above threshold). While oscillation frequencies increase monotonically with increasing $r^{\mathcal{E}}_{\mathrm{ext}}$, oscillation amplitudes increase initially for a small interval of $r^{\mathcal{E}}_{\mathrm{ext}}$ values and decrease over the following interval. For larger values of $r^{\mathcal{E}}_{\mathrm{ext}}$ oscillatory activity is destabilized and asynchronous states occur. Interestingly, an increase in a does not lead to oscillations. On the contrary, periodic population bursts are destabilized by a. The dependence of oscillation amplitude and frequency on τ_w is shown in **Figure 3B**. Stable oscillations exist for a large range of values of τ_w, where the frequencies decrease with increasing τ_w. Oscillations are unstable for small adaptation timescales in the range of the membrane time constant and for very large values of τ_w.

ADAPTATION MODULATES FREQUENCIES OF NETWORK-BASED OSCILLATIONS

Here we study the influence of adaptation on oscillations generated by recurrent synaptic excitation-inhibition ($\mathcal{E}$-$\mathcal{I}$) loops. The pace of such oscillations is believed to be largely determined by the decay of inhibition. To describe their dependence on the timescale of inhibition for various recurrent network regimes (from excitation dominated to inhibition dominated) we first consider networks of neurons without an adaptation current ($a = b = 0$), see **Figures 4A,B**. By varying the decay $\tau^{\mathcal{I}}_d$ of inhibition and its strength (by parameter g) across networks we find that stable oscillatory states occur if inhibition is sufficiently slow in comparison to excitation. The oscillation frequencies increase with increasing external input spike rate $r^{\mathcal{E}}_{\mathrm{ext}}$, increasing g and decreasing $\tau^{\mathcal{I}}_d$, respectively. A low value of $r^{\mathcal{E}}_{\mathrm{ext}}$ leads to frequencies in the low beta band (**Figure 4A**), for a higher value of $r^{\mathcal{E}}_{\mathrm{ext}}$ the frequencies span the beta and low gamma bands (**Figure 4B**). Note that the network parameters can be adjusted to obtain higher oscillation frequencies. The generating mechanism underlying the oscillations is a loop of recurrent synaptic excitation and inhibition, initiated by the excitatory external input. We verified this by removing the recurrent excitatory input to the inhibitory population, which lead to a destabilization of the oscillations. For larger values of g as the ones used in **Figure 4**, the

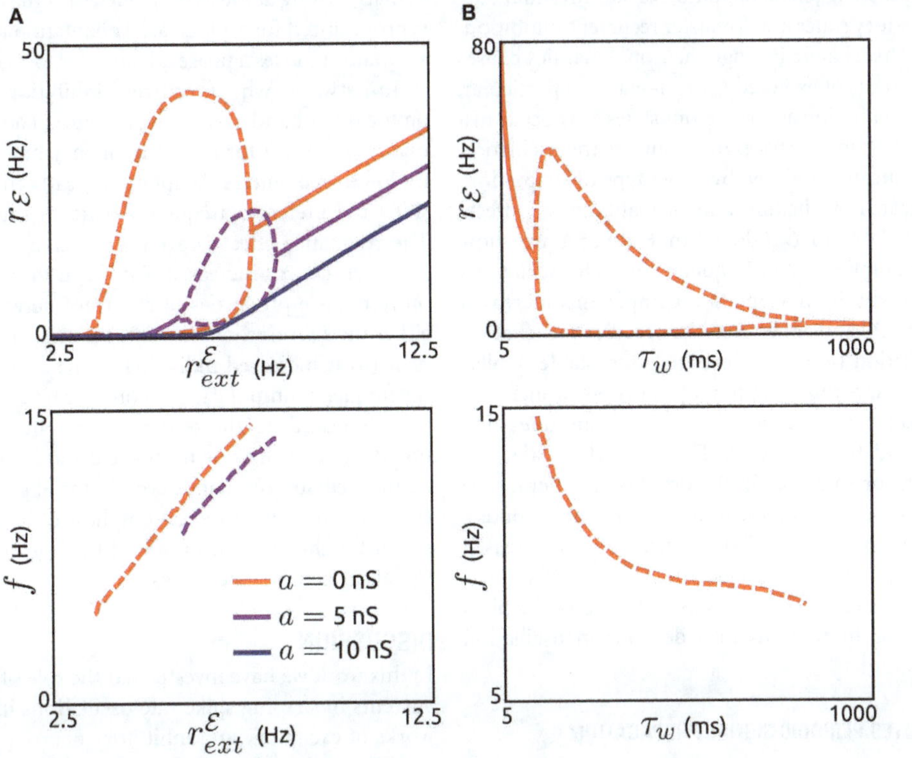

FIGURE 3 | Effects of subthreshold adaptation, external input, and adaptation timescale on population bursts. (A), Top: Spike rate $r_{\mathcal{E}}$ depending on the external input $r^{\mathcal{E}}_{\mathrm{ext}}$ for networks without subthreshold adaptation ($a = 0$, red) and with increased levels of a (5 nS, violet and 10 nS, dark blue). Maxima and minima of oscillating $r_{\mathcal{E}}$ are shown by dashed lines. Bottom: Corresponding frequencies f. $b = 0.05$ nA, $\tau_w = 200$ ms, $g = 1$, and other parameter values as in **Figure 2A**. **(B)**: Maxima and minima of $r_{\mathcal{E}}$ (top) and oscillation frequency as a function of the adaptation time constant τ_w. $a = 0$, $r^{\mathcal{E}}_{\mathrm{ext}} = 6.25$ Hz, and other parameter values as in **(A)**.

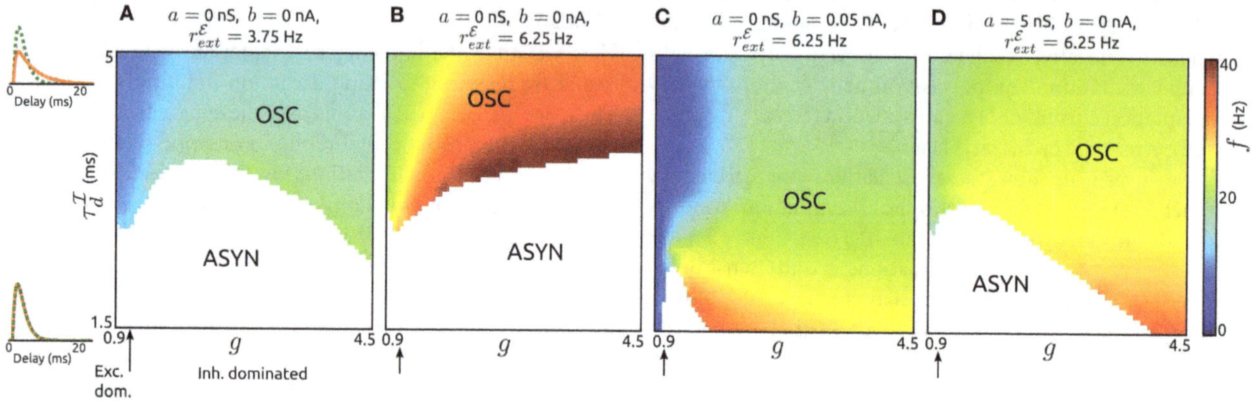

FIGURE 4 | Influence of synaptic inhibition and adaptation on network-based oscillations. (A–D): Existence of oscillatory states (OSC) and corresponding frequencies f as a function of the strength g and timescale $\tau^{\mathcal{I}}_d$ of synaptic inhibition for networks with adaptation parameters and external input strengths as specified. Asynchronous states (ASYN) are indicated by white regions in the parameter space. Arrows mark balance of recurrent excitation and inhibition. On the left $p^{\mathcal{E}}_d$ (green) and $p^{\mathcal{I}}_d$ (orange) are shown for $\tau^{\mathcal{I}}_d = 1.5$ ms, $\tau^{\mathcal{I}}_d = 5$ ms. $\tau^{\mathcal{I}}_r$ was chosen such that the peaks of $p^{\mathcal{E}}_d$ and $p^{\mathcal{I}}_d$ occur at the same delay value. $\tau_w = 200$ ms, $\tau^{\mathcal{E}}_r = 1.25$ ms, and $\tau^{\mathcal{E}}_d = 1.5$ ms. For other parameter values see the Methods section.

$\mathcal{E}$-$\mathcal{I}$-loop mechanism is replaced by an $\mathcal{I}$-$\mathcal{I}$-loop that does not depend on recurrent excitation (not shown). Since adaptation is only exhibited by excitatory neurons, we disregard the parameter space where $\mathcal{I}$-$\mathcal{I}$-loop-based rhythmic activity occurs and focus on $\mathcal{E}$-$\mathcal{I}$-loop-based oscillations instead.

An increase of spike-triggered adaptation or subthreshold current stabilizes oscillatory states also for faster recurrent inhibition, see **Figures 4C,D**. This change in single neuron dynamics causes oscillations in large parts of explored $(g, \tau^{\mathcal{I}}_d)$-space. In particular, for spike-triggered adaptation asynchronous states only occur in a small region of the parameter space. Interestingly, the oscillation frequencies are significantly reduced by either type of adaptation.

Next, we investigate how the timescale of adaptation τ_w affects oscillations mediated by an $\mathcal{E}$-$\mathcal{I}$-loop. In **Figure 5A** we show the dependence of amplitude and frequency of such oscillations on τ_w for networks with both adaptation components increased ($a = 5$ nS, $b = 0.05$ nA) and either dominant recurrent excitation ($g = 1.05$) or inhibition ($g = 1.5$). In both cases, stable oscillatory states exist for a large range of time constants. As τ_w increases the oscillation frequencies decrease while the amplitudes first increase abruptly and then decrease. The networks settle into asynchronous states for small τ_w (in the order of the membrane time constant) or large τ_w (several hundreds of milliseconds). Note that these effects of τ_w are similar if either a or b is increased individually (not shown). We validated these effects by simulations of aEIF neuron networks, see **Figure 5B**. The raster plots show that an increase in τ_w leads to a decrease in oscillation frequency and amplitude.

ADAPTATION PROMOTES PERIODIC SIGNAL PROPAGATION

To analyze how the resonance properties of recurrent networks in asynchronous states are influenced by adaptation currents, we here consider external Poisson-inputs with oscillatory rates with frequency f. Gain of input spike rate and phase difference between network and input spike rates as a function of input frequency for networks without ($a = b = 0$) and with adaptation ($a = 5$ nS, $b = 0.05$ nA) considering two adaptation time constants are presented in **Figures 6A,B**. Excitation dominated networks without adaptation do not exhibit resonance at any frequency and show only phase delays. The presence of an adaptation current leads to a significant amplification of oscillations in the input which is particularly strong at lower frequencies (of the beta band). This effect is pronounced for an increased adaptation timescale. In addition, adaptation causes a phase advance for low oscillation frequencies.

In networks where recurrent inhibition dominates excitation on the other hand even in the absence of adaptation currents resonance is shown for a high frequency band and phase advances for lower frequencies. Adaptation greatly enhances resonance and shifts the preferred frequency band to the high gamma range. The resonance effect is even stronger if the adaptation current is slower, i.e., τ_w increased. Although these effects of adaptation on resonance properties of recurrent networks are similar when either the subthreshold (a) or spike-triggered adaptation component (b) is increased individually, the dominant contribution to the frequency amplifications comes from b (not shown). We additionally examined the response of single neurons to oscillatory noisy inputs using our mean-field model and found that adaptation mediates resonance even in the absence of recurrent input (not shown). These results emphasize the importance of adaptation for the amplification and thus propagation of oscillatory signals in neuronal networks.

DISCUSSION

In this work we have investigated the role of neuronal adaptation currents in shaping spike rate oscillations in large recurrent networks of excitatory and inhibitory neurons. Based on a network of aEIF model neurons sparsely coupled through conductance-based synapses with heterogeneous delays and strengths driven by noisy external input, we used a mean-field method taking advantage of the FP equation. We simplified the problem by applying an adiabatic approximation and solved the resulting equations numerically. Using this method we obtain membrane potential

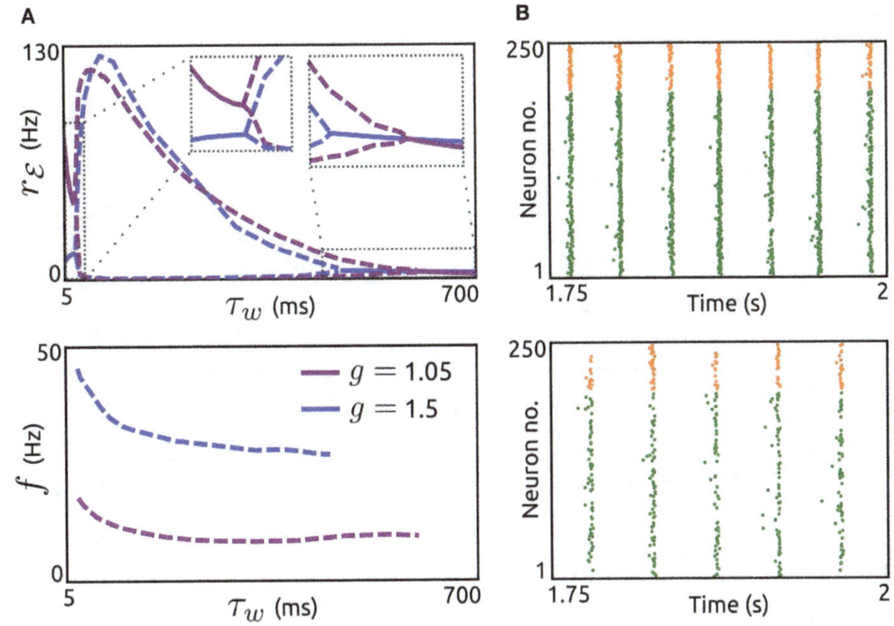

FIGURE 5 | Effects of adaptation timescale on network-based oscillations. (A) Top: Spike rate $r_\mathcal{E}$ as a function of the adaptation time constant τ_w for networks with dominant recurrent excitation ($g = 1.05$, violet) and inhibition ($g = 1.5$, blue). Dashed lines indicate maxima and minima of oscillating $r_\mathcal{E}$, solid lines represent constant $r_\mathcal{E}$. Bottom: Corresponding oscillation frequencies f. $a = 5$ nS and $b = 0.05$ nA. $r^\mathcal{E}_{ext} = 7.5$ Hz, $\tau^\mathcal{E}_r = 1.25$ ms, $\tau^\mathcal{E}_d = 1.55$ ms, $\tau^\mathcal{I}_r = 0.98$ ms, and $\tau^\mathcal{I}_d = 2$ ms. Other parameters as in **Figure 4**. **(B)**: Raster plots of simulated networks of size $N = 50{,}000$ with $g = 1.5$ and $\tau_w = 100$ ms (top) as well as $\tau_w = 400$ ms (bottom), showing the spike times of 200 excitatory and 50 inhibitory aEIF neurons. Other parameter values as in **(A)**.

distributions and population averages of spike rates and adaptation currents. At the same time, the dynamical properties of single neurons, i.e., the neuron model parameters, are retained in the derived mean-field network model.

Alternative mean-field methods have been developed for conductance-based model neurons (Robinson et al., 2008) and recurrent networks thereof in asynchronous states (Shriki et al., 2003), where spike rates are obtained without having to solve a PDE. Our approach based on the FP equation on the other hand treats noise in the synaptic inputs in more detail and allows for the calculation of membrane potential distributions in addition to spike rates.

We chose the aEIF model because it provides a rich yet low-dimensional description of neuronal dynamics and includes a proper phenomenological description of the M and AHP adaptation currents. The effects of subthreshold (a) and spike-triggered adaptation (b) on response properties of aEIF neurons (measured by spike rate-input current relationships and phase response curves) match those of M and AHP adaptation currents in a Hodgkin–Huxley type neuron model, respectively (Ladenbauer et al., 2012). Furthermore, fitting the aEIF model parameters to a detailed biophysical model using standard electro-physiological paradigms revealed a clear relationship between parameter a and the conductance for the M current as well as between parameter b and the AHP current (not shown).

Our method is based on several assumptions which allow to derive the mean-field equations. The Poisson approximation of spike train statistics is justified by experimental findings (Tolhurst et al., 1983; McAdams and Maunsell, 1999) although spiking seems to be more regular in some cortical areas (Maimon and Assad, 2009). The sparse random connectivity implies vanishing noise correlations between neurons in the large network limit and an experimental study in primary visual cortex of awake monkeys has reported almost zero noise correlations (Ecker et al., 2010). However, there is an ongoing debate about the strength of correlations in experimental data (Cohen and Kohn, 2011). We have used an adiabatic approximation, which relies on separable time scales of adaptation current and membrane voltage. Although this assumption is violated for small values of τ_w, numerically solving the unreduced FP system, Equations (18)–(24), showed that our results are robust regarding the violation of this assumption. The results we obtained by simulations of aEIF networks and the mean-field results show quantitative differences. However, the presented effects described using the mean-field model are validated qualitatively by the network simulations.

We have shown that spike-triggered adaptation provides a mechanism to generate spike rate oscillations in a low frequency range (alpha band and lower) if recurrent excitation is sufficiently strong. Increased subthreshold adaptation on the other hand does not contribute to this mechanism but rather dampens such oscillations. The type of adaptation current therefore strongly determines rhythmic activity in excitation dominated networks. The importance of activity-driven adaptation for slow oscillations is consistent with results from simulations of detailed (thalamo-)cortical spiking neuron network models (Bazhenov et al., 2002; Compte et al., 2003; Destexhe, 2009), mean-field

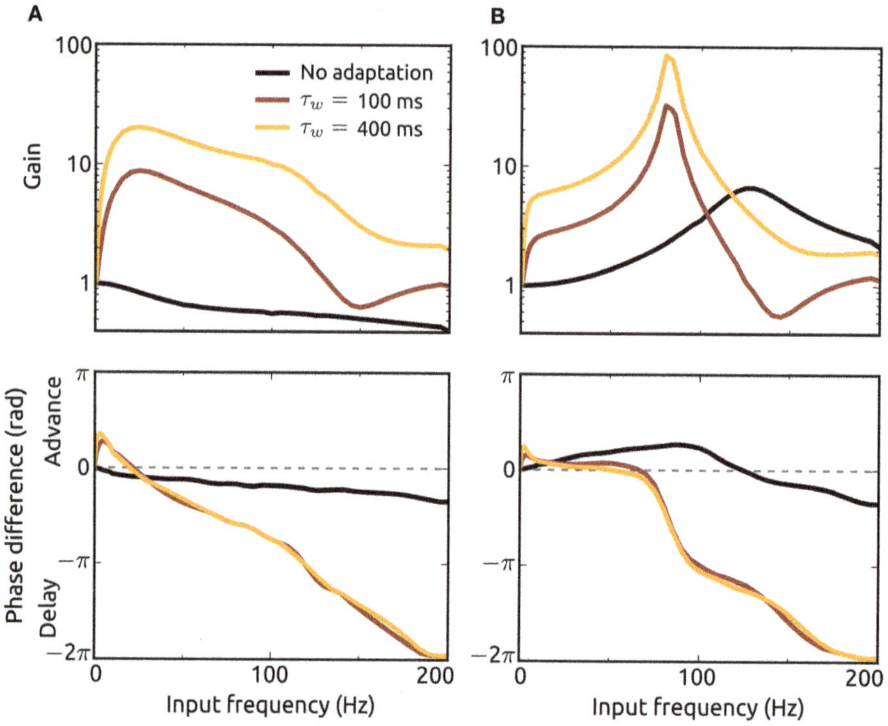

FIGURE 6 | Effects of adaptation on resonance properties of recurrent networks. Gain (top) and phase shift (bottom) of the spike rate $r_{\mathcal{E}}$ for networks with dominant recurrent excitation [$g = 1.05$, **(A)**] and inhibition [$g = 1.5$, **(B)**] as a function of the input frequency f. The gain is defined as the quotient of the oscillation amplitude in $r_{\mathcal{E}}$ for the input with frequency f and the amplitude for the lowest frequency ($f_{min} = 0.5$ Hz). Adaptation parameter values are $a = b = 0$ (black), $a = 5$ nS, $b = 0.05$ nA, $\tau_w = 100$ ms (dark red), and $a = 5$ nS, $b = 0.05$ nA, $\tau_w = 400$ ms (orange). Delay distributions are identically parameterized ($p_d^{\mathcal{E}} \equiv p_d^{\mathcal{I}}$) with $\tau_r = 1.25$ ms and $\tau_d = 1.5$ ms. The Poisson-input rates $r_{ext}^{\mathcal{E}}$, $r_{ext}^{\mathcal{I}}$ each consist of a baseline rate plus a sinusoidal component of small amplitude (1/1000th of the baseline) with frequency f. The baseline of $r_{ext}^{\mathcal{E}}$ is chosen to yield a steady-state spike rate $r_{\mathcal{E}}^{\infty}$ of 50 Hz with constant input rate. The baseline rate of $r_{ext}^{\mathcal{I}}$ is chosen as explained in the Methods section.

studies based on networks of excitatory neurons under the assumption sparse (Gigante et al., 2007b) and all-to-all connectivity (Nesse et al., 2008), as well as phenomenological rate models (Latham et al., 2000). We have further shown that reducing inhibitory synaptic strength leads to a reduction on oscillation frequency, which is in agreement with similar experimental findings (Sanchez-Vives et al., 2010).

The M and AHP K^+ currents, which mediate spike frequency adaptation in pyramidal neurons, are known to be deactivated by acetylcholine (McCormick, 1992), with the AHP current showing higher sensitivity. Since the adaptation parameter b is strongly related to AHP type adaptation, our results support the hypothesis that the cholinergically induced activating transition from slow-wave oscillations to asynchronous irregular states (Lee and Dan, 2012) is mediated (at least in part) by a reduction of spike-triggered adaptation (Destexhe, 2009).

We have demonstrated that an increase of either type of adaptation current leads to a reduction in the frequency of oscillations generated by a loop of recurrent excitation and inhibition. This shows that the dynamical properties of neurons in addition to coupling characteristics strongly affect the network frequency. Also the passive (integrative) membrane properties significantly influence such networks oscillations as has been described previously (Geisler et al., 2005). Our additional finding of decreased frequencies for increased adaptation time constants is consistent with the results from a computational study on clustering effects of spike-triggered adaptation in gamma oscillations (Kilpatrick and Ermentrout, 2011).

Low input frequencies have been shown to be suppressed in the output of single excitatory neurons with increased spike-triggered (Gigante et al., 2007a) or subthreshold adaptation (Richardson et al., 2003; Prescott and Sejnowski, 2008), which we confirmed using our aEIF-based mean-field model. Such a high pass property of single neurons has also been found using a more general model of adaptation (Benda and Herz, 2003). We have demonstrated that both adaptation currents cause spike rate resonance in excitation dominated recurrent networks. Inhibition dominated networks, on the other hand, exhibit resonance without adaptation and we have shown that increased adaptation of excitatory neurons strongly amplifies this resonance. A similar effect has been described for purely inhibitory networks (Richardson, 2009). In addition, our results show that adaptation shifts the resonance frequency to lower values.

In excitation dominated networks, adaptation further leads to phase advances for low input frequencies in addition to phase delays for higher frequencies as observed in previous studies on single excitatory neurons (Fuhrmann et al., 2002; Gigante et al., 2007a). These adaptation-induced phase advances enable synchronization of periodic activity between distant neurons (and populations of neurons) in different areas of the brain if the strength of adaptation is controlled appropriately, e.g., through cholinergic neuromodulation.

Here we have considered one adaptation current for each neuron of the excitatory population. To account for the multimodal distribution of adaptation timescales found experimentally (La Camera et al., 2006) our approach can be easily extended to include multiple adaptation currents.

ACKNOWLEDGMENTS

We thank Timm Lochmann for helpful comments on the manuscript. This work was supported by the DFG Collaborative Research Center SFB910.

REFERENCES

Abel, H. J., Lee, J. C. F., Callaway, J. C., and Foehring, R. C. (2004). Relationships between intracellular calcium and afterhyperpolarizations in neocortical pyramidal neurons. *J. Neurophysiol.* 91, 324–335.

Badel, L., Lefort, S., Brette, R., Petersen, C. C. H., Gerstner, W., and Richardson, M. J. E. (2008). Dynamic I-V curves are reliable predictors of naturalistic pyramidal-neuron voltage traces. *J. Neurophysiol.* 99, 656–666.

Bazhenov, M., Timofeev, I., Steriade, M., and Sejnowski, T. J. (2002). Model of thalamocortical slow-wave sleep oscillations and transitions to activated states. *J. Neurosci.* 22, 8691–8704.

Benda, J., and Herz, A. V. M. (2003). A universal model for spike-frequency adaptation. *Neural Comput.* 15, 2523–2564.

Brette, R., and Gerstner, W. (2005). Adaptive exponential integrate-and-fire model as an effective description of neuronal activity. *J. Neurophysiol.* 94, 3637–3642.

Brown, D. A., and Adams, P. R. (1980). Muscarinic suppression of a novel voltage-sensitive K+ current in a vertebrate neurone. *Nature* 283, 673–676.

Brunel, N. (2000). Dynamics of sparsely connected networks of excitatory and inhibitory spiking neurons. *J. Comput. Neurosci.* 8, 183–208.

Brunel, N., Hakim, V., and Richardson, M. (2003). Firing-rate resonance in a generalized integrate-and-fire neuron with subthreshold resonance. *Phys. Rev. E* 67, 051916.

Brunel, N., and Wang, X.-J. (2003). What determines the frequency of fast network oscillations with irregular neural discharges? I. Synaptic dynamics and excitation-inhibition balance. *J. Neurophysiol.* 90, 415–430.

Cohen, M. R., and Kohn, A. (2011). Measuring and interpreting neuronal correlations. *Nat. Neurosci.* 14, 811–819.

Compte, A., Sanchez-Vives, M. V., McCormick, D. A., and Wang, X.-J. (2003). Cellular and network mechanisms of slow oscillatory activity (<1 Hz) and wave propagations in a cortical network model. *J. Neurophysiol.* 89, 2707–2725.

Connors, B., Gutnick, M., and Prince, D. (1982). Electrophysiological properties of neocortical neurons *in vitro*. *J. Neurophysiol.* 48, 1302–1320.

Deco, G., Jirsa, V. K., Robinson, P. A., Breakspear, M., and Friston, K. (2008). The dynamic brain: from spiking neurons to neural masses and cortical fields. *PLoS Comput. Biol.* 4:e1000092. doi: 10.1371/journal.pcbi.1000092

Destexhe, A. (2009). Self-sustained asynchronous irregular states and up-down states in thalamic, cortical and thalamocortical networks of nonlinear integrate-and-fire neurons. *J. Comput. Neurosci.* 27, 493–506.

Destexhe, A., Rudolph, M., and Paré, D. (2003). The high-conductance state of neocortical neurons *in vivo*. *Nat. Rev. Neurosci.* 4, 739–751.

Ecker, A. S., Berens, P., Keliris, G. A., Bethge, M., Logothetis, N. K., and Tolias, A. S. (2010). Decorrelated neuronal firing in cortical microcircuits. *Science* 327, 584–587.

Engel, A., Fries, P., and Singer, W. (2001). Dynamic predictions: oscillations and synchrony in top-down processing. *Nat. Rev. Neurosci.* 2, 704–716.

Fourcaud-Trocme, N., Hansel, D., van Vreeswijk, C., and Brunel, N. (2003). How spike generation mechanisms determine the neuronal response to fluctuating inputs. *J. Neurosci.* 23, 11628–11640.

Fries, P. (2001). Modulation of oscillatory neuronal synchronization by selective visual attention. *Science* 291, 1560–1563.

Fuhrmann, G., Markram, H., and Tsodyks, M. (2002). Spike frequency adaptation and neocortical rhythms. *J. Neurophysiol.* 88, 761–770.

Geisler, C., Brunel, N., and Wang, X.-J. (2005). Contributions of intrinsic membrane dynamics to fast network oscillations with irregular neuronal discharges. *J. Neurophysiol.* 94, 4344–4361.

Ghazanfar, A., Chandrasekaran, C., and Logothetis, N. (2008). Interactions between the superior temporal sulcus and auditory cortex mediate dynamic face/voice integration in rhesus monkeys. *J. Neurosci.* 28, 4457–4469.

Gigante, G., Del Giudice, P., and Mattia, M. (2007a). Frequency-dependent response properties of adapting spiking neurons. *Math. Biosci.* 207, 336–351.

Gigante, G., Mattia, M., and Del Giudice, P. (2007b). Diverse population-bursting modes of adapting spiking neurons. *Phys. Rev. Lett.* 98, 1–4.

Goodman, D. F. M., and Brette, R. (2009). The brian simulator. *Front. Neurosci.* 3, 192–197. doi: 10.3389/neuro.01.026.2009

Hammond, C., Bergman, H., and Brown, P. (2007). Pathological synchronization in Parkinson's disease: networks, models and treatments. *Trends Neurosci.* 30, 357–364.

Isaacson, J. S., and Scanziani, M. (2011). How inhibition shapes cortical activity. *Neuron* 72, 231–243.

Jolivet, R., Schürmann, F., Berger, T. K., Naud, R., Gerstner, W., and Roth, A. (2008). The quantitative single-neuron modeling competition. *Biol. Cybern.* 99, 417–426.

Kilpatrick, Z. P., and Ermentrout, B. (2011). Sparse gamma rhythms arising through clustering in adapting neuronal networks. *PLoS Comput. Biol.* 7:e1002281. doi: 10.1371/journal.pcbi.1002281

Kumar, A., Schrader, S., Aertsen, A., and Rotter, S. (2008). The high-conductance state of cortical networks. *Neural Comput.* 20, 1–43.

La Camera, G., Rauch, A., Thurbon, D., Lüscher, H.-R., Senn, W., and Fusi, S. (2006). Multiple time scales of temporal response in pyramidal and fast spiking cortical neurons. *J. Neurophysiol.* 96, 3448–3464.

Ladenbauer, J., Augustin, M., Shiau, L., and Obermayer, K. (2012). Impact of adaptation currents on synchronization of coupled exponential integrate-and-fire neurons. *PLoS Comput. Biol.* 8:e1002478. doi: 10.1371/journal.pcbi.1002478

Latham, P. E., Richmond, B. J., Nelson, P. G., and Nirenberg, S. (2000). Intrinsic dynamics in neuronal networks. I. Theory. *J. Neurophysiol.* 83, 808–827.

Lee, S.-H., and Dan, Y. (2012). Neuromodulation of brain states. *Neuron* 76, 209–222.

LeVeque, R. (2002). *Finite Volume Methods for Hyperbolic Problems.* Cambridge: Cambridge University Press.

Maimon, G., and Assad, J. A. (2009). Beyond Poisson: increased spike-time regularity across primate parietal cortex. *Neuron* 62, 426–440.

Manuel, M., Meunier, C., Donnet, M., and Zytnicki, D. (2005). How much afterhyperpolarization conductance is recruited by an action potential? A dynamic-clamp study in cat lumbar motoneurons. *J. Neurosci.* 25, 8917–8923.

McAdams, C. J., and Maunsell, J. H. (1999). Effects of attention on the reliability of individual neurons in monkey visual cortex. *Neuron* 23, 765–773.

McCormick, D. A. (1992). Neurotransmitter actions in the thalamus and cerebral cortex and their role in thalamocortical activity. *Progr. Neurobiol.* 39, 337–388.

Melloni, L., Molina, C., Pena, M., Torres, D., Singer, W., and Rodriguez, E. (2007). Synchronization of neural activity across cortical areas correlates with conscious perception. *J. Neurosci.* 27, 2858–2865.

Naud, R., Marcille, N., Clopath, C., and Gerstner, W. (2008). Firing patterns in the adaptive exponential integrate-and-fire model. *Biol. Cybern.* 99, 335–347.

Nesse, W. H., Borisyuk, A., and Bressloff, P. C. (2008). Fluctuation-driven rhythmogenesis in an excitatory neuronal network with slow adaptation. *J. Comput. Neurosci.* 25, 317–333.

Nykamp, D. Q., and Tranchina, D. (2000). A population density approach that facilitates large-scale modeling of neural networks: analysis and an application to orientation tuning. *J. Comput. Neurosci.* 8, 19–50.

Pedarzani, P., Mosbacher, J., Rivard, A., Cingolani, L. A., Oliver, D., Stocker, M., et al. (2001). Control of electrical activity in central neurons by modulating the gating of small conductance Ca(2+)-activated K+ channels. *J. Biol. Chem.* 276, 9762–9769.

Pospischil, M., Piwkowska, Z., Bal, T., and Destexhe, A. (2011). Comparison of different neuron models to conductance-based post-stimulus time histograms obtained in cortical pyramidal cells using dynamic-clamp *in vitro*. *Biol. Cybern.* 105, 167–180.

Prescott, S. A., and Sejnowski, T. J. (2008). Spike-rate coding and spike-time coding are affected oppositely by different adaptation mechanisms. *J. Neurosci.* 28, 13649–13661.

Renart, A., Brunel, N., and Wang, X.-J. (2004). "Mean-field theory of irregularly spiking neuronal populations and working nemory in recurrent cortical networks," in *Computational Neuroscience: A Comprehensive Approach*, ed J. Feng (Boca Raton, FL: CRC Press), 431–490.

Richardson, M. (2004). Effects of synaptic conductance on the voltage distribution and firing rate of spiking neurons. *Phys. Rev. E* 69, 1–8.

Richardson, M. (2009). Dynamics of populations and networks of neurons with voltage-activated and calcium-activated currents. *Phys. Rev. E* 80, 1–16.

Richardson, M. J. E., Brunel, N., and Hakim, V. (2003). From subthreshold to firing-rate resonance. *J. Neurophysiol.* 89, 2538–2554.

Risken, H. (1996). *The Fokker–Planck Equation: Methods of Solutions and Applications.* Berlin: Springer.

Robinson, P. A., Wu, H., and Kim, J. W. (2008). Neural rate equations for bursting dynamics derived from conductance-based equations. *J. Theor. Biol.* 250, 663–672.

Saad, Y. (2003). *Iterative Methods for Sparse Linear Systems.* Philadelphia, PA: SIAM.

Sanchez-Vives, M. V., Mattia, M., Compte, A., Perez-Zabalza, M., Winograd, M., Descalzo, V. F., et al. (2010). Inhibitory modulation of cortical up states. *J. Neurophysiol.* 104, 1314–1324.

Shriki, O., Hansel, D., and Sompolinsky, H. (2003). Rate models for conductance-based cortical neuronal networks. *Neural Comput.* 15, 1809–1841.

Stocker, M. (2004). Ca(2+)-activated K+ channels: molecular determinants and function of the SK family. *Nat. Rev. Neurosci.* 5, 758–770.

Tamas, G., Buhl, E. H., and Somogyi, P. (1997). Fast IPSPs elicited via multiple synaptic release sites by different types of GABAergic neurone in the cat visual cortex. *J. Physiol.* 500, 715–738.

Tiesinga, P., and Sejnowski, T. J. (2009). Cortical enlightenment: are attentional gamma oscillations driven by ING or PING? *Neuron* 63, 727–732.

Tolhurst, D. J., Movshon, J. A., and Dean, A. F. (1983). The statistical reliability of signals in single neurons in cat and monkey visual cortex. *Vision Res.* 23, 775–785.

Touboul, J., and Brette, R. (2008). Dynamics and bifurcations of the adaptive exponential integrate-and-fire model. *Biol. Cybern.* 99, 319–334.

Uhlhaas, P. J., and Singer, W. (2010). Abnormal neural oscillations and synchrony in schizophrenia. *Nat. Rev. Neurosci.* 11, 100–113.

van der Vorst, H. A. (1992). Bi-CGSTAB: a fast and smoothly converging variant of Bi-CG for the solution of nonsymmetric linear systems. *SIAM J. Sci. Stat. Comput.* 13, 631–644.

Wang, X.-J. (2010). Neurophysiological and computational principles of cortical rhythms in cognition. *Phyiol. Rev.* 90, 1195–1268.

Williams, S. R., and Stuart, G. J. (2002). Dependence of EPSP efficacy on synapse location in neocortical pyramidal neurons. *Science* 295, 1907–1910.

Womble, M. D., and Moises, H. C. (1992). Muscarinic inhibition of M-current and a potassium leak conductance in neurones of the rat basolateral amygdala. *J. Physiol.* 457, 93–114.

Zijlmans, M., Jacobs, J., Zelmann, R., Dubeau, F., and Grotman, J. (2009). High-frequency oscillations mirror disease activity in patients with epilepsy. *Neurology* 72, 979–986.

11

Spatiotemporal imaging of complexity

Stephen E. Robinson[1]*, Arnold J. Mandell[2] and Richard Coppola[1]

[1] MEG Core Facility, National Institute of Mental Health, National Institutes of Health, Bethesda, MD, USA
[2] Department of Psychiatry, University California, San Diego, CA, USA

What are the functional neuroimaging measurements required for more fully characterizing the events and locations of neocortical activity? A prime assumption has been that modulation of cortical activity will inevitably be reflected in changes in energy utilization (for the most part) changes of glucose and oxygen consumption. Are such a measures complete and sufficient? More direct measures of cortical electrophysiological activity show event or task-related modulation of amplitude or band-limited oscillatory power. Using magnetoencephalography (MEG), these measures have been shown to correlate well with energy utilization sensitive BOLD fMRI. In this paper, we explore the existence of state changes in electrophysiological cortical activity that can occur independently of changes in averaged amplitude, source power or indices of metabolic rates. In addition, we demonstrate that such state changes can be described by applying a new measure of complexity, rank vector entropy (RVE), to source waveform estimates from beamformer-processed MEG. RVE is a non-parametric symbolic dynamic informational entropy measure that accommodates the wide dynamic range of measured brain signals while resolving its temporal variations. By representing the measurements by their rank values, RVE overcomes the problem of defining embedding space partitions without resorting to signal compression. This renders RVE-independent of absolute signal amplitude. In addition, this approach is robust, being relatively free of tunable parameters. We present examples of task-free and task-dependent MEG demonstrating that RVE provides new information by uncovering hidden dynamical structure in the apparent turbulent (or chaotic) dynamics of spontaneous cortical activity.

***Correspondence:**
Stephen E. Robinson, MEG Core Group, National Institute of Mental Health, 10 Center Drive, Bethesda, MD 20814, USA.
e-mail: robinsonse@mail.nih.gov

Keywords: magnetoencephalography, neuroscience, cognitive, beamformer, complexity, nonlinear, turbulence, mixing

INTRODUCTION

ENTROPY AND COMPLEXITY

The term "entropy" is commonly defined as a measure of the order or disorder in a physical system. In the context of time-varying electrophysiological brain signals we use the term "complexity" instead of "entropy" in order to emphasize the temporal fluctuations of information rate rather than the total information of that signal. Signals having low complexity include synchronous events and oscillations. Signals with high complexity appear more chaotic and correspond to a higher information rate.

The topographic characteristics of spatiotemporal fluctuations in cortical electrophysiological activity are analogous to those of non-laminar, turbulent flow as visualized by optical imaging using voltage sensitive dyes (Cohen et al., 1978). On a macroscopic scale, the activity of individual neurons is hidden from external non-invasive measures such as magnetoencephalography (MEG) (Cohen, 1968) or electroencephalography (EEG) (Berger, 1989), the ensemble behavior of the underlying cortical neural network exhibits complex emergent and traveling fronts of excitation and inhibition that are supported by both short-range inter-neuron connections and "small world" longer-range connections. There have been a variety of experimental approaches that have been developed to characterize the dynamics of turbulent fluid flow ranging from visualization of waves and eddies through the use of fluorescent dyes (Busse and Clever, 1979) and monitoring heat flux using cryogenic techniques (Swinney and Gollub, 1981) to laser Doppler techniques that allow measurement of local field velocities without perturbing the field significantly (Gollub and Steinman, 1981). The spatiotemporal patterns observed with changing parameter values include transitions from laminar (linear) flow via a Hopf bifurcation to periodic oscillations, followed by two or more simultaneous irrationally related periodic flows and finally the aperiodic oscillations of turbulent (chaotic) dynamics (Ruelle and Takens, 1971). The latter state is characterized by positive entropy generation (Eckmann and Ruelle, 1985) similar to that observed in the MEG record (Mandell et al., 2011a,b; Robinson et al., 2012).

Brain activity is most commonly modeled by narrow-band oscillatory regions that are coupled to one another via networks. Chaos theory is often used as a model to describe complex biological measurements for which linear theory is incomplete. The criteria for chaos modeling include sensitivity to initial conditions and topological mixing. Both of these conditions are satisfied by local measures of ongoing brain activity. This naturally leads to combining a measurement of local cortical signals such as a beamformer estimate derived from MEG to a sensitive and robust measure of the broad bandwidth non-linear properties of those signals such as RVE.

The lack of suitable existing complexity measures for MEG is our motivation for developing rank vector entropy. First, we require a method for observing the spatiotemporal structure of cortical non-linear dynamics. Retaining temporal resolution allows for the study of the entropy change time-course that is needed to characterize event and task-related brain activity. The focus of current MEG complexity measures has been long-term properties having no temporal resolution such as Lempel-Ziv complexity (Fernandez et al., 2011), transfer complexity (Vakorin et al., 2010), and comparisons of multiple entropy/complexity measures (Bruna et al., 2012). Although there are sliding block methods for observing temporal changes in entropy (Adler and Marcus, 1979), this is computationally inefficient when applied to thousands of voxels for functional brain imaging. The estimated source time-series from beamformed MEG is efficiently transformed into an entropy time-series by RVE.

The *rank vector entropy* (RVE) algorithm is a non-parametric partial analog to metric (Kolmogorov) entropy (ME) (Kolmogorov, 1958; Crutchfield and Feldman, 2003). Both methods estimate the entropy of a one-dimensional series of measurements (e.g., a neurophysiological signal) computed on probability distributions of short sequence "states" encountered in the time series. A unique property of the RVE as a metric entropy lies in its initial encoding of the time series using the topological property of sequence order (Cornfield et al., 1982; Bandt and Pompe, 2002). In the more conventional ME, a short sequence of lagged measurement values from a one-dimensional time-series are mapped into an N-dimensional phase space (Ott, 1993). This embedding space is then partitioned into N-dimensional hypercubes. Each partition represents a state that the signal can manifest in its trajectory through N-dimensional space. The metric entropy of the signal is a measure on the probability distribution of trajectories passing through possible partitioned spaces. The number of partitions in ME can be arbitrary and must be sufficient in number, and with sufficient continuity to accommodate the dynamic range of the signal. In some implementations, dynamic range compression of the measurements is required in order to limit the number of partitions to a manageable number. The classical criteria of a "generating partition"—no more than one entry per partitioned space (Eckmann and Ruelle, 1985) is impractical in the context of real biological data. In contrast, in the RVE algorithm the measurement values of a short sequence of samples extracted from the entire time series are converted to their rank ordered values. The number of states, as partitions of the one-dimensional sliding window is quantized according to the number of elements in the sequence of measurements. Each sequence, with the topological property of relative "nearness," is referred to as a "rank vector" which can also be thought of as a rank ordered one-dimensional embedding space. The RVE algorithm ignores the absolute signal amplitude in favor of its relative amplitude within the span of each sample window. A metric entropy is then computed on the probability distribution of the finite set of rank sequences. It will be shown that RVE is relatively free of arbitrarily tunable parameters (aside from selection of signal bandwidth, window length, and a decay time constant). The more conventional ME requires the investigator to use a variety of schemes, many involving the Whitney embedding theorem (Milnor, 1997; Temin, 1997), to determine the number of dimensions and lags for the embedding space and the size and number of partitions in embedding space.

We measure the spatiotemporal complexity of brain activity by applying the RVE analysis to sensor mediated brain signals. This could be accomplished by analyzing the signals from individual sensors (Vakorin et al., 2010; Gomez et al., 2011), pairs of sensors (Mandell et al., 2011a,b), or source estimates from MEG using a scalar LCMV beamformer (Robinson and Black, 1990; Robinson and Rose, 1993; Van Veen et al., 1997; Vrba and Robinson, 2002). The latter completes the analogy to characterization of time-series of turbulent chaotic fluid flow, sampled at multiple spatial points within the flow.

MAGNETOENCEPHALOGRAPHY

Spontaneous MEG signals are on the order of 10^{-13} Tesla peak-to-peak. Despite its small signal strength, MEG has been made practical by larger DC-SQUID based sensor arrays covering the entire head in combination with excellent rejection of environmental magnetic interference (Fife et al., 2002). The application of RVE to MEG signals is a natural one. The magnetoencephalogram is the magnetic counterpart of the electroencephalogram. MEG is a measure of the magnetic field arising from primary (impressed) neural currents, whereas EEG measures the electrical potentials on the scalp that arise from the volume currents and is therefore dependent on tissue conductivity and its boundaries (Plonsey, 1981). The major contributor to the observed primary currents is the potential difference between the dendritic tree and soma of neocortical pyramidal neurons. Because MEG is less dependent on tissue conductivity its measurements can be modeled using simple analytic solutions (Sarvas, 1987). The accuracy of such analytic solutions for MEG enables the use of beamformers (detailed in section "Scalar LCMV Beamformer") to estimate the source time series for any coordinate within the brain (Robinson, 1989). Application of the RVE transform (section "Rank Vector Entropy") to any source time series yields a corresponding complexity time series of that activity. The relationship of spatiotemporal RVE to sensorimotor events and cognitive tasks can then be determined by signal averaging or by comparison of the RVE signals that have been parsed into active and control state time segments.

EXAMPLE MEG STUDIES

We have selected four different examples of MEG studies to explore the properties of spatiotemporal RVE analysis. These datasets were selected from an archive of normal control studies. The task-free (resting) MEG dataset was chosen to compare the spatial distribution and timing relationships of RVE complexity to power in a 4–150 Hz bandpass. The P300 study, also referred to as the mismatch negativity (MMN), demonstrates the properties of evoked signals to frequent and deviant auditory stimuli. In the EEG, comparison of the frequent to deviant tone signal averages is characterized by a slow wave after about 250 ms (Naatanen et al., 1978). The same protocol is also referred to as a P_{300} study when a response is required for the deviant tones (Donchin, 1981).

The working memory (n-back) study is used to compare broadband RVE with power in an effortful short-term memory task (Kirchner, 1958). Lastly, we present a MEG study of self-paced voluntary finger movement to compare complexity with SCP. Self-paced voluntary movement is preceded by a slow "readiness" potential (Bereitschaftspotential) (Kornhuber and Deecke, 1964) and a corresponding "readiness" field (Bereitschaftsfield) (Deecke et al., 1982).

METHODS

RANK VECTOR ENTROPY

The RVE algorithm can be described as follow: first, consider a one-dimensional discretely sampled time series of length K samples: $\mathbf{X} = [x_1, x_2, \ldots, x_K]$. Let the sample rate and low-pass "corner" frequency of $\mathbf{X}$ be denoted by f_S and f_C, respectively. For any given low-pass frequency, $\mathbf{X}$ is completely determined at $2f_C$ samples per second. It is unnecessary for the rank vector to represent every sample, sequentially. It is sufficient to define the lag ξ required to avoid oversampling as:

$$\xi = \frac{f_S}{2f_C}. \tag{1}$$

Thus, for any specified low-pass cutoff and sample rate we need only process every ξth sample (ξ is rounded up to the nearest integer). Note the analogy of ξ to the sample lags that are used to define the dimensionality of the embedding space in conventional ME computations (Eckmann and Ruelle, 1985; Crutchfield and Feldman, 2003). The selection of lags in ME is usually based upon the mixing length reflected in the decay of the autocorrelation function (Walters, 1982). In this way it is biased in favor of the dominant signal and its ordering. These methods characteristically assume that the signal is stationary (which it is not) and it may also have the unfortunate side effect of aliasing information. Furthermore, it appears that with real biological data, some investigators have been occasionally arbitrary in their selection of lags (evaluating several different lags so as to obtain results more consistent with their expectations). In the RVE algorithm, the lags are rigorously defined by sample rate and low-pass corner frequency, thus not justifying any further modification. If the frequency band of interest is below the data acquisition bandwidth, the investigator can set the low-pass frequency accordingly, from which the lags are again automatically determined.

Let us select a sub-window of W samples (at integer ξ intervals) from $\mathbf{X}$, with the window beginning with the kth sample: $\mathbf{W}_k = [x_k, x_{k+\xi}, \ldots, x_{k+(W-1)\xi}]$. The measured signal for each lagged sample within sub-window $\mathbf{W}_k$ is initially converted to its integer rank values, forming a rank vector $\mathbf{R}_k$ of length W: $\mathbf{R}_k = [rank_1, rank_2, \ldots, rank_W]$. For a window of length W there are $W!$ (factorial) unique rank vectors (i.e., vectors of length W for which the ordered rank values do not repeat). Let there be a table $\mathbf{S}$ to map rank vector sequences to symbols, where the symbol value is obtained from a "look up" table indexed for matching rank vectors. For example, let us consider a window length of $W = 5$ for which there are $5! = 120$ unique rank vectors from which we derive 120 state symbols, s_n. Counting and normalizing the number of occurrences of each unique symbol can then generate a probability histogram. Counting these symbols in RVE is analogous to counting visits of the signal to the higher dimensional hypercube partitions in ME (Ott, 1993). For this example, we use $W = 5$, $f_S = 600$ Hz, $f_C = 100$ Hz, and $\xi = 3$. For example, let the measured values of x_k through $x_{k+4\xi}$ (i.e., $\mathbf{W}_k$) be (4.07, −3.12, 3.95, 8.51, −1.21). Its rank vector and symbol value are (2, 5, 3, 1, 4) and 45, respectively (a symbol value of 45 indicates its place in an ascending numerical order of rank vectors).

As the sub-window of W samples is advanced through $\mathbf{X}$ one sample at a time, a new rank vector R_k and new symbolic representation s_n is generated. The frequency of occurrence of each of these symbols is accumulated in a corresponding state histogram: $\mathbf{F}_k = [f_1(k), f_2(k), \ldots, f_{W!}(k)]$. The resulting histogram contains the cumulative counts of each rank vector (state). Since our primary interest is in observing the time-dependent, event-related changes in the rank vector informational entropy, it is necessary to avoid the reduction in relative temporal sensitivity by saturation. We prevent this by introducing a time-constant determining the rate of decay of histogram counts with time. The integrator decay rate τ ($1/e$ time) is required in order to measure the fluctuations in entropy over time. The amplitude of the entropy fluctuations depends on the decay rate (longer τ yields smaller peak-to-peak fluctuations). The relative rather than the absolute changes in entropy are of interest for event or task-related functional imaging (including ICA or resting state MEG). Provided that τ is longer than the time required to completely fill all states, the entropy waveform will be independent of τ—except for its amplitude. As a practical matter, we select a time constant such that the $1/e$ time (in samples) corresponds to three times the number of states. This is implemented by defining constant α:

$$\alpha = e^{-1/(\tau f_S)}, \tag{2}$$

in which τ is the time for the counts to decay to $1/e$ of their initial values, such that for each time step:

$$\mathbf{F}_k = \alpha \mathbf{F}_{k-1}. \tag{3}$$

This constitutes what is termed a "leaky integrator." The histogram count corresponding to the current state symbol is the incremented by one. Based upon the revised count frequencies, there will be a corresponding set of probabilities for each state:

$$\mathbf{P}_k = [p_1(k), p_2(k), \ldots, p_{W!}(k)]. \tag{4}$$

If the cumulative entropy over all samples of $\mathbf{X}$ is required, then $\alpha = 1$. Otherwise, the entropy is estimated as time-dependent. Finally, for each step k, we compute the Shannon entropy (Shannon, 1963) over all state probabilities greater than zero, as normalized by its maximum value, constraining entropy to the range 0–1:

$$h(k) = \frac{1}{\log_2 W!} \sum_{n=1}^{W!} -p_n(k) \log_2 p_n(k). \tag{5}$$

The steps in the algorithmic procedure for computing the time series of RVEs are as follows:

1. Initialize the state count histogram **F** (set all f_n values to 1.0).
2. For each sample index k in time series **X**, generate a length W rank vector $\mathbf{R}_k$ with lags of ξ samples.
3. Look up state symbol index n corresponding to $\mathbf{R}_k$.
4. Multiply all elements of histogram **F** by α, thus allowing the count histories to decay (Equation 3).
5. Increment the corresponding histogram count f_n by one (where n is the index in **S** corresponding to $\mathbf{R}_k$).
6. Compute the probabilities of each state from the histogram of counts (Equation 4).
7. Compute the RVE metric entropy for this time step (Equation 5).
8. Advance sample index by one sample and continue to repeat steps 2 through 7 and in this way generating a new entropy value for each cycle of the algorithmic process.

SCALAR LCMV BEAMFORMER

Synthetic aperture magnetometry (SAM) is a scalar linearly constrained minimum variance (LCMV) beamformer estimating source activity from MEG signals for specified coordinates in the brain. The mathematics of the beamformer procedure can be traced to the minimum variance estimator first described by Gauss (1823). SAM minimizes the variance (power) of all correlated signals observed by an array of SQUID sensors, subject to a unity gain constraint for a specified coordinate. As such, the action of the SAM may be regarded as spatially selective noise reduction, where noise is defined as unwanted environmental or biological magnetic signals.

The computational procedure has been described in detail elsewhere but can be summarized briefly, as follows: consider measured MEG from an array of sensors. Let the signal space vector at time sample k be denoted by $\mathbf{M}(k)$. Given a sufficient number of time samples, we construct a source estimate $\hat{S}_{\mathbf{r}}$ for coordinate **r** as the weighted sum MEG measurements.

$$\hat{S}_{\mathbf{r}}(k) = \mathbf{W}_{\mathbf{r}}^T \mathbf{M}(k). \tag{6}$$

To compute the weights using the method of Gauss, we use the quadratic form:

$$\left[\hat{S}_{\mathbf{r}}(k) = \mathbf{W}_{\mathbf{r}}^T \mathbf{M}(k)\right]^2, \tag{7}$$

for which, after integrating over time, we obtain:

$$\hat{S}_{\mathbf{r}}^2 = \mathbf{W}_{\mathbf{r}}^T \mathbf{C} \mathbf{W}_{\mathbf{r}}, \tag{8}$$

where **C** is the covariance matrix computed over the integration time:

$$\mathbf{C} = \left\langle \mathbf{M}\mathbf{M}^T \right\rangle, \tag{9}$$

where <.> denotes the expectation value. We solve for **W** by introducing a constraint such that $\hat{S}_{\mathbf{r}}^2$ (power or variance) is minimized subject to unit gain for a specified coordinate. One such constraint is:

$$\mathbf{W}_{\mathbf{r}}^T \mathbf{B}_{\mathbf{r}} = 1, \tag{10}$$

where $\mathbf{B}_{\mathbf{r}}$ is the *a priori* forward solution for the field observed by an array of M sensors generated by a current dipole source located at **r**. That is:

$$\mathbf{B}_{\mathbf{r}} = \begin{bmatrix} b_1(\mathbf{r}) \\ b_2(\mathbf{r}) \\ \vdots \\ b_M(\mathbf{r}) \end{bmatrix}. \tag{11}$$

Suitable methods for computing forward solutions include the current dipole in a homogeneously conducting sphere model (Grynszpan and Geselowitz, 1973; Sarvas, 1987; Hari et al., 1988), multiple local spheres fitted to the surface of the head (Huang et al., 1999), boundary element methods (De Munck, 1992) or perturbative solutions derived from the spherical harmonic expansion of the conductive boundary (Nolte et al., 2004). However, to compute $\mathbf{B}_{\mathbf{r}}$ we must first estimate the dipole orientation. We do this by finding the dipole orientation yielding the highest signal-to-noise ratio (SNR) at location **r**. We define $\mathbf{L}_{\mathbf{r}}$, the matrix of forward solutions for dipoles oriented in the three cardinal directions as:

$$\mathbf{L}_{\mathbf{r}} = \begin{bmatrix} b_{11} & b_{12} & b_{13} \\ b_{21} & b_{22} & b_{23} \\ \vdots & \vdots & \vdots \\ b_{M1} & b_{M2} & b_{M3} \end{bmatrix}. \tag{12}$$

We also define a diagonal matrix $\mathbf{\Sigma}$ of uncorrelated sensor instrumental noise power σ_{m}^2:

$$\Sigma = \begin{bmatrix} \sigma_1^2 & & & 0 \\ & \sigma_2^2 & & \\ & & \ddots & \\ 0 & & & \sigma_M^2 \end{bmatrix} \cong \bar{\sigma}^2 \mathbf{I}. \tag{13}$$

The source power **S** in each of three cardinal directions is given by:

$$\mathbf{S}_{\mathbf{r}}^2 = \left[\mathbf{L}_{\mathbf{r}}^T C^{-1} \mathbf{L}_{\mathbf{r}}\right]^{-1}, \tag{14}$$

and the noise power **N** by:

$$\mathbf{N}_{\mathbf{r}}^2 = \left[\Sigma\, \mathbf{L}_{\mathbf{r}}^T \mathbf{C}^{-2} \mathbf{L}_{\mathbf{r}}\right]^{-1}. \tag{15}$$

The SNR is given by a generalized eigensystem of these two 3 × 3 matrices (Sekihara and Nagarajan, 2008). By assuming that the SQUID noise is nearly equal in all sensors, we can neglect $\mathbf{\Sigma}$, as it represents a scalar ($\bar{\sigma}^2 I$) that will not affect determination of the moment vector. The dipole orientation maximizing SNR is given by the eigenvector $\mathbf{e}_{max}$ corresponding to the maximum eigenvalue λ_{max} of the generalized eigensystem:

$$\mathbf{L}_{\mathbf{r}}^T \mathbf{C}^{-2} \mathbf{L}_{\mathbf{r}} e_k = \lambda_k \mathbf{L}_{\mathbf{r}}^T \mathbf{C}^{-1} \mathbf{L}_{\mathbf{r}} \mathbf{e}_k. \tag{16}$$

The forward solution for the dipole vector for the highest SNR is therefore:

$$\mathbf{B}_\mathbf{r} = \mathbf{L}_\mathbf{r}\mathbf{e}_{\max}. \quad (17)$$

Solving for the optimum scalar LCMV beamformer weights using Lagrange multipliers results in:

$$\mathbf{W}_\mathbf{r} = \frac{\mathbf{C}^{-1}\mathbf{B}_\mathbf{r}}{\mathbf{B}_\mathbf{r}^T\mathbf{C}^{-1}\mathbf{B}_\mathbf{r}}. \quad (18)$$

Substituting $\mathbf{W}_\mathbf{r}$ into Equation (6) yields an estimate of the source time series.

APPLICATION OF RVE TO MEG DATA

Subjects

MEG data from four healthy normal control subjects, one per example study, were randomly selected from a larger group of NIMH study subjects of both genders, mean age 27.6 years. All subjects gave written informed consent according to protocols approved by the NIH CNS Institutional Review Board.

Data acquisition

MEG data were acquired using a 275-channel whole head MEG (CTF Systems, Inc.) housed within a three layer magnetically shielded room (Vacuumschmelze AK-3). Three head localization coils were affixed to subjects at the nasion, right preauricular, and left preauricular points. The acquisition software energizes these coils with sinusoidal currents at three different frequencies before and after data acquisition in order to localize and establish each subject's head position relative to the MEG sensors. Data were sampled continuously, without breaking it into epochs or trials at 600 Hz in a bandpass of DC to 150 Hz, with the subjects in seated position. Stimulus and response trigger markers for each study were recorded with the data. Synthetic 3rd-gradient mode was used during data acquisition to obtain further reduction in magnetic noise (Vrba and Robinson, 2002). Raw data were archived on disk for subsequent analysis.

RVE analysis parameters for all studies were fixed at a 4–150 Hz bandpass, $W = 5$ (120 states), lags every two samples, and an integrator decay time constant of 0.6 s.

All subjects were given a T1-weighted volumetric MRI. Radiological markers were affixed to the identical fiducial points as were used for the head localization coils used during MEG acquisition. Markers were used to transform the MRI to the MEG head frame for subsequent processing, including segmentation of the cortical boundary, and coregistration of functional and anatomical data.

Data analysis

Analyses were applied to the unaveraged continuous data. We use the single-layer realistic head model (Nolte et al., 2001) to compute the forward solutions. The scalar beamformer processing includes the steps:

1. Coregister a T1-weighted MRI to the MEG frame and segment the MRI to extract subject's brain hull, using AFNI software (Cox, 1996).
2. Compute the outward-pointing normal vectors for the brain hull.
3. Estimate the MEG measurement covariance matrix for the required time segments and frequency bandpass (Equation 9).
4. Compute points (voxel coordinates) on a regular three-dimensional grid at 5 mm intervals within the head.
5. For each voxel within the hull boundary:
   a. Compute the lead-field matrix (Equation 12) using the brain hull as a single-layer realistic head model (Nolte et al., 2001).
   b. Compute the beamformer coefficients (Equation 18).
   c. Estimate the source time series (Equation 6).

The RVE voxel time-series is computed for a 4–150 Hz bandpass (Equation 1–5). No additional filtering or smoothing is required as the RVE time-series is inherently smooth. Source power time-series are computed from the smoothed envelope of a Hilbert transform following bandpass filtering of the MEG data. The Hilbert envelope was smoothed using lowpass filter corresponding to the lowpass corner frequency of each selected bandpass.

The fluctuations in RVE are relatively small (on the order of 5–15% for $\alpha = 0.6$ s). RVE deviation relative to its statistical mode is used for analysis of the task-free data. For the remaining studies, we compute the Student's T-value for each latency in the RVE time, relative to a selected baseline. Static (3D) and spatiotemporal images (3D + time) were assembled and displayed using AFNI software (Cox, 1996).

Task-free (resting) protocol

Two hundred and forty seconds of task-free ("resting') MEG data were recorded from a normal subject (eyes opened), using data acquisition procedures outlined in section "Data Acquisition." Beamformer weights were computed as above for the entire duration at 5 mm voxel intervals on a three-dimensional grid occupying the entire head. The envelope of the source power S^2 and the RVE were then computed for each voxel and the results mapped as three dimensions plus time images at 50 ms intervals. Because RVE is a measure on temporally hierarchical brain signals, it is studied using a broad bandwidth of 4–150 Hz. In this way we avoid the potential reduction in complexity that would accompany our narrowing the bandwidth of observation. In comparing RVE, with the simultaneously studied envelopes of band width power, the latter was computed using a smoothed Hilbert transform for a sequence of bandwidths that included: 4–150 Hz, 4–8 Hz (theta), 8–13 Hz (alpha), 15–30 Hz (beta), 35–70 Hz (low gamma), and 70–150 Hz (high gamma). The RVE time series is inherently smooth and required no additional filtering.

Auditory P300 (Mismatched Negativity) protocol

The auditory P300 protocol consisted of random presentation of 200 frequent (1.0 kHz) and 50 rare (1.5 kHz) 50 ms duration tone bursts delivered binaurally via non-magnetic earphones (Etymotic), with a 1.0–1.5 s pseudo-random interstimulus interval (ISI). Subjects were instructed to respond to the rare tones by pressing a response button. MEG data were acquired as noted in section "Data Acquisition" and stored to disk together with trigger markers for identifying the onset of the rare and frequent tone bursts, along with the button response.

Beamformer weights were computed from the *unaveraged* MEG data for each of three conditions: (1) both frequent and rare tones, (2) frequent tones, and (3) rare tones. The weights were computed in a 4–150 Hz bandpass. Three-dimensional images of RVE were then computed at 5 ms intervals over a time window from −0.2 to +0.8 s relative to the markers for each of the three conditions. Image maxima and minima coordinates were determined and additional beamformer weights computed for a DC to 100 Hz bandpass. These weights were then applied to the averaged RVE signal of the three conditions in order to show the time course of the entropy waveforms. Note that we compute the average of the entropy and *not* the entropy of the averaged signal. The RVE functional images and time series are displayed as Student's T-values for each voxel, relative to the selected pre-stimulus baseline.

Working memory (N-back) protocol

The numerals 1 through 4 were randomly presented to the subject at 1.4-s intervals in 18 blocks of 11 trials each, using a DLP projector. Preceding each block the subject received instructions how to respond to via four numbered buttons, that corresponds to the numbers 1 through 4. For 0-back blocks, the subject simply pressed the button corresponding to the number presented. For 1 and 2-back conditions, the subject pressed the button corresponding to the numbers that were presented one or two trials back, respectively. MEG was recorded, along with trigger markers indicating the task (i.e., respond to 0, 1, or 2-back), which number was displayed and which response button was depressed, using the settings in section "Data acquisition."

The RVE was applied to the continuous source time series of each voxel, resulting in an RVE time series. The RVE voxel time series was then parsed into 0.5-s segments (± 0.25 s relative to the button response) for the 0, 1, and 2-back conditions. The RVE was integrated over each segment. A Student's T-test was used to compare the difference in integrated RVE signal for pairs of each condition (i.e., 2 vs. 0-back, 2 vs. 1-back) for each individual voxel. The results were displayed as p-values using AFNI.

In a similar manner, we computed and displayed the comparisons for beta-band (14–30 Hz) power using the same conditions.

Self-paced voluntary movement protocol

Subjects performed self-paced button presses at intervals of at least 10 s while continuous MEG was recorded together with time markers for each button press, as outlined in section "Data acquisition." No cues were given to the subjects as to when to press the button.

Scalar beamformer weights were computed for the entire unaveraged dataset in a bandpass of 4–150 Hz. Weights were then applied to the measured MEG data yielding a source estimate time series for each voxel. The voxel time series was then transformed to a RVE time series. The mean entropy value over the interval from −3.0 to −2.5 s prior to the button press was designated as a baseline for comparison of later entropy changes; the RVE time-series was averaged relative to the voluntary button press, at 5 ms intervals from −3.0 to 2.0 s. The RVE averaged response is displayed as its Student's T-value relative to the selected baseline. The voxel having the maximum relative RVE prior to the button press was also used to compute the averaged source strength time-series.

RESULTS

TASK-FREE (RESTING) PROTOCOL

Comparison of the spatial and temporal patterns in the 4–150 Hz bandpass reveals very little apparent correlation between RVE and the Hilbert envelope of power. The fluctuations in entropy are noticeably slower than that of power. In many cortical locations the RVE shows transient decreases from its modal value; spontaneous entropy increases are not as prominent in the resting condition (**Figure 1** top panel). Changes in power relative to its modal value (**Figure 1** center panel) are much more rapid than those of the RVE. The spatial distribution of RVE and power also are seen to differ (**Figure 1** bottom panel).

An expanded 30-s view of the time course of the smoothed Hilbert envelope of power and across multiple frequency bands shows no apparent correlation with RVE 4–150 Hz (**Figure 2**). Changes in entropy clearly show slower, longer wavelength features that are not evident in measures of power.

AUDITORY P300 TASK

In this characteristic example, we observed a reduction in entropy coinciding with the N_{100M} peak (**Figure 3B**) for frequent and combined frequent and rare trials (**Figure 3A**). The reduction in entropy at 100 ms was much smaller for the rare tones, alone (**Figure 3B**). The reduction in entropy was maximal in the vicinity of the left Heschl's gyrus (**Figures 3C,D,E**), with a much smaller reduction in the right hemisphere. Although a flat baseline was seen in the pre-stimulus interval of −0.2 to 0.0 s in the averaged overlay of all sensors (**Figure 3B**), it is absent from the combined and frequent trial averages (**Figure 3A**). We also observed an increase in the entropy T-value after 100 ms for the rare tones (**Figure 3A**). At 700 ms this increase was maximal in anterior cingulate and left temporal cortex (**Figure 3F**). The increase does not appear in the sensor signal averaged overlay.

WORKING MEMORY TASK

In the 2 vs. 0-back comparison, we observe a reduction in beta-band power in the 2-back task relative to the 0-back task, ERD, in dorsolateral prefrontal cortex (DLPFC) and an increase in power, ERS, in inferior occipital cortex (**Figure 4A**). For the identical comparison, there is a significant increase in entropy ($p < 10^{-5}$) in the 2-back condition that is widely distributed throughout the brain, with the largest changes in the left hemisphere (**Figure 4B**).

In the 2 vs. 1-back comparison, beta-band ERD is seen in DLPFC and bilaterally near the inferior temporal pole (**Figure 5A**). The same comparison for RVE shows an increase in entropy in anterior cingulate cortex and a decrease in the right inferior temporal pole (**Figure 5B**).

SELF-PACED VOLUNTARY FINGER MOVEMENT

The Bereitschaftsfield (BF), average of 29 trials, appears as a slow low frequency rise in the source moment in premotor cortex

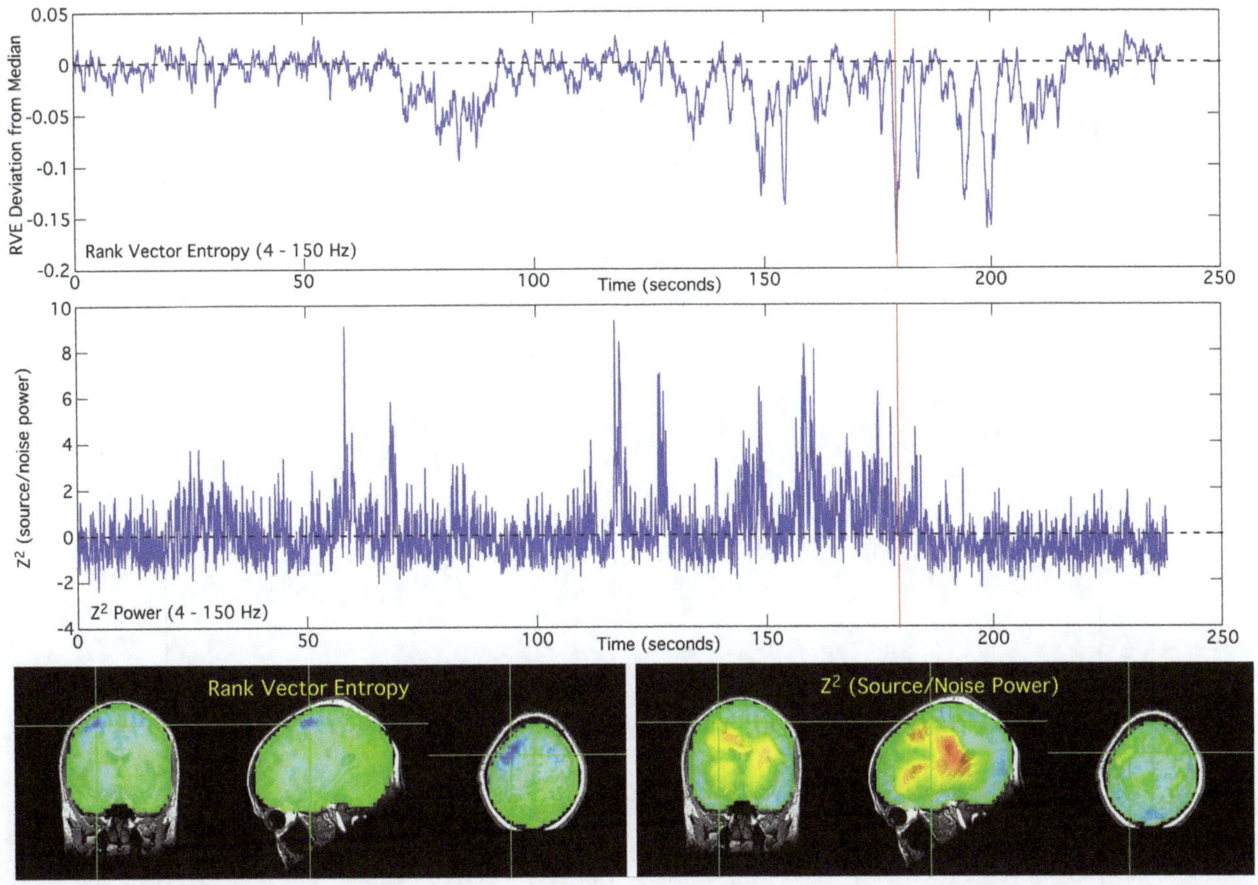

FIGURE 1 | Rank vector entropy and noise-normalized source power differed in both locations and dynamical patterns, i.e., in both time and space. The time-courses of RVE and power for the 4–150 Hz bandwidth are shown for a single location in the brain, as indicated by the cross-hairs in the functional images. The functional images of RVE and power correspond to activity at the time indicated by the red cursor.

that occurs over the time span from −2.5 s to 0 s, relative to the button press (**Figure 6** top). We observed a peak dipole moment of about 10 nA -m relative to a mean baseline over the interval −3.0 to −2.5 s. Signal-to-noise ratio for this source is low, requiring a lowpass filter of 5 Hz in order to see the slow changes. By contrast, the averaged RVE (4–150 Hz), displayed as a T-value relative to baseline, has excellent signal-to-noise and spans −1.75 to 0 s (**Figure 6** bottom). We refer to this wave as the "Bereitschaftskomplexität" (BK), to emphasize its relationship to the BF. Both the BF and BK waveforms are similar.

DISCUSSION

Our single most important finding is that the RVE measure of complexity adds new information about brain dynamics that was previously hidden within the apparent chaos of spontaneous cortical signals. Moreover, RVE, when combined with a scalar beamformer, reveals an underlying spatiotemporal complexity pattern that is modulated by stimuli and tasks. We have presented experimental evidence demonstrating that these patterns of complexity are decoupled from conventional measures of amplitude and oscillatory power. Thus, RVE reveals new information on the dynamics of brain activity.

Next, we will examine the experimental evidence regarding what directional changes in entropy signify. MEG measures such as band-limited oscillatory power or amplitude have been shown to be concordant with functional imaging by BOLD fMRI (Singh et al., 2002; Coppola et al., 2004). Induced changes in cortical activity, particularly for movement, are signaled by event-related desynchronization (ERD) of power (Taniguchi et al., 2000) and also by increases in the BOLD signal relative to a resting or control state. How does one interpret event-related changes in RVE? The answer is not straightforward. We show that a simple auditory stimulus induces a decrease in the RVE at a latency corresponding to the N_{100}m and location corresponding to primary auditory cortex in the left hemisphere. Comparable MEG studies also show ERD in the beta and alpha bands at the latency and locations corresponding to the N_{100}m, and fMRI shows a corresponding increase in the BOLD signal.

In our auditory P_{300} study the response to the rare tones elicited later increases in the RVE signal that persisted for over 1 s. The increase was seen broadly in anterior cingulate cortex and in left temporal cortex in a wide area centered on where the N_{100}m response appeared. These late responses are not visible in the averaged overlay of sensors and in the event-related changes

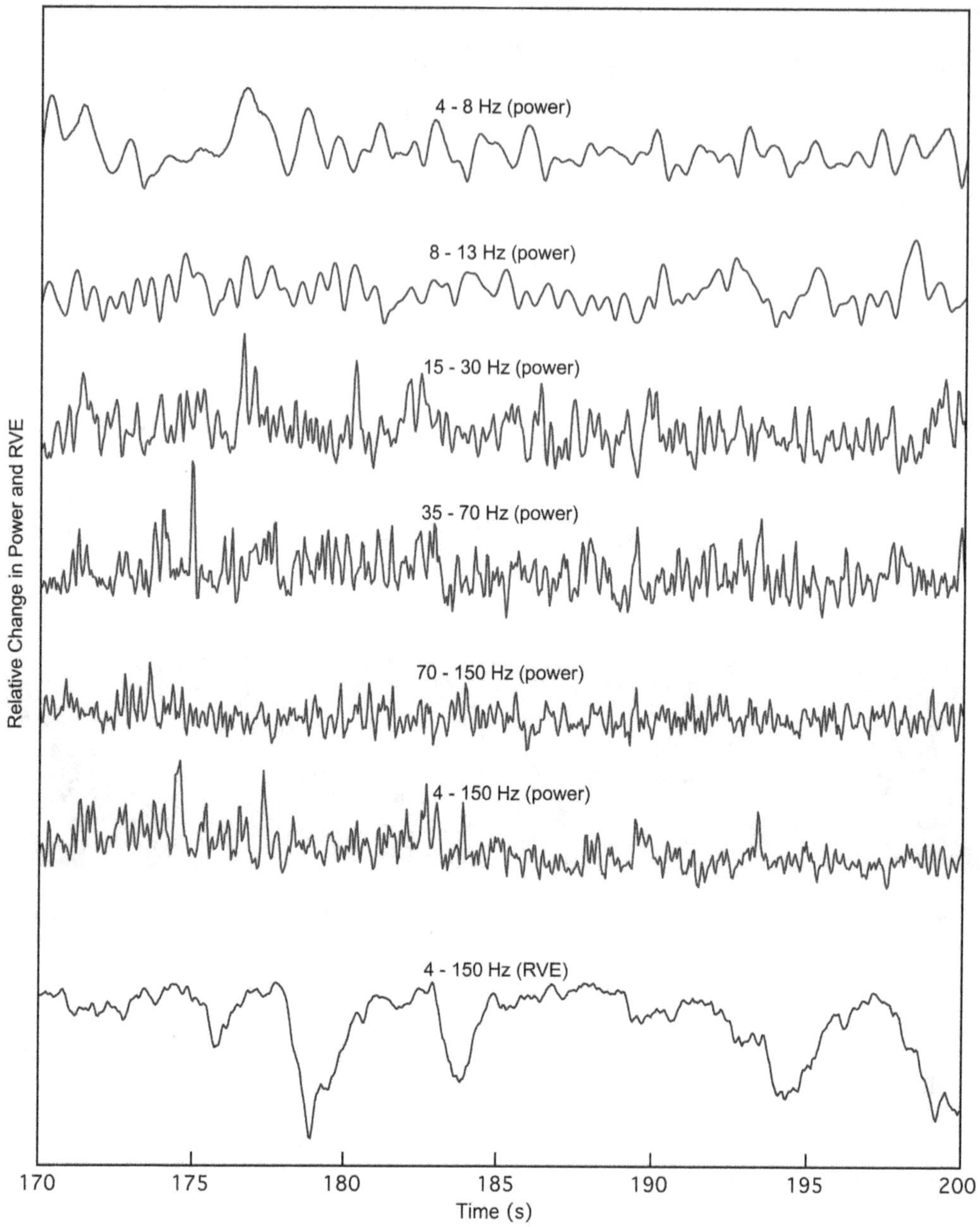

FIGURE 2 | The time course of rank vector entropy, *h*(*k*) (blue trace), is apparently uncorrelated with changes in the envelope of source power, in any bandpass. The 4–150 Hz RVE is compared with source power at the same location in multiple bandwidths for a 30 s expanded view derived from the waveforms shown in **Figure 1**.

in power. We see that the absence of a stable baseline for the frequent tones is a consequence of the slow return to baseline of the entropy increase evoked by the rare tones. That is, the 1.0–1.5 s ISI is not sufficient for the induced RVE increase to return to its resting value.

These P_{300} results demonstrate that stimuli and tasks can induce either in increase or a decrease in entropy relative to its resting value. The RVE of task-free MEG is characterized by transient decreases in entropy from its modal value of ~0.92, lasting two or more seconds. Increases above the modal value are not as prominent and are more rapid—suggesting that bidirectional modulation of RVE reflects the parabolic character of the entropy function and/or its governance by at least two different mechanisms. The N_{100} evoked component of frequent tones corresponds to a transient decrease in the RVE signal that is much shorter than the observed transients in the task-free MEG recordings. The localization of decrease was centered on the left auditory cortex, but included perisylvian areas. The broad distribution of the induced entropy changes confirm that the auditory N_{100} component arises from multiple regions and not simply primary

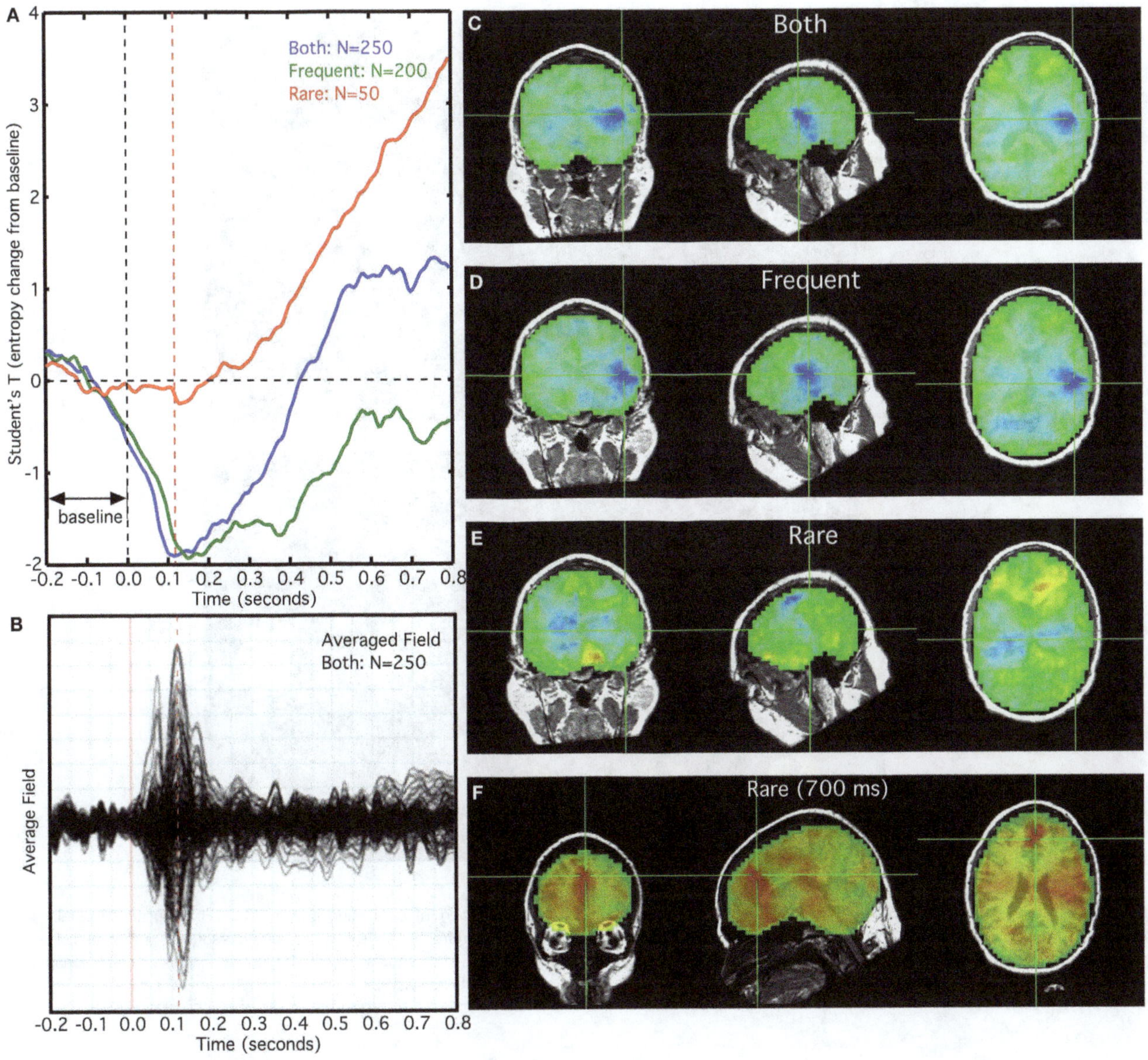

FIGURE 3 | Relationship of rank vector entropy to the auditory evoked response to rare and frequent tone bursts. (A) Average of entropy time series for left primary auditory cortex; **(B)** average overlay of 275 MEG sensors; **(C)** RVE image of combined rare and frequent tones at 100 ms; **(D)** RVE image of frequent tones at 100 ms; **(E)** RVE image of rare tones at 100 ms; **(F)** RVE image of rare tones at 700 ms latency.

auditory cortex (Naatanen and Picton, 1987). Although the averaged evoked response to the rare tones showed only a small peak corresponding to the P_{300} response, there was a profound slow increase in the RVE signal starting at about 250 ms. This slow increase is concordant with the mismatch negativity signal that is observed in similar protocols involving frequent and deviant tones. It appears that synchronized cortical activity, such as that leading to an averaged evoked response component, induces a transient decrease in entropy in the corresponding regions. By contrast, the slow and prolonged rise in entropy induced by the rare tones suggests an increase in asynchronous cortical activity that signifies attentional mechanisms. It should be noted that the frequent tone average (**Figure 3A**) shows what appears to be activity where the pre-stimulus baseline should instead be flat. This is an artifact due to the long duration of the slow RVE component of the rare tones and the relatively short 1.5 s interstimulus interval.

RVE's relatively long time scales (in seconds) and the continuity and differentiability in its time-dependent changes suggests a relationship of this measure to the family of slow cortical potentials (SCPs), including the contingent negative variation (CNV) and the Bereitschaftsfield (Birbaumer et al., 1990). This is particularly evident when comparing BF and BK waveforms seen in **Figure 6**. The slow changes in entropy are only partially due to integration of symbolic state counts. The decay time constant incorporated into the integrator permits RVE to respond rapidly

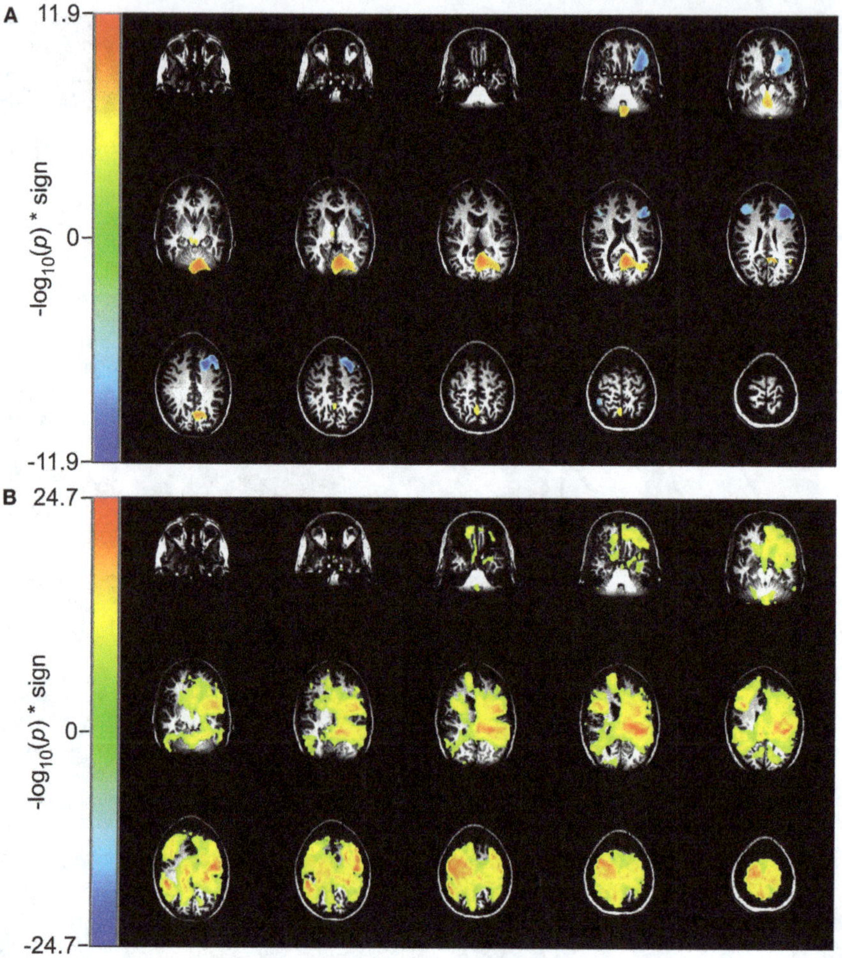

FIGURE 4 | Comparison of event-related changes in beta-band power and in rank vector entropy for 2 vs. 0-back working memory task centered on the response. Images are univariate *p*-values for a Student's *T*-test, with a threshold of 10^{-5}. **(A)** Event-related desynchronization of beta band power (14–30 Hz) appears bilaterally in dorsolateral prefrontal cortex and in left supraorbital prefrontal cortex. **(B)** RVE (4–150 Hz) shows widely distributed increases that overlap with regions of beta-band ERD.

to changing complexity. The observed slow changes in RVE are significantly longer than the 0.6-s $1/e$ integration decay time constant used in these analyses. Thus, the slow shifts in entropy are not an artifact of the analysis but rather reflect cortical processes. Further studies will be needed to compare RVE with other SCP phenomena (e.g., the contingent negative variation paradigm and orienting responses).

The working memory task lends additional insight into how the RVE complexity measure is modulated by cognitive effort. The contrast for the 2-back to the 0-back condition for RVE (**Figure 4**) shows widespread and highly significant ($p < 10^{-5}$) increases in entropy throughout the brain. The 2-back task engages working memory whereas the 0-back task does not. Although the RVE spatial distribution is not uniform, it suggests greater and more significant changes than does event-related beta-band power. These same conditions viewed as beta-band power show the expected focal changes in DLPFC. The difference between RVE and beta-band power images suggests that there vast tracts of cortex that have changed into an "up" state (i.e., activation of the thalamo-cortical attention circuit), without significant expenditure of energy. Is this arousal? Is it readiness? One might speculate that this widespread *increase* in entropy represents a decrease in the cortical excitability threshold—necessary for the efficient performance of the 2-back task. Such a mechanism would be concordant with our observations of other slow changes in RVE, such as that seen in the self-paced voluntary finger movement study and late P_{300} components for the rare tones. By contrast, the 2-back and 1-back conditions both engage working memory but with different levels of effort. For this comparison the RVE demonstrates a number of focal increases bilaterally in anterior cingulate gyri, supraorbital prefrontal cortex, and a focal decrease in the left inferior temporal pole ($p < 10^{-11}$) as shown in **Figure 5**. Thus, the contrast for increasing memory workload can result in both increases and decreases in RVE. The RVE results are qualitatively different from the same contrasts in task-related beta-band power (**Figures 4** and **5**). Beta-band changes appear

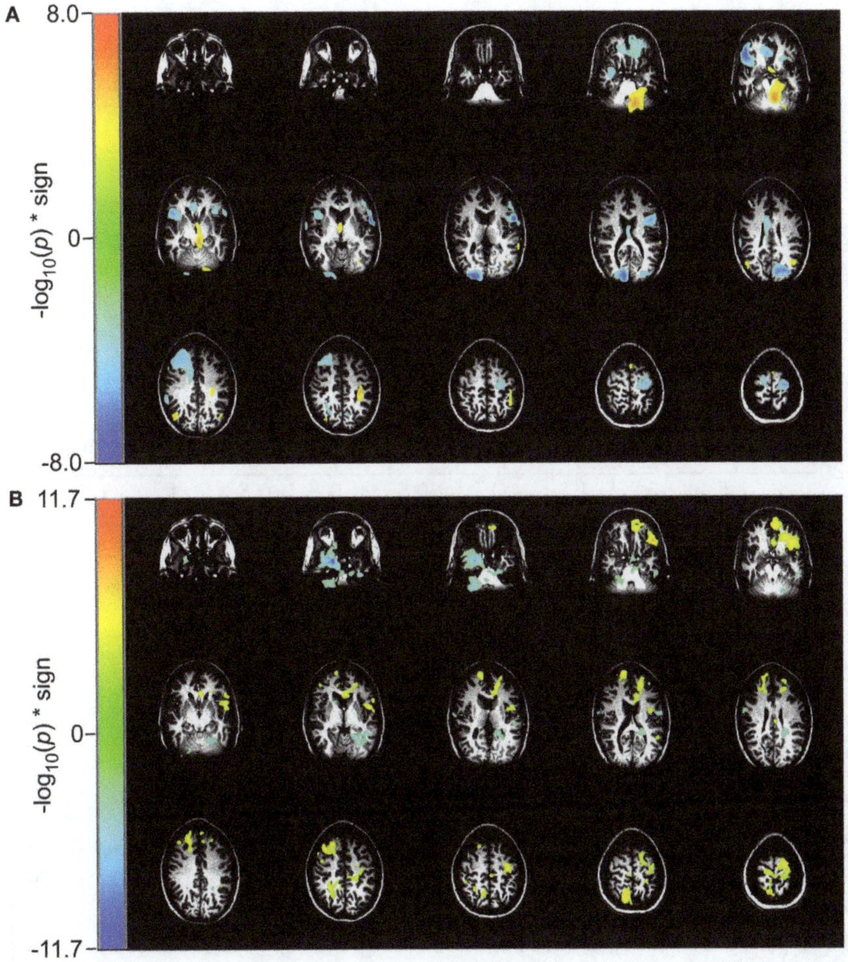

FIGURE 5 | Comparison of event-related changes in beta-band power and in entropy for 2 vs. 1-back working memory task centered on the response. Images are univariate *p*-values for a Student's *T*-test, with a threshold of 10^{-3}. **(A)** Event-related desynchronization of beta band power (14–30 Hz) and **(B)** RVE (4–150 Hz).

mainly as ERD in dorsolateral prefrontal and parietal cortex for both 2 vs. 0-back and 2 vs. 1-back. The *p*-values for these regions are smaller than those for the RVE. Overall, the working memory task suggests the higher cognitive load is associated with increases in RVE.

The results obtained from these MEG studies provide evidence that RVE—specifically increases in complexity—are measures of attention and intention. The neurophysiological basis of attentional arises from the non-specific projections from the centromedian thalamic nucleus to the neocortex (Steriade, 1995). Activation of these projections depolarizes the apical dendrites of neocortical pyramidal neurons resulting in a decrease in the excitability threshold. An increase in asynchronous firing rate of these neurons will be reflected by an increase in complexity, as seen in the RVE signal. It should also be noted that this same mechanism is responsible for the low frequency negative signal appearing in the scalp EEG—the so-called SCP (Birbaumer et al., 1990). Detection of the EEG SCP signals requires careful removal of motion artifacts, eye-blinks, and higher frequency signals and rhythms. By contrast the RVE signals corresponding to attention are readily measured in a broad bandwidth with little or no filtering. Thus RVE is a more sensitive measure of attentional mechanisms than is the SCP.

The complexity decrease associated with synchronous and evoked events such as the auditory N100 implies a *low information rate*. This calls to question the model that synchronous events represent transfer of information. Instead, we suggest a new model in which synchronous activity signifies degradation of the current cognitive context in a cortical region so that new information from sensory or associative sources can be incorporated into a new cognitive context. Exploration of this model is the subject of our ongoing research.

The RVE combines some properties of topological (relative nearness as non-numeric sequences) and metric (probability measure theoretic) entropies (Cornfield et al., 1982; Ornstein, 1989; Milnor, 1997). The log density of states (Equation 7) is a metric entropy. These states are a consequence of mapping topologically ordered sequences to vectorial states, then mapping these

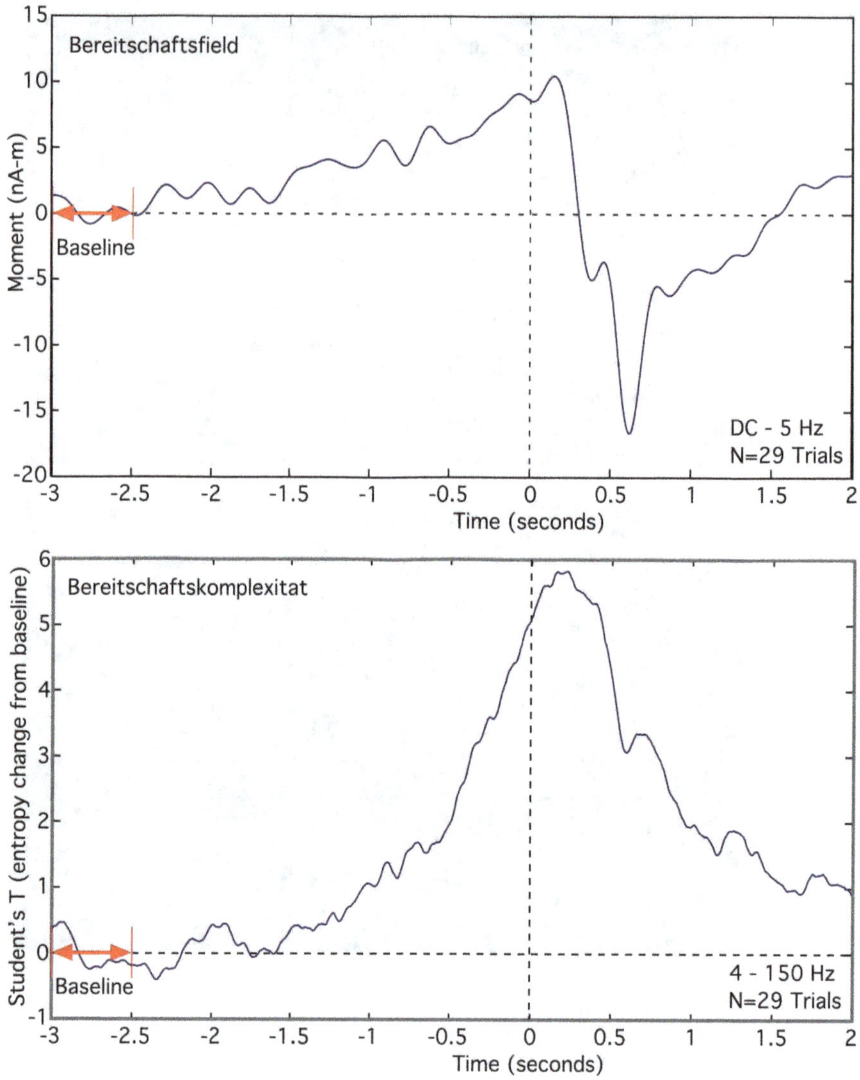

FIGURE 6 | Comparison of the averaged Bereitschaftsfield (DC to 5 Hz) to the averaged Bereitschaftskomplexität RVE (4–150 Hz) for a single voxel in premotor cortex contralateral to a self-paced voluntary finger movement (button press).

states into a symbolic dynamic topology, eventuating in the metric transformation of the density distribution of these symbolic states (Pollicott and Yuri, 1998).

The RVE is distinguished from ME in the order of operations. In ME, the states are defined by discrete partitions in the embedding space of *measured values* and the probabilities are derived from the number of counts in each n-dimensional partition. It can be difficult to define the boundaries of each partition—particularly when signals cover a wide dynamic range. In such cases, signal amplitude compression may be required. By contrast, RVE reduces the measurements to their rank values for each length W window. Each rank vector represents a state symbol (Adler et al., 1977) and partitions, as such, are no longer required; it only necessary to count the instances of each symbol. This step not only defines a finite number of available states but also renders the entropy measure-independent of absolute signal amplitude.

As a consequence of the integrator decay time constant, the mean of the entropy time series will be smaller than in the limit of $\alpha = 1$ for which integration takes place over all samples. A similar decrement from the maximum entropy was also found in older methods (Walters, 1982). This decay time constant is required in order to maintain sensitivity to entropy changes over time. As expected, RVE approaches its limiting value as the decay constant is increased. At long decay constants fluctuations will be very small due to the accruing "memory" of the state counts. For MEG data sampled at 600 Hz and $W = 5$, we choose a $1/e$ time constant 0.6 s—corresponding to three times the number of states, in samples. This is more efficient than the sliding block methods for which entropy is computed for the number of samples in each block, and the blocks are advanced one sample at a time (Adler and Marcus, 1979). It should be mentioned here that altering the decay time constant changes the peak-to-peak amplitude of the entropy fluctuations, but not its waveform (thus the RVE measure)—provided the time constant is sufficiently long to allow the state counts to fully populate.

There is an inherent frequency bias in the RVE method. The duration of the sub-window from which the rank vector is obtained constitutes a highpass filter on the signal. To a measureable extent the contribution of the entropy of signals with wavelengths longer than this sub-window is reduced. This suggests future innovations of the RVE algorithm for the purpose of better conserving the range of broadband responses. For example, one could apply a 6 dB per octave increase in the measured signal for frequencies below the window cutoff to compensate for the decline in sensitivity.

The tunable parameters for RVE analysis are the rank vector length, signal lowpass frequency, and integration decay rate. We here note practical limitations of rank vector length. Since the number of possible states is exactly determined by the length of the rank vector, if $W = 4$, 5, and 6 there are 24, 120, and 720 possible states, respectively. As a compromise, $W = 5$ seems most attractive because it allows for a sufficient number of states to reflect the probabilities without too many or too few states to be impractical (i.e., to not fully represent the latent structure in the time-series). For example, when $W = 3$, there are only 6 allowable states and when $W = 7$ there are 5040 allowable states. The latter would require a very large number of samples to accurately reflect the probabilities of each state, while the former would provide very poor state resolution. The lags defining the phase space are determined by the signal lowpass frequency. Since signal complexity decreases as bandwidth is reduced, it defeats the purpose of complexity analysis to limit the bandwidth. Therefore, the low pass should reflect the information content of the measured signal. Lastly, the integrator decay rate is selected so as to allow the state count histogram to be well-populated (a sufficient number symbol counts for obtaining a good estimate of the entropy) and have a short lead-in time (i.e., the time required for the entropy to approach its asymptotic value). For 120 states, and a sample rate of 600 Hz, a $1/e$ time of 0.6 s is sufficient. Note that, as indicated above, the integrator decay does not lowpass filter the entropy waveform. It only affects the relative amplitude of the entropy fluctuations around the asymptotic value.

The normal cerebral cortex is never quiescent—even when not engaged in specific tasks. We have shown that stimuli and tasks modulate the regional entropy of cortical activity, inducing either increases or decreases in our RVE measure. The question posed initially was whether RVE provides new information on brain activity that is not obvious when observing only changes in source power. We conclude that RVE is a sensitive measure of brain signal complexity that complements other MEG functional imaging techniques including event and task-related changes in power.

ACKNOWLEDGMENTS

The authors wish to thank Tom Holroyd for software for extracting the hull model from the MRI, and Frederick Carver and Judy Mitchell-Francis for access to the many archived MEG studies, and to Surjo Soekedar and Matthias Witkowski for the self-paced finger movement datasets. This work is supported by the Intramural Research Program of the National Institute of Mental Health, with additional support for Arnold J. Mandell from the Franklin-Fetzer Fund.

REFERENCES

Adler, R. L., Goodwyn, L. W., and Weiss, B. (1977). Equivalence of topographic Markov shifts. *Israel. J. Math.* 27, 49–63.

Adler, R. L., and Marcus, B. (1979). Topological entropy and equivalence of dynamical systems. *Mem. Am. Math. Soc.* 219, 114–126.

Bandt, C., and Pompe, B. (2002). Permutation entropy: a natural complexity measure for time series. *Phys. Rev. Lett.* 88:174102. doi: 10.1103/PhysRevLett.88.174102

Berger, S. (1989). "On the electroencephalogram of man. The fourteen original reports on the human electroencephalogram," in *Electroencephalography and Clinical Neurophysiology,* Trans. from the German and ed P. Gloor (1969) (New York, NY: Elsevier), xii + 350, (Suppl. 28), 151–171.

Birbaumer, N., Elbert, T., Canavan, A. G., and Rockstroh, B. (1990). Slow potentials of the cerebral cortex and behavior. *Physiol. Rev.* 70, 1–41.

Bruna, R., Poza, J., Gomez, C., Garcia, M., Fernandez, A., and Hornero, R. (2012). Analysis of spontaneous MEG activity in mild cognitive impairment and Alzheimer's disease using spectral entropies and statistical complexity measures. *J. Neural Eng.* 9:036007. doi: 10.1088/1741-2560/9/3/036007

Busse, F. H., and Clever, R. M. (1979). Instabilities of convection rolls in a fluid of moderate Prandl number. *J. Fluid Mech.* 91, 319–327.

Cohen, D. (1968). Magnetoencephalography: evidence of magnetic field produced by alpha rhythm currents. *Science* 161, 784–786

Cohen, L. B., Salzberg, B. M., and Grinvald, A. (1978). Optical methods for monitoring neuron activity. *Annu. Rev. Neurosci.* 1, 171–182.

Coppola, R., Callicott, J. H., Holroyd, T., Verchinski, B. A., Sust, S., and Weinberger, D. R. (2004). "MEG activation comparison to fMRI BOLD for a working memory task," in *Proceedings of the 14th International Conference on Biomagnetism*, eds E. Halgren, S. Ahlfors, M. Hämäläinen, and D. Cohen (Boston, MA), 7.

Cornfield, B. R., Fomin, V., and Sinai, Y. (1982). *Ergodic Theory.* Berlin: Springer-Verlag.

Cox, R. W. (1996). AFNI: software for analysis and visualization of functional magnetic resonance neuroimages. *Comput. Biomed. Res.* 29, 162–173.

Crutchfield, J. P., and Feldman, D. P. (2003). Regularities unseen, randomness observed: levels of entropy convergence. *Chaos* 13, 25–54.

Deecke, L., Weinberg, H., and Brickett, P. (1982). Magnetic-fields of the human-brain accompanying voluntary movement – Bereitschaftsmagnetfeld. *Exp. Brain Res.* 48, 144–148.

De Munck, J. C. (1992). A linear discretization of the volume conductor boundary integral equation using analytically integrated elements. *IEEE Trans. Biomed. Eng.* 39, 986–990.

Donchin, E. (1981). Presidential address, 1980. Surprise!... Surprise? *Psychophysiology* 18, 493–513.

Eckmann, J. P., and Ruelle, D. (1985). Ergodic theory of chaos and strange attractors. *Rev. Mod. Phys.* 57, 617–656.

Fernandez, A., Lopez-Ibor, M. I., Turrero, A., Santos, J. M., Moron, M. D., Hornero, R., et al. (2011). Lempel-Ziv complexity in schizophrenia: a MEG study. *Clin. Neurophysiol.* 122, 2227–2235.

Fife, A. A., Vrba, J., Haid, G., Hoang, T., Kubik, P. R., Lee, S., et al. (2002). "A 275-channel whole cortex MEG system," in *Proceedings of the 13th International Conference on Biomagnetism*, eds H. Nowak, J. Hauesen, F. Gießler, and R. Huonker (Berlin: VDE Verlag GMBH), 912–914.

Gauss, C. F. (1823). "Theoria combinationis observationum erroribus minimus obnoxiae," Trans. Stewart, G. W. (1995). "Theory of the combination of observations least subject to errors," in *Classics in Applied Mathematics, Chap. 4* (Philadelphia, PA: SIAM), 30.

Gollub, J., and Steinman, J. (1981). Doppler imaging of the onset of turbulent convection. *Phys. Rev. Lett.* 47, 505–509.

Gomez, C., Poza, J., Garcia, M., Fernandez, A., and Hornero, R. (2011). Regularity analysis of spontaneous MEG activity in Attention-Deficit/Hyperactivity

Disorder. *Conf. Proc. IEEE Eng. Med. Biol. Soc.* 2011, 1765–1768.

Grynszpan, F., and Geselowitz, D. B. (1973). Model studies of the magnetocardiogram. *Biophys. J.* 13, 911–925.

Hari, R., Joutsiniemi, S. L., and Sarvas, J. (1988). Spatial resolution of neuromagnetic records: theoretical calculations in a spherical model. *Electroencephalogr. Clin. Neurophysiol.* 71, 64–72.

Huang, M. X., Mosher, J. C., and Leahy, R. M. (1999). A sensor-weighted overlapping-sphere head model and exhaustive head model comparison for MEG. *Phys. Med. Biol.* 44, 423–440.

Kirchner, W. K. (1958). Age differences in short-term retention of rapidly changing information. *J. Exp. Psychol.* 55, 352–358.

Kolmogorov, A. N. (1958). A new metric invariant of transitive dynamical systems and automorphisoms of Lebesgue spaces. *Dokl. Russ. Acad. Sci.* 119, 861–864.

Kornhuber, H. H., and Deecke, L. (1964). Hirnpotentialanderungen beim Menschen vor und nach Willkurbewegungen dargestellt mit Magnetbandspeicherung und Ruckwartsanalyse. *Pflugers Arch. Eur. J. Physiol.* 281, 52.

Mandell, A. J., Selz, K. A., Aven, J., Holroyd, T., and Coppola, R. (2011a). "Daydreaming, thought blocking and strudels in the taskless, resting human brain's magnetic fields," in *International Conference on Applications in Nonlinear Dynamics (ICAND 2010)*, eds V. In, P. Longhini, and A. Palacios (Lake Louise; Melville: American Institute of Physics), 7–24.

Mandell, A. J., Selz, K. A., Holroyd, T., and Coppola, R. (2011b). "Intermittent vorticity, power spectral scaling and dynamical measures on resting brain magnetic field fluctuations," in *Neuronal Variability and Its Functional Signficance*, eds D. Glanzman and M. Ding (New York, NY: Oxford University Press), 328–390.

Milnor, J. (1997). *Topology from the Differential Viewpoint.* Princeton, NJ: Princeton University Press.

Naatanen, R., Gaillard, A. W., and Mantysalo, S. (1978). Early selective-attention effect on evoked potential reinterpreted. *Acta Psychol. (Amst.)* 42, 313–329.

Naatanen, R., and Picton, T. (1987). The N1 wave of the human electric and magnetic response to sound: a review and an analysis of the component structure. *Psychophysiology* 24, 375–425.

Nolte, G., Fieseler, T., and Curio, G. (2001). Perturbative analytic solutions of the magnetic forward problem for realistic volume conductors. *J. Appl. Phys.* 89, 2360–2369.

Nolte, G., Holroyd, T., Carver, F., Coppola, R., and Hallett, M. (2004). Localizing brain interactions from rhythmic EEG/MEG data. *Conf. Proc. IEEE Eng. Med. Biol. Soc.* 2, 998–1001.

Ornstein, D. S. (1989). Ergodic theory, randomness, and "chaos." *Science* 243, 182–187.

Ott, E. (1993). *Chaos in Dynamical Systems.* Cambridge: Cambridge University Press.

Plonsey, R., (1981). "Generation of magnetic fields by the human body (theory)," in *Proceedings Third International Workshop on Biomagnetism*, eds S. N. Erné, H.-D. Halbohm, and H. Lübbig (Berlin; New York: Walter de Gruyter), 177–205.

Pollicott, M., and Yuri, M. (1998). *Dynamical Systems and Ergodic Theory.* Cambridge: Cambridge University Press.

Robinson, S. E. (1989). "Theory and properties of lead field synthesis analysis," in *Advances in Biomagnetism*, eds H. Manfried, S. J. Williamson, M. Kotani, and G. Stroink (New York, NY: Plenum Press), 599–602.

Robinson, S. E., and Black, W. C. Jr. (1990). *Analysis of Biological Signals Using Data from Arrays of Sensors.* USA patent application 07/359, 640. December 18, 1990.

Robinson, S. E., Mandell, A. J., and Coppola, R. (2012). "Imaging complexity," in *18th Annual Meeting of the Organization for Human Brain Mapping.* (Beijing).

Robinson, S. E., and Rose, D. F. (1993). "Current source image estimation by spatially filtered MEG," in *Biomagnetism: Clinical Aspects*, eds M. Hoke, S. N. Erne, Y. C. Okada, and G. L. Romani (Muenster, Germany: Elsevier Science Publishers, B.V.), 761–765.

Ruelle, D., and Takens, F. (1971). On the nature of turbulence. *Commun. Math. Phys.* 82, 137–151.

Sarvas, J. (1987). Basic mathematical and electromagnetic concepts of the biomagnetic inverse problem. *Phys. Med. Biol.* 32, 91–97.

Sekihara, K., and Nagarajan, S. S. (2008). "Scalar adaptive spatial filter: deriving the optimum source orientation," in *Adaptive Spatial Filters for Electromagnetic Brain Imaging*, ed J. H. Nagel (Berlin, Heidelberg: Springer-Verlag), 89–92.

Shannon, C. E. (1963). *A Mathematical Theory of Communication.* Champaign-Urbana, IL: University of Illinois Press.

Singh, K. D., Barnes, G. R., Hillebrand, A., Forde, E. M., and Williams, A. L. (2002). Task-related changes in cortical synchronization are spatially coincident with the hemodynamic response. *Neuroimage* 16, 103–114.

Steriade, M. (1995). Neuromodulatory systems of thalamus and neocortex. *Sem. Neurosci.* 7, 361–370.

Swinney, H., and Gollub, J. (eds.). (1981). *Hydrodynamic Instabilities and the Transition to Turbulence.* Berlin: Springer.

Taniguchi, M., Kato, A., Fujita, N., Hirata, M., Tanaka, H., Kihara, T., et al. (2000). Movement-related desynchronization of the cerebral cortex studied with spatially filtered magnetoencephalography. *Neuroimage* 12, 298–306.

Temin, R. (1997). *Infinite Dimensional Dynamical Systems in Mechanics and Physics.* Applied mathematical sciences, 2nd Edn. (Berlin: Springer), 648.

Vakorin, V. A., Ross, B., Krakovska, O., Bardouille, T., Cheyne, D., and McIntosh, A. R. (2010). Complexity analysis of source activity underlying the neuromagnetic somatosensory steady-state response. *Neuroimage* 51, 83–90.

Van Veen, B. D., Van Drongelen, W., Yuchtman, M., and Suzuki, A. (1997). Localization of brain electrical activity via linearly constrained minimum variance spatial filtering. *IEEE Trans. Biomed. Eng.* 44, 867–880.

Vrba, J., and Robinson, S. E. (2002). SQUID sensor array configurations for magnetoencephalography applications. *Supercond. Sci. Technol.* 15, R51–R89.

Walters, P. (1982). *An Introduction to Ergodic Theory.* Berlin: Springer.

12

Inferring network properties of cortical neurons with synaptic coupling and parameter dispersion

Dipanjan Roy[1,2,3]* and Viktor Jirsa[1]

[1] Theoretical Neuroscience Group, Faculté de Médecine, Institut de Neurosciences des Systèmes, Inserm UMR1106, Aix-Marseille Université, Marseille, France
[2] Bernstein Center for Computational Neuroscience, Berlin, Germany
[3] Department of Software Engineering and Theoretical Computer Science, Technische Universität Berlin, Berlin, Germany

Correspondence:
Dipanjan Roy, Department of Software Engineering and Theoretical Computer Science, Technische Universität Berlin, Neural Information Processing Group, Marchstrasse 23, MAR 5-6, 10587 Berlin, Germany.
e-mail: dipanjan@ni.tu-berlin.de

Computational models at different space-time scales allow us to understand the fundamental mechanisms that govern neural processes and relate uniquely these processes to neuroscience data. In this work, we propose a novel neurocomputational unit (a mesoscopic model which tell us about the interaction between local cortical nodes in a large scale neural mass model) of bursters that qualitatively captures the complex dynamics exhibited by a full network of parabolic bursting neurons. We observe that the temporal dynamics and fluctuation of mean synaptic action term exhibits a high degree of correlation with the spike/burst activity of our population. With heterogeneity in the applied drive and mean synaptic coupling derived from fast excitatory synapse approximations we observe long term behavior in our population dynamics such as partial oscillations, incoherence, and synchrony. In order to understand the origin of multistability at the population level as a function of mean synaptic coupling and heterogeneity in the firing rate threshold we employ a simple generative model for parabolic bursting recently proposed by Ghosh et al. (2009). Further, we use here a mean coupling formulated for fast spiking neurons for our analysis of generic model. Stability analysis of this mean field network allow us to identify all the relevant network states found in the detailed biophysical model. We derive here analytically several boundary solutions, a result which holds for any number of spikes per burst. These findings illustrate the role of oscillations occurring at slow time scales (bursts) on the global behavior of the network.

Keywords: multispikes, self-organization, transients, firing rate, parabolic burst, network synchrony, generative model, oscillations

1. INTRODUCTION

The neuronal spike-burst activity is characterized by recurrent transitions between rest state and firing state where bursts are temporal groupings of multiple spikes. Certain cells in the mammal brain, for example, neurons in the thalamus during periods of drowsiness, attentiveness, and sleep are known to exhibit this type of spike-burst behavior (Sherman and Koch, 1986; Steriade and Llinás, 1988; McCormick and Feeser, 1990; Steriade et al., 1993; Amzica and Steriade, 1998). Autonomously bursting neurons are found in a variety of neural systems, from the mammalian cortex (Morris and Lecar, 1981; Dhamala et al., 2004a,b) to brainstem (Hindmarsh and Rose, 1984; Wang, 1994; Izhikevich, 2007; Jirsa and McIntosh, 2007; Jirsa, 2008). When neurons are coupled with each other, they produce different modes of behavior, including synchrony and phase-locking, which have been implicated in memory, cognition, sensory processing, motor planning, and execution (McCormick and Feeser, 1990; Wang, 1994; Jirsa and McIntosh, 2007). Many neurological diseases, on the other hand, including Parkinson, schizophrenia, and epilepsy, are the result of abnormal synchronization (Uhlhaas and Singer, 2006; Jensen et al., 2007), which suggests that a better understanding of the basic mechanisms producing synchrony and phase locking will be a stepping stone toward the repair of brain function. Modeling attempts using large scale networks to understand emergence of cognitive states rely heavily on the approximation of the dynamics as a neural ensemble. The concept of a neural mass like abstraction (Hebb, 1949; Beurle, 1956) designates a group of Co-activated neurons capable of acting like a closed system when performing a certain function. A small scale network of this kind is sometimes referred to as a "neurocomputational unit." In large scale brain networks, these mesoscopic units of operation serve as the network nodes (see for instance, Deco et al., 2008, 2011; Ghosh et al., 2008). On intermediate spatial scales of few cm, neural activations along the spatially continuous cortical sheets are described by neural fields, for which the connectivity is assumed to be translationally invariant (see, Wilson and Cowan, 1972; Nunez, 1974; Amari, 1977; Jirsa and Haken, 1997; Feng et al., 2006; Jirsa, 2009; Robinson, 2011). To define such small neurocomputational units, simplified neuron models, known as phase models, offer an attractive tool for the study of network modes, since they allow for detailed mathematical analysis of network dynamics (Breakspear et al., 2010). As an example, Carbal et al. have explored the role of local network oscillations in resting-state functional connectivity by using such phase oscillators in the respective nodes of the simulated network. They have shown when these oscillatory units are integrated in the network, they behave as weakly coupled oscillators. Moreover, for a set of network parameters they found subsets of nodes tend to synchronize although the network is not globally synchronized (Cabral et al., 2011). For the present work we use a recently proposed phenomenological model that admits parabolic bursting in one dimension, which is a type of bursting observed in the R-15 neuron in abdominal ganglion of aquatic mollusc Aplysia Californica (Ermentrout and Kopell, 1986; Izhikevich, 2000; Ghosh et al., 2009). This type of bursting can arise even without bistability in the generation of spikes. The investigation carried out in this work with a detailed neuron model capable of displaying spiking and bursting behavior and a minimal model that not only reproduces the mean field amplitude of the original networks but also capture the most important temporal features of its dynamics. The detailed model used here is extensively discussed in Rinzel and Ermentrout (1989). On the other hand, our phase model is a minimal model that captures the generality of the mechanism of bursting present in the detailed model. As we vary network parameters including mean field coupling strength and dispersion, both networks display various temporal dynamics. In order to understand these states in mathematically tractable terms we take advantage of the mean field coupled network of phase model. Our goal is to identify to what degree this mean field model serves as a reliable neurocomputational unit and captures the qualitative features of temporal dynamics of the full network as a function of the investigated network parameters. Mean field analysis for singleton burst reveals solutions such as incoherence and partial oscillation which can be completely described analytically. However, as we are interested in a multispike system where analytical calculation is rather non-trivial and therefore, we combine semi-analytical approach with numerics to derive the stability diagram. Mean field phase network allow us to identify the mechanism of transitions between various network states that appear as solutions of the full network. Stability diagram is independent of number of spikes per burst and qualitatively commensurates well with the findings in our full network. The paper is structured as follows. In the next section, we introduce the Rinzel–Ermentrout model (Rinzel and Ermentrout, 1989) for parabolic bursting and describe the model in details. In the following section, we couple individual neurons via global coupling and present our analysis of this network model. In the subsequent section, we set up a generic network of bursters coupled to their mean field and derive semianalytically all the network states and corresponding phase transition boundaries. In the next section, we derive numerically a stability diagram using global phase coherence measure. In the final section, we summarize the results obtained from mean field descriptions and link them systematically with the network states obtained from biophysical model network.

2. MATERIALS AND METHODS

2.1. SINGLE NEURON MODEL

A dynamical system with multiple time scales (for example, a neuron with spiking-bursting behaviors) can be written in a singularly perturbed form: $\dot{\mathbf{x}} = f(x, y)$, $\dot{\mathbf{y}} = rg(x, y)$, where $\mathbf{x}$ is the vector of fast variables, $\mathbf{y}$ the vector of slow variables that modulate the fast activity, and $r \ll 1$ is a ratio of fast/slow time scales. A system which has been proposed to describe parabolic bursting behavior is known as Rinzel model (1989). Single neuron model parameters used here are exactly as described in Rinzel and Ermentrout (1989).

$$\begin{aligned}
\dot{V} &= (I - I_{Ca} - (g_K w + g_{kca} z)(V - V_K) - g_l(V - V_l))/c \\
\dot{w} &= \phi(w_\infty - w)/\tau_w \\
\dot{Ca} &= \epsilon(-\mu I_{Ca} - Ca) \\
\dot{n} &= \epsilon(n_\infty(V) - n)/\tau_n
\end{aligned} \tag{1}$$

where $I_{Ca} = (g_{Ca} m_\infty(V) + g_{sCa} n)(V - V_{Ca})$, $z = \frac{Ca}{Ca + Ca_0}$ and gating functions are

$$\begin{aligned}
m_\infty(V) &= 0.5(1 + \tan h((V - v_1)/v_2)) \\
w_\infty(V) &= 0.5(1 + \tan h((V - v_3)/v_4)) \\
n_\infty(V) &= 0.5(1 + \tan h((V - v_5)/v_6)) \\
\tau_w(V) &= 0.5(1 + \tan h((V - v_3)/2v_2))
\end{aligned} \tag{2}$$

where V is the membrane potential, w is associated with the fast current, Na^+ or K^+, Ca and n are the two slow currents, Model parameters which are held fixed throughout our simulations are, $V_K = -84$, $V_l = 60$, $V_{Ca} = 120$, $g_K = 8$, $g_l = 2$, $c = 20$, $v_1 = 1.2$, $v_2 = 18$, $v_6 = 24$, $v_5 = 12$, $v_3 = 12$, $v_4 = 17.4$, $\tau_n = 0.05$, $\phi = 0.06666666$, $gCa = 4.0$, $\mu = 0.025$, $Ca_0 = 1$, $\epsilon = 0.0005$, and $g_{kCa} = 1$, $g_{sCa} = 1$.

I is the applied input current. The ionic currents are given by an ohmic leak current, determined by the leak conductance g_l and leak reversal potential V_l, and a Na^+ current which is responsible for the generation of spikes. The dynamics of this model which is relevant to our study is outlined as follows. When the input current I exceeds a critical value I_c a single neuron described by Equation (1) undergoes a Saddle-node bifurcation on an invariant circle (SNIC). This same system for two different parameterization of I and in the presence of the slow currents can exhibit both spiking as well as parabolic bursting behavior. Spiking behaviors are elicited for a slightly higher value of the external drive. For example, to observe a typical burst-like pattern in this system we held the input current to the values $I = 68$ and for spikes $I \geq 70$. **Figure 1** displays the relationship between the applied input current and a parabolic bursting pattern that is observed in the single neuron dynamics.

2.2. PHASE MODEL

The generality of the underlying mechanism for parabolic bursting is investigated in details by numerous authors (Ermentrout and Kopell, 1986; Baer et al., 1995; Izhikevich, 2000). In many such formulations, parabolic bursting neurons are typically in their canonical form described as:

$$\begin{aligned}
\dot{\theta} &= [1 - \cos(\theta) + f(x, y)] \\
\dot{x} &= \mu_x[x_\eta(\theta) - x] \\
\dot{y} &= \mu_y[y_\eta(\theta) - y]
\end{aligned} \tag{3}$$

where function $f(x, y)$ in the above equation couples to spike generative mechanism depending on the slow variables x, y dynamics, respectively. The function $f(x, y)$ is a smoothly varying periodic function alternating signs such that the system undergoes a SNIC to generate parabolic burst at the single neuron level. Recently Ghosh et al. (2009) has also proposed a simpler model that in principle captures the underlying mechanism of parabolic bursting involving only a circular phase variable θ and moreover, involve only one slow term to allow the fast dynamics to enter or get out of repetitive firing. Motivation for using such a model is primarily mathematical tractability. Parameter space of this model cannot be directly linked to the biophysical parameters, however, qualitatively it may account for the transient and longterm behavior of more detailed biophysical models. In this model a single neuron is described by the following equation,

$$\dot{\theta} = I - \cos\theta - \cos\frac{\theta}{n} \tag{4}$$

In Equation (4) a slow variable activation term is represented by a modulation term $\cos(\frac{\theta}{n})$ which mimics the entire slow subsystem instead of describing it as a separate dynamical system, I is the applied input current and n is an integer, which determines the number of spikes per burst. In our simulation with this model all the results are for $n = 5$ spikes per burst unless otherwise specified.

2.3. FULL NETWORK MODEL

Golomb and Rinzel (1993) considered a heterogeneous network of all-to-all coupled inhibitory bursting neurons and found regimes of synchronous, anti-synchronous and asynchronous behavior when the width of the heterogeneity was changed (Golomb and Rinzel, 1993; Stefanescu and Jirsa, 2008, 2011; Smeal et al., 2010; Jirsa and Stefanescu, 2011). We describe our network equations via a fast instantaneous coupling. N synaptically coupled (all-to-all) parabolic bursting neurons are described by a similar set of non-linear differential equations with fast chemical synapse. To this end we formally describe:

$$\begin{aligned}
\dot{V}_i &= (bI_i - I_{Ca} - (g_K w + g_{kca} z)(V_i - V_k) \\
&\quad - g_l(V_i - V_l) + KS(V_i - V_{\text{th}}))/c \\
\dot{w}_i &= \phi(w_\infty - w_i)/\tau_w \\
\dot{Ca}_i &= \epsilon(-\mu I_{ca} - Ca_i) \\
\dot{n}_i &= \epsilon\,(n_\infty(V) - n_i)\,/\tau_n \\
\dot{s}_i &= a_s(V_i)(1 - s_i) - \frac{s_i}{\beta}
\end{aligned} \tag{5}$$

where all the parameters and the gating variables inherit from the single neuron model Equation (1, 2) and b is a rescaling factor to applied drive to cross the threshold and elicit spike/burst in the uncoupled system. Stimulus that all the neurons see $I_i > 0$ are drawn from a uniform distribution assumed to be symmetrically distributed over the interval $I_i \in [2.1 - \Delta I, 2.1 + \Delta I]$. Where ΔI is the spread of the applied stimulus parameter. ΔI introduces a heterogeneity in the spike threshold. The synaptic coupling appears as an ensemble average given by $S = \frac{1}{N}\sum_{i=1}^{N} s_i$, where $a_{s_i}(V_i) = \frac{1}{(1+\exp(-V_i/2))}$ is a sigmoidal activation function. The synaptic strength K is the same for all the neurons. For the entire simulation, we fixed the reversal potential of potassium ions to $v_{\text{th}} \approx 0.0$ (for purely excitatory connectivity).

Analysis is carried out for a fast synapse (AMPA-type glutamate receptors), such as those found in the auditory system, the rise time is instantaneous, and post-synaptic responses commence almost instantaneously after the start of presynaptic action potential (Nunez, 1974; Morris and Lecar, 1981). This brisk communication is a consequence of rapid calcium-channel kinetics, which allows significant calcium entry during the upstroke of the presynaptic action potential (Sabatini and Regehr, 1996). Under the fast synapse approximation the variable s_i relaxes much more rapidly than V_i, in which case we may apply a quasi-static approximation to (Equation 5) (e), $\dot{s}_i \approx 0$, allowing us to adiabatically eliminate the synaptic variable via $s_i = \frac{\beta}{(1+\beta+\exp(-V_i/2))}$. The time course of the postsynaptic conductivity caused by an activation of AMPA receptors can be captured by a rise time $\beta_{\text{rise}} = 0.09$ ms and decay time $\beta_{\text{decay}} = 1.5$ ms (Gabbiani et al., 1994; Parnas and Parnas, 1994). Numerical results in **Figure 3** provides a good approximation for β in the range between [0.01 ms, 0.5 ms]. Although, we have provided here the details about the fast excitatory synaptic connectivity, our approach can be readily extended to inhibitory connectivity as well. In the continuum limit, a mean field formulation with inhibitory synaptic coupling is provided in details in Appendix.

2.4. MEAN FIELD COUPLED PHASE MODEL

Each generic neuron is coupled to this mean field and typically their response to the mean field expressed as $R(\theta)$ explicitly dependent on θ, and implicitly on time. In absence of any coupling, their vector field flow on a real line is governed by $F(\theta) = \omega - \cos(\theta) - \cos(\theta)/n$. In the absence of the term $\cos(\theta)/n$ expression reduces to a mathematical description used in Roy et al. (2011). Together, we can write for N (still finite) such neurons:

$$\dot{\theta}_i = F(\theta_i) - \Gamma R(\theta_i), \tag{6}$$

Recently, we have proposed a formulation for mean synaptic activation term under fairly general setting and taking advantage of instantenous activation, deactivation between pre and postsynaptic events. It allows one to describe synaptic activation variable $s_i = \frac{\beta}{1+\beta+\exp\left(\frac{-V_i}{2}\right)}$ as a non-linear transfer function of membrane voltage (Roy et al., 2011). Moreover, we have described how the mean field coupled spiking neurons can be described mathematically with this synaptic coupling. Details of this formulation is described elsewhere, (Roy et al., 2011). Collective activity of synapses is described by a mean field. For a given population of neurons is expressed more formally as,

$$\Gamma = \frac{K}{N}\sum_{l=1}^{N} \frac{\beta}{\left(1 + \beta + \exp\left(-\frac{\cos\theta_l}{2}\right)\right)}, \quad i \neq l. \tag{7}$$

where Γ is the mean field influence function. Coupling K is the same for all the neurons. In our previous work, response to such mean field coupling explicitly described as $R(\theta_i) = \sin\theta_i(\cos\theta_i - \nu_{\text{th}})$,

$$\dot{\theta}_i = F(\theta_i) - \Gamma\sin\theta_i(\cos\theta_i - \nu_{\text{th}}) + O(\epsilon), \quad (8)$$

where $O(\epsilon)$ contains non-circular deviations of the order ϵ that results due to perturbations. $\nu_{\text{th}} \approx 0.0$ for all simulations and analytical calculations unless mentioned otherwise. It is important to note that the couplings in the phase descriptions retain their mathematical expression in the full model plus some linearly added correction terms, which scale with the degree of order of deviation from the circle (Roy et al., 2011). Hence, in application it is rather suitable when phase perturbations are close to the circular orbit. The above equation further can be written combining the terms containing a single Fourier harmonic in the coupling plus the higher order Fourier terms.

$$\dot{\theta}_i = \omega_i - \sin\theta_i - \sin(\theta_i/n) + P(\theta_l)\sin\theta_i\nu_{\text{th}} + O(2\theta_i) + O(\epsilon), \quad (9)$$

$$P(\theta_l) = \frac{K}{N}\sum_{l=1}^{N}\frac{\beta}{\left(1+\beta+\exp\left(-\frac{\cos\theta_l}{2}\right)\right)}, \quad i \neq l. \quad (10)$$

See for details (Roy et al., 2011). Where, in Equation (6) the frequencies $I_i \geq 0$ are assumed to be symmetrically distributed over the interval $I_i \in [I - \Delta I, I + \Delta I]$ according to a uniform probability distributions.

2.5. CHARACTERIZATION OF SPIKE/BURST COHERENCE IN BIOPHYSICAL NETWORK MODEL WITH MEAN FIELD COUPLING

The bursting coherence and incoherence is quantitatively characterized in terms of a statistical-mechanical spike-based measure. We consider an excitatory population of neurons coupled to a common mean field drive and heterogeneity in their threshold for spikes/bursts. By varying the strength of the coupling K and the stimulus spread ΔI we investigate the emergence of spike/burst coherence. Emergence of collective spiking/bursting coherence may be well described by the (population-averaged) global potential,

$$V_{\text{mean}}(t) = \frac{1}{N}\sum_{i=1}^{N} V_i \quad (11)$$

In the thermodynamic limit ($N \to \infty$), a collective state becomes coherent if $\delta V_{\text{mean}}(t) \equiv [V_{\text{mean}}(t) - \overline{V_{\text{mean}}}(t)]$ is non-stationary (i.e., an oscillating global potential V_{mean} appears for a coherent case), where the overbar represents the time average, and also, the correlated mean field $\Gamma(t)$ activity appears oscillatory. Otherwise (i.e., when V_{mean} is time independent or stationary), it either becomes incoherent (IN) or partial oscillatory (PO). In $N \to \infty$ limit both these states converges to a stationary solution. Thus, the mean square deviation of the global potential is a global marker for mean burst coherence for the entire population described here. More formally one can write it as (i.e., time-averaged fluctuations of V_{mean}),

$$R(t) = \bar{(}V_{\text{mean}}(t) - \overline{V_{\text{mean}}}(t))^2 \quad (12)$$

plays the role of an order parameter used for describing the coherence-incoherence transition (Manrubia et al., 2004). For the coherent (IN) state, the order parameter $R(t)$ approaches a non-zero (zero) limit value as N goes to the infinity. We compute $R(t)$ in Equation (12) as a function of mean field coupling strength K and dispersion parameter ΔI for the full system. We vary both K, ΔI from 0 to 1 in a step size of 0.01. Subsequently, computed values of $R(t)$ is plotted in grid size of 100×100. Contour plot is colorcoded from low values at zero (blue) to high values at 1 (red). Nearly (in phase or anti phase) synchronized population spike/burst activity is lumped into a regime with labeled as SR and IN population spike/burst activity is lumped into a regime called IN activity. In the IN regime as described above $R(t)$ values stays close to zero with substantial subthreshold fluctuations. Partial bursty regime is labeled as PO observed for $R(t)$ values stationary and close to values other than zero. This regime displays dynamical behaviors far from synchrony, such as multi-clustering (some of the neurons are firing incoherently while others are not firing at all) in the phase for instance. Depending on the heterogeneity in stimulus spread we get random distribution of phases such that individual members can exhibit cluster hopping. Multiclustering in our model can reliably be captured using an ensemble average quantity rotation number ρ_i given by Equation (14).

2.6. CHARACTERIZATION OF SPIKE/BURST COHERENCE IN PHASE NETWORK MODEL WITH MEAN FIELD COUPLING

The bursting coherence and incoherence is quantitatively characterized in terms of statistical mechanical order parameter coherence measure. As an alternative to storing and plotting many time series data $\theta_i(t), i = 1, \ldots, N$ for all $N = 1000$ variables, we define an order parameter

$$R_\theta(t) = \frac{1}{N}\sum_{i=1}^{N}\cos\theta_i \quad (13)$$

Equation (13) measures the population dynamics. The advantage of using such a formulation becomes apparent immediately. Let's say our model system has periodic orbit then $\theta_i(t)$ $\theta_i(t+T)$, where T periodic pacing spikes or bursts (latency). Then in order parameter space one can can detect this state in a straight forward manner as a solution $R_\theta(t)R_\theta(t+T)$. This result holds for all i, t. In this case, R_θ dynamics is dominated mostly by the x co-ordinate dynamics. Absolute values of mean order parameter mod $R_\theta \leq 1$. There is a mathematical relationship of macroscopic global phase measure with macroscopic $V_{\text{mean}}(t)$ in Equation (11). The interval between each microscopic spike/burst in an arbitrary ith stripe of spike/burst can be determined in a statistical-mechanical way by taking into consideration its contribution to the macroscopic global membrane potential $V_{\text{mean}}(t)$. In this interpretation, the time series of the global potential $V_{\text{mean}}(t)$ has a local maxima and minima, respectively and strictly bounded between [0,1]. The global cycle in the suprathreshold regime starting from the minimum of $V_{\text{mean}}(t)$ which appears first after the transient time is regarded as the first global cycle, which is denoted by G_1. The 2nd global cycle G_2 begins from the next following right minimum of G1, and so on. Then, we can introduce an instantaneous global phase measure

$\theta(t)$ of $V_{mean}(t)$ via a linear interpolation in the two successive subregions forming a complete global cycle (Lim and Kim, 2011). A microscopic spike makes the most constructive (inphase) contribution to V_{mean} when the corresponding global phase θ_k for kth cycle of spikes/burst is $2n\pi$ ($n = 0, 1, 2, \ldots$), while it makes the most destructive (anti-phase) contribution to $V_{mean}(t)$ when θ_i for an arbitrary ith cycle of burst is $2(n1/2)\pi$. By averaging the contributions of all microscopic spikes within a burst in the ith burst stripe to V_{mean}, we can obtain the following degree of ordering of spikes/bursts. Hence, the contribution of kth microscopic burst occurring at the time t_k is ordered by $R_\theta(t_k)$. If the degree of synchrony is high between the bursts/spikes then $R_\theta(t_k) \to 1$. We quantify the average firing frequency to compare the long-term behavior of individual neurons in the population model. We compute the average frequency (also known as the rotation number) of population of neurons using

$$\rho_i = \lim_{t \to \infty} \frac{\theta_i}{t}, \quad i = 1, \ldots, N. \tag{14}$$

Averaging is carried out over about 1000 neurons starting from random initial conditions after the transient have died out. Collective states of ensemble of $N = 1000$ neurons with spikes per burst $n = 5$ as indicated by their rotation numbers with uniform distribution of frequency I in the interval $[2.1 - \Delta I, 2.1 + \Delta I]$. Different branch of rotation index indicate different dynamical states of the network as a function of mean field coupling strength K, ΔI. We carry out a grid search in the 2D parameter space K, ΔI. Our goal is to obtain a phase transition diagram to understand long-term collective behavior of Equation (8) for large N, as a function of the coupling strength $K \geq 0$ and the stimulus spread $\Delta I \in [0, 1)$. Global order parameter $R_\theta(t)$ is computed for different parameterization of K, ΔI and embedded on a contour plot. Color spectrum is the same as the one used for displaying phase diagram in the full network. The values which are high and close to 1 are indicated by red and the values which are close to zero are indicated by blue.

2.7. CLUSTERING ANALYSIS IN N COUPLED FULL AND PHASE NETWORK MODEL

We describe firing patterns in large networks (finite N) with excitatory mean field coupling in terms of array diagrams. Array diagrams are obtained by simulating a coupled system consisting of mean field coupled biophysical neurons ($N = 100$) governed by the Equation (5). All the coupling coefficients are the same K where $i = 1, \ldots, N$. In the arrays the intensity of the voltage variables $V_1, \ldots, V_i$ have been encoded in color spectrum. Two different color spectrums are used for the biophysical network (see **Figure 4**). In the first color spectrum blue part of the array values implies the quiescent activity of the spikes where the voltage variables have relatively lower values. All the other colors in the spectrum indicates the higher values for the voltage variables, consequently these pixels in the array imply the spike activity. The horizontal line of the array shows the time with increasing epoches of activity. The second color spectrum used here shows burst depiction in the nearly coherent parameter regime. Green colors in the array indicate completely silent neurons. Purple pixels on the green background shows burst activity. On the vertical axis neuron index are aligned and again, on the horizontal axis gives the direction of time. These diagrams were obtained from a phase network by monitoring phases of individual neurons $i = 1, \ldots, N$ and aligning them on the vertical axis. The choice of the color spectrum used for phases is given by a colorbar with uniformly distributed phase values. In **Figure 9** red color index in the spectrum corresponds to higher phase values of θ (close to π) and orange color index are for lower phase values (close to $-\pi$). First initial conditions $\theta_i(0)$ is generated randomly and then they are sorted according to their neuron index and subsequently distributed uniformly about $[-\pi, \pi]$. The parameters K, ΔI, for both realizations are chosen from SR, IN regime of the respective phase diagrams.

2.8. NUMERICAL PROCEDURES AND VISUALIZATION OF THE SYSTEM DYNAMICS

Two network models were implemented in Matlab, numerically integrated using second order Runge Kutta routine and Euler–Maruyama (EM) method (Higham, 2001). The simulations were performed with a fixed time step of $dt = 0.05$. The first 200 time points of the simulation are disregarded to set the network to a steady state. Thus, the results within this time were ignored. The membrane potential $V(t)$, standard deviation of membrane potential std V, mean field $\Gamma(t)$, order parameters $R(t)$, $R_\theta(t)$ are captured for the entire population. For full network, simulation is carried out for $N = 100$ neurons and for the phase network for $N = 1000$ neurons. Numerical Phase diagrams are obtained using parallel for loops implemented in Matlab. Coupled mean field Phase model represented in Equation (8) can be visualized as a collection of N points rotating around the unit circle, where the estimated phase for each neuron $\theta_i(t)$ denotes their position on a ring or a circle at time t. This alternate representation of the dynamical system (as N points moving along a circular reference frame, instead of a single point tracing out a trajectory in an N-dimensional phase space) is possible because the system's state space, the N-torus, is equivalent to N copies of the unit circle. It is worth noting that for most other N-dimensional state spaces such a reduced representation is not feasible. In order to distinguish between oscillators with different natural frequencies, we color the dots according to the standard color spectrum: the neurons correspond to the low end of the spectrum (close to $-\pi$)(red), neurons at the high end (close to π) (blue), while those in between occupy the middle part of the spectrum (orange/yellow/green). To show how the system evolves from one instant to the next, we plot a series of snapshots of the system at different times (see **Figures 11B–D**, for example). This allows us to observe the behavior of individual neurons at the same time as we witness the collective evolution of the system toward an attractive state.

3. RESULTS

3.1. SINGLE NEURON BURST DYNAMICS

We first examine the behavior of single neuron model Equation (2.1) as the applied input current I is brought close to the threshold for generating spikes or bursts. For the given parameters In Equation (2.1) a neuron is excitable. **Figure 1** depicts the relationship between applied input and parabolic bursting pattern. We are only interested in the behavior of this

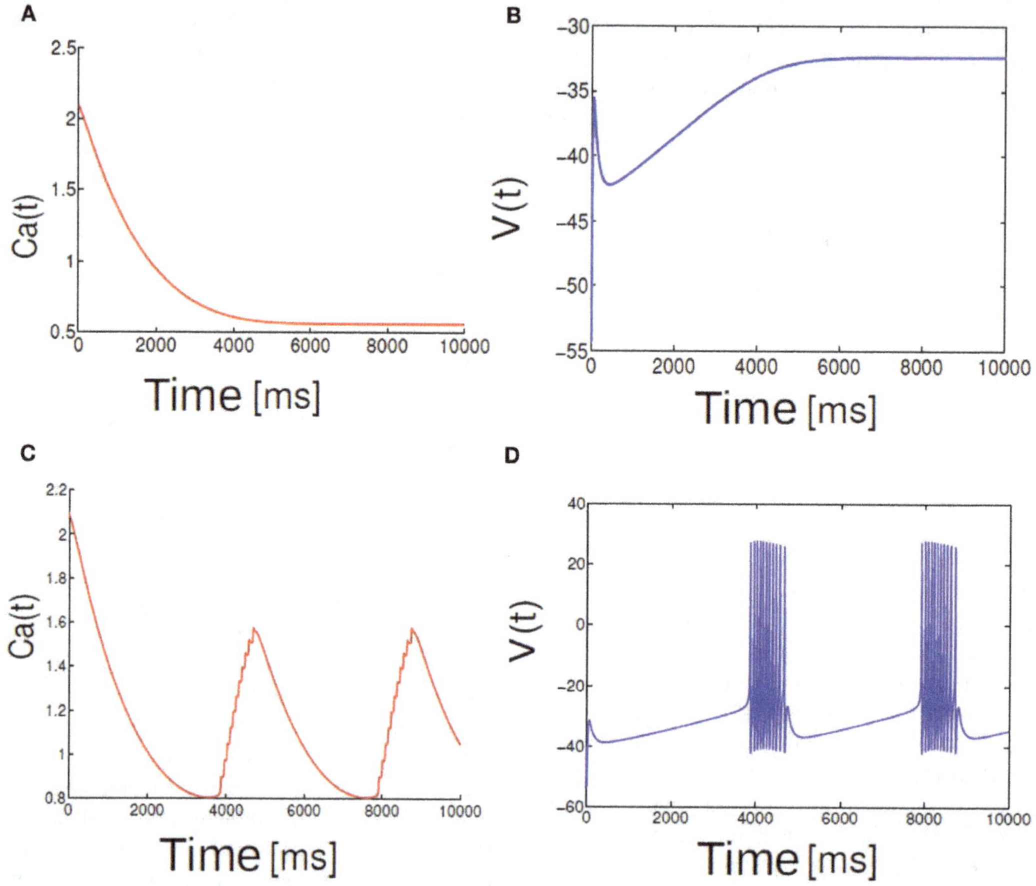

FIGURE 1 | Shown here trace of membrane potential and calcium dynamics. Fast spikes rides on a slow modulation of calcium. Slow subsystem moves Ca back and forth across SNIC bifurcation points **(A,C)**. In **(B,D)** membrane potential dynamics is shown for two different cases **(A)** $I < I_c$ and **(B)** $I > I_c$ in the single neuron model.

system for low current values where the resting state of membrane voltage is sufficiently depolarized below −40 mV. When the applied input current I is below a critical value membrane potential $V(t)$ maintains their steady state value and for values greater than the threshold exhibits bursting behavior. For the parameterization used here we find that at $I \geq 60$ steady state destabilizes exhibiting multispikes. When the applied input current is further increased a neuron make transition from bursting to spiking behavior. In order to observe a typical spiking behavior we set $I \geq 70$. To get an intuitive understanding about the relationship between slow and fast subsystems, Rinzel and Lee analyzed this model by varying *ca* (a variable in the slow subsystem) as a bifurcation parameter to report that parabolic bursting is obtained from an oscillation in the slow subsystem that periodically moves the *ca* variable back and forth across the SNIC bifurcation, to link the steady state solution of this system to (quiescence state in **Figure 1A**) the branch of periodic solutions (**Figure 1B**) and vice versa. Time series of fast variable shows that the interspike interval is relatively longer at the beginning and end of each burst. As has been shown by numerous authors oscillation for the fast dynamics is obtained when the slow variables are held fixed; it is where the saddle-node-loop bifurcation occurs. There is a clear threshold below which there is a unique stable fixed point. Parabolic bursting can occur without having any bistability in the spike generating process. One way to achieve parabolic bursting behavior without requiring any bistability in the generating process and moreover, mathematically tractable would require a generic description like the one shown in Equation (2.2) (see section 2). From numerical results we find that as the applied input current $I \to 2$, time period $T \to \infty$. Applied input current can be tuned such that it is possible to obtain parabolic bursts of desired interburst gap. The time evolution of a single neuron activity is shown in **Figure 2**, where a membrane potential like variable $V(t) = -\cos[\theta(t)]$ is plotted by numerically integrating Equation (2.2). Temporal dynamics shows regular parabolic bursting behavior. For $I < I_c$ a neuron fires few spikes before it settles into a steady state. For $I > I_c$ ($I = 2.01$, $n = 5$) neurons exhibits parabolic bursting behavior. Based on the qualitative similarity in the burst pattern with parabolic bursting neurons (At the start and the end of the active phase the spike frequency is smaller compared to the middle of the active phase as can be seen in **Figure 2** detailed model is substituted to investigate the network effects.

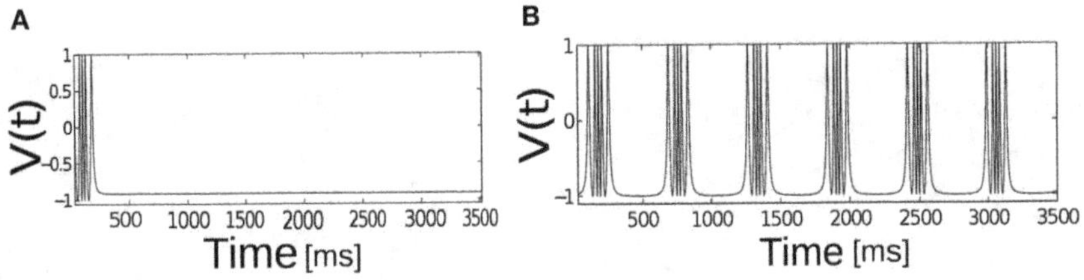

FIGURE 2 | The temporal dynamics of the phase model of spike-burst neuron. $V(t) = -\cos[\theta]$ is plotted as a function of time, $I_c = 2.01$, $n = 5$, for **(A)** $I < I_c$ and for **(B)** $I > I_c$.

3.2. NETWORK DYNAMICS OF PARABOLIC BURSTING NEURONS WITH HETEROGENEITY

To understand the influence of heterogeneity in the applied input current and the coupling strength in a network of single neurons exhibiting parabolic bursting we use Equation (5) and parameters as described in section 2.4. We use fast excitatory synapses to couple these units. When the synaptic coupling is sufficiently fast, the coupling tends to push the neurons toward anti-synchrony (Wang and Rinzel, 1992; Friesen, 1994; Van Vreeswijk et al., 1994). Moreover, several studies have observed emergence of multistable solutions in their mean field network with parameter heterogeneity (Assisi et al., 2005; Jirsa and Stefanescu, 2011). Our motivation is to go toward this particular direction to capture the relevant network dynamics at the population level. In particular to understand the combined effect of heterogeneity in the firing rate threshold (biophysical model) with the fast time scale of activation-deactivation of synapses in the coupling; the interplay between these two critical factors in spike/burst timing at the population level is largely unknown. In our formalism their individual and combined influence on the network dynamics become clearly visible. Typical time course of such responses of synaptic variable in our model simulation are shown in **Figure 2**). Fast synapse approximation holds as long as the variable s_i relaxes much more rapidly than V_i, in which case we may apply a quasistatic approximation to reduce s_i further in Equation (5), $s_i \simeq 0$ allowing us to adiabatically eliminate β, and set the synaptic variable via an approximation as $s_i = \frac{\beta}{1+\beta+\exp\left(\frac{-V_i}{2}\right)}$. The mean synaptic action can be formulated as $\Gamma = \frac{1}{N}\sum_{i=1}^{N} s_i$, where $a_s(V_i) = \frac{1}{(1+\exp(-V_i/2))}$. The synaptic constant K is the same for all the neurons. **Figures 3A–D** shows kinetics of excitatory synaptic variable s_i (plotted with black solid lines) for different β values. Mean synaptic variable (plotted with dotted lines) for the same set of values of time constant β shows dissimilar temporal response compared to s_i for higher time constant values. For smaller time constant values simulation provides relatively better aggrement as can be seen from **Figure 3**. We numerically integrate the above network to investigate how the mean population burst changes with time as a function of spread of applied stimulus ΔI and mean field coupling strength K. Firing patterns in this network are shown with array diagrams in **Figures 4A,B**. For small spread in the applied stimulus and sufficient coupling strength $\Delta I = 0.001$, $K = 0.7$ nearly burst synchronization takes place. Moreover, in the array diagram we detect clusters of synchronous states which fires in a wave-like pattern. Corresponding time series of mean quantities such as the membrane potential $V_{mean}(t)$ in Equation (11), mean field $\Gamma(t)$ shows periodic activity in **Figure 4C**. Membrane potential spiking activity is nearly synchronized across population of neurons in **Figure 4**. On the other hand, for the IN state mean membrane potential fast decays to zero and shows subthreshold fluctuations about mean zero. Response of mean membrane potential is more suppressed compared to their mean field oscillations between [0,1]. Amplitude of mean field $\Gamma(t)$ changes in time systematically but fluctuates about the mean value of 0.5 instead of approaching zero values as can be seen in **Figure 4D**. Population burst synchrony is observed for many different parameterization, for one such choice of parameter $\Delta I = 0.002, K = 0.8$, an array diagram is computed and plotted in **Figure 5A**. As can be seen in the figure a wave-like spread of activity. In **Figure 5B** various time series plots of population burst synchrony is shown across 10 neurons. In order to identify different network states for all possible combination

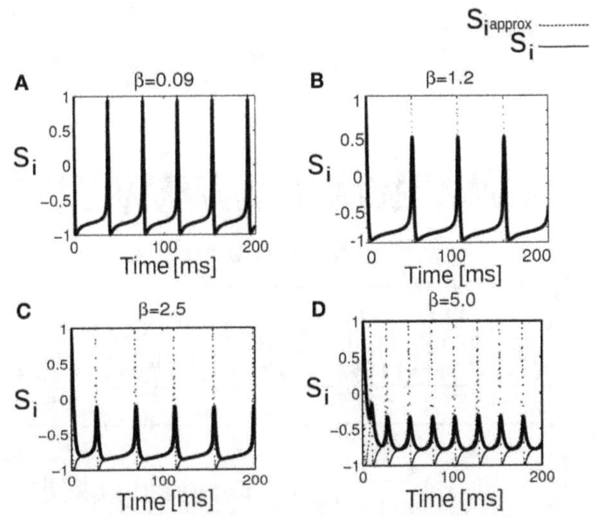

FIGURE 3 | Shown here trace of synaptic variable and approximated synaptic variable. Traces are plotted for a spiking regime of our network at $I = 80$, this external current is applied to each neurons in this population. Panels **(A–D)** are generated for low to high β synaptic time constant values. figure shows approximation breaks down progressively as we go to higher β values or access slower time scale. Approximation holds for faster time scale of oscillations.

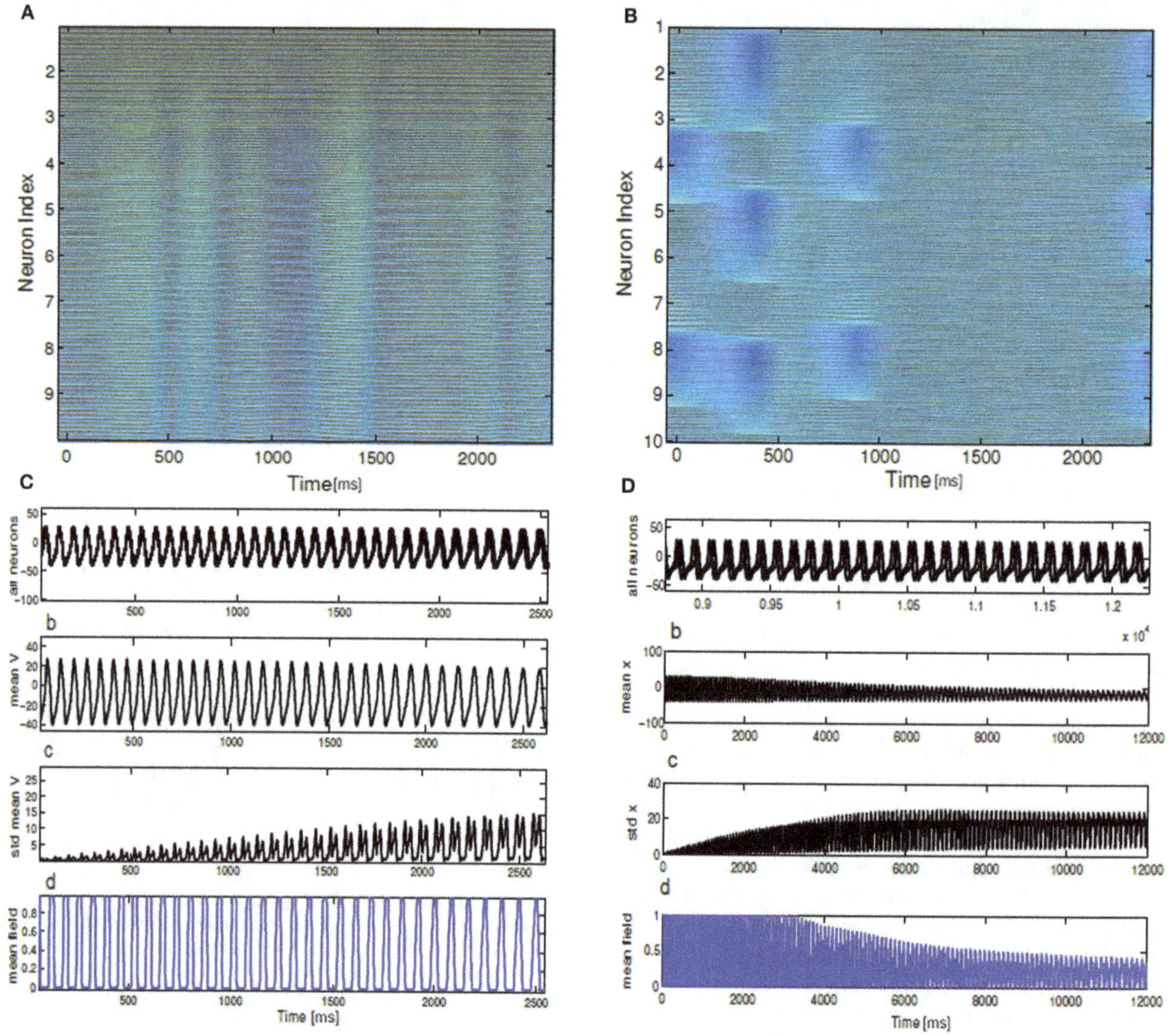

FIGURE 4 | Array diagrams are shown in (A,B) for two distinct network states. In a nearly coherent states with clusters of synchronous bursting activity $\Delta I = 0.001$, $K = 0.7$, in **(B)** incoherent states for $\Delta I = 0.12$, $K = 0.01$. Nearly coherent states showing dynamical clustering effects and wave-like activity spread. Membrane potential time series is shown for all the neurons exhibiting spiking dynamics both in the coherent and incoherent states. Mean membrane potential amplitude decreases and converge to a stationary solution. Standard deviation shown in **(C,D)** shows growth in time. Mean field traces shows periodic activation and deactivation in the coherent state. In the incoherent state mean field amplitude systematically decrease in time.

of two parameters K, ΔI we carry out a grid search and compute the values of R in Equation (12). Global order parameter measure identifies three distinct network states in the parameter space as shown in **Figure 6A**. For low coupling values K, order parameter shows fluctuations about mean zero. In this regime each neurons activity is mainly driven by their firing rate threshold and displays largely incoherence. For medium values of both coupling strength K and stimulus spread ΔI network exhibits a hybrid state (some neurons are firing and some of them are silent). For very small values of stimulus spread and medium to high K values nearly burst synchrony appears. Temporal dynamics of membrane potential activity $V(t)$ for four neurons are plotted in **Figures 6B–D** for three arbitrary parameterization of our network model. In **Figures 6B,D** PO state is shown where one neuron is spiking or bursting and three neurons are silent. In **Figure 6C** all neurons are showing nearly synchronized parabolic bursting behavior.

3.3. NETWORK DYNAMICS OF PARABOLIC BURSTING PHASE MODEL WITH HETEROGENEITY

In this section, we use a phase network with mean field coupling to get some insights about the novel network states observed in (K, ΔI) the parameter space of the full network model. Coupling between each phase neuron via a mean field is formulated in section 2.4. Numerically we integrate Equation (6) to compute time averaged membrane potential, mean field Γ as in Equation (10) (see section 2), global measure of coherence R_θ as a function of K, ΔI a parameter combination which is used in

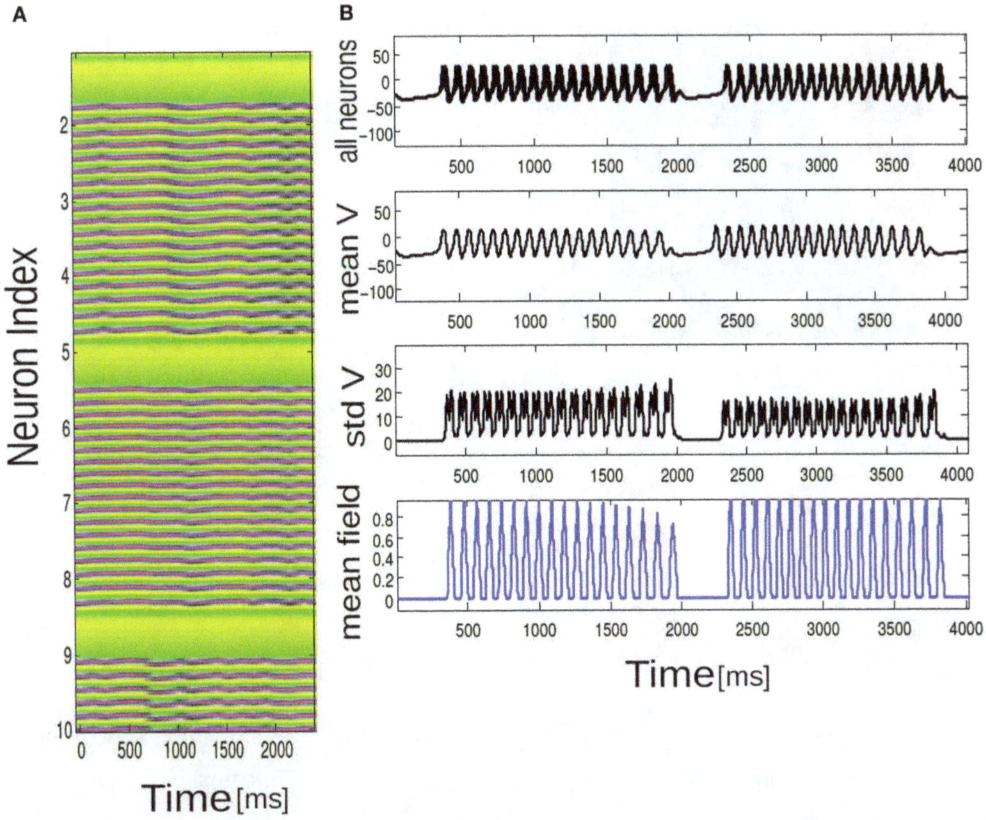

FIGURE 5 | In (A) array diagram showing firing pattern in a population of 100 neurons. Only 10 neuron index are shown for clarity. Horizontal axis is always time and vertical axis is labeled as neuron index. Green color corresponds to no firing activity or quiescence. Purple pixels corresponds to parabolic bursting activity of each individual neurons which are locked in time. In **(B)** time series data for membrane potential of $V(t)$, $V_{mean}(t)$, $\Gamma(t)$, and std $V_{mean}(t)$ are plotted for 10 neurons. Mean population burst synchronizes in time.

the detailed network model. Time evolution of the above quantiles are shown in **Figure 7** for a parameterization $K = 0.8$, $\Delta I = 0.001$. The parameter choice is the same as the full network investigations. With this combination of parameters all the neurons synchronously spikes. Mean membrane potential-like quantity $V_{mean}(t)$ oscillates in phase with synchronized spike activity as plotted in **Figure 7B**. Here, n a quantity which determines the number of spikes per burst is kept at $n = 1$. Mean field Γ also shows up and down states (Locked in time) and act as an oscillating drive to each individual neurons. The time series of the global order parameter $R_\theta(t)$ for synchronized spiking is periodic in **Figure 7E**. Next, we show in **Figure 8** temporal evolution of the mean quantities for the choice of $K = 0.8$, $\Delta I = 0.5$. For medium values of mean field coupling strength and stimulus spread network shows PO behavior, where some of the neurons are firing incoherently and others are completely silent. This means for some parameterization network has two stable branches of solutions. It is important to note PO state of the network was observed in the full network for a comparable parameterization (see **Figure 6**). Time series for 10 neurons and their order parameter evolution in time is plotted in **Figure 8**. Three neurons are completely silent while other seven neurons are bursting with variable inter-burst intervals. As there is no noise in this system and coupling magnitude is set at high values as in the case of sync, this variability must be introduced by the heterogeneity in their individual firing rate threshold via stimulus spread.

Figure 6 shows the parameter space diagram for the full and phase models presented in Equations (5) and (6–9). Phase boundaries are calculated by computing the mean field for both full and the phase model for different combination of (K, I) values on a two-dimensional grid. In the following subsection we would lay out the details for obtaining the phase transition boundaries semi analytically. Interestingly, Over a wide range of $(K - \Delta I)$ values the collective dynamics of the two networks primarily show three distinct regions of interest which are close to each other in the parameter space. For sufficiently large K values holding ΔI fixed to a narrow range of values near zero, the system converges to a state of partial oscillations in which the some of the neurons are not firing altogether, while the others display IN oscillations. Very large K values result in damping of oscillation activity and all the neurons stops firing altogether. The stability state of locking is much more difficult to achieve and infact we found distinct branches in their rotation number, these states should all be regarded as variants of 1:1 locking, and therefore we lump them together in the locked region of the stability diagram. With further increase in ΔI, parameter heterogeneity,

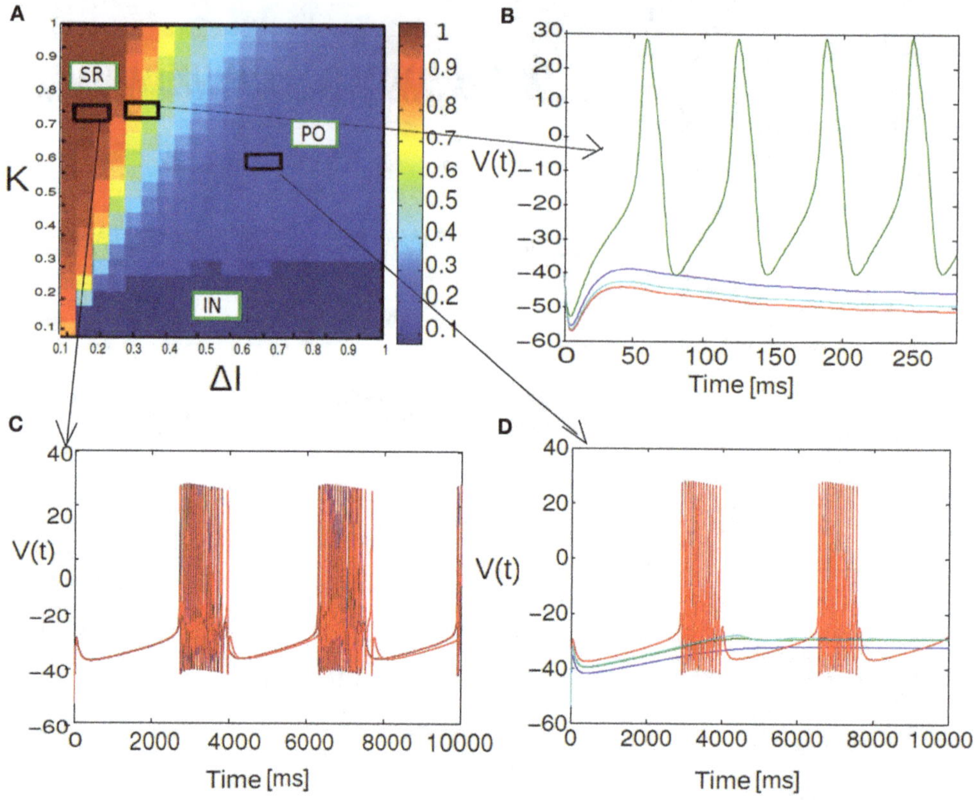

FIGURE 6 | Phase diagram of mean synaptic action variable is shown as a function of 2D parameter space of stimulus spread ΔI and excitatory coupling strength K. In the partial burst regime labeled as PO in **(A)**, a subset of neurons are not firing at all as their respective drives are below their individual firing thresholds. Heterogeneous dynamics between synchronized population spiking activity and oscillation frequency death response for PO state is displayed in **(B)**. Nearly synchronized population of spike/burst activity lumped in a regime labeled as SR [corresponding time series is displayed in **(C)**] and incoherent population spike/burst activity is lumped into a regime called IN. In the incoherent regime mean field values stay close to zero with substantial subthreshold fluctuations. In **(D)** multi stability of PO state is displayed again; now between population burst and fixed point dynamics for an entirely different parameterization.

successively more neurons peel away until eventually the entire population is IN.

4. PHASE DIAGRAM USING SEMI ANALYTICAL METHODS FOR MEAN FIELD PHASE MODEL

Mean field coupled neurons in phase model is described in Equation (6). Let's rewrite the mean field equation explicitly.

$$\dot{\theta}_i = (F(\theta_i) - \Gamma \sin\theta_i(\cos\theta_i - V_{\text{th}})) \tag{15}$$

where $\Gamma = \frac{K}{N}\sum_{j=1}^{N} \frac{\beta}{\left(1+\beta+\exp\left(-\frac{\cos\theta_j}{2}\right)\right)}$.

In a semianalytical approach we would like to understand the phase transitions between three distinct network states discovered in two networks. For the IN states where the average firing frequency increases monotonically plotted in **Figure 10**, the θ_i are all distributed across the closed orbit in a unit circle. This leads to the following phase evolution equation SR state may undergo instability either through parameter changes of K or ΔI and make phase transition to either IN or PO state. Mean field Γ approaches a stationary density as the number of neurons are increased in both PO and IN state (see **Figure 4D**). Hence, Γ approaches some positive real number for these two states. When varying K, we consider small perturbations μ to the SR solution $\theta = \theta_i = 0$. With $\theta = \theta_i = 0 + \mu$ Equation (15) becomes $\dot{\theta}_i = \dot{\mu} = F(\mu) + \frac{\Gamma}{2}\sin(2\mu)$ and linearization yields $\dot{\theta}_i = (F'(0) + \Gamma)\mu$. Moreover, SR state may gets phase locked at $\theta = \pi$ (subpopulation clusters). Hence, $\theta = \pi$ may get destabilized as we changed the width of heterogeneity by changing ΔI or the coupling strength K. Similarly, we consider small perturbations μ about solution $\theta = \pi$. Hence, we can write $\theta_i = \pi + \mu$, $\dot{\theta}_i = \dot{\mu} = F(\pi + \mu) + \frac{\Gamma}{2}\sin(2\pi + 2\mu)$ and linearization yields $\dot{\theta}_i = (F'(\pi) + \Gamma)\mu$. With $F(\theta) \approx I - \cos\theta - \cos\frac{\theta}{n}$ for the SR state, we find that $F'(\theta) \approx -\sin(\theta) - \frac{1}{n}\sin\frac{\theta}{n}$ will be generally small for $\theta = 0, \pi$. SR state solution hence becomes unstable when $F'(0, \pi) + \Gamma = 0$, which suggest almost a vertical critical line between SR and PO, IN state. The bifurcation route from PO (multistable state) to IN solutions as the parameter ΔI increases is less conclusive in the framework of the circular approximation, since in the previous stability analysis the only I-dependent term is $F'(0, \pi)$, which is very small, hence higher orders of the approximation must be considered. We use the following ansatz: If r is the radius of a unit circle, any smooth deformation from a unit circle can be approximated as, $r(\theta_i) = 1 + \epsilon h(\theta_i)$. Hence we can

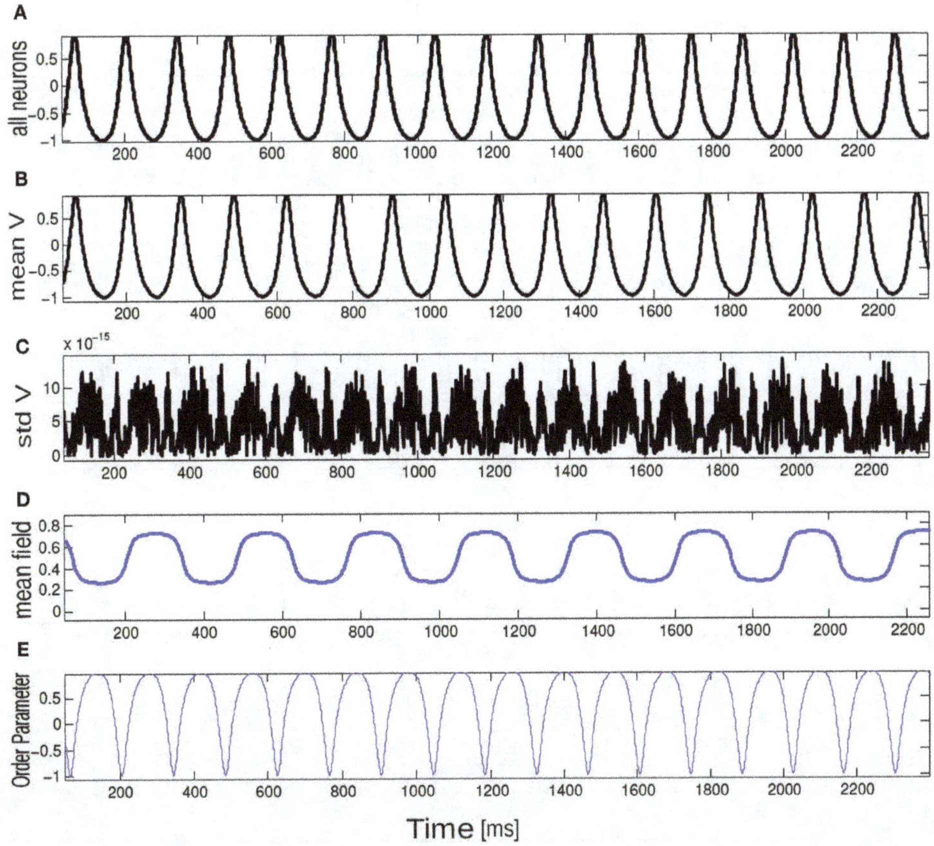

FIGURE 7 | Time series of (A) $V(t) = -\cos\theta_i(t)$, (B) $V_{mean}(t)$, (C) std $V_{mean}(t)$, (D) mean field Γ, and (E) order parameter $R_\theta(t)$ are plotted for 10 neurons. All neurons are spiking in synchrony and time locked. The parameter values are $K = 0.8$, $\Delta I = 0.001$.

compute the non-linear flow contribution with the above first order correction term as $F(\theta_i) + \epsilon H(\theta_i)$. It is possible to explicitly determine $H(\theta_i)$ for a certain choice of $h(\theta_i)$ and moreover, $H(\theta_i)$ has a periodicity of π, that is $H(\theta + \pi) = H(\theta)$. Thus the linear stability analysis about the fixed point $\theta_i^* = 0 + \mu$ gives

$$\dot{\mu} = (F'(0) + \epsilon H'(0) + \Gamma)\mu = (F'(\pi) + \epsilon H'(\pi) + \Gamma)\mu \quad (16)$$

From the above equation with $F'(0) \approx 0$ and the π-periodicity of $H(\theta_i)$, we find that the two fixed points at $0, \pi$ lose stability at the same time for increasing ΔI and as a result leads directly to the IN state. Since $H'(\theta_i) \sim I$, scales linearly for fixed μ, we can also estimate the critical line of transition in the parameter space in **Figure 11** which separates PO state from IN state. For the critical line: $H'(\theta_i) = m(I - I_c)^p$ where m is the slope of this line and $m > 0$ allows for destabilization. Hence the critical condition is $\epsilon H'(0) + \Gamma = 0$. By substituting the dependence of $H'(\theta_i)$ on (I, I_c) and in turn dependence on ΔI one can write $\epsilon m(I - I_c)^p + \Gamma = 0$. This implies coupling strength $K = -\epsilon(\Delta I + \Delta I_c)^p$ for $(m > 0)$ and p is some exponent representing a scaling relationship near saddle-node bifurcation. Thus the critical condition is $|K| = \epsilon m(\Delta I - \Delta I_c)$, which serves as a convenient guide to numerically compute the stability line separating PO region from IN. Next we try to obtain analytically the stability boundary between INC and PO oscillation states in the infinite-N limit. it turns out that the IN and partial oscillation states can be made steady in our system. The possibility of doing so was suggested by the numerical results. In numerics we observed that as the number of neurons N is increased, the order parameter R_t approaches a constant for both these states **Figure 8** and the oscillators tend to arrange themselves in a stationary distribution around the circle **Figure 11**. The way to approach these two states analytically, therefore, is to first write down the appropriate infinite-N analog of our model.

$$\frac{\partial}{\partial t}f + \frac{\partial}{\partial \theta}\left\{\left[F(\theta) - \left(\left(\int_0^{2\pi}\int_{I-\Delta I}^{I+\Delta I} \Gamma p(\theta', t, I')g(I')dI'd\theta'\right)\right) \times \sin(2\theta)\right]p\right\} = 0 \quad (17)$$

The above equation is the infinite-N analog of continuity equation introduced earlier. It is a non-linear partial integro-differential equation for the number density $f(\theta, t, \omega)$. In addition we demand f to be non-negative, 2π periodic in θ, and we impose the normalization

$$\int_0^{2\pi} f(\theta, t, I)d\theta = 1, \quad (18)$$

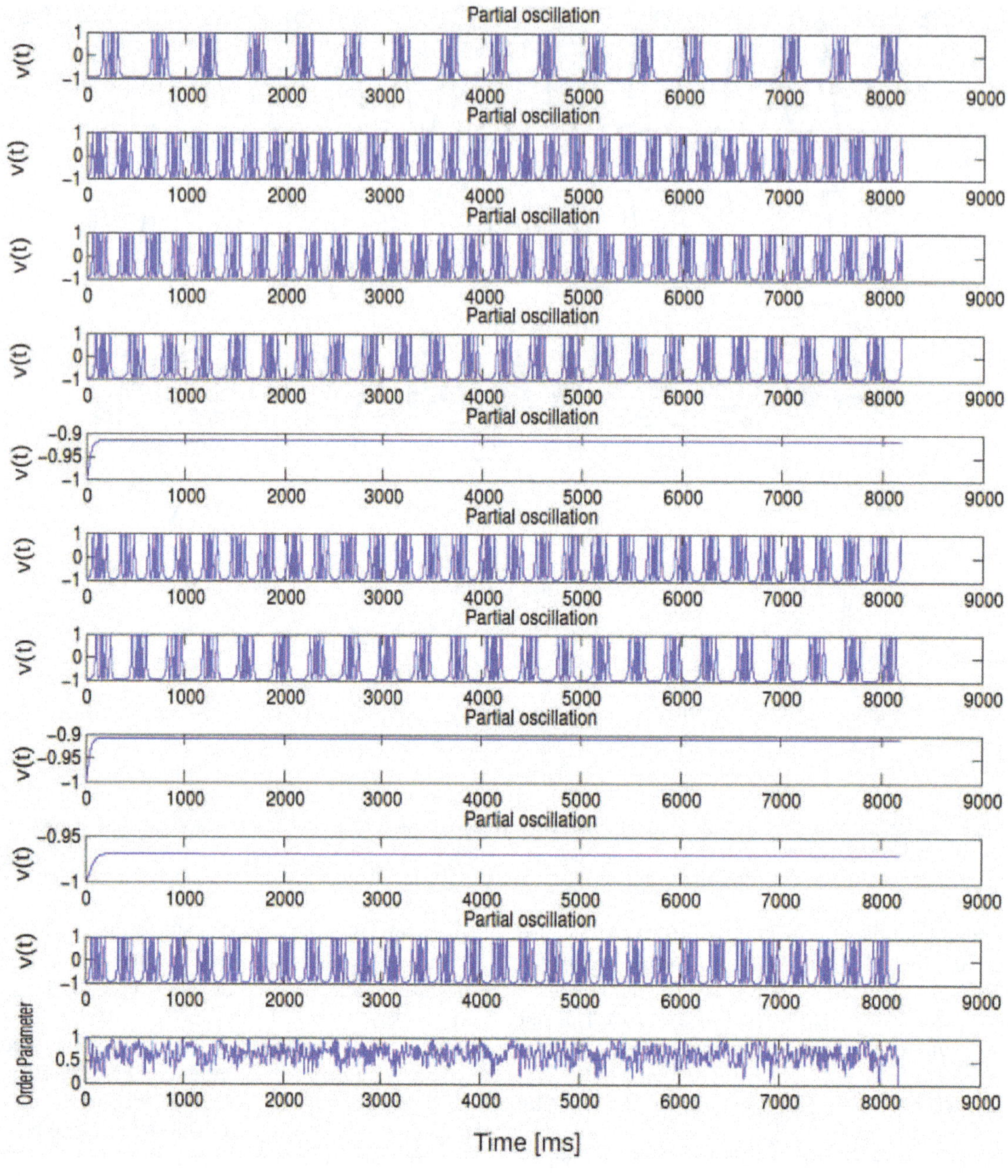

FIGURE 8 | Temporal evolution $V_i(t)$ for $N = 10$ neurons are shown here for an arbitrary parameterization $K = 0.8$, $\Delta I = 0.5$. K value is unchanged from previous figure. Stimulus spread ΔI is changed. Time series of order parameter $R_0(t)$ undergoes statistical fluctuations of magnitude $O(\frac{1}{\sqrt{(N)}})$ about some positive constant value. After 8000 time points, dynamics is truncated assuming network dynamics settles into a steady state.

For incoherence and partial oscillation the above system tends toward a stationary distribution of phases in time. The above two states are the fixed points of the stationary density in the continuum limit. To solve for the fixed points we set $\frac{\partial}{\partial t}f = 0$ in Equation (10). let's assume that $f_0(\theta, \omega)$ be the stationary phase density and $v_0 = [F(\theta) - ((\int_0^{2\pi} \int_{I-\Delta I}^{I+\Delta I} \Gamma f(\theta', t, I')g(I')dI'd\theta')) \sin(2\theta)]$ be the velocity field. Then one can write

$$\frac{\partial}{\partial\theta}(f_0 v_0) = 0 \Rightarrow f_0 v_0 = L(I) \tag{19}$$

where $L(I)$ is a constant which is determined exactly by using normalization condition. Depending on it's applied drive I, neuron's steady state behavior falls in the following two categories:

Case (i) When $I << \Gamma$ implies

$$v_0(\theta, I) = F(\theta) - \Gamma \sin(2\theta) = 0 \tag{20}$$

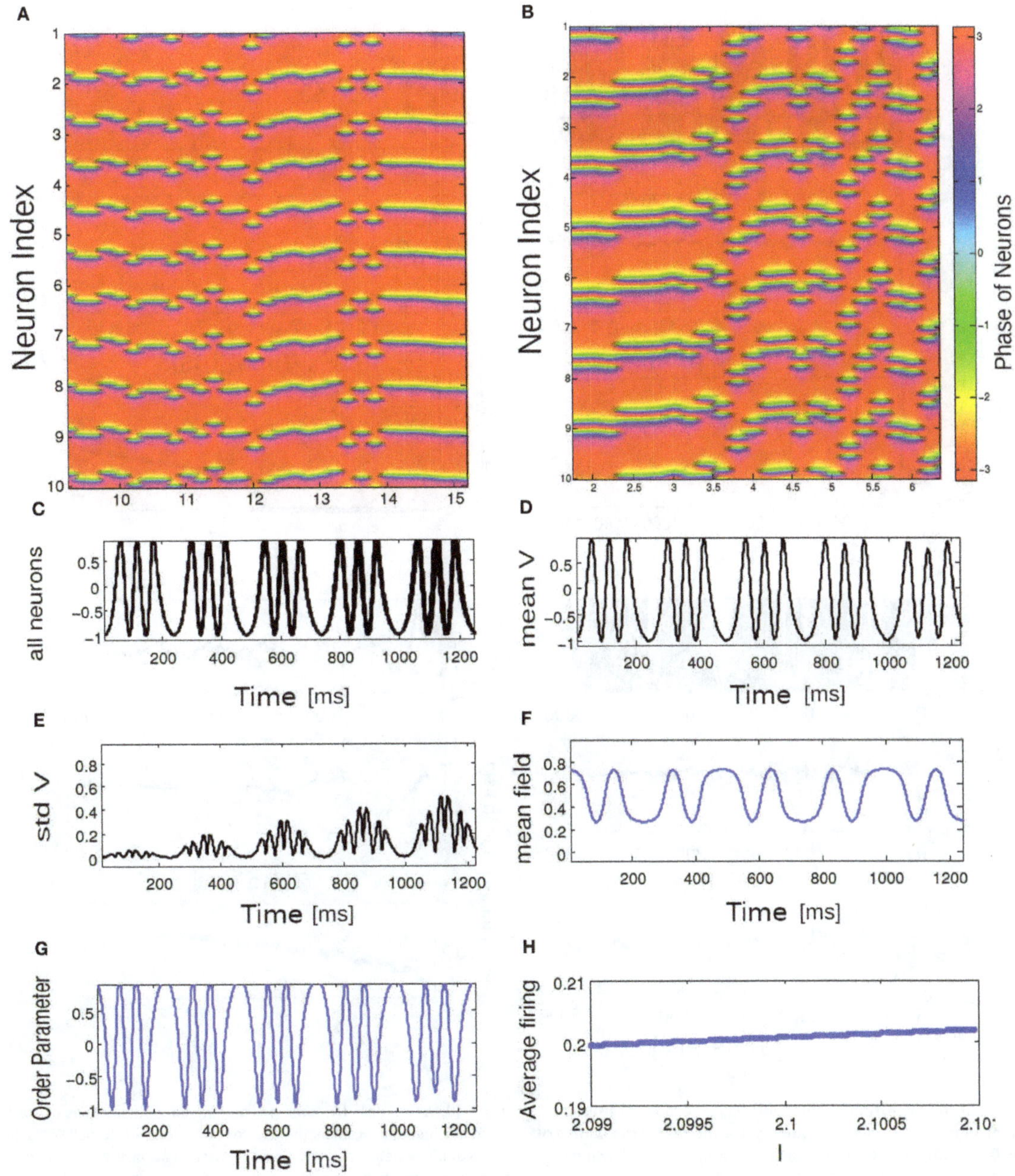

FIGURE 9 | In (A,B) an array diagram is shown for phase network model for a parameter combination. In **(A)** $K = 0.61$, $\Delta I = 0.001$, $n = 1$ spikes only and in **(B)** $K = 0.001$, $\Delta I = 0.15$, $n = 3$ bursts only. Almost always, near synchronous burst states are observed for high K and low ΔI values. In **(C)** corresponding time evolution of $V_i(t)$ is shown for all 10 bursting neurons. In **(D)** temporal response of V_{mean} is shown for the coherent state of our network. In **(E)** standard deviations of V_{mean} is plotted as a function of time. In **(F)** mean field Γ vs. time for the coherent state is shown. **(G)** displays temporal dynamics of order parameter. Average firing frequency as described in Equation (14) is plotted in **(H)** for the parameter combination of $K = 0.001$, $\Delta I = 0.15$. Panel **(H)** further demonstrates phase locking behavior among all the neurons.

Case (ii) When $I >> \Gamma$ neuron fires incoherently and typically individual phases follows an uniform distribution about the unit circle. In this case the velocity field turns out to be,

$$v_0(\theta, I) = F(\theta) - \Gamma \sin(2\theta) \tag{21}$$

Fixed point solution demands that the density must be inversely proportional to the velocity:

$$f_0(\theta, I) = \frac{L(I)}{F(\theta) - \Gamma \sin(2\theta)} \tag{22}$$

In the IN state, neurons driven by different external drives are firing at different phases, however, their collective state is close to being stationary. Every neuron belong to Case (ii) as described above. Further, it is possible to derive nearly an exact relationship between $K, \Delta I$ that gives the transition from case (i) to

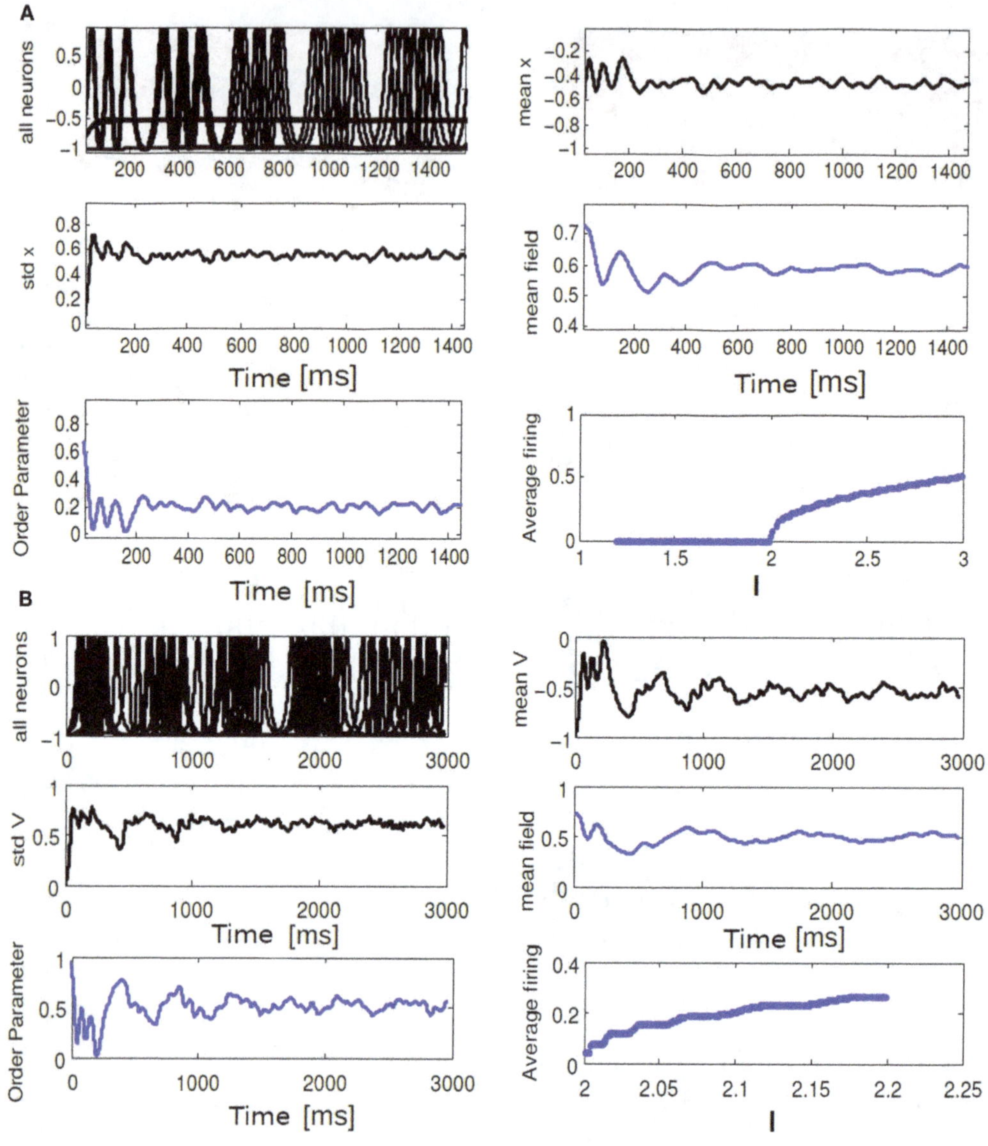

FIGURE 10 | In (A) time evolution of $V_i(t)$, std V_{mean}, order parameter $R_\theta(t)$, V_{mean}, mean field Γ, Average frequency are shown for the choice of $K = 0.6$, $\Delta I = 0.3$. In **(B)** time evolution of the same quantities are shown for $K = 0.01$, $\Delta I = 0.1$. In **(A)**, average firing frequency plot shows clusters of neurons firing incoherently while another cluster of neurons are completely silent. In **(B)** same subfigure shows a monotonic increase in average firing frequency.

case (ii) as described above. As shown before, in case of a finite size network such a relationship in the first order perturbation $\epsilon m(I - I_c)^p + \Gamma = 0$ does exist. In this scenario those neurons with a minimum bound on their applied drive $I_{\min}$ reach cessation of firing as we find from numerical simulations. They then fall into the Case (i) above where mean field Γ exerts much bigger influence on the dynamics and overall effect is damping of firing activity. The first neurons to stop firing are the ones which do not cross the threshold for firing which in this case $I > 2$. Then the boundary that separates IN from PO in the phase diagram is almost a straight line given by,

$$|K| = \epsilon m(\Delta I - \Delta I_c) \tag{23}$$

Hence, both finite and infinite analog of our network identifies the putative transition boundary between IN and PO states. Now from numerical simulations we find Andronov–Hopf (AH) bifurcations leads to the transition from INC to SR solutions in the **Figure 6** near K, I values close to zero. It is equivalent to look at the imaginary eigensolutions that arise due to the instability of the IN state. This instability requires calculation of higher order perturbation terms of the stationary density obtained at the IN state of our network. This is out of the scope of our paper, however, we show a numerical fitting result which gives an empirical relationship between K and ΔI to quantify the transition boundary between IN and SR states. Assuming ϵ is the perturbation to the IN

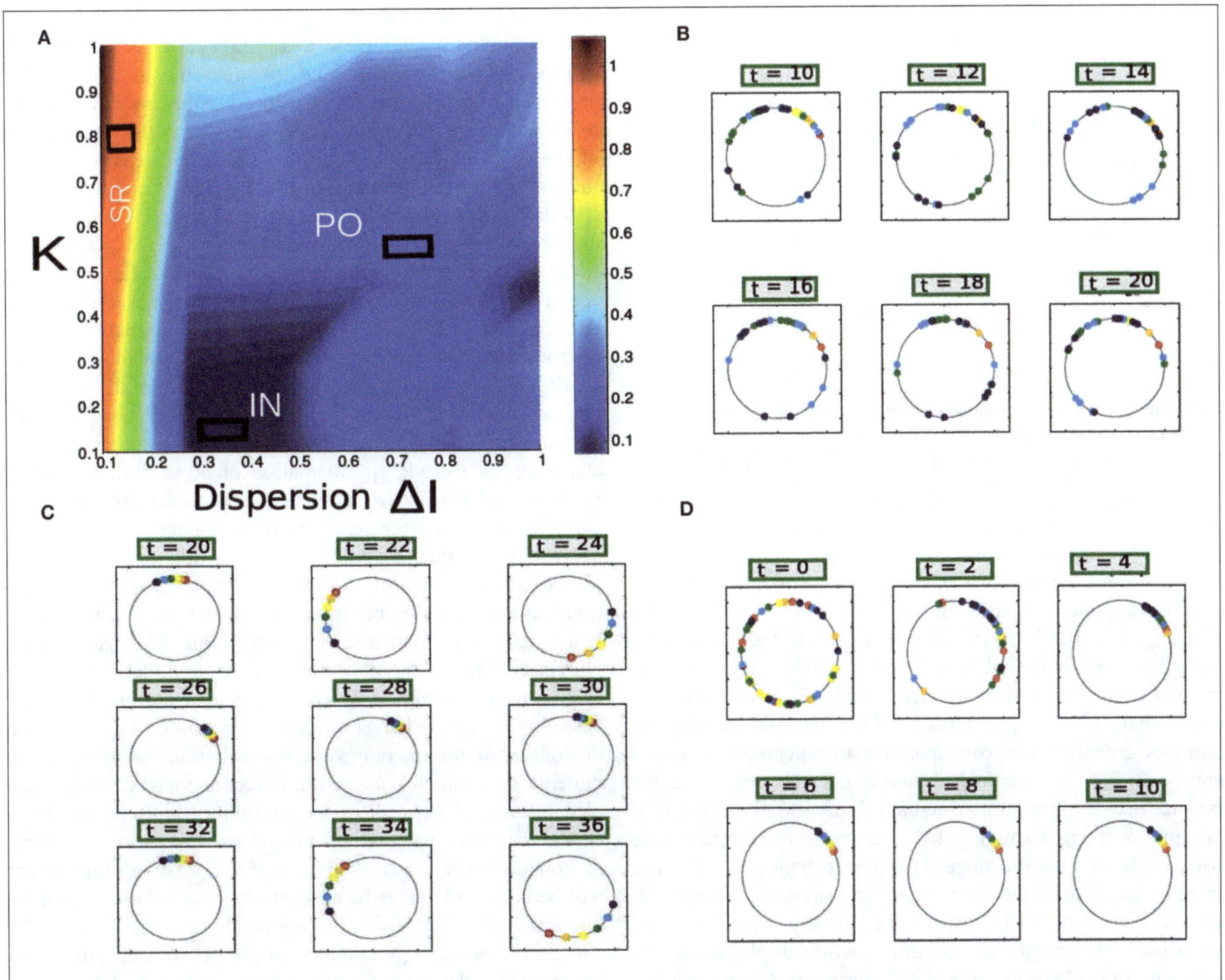

FIGURE 11 | (A) Parameter space diagram for K, ΔI are shown. Color coded computed values of R_θ shows primarily three distinct network states, labeled as SR, PO, and IN. **(B–D)** For three arbitrary pixel values corresponding firing frequency of individual neurons are shown in a unit circle. Each position in a circle corresponds to a particular phase and color coded according to the scheme described in section 2.8.

solution we can express a relationship between K and ΔI as follows,

$$|K| = a_0\epsilon + a_1\epsilon^2 + a_2\epsilon^3 + O(\epsilon^4) \tag{24}$$

Equation (24) gives us an empirical relationship between parameters upto fourth order perturbations for the bifurcation of a limit cycle. Optimization of the above equation gives coefficients $a_0 = \frac{8}{\pi}, a_1 = 0, a_2 = \frac{128}{\pi^3}$, respectively. Next, we substitute the amount of dispersion ΔI into the perturbative term ϵ to obtain the boundary between IN and SR state. Taken together we can write,

$$|K| = \frac{8}{\pi}\Delta I + \frac{128}{\pi^3}\Delta I^3 + O(\Delta I^4) \tag{25}$$

Results are shown in **Figure 12** in the $(K, \Delta I)$ plane using Equations (25) and 23. Critical lines obtained semi analytically qualitatively agrees well with the numerical results that captures various network states in both these models with purely excitatory coupling. In Appendix, we show a stability calculation for an inhibitory coupled mean field network in the infinite analog limit. From numerical simulations we find that the results are independent of the number of spikes n per burst.

5. DISCUSSION

One of the most frequent assumption employed in simulations of large neural networks is that the whole network can be lumped into small aggregates of collective unit (sometimes called a "neurocomputational unit") exhibit a sufficiently similar dynamical behavior. Consequently, the network that instantiates this ensemble, consisting of thousands of excitatory and inhibitory neurons, it is considered to display a synchronized behavior with no other significant temporal features for the dynamics of the large scale network. The main reason for this assumption, is the impractical large computational time arising from too many details considered in the large network properties. In this paper, we

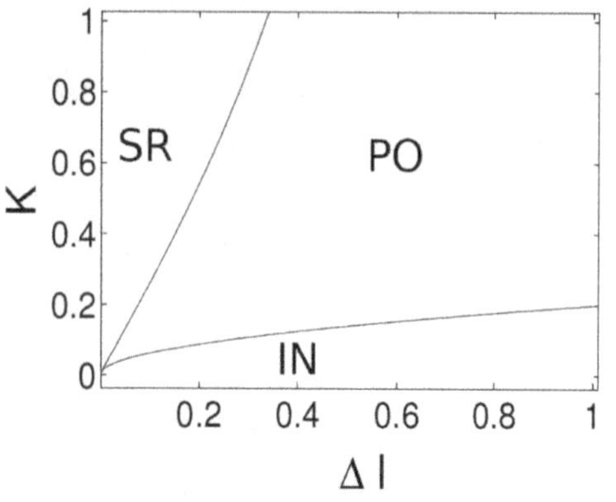

FIGURE 12 | Parameter boundaries are shown in (K, ΔI) parameter space using analytic results. Critical lines separates three distinct network states, labeled as SR, PO, and IN. Critical line separating PO, IN states corresponds to a saddle-node bifurcation and the line that separates IN, SR states corresponds to a Hopf bifurcation.

have analyzed the behavior of a neural network that serves as a good example of such a unit, namely a mean field coupled bursting ensemble. First, we have investigated a Hodgkin–Huxley type detailed biophysical model widely employed in theoretical and computational neuroscience with global coupling. We found that the dynamical features of the network are far more complex then the ones corresponding to synchronized or rest state behavior. The network dynamics depends critical on the balance between firing rate threshold dispersion and mean field synaptic coupling strength; in fact, the synchronized state can be found only for a specific range of parameters typically involving a large or medium values for the coupling strength and low values of dispersion. On the other hand, for large dispersion and weak coupling strength values both networks display purely IN behavior. In the IN state, individual neurons are driven by different external drives results in firing at different phases, however, their collective state is close to being stationary. This stationarity in the density distribution led us to formulate scaling relationship between coupling strength and dispersion parameter. One interesting finding is that, when mean field exerts a greater influence than parameter dispersion; it causes shutting down of the neural activity in some neurons. In this parameter range, we find interesting dynamical behavior such as partial activity. In order to address the problem of the high computational cost of such an implementation, we have further developed a self-consistent mathematically tractable mean field coupled phase model following (Assisi et al., 2005; Ghosh et al., 2009; Jirsa and Stefanescu, 2011), but incorporating a higher degree of realism. Rather than finding the most appropriate type and number of dimensions that could minimize certain error functions or capture statistical variance in the full network, we have focused our attention on understanding a phenomenological burst generation model system which captures the most important network dynamics of bursting units at the population level. Collective activity of synapses is described by a mean field which relies on instantaneous rise and decay time (Roy et al., 2011). This mean field is then employed in the coupling to individual neurons to describe phase network. Together, we investigate this population of neurons coupled to a common mean field drive and heterogeneity in their threshold for spikes/bursts. Our detailed analysis demonstrated that the reduced representation manages to recreate correctly the topology of the mean field amplitudes of the original system for various parameter scenarios. In the full network, In the thermodynamic limit ($N \rightarrow \infty$), a collective state becomes coherent if $\delta V_{\text{mean}}(t) \equiv [V_{\text{mean}}(t) - \overline{V_{\text{mean}}(t)}]$ is non-stationary (i.e., an oscillating global potential V_{mean} appears for a coherent case) and also, the correlated mean field $\Gamma(t)$ activity appears oscillatory. In the phase network, global order parameter is computed by averaging the contributions of all microscopic spikes within a burst in order to obtain a similar degree of ordering of spikes/bursts as in the full model for identical parameterization. Hence, for a dynamical behavior such as coherence-incoherence transition macroscopic order parameter gives us a crude approximation of burst timing. From a more general perspective, despite its limitations because of the consideration of purely excitatory or inhibitory network, it can be readily extended to study networks with mixed coupling. Moreover, the analytical approach to estimate the scaling relationship and transition boundaries between the IN-PO-SR states is not restricted to small scale network only. With global coupling, as the size of the network grows the boundaries may shift leading to a different parameterization than the one displayed here; however, underlying bifurcations remain the same. We have demonstrated this in our work by analytically deriving a low dimensional mean field amplitude reduction for a inhibitory coupled mean field network in the continuum limit. In this case, all the relevant dynamics of an infinite dimensional network in Equations (29) and (30) is captured by a two dimensional representation of the reduced mean field population given by Equation (40). Thus, using this approach, we derive analytically a low dimensional representation of the network dynamics and we show that the main features of the neural population's collective behavior can be captured well by the dynamics of a few cortical nodes exhibiting spiking as well as bursting behavior. While it is true that strong reductionist assumptions are common (sacrificing many of the biological realism of a network node's dynamics) in large-scale network modeling, these assumptions are usually made *ad-hoc* on the network node's dynamics and limit the network dynamics to a small range. We emphasize here that because of the "near to synchrony" assumption, neural mass models cannot capture complex dynamical features such as multi-clustering, oscillator death or multi-time scale synchronization. Evidently a reduced small scale network model is desirable to serve as a node in a large scale network simulation whereby displaying a sufficiently rich dynamic repertoire. Here it is of less importance to find a quantitatively precise reduced description of a neural population; rather more importantly, we seek a computationally inexpensive population model (this means typically low-dimensional) which is able to display the major qualitative dynamic behaviors (synchronization, rest state, multi-clustering, etc.) for realistic parameter ranges as observed in the total population of neurons. Our approach may offer a viable alternative to the neural mass models currently used in the literature. By comparison, our model offers the possibility to account for such features (temporal details of their spiking activity considered irrelevant for the dynamics of the large network) at a very low computational cost. Therefore, the type of reduced representation discussed in this paper qualifies as a good candidate for a "neural unit" in computational simulations of large scale neural networks.

ACKNOWLEDGMENTS

We would like to thank Anandamohan Ghosh and Mohit Adhikari for the helpful corrections on this manuscript. The research reported herein was supported by the Brain Network Recovery Group through the James S. McDonnell Foundation and the FP7-ICT BrainScales.

REFERENCES

Amari, S. (1977). Dynamics of pattern formation in lateral-inhibition type neural fields. *Biol. Cybern.* 27, 77–87.

Amzica, F., and Steriade, M. (1998). Electrophysiological correlates of sleep delta waves. *Electroencephalogr. Clin. Neurophysiol.* 107, 69–83.

Antonsen, T. M., Faghih, R. T., Girvan, M., Ott, E., and Platig, J. (2008). External periodic driving of large systems of globally coupled phase oscillators. *Chaos* 18:037112. doi: 10.1063/1.2952447

Assisi, C. G., Jirsa, V. K., and Kelso, J. A. S. (2005). Synchrony and clustering in heterogeneous networks with global coupling and parameter dispersion. *Phys. Rev. Lett.* 94:018106. doi: 10.1103/PhysRevLett.94.018106

Baer, S. M., Rinzel, J., and Carrillo, H. (1995). Analysis of an autonomous phase model for neuronal parabolic bursting. *J. Math. Biol.* 33, 309–333.

Beurle, R. L. (1956). Properties of a mass of cells capable of regenerating pulses. *Philos. Trans. R Soc. Lond. B Biol. Sci.* 240, 55–94.

Breakspear, M., Heitmann, S., and Daffertshofer, A. (2010). Generative models of cortical oscillations: neurobiological implications of the Kuramoto model. *Front. Hum. Neurosci.* 4:190. doi: 10.3389/fnhum.2010.00190

Cabral, J., Hugues, E., Sporns, O., and Deco, G. (2011). Role of local network oscillations in resting-state functional connectivity. *Neuroimage* 57, 130–139.

Deco, G., Jirsa, V. K., and McIntosh, A. R. (2011). Emerging concepts for the dynamical organization of resting-state activity in the brain. *Nat. Rev. Neurosci.* 12, 43–56.

Deco, G., Jirsa, V. K., Robinson, P. A., Breakspear, M., and Friston, K. (2008). The dynamic brain: from spiking neurons to neural masses and cortical fields. *PLoS Comput. Biol.* 4:e1000092. doi: 10.1371/journal.pcbi.1000092

Dhamala, M., Jirsa, V., and Ding, M. (2004a). Enhancement of neural synchrony by time delay. *Phys. Rev. Lett.* 92, 6–9.

Dhamala, M., Jirsa, V. K., and Ding, M. (2004b). Transitions to synchrony in coupled bursting neurons. *Phys. Rev. Lett.* 92, 2–5.

Ermentrout, G. B., and Kopell, N. (1986). Parabolic bursting in an excitable system coupled with a slow oscillation. *SIAM J. Appl. Math.* 46, 233–253.

Feng, J., Jirsa, V. K., and Ding, M. (2006). Synchronization in networks with random interactions: theory and applications. *Chaos* 16:015109. doi: 10.1063/1.2180690

Friesen, W. O. (1994). Reciprocal inhibition: a mechanism underlying oscillatory animal movements. *Neurosci. Biobehav. Rev.* 18, 547–553.

Gabbiani, F., Midtgaard, J., and Knöpfel, T. (1994). Synaptic integration in a model of cerebellar granule cells. *J. Neurophysiol.* 72, 999–1009.

Ghosh, A., Roy, D., and Jirsa, V. K. (2009). Simple model for bursting dynamics of neurons. *Phys. Rev. E Stat. Nonlin. Soft Matter Phys.* 80(4 Pt 1):041930. doi: 10.1103/PhysRevE.80.041930

Ghosh, A., Rho, Y., McIntosh, A. R., Kötter, R., and Jirsa, V. K. (2008). Cortical network dynamics with time delays reveals functional connectivity in the resting brain. *Cogn. Neurodyn.* 2, 115–120.

Golomb, D., and Rinzel, J. (1993). Dynamics of globally coupled inhibitory neurons with heterogeneity. *Phys. Rev. E* 48, 4810–4814.

Hebb, D. O. (1949). *The Organization of Behavior: A Neuropsychological Theory*. Vol 44. New York, NY: Wiley.

Higham, D. J. (2001). An algorithmic introduction to numerical simulation of stochastic differential equations. *SIAM Rev.* 43, 525–546.

Hindmarsh, J. L., and Rose, R. M. (1984). A model of neuronal bursting using three coupled first order differential equations. *Proc. R Soc. Lond B* 221, 87–102.

Izhikevich, E. M. (2000). Neural excitability, spiking and bursting. *Int. J. Bifurcat. Chaos* 10, 1171–1266.

Izhikevich, E. M. (2007). *Dynamical Systems in Neuroscience: The Geometry of Excitability and Bursting*. Vol 25. Cambridge: MIT press.

Jensen, O., Kaiser, J., and Lachaux, J. P. (2007). Human gamma-frequency oscillations associated with attention and memory. *Trends Neurosci.* 30, 317–324.

Jirsa, V. K. (2008). Dispersion and time delay effects in synchronized spike-burst networks. *Cogn. Neurodyn.* 2, 29–38.

Jirsa, V. K. (2009). Neural field dynamics with local and global connectivity and time delay. *Philos. Trans. R Soc. A Math. Phys. Eng. Sci.* 367, 1131–1143.

Jirsa, V. K., and Haken, H. (1997). A derivation of a macroscopic field theory of the brain from the quasi-microscopic neural dynamics. *Physica D* 99, 503–526.

Jirsa, V. K., and McIntosh, A. R. (2007). *Handbook of Brain Connectivity*. Berlin: Springer.

Jirsa, V. K., and Stefanescu, R. A. (2011). Neural population modes capture biologically realistic large scale network dynamics. *Bull. Math. Biol.* 73, 325–343.

Lim, W., and Kim, S.-Y. (2011). Statistical-mechanical measure of stochastic spiking coherence in a population of inhibitory subthreshold neurons. *J. Comput. Neurosci.* 31, 667–677.

Manrubia, S. C., Mikhailov, A. S., and Zanette, D. H. (2004). *Emergence of Dynamical Order. Synchronization Phenomena in Complex Systems*, Singapore: World Scientific Publishing Co.

McCormick, D. A., and Feeser, H. R. (1990). Functional implications of burst firing and single spike activity in lateral geniculate relay neurons. *Neuroscience* 39, 103–113.

Morris, C., and Lecar, H. (1981). Voltage oscillations in the barnacle giant muscle fiber. *Biophys. J.* 35, 193–213.

Nunez, P. L. (1974). The brain wave equation: a model for the eeg. *Math. Biosci.* 21, 279–297.

Ott, E., and Antonsen, T. M. (2009). Long time evolution of phase oscillator systems. *Chaos* 19:023117. doi: 10.1063/1.3136851

Parnas, H., and Parnas, I. (1994). Neurotransmitter release at fast synapses. *J. Mem. Biol.* 142, 267–279.

Rinzel, J., and Ermentrout, G. (1989). *Analysis of Neural Excitability and Oscillations*. Cambridge, MA: MIT Press.

Robinson, P. A. (2011). Neural field theory of synaptic plasticity. *J. Theor. Biol.* 285, 156–163.

Roy, D., Ghosh, A., and Jirsa, V. K. (2011). Phase description of neural oscillators with global electric and synaptic coupling. *Phys. Rev. E Stat. Nonlin. Soft Matter Phys.* 83, 1–10.

Sabatini, B. L., and Regehr, W. G. (1996). Timing of neurotransmission at fast synapses in the mammalian brain. *Nature* 384, 170–172.

Sherman, S. M., and Koch, C. (1986). The control of retinogeniculate transmission in the mammalian lateral geniculate nucleus. *Exp. Brain Res.* 63, 1–20.

Smeal, R. M., Ermentrout, G. B., and White, J. A. (2010). Phase-response curves and synchronized neural networks. *Philos. Trans. R Soc. Lond. B Biol. Sci.* 365, 2407–2422.

Stefanescu, R. A., and Jirsa, V. K. (2008). A low dimensional description of globally coupled heterogeneous neural networks of excitatory and inhibitory neurons. *PLoS Comput. Biol.* 4:e1000219. doi: 10.1371/journal.pcbi.1000219

Stefanescu, R. A., and Jirsa, V. K. (2011). Reduced representations of heterogeneous mixed neural networks with synaptic coupling. *Phys. Rev. E* 83, 1–12.

Steriade, M., and Llinás, R. R. (1988). The functional states of the thalamus and the associated neuronal interplay. *Physiol. Rev.* 68, 649–742.

Steriade, M., McCormick, D., and Sejnowski, T. J. (1993). Thalamocortical oscillations in the sleeping and aroused brain. *Science* 262, 679–685.

Uhlhaas, P. J., and Singer, W. (2006). Neural synchrony in brain disorders: relevance for cognitive dysfunctions and pathophysiology. *Neuron* 52, 155–168.

Van Vreeswijk, C., Abbott, L. F., and Ermentrout, G. B. (1994).

When inhibition not excitation synchronizes neural firing. *J. Comput. Neurosci.* 1, 313–321.

Wang, X. J. (1994). Multiple dynamical modes of thalamic relay neurons: rhythmic bursting and intermittent phase-locking. *Neuroscience* 59, 21–31.

Wang, X. J., and Rinzel, J. (1992). Alternating and synchronous rhythms in reciprocally inhibitory model neurons. *Neural Comput.* 4, 84–97.

Wilson, H. R., and Cowan, J. D. (1972). Excitatory and inhibitory interactions in localized populations of model neurons. *Biophys. J.* 12, 1–24.

APPENDIX

MEAN FIELD REDUCTION FOR INHIBITORY SYNAPTIC COUPLING

Here, we extend our network in the continuum limit in the presence of inhibitory coupling. V_{th} is held negative. $(N \to \infty)$, where the state of the coupled system can be described by a density function $f(\theta, I, t)$, where f is defined such that the fraction of neurons with phases lying between θ and $d\theta$ and applied drive between I and dI is given by $f(\theta, I, t)d\theta dI$ (Antonsen et al., 2008; Ott and Antonsen, 2009). The applied stimulus are drawn from a distribution $g(I)$ such that

$$\int_{-\infty}^{\infty}\int_{0}^{2\pi} f(\theta, I, t)d\theta dI = 1 \qquad (26)$$

$$\int_{0}^{2\pi} f(\theta, I, t)d\theta = g(I) \qquad (27)$$

For the conservation of currents I the continuity equation is written as

$$\frac{\partial f}{\partial t} + \frac{\partial(f\,v)}{\partial \theta} = 0. \qquad (28)$$

In order to make the coupling amenable to analytical study we use a pulse-like function for the mean field $\Gamma = a1 + b1(1 + \cos\theta)$. Response to the mean field by individual neuron's $R(\theta) = V_{th}\sin(\theta)$, containing only single Fourier component, a choice motivated primarily due to the tractability of the resulting model. Further, $V_{th} = -1$ for the convenience of calculations without losing any generality of our results. The velocity $v(\theta, I, t)$ in Equation (28) is now written as

$$v(\theta, I, t) = a + \epsilon \int_{-\infty}^{\infty}\int_{0}^{2\pi} (1 + \cos(\hat{\theta}))(-\sin\theta) f(\hat{\theta}, \hat{I}, t)d\hat{\theta}d\hat{I} - F\sin(\theta) - F\sin(\theta/n) \qquad (29)$$

where without loss of any generality we are using sin functions instead of cos functions in Equation (6).

In the continuum limit the order parameter z can be defined as

$$z(t) = \int_{-\infty}^{\infty}\int_{0}^{2\pi} \frac{(e^{i\theta} + e^{-i\theta})}{2} f(\theta, I, t)d\theta dI \qquad (30)$$

It's a linear sum of two complex order parameters and one could in principle unfold the entire dynamics of the network in any one of the manifold given above. Here,

$$z1(t) = \int_{-\infty}^{\infty}\int_{0}^{2\pi} e^{i\theta} f(\theta, I, t)d\theta dI \qquad (31)$$

$$z2(t) = \int_{-\infty}^{\infty}\int_{0}^{2\pi} e^{-i\theta} f(\theta, I, t)d\theta dI \qquad (32)$$

Using the above it is easy to see that the expression for velocity becomes

$$v(\theta, I, t) = I + \frac{1}{2i}\left[\left(1 + \frac{\epsilon}{2}(z2 + z1^*) + F\right)e^{-i\theta} - \left(1 + \frac{\epsilon}{2}(z1 + z2^*) + F\right)e^{i\theta}\right] - F\left(\frac{e^{i\theta/n}}{2i} - \frac{e^{-i\theta/n}}{2i}\right) \qquad (33)$$

$*$ indicates the complex conjugate. The distribution function can be expressed as a Fourier series

$$f(\theta, I, t) = \frac{g(I)}{2\pi}\left[1 + \sum_{k=1}^{\infty} f_k(I, t)e^{ik\theta} + c.c.\right] \qquad (34)$$

The above infinite dimensional system is difficult to analyze. However, the "amazing" anstaz of Ott and Antonsen (2009) has been shown to be successful in obtaining the low-dimensional description of the globally coupled phase oscillators. The anstaz impose a restriction on the fourier coefficients:

$$f_k(I, t) = (\psi(I, t))^k \qquad (35)$$

for $k \geq 1$ and has been shown to be a reasonable guess under different scenariors (Ott and Antonsen, 2009). This restricted class of functions readily reduces our continuity equation to an θ-independent form

$$\frac{d\psi}{dt} = \frac{1}{2}\left(1 + \frac{\epsilon}{2}z1 + F\right)^* - iI\psi - \frac{1}{2}\left(1 + \frac{\epsilon}{2}z1 + F\right)\psi^2 - F\left(\frac{\psi^{1+1/n}}{2} - \frac{\psi^{1-1/n}}{2}\right) \qquad (36)$$

with $z1$ satisfying

$$z1(t) = \int_{-\infty}^{\infty} \psi^*(I, t)g(I)dI. \qquad (37)$$

If we assume that $g(I)$ is a Lorentzian distribution function

$$g(I) = \frac{1}{\pi[(I - I_0)^2 + 1]}. \qquad (38)$$

$z(t)$ can be evaluated by contour integration with poles at $I = I_0 - i$ and we obtain the exact evolution equation of order parameter z

$$\frac{dz1}{dt} = iI_0 z1 - z1 + \frac{1 + \frac{\epsilon}{2}z1 + F}{2} - \frac{1 + \frac{\epsilon}{2}z1^* + F}{2} - F\left(\frac{z1^{1+1/n}}{2} - \frac{z1^{1-1/n}}{2}\right) \qquad (39)$$

The above equation can be expressed in polar coordinates if we substitute $z1 = \rho_1 \exp(i\phi_1)$ giving evolution equations for ρ_1 and ϕ_1

$$\frac{d\rho_1}{dt} = \frac{\epsilon}{2}\rho_1\left(1-\rho_1^2\right) - \rho_1 + \frac{F}{2}\left(1-2\rho_1^2\right)\cos\phi_1 + \frac{1}{2}\cos(\phi_1) + \frac{F\rho_1}{2}\left(\rho_1^{-1/n} - \rho_1^{1/n}\right)\cos(\phi_1/n) \tag{40}$$

$$\frac{d\phi_1}{dt} = I_0 - \frac{F}{2}\left(\rho_1 + \frac{1}{\rho_1}\right)\sin\phi_1 - \frac{\rho_1}{2}\sin(\phi_1) - \frac{F}{2}\left(\rho_1^{1/n} + \frac{1}{\rho_1^{1/n}}\right)\sin(\phi_1/n). \tag{41}$$

For the Lorentzian distribution function the above equation is exact, However, we do not find any deviation of the above results for any other unimodal distributions of our firing threshold (such as uniform distribution) such as the one considered in the numerical simulations with excitatory coupling. The above two dimensional system can be solved numerically to identify the full network states and the corresponding transition boundaries.

13

Top-down influences on local networks: Basic theory with experimental implications

Ramesh Srinivasan[1,2,3]*, Samuel Thorpe[3] and Paul L. Nunez[4]

[1] Department of Cognitive Sciences, University of California, Irvine, CA, USA
[2] Department of Biomedical Engineering, University of California, Irvine, CA, USA
[3] Institute for Mathematical Behavioral Sciences, University of California, Irvine, CA, USA
[4] Cognitive Dissonance, LLC, San Diego, CA, USA

***Correspondence:**
Ramesh Srinivasan, Department of Cognitive Sciences, University of California, 3151 SSPA, Irvine, CA 92617, USA.
e-mail: r.srinivasan@uci.edu

The response of a population of cortical neurons to an external stimulus depends not only on the receptive field properties of the neurons, but also the level of arousal and attention or goal-oriented cognitive biases that guide information processing. These top-down effects on cortical neurons bias the output of the neurons and affect behavioral outcomes such as stimulus detection, discrimination, and response time. In any physiological study, neural dynamics are observed in a specific brain state; the background state partly determines neuronal excitability. Experimental studies in humans and animal models have also demonstrated that slow oscillations (typically in the alpha or theta bands) modulate the fast oscillations (gamma band) associated with local networks of neurons. Cross-frequency interaction is of interest as a mechanism for top-down or bottom up interactions between systems at different spatial scales. We develop a generic model of top-down influences on local networks appropriate for comparison with EEG. EEG provides excellent temporal resolution to investigate neuronal oscillations but is space-averaged on the cm scale. Thus, appropriate EEG models are developed in terms of population synaptic activity. We used the Wilson–Cowan population model to investigate fast (gamma band) oscillations generated by a local network of excitatory and inhibitory neurons. We modified the Wilson–Cowan equations to make them more physiologically realistic by explicitly incorporating background state variables into the model. We found that the population response is strongly influenced by the background state. We apply the model to reproduce the modulation of gamma rhythms by theta rhythms as has been observed in animal models and human ECoG and EEG studies. The concept of a dynamic background state presented here using the Wilson–Cowan model can be readily applied to incorporate top-down modulation in more detailed models of specific cortical systems.

Keywords: EEG, population dynamics, neural mass models, top-down control, ECoG

INTRODUCTION

A fundamental question in any neurophysiological study is whether observed modulations of neural responses in cortex by cognitive processes are the result of the action of a *local* network or due to the interactions between this local network and the rest of the brain in *global* networks. This conceptual framework of local and global networks interacting in cognitive processes is salient to the interpretation of physiological signals obtained from the brain with any technique – EEG, MEG, fMRI, LFPs, or unit activity and to models of the underlying cognitive processes. That is, even when signals are recorded from a small number of neurons (or even just one neuron) the observed dynamics result both from the intrinsic properties of the local network and from the influence of other neurons located in nearby or even distant cortex (Mountcastle, 1997). This simple distinction can be understood in terms of behavior – the response of neurons to inputs depends not only on the receptive field of the neurons but also on the level of arousal, typically by the action of neuromodulators, and attention or goal-oriented cognitive biases that guide information processing. The latter are sometimes called top-down effects (Engel et al., 2001), which bias the output of the neurons and affect behavioral outcomes such as stimulus detection, short term memory, and reaction time.

The objective of this paper is to develop a model of local networks with which we can investigate the effect background brain state or top-down signaling on the local network. In order to develop this model, we have to make choices of spatial scale and physiological detail to incorporate into the model. Very detailed models have the potential to provide more information about specific neural systems, e.g., details models of the visual system (Lumer et al., 1997). However, detailed model parameters are not available in humans, where the competition/interaction between global and local dynamics is expected to be the most robust (Nunez, 1995, 2000; Nunez and Srinivasan, 2006). In addition, detailed models may not lead to generalized principles that can potentially guide experimental studies in a variety of behavioral contexts; detailed cellular models are not easily compared to electrocorticogram (ECoG) and electroencephalogram (EEG) data obtained in humans.

Electroencephalogram is uniquely positioned to differentiate local and global processes and to examine their interactions in human subjects. EEG provides excellent temporal resolution allowing us to separate processes at different time scales at electrodes over cortex while allowing for sufficient spatial coverage to investigate interactions of sensory neurons with neural processes in other areas of the brain. The main limitation of EEG is spatial resolution; EEG signals are space-averaged on the cm scale (Nunez, 1981; Nunez and Srinivasan, 2006) by volume conduction through the tissues of the head. An active area of research is to improve our understanding of the structure of cortical sources and connectivity from EEG data (Pinotsis et al., 2012). ECoG in humans combines the temporal dynamics of EEG with the greater spatial detail and (depending on the patient) partial coverage of the cortex (Schalk and Leuthardt, 2011). Although ECoG is only available in limited cases in patients with intractable epilepsy, these data are a useful source of information on the nature of dynamics of localized population of neurons.

EEG signals span a frequency range of 1–50 Hz while ECoG signals span a broader frequency range of 1–150 Hz (Canolty et al., 2010; Schalk and Leuthardt, 2011). The lower portion of this spectrum (below 20 Hz) has strongly global properties with spatial distribution across the brain that depends strongly on the frequency (von Stein and Sarnthein, 2000; Nunez et al., 2001; Nunez and Srinivasan, 2006). For example human alpha rhythms, which are quite robust in alert subjects, may be recorded over nearly all of the upper scalp or cortex with a visible peak in the power spectrum near 10 Hz. Alpha rhythm power and phase synchronization (usually measured as coherence) are modulated in specific large-scale cortical networks by a wide variety of different cognitive processes including attention (Thut et al., 2006; Thorpe et al., 2012) and working memory (Sarnthein et al., 1998; Sauseng et al., 2005). Consistent with this "global" picture of low frequency EEG signals are studies using periodic visual input to elicit steady-state visual evoked potentials (SSVEPs). SSVEPs are responses to visual flicker at the flicker frequency (and harmonics). Low frequency (<20 Hz) SSVEPs elicit "resonant" responses in large-scale networks whose spatial distribution depends strongly on the input temporal frequency (Ding et al., 2006; Srinivasan et al., 2006). These large-scale networks have both distinct characteristic frequencies and functional properties (Ding et al., 2006; Bridwell and Srinivasan, 2012).

At higher frequencies (>30 Hz) the spatial distribution of EEG and ECoG signals is (apparently) localized at the cm scale. EEG studies have shown task dependent modulations of gamma networks in networks localized in sensory and motor cortex. These studies were inspired by single-unit and LFP studies in animal models, most notably by Singer and colleagues (Engel and Singer, 2001; Fries et al., 2007) that demonstrate localized networks synchronizing at gamma band frequencies. This local view of the origin of gamma rhythms is supported by ECoG studies that show relatively low coherence between electrodes at gamma band frequencies (Menon et al., 1996). SSVEP data at gamma band frequencies are consistent with this localized picture of fast EEG rhythms – γ-SSVEPs appear to be local processes in the visual cortex (Thorpe et al., 2011).

The distinct spatial and dynamical property of EEG oscillations in low (<20 Hz) and high (>20 Hz) frequency bands suggests the need for different types of models to explain these phenomena. Given any unknown physical or biological system that produces oscillations at some preferred (or resonant) frequency $f = \omega/2\pi$, a reasonable starting point for developing a model is the origin of the implied underlying time delay τ roughly estimated as

$$\tau \sim \omega^{-1} \tag{1}$$

The implied physiological time scale for the (8–13 Hz) alpha rhythm is $\tau = 12$–20 ms. More generally, the most robust human EEG rhythms recorded from the scalp (1–20 Hz) correspond to time delays $\tau = 8$–160 ms. How does this delay range compare with mammalian physiology? Whereas early studies of membrane time constants in mammalian cortex were very short, typically less than 10 ms, more modern studies with improved recording methods report a wider range up to 100 ms (Koch et al., 1996). While synaptic delays (PSP rise and decay times) lie in a general range (within a factor of perhaps 5 or 10) that might account for dominant EEG frequencies, claims of close agreement between the *details* of observed EEG spectra and dynamic theories based on membrane time constants are not by themselves a critical validation of a model. Model parameters can always be chosen to "match" EEG data, which, in any case, varies widely between brain states.

Local network theories refers to models of cortical or thalamocortical interactions in which signal propagation delays in axons are neglected. For example, coupled non-linear oscillators interact without any transmission delay in a local theory. In contrast, models that incorporate the spatial extent of the cortex and the transmission delays between neural populations are *global* theories. Global theories predict spatially coherent oscillations over the surface of the cortex with wave-like properties that depend primarily on the transmission delays between cortical populations and the size (surface area) of the cortex (Nunez, 1981, 1995, 2000). The dominant modes of these spatially distributed oscillations are predicted to lie below 15 Hz in the theta and alpha bands. While both global and local network theories have been developed independently, their interaction across spatial and temporal scales is less well understood. Previous studies have focused on how local networks influence global networks (Jirsa and Haken, 1996; Nunez, 2000), and a recent study investigates the interaction between local connectivity and long-range interactions (Pinotsis et al., 2013). In this paper we consider how global network dynamics may influence local networks.

The underlying time scales in local network theories are typically postsynaptic potential rise and decay times due to membrane capacitive-resistive properties (Wilson and Cowan, 1972, 1973). Local theories typically predict EEG signals with frequencies above 20 Hz. These results are consistent with more detailed studies of spiking neuron models (Izhikevich, 2006; Izhikevich and Edelman, 2008) that predict fast frequency oscillations in cortical populations unless coupled with delays as in a global network. Physiologically realistic compartment models incorporating the interactions between excitatory and inhibitory populations in cortex give rise to fast oscillations at gamma band frequencies (Bush and Sejnowski, 1996; Traub et al., 1997; Whittington et al., 2000). In these types of model, the dynamics are determined primarily by the synaptic rise and decay times and the strength of excitatory and inhibitory synaptic connections. More specific local models in sensory systems incorporate the essential spiking dynamics and connectivity of thalamocortical networks (Lumer et al., 1997) also giving rise to gamma band oscillations. While the physiological detailed models are useful to compare to data in animal models, comparisons to EEG and ECoG require model development in macroscopic variables that describe synaptic mass action.

The Wilson–Cowan model is one of the earliest and most often cited dynamic models based on local (PSP rise and decay) delays (Wilson and Cowan, 1972, 1973). The Wilson–Cowan model produces either sustained (limit cycle) or damped oscillations over a broad range of physiologically realistic parameter space in response to a step function input to the excitatory population. The oscillations in all parts of the network are highly correlated, as there is no independent noise in each population. The rate of damping of the oscillations is largely determined by the ratio of excitatory to inhibitory weights with higher inhibition leading to damped oscillations. The frequency of the oscillation is determined primarily by the membrane time constants and connectivity strength.

In this paper, we will make use of the Wilson–Cowan model to investigate how properties of high frequency (gamma band) oscillations generated by a local network in response to input is influenced by modulation of the background state by top-down influences. Our objective here is to formalize the general principles by which local networks in cortex are influenced by modulatory signals. For this purpose, we have modified the Wilson–Cowan equations to make more physiologically realistic by incorporating background state parameters into the model. In any physiological study neural dynamics are observed in a specific brain state (e.g., asleep, awake, alert, attentive, etc.) determined partly by neuromodulatory action at much longer time scales. As brain state changes, the background state partly determines the excitability of the network (Fellous and Linster, 1998; Romei et al., 2008). Experimental studies in humans and animal models have also demonstrated that top-down influences in cognitive processes involve the action of slower oscillations typically in the alpha or theta bands which appear to reflect the coherent behavior of global networks distributed across the cortex. We believe that the mostly likely underlying time scale for such global oscillations is transmission delays in corticocortical axons, and we have proposed a specific global model that predicts global standing waves with frequencies in the general range at the slower end of the EEG spectrum (Nunez, 1995, 2000; Nunez and Srinivasan, 2006). Our analysis here depends only on the existence of such global, low frequency oscillations as has been commonly observed for almost 100 years with scalp EEG and not any specific global field theory of EEG. Using the modified Wilson–Cowan model, we identify cross-frequency coupling as an EEG or ECoG signature of the effects of background state changes by top-down signals on local network dynamics.

MATERIALS AND METHODS

THE MODIFIED WILSON–COWAN MODEL

Wilson and Cowan (1972) derived a model neural population containing both excitatory and inhibitory neurons with dynamics described by a set of coupled, non-linear differential equations, herein labeled WC. The solution of these equations gives the proportion of cells in each subpopulation (excitatory/inhibitory) that become active per unit time. The cells comprising the population are assumed to be in close spatial proximity, with interconnections dense enough so that any two cells within it are path-connected. Furthermore, the model assumes that local interactions between neurons within the population are largely random, but that this local randomness gives rise to structure at larger spatial scales. The situation is analogous to an example taken from thermodynamics, in which a fluid with a macroscopically structured flow can be observed to be undergoing stochastic Brownian motion at the molecular level. The same framework set forth by Wilson and Cowan has been extended in a number of straightforward ways to models with more general connectivity, and an arbitrary number of spatially distinct neural populations (Campbell and Wang, 1996; Borisyuk et al., 2000). Extensions of the WC framework have been developed to model interacting thalamic (reticular formation) and cortical structures involved in the generation of spindle oscillations (7–14 Hz) in early sleep stages (Yousif and Denham, 2005). Jirsa and Haken (1997), used a WC model interacting with a global model to interpret MEG data in a syncopated tapping audio-motor task. Other model developments related to the WC model have incorporated spatially extended models with axonal delays and more detailed physiological parameters (Jirsa and Haken, 1996, 1997; Robinson et al., 1997; Liley et al., 1999).

Here we adopt a modified version of WC to make it more physiologically realistic as outlined in the Appendix. The basic dependent variables are the *fractions of excitatory and inhibitory active cells* (action potential densities) $E(t)$, $I(t)$, which can evidently exhibit high frequency jitter not treated in this analysis. Rather, the WC equations are expressed in terms of coarse grained excitatory $\langle E(t)\rangle$ and inhibitory $\langle I(t)\rangle$ action potential densities. The basic model is illustrated in **Figure 1**. We introduce the new dependent variables $X_E(t)$, $X_I(t)$, which provide perturbations about the critical (equilibrium) point (E_0, I_0), which we have interpreted as the background brain state which is controlled by various neuromodulators or top-down signaling. Thus, we express

$$\begin{aligned}\langle E(t)\rangle &= E_0 + X_E(t)\\ \langle I(t)\rangle &= I_0 + X_I(t)\end{aligned} \tag{2}$$

Since the excitatory action potential densities are defined as fractions of the total cell populations, we require

$$\begin{aligned}0 \le E_0 + X_E(t) \le 1\\ 0 \le I_0 + X_I(t) \le 1\end{aligned} \tag{3}$$

The basic WC equations then become

$$\begin{aligned}\frac{dX_E}{dt} &= -E_0 - X_E + (1 - E_0 - X_E)\, S_E\,(X_E, X_I, P)\\ A\frac{dX_I}{dt} &= -I_0 - X_I + (1 - I_0 - X_I)\, S_I\,(X_E, X_I)\end{aligned} \tag{4}$$

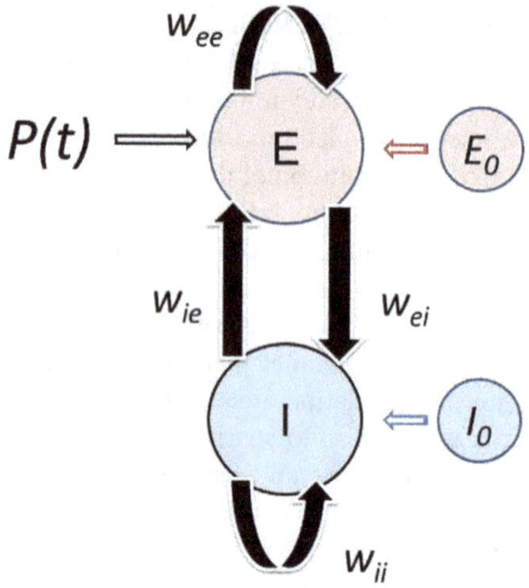

FIGURE 1 | Schematic of the modified Wilson–Cowan model. The localized population consists of excitatory and inhibitory neurons that interact with each other with negligible transmission delays. The population receives afferent input $P(t)$. Simultaneously, the population is subject to influences from both nearby and distant cortex. This top-down modulation of the neural population is the result of feedback from large-scale networks and/or global synaptic fields spanning the cortex. The model consists of an Excitatory (E) and Inhibitory (I) subpopulations with membrane time constants τ_E and τ_I, which interact with each other via the connection weights w_{EI} and w_{IE}. The neurons within each subpopulation also interact with each other, reflected in the self-excitation w_{EE} and self-inhibition w_{II} weights. The influence of other cortical areas on the population is reflected in the background state of the excitatory E_0 and inhibitory I_0 subpopulation. The Wilson–Cowan model was modified to incorporate the background state variables (see Appendix).

Here $A = \frac{\tau_I}{\tau_E}$ is the ratio of inhibitory to excitatory time constants, and $P(t)$ is an excitatory external (driving) input from another cortical population or potentially input to the population from the thalamus. The set of parameters (w_{EE}, w_{IE}, w_{EI}, w_{II}) are gain parameters that give the strength of connections between the excitatory and inhibitory populations as indicated in **Figure 1**. As shown in the Appendix for the special case $P(t) = 0$, the sigmoid functions S_E, S_I in Eq. 4 then take the forms

$$S_E = \frac{1}{1 + \left(\frac{1}{E_0} - 2\right) \exp\left(-w_{EE}X_E + w_{IE}X_I - P\right)} \qquad E_0 < \frac{1}{2} \quad (5)$$

$$S_I = \frac{1}{1 + \left(\frac{1}{I_0} - 2\right) \exp\left(-w_{EI}X_E + w_{II}X_I\right)} \qquad I_0 < \frac{1}{2} \quad (6)$$

PARAMETER CHOICES

For our simulations the main parameters of interest are the background state variables E_0 and I_0, which we will vary as described in the following sections. The free parameters in our analysis are the set of connection weights (w_{EE}, w_{EI}, w_{IE}, w_{II}) which are determined by the following physiological considerations: (1) In the cortex, excitatory connections are estimated to be 4–5 times more common than inhibitory connections (Bush and Sejnowski, 1996) and (2) Inhibitory connections are more typically found on the cell body possibly increasing their effectiveness in comparison to excitatory connections on dendritic trees (Mountcastle, 1997). Taking these two points into consideration we first fixed the two parameters $w_{EI} = 50$ and $w_{IE} = 15$. We set the self-inhibition $w_{II} = 0$, as we found little practical effect for the small values of this parameter, other than to increase damping in the system, and shift the critical point for transition from a damped oscillation to a limit cycle regime.

Equation 4 produce stable limit cycle solutions about the critical point (E_0, I_0) for a wide range of the parameters. For example, setting $A = 1$ and $E_0 = I_0$ the necessary condition for oscillatory solutions about E_0, I_0 is

$$w_{EE} < 2\sqrt{w_{IE} w_{EI}} \quad (7)$$

This oscillatory solution is unstable (e.g., an unstable spiral allowing for a stable limit cycle) if

$$w_{EE} > \frac{2}{E_0 (1 - 2E_0)} \quad (8)$$

From Eq. 8 we were always able to find the critical value of w_{EE} below which the system produced damped oscillations in response to a step function input, while above this value the system produced limit cycle oscillations.

TOP-DOWN (GLOBAL) INFLUENCES ON A LOCAL WC NETWORK

We explicitly consider two types of top-down influences on the local WC network developed in section "The Modified Wilson–Cowan Model": (1) the effect of neuromodulators setting the background state (E_0, I_0) of the population. For the purpose of the analysis here we consider this effect on the background state to be static as it takes place at very long time scales as compared to the frequency of the oscillations and (2) the effect of dynamic modulation of the background state of the local network (top-down) by oscillations in larger scale networks that incorporate the cells that constitute the local network. For simplicity of analysis we presume that the larger scale networks (or global synaptic fields) generate oscillations at frequency ω_α that modulate the background state of the WC oscillator; that is

$$\begin{aligned} E_0 &\rightarrow E_0 + \alpha_E \cos(\omega_\alpha t) \\ I_0 &\rightarrow I_0 + \alpha_I \cos(\omega_\alpha t + \phi_\alpha) \end{aligned} \quad (9)$$

Here the amplitudes (α_E, α_I) of the background modulations are constrained to be less than the constant background (E_0, I_0). We introduce a phase offset ϕ_α to allow for differences in local processing of the modulatory input by the excitatory and inhibitory subpopulations, as might occur if they have different membrane time constants.

SIMULATIONS AND DATA ANALYSIS

All of the simulations carried out here were performed using the built in ode solver in MATLAB (Natick, MA, USA), *ode23*. We considered several types of inputs $P(t)$ – step function, impulse, sinusoidal, and random noise and found the essential characteristics of the system response were represented by the step function input. The spectrum of the model output was analyzed using a

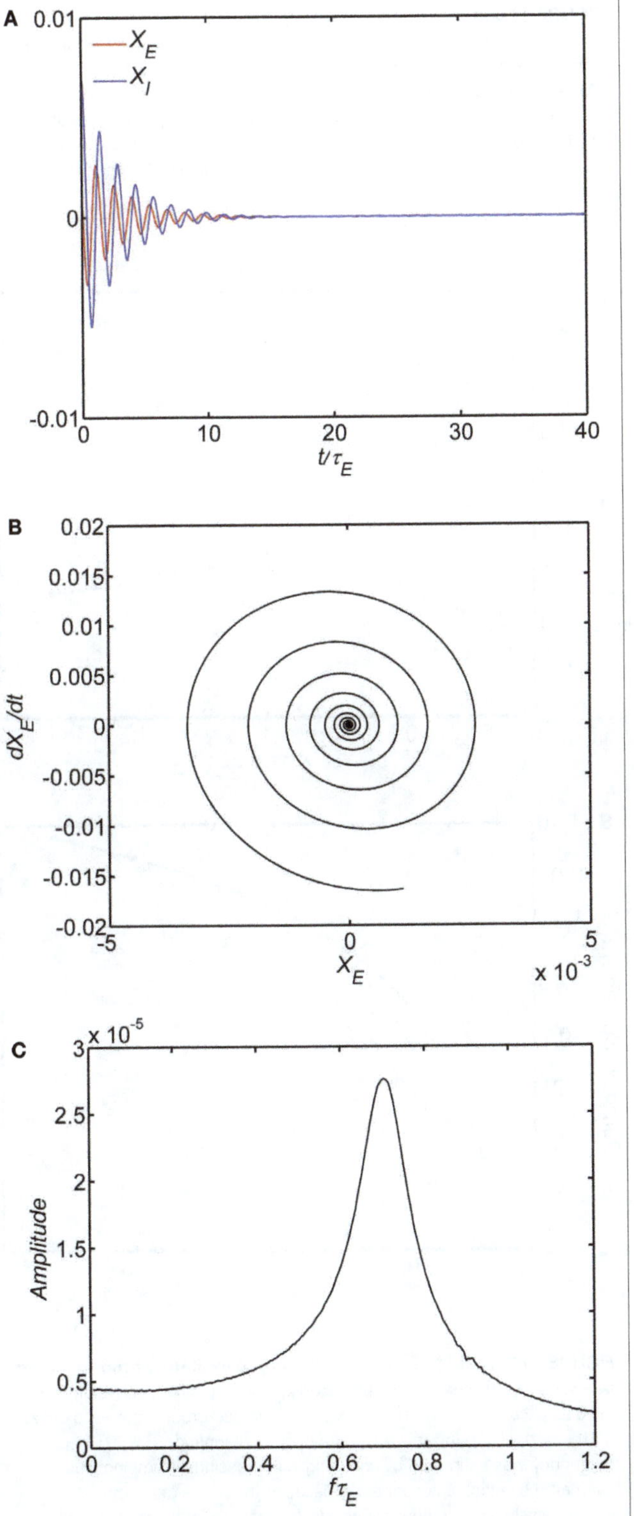

FIGURE 2 | Damped oscillation regime of the model. In all of the simulations, the following parameters are fixed: (1) The ratio of time constants $A = \tau_I/\tau_E = 1$, (2) the background state $E_0(t) = I_0(t) = 0.25$, (3) the connection weights are $(w_{EI}, w_{IE}, w_{II}) = (50, 15, 0)$ and (4) the input $P(t) = 0.1$ is a step function at time 0. Damped oscillation observed with *(Continued)*

FIGURE 2 | Continued
self-excitation $w_{EE} = 12$. The time series of the excitatory and inhibitory subpopulations are shown in **(A)**. In these plots time is normalized by excitatory membrane time constant τ_E. Phase-plane plots for the excitatory. subpopulation are shown in **(B)**. Amplitude spectra obtained by the FFT are shown in **(C)**. Normalized frequency is $f\tau_E$. If $\tau_E = 20$ ms, a normalized frequency of 1 corresponds to 50 Hz.

FFT in MATLAB (Mathworks, Natick, MA, USA). For sustained oscillations in the limit cycle regime, we also analyzed the model outputs either by using Hilbert Transforms to estimate the frequency and amplitude of the oscillation or by a complex Morlet wavelet transform. For the damped oscillations, we fit the oscillation to a damped sinusoid $\exp(j2\ \pi ft(1 + j\gamma))$ where f is the frequency of the oscillation and γ is the damping coefficient. We obtained direct estimates of frequency using zero crossings and estimated the damping coefficient by fitting an exponential to the decay of amplitude across cycles of the oscillation.

RESULTS

BASIC RESPONSE PROPERTIES OF WC OSCILLATOR

We first examined the behavior of the system with identical excitatory and inhibitory time constants ($A = \tau_I/\tau_E = 1$) and a fixed background state ($E_0 = I_0 = 0.25$). The specific value of w_{EE} separating limit cycle from damped oscillations depends on the background excitability as in Eq. 8; with $E_0 = I_0 = 0.25$ the critical value is $w_{EE} = 15$. The limit cycle is observed if the self-excitation is sufficiently large ($w_{EE} > 15$); smaller values lead to damped oscillations of higher frequency. An example of numerical solutions for the model with the self-excitation (w_{EE}) parameter in the damped oscillation range is shown in **Figure 2**. In the time series plot (**Figure 2A**), the time variable is normalized with respect to the excitatory membrane time constant τ_E and in the amplitude spectra (**Figure 2C**) the frequency variable f is normalized as $f\tau_E$ For example, if τ_E falls in the range of 10–20 ms range, the damped oscillation corresponds to a gamma band oscillation in the 35–70 Hz band. The limit cycle is observed if the self-excitation is sufficiently large (**Figure 3**). The limit cycle has a lower fundamental frequency as shown in the spectrum in **Figure 3C**; if τ_E falls in the range of 10–20 ms range, the dominant frequency is in the 25–50 Hz range and also exhibits harmonics (Second harmonic shown).

The ratio of inhibitory to excitatory time constants A influences both the frequency and damping of the oscillations. **Figures 4A,B** show the oscillation frequency and damping coefficient in the damped oscillation regime for self-excitation in the damped oscillation range ($w_{EE} = 12$). When the inhibitory time constant is smaller than the excitatory time constant ($A < 1$) the oscillations are highly damped, but if the inhibitory time is constant is larger than the excitatory time constant ($A > 1$) the oscillations are weakly damped. Thus, in order to observe the damped oscillations, it must be the case that inhibitory time constants are longer than the excitatory time constant. As the ratio A increases further the system will eventually transition to a limit cycle oscillation.

Figures 5A,B shows an example with the self-excitation parameter in the limit cycle regime ($w_{EE} = 18$). As A increases the frequency of the oscillation decreases and the amplitude increases

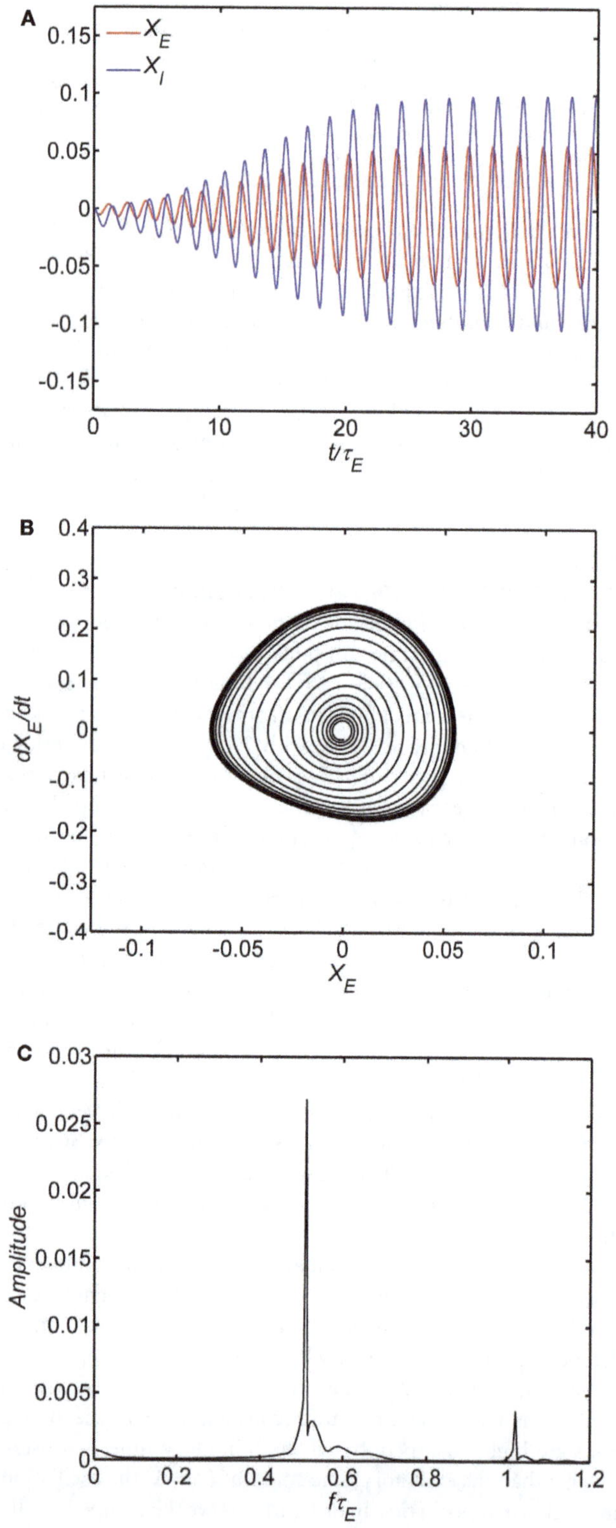

FIGURE 3 | Limit cycle regime of the model. In all of the simulations, the following parameters are fixed: (1) The ratio of time constants $A = \tau_I/\tau_E = 1$, (2) the background state $E_0(t) = I_0(t) = 0.25$, (3) the connection weights are $(w_{EI}, w_{IE}, w_{II}) = (50,15,0)$ and (4) the input $P(t) = 0.1$ is a step function at

(Continued)

FIGURE 3 | Continued
time 0. Limit cycle oscillation observed with self-excitation $w_{EE} = 20$. The time series of the excitatory and inhibitory subpopulations are shown in **(A)**. In these plots time is normalized by excitatory membrane time constant τ_E. Phase-plane plots for the excitatory subpopulation are shown in **(B)**. Amplitude spectra obtained by the FFT are shown in **(C)**. Normalized frequency is $f\tau_E$. If $\tau_E = 20$ ms, a normalized frequency of 1 corresponds to 50 Hz.

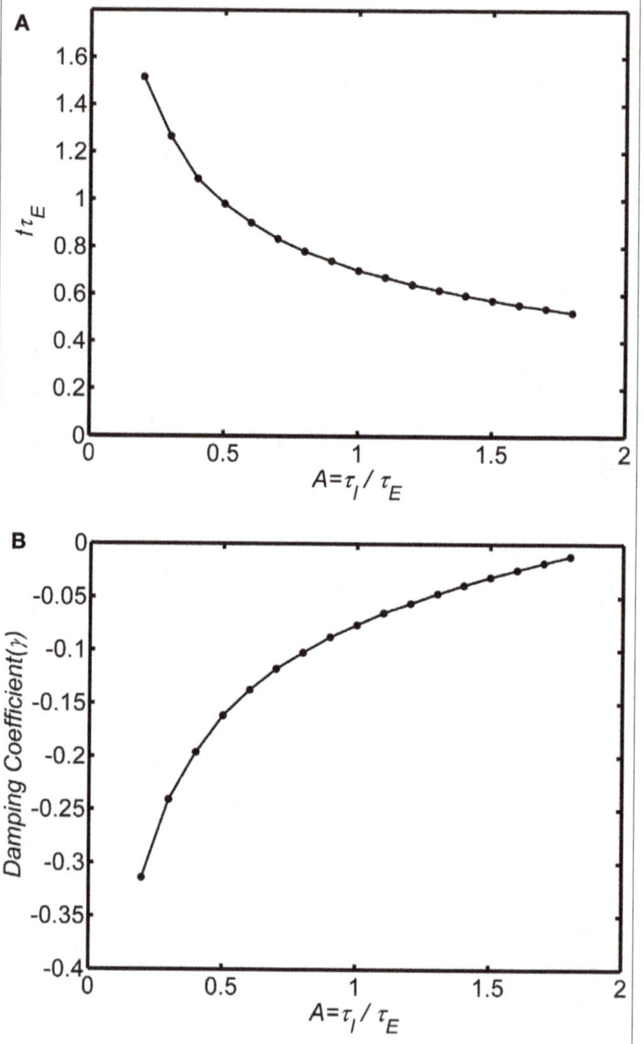

FIGURE 4 | Effect of the ratio of inhibitory to excitatory time constants ($A = \tau_I/\tau_E$) on the damped oscillations. System connection weights are fixed as $(w_{EI}, w_{IE}, w_{II}, w_{EE}) = (50,15,0, 12)$. The background state is fixed as $E_0(t) = I_0(t) = 0.25$. Input is a step function of magnitude $P(t) = 0.1$. Frequency was estimated by analyzing zero crossings. Damping was estimated by fitting an exponential decay to the peaks of a rectified (absolute value) of the time series. **(A)** Normalized frequency is $f\tau_E$. If $\tau_E = 10$ ms, a normalized frequency of 1 corresponds to 100 Hz. **(B)** Damping coefficient.

consistent with reduced damping in the system. Essentially, for any level of self-excitation w_{EE}, as inhibitory time constant increases, damping is reduced, and frequency decreases. The frequency range

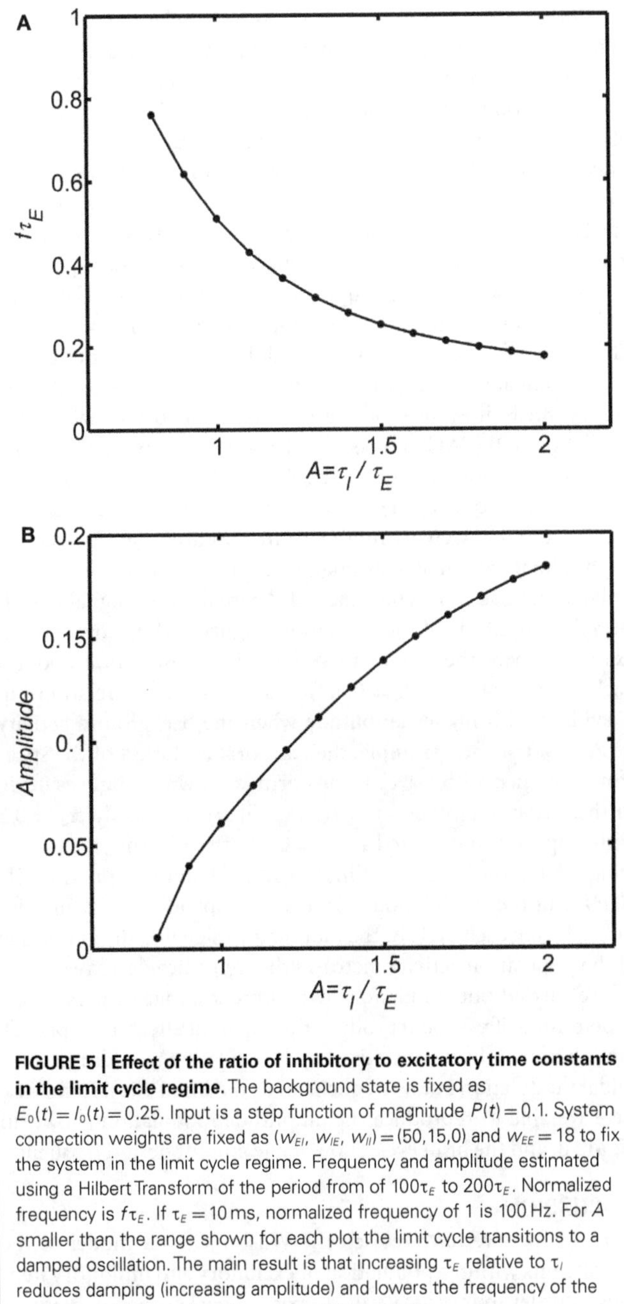

FIGURE 5 | Effect of the ratio of inhibitory to excitatory time constants in the limit cycle regime. The background state is fixed as $E_0(t) = I_0(t) = 0.25$. Input is a step function of magnitude $P(t) = 0.1$. System connection weights are fixed as $(w_{EI}, w_{IE}, w_{II}) = (50,15,0)$ and $w_{EE} = 18$ to fix the system in the limit cycle regime. Frequency and amplitude estimated using a Hilbert Transform of the period from of $100\tau_E$ to $200\tau_E$. Normalized frequency is $f\tau_E$. If $\tau_E = 10$ ms, normalized frequency of 1 is 100 Hz. For A smaller than the range shown for each plot the limit cycle transitions to a damped oscillation. The main result is that increasing τ_E relative to τ_I reduces damping (increasing amplitude) and lowers the frequency of the oscillation. **(A)** Normalized frequency **(B)** Amplitude.

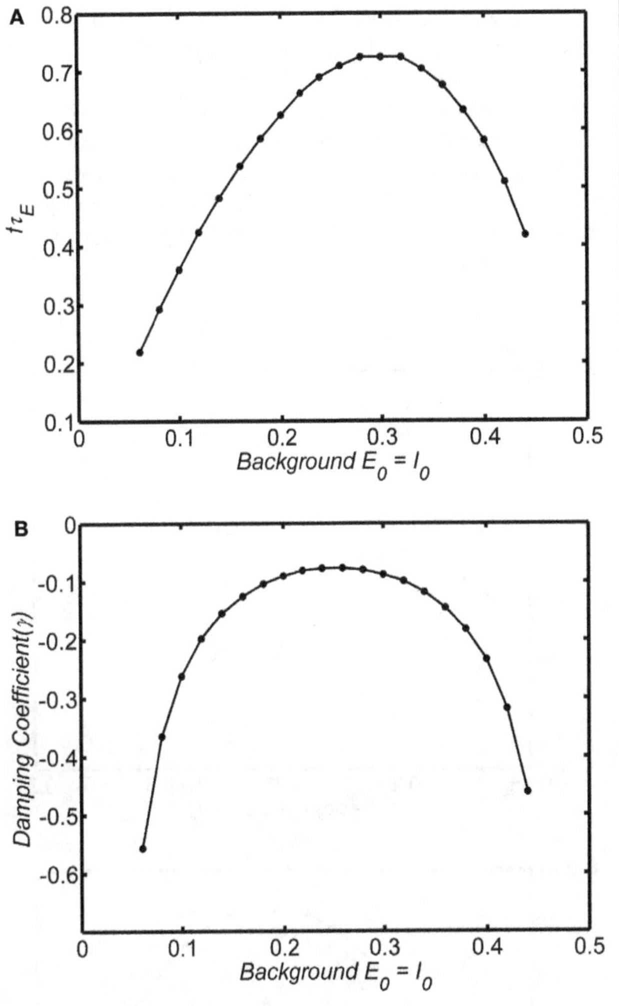

FIGURE 6 | Dependence of frequency and damping on background state for the damped oscillations. System connection weights are fixed as $(w_{EI}, w_{IE}, w_{II}, w_{EE}) = (50,15,0, 15)$. Input is a step function of magnitude 0.1. We have verified that the curves are the same for step functions up to 0.3 Frequency was estimated by analyzing zero crossings. Damping was estimated by fitting an exponential decay to the peaks of a rectified (absolute value) of the time series. Normalized frequency is $f\tau_E$. If $\tau_E = 20$ ms, normalized frequency of 1 corresponds to a 50 Hz oscillation. **(A)** Normalized frequency **(B)** Damping coefficient.

of the limit cycle oscillations is much lower than the damped oscillation. For $\tau_E = 10$ ms the damped oscillations are in the high gamma band frequency range (60–100 Hz) when A ranges from 0.5–1.5. In contrast, for the same range of τ_E and A ranging from 1–2 the limit cycle oscillations range is in the lower gamma frequency range (20–50 Hz).

EFFECT OF BACKGROUND STATE

The frequency and damping of the WC oscillator is strongly influenced by the background state. **Figures 6A,B** shows the frequency and damping as a function of background state variables $E_0 = I_0$ for an example in the damped oscillation regime ($w_{EE} = 12$; $A = 1$). At very low levels of background activity the system exhibits low frequency rapidly damped oscillations. As the background activity increases above $E_0 = I_0 = 0.1$ the oscillations become weakly damped and frequency increases as damping decreases. Damping reaches a minimum at $E_0 = I_0 = 0.25$ and the frequency of the oscillation reaches a peak at $E_0 = I_0 = 0.3$. At higher levels of background activity, the oscillations decrease in frequency and are again highly damped. Thus only at the center of the range, at around 0.2–0.3 can we observe high frequency weakly damped oscillations.

If the system is in the limit cycle regime the same essential damping behavior is observed as shown for an example in

Figures 7A,B ($w_{EE} = 18$; $A = 1$). The limit cycle amplitude is suppressed above and below $E_0 = I_0 = 0.25$; at very large or very small values of the background state the limit cycle disappears and is replaced by a damped oscillation. The range of background activity over which the limit cycle is observed can be expanded by increasing the self-excitation parameter (w_{EE}). However, in contrast to the damped oscillation regime, in the limit cycle the frequency of the oscillations is much less dependent on the background activity level, remaining stable over the range of background states with the high amplitude.

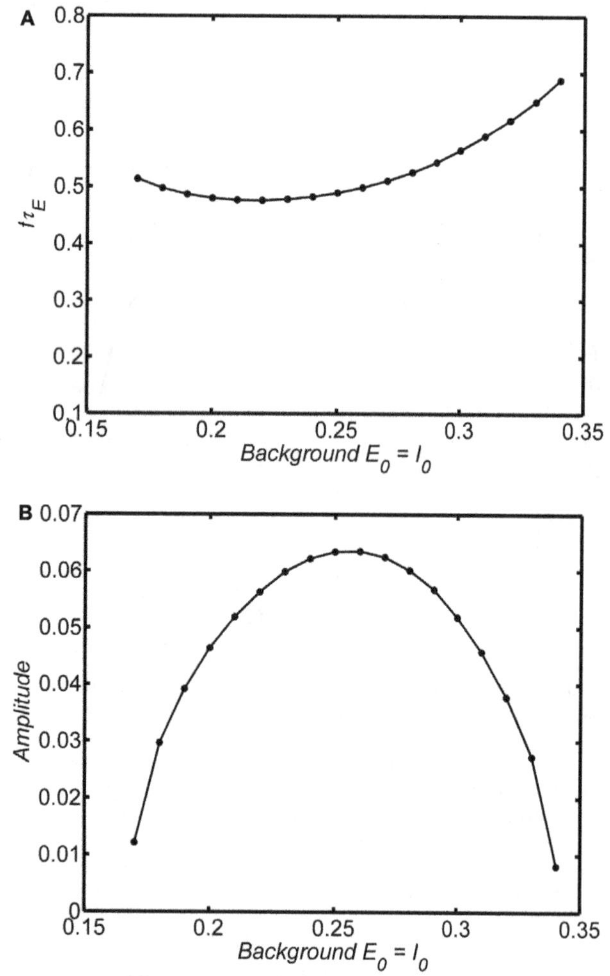

FIGURE 7 | Dependence of frequency and amplitude of limit cycle oscillations on the background state. System connection weights are fixed as (w_{EI}, w_{IE}, w_{II}, w_{EE}) = (50,15,0, 20) (dashed line) or (w_{EI}, w_{IE}, w_{II}, w_{EE}) = (50,15,0, 25) (solid line). Input is a step function of magnitude 0.1. Frequency and amplitude estimated using a Hilbert Transform of the period from of $100\tau_E$–$200\tau_E$. Normalized frequency is $f\tau_E$. If $\tau_E = 20$ ms, normalized frequency of 1 corresponds to a 50 Hz oscillation. Outside the range of background states shown there are no limit cycle oscillation for each level of w_{EE} and the oscillations damp out. The main point is that the amplitude of the limit cycle oscillations depend strongly on the background state. Compared to the damped oscillations (**Figure 6**) the limit cycle frequency does not depend strongly on the background state. **(A)** Normalized frequency **(B)** Amplitude.

EFFECTS OF TOP-DOWN SIGNALING

It is increasingly appreciated that neural populations are subject to top-down signals reflected in oscillations in large-scale cortical networks. We modified the WC system equations to incorporate dynamic modulation of background state as in Eq. A12. For simplicity we modulated the background state variables (E_0, I_0) with a sinusoidal signal of fixed frequency; these modulatory frequencies are much slower than the intrinsic frequencies of the WC oscillator. The presence of the modulatory signal alone was not sufficient to drive the system – excitatory input $P(t)$ was always required.

Figure 8 shows some example simulations of the model with the self-excitation parameter set in the limit cycle regime ($w_{EE} = 18$). The main effect of the dynamic modulation of background state is to modulate the amplitude and frequency of the oscillation. **Figures 8A,B** show the time course of a modulatory signal and the oscillation in the WC model. In this example, the modulatory signal is an oscillation about a background state $E_0 = I_0 = 0.2$ with normalized frequency $f\tau_E = 0.03$. The oscillation in population activity can be seen to modulate in amplitude at the rate of the modulatory signal, with higher amplitude when background activity increases. Thus the phase of the modulatory signal modulates the amplitude of the oscillation. **Figures 8D,E** show another example where the modulatory signal is an oscillation about a background state $E_0 = I_0 = 0.3$. Here a different phase relationship is evident with higher amplitude when the background activity decreases. For each example, the temporal evolution of the spectrum obtained with wavelet transform is shown in **Figures 8C,F**. In these examples, the population oscillates at roughly $f\tau_E = 0.5$ with amplitude modulated at $f\tau_E = 0.03$. If $\tau_E = 10$ ms, the underlying oscillation frequency is in the gamma band at approximately 50 Hz and the modulation is in the theta band at 3 Hz. In both cases, during each cycle of the modulatory signal as the amplitude of the population activity increases the frequency decreases.

We carried out simulations over a broad range of parameters to determine if we could produce the apparent effect of amplitude modulation of the intrinsic limit cycle oscillation by adding a sinusoidal modulation at low frequencies to the input $P(t)$. In no case were we able to reproduce the amplitude modulation shown in **Figure 8**, and the limit cycle show stable amplitude and frequency.

DISCUSSION

In this paper we have revised the Wilson–Cowan model of the interactions within a population of excitatory and inhibitory neurons in order to investigate the impact of background activity on the dynamics of neural populations. In our model this background state is determined statically at very long time scales (presumably by neuromodulator systems) and dynamically at faster time scales by the activity of other cortical systems that exert top-down control on the neural population. We find that our model formalizes the mechanisms by which background state can influence local population dynamics consistent with observations in experimental studies in different behavioral contexts and recording methods.

DYNAMICS OF THE WILSON–COWAN SYSTEM

The basic response properties of the system around a fixed background state indicate that the system produced damped oscillations or sustained limit cycle oscillations depending on the

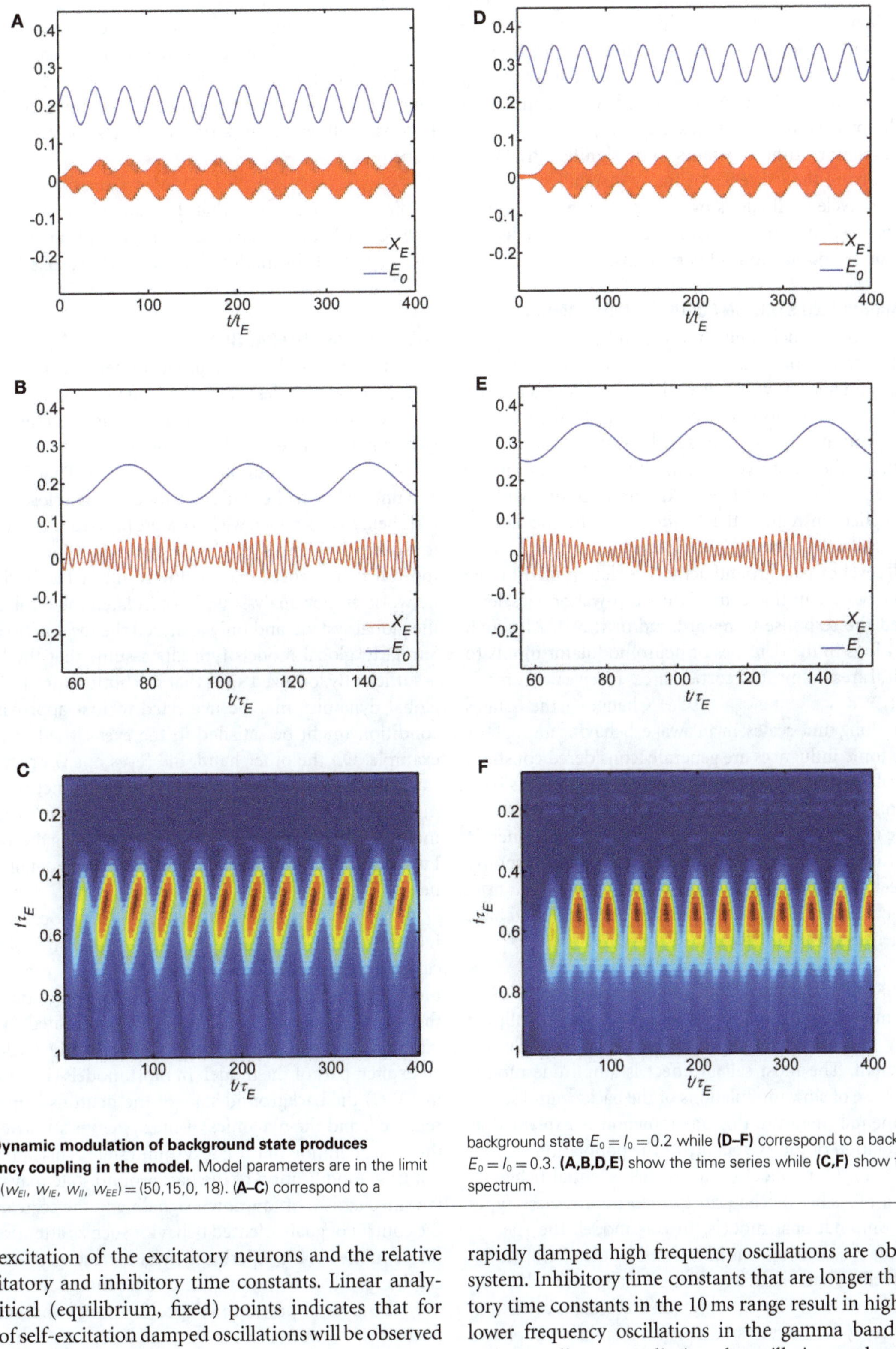

FIGURE 8 | Dynamic modulation of background state produces cross-frequency coupling in the model. Model parameters are in the limit cycle regime (w_{EI}, w_{IE}, w_{II}, w_{EE}) = (50,15,0, 18). **(A–C)** correspond to a background state $E_0 = I_0 = 0.2$ while **(D–F)** correspond to a background state $E_0 = I_0 = 0.3$. **(A,B,D,E)** show the time series while **(C,F)** show the wavelet spectrum.

level of self-excitation of the excitatory neurons and the relative value of excitatory and inhibitory time constants. Linear analysis about critical (equilibrium, fixed) points indicates that for lower values of self-excitation damped oscillations will be observed while at higher values of self-excitation limit cycle oscillations are observed. In addition, sustained oscillations are more likely to be observed within local populations with longer inhibitory time constants than excitatory time constants. When excitatory time constants are longer than the inhibitory time constants, rapidly damped high frequency oscillations are observed in the system. Inhibitory time constants that are longer than the excitatory time constants in the 10 ms range result in higher amplitude lower frequency oscillations in the gamma band (30–100 Hz) and generally support limit cycle oscillations rather than damped oscillations. In cases where the inhibitory time constants are much longer these sustained oscillations can be produced at even lower frequencies in the beta (13–30 Hz) and alpha (8–12 Hz) ranges.

Whereas early studies of membrane time constants in mammalian cortex were very short, typically less than 10 ms, more modern studies with improved recording methods report the wide range up to 100 ms (Koch et al., 1996). In particular, very long inhibitory time constants have been reported for thalamic and cortical populations. Thus, we can reasonably expect the ratio of inhibitory to excitatory time constants to be significantly larger than one, supporting the existence of linear instability and corresponding limit cycle oscillations over a broad range of model parameters. Such self-sustained dynamics may contribute locally to the generation of spontaneous EEG rhythms.

EFFECTS OF BACKGROUND STATE ON POPULATION DYNAMICS

The dynamics of the model population depend very strongly on the background state in both limit cycle and damped oscillation ranges of the parameters. At very low levels of background activity (E_0, $I_0 < 0.2$), the population does not respond to the external input. As background activity increases the system responds to external input. In the limit cycle regime, the *amplitude* of the oscillation depends strongly on the background activity while in the damped oscillation regime the *frequency* of the oscillations depends strongly on the background activity.

The overall level of background activity is determined by the neuromodulatory systems that control the sleep-wake cycles, level of arousal, and the response to reward and/or threat. Although there are variations in the densities of neuromodulator inputs to different cortical areas, almost all cortical areas receive neuromodulatory input (Goldman-Rakic et al., 1990). Changes in these states occur over very long time scales; in an awake, behaving animal (or human) these tonic influences are generally considered constant. Thus in general, we can expect that the background level is constant over a responsive level of the population, although there are also phasic modulations of the cholinergic and dopaminergic neuromodulator systems that may play a role in stimulus response and reward seeking behavior (Sarter and Bruno, 1997; Chuhma et al., 2004; Zhang and Sulzer, 2004), and can be expected to have dynamic influences on local networks.

MODULATION OF POPULATION DYNAMICS BY TOP-DOWN SIGNALS

The dynamic modulation of background state creates amplitude and frequency modulation of the intrinsic gamma oscillations of the WC system. The most salient effect is amplitude modulation by the phase of slow modulations of the background states. In the experimental literature this phenomenon is explained as dynamic modulation of the excitability of the population (Jensen and Colgin, 2007). Our model captures this essential behavior, and provides a plausible mechanism to incorporate these types of effects in computational models. In our model, the specific phase/amplitude relationship was influenced by the overall activity level; the specific phase of the modulation that produced robust oscillations was arbitrary. The experimental literature is consistent with this picture, with different studies reporting different phases of the modulation signal for peak amplitude of the local oscillation as shown in **Figure 1** of (Lisman and Buzsaki, 2008).

This essential phenomenon of cross-frequency coupling has been observed in animal models in a number of experimental contexts (Buzsaki and Draguhn, 2004; Scheffzuk et al., 2011) and human ECoG recordings (Canolty and Knight, 2010; Voytek et al., 2010). These findings have since been confirmed in human EEG where the phase of the theta rhythm is shown to modulate the amplitude of the gamma rhythm (Demiralp et al., 2007). It has long been known that the phase of the alpha rhythm at stimulus onset influences amplitude and phase of the evoked potential (Dustman and Beck, 1965; Jansen and Brandt, 1991; Gruber et al., 2005; Hanslmayr et al., 2007). Moreover, there are a number of studies that have shown that the state of the cortex (as measured by EEG oscillations) can predict the perception of a sensory stimulus, presumably by modulating the sensory evoked response (Haig and Gordon, 1998; Hanslmayr et al., 2007).

LOCAL-GLOBAL INTERACTIONS

We have proposed a conceptual framework in which local networks (cell assemblies) are embedded in a global environment that produces standing waves due to propagation in the corticocortical (white matter) fibers and periodic boundary conditions (Nunez, 1995, 2000; Nunez and Srinivasan, 2006). That is, the neocortex and underlying white matter are modeled as a closed loop or spherical shell. In this paper, we have a proposed a method to model the top-down influences of such systems on a local network. These top-down influences may be the result of feedback from global network. In our analysis we have isolated the local network from the global system, and only analyzed the local network dynamics. Similarly, global models typically assume that the local network is sufficiently localized such that its (bottom up) influence on the global dynamics may be neglected to first approximation. This condition might be satisfied in the eyes closed resting state, for example. On the other hand, the (eyes open) processing of substantial visual input or complex cognitive functions may involve multiple local thalamocortical networks that act (bottom up) to modify the global networks that are influencing the local networks. Future work must explicitly consider in more detail how the local networks and global networks interact.

Our study suggests that models of these local networks must incorporate the idea that the response properties of the networks can be modified by modulatory inputs. In our modified WC model, the addition of oscillatory afferent input does not modify the system dynamics. We explicitly incorporated dynamic modulation of the system properties by making the background state an explicit part of the model. In most models (including the original WC) the background state of the neurons is mathematically removed, and the dynamics of the system is studied without further consideration of the background state. This approximation is limiting; modification of the background state may be an important mechanism of top-down signaling in the cortex, especially in the control of goal-oriented behavior such as attention. Local networks in the cortex experience dynamic background states which can be readily incorporated into most model formulations. This may also have importance in specific models that seek to make a distinction between feedforward and feedback connections in sensory systems (Mountcastle, 1997; Lamme and Roelfsema, 2000).

CONCLUSIONS

Since the first human recording in the early 1920s the physiological bases for the wide range of rhythmic EEG activity has been somewhat of a mystery. As one important "window on the mind," EEG has long provided a critical tool in pursuit of connecting neural dynamics to cognitive processes. Human brains produce a proverbial "spectral zoo" that is closely correlated to behavior and cognition. A major obstacle in this quest is a shortage of robust and widely appreciated theoretical support for EEG's dynamic behavior in time and spatial location over the scalp. The conceptual framework facilitated by such theory could have a substantial influence on the design of new EEG-cognitive experiments. In this paper, we propose an approach to incorporate global (top-down) influences on local networks. The essence of our approach is to immerse the local network in a dynamic background state. These dynamics could be generated by a global model of interactions across the cortex; they could also be modeled from experimental EEG data. This approach is sufficiently general to be applied to other theoretical formulations of population dynamics in neural populations and to models of specific cognitive influences on local circuit dynamics.

REFERENCES

Borisyuk, R., Denham, M., Hoppensteadt, F., Kazanovich, Y., and Vinogradova, O. (2000). An oscillatory neural network model of sparse distributed memory and novelty detection. *BioSystems* 58, 265–272.

Bridwell, D. A., and Srinivasan, R. (2012). Distinct attention networks for feature enhancement and suppression in vision. *Psychol. Sci.* 23, 1151–1158.

Bush, P., and Sejnowski, T. (1996). Inhibition synchronizes sparsely connected cortical neurons within and between columns in realistic network models. *J. Comput. Neurosci.* 3, 91–110.

Buzsaki, G., and Draguhn, A. (2004). Neuronal oscillations in cortical networks. *Science* 304, 1926–1929.

Campbell, S., and Wang, D. (1996). Synchronization and desynchronization in a network of locally coupled Wilson–Cowan oscillators. *IEEE Trans. Neural Netw.* 7, 541–554.

Canolty, R. T., Ganguly, K., Kennerley, S. W., Cadieu, C. F., Koepsell, K., Wallis, J. D., et al. (2010). Oscillatory phase coupling coordinates anatomically dispersed functional cell assemblies. *Proc. Natl. Acad. Sci. U.S.A.* 107, 17356–17361.

Canolty, R. T., and Knight, R. T. (2010). The functional role of cross-frequency coupling. *Trends Cogn. Sci. (Regul. Ed.)* 14, 506–515.

Chuhma, N., Zhang, H., Masson, J., Zhuang, X., Sulzer, D., Hen, R., et al. (2004). Dopamine neurons mediate a fast excitatory signal via their glutamatergic synapses. *J. Neurosci.* 24, 972–981.

Demiralp, T., Bayraktaroglu, Z., Lenz, D., Junge, S., Busch, N. A., Maess, B., et al. (2007). Gamma amplitudes are coupled to theta phase in human EEG during visual perception. *Int. J. Psychophysiol.* 64, 24–30.

Ding, J., Sperling, G., and Srinivasan, R. (2006). Attentional modulation of SSVEP power depends on the network tagged by the flicker frequency. *Cereb. Cortex* 16, 1016–1029.

Dustman, R. E., and Beck, E. C. (1965). Phase of Alpha Brain Waves. *Electroencephalogr. Clin. Neurophysiol.* 18, 433–440.

Engel, A. K., Fries, P., and Singer, W. (2001). Dynamic predictions: oscillations and synchrony in top-down processing. *Nat. Rev. Neurosci.* 2, 704–716.

Engel, A. K., and Singer, W. (2001). Temporal binding and the neural correlates of sensory awareness. *Trends Cogn. Sci. (Regul. Ed.)* 5, 16–25.

Fellous, J. M., and Linster, C. (1998). Computational models of neuromodulation. *Neural Comput.* 10, 771–805.

Fries, P., Nikolic, D., and Singer, W. (2007). The gamma cycle. *Trends Neurosci.* 30, 309–316.

Goldman-Rakic, P. S., Lidow, M. S., and Gallager, D. W. (1990). Overlap of dopaminergic, adrenergic, and serotoninergic receptors and complementarity of their subtypes in primate prefrontal cortex. *J. Neurosci.* 10, 2125–2138.

Gruber, W. R., Klimesch, W., Sauseng, P., and Doppelmayr, M. (2005). Alpha phase synchronization predicts P1 and N1 latency and amplitude size. *Cereb. Cortex* 15, 371–377.

Haig, A. R., and Gordon, E. (1998). Prestimulus EEG alpha phase synchronicity influences N100 amplitude and reaction time. *Psychophysiology* 35, 591–595.

Hanslmayr, S., Aslan, A., Staudigl, T., Klimesch, W., Herrmann, C. S., and Bauml, K. H. (2007). Prestimulus oscillations predict visual perception performance between and within subjects. *Neuroimage* 37, 1465–1473.

Izhikevich, E. M. (2006). Polychronization: computation with spikes. *Neural. Comput.* 18, 245–282.

Izhikevich, E. M., and Edelman, G. M. (2008). Large-scale model of mammalian thalamocortical systems. *Proc. Natl. Acad. Sci. U.S.A.* 105, 3593–3598.

Jansen, B. H., and Brandt, M. E. (1991). The effect of the phase of prestimulus alpha activity on the averaged visual evoked response. *Electroencephalogr. Clin. Neurophysiol.* 80, 241–250.

Jensen, O., and Colgin, L. L. (2007). Cross-frequency coupling between neuronal oscillations. *Trends Cogn. Sci. (Regul. Ed.)* 11, 267–269.

Jirsa, V. K., and Haken, H. (1996). Field theory of electromagnetic brain activity. *Phys. Rev. Lett.* 77, 960–963.

Jirsa, V. K., and Haken, H. (1997). A derivation of a macroscopic field theory of the brain from the quasi-microscopic neural dynamics. *Physica D* 99, 503–526.

Koch, C., Rapp, M., and Segev, I. (1996). A brief history of time (constants). *Cereb. Cortex* 6, 93–101.

Lamme, V. A., and Roelfsema, P. R. (2000). The distinct modes of vision offered by feedforward and recurrent processing. *Trends Neurosci.* 23, 571–579.

Liley, D. T. J., Cadusch, P. J., and Wright, J. J. (1999). A continuum theory of electrocortical activity. *Neurocomputing* 26, 795–800.

Lisman, J., and Buzsaki, G. (2008). A neural coding scheme formed by the combined function of gamma and theta oscillations. *Schizophr. Bull.* 34, 974–980.

Lumer, E. D., Edelman, G. M., and Tononi, G. (1997). Neural dynamics in a model of the thalamocortical system. *Cereb. Cortex* 7, 207–227.

Menon, V., Freeman, W. J., Cutillo, B. A., Desmond, J. E., Ward, M. F., Bressler, S. L., et al. (1996). Spatio-temporal correlations in human gamma band electrocorticograms. *Electroencephalogr. Clin. Neurophysiol.* 98, 89–102.

Mountcastle, V. B. (1997). *Perceptual Neuroscience: The Cerebral Cortex.* Cambridge: Harvard University Press.

Nunez, P. L. (1974). The brain wave equation: a model for the EEG. *Math. Biosci.* 21, 279–297.

Nunez, P. L. (1981). *Electric Fields of the Brain: The Neurophysics of EEG.* New York: Oxford University Press.

Nunez, P. L. (1995). *Neocortical Dynamics and Human EEG Rhythms.* New York: Oxford University Press.

Nunez, P. L. (2000). Toward a quantitative description of large-scale neocortical dynamic function and EEG. *Behav. Brain Sci.* 23, 371–398; discussion 399–437.

Nunez, P. L., and Srinivasan, R. (2006). *Electric Fields of the Brain: The Neurophysics of EEG,* 2nd Edn. New York: Oxford University Press.

Nunez, P. L., Wingeier, B. M., and Silberstein, R. B. (2001). Spatial-temporal structures of human alpha rhythms: theory, microcurrent sources, multiscale measurements, and global binding of local networks. *Hum. Brain Mapp.* 13, 125–164.

Pinotsis, D. A., Hansen, E., Friston, K. J., and Jirsa, V. K. (2013). Anatomical connectivity and the resting state activity of large cortical networks. *Neuroimage* 65, 127–138.

Pinotsis, D. A., Schwarzkopf, D. S., Litvak, V., Rees, G., Barnes, G., and Friston, K. J. (2012). Dynamic causal modelling of lateral interactions in the visual cortex. *Neuroimage* 66C, 563–576.

Robinson, P. A., Rennie, C. J., and Wright, J. J. (1997). Propagation and stability of waves of electrical activity in the cerebral cortex. *Phys. Rev. E* 55, 826–840.

Romei, V., Rihs, T., Brodbeck, V., and Thut, G. (2008). Resting electroencephalogram alpha-power over posterior sites indexes baseline visual cortex excitability. *Neuroreport* 19, 203–208.

Sarnthein, J., Petsche, H., Rappelsberger, P., Shaw, G. L., and Von Stein, A. (1998). Synchronization between prefrontal and posterior association cortex during human working memory. *Proc. Natl. Acad. Sci. U.S.A.* 95, 7092–7096.

Sarter, M., and Bruno, J. P. (1997). Cognitive functions of cortical acetylcholine: toward a unifying hypothesis. *Brain Res. Brain Res. Rev.* 23, 28–46.

Sauseng, P., Klimesch, W., Doppelmayr, M., Pecherstorfer, T., Freunberger, R., and Hanslmayr, S. (2005). EEG alpha synchronization and functional coupling during top-down processing in a working memory task. *Hum. Brain Mapp.* 26, 148–155.

Schalk, G., and Leuthardt, E. C. (2011). Brain-computer interfaces using electrocorticographic signals. *IEEE Rev. Biomed. Eng.* 4, 140–154.

Scheffzuk, C., Kukushka, V. I., Vyssotski, A. L., Draguhn, A., Tort, A. B., and Brankack, J. (2011). Selective coupling between theta phase and neocortical fast gamma oscillations during REM-sleep in mice. *PLoS ONE* 6:e28489. doi:10.1371/journal.pone.0028489

Srinivasan, R., Bibi, F. A., and Nunez, P. L. (2006). Steady-state visual evoked potentials: distributed local sources and wave-like dynamics are sensitive to flicker frequency. *Brain Topogr.* 18, 167–187.

Thorpe, S., D'zmura, M., and Srinivasan, R. (2012). Lateralization of frequency-specific networks for covert spatial attention to auditory stimuli. *Brain Topogr.* 25, 39–54.

Thorpe, S. D. S., Garcia, J. O., Lee, R. R., Huang, M., and Srinivasan, R. (2011). Spatial attention enhances steady-state visual evoked potentials in the gamma band. *Int. J. Bioelectromagn.* 13, 233–238.

Thut, G., Nietzel, A., Brandt, S. A., and Pascual-Leone, A. (2006). Alpha-band electroencephalographic activity over occipital cortex indexes visuospatial attention bias and predicts visual target detection. *J. Neurosci.* 26, 9494–9502.

Traub, R. D., Jefferys, J. G., and Whittington, M. A. (1997). Simulation of gamma rhythms in networks of interneurons and pyramidal cells. *J. Comput. Neurosci.* 4, 141–150.

von Stein, A., and Sarnthein, J. (2000). Different frequencies for different scales of cortical integration: from local gamma to long range alpha/theta synchronization. *Int. J. Psychophysiol.* 38, 301–313.

Voytek, B., Canolty, R. T., Shestyuk, A., Crone, N. E., Parvizi, J., and Knight, R. T. (2010). Shifts in gamma phase-amplitude coupling frequency from theta to alpha over posterior cortex during visual tasks. *Front. Hum. Neurosci.* 4:191. doi:10.3389/fnhum.2010.00191

Whittington, M. A., Traub, R. D., Kopell, N., Ermentrout, B., and Buhl, E. H. (2000). Inhibition-based rhythms: experimental and mathematical observations on network dynamics. *Int. J. Psychophysiol.* 38, 315–336.

Wilson, H. R., and Cowan, J. D. (1972). Excitatory and inhibitory interactions in localized populations of model neurons. *Biophys. J.* 12, 1–24.

Wilson, H. R., and Cowan, J. D. (1973). A mathematical theory of the functional dynamics of cortical and thalamic nervous tissue. *Kybernetik* 13, 55–80.

Yousif, N. A., and Denham, M. (2005). A population-based model of the nonlinear dynamics of the thalamocortical feedback network displays intrinsic oscillations in the spindling (7–14 Hz) range. *Eur. J. Neurosci.* 22, 3179–3187.

Zhang, H., and Sulzer, D. (2004). Frequency-dependent modulation of dopamine release by nicotine. *Nat. Neurosci.* 7, 581–582.

APPENDIX

THE BASIC WC ANALYSIS

The classical WC model (Wilson and Cowan, 1972, 1973) applies to populations of interacting excitatory and inhibitory neurons in some local neocortical region as indicated in **Figure 1**. An important WC assumption is that axon propagation delays are negligible; that is, all WC delays are due to PSP rise and decay times. WC is then a strictly local model and represents the opposite limiting case to global models in which delays are axonal, especially in the longer corticocortical axons forming most of human white matter (Nunez, 1974; Nunez and Srinivasan, 2006). These distinct local and global models have been shown to be fully compatible and may be combined into local/global models (Jirsa and Haken, 1996; Nunez, 2000).

The basic WC dependent variables are the *fractions of excitatory and inhibitory active cells* (dimensionless action potential densities) $E(t)$, $I(t)$, which can evidently exhibit very high frequency jitter not treated in the analysis. Rather, the WC equations are expressed in terms of coarse grained (in time) excitatory $\langle E(t)\rangle$ and inhibitory $\langle I(t)\rangle$ action potential densities, where the critical point $\langle E(t)\rangle, \langle I(t)\rangle = (0,0)$ is considered by WC to be an equilibrium background state occurring when the external (afferent) driving function $P(t) = 0$. Thus, the variables $\langle E(t)\rangle$, $\langle I(t)\rangle$ are allowed to take on negative values by WC, an inaccurate and (as we show here) unnecessary approximation to their physiological interpretation as fractions of active cells. The WC equations (1.3.1 and 1.3.2 from the 1973 paper) are

$$\begin{aligned}\tau_E \frac{d\langle E(t)\rangle}{dt} &= -\langle E(t)\rangle + [1 - r_E\langle E(t)\rangle]\, S_E\,[P(t) \\ &\quad + w_{EE}\langle E(t)\rangle - w_{IE} I(t)] \\ \tau_I \frac{d\langle I(t)\rangle}{dt} &= -\langle I(t)\rangle + [1 - r_I\langle I(t)\rangle]\, S_I\,[w_{EI}\langle E(t)\rangle \\ &\quad - w_{II}\langle I(t)\rangle] \end{aligned} \quad \text{(A1)}$$

Here we drop the spatial dependence x of all variables since axon speeds are assumed to be infinite implying that neural spatial separations have no effect on dynamic behaviors in this approximation. We also distinguish between the excitatory and inhibitory membrane time constants τ_E, τ_I. In addition, we only allow excitatory afferent input $P(t)$.

SOME ISSUES WITH THE ORIGINAL WC ANALYSIS

1. WC write *the proportion of sensitive excitatory cells* (neurons currently firing or in their refractory periods r_E) as $R_E(t) = 1 - \int_{t-r_E}^{t} E(t')dt'$. This is not dimensionally correct and leads to the dimensionally incorrect Eq. A1. The WC equation also yields the incorrect result $R_E(t) \to 1$ as the refractory period $r_E \to 0$. The correct expression is

$$\begin{aligned} R_E(t) &= 1 - \frac{1}{r_E}\int_{t-r_E}^{t} E(t')dt' \\ R_E(t) &\to 1 - E(t) \text{ when } r_E \to 0 \end{aligned} \quad \text{(A2)}$$

In this limit, the sensitive population $R_E(t)$ consists of all cells not firing at time t. The excitatory and inhibitory integrals should have been divided by the refractory times r_E, r_I, equivalent to setting $r_E, r_I = 1$, in Eq. A1, a simple corrective step often adopted by others using the WC model.

2. Negative values of $\langle E(t)\rangle$, $\langle I(t)\rangle$ are not realistic physiologically for essentially the same reason. During times when $E(t)$, $I(t) < 0$, the fractions of sensitive cells $R_E(t), R_I(t) > 1$, which is also inconsistent with realistic physiology. By contrast, the modified WC model presented here forces

$$\langle E(t)\rangle, \langle I(t)\rangle \geq 0, \text{ for } -\infty < t < +\infty.$$

3. WC choose sigmoid response functions such that $S_E(0) = S_I(0) = 0$ in order to force (0,0) to be a critical (equilibrium) point where the variable time derivatives equal zero. Such critical points may be either state or unstable. If a critical point is stable, any brain dynamic state coming sufficiently close to this point will become fixed (forever static or "brain dead"). Of more interest to us are unstable critical points associated with on-going oscillations (limit cycles), possibly underlying EEG. In WC, the tissue response functions can become negative, a physiological impossibility; thus, in our following modified analysis, the WC conditions are replaced by

$$\begin{aligned} S_E[P(t), \langle E(t)\rangle, \langle I(t)\rangle] &\geq 0 \\ S_I[\langle E(t)\rangle, \langle I(t)\rangle] &\geq 0 \end{aligned} \quad \text{(A3)}$$

4. WC interpret the WC parameter μ as a single membrane time constant. Based on the classic solution of the cable equation and the distribution of excitatory synapses on dendrites with inhibitory synapses typically near cell bodies and our increased appreciation of wide ranges of excitatory and inhibitory time constants τ_E, τ_I, we consider cases $\tau_E \neq \tau_I$.

A MODIFIED VERSION OF THE WC ANALYSIS

Define the non-dimensional time $t_1 = \frac{t}{\tau_E}$ and time constant ratio $A = \frac{\tau_I}{\tau_E}$ so that with rescaled variables Eq. A1 become

$$\begin{aligned} \frac{d\langle E\rangle}{dt_1} &= -\langle E\rangle + (1 - \langle E\rangle)\, S_E\,(P + w_{EE}\langle E\rangle - w_{IE}\langle I\rangle) \\ A\frac{d\langle I\rangle}{dt_1} &= -\langle I\rangle + (1 - \langle I\rangle)\, S_I\,(w_{EI}\langle E\rangle - w_{II}\langle I\rangle) \end{aligned} \quad \text{(A4)}$$

Here the non-dimensional parameter A may range from somewhat less than one to as high as perhaps 5. For convenience we drop the subscript 1 on the non-dimensional time variable. We introduce the new dependent variables $X_E(t), X_I(t)$, which provide perturbations about the critical point (E_0, I_0)

$$\begin{aligned} \langle E(t)\rangle &= E_0 + X_E(t) \\ \langle I(t)\rangle &= I_0 + X_I(t) \end{aligned} \quad \text{(A5)}$$

We assume that the input function $P(t)$ is exclusively excitatory such that $P(t) \geq 0$ at all times. The following conditions follow from the variable definitions

$$0 \le E_0 + X_E(t) \le 1$$
$$0 \le I_0 + X_I(t) \le 1 \quad \text{(A6)}$$

Equations (A4) then yield

$$\frac{dX_E}{dt} = -E_0 - X_E + (1 - E_0 - X_E)\, S_E\, [P + w_{EE}(E_0 + X_E) - w_{IE}(I_0 + X_I)]$$
$$A\frac{dX_I}{dt} = -I_0 - X_I + (1 - I_0 - X_I)\, S_I\, [w_{EI}(E_0 + X_E) - w_{II}(I_0 + X_I)] \quad \text{(A7)}$$

The sigmoid functions S_E, S_I are chosen here such that (E_0, I_0) is a critical point when $P(t) = 0$. Thus, we choose the following alternate sigmoid tissue response functions.

$$S_I = \frac{1}{1 + \exp[-w_{EI}(E_0 + X_E) + w_{II}(I_0 + X_I) + K_I]} \quad \text{(A8)}$$
$$S_E = \frac{1}{1 + \exp[-w_{EE}(E_0 + X_E) + w_{ie}(I_0 + X_I) + K_E]} \quad \text{(A9)}$$

The constants K_E, K_I are added to the original WC sigmoid functions, thereby determining the response range during oscillations about fixed points. This choice of the forms of the sigmoid response functions insures that (1) (E_0, I_0) or $(X,Y) = (0,0)$ is a critical point and (2) $0 \le S_E \le 1$ and $0 \le S_I \le 1$. Substitution of Eqs A8 and A9 into Eq. A7 and setting $X_E(t) = X_I(t) = 0$ yields the sigmoid constants in terms of the critical point

$$K_I = w_{EI} E_0 - w_{II} I_0 + Log\left[\frac{1}{I_0} - 2\right] \quad \text{(A10)}$$
$$K_E = w_{EE} E_0 - w_{IE} I_0 + Log\left[\frac{1}{E_0} - 2\right] \quad \text{(A11)}$$

Substitution of Eqs A10 and A11 into Eqs A8 and A9 yields

$$S_I\,[w_{EI}(E_0 + X_E) - w_{II}(I_0 + X_I)] = \frac{1}{1 + \left(\frac{1}{I_0} - 2\right)\exp(-w_{EI}X_E + w_{II}X_I)} \quad I_0 < \frac{1}{2} \quad \text{(A12)}$$
$$S_E\,[w_{EE}(E_0 + X_E) - w_{IE}(I_0 + X_I)] = \frac{1}{1 + \left(\frac{1}{E_0} - 2\right)\exp(-w_{EE}X_E + w_{IE}X_I)} \quad E_0 < \frac{1}{2} \quad \text{(A13)}$$

PHASE-PLANE ANALYSIS

We assume $w_{II} \cong 0$ in all of the following analyses based on our preliminary studies: In simulations with non-zero w_{II} the effect is only to set the activity level of the system and has no significant influence on the dynamics. The first step in the analysis of Eq. A7 is to find the nature of the critical point (0,0). To accomplish this we expand the functions $F(X_E, X_I)$ and $G(X_E, X_I)$ about (0,0), where these functions are the expressions on the right sides of Eq. A7, that is

$$F(X_E, X_I) = -E_0 - X_E + (1 - E_0 - X_E)\, S_e$$
$$G(X_E, X_I) = [-I_0 - X_I + (1 - I_0 - X_I)\, S_i]/A \quad \text{(A14)}$$

Taylor expansion about the critical point (0,0) yields equations of the general form

$$\frac{dX_E}{dt} = F(X_E, X_I) \cong F(0,0) + \left(\frac{\partial F}{\partial X_E}\right)_0 X_E + \left(\frac{\partial F}{\partial X_I}\right)_0 X_I \equiv aX_E + bX_I$$
$$\frac{dX_I}{dt} = G(X_E, X_I) \cong G(0,0) + \left(\frac{\partial G}{\partial X_E}\right)_0 X_E + \left(\frac{\partial G}{\partial X_I}\right)_0 X_I \equiv cX_E + dX_I \quad \text{(A15)}$$

Here we have forced $F(0,0) = G(0,0) = 0$ by proper choice of the constants K_E, K_I in Eqs A10 and A11. The partial derivatives are evaluated at (0,0) yielding the parameters (a, b, c, d). Eq. A15 then consist of two first order linear equations governing the dynamic behavior of the non-linear system close to (0,0). Define the parameters $\beta = a + d$ and $\gamma = ad - bc$; the eigenvalues $\lambda_{1,2}$ of the linear system satisfy $\lambda^2 - \beta\lambda + \gamma = 0$ with solution

$$\lambda_{1,2} = \frac{1}{2}\left(\beta \pm \sqrt{\beta^2 - 4\gamma}\right) \quad \text{(A16)}$$

We are mainly interested in oscillatory solutions about the critical point (0,0); that is, stable limit cycle solutions. These are expected when (0,0) is an *unstable* spiral, which occurs when $\beta > 0$ and $\beta^2 < 4\gamma$. By contrast, stable spirals result in damped oscillations. Saddle points and nodes result in non-oscillatory solutions (stable or unstable) that are of minimal interest here.

Consider the following example with $E_0 = I_0$. The critical point (E_0, I_0) is unstable if the following condition is met

$$w_{EE} > \frac{A + 1}{AE_0(1 - 2E_0)} \quad 0 < E_0 < \frac{1}{2} \quad \text{(A17)}$$

Note that $A = \frac{\tau_I}{\tau_E}$ so if inhibitory time constants are much shorter than excitatory time constants, larger values of w_{EE} are required to produce linear instability. For the physiologically interesting range $0.1 < E_0 < 0.4$ and $A = 1$, all $w_{EE} > 25$ cause the fixed point to be unstable.

For the case $E_0 = I_0$ and $A = 1$, the fixed point is a spiral if

$$w_{EE} < 2\sqrt{w_{IE} w_{EI}} \quad \text{(A18)}$$

By combining Eqs A17 and A18 we find the necessary (but possibly not sufficient) conditions for a stable limit cycle about (E_0, E_0) when $A = 1$, that is

$$\frac{2}{E_0(1 - 2E_0)} < w_{EE} < 2\sqrt{w_{IE} w_{EI}} \quad \text{(A19)}$$

If this condition is met, the corresponding spiral frequency is

$$\omega_{spiral} = N(E_0)\sqrt{4 w_{IE} w_{EI} - w_{EE}^2} \quad \text{(A20)}$$

Here the numerical factor lies in the range $0.00790 < N(E_0) < 0.0294$ if $0.1 < E_0 < 0.4$. An *unstable* spiral point at (E_0, I_0)

suggests a likely *stable limit cycle*, but the limit cycle frequency will not generally equal the (linear) spiral frequency. If w_{EE} exceeds the upper limit in Eq. A19 an unstable node or saddle point will occur. In this case the solutions $X_E(t)$, $X_I(t)$ are likely to grow beyond physiologically realistic ranges, implying that the basic WC equations are no longer valid.

14

Neural mass modeling of power-line magnetic fields effects on brain activity

J. Modolo[1,2,3]*, A. W. Thomas[1,2,3] and A. Legros[1,2,3,4]

[1] Human Threshold Research Group, Lawson Health Research Institute, London, ON, Canada
[2] Department of Medical Biophysics, Western University, London, ON, Canada
[3] Department of Medical Imaging, Western University, London, ON, Canada
[4] School of Kinesiology, Western University, London, ON, Canada

***Correspondence:**
J. Modolo, Human Threshold Research Group, Lawson Health Research Institute, 268 Grosvenor Street, London, ON N6A4V2, Canada.
e-mail: jmodolo@lawsonimaging.ca

Neural mass models are an appropriate framework to study brain activity, combining a high degree of biological realism while being mathematically tractable. These models have been used, with a certain success, to simulate brain electric (electroencephalography, EEG) and metabolic (functional magnetic resonance imaging, fMRI) activity. However, concrete applications of neural mass models have remained limited to date. Motivated by experimental results obtained in humans, we propose in this paper a neural mass model designed to study the interaction between power-line magnetic fields (MFs) (60 Hz in North America) and brain activity. The model includes pyramidal cells; dendrite-projecting, slow GABAergic neurons; soma-projecting, fast GABAergic neurons; and glutamatergic interneurons. A simple phenomenological model of interaction between the induced electric field and neuron membranes is also considered, along with a model of post-synaptic calcium concentration and associated changes in synaptic weights Simulated EEG signals are produced in a simple protocol, both in the absence and presence of a 60 Hz MF. These results are discussed based on results obtained previously in humans. Notably, results highlight that (1) EEG alpha (8–12 Hz) power can be modulated by weak membrane depolarizations induced by the exposure; (2) the level of input noise has a significant impact on EEG power modulation; and (3) the threshold value in MF flux density resulting in a significant effect on the EEG depends on the type of neuronal populations modulated by the MF exposure. Results obtained from the model shed new light on the effects of power-line MFs on brain activity, and will provide guidance in future human experiments. This may represent a valuable contribution to international regulation agencies setting guidelines on MF values to which the general public and workers can be exposed.

Keywords: neural mass models, power-line magnetic fields, electroencephalogram (EEG), synaptic plasticity, brain stimulation

INTRODUCTION

Since the pioneering work of Wilson and Cowan (1973) and Amari (1977), neural field models have been increasingly used, expanded and studied by a developing multidisciplinary community including: mathematicians, physicists, neuroscientists, medical imaging scientists *etcetera*. Neural field models provide a concise, yet insightful description of cortical activity. This theory has not only led to successful reproduction of numerous experimental results, but also to the prediction of a certain number of phenomena that have been observed *in vivo* (for a review of these phenomena, see Modolo et al., 2010). A popular simplification of neural field models consists in neglecting the role of space, consider neural populations present in cortical columns (such as pyramidal neurons) and to consider a connectivity matrix between the different neural masses considered (Wendling et al., 2002; Sotero and Trujillo-Barreto, 2008; Bojak et al., 2010). This approach has been used to build large-scale models of brain activity, including models simulating the electroencephalogram (EEG), or the blood oxygen level-dependent signal (BOLD) reflecting metabolic activity of brain tissue (Wendling et al., 2002; Sotero and Trujillo-Barreto, 2008; Bojak et al., 2010). Indeed, since neural mass models are tractable and make the link between local variables and observables, these models appear as an excellent comprise between biological realism and computational complexity. Therefore, here we present an application of neural mass model to a specific question that many teams over the world have been tackling for a number of years using various neuroimaging modalities: how do power-line frequency (60 Hz in North America) magnetic fields (MFs) interact with human brain activity (interaction mechanisms), and how does it translate into observable outcomes (neuroimaging data such as EEG, motor/cognitive performance)?

The effects of extremely low-frequency (categorized as being <300 Hz) MF such as power-line MF on human neurophysiology have been studied for several decades. Despite an impressive amount of experimental data *in vitro*, *in vivo*, and in humans, a complete understanding of the interaction mechanisms and associated effects is still to be achieved. One complication in comparing outcomes from these studies is the wide range of MF flux densities, MF exposure setups, and exposure protocols used (Crasson, 2003). First, significant work has been done has been done *in vivo* and *in vitro* in order to characterize the effects of electric fields in terms of membrane potential perturbation, excitability and neural network oscillations (Jefferys et al., 2003; Bikson et al., 2004; Deans et al., 2007; Fröhlich and McCormick, 2010; Reato et al., 2010). These studies have highlighted the role of neuronal morphology and orientation were critical in understanding the interaction with electric field, but also that membrane depolarization far below the firing threshold can influence the activity of neuronal networks. Second, among the reported effects in humans, let us mention the modulation of pain threshold (Ghione et al., 2005), effects on resting tremor (Legros and Beuter, 2005), modulations in functional brain activity as measured by BOLD (Legros et al., 2011), interference with learning in a short-term memory test (Corbacio et al., 2011). The most established interaction mechanism of MF exposure consists in induced currents, resulting from Faraday's law of induction, stating that a time-varying MF induces a time-varying electric field. This electric field will induce charge movement, creating a current. This is termed as the *induced current mechanism* (National Institute of Environmental Health Sciences of the National Institutes of Health, 1998). The induced current mechanism will be the mechanism considered in this paper. Interestingly, several studies have reported lasting effects associated with ELF MF exposure, i.e., an effect that is still detectable after cessation of the exposure. Using a specific pulsed MF, modulations of the EEG have been observed post-exposure (Cook et al., 2004, 2005). In the case of 60 Hz MF in the millitesla range (1.8 and 3 mT), modulations of the BOLD signal measured in humans during motor (finger tapping) and cognitive (mental rotation) tasks (Legros et al., 2010; Miller et al., 2010) have been found to be modulated post-exposure.

The interest for the interaction between power-line MF and human neurophysiology is twofold. First, there is a growing concern from the general public regarding the possible deleterious effects of power-line MF on human health, even if such negative effects remain to be demonstrated. Second, international regulation agencies such as ICNIRP (International Commission on Non-Ionizing Radiation Protection, http://www.icnirp.de) need results from the scientific literature to set their exposure guidelines (ICNIRP, 2010), aiming to protect the general public and workers, that are used by governments. One of the most long awaited data is the threshold in MF flux density at 60 Hz resulting in detectable effects in humans. One well-known effect of ELF MF exposure is magnetophosphenes, the perception of flickering lights in the visual field in the presence of a sufficiently strong MF. ICNIRP states that: "*Since the perception of magnetophosphenes constitutes the most reliable effect of MF exposure on human biology, this serves as a basis for the ICNIRP guidelines*" (ICNIRP, 2010). However, no data is available at 60 Hz regarding threshold values, therefore new approaches that could assist in the interpretation of existing experimental results, but also in the prediction of new results such as an estimation of threshold values that could be tested experimentally, would constitute significant advances in the field.

In order to shed light on the mechanisms involved in lasting effects of 60 Hz MF exposure on human neurophysiology, and also provide an estimate of the threshold value resulting in detectable changes in EEG caused by 60 Hz MF exposure, we present in this paper a neural mass model aiming to model brain tissue dynamics at different time scales, bridging biophysical mechanisms with changes in observables. Among the panel of brain tissue dynamics models available, the approach initiated by Jansen and Rit (1995), consisting in considering sub-populations of neurons synaptically connected; later extended and improved by Wendling et al. (2002), provides a meaningful and accurate description of cortical dynamics. Indeed, such models have been successfully applied to understand the transition between baseline EEG and epileptic activity (Wendling et al., 2002, 2005; Molaee-Ardekani et al., 2010). First, we present an extension of the neural mass model developed by Sotero and Trujillo-Barreto (2008), by including a population of fast GABAergic neurons as suggested by Wendling et al. (2002). Second, we include a simple biophysical model of interaction between the 60 Hz MF and neuronal activity, along with a model of synaptic plasticity changes related to post-synaptic calcium concentration levels (Shouval et al., 2002a,b). Third, we use this model to investigate *in silico* the effects of 60 Hz MF on cortical dynamics, notably to evaluate the threshold in MF flux density resulting in detectable changes in variables of interest. The role of synaptic input noise, neuronal populations modulated by the exposure, and synaptic plasticity are also explored. Finally, we discuss future directions of research using this modeling approach.

MATERIALS AND METHODS

NEURAL MASS MODEL

In order to develop a biologically grounded model to study the effect of 60 Hz MF on neuronal activity, we have extend the thalamo-cortical model proposed by Sotero and Trujillo-Barreto (2008) by including a population of soma-projecting, fast inhibitory γ-amino-butyric acid (GABA) interneurons to extend the possible dynamical repertoire of the model [as shown by Wendling et al. (2002)]. The proposed modification of the block diagram proposed by Sotero and Trujillo-Barreto (2008) used to describe the thalamo-cortical model is the following:

Model equations are obtained by using the fact that the synaptic response function (Green's function) for a type of synapse i (e.g., glutamatergic) writes as $V_i(t) = A_i.a_i.t.\exp(-a_i.t)$, where A_i is the response amplitude and a_i the response time constant. Considering the temporal operator $\hat{L} = \frac{d^2}{dt^2} + 2a_i\frac{d}{dt} + a_i^2$, and using the fact that the synaptic response is a Greens' function for the temporal operator, we can use $\hat{L}V_i(t) = \delta(t)$ to write the following neural mass equation:

$$\frac{d^2}{dt^2}V_i(t) + 2.a.\frac{d}{dt}V_i(t) + a^2.V_i(t) = A.a.\upsilon_i(t) \tag{1}$$

where $\upsilon_i(t)$is the incoming firing rate. It is often practical to write Equation (1) under the form of a system of two first-order differential equations:

$$\begin{aligned}\frac{d}{dt}V_i(t) &= y_i(t)\\ \frac{d}{dt}y_i(t) &= A.a.\upsilon_i(t) - 2.a.\frac{d}{dt}y_i(t) + a^2.V_i(t)\end{aligned} \tag{2}$$

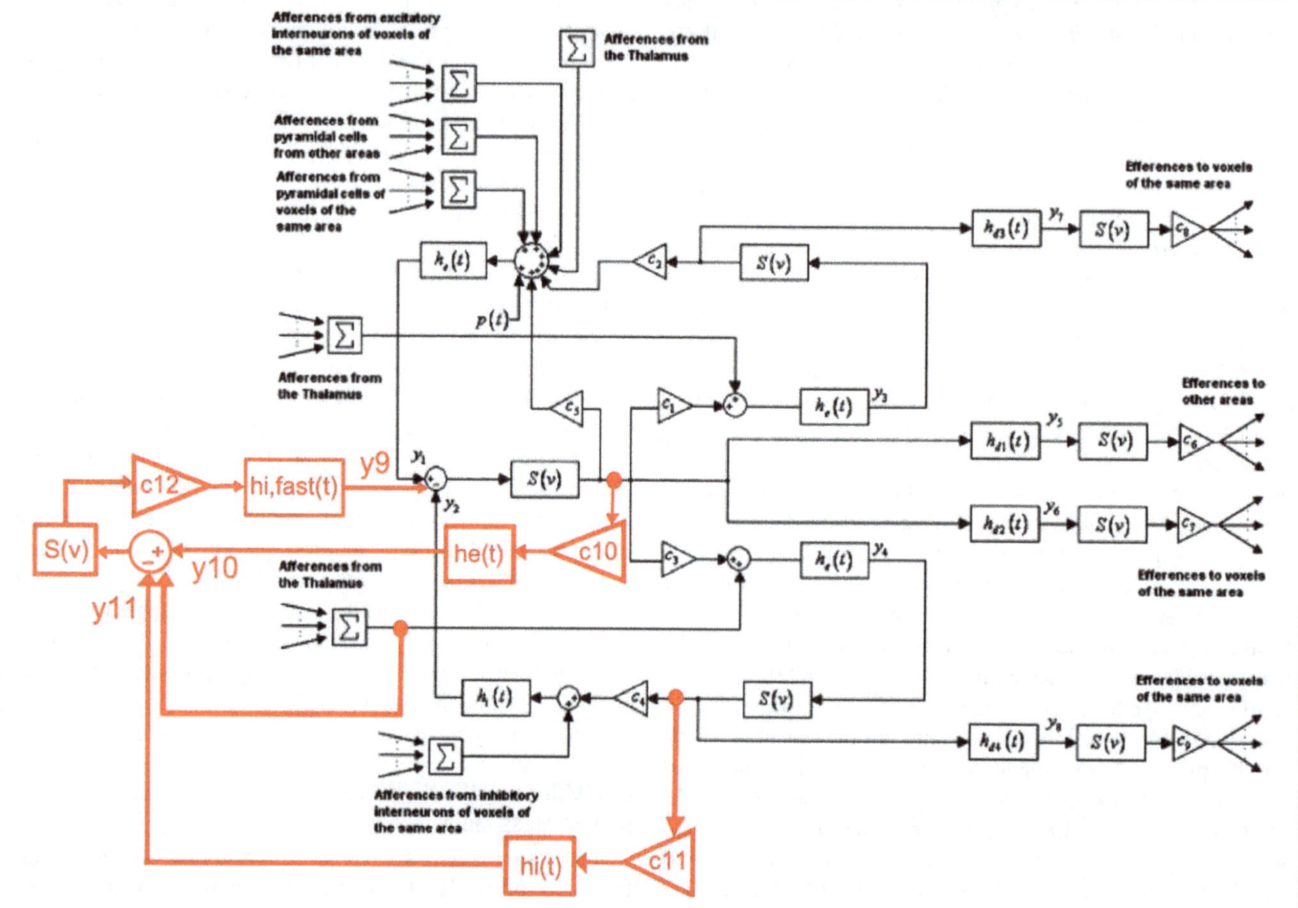

FIGURE 1 | Proposed extension of the Sotero et al. model of cortical dynamics (figure modified from (Sotero and Trujillo-Barreto, 2008); with permission). The inclusion of the new population of fast GABAergic neurons and its connectivity with other neuronal populations is highlighted in red.

Using this principle for each block of EPSP/IPSP presented in **Figure 1**, it is possible to formulate our extended thalamo-cortical model as a system of 22 differential equations (6 new equations corresponding to the new population of fast inhibitory interneurons, its feedback loop with pyramidal neurons, and its inhibitory input from slow inhibitory interneurons) presented below:

$$
\begin{aligned}
\dot{y}_1^{nj}(t) &= y_{12}^{nj}(t)\\
\dot{y}_2^{nj}(t) &= y_{13}^{nj}(t)\\
\dot{y}_3^{nj}(t) &= y_{14}^{nj}(t)\\
\dot{y}_4^{nj}(t) &= y_{15}^{nj}(t)\\
\dot{y}_5^{nj}(t) &= y_{16}^{nj}(t)\\
\dot{y}_6^{nj}(t) &= y_{17}^{nj}(t)\\
\dot{y}_7^{nj}(t) &= y_{18}^{nj}(t)\\
\dot{y}_8^{nj}(t) &= y_{19}^{nj}(t)\\
\dot{y}_9^{nj}(t) &= y_{20}^{nj}(t)\\
\dot{y}_{10}^{nj}(t) &= y_{21}^{nj}(t)\\
\dot{y}_{11}^{nj}(t) &= y_{22}^{nj}(t)\\
\dot{y}_{12}^{nj}(t) &= A.a.\left\{c_5.S\left[y_1^{nj}(t) - y_2^{nj}(t) - y_9^{nj}(t)\right] + c_2.S\left[y_3^{nj}(t)\right] + K^{th,n}c_3^t.S\left[x_4(t)\right]\right\}\\
&\quad + A.a.\left\{\sum_{\substack{m=1\\ m\neq j}}^{M_n}\left(k_{e1}^{mj}.c_7.S\left[y_6^{mn}(t)\right] + k_{e2}^{mj}.c_8.S\left[y_7^{mn}(t)\right]\right) + \sum_{\substack{i=1\\ i\neq n}}^{N} K^{i,n}\sum_{m=1}^{M_i} c_6.S\left[y_5^{im}(t)\right]\right\}\\
&\quad - 2.a.y_{12}^{nj}(t) - a^2 y_1^{nj}(t) + A.a.p^{nj}(t)
\end{aligned}
\tag{3}
$$

$$\dot{y}_{13}^{nj}(t) = B.b.\left\{ c_4.S\left[y_4^{nj}(t)\right] + \sum_{\substack{m=1 \\ m \neq j}}^{M_n} \left(k_i^{mj}.c_9.S\left[y_8^{mn}(t)\right]\right) \right\}$$

$$-2.b.y_{13}^{nj}(t) - b^2 y_2^{nj}(t)$$

$$\dot{y}_{14}^{nj}(t) = A.a.\left\{c_1.S\left[y_1^{nj}(t) - y_2^{nj}(t) - y_9^{nj}(t)\right] + K^{th,n}.c_4^t S\left[x_5(t)\right]\right\}$$

$$-2.a.y_{14}^{nj}(t) - a^2 y_3^{nj}(t)$$

$$\dot{y}_{15}^{nj}(t) = A.a.\left\{c_3.S\left[y_1^{nj}(t) - y_2^{nj}(t) - y_9^{nj}(t)\right] + K^{th,n}.c_5^t S\left[x_6(t)\right]\right\}$$

$$-2.a.y_{15}^{nj}(t) - a^2 y_4^{nj}(t)$$

$$\dot{y}_{16}^{nj}(t) = A.a_{d1}.\left\{S\left[y_1^{nj}(t) - y_2^{nj}(t) - y_9^{nj}(t)\right]\right\}$$

$$-2.a_{d1}.y_{16}^{nj}(t) - a_{d1}^2 y_5^{nj}(t)$$

$$\dot{y}_{17}^{nj}(t) = A.a_{d2}.\left\{S\left[y_1^{nj}(t) - y_2^{nj}(t) - y_9^{nj}(t)\right]\right\}$$

$$-2.a_{d2}.y_{17}^{nj}(t) - a_{d2}^2 y_6^{nj}(t)$$

$$\dot{y}_{18}^{nj}(t) = A.a_{d3}.\left\{S\left[y_3^{nj}(t)\right]\right\} - 2.a_{d3}.y_{18}^{nj}(t) - a_{d3}^2 y_7^{nj}(t)$$

$$\dot{y}_{19}^{nj}(t) = B.b_{d4}.\left\{S\left[y_4^{nj}(t)\right]\right\} - 2.b_{d4}.y_{19}^{nj}(t) - b_{d4}^2 y_8^{nj}(t)$$

$$\dot{y}_{20}^{nj}(t) = G.g.\left\{c_{12}.S\left[y_{10}^{nj}(t) - y_{11}^{nj}(t)\right] + K^{th,n}.c_5^t S\left[x_6(t)\right]\right\}$$

$$-2.g.y_{20}^{nj}(t) - g^2 y_9^{nj}(t)$$

$$\dot{y}_{21}^{nj}(t) = A.a.\left\{c_{10}.S\left[y_1^{nj}(t) - y_2^{nj}(t) - y_9^{nj}(t)\right]\right\}$$

$$-2.a.y_{21}^{nj}(t) - a^2 y_{10}^{nj}(t)$$

$$\dot{y}_{22}^{nj}(t) = B.b.\left\{c_{11}.S\left[y_4^{nj}(t)\right]\right\} - 2.b.y_{22}^{nj}(t) - b^2 y_{11}^{nj}(t)$$

The equations describing the activity of the thalamus, composed of a population of thalamocortical cells and a population of reticular cells are [modified from Sotero and Trujillo-Barreto (2008)]:

$$\dot{x}_1(t) = x_7(t)$$

$$\dot{x}_2(t) = x_8(t)$$

$$\dot{x}_3(t) = x_9(t)$$

$$\dot{x}_4(t) = x_{10}(t)$$

$$\dot{x}_5(t) = x_{11}(t)$$

$$\dot{x}_6(t) = x_{12}(t)$$

$$\dot{x}_7(t) = A_t.\grave{a}_t.\left\{\sum_{i=1}^{N} K^{th,i} \sum_{m=1}^{M_i} c_6.S\left[y_5^{im}(t) + p_{th}(t)\right]\right\}$$

$$-2.a_t.x_7(t) - a_t^2 x_1(t)$$

$$\dot{x}_8(t) = B_t.b_t.c_{2t}.S\left[c_{1t}x_3(t)\right] - 2.b_t.x_8(t) - b_t^2 x_2(t)$$

$$\dot{x}_9(t) = A_t.a_t.S\left[x_1(t) - x_2(t)\right] - 2.a_t.x_9(t) - a_t^2 x_3(t)$$

$$\dot{x}_{10}(t) = A_t.a_{d1t}.S\left[x_1(t) - x_2(t)\right] - 2.a_{d1t}.x_{10}(t) - a_{d1t}^2 x_4(t)$$

$$\dot{x}_{11}(t) = A_t.a_{d2t}.S\left[x_1(t) - x_2(t)\right] - 2.a_{d2t}.x_{11}(t) - a_{d2t}^2 x_5(t)$$

$$\dot{x}_{12}(t) = A_t.a_{d3t}.S\left[x_1(t) - x_2(t)\right] - 2.a_{d3t}.x_{12}(t) - a_{d3t}^2 x_6(t) \quad (4)$$

The physical meaning and values of model parameters are detailed in **Table A1** (Appendix section). For more details, the reader can refer to Sotero and Trujillo-Barreto (2008). Overall, the model is composed of 22 differential equations describing cortical dynamics of four different neuronal populations (pyramidal neurons, glutamatergic interneurons, fast/slow GABAergic neurons, and 12 differential equations defining thalamic activity). Therefore, this set of 34 differential equations describes the thalamocortical activity including time delays between cortical areas, connectivity parameters, synaptic responses derived from neurophysiology, and a biologically plausible (even if it is obviously simplified) circuitry between the neuronal populations considered. **Table A1** provided in Appendix summarizes the parameters used in the model, with new parameters added due to the population of fast inhibitory interneurons that have been highlighted.

MODEL OF INTERACTION BETWEEN 60 Hz EXPOSURE AND NEURON MEMBRANES

In order to model the interaction between the electric field induced by 60 Hz MF exposure and neural tissue, we have used the ≪ $\lambda \cdot E$ ≫ model in order to simulate the modulation of neuron membrane polarization (Molaee-Ardekani et al., 2013). In this model, the membrane depolarization dV in the presence of an electric field **E** is a function of a constant $\boldsymbol{\lambda}$ termed "polarization length" (Radman et al., 2009). More precisely, the membrane depolarization is expressed as $dV = \boldsymbol{\lambda} \cdot \boldsymbol{E}$, where $\boldsymbol{\lambda}$ is a vector oriented along the neuron fibre, and $\boldsymbol{E}$ is the electric field vector. This expression is valid for a static electric field. In the case of a time-varying electric field (such as the electric field induced by 60 Hz MF), a frequency-dependent term needs to be included (Gianni et al., 2006), resulting in:

$$dV = \frac{\lambda \cdot E}{\sqrt{1 + \omega^2 \tau^2}} \quad (5)$$

where $\omega = 2\pi f$, f being the frequency (in our case, $f = 60$ Hz), and τ is the polarization time constant. In order to use Equation (5), describing membrane depolarization induced by the induced electric field, at the level of a neuronal population, we made the following assumptions: (1) the induced 60 Hz electric field is homogeneous in space at the level of the neural mass (i.e., the MF flux density is constant at each point of the cortical column); (2) the MF-induced membrane depolarization is applied to pyramidal neurons only because of their large size compared to other types of neurons in the human cortex; (3) pyramidal neurons in a given neural mass all have the same spatial orientation. Taken together, assumptions (1) and (3) result in identical dV values for all pyramidal neurons in a neural mass at a given time. These assumptions lead to the use Equation (3) in the context of a neural mass model.

This was achieved by modifying the expression of the total post-synaptic potential at the level of pyramidal neurons:

$$y_1(t) - y_2(t) - y_9(t) \rightarrow y_1(t) - y_2(t) - y_9(t) + dV(t) \quad (6)$$

As it is commonly calculated in neural mass model, the EEG signal was computed as the summation of excitatory and inhibitory post-synaptic potential at the level of pyramidal neurons:

$$EEG(t) = y_1(t) - y_2(t) - y_9(t) + dV(t) \quad (7)$$

Let us mention that, even if the MF-induced depolarization is included in the model as a simple additive perturbation, it has the potential to induce non-linear effects. Indeed, the effective potential at the level of pyramidal neurons (7) is used as an input for other neuronal populations, and is transformed from a potential to a firing rate using a sigmoid function, which is fundamentally non-linear. In the "Results" section, we have used arbitrary values for the field-induced membrane depolarization dV, guided by preliminary simulation results. Based on dV values resulting in significant changes in the EEG alpha power with or without synaptic plasticity in the model, we will provide an estimate of the corresponding level of 60 Hz MF flux density. This will provide us with an order of magnitude of the 60 Hz MF flux density threshold value that should result in effects detectable experimentally in humans.

In our simulations, we focused specifically on the EEG alpha rhythm (8–12 Hz). The reason of this choice is twofold. First, as mentioned in the Introduction, there is converging evidence that extremely low-frequency MF in the millitesla range, such as 60 Hz MF, can induce EEG alpha activity modulation. Second, the model we have developed is basically an extension of the Jansen and Rit model, designed to model EEG alpha activity. It is possible to reproduce other types of EEG rhythms (e.g., beta −13 to 30 Hz), for example by introducing heterogeneity in the time constant of neural populations over different neural masses (Wendling et al., 2002), which exceeds the scope of this paper.

BIOPHYSICAL MODEL OF SYNAPTIC PLASTICITY

In order to investigate the hypothesis that 60 Hz MF exposure might modulate with human neurophysiology by modulating synaptic plasticity, we have implemented a simplified model of synaptic plasticity, based on the biophysical model developed by Shouval et al. (2002a,b). It is now well accepted that the mechanisms of long-term synaptic potentiation and depression (LTP/LTD, respectively) involve changes in post-synaptic calcium concentration and the trafficking of α-amino-3-hydroxy-5-methyl-4-isoxazole-propionic acid (AMPA) glutamate receptors between the intracellular medium and the synapse site. Depending on the calcium concentration, AMPA receptors can either insert into the membrane at the level of the synaptic cleft, or undergo an endocytosis, which is termed *receptor trafficking* (Collingridge et al., 2004). An increase in the number of AMPA receptors at the synaptic level will increase the number of glutamate molecules that can bind on post-synaptic membranes, thereby increasing membrane depolarization during a synaptic event. Consequently, the number of post-synaptic AMPA receptors is directly proportional to the synaptic weight. The model proposed by Shouval et al. (2002a,b) has been a significant progress in the modeling of the biophysical processes at play during LTP/LTD. This model is based on the "calcium control hypothesis," according to which the level of post-synaptic calcium is the main factor regulating the exocytosis/endocytosis rate of AMPA receptors, and therefore the dynamics of synaptic plasticity changes.

We have adapted the model by Shouval et al. (2002a,b) to our neural mass model, and despite some simplifications with respects to the original model; our synaptic plasticity model captures some of its essential features. Based on the experimental literature on 60 Hz MF exposure effects on the EEG alpha rhythm, we assume that (1) no qualitative changes of EEG dynamics will occur due to 60 Hz MF exposure, changes will be purely quantitative (i.e., EEG alpha rhythm amplitude/spectral power changes, but no qualitative change in dynamical regime such as a transition toward high-amplitude, low-frequency spiking); (2) the coupling between the synaptic plasticity model and the 60 Hz MF is *via* the equation linking the EEG with the post-synaptic calcium concentration, occurring on long timescales (depending on the opening of N-methyl-D-aspartate (NMDA) glutamate receptors, not represented in the model). Therefore, the model offers the possibility to test the hypothesis that 60 Hz MF exposure can modulate synaptic plasticity by interfering with the calcium fluxes at the level of synapses. However, it does not take into account possible effects of 60 Hz MF exposure on spike timing (see the "Discussion" section).

Let us consider the average calcium post-synaptic concentration in a neural mass. The model proposed by Shouval et al. (2002a,b) links the calcium current at the level of NMDA receptors with the calcium concentration, and finally to a differential equation describing the dynamics of synaptic weight change as a function of two different calcium-dependent functions. The time constant of calcium concentration dynamics is long (on the order of minutes), and the calcium concentration increases with the membrane potential. Therefore, it appears reasonable to approximate calcium dynamics by a low-pass filtering of the mean potential of a given neural mass:

$$\tau_{Ca^{2+}} \frac{d}{dt}[Ca^{2+}] + [Ca^{2+}] = \gamma(y_1 - y_2 - y_9) \quad (8)$$

where $y_1 - y_2 - y_9$ is the "EEG" signal at the level of a neural mass (e.g., summation of post-synaptic potentials at the level of pyramidal neurons as defined previously). Once the post-synaptic dendritic calcium concentration is obtained, it is possible to evaluate the calcium-dependent functions η and Ω present in the Shouval et al. (2002a,b) model, used to express the dynamics of the synaptic weight c_i (i denoting the type of synapse in the neural mass, e.g., afferent glutamatergic synapses on pyramidal neurons) at the level of a given neural mass:

$$\frac{dc_i(t)}{dt} = \eta(t) \cdot [\Omega_{Ca^{2+}}(t) - c_i(t)] \tag{9}$$

The function Ω was approximated by a combination of piecewise-linear and quadratic functions (see Appendix, **Figure A1** for details) similar to the function proposed in Shouval et al. (2002b). The function Ω used in our model differs quantitatively from the one proposed in Shouval et al. (2002a,b), since the authors were linking with this function the level of post-synaptic calcium concentration with the relative change in synaptic weight, where we directly link the post-synaptic calcium concentration with the synaptic weight itself. Nevertheless, the Ω used in this paper captures the most important qualitative properties proposed by Shouval et al. (2002a,b). In our simulations, we have assumed that was $\eta(t)$ a constant, $[Ca^{2+}(t)]$ being bounded between 0 and 1 μM. We assumed that the synapses modulated were the synapses terminating on pyramidal neurons, pooled in the constant c_5, becoming the variable $c_5(t)$ in our model. Numerical implementation for the neural mass model was performed using Matlab 2010 (The Mathworks, USA) on a quad-core Apple iMac (2.66 GHz/CPU) with 8 GB of RAM. The simulation of a neural mass using the complete model during 2 h with a time step of $dt = 1$ ms took typically 8 min.

60 Hz MF EXPOSURE PROTOCOL

In order to study the effects of 60 Hz MF on the simulated EEG, we used the following protocol: the neural mass was simulated during 2 h overall with a 1 ms resolution, which was decomposed as (1) 30 min without 60 Hz MF exposure (termed "sham," of sufficient duration to reach a steady state); (2) 60 min with 60 Hz MF exposure (sufficient to reach the new steady state); and (3) 30 min without 60 Hz MF exposure. Previous research in our team using fMRI to image the functional changes in brain activity due to 60 Hz MF exposure involved comparable durations (notably, a 60 min exposure period and fMRI acquisitions performed before and after, see Legros et al., 2010). Simulations were performed both (1) using the synaptic plasticity model, and (2) using a fixed synaptic weight value taken as the steady state value when synaptic plasticity was taken into account. By doing so, we aimed at decomposing the respective contribution of the 60 Hz sinusoidal perturbation in membrane potential one the one hand, and of possible calcium-related synaptic plasticity modulations on the other hand.

RESULTS

EFFECT OF 60 Hz MF ON THE EEG IN THE MODEL

As an example, we present in **Figure 2** an example of simulated EEG data, and associated mean post-synaptic calcium concentration and synaptic weight obtained by solving Equations (3, 4, 8, 9).

We have investigated the effect of increasing values (125, 250, 500, and 1000 μV) for the MF-induced membrane depolarization on the EEG alpha power. EEG alpha spectral power was computed before, during and after the 1-h 60 Hz MF exposure. 10 runs of 7200 s were performed for each tested value of dV. The averaged EEG alpha power for each condition (before, during, and after exposure) is presented in **Figure 3**.

From the results presented in **Figure 3**, it appears that increasing values of dV gradually decreases EEG alpha power during

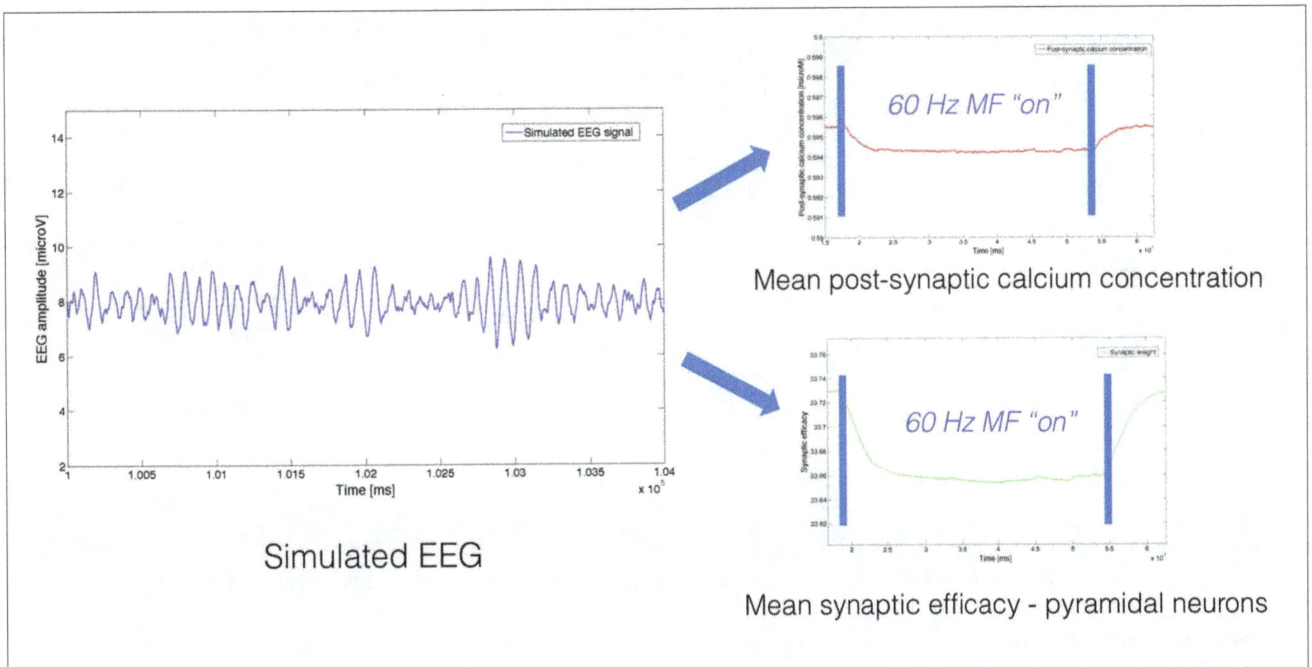

FIGURE 2 | Example of neurophysiological signals (EEG, post-synaptic calcium concentration, synaptic weight) simulated using the model, both without and with exposure to a 60 Hz MF.

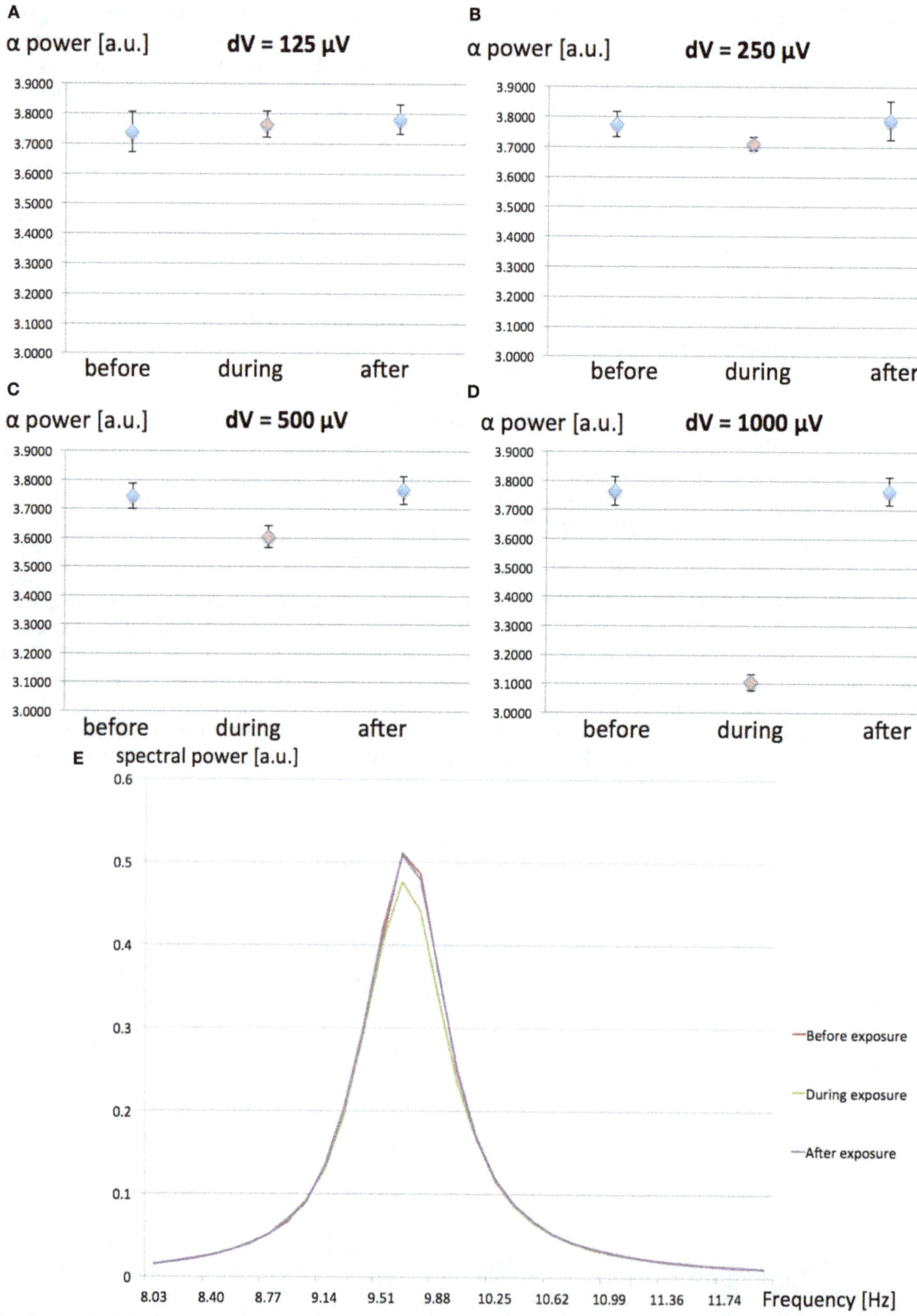

FIGURE 3 | (A–D): Spectral power in the EEG alpha (8–12 Hz) band as a function of the MF-induced membrane polarization *dV*; before (blue), during (red) and after (blue) the 1-h 60 Hz MF exposure period. **(A)** $dV = 125\,\mu V$; **(B)**, $dV = 250\,\mu V$; **(C)** $dV = 500\,\mu V$; **(D)** $dV = 1000\,\mu V$. A decrease in EEG alpha power is observed as the value of *dV* (proportional to the MF flux density) increases. **(E)** Example of average power spectrum before, during and after exposure to the 60 Hz MF, for $dV = 500\,\mu V$.

exposure. In order to test the significance of the amplitude of dV on the EEG alpha power during 60 Hz MF exposure, we conducted a statistical analysis of the results. We performed a $4 \times 3 \times 2$ ANOVA for repeated measures (SPSS 21, IBM, USA), respectively testing for the effects of "dV" (125, 250, 500, and 1000 μV), "time" (before, during and after), and "plasticity" (with/without synaptic plasticity). The standard p-value of 0.05 (Greenhouse-Geisser) was chosen as the threshold for significance, and p-values were corrected for multiple comparisons. The statistical results reveal a significant decrease of the EEG alpha power for $dV = 500$ μV as compared to the other values of dV ($p < 0.001$). This indicates that the threshold for a significant decrease of EEG alpha power due to 60 Hz MF exposure lies between induced membrane depolarization values of 250–500 μV. In the next section, we attempt to link the membrane depolarization values to the corresponding MF flux density at 60 Hz.

Due to the possibility that the weak 60 Hz membrane depolarization can be seen as an additive noise, we have tested the influence of the input noise level [$p(t)$ in the model, see **Table A1** of the Appendix] variance on EEG alpha power modulation due to the exposure. Since the dynamics of the model itself depend critically on the input noise level, we have indeed investigated the possibility that the 60 Hz MF exposure has an effect of variable amplitude depending on input noise. The interest is that model predictions could be tested experimentally (e.g., in an experimental setting where different levels of visual input would be tested). Therefore, the objective was not to study the influence of the noise level on the model dynamics, but rather how the effects of the 60 Hz MF on model dynamics are dependent on the noise level. Four different values of noise variance were tested ($\sigma = 120$, 150, 180, and 210 spikes/s) for the same maximal dV value of 0.5 mV. 10 runs of 7200 s following the same protocol than previously were run for each noise level value (40 runs total). The influence of the input noise level on EEG alpha power modulation by the 60 Hz MF is presented in **Figure 4**.

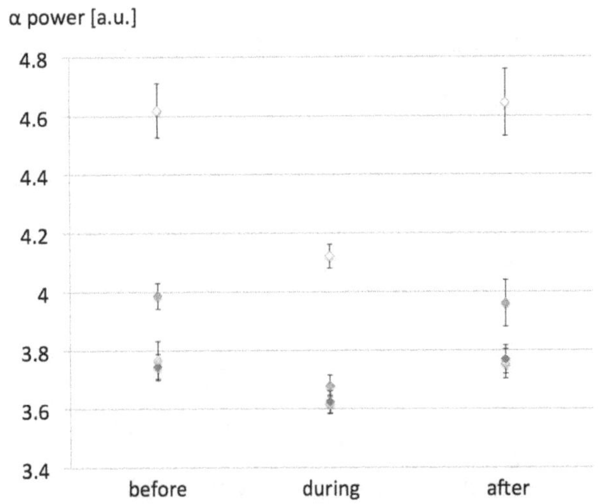

FIGURE 4 | Effect of the input noise level variance on EEG alpha power modulation caused by the 60 Hz MF exposure in the presence of the simplified synaptic plasticity model. Noise variance σ was varied as follows: yellow, 120 spikes/s; orange: 150 spikes/s; red, 180 spikes/s; blue: 210 spikes/s. The value of dV was fixed to 500 μV in all simulations. The EEG alpha power is presented for each noise variance value before, during and after 60 Hz MF exposure. The impact of the 60 Hz MF exposure on EEG alpha power decreases with increased input noise amplitude, likely since the weak 60 Hz membrane potential perturbation becomes "buried" in noise.

The results presented in **Figure 4** highlight the importance of the input noise level of the model. If the input $p(t)$, representing external noisy input to the neural mass, is too high; then the effect induced by the 60 Hz MF on EEG alpha power modulation decreases. This has an immediate consequence on threshold values of MF flux density resulting in detectable effects in brain activity: the MF flux density needed to elicit a response in brain tissue will be lower in the presence of a low level of noise. Interestingly, there is experimental evidence that the visual input can play a role on the effects of MF exposure in humans, with an higher effect when the eyes are closed (Legros et al., 2011). EEG alpha oscillations increase dramatically eyes closed, and decrease in the presence of a visual input, that increases the input noise to the occipital cortex. Therefore, even if there is a considerable gap between the model and human data, it is tempting to make a parallel between smaller effects of 60 Hz MF in the model with high levels of noise, and smaller effects of 60 Hz MF exposure eyes open with an increased input noise level. One advantage of using our neural mass over interpreting experimental results is the possibility to point at precise mechanisms by which the observed decrease in EEG alpha activity occurs due to the 60 Hz MF exposure. From a physiological point of view, it is relevant to investigate which neuronal pathways are mainly modulated by the exposure. In the model, we observe an immediate decrease in the activity of the loop between pyramidal neurons and slow GABAergic neurons, likely increasing the effect of excitatory input. To complement this observation, it is relevant to note that, using a bifurcation theory analysis of the Jansen and Rit model (the core of our model), Grimbert and Faugeras (2006) have shown that increasing the input noise level at the level of pyramidal neurons in the alpha oscillations regime (corresponding to a Hopf bifurcation) had the effect to decrease the amplitude of alpha oscillations. Therefore, the 60 Hz MF stimulus used in our model seems to have a similar effect than an additive, positive constant membrane depolarization on pyramidal neurons. This results physiologically speaking from an efficiency decrease of the slow inhibitory GABAergic feedback at the pyramidal neurons level. In terms of dynamical systems theory, this seems to be the natural result of increased input level in a specific dynamical system on a Hopf cycle.

In order to distinguish between the contribution of the MF-induced membrane polarization on the one hand, and changes in synaptic plasticity on the other hand, we ran the same simulations than previously for four different values of dV (125, 250, 500, and 1000 μV), with a constant value for the synaptic weight c_5. The objective was to identify if synaptic plasticity was affecting the direction (increase/decrease of EEG alpha spectral power) or amplitude of the effects. In the following, the value c_5 of was chosen as the steady-state value in the case where synaptic plasticity was considered. 10 simulations of 7200 s were ran for each value of dV. The results are presented in **Figure 5**.

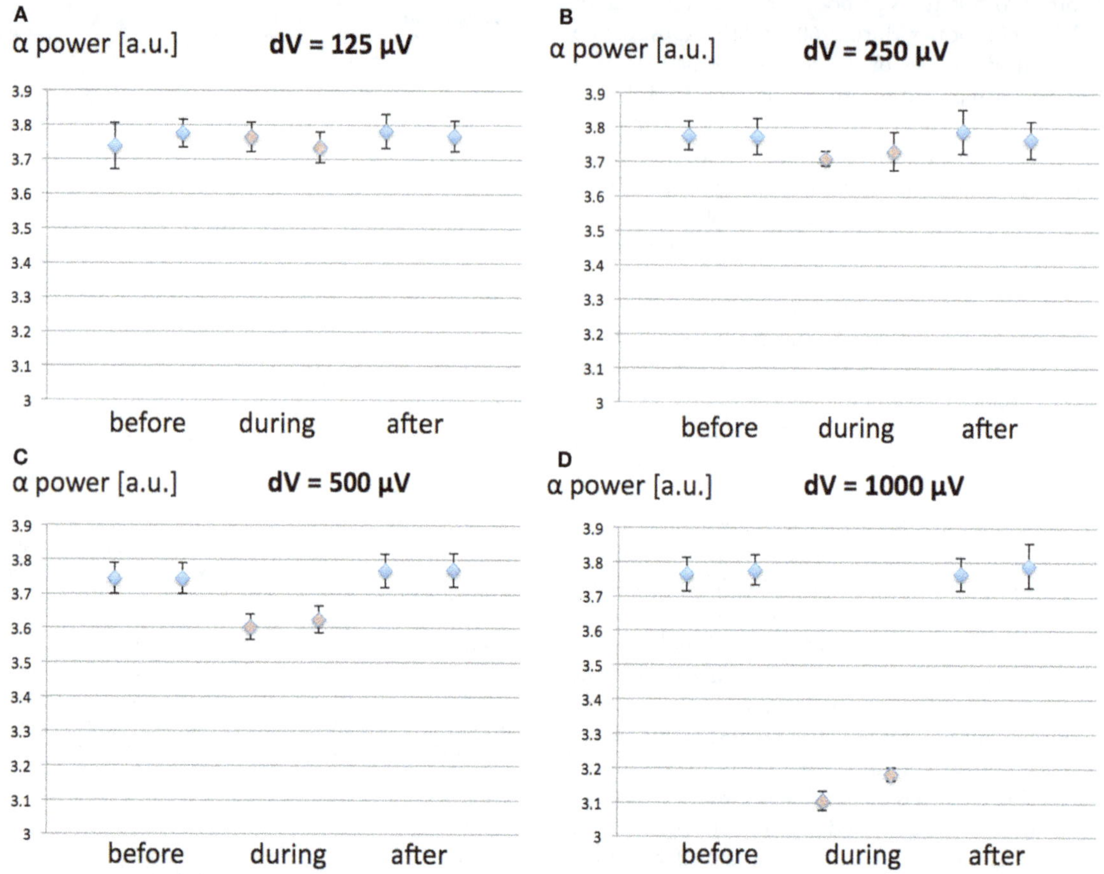

FIGURE 5 | Effect of synaptic plasticity on EEG alpha power modulation by 60 Hz MF exposure compared to the case where synaptic plasticity is not taken into account. The conditions are Before, During, and After 60 Hz MF exposure, with (1, 3, 5) and without (2, 4, 6) synaptic plasticity. **(A)** dV = 125 µV; **(B)** dV = 250 µV; **(C)** dV = 500 µV; **(D)** dV = 1000 µV.

From the results in **Figure 5**, it appears that the modulation of post-synaptic calcium concentration and corresponding changes in synaptic weight plays a minimal role in EEG alpha power modulation due to the 60 Hz MF exposure, and does not impact qualitatively the result (the direction of the effects is the same, and the amplitude of the effects is minimally affected). Indeed, the results from the ANOVA shows no significant interaction effect between synaptic plasticity and dV values ($p = 0.253$). This indicates that the presence of the synaptic plasticity mechanisms included in the model does not significantly change the effect of the membrane depolarization. It seems however to induce a non-significant increase the amplitude of the 60 Hz MF exposure effect. Different choices for the function linking the post-synaptic calcium concentration level with the updated synaptic weight Ω lead to similar results (not shown). Therefore, it seems that, if a modulation of synaptic plasticity explains lasting effects of 60 Hz MF exposure, it does not occur primarily by the modulation of post-synaptic calcium currents. However, it is still plausible that receptor trafficking and synaptic plasticity could be impacted by a perturbation of spike timing due to the 60 Hz MF exposure, a mechanism not included in the present model, which we discuss later.

In the model develop by Molaee-Ardekani et al. (2013), investigating the effects of transcranial direct current stimulation (tDCS), the neurons being modulated by the induced field were pyramidal neurons and inhibitory interneurons. Since the simulated EEG could result in different outcomes due to the exposure depending on the neuronal populations simulated, possibly assisting in discriminating between different interaction mechanisms; we have also simulated the EEG in the case of a 60 Hz MF exposure modulating the activity of different populations of inhibitory interneurons. To do so, in a similar fashion to Equation (7) describing the membrane depolarization of pyramidal neurons, we simulated different scenarios: (1) slow and fast GABAergic interneurons are involved, (2) slow GABAergic interneurons are involved, and (3) fast inhibitory neurons are involved. Depending on the scenario, we also added the variable $dV(t)$ to $y_4(t)$ (slow GABAergic interneurons), or to $y_{10}(t)$-$y_{11}(t)$ (fast GABAergic interneurons), and to both of these quantities for scenario (1). We have simulated the EEG for a similar protocol than previously (30 min without exposure, 1 h of exposure, 30 min without exposure), with a maximal value of $dV =$ 1000 µV. The resulting EEG alpha power before, during and after exposure for each of these scenarios is presented in **Figure 6**.

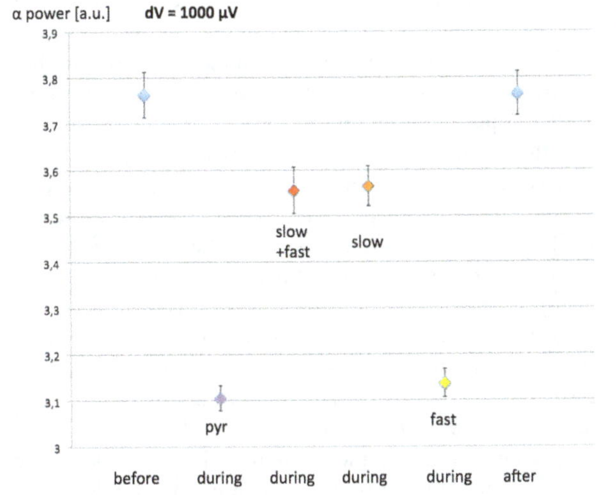

FIGURE 6 | Effect of the 60 Hz MF exposure on EEG alpha power depending on which populations of neurons are modulated by the induced electric field. The exposure protocol is the same than previously (1-h exposure, with 30 min before and after without exposure). The maximal value of the MF-induced membrane depolarization was $dV = 1$ mV. Pyramidal neurons are considered to be modulated in each scenario. Pyr, pyramidal neurons only; slow+fast, pyramidal neurons, slow and fast GABAergic interneurons; slow, pyramidal neurons, slow GABAergic neurons; fast, pyramidal neurons, fast GABAergic neurons.

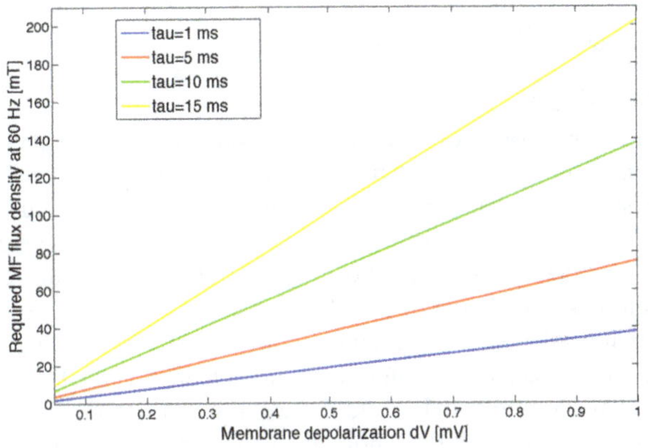

FIGURE 7 | MF flux density curves as a function of the MF-induced membrane depolarization *dV*, computed for different values of the polarization time constant τ. The input noise variance to the model was taken as 180 spikes/s. Different noise variance values will result in different MF threshold curves.

The results presented in **Figure 6** show that, if the fast GABAergic interneurons are modulated by the 60 Hz MF in addition to pyramidal neurons, the difference in the EEG is minimal. However, if the slow GABAergic interneurons are modulated, the decrease in EEG alpha power is much smaller, dropping from 17% (pyramidal neurons only) to 5%. Therefore, if the slow GABAergic interneurons are also modulated by the induced electric field due to the 60 Hz MF exposure, the threshold leading to a systematic EEG alpha power modulation will be higher. From the interpretation on the decrease in EEG alpha power when the pyramidal neurons alone are stimulated, where a decrease in the efficiency of the loop between pyramidal neurons and slow inhibitory interneurons is observed, we can speculate that the effect of modulating the slow GABAergic interneurons in addition to pyramidal neurons has an opposite effect of increasing the activity of this loop. Consequently, if slow GABAergic interneurons are modulated by the exposure to the 60 Hz MF exposure, the model suggests that it would result in a compensation of the modulation of pyramidal neurons' activity alone, thereby increasing the threshold in MF flux density leading to a systematic decrease in alpha. In other words, the modulation of pyramidal neurons and slow GABAergic interneurons activity would have competing effects regarding the decrease in EEG alpha power.

THRESHOLD OF 60 Hz MF FLUX DENSITY RESULTING IN DETECTABLE EFFECTS

Based on the expression of the electric field induced by a time varying MF at the level of a sphere of radius R (approximating the brain in that scenario), we can obtain an estimate of the corresponding MF flux density at 60 Hz. Let us approximate the head as a sphere of radius R, and let us write the 60 Hz MF as $B(t) = B_0 \sin(\omega t + \phi)$. From Maxwell-Faraday's law of magnetic induction, the induced electric field expresses as $E = \frac{R}{2}\frac{dB}{dt} = \pi R f B_0$. By using this expression in Equation (5), we obtain $B = \frac{dV(1+\omega^2\tau^2)^{1/2}}{\lambda \pi R f}$, linking the MF-induced membrane depolarization to the MF flux density. We used the following values to estimated the threshold values: $R = 0.15$ m, $\lambda = 10^{-3}$ m, and $f = 60$ Hz. The MF flux density value as a function of the MF-induced membrane depolarization dV, depending on different τ values, is shown in **Figure 7**.

We have shown based on our statistical analysis that a significant EEG alpha power modulation occurs in the model for a dV value between 250 and 500 µV. Given the uncertainty on the polarization time constant, it is only possible to provide an estimate of the MF flux density threshold at 60 Hz which should result in a significant decrease of EEG alpha activity. Assuming an intermediate dV value as a threshold value (375 µV), the corresponding threshold MF flux density would range between 15 and 75 mT, for polarization time constants between 1 and 15 ms. Let us also mention that this threshold value is, as shown above, depending on the input noise level. Uncertainties on the values of the polarization time constant and on the input noise level are problematic to estimate a more precise MF flux density threshold value. Depending on the neural elements activated by the induced electric field, this polarization time constant can be very different (higher for the whole soma than for fibers for example). For a neuron soma, the polarization time constant would be of several milliseconds; whereas if the membrane depolarization occurs at the level of Ranvier nodes, than the polarization time constant is considerably smaller, around 20 µs (Gianni et al., 2006). Therefore, it is reasonable to assume that the polarization time constant is in the low millisecond range. As an example, a polarization time constant between 1 and 5 ms would result in a threshold value between 15 and 25 mT for a 60 Hz MF. The validation of these values will require experimental recordings performed in humans, which will be performed in the near future in our group (Legros et al., 2012a,b).

DISCUSSION

In this paper, we have developed an innovative application of neural mass models, i.e., the study of how extremely low-frequency MF such as power-line MF interact with brain activity. Indeed, this is the first time that this problem is tackled using neural mass modeling. We have shown that 60 Hz MF exposure can result in a modulation of the EEG alpha rhythm, even for small membrane depolarization values (<1 mV). For reasonable polarization time constant values, the model predicts that 60 Hz MF between 15 and 25 mT could induce a systematic decrease in EEG alpha power. Furthermore, the neural mass model that we have developed includes, in a simplified manner, a contribution of synaptic plasticity processes. To our knowledge, this is the first attempt to include a contribution of calcium-related processes into changes of effective connectivity in neural mass models. The contribution of calcium currents on synaptic weights changes is obviously overly simplified in our model since the calcium concentration is modeled as a low-pass filtered version of the EEG. Nevertheless, it represents a first step that could serve as a basis in future models integrating more biophysically detailed models of synaptic plasticity. Let us mention that Robinson (2011) proposed a neural field model including synaptic plasticity, though in a different manner. Indeed, this model used the relative phase between pre- and post-synaptic neural populations to compute the synaptic weight changes due to an STDP rule. In the present paper, we have intended to provide the bases for mechanism-based neural mass models, on the grounds of a reliable synaptic plasticity model (Shouval et al., 2002a,b). Expanding our model using modeling principles of Robinson (2011) could be a solution so include the effect of spike timing perturbation induced by 60 Hz MF on neural mass activity.

One hypothesis investigated was that changes in post-synaptic calcium concentration could modulate synaptic weights, resulting in a lasting modulation of brain tissue dynamics. Obviously, our model of synaptic plasticity is still simplified and does not explicitly model the voltage-dependence of calcium currents through NMDA receptors. From our results, it appears that, despite a modulation in post-synaptic calcium concentration taking some time to build up, and lasting several minutes after the exposure, these changes are too small to impact neural mass dynamics. However, there is another important mechanism by which receptor trafficking and synaptic plasticity could be modulated by 60 Hz MF exposure. There is indeed a convergence of theoretical (Reato et al., 2010; Stodilka et al., 2011) and experimental (Radman et al., 2007) studies that illustrate the possibility for weak membrane depolarizations induced by electric fields to impact spike timing. Indeed, Radman et al. (2007) have shown that, due to the non-linear properties of neuron membranes, small membrane depolarizations can modulate spike timing. Since post-synaptic calcium currents play the role of "coincidence detector" between pre- and post-synaptic spikes, a perturbation of spike timing could impact receptor trafficking and synaptic weight changes. The challenge is to consider these mechanisms in neural mass or neural field models, which are rate-coding based and not time-coding based. A recent study proposed how to consider plasticity rules based on spike timing in neural field theory (Robinson, 2011), providing a possibility to investigate the impact of 60 Hz MF perturbation on spike timing at a mesoscopic scale. The perturbation of spike timing by 60 Hz MF exposure will be considered in a future extension of the model presented in this paper, since this synaptic plasticity pathway could be more prone to small membrane perturbations due to the 60 Hz MF exposure, and could induce lasting effects in neural dynamics.

Using our model, we have also investigated the effect of the small 60 Hz membrane depolarization induced by 60 Hz MF exposure depending of the input noise level of the model. Our suggests that the threshold value in MF flux density for which significant changes can be detected in the EEG alpha frequency band is a function of the model input noise level. More specifically, for lower values of input noise level, the decrease in EEG alpha power is higher than for higher input noise level values. However, these results do not imply that stochastic resonance effects are present, which could be tested however by testing many different values of dV, and identify a range of dV values for which the modulation of EEG alpha power would be present. The stochastic resonance mechanism has been already explored in the literature to explain the effects of 60 Hz MF exposure, and constitutes a possibility of future study using our model. This result on the importance of the input noise level has also important implications for the detection of EEG alpha power modulation in humans due to 60 Hz MF exposure. We predict that the threshold in MF flux density at 60 Hz, required to modulate systematically the EEG in the occipital cortex, is lower a condition when the ambient light is low, compared to the effects of the same exposure using a high ambient light level. Indeed, EEG alpha oscillations decrease in the occipital cortex in humans due to the higher input noise level. Therefore, it might be relevant to study a variation of 60 Hz MF threshold values in humans at the level of the occipital cortex using different intensities of ambient light. If such experimental evidence was provided, that would be a precious piece of information that could be of interest to agencies such as ICNIRP. Another indication that the prediction that the level of input is important in the physiological outcome is that the perception of magnetophosphenes and the threshold at which they can be observed is light intensity-dependent (Lövsund et al., 1980). This motivates a future human experimental study using in parallel our neural mass model in order to provide an improved knowledge on the underlying interaction mechanisms. Another valuable insight from the model is the differential effect observed on EEG alpha activity depending on the neuronal populations modulated (pyramidal neurons only, or pyramidal neurons and slow/fast inhibitory interneurons). Since the model predicts a different outcome in the case where slow inhibitory interneurons are also modulated (smaller decrease in alpha activity), this offers a possibility to discriminate in future EEG data acquired in humans which neuronal populations are modulated by the MF exposure. This adds further support for the use of neural mass models to study the effects of power-line MF on human brain activity, since they can offer a deeper insight into the experimental data in order to clarify the interaction mechanisms involved.

Among the limitations of our approach, let us mention first the absence of ephactic interactions. It has been indeed demonstrated that post-synaptic potentials can induce in neighboring cells a small but measurable polarization (for a review, see Weiss and Faber, 2010). In the cortex, where the axons of pyramidal axons have a similar and consistent orientation, it is likely that ephactic interactions could enhance the effect of weak membrane depolarizations. Therefore, the presence of ephactic interactions should lower the threshold for detectable modulations of neuronal activity, and should be included in future biophysical models studying the effects of low-frequency MF on cortical activity. Second, our model of synaptic plasticity is a significant simplification compared to the biophysically detailed model by Shouval et al. (2002a,b). The present model could be extended by including a more detailed model of the detailed processes underlying receptor trafficking at the synaptic level. Third, the exact orientation of pyramidal axons with respect to the induced electric field was not taken into account, since it was assumed that the orientation was "ideal" (electric field parallel to pyramidal neuron axons). Fourth, we assumed that the power-line MF interacts with brain tissue *via* the induced electric field. However, there is evidence that the MF itself could interact with cellular signaling, and induce biological effects (Pilla, 2012). Studying such phenomena appears however out of reach with our proposed model. Let us note that the possibility that either the MF or the induced electric field modulate neuronal activity is not exclusive, and both mechanisms might even turn out to be complementary and have effects on different cellular components.

Finally, let us mention that, in most studies investigating the effects of low-frequency MF on the human EEG, the data analyzed is from before or after exposure, not during. There is indeed an experimental difficulty in recording the EEG during exposure to low-frequency MF. However, it is possible to compensate using specific signal processing techniques, such as wavelet-based methods (Modolo et al., 2011). We believe that such signal processing techniques applied to EEG acquired during 60 Hz MF exposure, combined with the neural mass model proposed in this paper, could provide an integrated framework for a thorough understanding of power-line frequency MF on human brain activity.

CONCLUDING REMARKS

We have presented a novel application of neural field models, in the context of brain exposure to 60 Hz MF. The model takes into account different neural populations in cortical tissue, synaptic kinetics proper to each type of synapse considered, synaptic connectivity patterns inspired from neuroanatomy, and a simplified model of synaptic plasticity based on the "calcium-control" hypothesis. The model includes the interaction with the electric field induced by 60 Hz MF exposure, and results in a time-varying membrane depolarization. Using this model, we have shown that membrane depolarization between 250 and 500 μV at 60 Hz is sufficient to induce a significant decrease in EEG alpha power. We also conclude that the modulation of post-synaptic calcium currents by 60 Hz MF exposure does not appear to predict the lasting effects observed experimentally. Future work should investigate the role of spike timing perturbation by the induced electric field during 60 Hz MF exposure, which is another candidate mechanism to induce plastic changes and lasting changes in neuronal activity. The models provides predictions that can, and will be, tested in experimental protocols during which humans will be exposed to increasing levels of 60 Hz MF exposure up to 50 mT (Legros et al., 2012a,b). Thorough comparison of experimental data with model predictions will constitute a unique opportunity for the validation and calibration of this neural mass model, which might become a relevant tool in the assessment of public and workers exposure to environmental MF, and assisting in the development and evaluation of guidelines developed by ICNIRP.

ACKNOWLEDGMENTS

This work is supported by an Elevate Post-Doctoral Fellowship from Mitacs, Hydro-Québec/Electricité de France/Réseau de Transport d'Electricité, and the Canadian Institutes of Health Research.

REFERENCES

Amari, S. (1977). Dynamics of pattern formation in lateral-inhibition type neural fields. *Biol. Cybern.* 27, 77–87.

Bikson, N., Inoue, M., Akiyama, H., Deans, J. K., Fox, J. E., Miyakawa, H., et al. (2004). Effects of uniform extracellular DC electric fields on excitability in rat hippocampal slices *in vitro*. *J. Physiol.* 557(Pt 1), 175–190.

Bojak, I., Oostendorp, T. F., Reid, A. T., and Kotter, R. (2010). Connecting mean field models of neural activity to EEG and fMRI data. *Brain Topogr.* 23, 139–149.

Collingridge, G. L., Isaac, J. T., and Wang, Y. T. (2004). Receptor trafficking and synaptic plasticity. *Nat. Rev. Neurosci.* 5, 952–962.

Cook, C. M., Thomas, A. W., Keenliside, L., and Prato, F. S. (2005). Resting EEG effects during exposure to a pulsed ELF magnetic field. *Bioelectromagnetics* 26, 367–376.

Cook, C. M., Thomas, A. W., and Prato, F. S. (2004). Resting EEG is affected by exposure to a pulsed ELF magnetic field. *Bioelectromagnetics* 25, 196–203.

Corbacio, M., Brown, S., Dubois, S., Goulet, D., Prato, F. S., Thomas, A. W., et al. (2011). Human cognitive performance in a 3 mT power-line magnetic field. *Bioelectromagnetics* 23, 620–633.

Crasson, M. (2003). 50-60 Hz electric and magnetic field effects on cognitive function in humans: a review. *Radiat. Prot. Dosimetry* 106, 333–340.

Deans, J. K., Powell, A. D., and Jefferys, J. G. (2007). Sensitivity of coherent oscillations in rat hippocampus to AC electric fields. *J. Physiol.* 583(Pt 2), 555–565.

Fröhlich, F., and McCormick, D. A. (2010). Endogenous electric fields may guide neocortical network activity. *Neuron* 67, 129–143.

Ghione, S., Seppia, C. D., Mezzalma, L., and Bonfglio, L. (2005). Effects of 50 Hz electromagnetic fields on electroencephalography alpha activity, dental pain threshold and cardiovascular parameters in humans. *Neurosci. Lett.* 382, 112–117.

Gianni, M., Liberti, M., Appollonio, F., and D'Inzeo, G. (2006). Modeling electromagnetic fields detectability in a HH-like neuronal system: stochastic resonance and window behavior. *Biol. Cybern.* 94, 118–127.

Grimbert, F., and Faugeras, O. (2006). Bifurcation analysis of Jansen's neural mass model. *Neural Comput.* 18, 3052–3068.

ICNIRP—International Commission on Non-Ionizing Radiation Protection. (2010). Guidelines for Limiting Exposure to Time-Varying Electric and Magnetic Fields (1 Hz – 100 kHz). *Health Phys.* 99, 818–836.

Jansen, B. H., and Rit, V. G. (1995). Electroencephalogram and visual evoked potential generation in a mathematical model of coupled cortical columns. *Biol. Cybern.* 73, 357–366.

Jefferys, J. G., Deans, J., Bikson, M., and Fox, J. (2003). Effects of weak electric fields on the activity of neurons and neuronal networks. *Radiat. Prot. Dosimetry* 106, 321–323.

Legros, A., and Beuter, A. (2005). Effect of a low intensity magnetic field on human motor behavior. *Bioelectromagnetics* 26, 657–669.

Legros, A., Corbacio, M., Beuter, A., Modolo, J., Goulet, D., Prato, F. S., et al. (2012a). Neurophysiological and behavioral effects of a 60 Hz, 1800 microtesla magnetic field in humans. *Eur. J. Appl. Physiol.* 112, 1751–1762.

Legros, A., Modolo, J., Goulet, D., Plante, M., Souques, M., Deschamps, F., et al. (2012b). "Threshold for a systematic neurophysiological response to 50 and 60 Hz magnetic fields up to 50 millitesla," *34th Annual Conference of the Bioelectromagnetics Society* (Brisbane, QLD).

Legros, A., Miller, J. E., Modolo, J., Corbacio, M., Robertson, J. R., Goulet, D., et al. (2010). "Is finger tapping induced brain activation modulated by an exposure to a 60 Hz, 3000 μT magnetic field?" in *32nd Annual Conference of the Bioelectromagnetics Society* (Seoul).

Legros, A., Miller, J., Modolo, J., Corbacio, M., Robertson, J., Goulet, D., et al. (2011). Multi-modalities investigation of 60 Hz magnetic field effects on the human central nervous system. *Electra* 256, 14–18.

Lövsund, P., Oberg, P. A., Nilsson, S. E., and Reuter, T. (1980). Magnetophosphenes: a quantitative analysis of thresholds. *Med. Biol. Eng. Comput.* 18, 326–334.

Miller, J. E., Modolo, J., Robertson, J. R., Corbacio, M., Dubois, S., Goulet, D., et al. (2010). "Effects of a 60 Hz magnetic field exposure on human brain activity during a mental rotation task as measured by fMRI," *32nd Annual Conference of the Bioelectromagnetics Society* (Seoul).

Modolo, J., Bhattacharya, B., Edwards, R., Campagnaud, J., Legros, A., and Beuter, A. (2010). Using a virtual cortical modulate implementing a neural field model to modulate brain rhythms in Parkinson's disease. *Front. Neurosci.* 4:45. doi: 10.3389/fnins.2010.00045

Modolo, J., Juen, N., Robertson, J. A., Thomas, A. W., and Legros, A. (2011). "EEG frequency analysis of 60 Hz magnetic field exposure within the MRI," *Conference of the Conseil International des Grands Réseaux Electriques (CIGRE)* (Paris).

Molaee-Ardekani, B., Benquet, P., Bartolomei, F., and Wendling, F. (2010). Computational modeling of high-frequency oscillations at the onset of neocortical partial seizures: from "altered structure" to "dysfunction". *Neuroimage* 52, 1109–1122.

Molaee-Ardekani, B., Márquez-Ruiz, J., Merlet, I., Leal-Campagnario, R., Gruart, A., Sánchez-Campusano, R., et al. (2013). Effects of transcranial direct current stimulation (tDCS) on cortical activity: a computational modeling study. *Brain Stimul.* 6, 25–39.

National Institute of Environmental Health Sciences of the National Institutes of Health. (1998). *Assessment of Health Effects From Exposure to Power-Line Frequency Electric and Magnetic Fields*, eds C. J. Protier and M. S. Wolfe (Research Triangle Park, NC: NIH publication No. 98-3981).

Pilla, A. (2012). Electromagnetic fields instantaneously modulate nitric oxide signaling in challenged biological systems. *Biochem. Biophys. Res. Commun.* 426, 330–333.

Radman, T., Ramos, R. L., Brumberg, J. C., and Bikson, M. (2009). Role of cortical cell type and morphology in subthreshold and suprathreshold uniform electric field stimulation *in vitro*. *Brain Stimul.* 2, 215–228.

Radman, T., Su, Y., An, J. H., Parra, L. C., and Bikson, M. (2007). Spike timing amplifies the effects of electric fields on neurons: implications for endogenous field effects. *J. Neurosci.* 27, 3030–3036.

Reato, D., Rahman, A., Bikson, M., and Parra, L. C. (2010). Low-intensity electrical stimulation affects network dynamics by modulating population rate and spike timing. *J. Neurosci.* 30, 15067–15079.

Robinson, P. A. (2011). Neural field theory of synaptic plasticity. *J. Theor. Biol.* 285, 156–163.

Shouval, H. Z., Castellani, G. C., Blais, B. S., Yeung, L. C., and Cooper, L. N. (2002a). Converging evidence for a simplified biophysical model of synaptic plasticity. *Biol. Cybern.* 87, 383–391.

Shouval, H. Z., Bear, M. F., and Cooper, L. N. (2002b). A unified model of NMDA receptor-dependent bidirectional synaptic plasticity. *Proc. Natl. Acad. Sci. U.S.A.* 99, 10831–10836.

Stodilka, R. Z., Modolo, J., Prato, F. S., Robertson, J. A., Cook, C., Patrick, J., et al. (2011). Pulsed magnetic field exposure induces lasting changes in neural network dynamics. *Neurocomputing* 74, 2164–2175.

Sotero, R. C., and Trujillo-Barreto, N. J. (2008). Biophysical model for integrating neuronal activity, EEG, fMRI and metabolism. *Neuroimage* 39, 290–309.

Weiss, S. A., and Faber, D. S. (2010). Field effects in the CNS play functional roles. *Front. Neural Circuits* 4:15. doi: 10.3389/fncir.2010.00015

Wendling, F., Bartolomei, F., Bellanger, J. J., and Chauvel, P. (2002). Epileptic fast activity can be explained by a model of impaired GABAergic dendritic inhibition. *Eur. J. Neurosci.* 15, 1499–1508.

Wendling, F., Hernandez, A., Bellanger, J. J., Chauvel, P., and Bartolomei, F. (2005). Interictal to ictal transition in human temporal lobe epilepsy: insights from a computational model of intracerebral EEG. *J. Clin. Neurophysiol.* 22, 343–356.

Wilson, H. R., and Cowan, J. D. (1973). A mathematical theory of the functional dynamics of cortical and thalamic nervous tissue. *Kybernetik* 13, 55–80.

APPENDIX

Table A1 | Summary of the parameters used in the model with their physiological meaning and their values.

Parameter	Physiological significance	Value
c_1	Number of synaptic contacts from pyramidal to exc. Interneurons	135
c_2	Number of synaptic contacts from exc. interneurons to exc. interneurons	$0.8 \times c_1$
c_3	Number of synaptic contacts from pyramidal to slow inh. Interneurons	$0.25 \times c_1$
c_4	Number of synaptic contacts from slow inh. interneurons to pyramidal cells	$0.25 \times c_1$
c_5	Number of synaptic contacts between pyramidal cells in the same cortical column	$0.25 \times c_1$
c_6	Number of synaptic contacts from pyramidal cells to other areas	200
c_7	Number of synaptic contacts from pyramidal cells to pyramidal cells in the same brain area	100
c_8	Number of synaptic contacts from exc. interneurons to pyramidal cells in the same brain area	100
c_9	Number of synaptic contacts from slow inh. interneurons to pyramidal cells in the same brain area	100
c_{10}	Number of synaptic contacts from pyramidal cells to fast inh. interneurons	$0.3 \times c_1$
c_{11}	Number of synaptic contacts from slow inh. interneurons to fast inh. interneurons	$0.8 \times c_1$
c_{12}	Number of synaptic contacts from fast inh. interneurons to pyramidal cells	$0.1 \times c_1$
r	Slope of the sigmoidal function	0.56
e_0	Maximum of the sigmoid function	2.5 Hz
v_0	Threshold of the sigmoid function	6 mV
A	Amplitude of glutamatergic EPSPs	3.25 mV
B	Amplitude of $GABA_a$ slow and $GABA_b$ IPSPs	22 mV
G	Amplitude of $GABA_a$ fast IPSPs	10 mV
a	Synaptic time constant for excitatory connections	100/s
b	Synaptic time constant for slow inhibitory connections	50/s
g	Synaptic time constant for fast inhibitory connections	350/s
a_{d1}	Time constant of efferent connections	33/s
a_{d2}	Time constant of efferent connections	100/s
a_{d3}	Time constant of efferent connections	100/s
b_{d4}	Time constant of efferent connections	40/s
c_{1t}	Number of synaptic contacts from TC to RE cells	50/s
c_{2t}	Number of synaptic contacts from RE to TC cells	50/s
c_{3t}	Number of synaptic contacts from TC to pyramidal cells	80/s
c_{4t}	Number of synaptic contacts from TC to exc. Interneurons	100/s
c_{5t}	Number of synaptic contacts from TC to inh. Interneurons	80/s
A_t	Amplitude of thalamic excitatory EPSPs (TC cells)	3.25 mV
A_t	Amplitude of thalamic excitatory EPSPs (TC cells)	3.25 mV
B_t	Amplitude of thalamic inhibitory IPSPs (RE cells)	22 mV
a_t	Synaptic time constant of TC cells	200/s
b_t	Synaptic time constant RE cells	40/s
$p(t)$	Input noise to pyramidal cells	120 pulses/s
K	Coupling constant between the thalamic and cortical modules of the model	0.2
K_{Cx}	Coupling constant between the cortical and thalamic modules of the model	10
K	Coupling constant between different areas	3.33
τ_{Ca}	Time constant of calcium current dynamics	0.05 s
γ	Sensitivity of calcium concentration to EEG changes	0.055
η	Time constant of synaptic weight changes	0.054 ms

Novel parameters compared to Sotero and Trujillo-Barreto (2008) are highlighted in red.

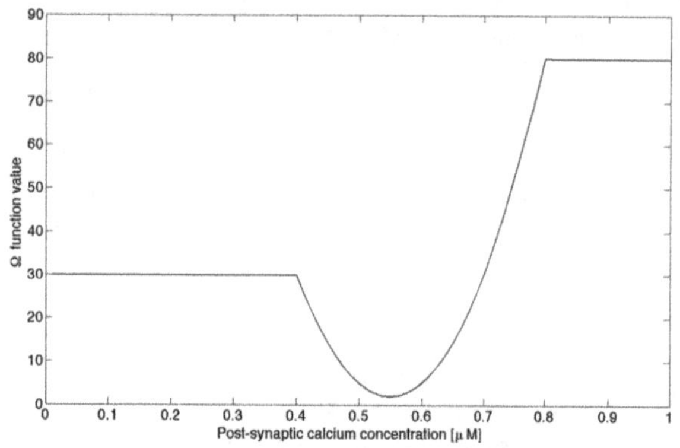

FIGURE A1 | Function Ω used in our model as a piecewise-linear approximation of the function used by Shouval et al. (2002b), preserving the main properties of this function, i.e., the level of post-synaptic calcium concentration regulating LTP and LTD processes.

15

Cortical information flow in Parkinson's disease: A composite network/field model

Cliff C. Kerr[1,2,3]*, Sacha J. Van Albada[4], Samuel A. Neymotin[1,5], George L. Chadderdon[1], P. A. Robinson[2,3] and William W. Lytton[1,6]

[1] Department of Physiology and Pharmacology, State University of New York Downstate Medical Center, Brooklyn, NY, USA
[2] School of Physics, University of Sydney, NSW, Australia
[3] Brain Dynamics Centre, Westmead Millennium Institute, Westmead, NSW, Australia
[4] Institute of Neuroscience and Medicine (INM-6) and Institute for Advanced Simulation (IAS-6), Jülich Research Centre and JARA, Jülich, Germany
[5] Department of Neurobiology, Yale University, New Haven, CT, USA
[6] Department of Neurology, Kings County Hospital, Brooklyn, NY, USA

Correspondence:
Cliff C. Kerr, Department of Physiology and Pharmacology, State University of New York Downstate Medical Center, 450 Clarkson Avenue, Po Box 31, Brooklyn, NY 11203, USA.
e-mail: ckerr@physics.usyd.edu.au

The basal ganglia play a crucial role in the execution of movements, as demonstrated by the severe motor deficits that accompany Parkinson's disease (PD). Since motor commands originate in the cortex, an important question is how the basal ganglia influence cortical information flow, and how this influence becomes pathological in PD. To explore this, we developed a composite neuronal network/neural field model. The network model consisted of 4950 spiking neurons, divided into 15 excitatory and inhibitory cell populations in the thalamus and cortex. The field model consisted of the cortex, thalamus, striatum, subthalamic nucleus, and globus pallidus. Both models have been separately validated in previous work. Three field models were used: one with basal ganglia parameters based on data from healthy individuals, one based on data from individuals with PD, and one purely thalamocortical model. Spikes generated by these field models were then used to drive the network model. Compared to the network driven by the healthy model, the PD-driven network had lower firing rates, a shift in spectral power toward lower frequencies, and higher probability of bursting; each of these findings is consistent with empirical data on PD. In the healthy model, we found strong Granger causality between cortical layers in the beta and low gamma frequency bands, but this causality was largely absent in the PD model. In particular, the reduction in Granger causality from the main "input" layer of the cortex (layer 4) to the main "output" layer (layer 5) was pronounced. This may account for symptoms of PD that seem to reflect deficits in information flow, such as bradykinesia. In general, these results demonstrate that the brain's large-scale oscillatory environment, represented here by the field model, strongly influences the information processing that occurs within its subnetworks. Hence, it may be preferable to drive spiking network models with physiologically realistic inputs rather than pure white noise.

Keywords: neural field model, spiking neural networks, Parkinsons's disease, thalamus, cortex, basal ganglia, Granger causality, interlaminar processing

1. INTRODUCTION

Parkinson's disease (PD) is a multiscale phenomenon, encompassing pathology at the level of single neurons, local networks, large neuronal ganglia, and the complex interactions between these ganglia and the cortex. PD is caused by the degeneration of dopaminergic neurons in the substantia nigra pars compacta, with the damage later spreading to dopaminergic neurons in the ventral tegmental area (Cools, 2006). The loss of dopaminergic input alters the dynamics of the striatum, which then affects the dynamics of large portions of the thalamus and cortex, which in turn affects the spinal cord and muscles (Bolam et al., 2002). Striatal dynamics are crucial to several large-scale projection pathways, including the well-characterized direct and indirect pathways. Dopaminergic input to the striatum increases transmission in D1-expressing striatal neurons involved in the direct pathway. These neurons inhibit the globus pallidus internal segment (GPi). Dopaminergic input also decreases input to D2-expressing striatal neurons involved in the indirect pathway. These neurons inhibit the globus pallidus external segment (GPe), which in turn inhibits the GPi. Thus, alterations to the direct and indirect pathways in PD are both thought to increase the firing rate of the GPi, which in turn inhibits the thalamus. There is also a hyperdirect pathway from the cortex to the GPi via the subthalamic nucleus (STN), as well as other lesser pathways (**Figure 1**).

Numerous models of PD and the basal ganglia have been proposed, using either field or network approaches. Van Albada and Robinson (2009) developed a field-based model of the basal

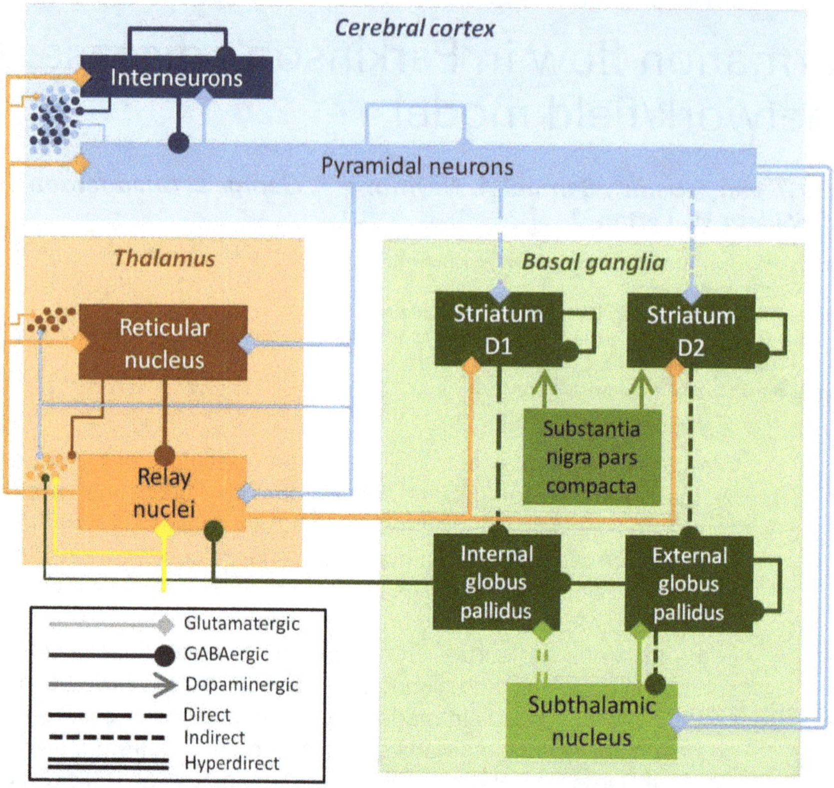

FIGURE 1 | Schematic of the field model, showing excitatory populations and connections (light colors, diamond arrows) and inhibitory ones (dark colors, round arrows). The key efferent nucleus of the basal ganglia is the internal globus pallidus (GPi), which receives cortical input via direct, indirect, and hyperdirect pathways. The field model drives a spiking network model, shown here schematically (dots at left); the inputs from the field model to the spiking model are indicated by the thin lines. The substantia nigra pars compacta modulates parameters, but is not explicitly modeled. Inputs to the thalamus (yellow arrow) were modeled as white noise.

ganglia/thalamocortical system. This model was shown to reproduce realistic firing rates of each neuronal population in both healthy and PD states. One early network model was that of Terman et al. (2002), which represented a small network of neurons in the GPe and STN. A considerably larger and more complex (non-spiking) network model was developed by Leblois et al. (2006). This model explored both basal ganglia and thalamocortical cell populations, looking at competition between the direct and hyperdirect pathways. They suggested that PD disrupted this competitive balance, resulting in loss of the network's ability to select motor programs. Another network model focusing on motor-selection abilities was developed by Humphries et al. (2006), who also found that decreased dopamine interfered with the basal ganglia's capacity for selecting actions. Network models have also been used to analyze and predict the effects of deep brain stimulation on basal ganglia nuclei (Hahn and McIntyre, 2010; Guo and Rubin, 2011; Dovzhenok et al., 2013).

Previous neuronal network models of PD have either not included a cortex at all (Terman et al., 2002; Rubchinsky et al., 2003; Park et al., 2011), approximated it as a random Poisson process (Humphries et al., 2006), or considered it as a single layer with a single cell type (Leblois et al., 2006). The thalamus has also either been omitted or treated as a single population. In this work, we sought to fill this gap by exploring the interactions of the large-scale dynamics of basal ganglia, represented by a field model, with a far smaller but more spatially detailed network model of the thalamus and six-layered cortex.

1.1. COMPOSITE MODEL

The primary aim of this paper is to determine how the large-scale dynamics of the brain affect the information flow in small networks of neurons. Most previous brain modeling efforts have been directed at one of these two scales, rather than their interaction. These efforts have consisted of either (1) neural field models that describe the dynamics of the whole brain, without explicitly modeling the activity of individual neurons (Nunez, 1974; Jirsa and Haken, 1996; Robinson et al., 1997; Destexhe and Sejnowski, 2009), or (2) spiking neuronal network models that capture individual neurons' dynamics, but are many orders of magnitude smaller than the brains of even the simplest vertebrates (Lumer et al., 1997; Neymotin et al., 2011b). Several large network models have also been published that have roughly as many "neurons" as the full mammalian brain (Izhikevich and Edelman, 2008; Ananthanarayanan et al., 2009). However, these models have not yet reproduced large-scale dynamics with the same degree of fidelity as neural field models. For example, the model of

Izhikevich and Edelman (2008) showed simultaneous peaks in the delta and alpha bands, whereas experimentally these peaks are characteristic of sleep and wakefulness, respectively, and are hence rarely observed simultaneously (Niedermeyer and Lopes da Silva, 1999). Such infidelity may be because the enormous computational resources required to run these models makes it impractical to constrain their parameters by fitting their dynamics to experimental data.

Recently, both Deco and Jirsa (2012) and Wilson et al. (2012) described approximations that allow small and large spatial scales to be spanned at a mesoscopic level of description, allowing large-scale dynamics (e.g., BOLD signals) to be related to small-scale network properties (e.g., criticality). Robinson and Kim (2012) took a different approach: they described the theoretical basis of combining spiking network and neural field components into a single model. The fundamental challenge in combining these two modeling approaches is to create a common representation of neuronal activity, since individual spikes are used in network models, while field models use average firing rates. Converting individual spikes into an average firing rate is a straightforward reduction of dimensionality: one simply needs to average over multiple neurons in the model. In contrast, converting an average population firing rate into individual spikes in multiple neurons requires an increase in dimensionality. This is a degenerate problem, so additional assumptions must be made. One approach, described in Robinson and Kim (2012), is to treat each neuron as a phase oscillator. The average firing rate then represents the instantaneous rate of phase change, with a given neuron firing whenever its phase advances by 2π radians. However, here we used an alternative approach, in which the average firing rate is taken as the instantaneous rate for an ensemble of Poisson processes. These are then used to generate individual spike times (Dayan and Abbott, 2001; Leblois et al., 2006; Chadderdon et al., 2012). This approach produces variability in spike timings even with a constant average firing rate, as is seen in real neuronal populations.

2. METHODS

The model we used consisted of a network of spiking neurons that was "embedded" in a neural field model. The embedding consisted of having the field model generate spikes (via an ensemble of Poisson processes) that were used to drive the network model. Except where otherwise noted, all analyses were performed on the network model. The complete model is publicly available via ModelDB: https://senselab.med.yale.edu/modeldb/ShowModel.asp?model=147366.

2.1. NEURAL FIELD MODEL

The neural field model was based on the work of Van Albada and Robinson (2009) and Van Albada et al. (2009). The neuronal populations and connections that constitute this model are shown in **Figures 1** and **3A** respectively. The basal ganglia nuclei modeled were the striatum, internal and external pallidal segments, and STN. The internal pallidal population can be thought of as including the substantia nigra pars reticulata, which has very similar connections and properties. The substantia nigra pars compacta was not explicitly modeled, except through its effects on the other nuclei. The thalamus was modeled as two populations: the inhibitory thalamic reticular nucleus (TRN) and the excitatory thalamocortical relay nuclei (TCR). The cortex was also modeled as two populations, representing inhibitory interneurons and excitatory pyramidal neurons. Since together these neuronal populations comprise a large portion of the brain, a network formulation would be computationally intractable. Except for a unitless normalization constant, all parameter values were based on anatomical and physiological data, as listed in Table 2 of Van Albada and Robinson (2009).

In neural field models, neuronal properties are spatially averaged. The dynamics are then governed by a set of equations relating the mean firing rates of populations of neurons to changes in mean cell-body potential, which are in turn triggered by mean rates of incoming spikes. The neural field model used here was based on a previously published model of the electrophysiology of the thalamocortical system (Robinson et al., 1997, 2001, 2002, 2005; Rennie et al., 1999), which in turn was based on earlier field models (Wilson and Cowan, 1973; Nunez, 1974; Freeman, 1975; Steriade et al., 1990; Wright and Liley, 1996).

The first component of the model is the description of the average response of populations of neurons to changes in mean cell-body potential. The mean firing rate Q_a of each population a is the maximum attainable firing rate $Q_a^{\max}$ times the proportion of neurons with a membrane potential V_a above the mean threshold potential θ_a. This can be approximated by the sigmoid function

$$Q_a(\mathbf{r}, t) = \frac{Q_a^{\max}}{1 + e^{-[V_a(\mathbf{r},t)-\theta_a]/\sigma'}}, \quad (1)$$

where $\mathbf{r}$ is the spatial coordinate, t is time, and σ' is $\sqrt{3}/\pi$ times the standard deviation of the distribution of firing thresholds (Wright and Liley, 1995). This function increases smoothly from 0 to $Q_a^{\max}$ as V_a changes from $-\infty$ to ∞.

The change in the mean cell-body potential due to afferent activity depends on the mean number of synapses N_{ab} from neurons of population b to neurons of population a (note that the direction of projection $b \to a$ follows the conventions of control theory and matrix multiplication). The change in potential also depends on s_{ab}, the time-integrated change in cell-body potential per incoming spike. Defining $\nu_{ab} = N_{ab}s_{ab}$, the change in the mean cell-body potential in neurons of population a is (Robinson et al., 2004).

$$D_{\alpha\beta}(t)V_a(t) = \sum_b \nu_{ab}\phi_b(t - \tau_{ab}), \quad (2)$$

$$D_{\alpha\beta}(t) = \frac{1}{\alpha\beta}\frac{d^2}{dt^2} + \left(\frac{1}{\alpha} + \frac{1}{\beta}\right)\frac{d}{dt} + 1. \quad (3)$$

Here, $\phi_b(t - \tau_{ab})$ is the incoming firing rate, τ_{ab} represents the axonal time delay for signals traveling from population b to population a neurons, and α and β are the decay and rise rates of mean cell-body potential. The differential operator $D_{\alpha\beta}(t)$ represents dendritic and synaptic integration of incoming signals (Robinson et al., 1997; Rennie et al., 2000). The synapses and dendrites form an effective low-pass filter with a cut-off frequency between $1/\alpha$ and $1/\beta$.

In this model, neuronal activity spreads along the cortex in a wavelike fashion. This reflects previous models (Nunez, 1995; Jirsa and Haken, 1996; Bressloff, 2001) as well as experimental observations of such waves following cortical stimulation (Burns, 1951; Nunez, 1974; Rubino et al., 2006). Estimates of characteristic axonal ranges and propagation speeds suggest that these waves are significantly damped on the scale of the human cortex (Robinson et al., 2001, 2004; Wright and Liley, 1995). Assuming that the range distribution of corticocortical fibers decays exponentially at large distances, activity propagates according to a 2D damped-wave equation of the form (Robinson et al., 1997)

$$Q_a(\mathbf{r}, t) = \left[\frac{1}{\gamma_a^2}\frac{\partial^2}{\partial t^2} + \frac{2}{\gamma_a}\frac{\partial}{\partial t} + 1 - r_a^2\nabla^2\right]\phi_a(\mathbf{r}, t), \quad (4)$$

where $\gamma_a = v_a/r_a$ is the damping rate, consisting of the average axonal transmission speed v_a ($\simeq 10\,\text{m}\cdot\text{s}^{-1}$) and the characteristic axonal range r_a. In practice, most types of axons are short enough to justify setting $\gamma_a = \infty$, which has been termed the local interaction approximation (Robinson et al., 2004). We therefore take only γ_e, the damping rate of cortical pyramidal neurons, to be finite. This turns all wave equations except the cortical one into delayed one-to-one mappings. The model was implemented on a 5×5 grid of nodes with coupling to nearest-neighbor nodes via this damped-wave equation.

2.2. SPIKING NETWORK MODEL

The spiking network was based on several previous models developed by our group (Lytton and Stewart, 2005; Lytton et al., 2008b; Neymotin et al., 2011b; Kerr et al., 2012; Song et al., 2013). It consisted of 4950 event-driven integrate-and-fire neurons. These were divided into three types (excitatory pyramidal cells *E*, fast-spiking inhibitory interneurons *I*, and low-threshold spiking interneurons *IL*), which were in turn distributed across the six layers of the cortex, plus two thalamic cell populations (excitatory thalamocortical relay *TCR* and inhibitory thalamic reticular *TRN*), for 15 distinct neuronal populations in total. The numbers and locations of each neuronal population are illustrated in **Figure 2**, and were as follows: E2 (i.e., excitatory pyramidal neurons of layer 2/3), 1500; I2, 250; IL2, 150; E4, 300; I4, 200; IL4, 150; E5R, 650; E5B, 150; I5, 250; IL5, 150; E6, 600; I6, 250; IL6, 150; TCR, 100; and TRN, 100. The pyramidal neurons

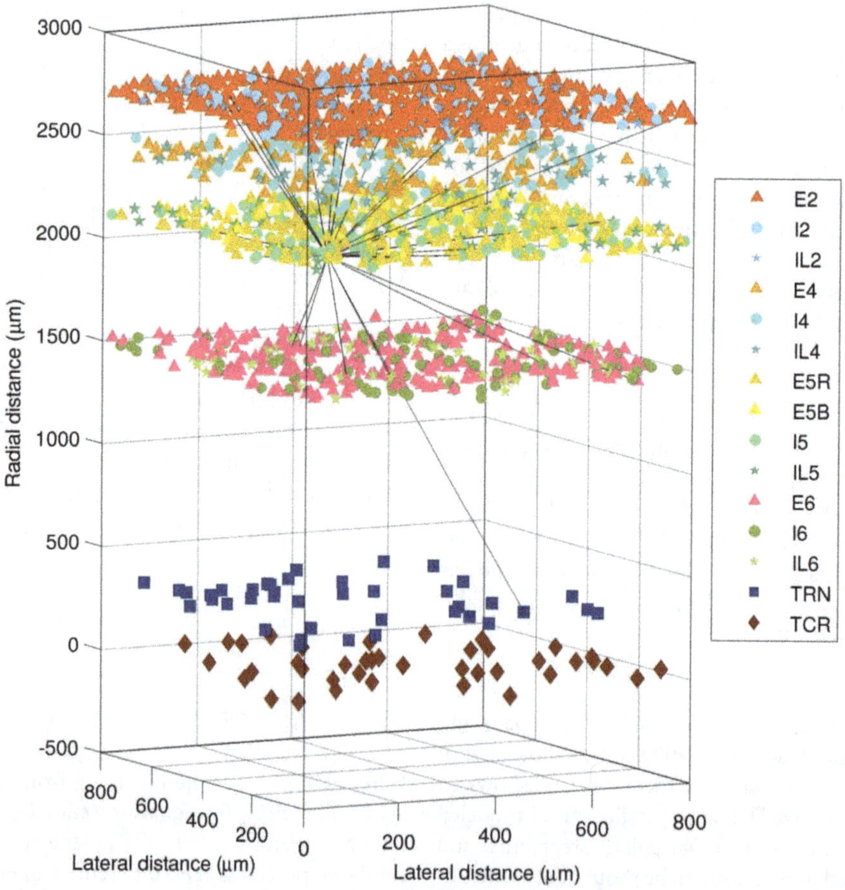

FIGURE 2 | Layout of the 4950 neurons in the spiking network model (1980 cells shown). Shapes show type (triangle = excitatory pyramidal, E; circle = fast-spiking interneuron, I; star = low-threshold spiking interneuron, IL; square = thalamic reticular, TRN; diamond = thalamocortical relay, TCR). The 28 efferent connections from a single layer 5 pyramidal neuron are shown (black lines). The distance from the thalamus to the cortex is not shown to scale.

in layer 5 are divided into two populations, *R* (regular firing) and *B* (bursting), since these have different cellular properties and connectivity patterns.

Connectivity (shown in **Figure 3B**) and the relative numbers of neurons per layer were based on published models (Traub et al., 2005; Neymotin et al., 2011a,b) and anatomical studies (Thomson et al., 2002; Binzegger et al., 2004; Song et al., 2005; Lefort et al., 2009; Adesnik and Scanziani, 2010). Connectivity was strongest between populations within a given layer, as seen from the four clusters visible along the diagonal of **Figure 3B**. Overall, excitatory neurons had more projections than inhibitory ones, but inhibitory projections were typically stronger. This balanced excitation and inhibition such that the overall gain of the system (the number of additional output spikes for every additional input spike) was close to unity. Such balance is necessary for avoiding the stable but undesirable states of seizure (pathologically high firing) and quiescence (pathologically low firing).

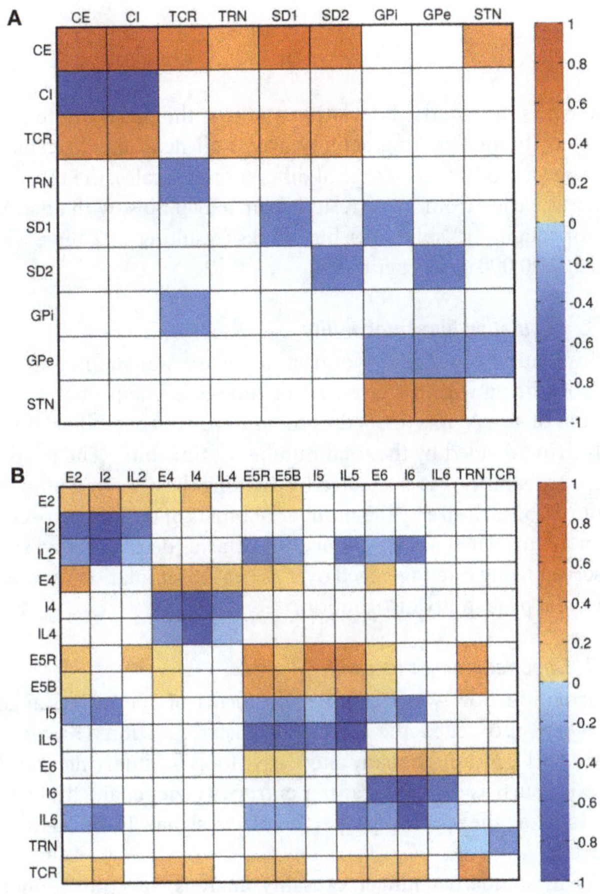

FIGURE 3 | Connectivity of the models. Color shows normalized effective connectivity (probability × weight) from rows to columns, with red denoting excitation and blue denoting inhibition. **(A)** Connections in the field model (CE, cortical excitatory; CI, cortical inhibitory; TCR, thalamocortical relay; TRN, thalamic reticular nucleus; SD1, striatal D1; SD2, striatal D2; GPi, internal globus pallidus; GPe, external globus pallidus; STN, subthalamic nucleus). **(B)** Connections in the network model. Approximate diagonal symmetry shows that most connections are reciprocal; relatively strong connections along the diagonal indicate high intralaminar connectivity.

Individual neurons were modeled as event-driven, rule-based units. Since computing resources are finite, a tradeoff must be made between the complexity of neurons vs. the complexity of the network. The neuron model used was complex enough to replicate key features found in real neurons, including adaptation, bursting, depolarization blockade, and voltage-sensitive NMDA conductance (Lytton and Stewart, 2005, 2006; Lytton and Omurtag, 2007; Lytton et al., 2008a,b; Neymotin et al., 2011b), yet was simple enough to connect into large (10^3–10^6 neuron) networks.

Each neuron had a membrane voltage state variable (V_m) with a baseline value determined by a resting membrane potential parameter (V_{RMP}, set at −65 mV for pyramidal neurons and low-threshold-spiking interneurons, and at −63 mV for fast-spiking interneurons). This membrane voltage was updated by one of three events: synaptic input, threshold spike generation, and refractory period. These events are described briefly below; further detail can be found in the papers and code cited above.

2.2.1. Synaptic input

The response of the membrane voltage to synaptic input was modeled as an instantaneous rise and exponential decay: $V_n(t) = V_n(t_0) + w_s(1 - V_n(t_0)/E_i)e^{-\frac{t-t_0}{\tau_i}}$, where V_n is the membrane voltage of neuron *n*; t_0 is the synaptic event time (i.e., $t - t_0$ is the time since the event); w_s is the weight of synaptic connection *s*; E_i is the reversal potential of ion channel *i*, relative to resting membrane potential (where i = AMPA, NMDA, or $\mathrm{GABA_A}$; and $E_{\mathrm{AMPA}} = 65$ mV, $E_{\mathrm{NMDA}} = 90$ mV, and $E_{\mathrm{GABA_A}} = -15$ mV); and τ_i is the receptor time constant for ion channel *i* (where $\tau_{\mathrm{AMPA}} = 20$ ms; $\tau_{\mathrm{NMDA}} = 30$ ms; and $\tau_{\mathrm{GABA_A}} = 10$ or 20 ms for somatic and dendritic $\mathrm{GABA_A}$, respectively).

2.2.2. Action potentials

A neuron fires an action potential at time *t* if $V_n(t) > T_n(t)$ and $V_n(t) < B_n$, where V_n, T_n, and B_n are the membrane voltage, threshold voltage (−40 mV for pyramidal neurons and fast-spiking interneurons, −47 mV for low-threshold-spiking interneurons), and blockade voltage (−10 mV for interneurons and −25 mV for pyramidal neurons), respectively, for neuron *n*. Action potentials arrive at target neurons at time $t_2 = t_1 + l(n_1, n_2)/v + \tau_s$, where t_1 is the time the first neuron fired, τ_s is the delay due to synaptic conduction effects, $l(n_1, n_2)$ is the axon length between neurons n_1 and n_2, and v is the axonal conduction velocity ($\simeq 1\ \mathrm{m \cdot s^{-1}}$, which is smaller than in the field model, since long-range fibers tend to be more heavily myelinated).

2.2.3. Refractory period

After firing, a neuron cannot fire during the absolute refractory period, τ_A (10 ms for interneurons and 50 ms for pyramidal neurons). Firing is reduced during the relative refractory period by two effects: first, an increase in threshold potential, $T_n(t) = \left(1 + Re^{-\frac{t-t_0}{\tau_R}}\right) T_n(t_0)$, where *R* is the fractional increase in threshold voltage due to the relative refractory period (0.25 for interneurons and 0.75 for pyramidal neurons) and τ_R is its time constant (1.5 ms for interneurons and 8 ms for pyramidal neurons); and second, by hyperpolarization, $V_n(t) = V_n(t_0) - He^{-\frac{t-t_0}{\tau_H}}$, where H is the amount of hyperpolarization (0.5 mV for interneurons and 1 mV for pyramidal neurons) and τ_H is its time constant (50 ms for interneurons and 400 ms for pyramidal neurons).

Local field potentials (LFPs) were computed for each cortical layer as the average membrane voltage across all neurons in that layer; after baseline removal and normalization, this approach is roughly equivalent to summing over all synaptic currents (Mazzoni et al., 2010). While this approach does not take into consideration synaptic and dendritic geometry, this is not possible in the event-driven point-neuron model used here.

Simulations were run in NEURON 7.3 (Hines and Carnevale, 2001; Carnevale and Hines, 2006) on a Linux workstation with an Intel Xeon 2.7 GHz CPU; each 20 s simulation took approximately 10 min to run on a single core. To avoid edge effects, the first and last 2 s of simulated data were discarded. All analyses were performed on the remaining 16 s of simulated data. Since the model is at steady-state and does not incorporate plasticity effects, longer runs produced similar results (data not shown). Model parameters were tuned manually (within physiological limits) to match experimentally observed firing rates, dynamics, and information-theoretic properties, as described in Song et al. (2013).

2.3. INPUT DRIVE

The composite model consisted of the spiking network model being driven by ("embedded in") the activity of the field model. Since the field model represents a brain region much larger than the network model, the field causally influences the network, but not vice versa. The key methodological novelty of this work is that the spiking network model is thus embedded in an environment with physiologically realistic dynamics (as provided by the field model), rather than the white noise environment such models are typically embedded in.

To obtain realistic firing rates in the network model, the input spiking rate each neuron receives must be bounded. Hence, the firing rate from each neuronal population in the field model was normalized so that the minimum and maximum input spiking rates were 225 and 1125 s^{-1} for excitatory neurons and 30% lower for inhibitory neurons. The input drive was obtained by treating each of these normalized instantaneous firing rates as the rate of an ensemble of Poisson processes for generating spikes. These spikes were then used to drive each population of spiking neurons, using the same connections as used in the field model itself (e.g., excitatory cortical neurons in the network model received input from the excitatory cortical field, the inhibitory cortical field, and the thalamic field); relative connection weights were also set to match those of the field model. Thus, each neuron belonging to a given population in the network model receives the same average rate of input from the field model, but from a separate Poisson process, thereby avoiding artificial correlations in input spike times between neurons.

Four different inputs were explored in this work. First, all neurons in the network were driven by spikes drawn from a spectrally white distribution ("WN", the white noise model). This represents the control condition, and is identical to the approach used in previous work with the network model (Neymotin et al., 2011b). Second, neurons were driven by the thalamocortical version of the field model ("TC", the thalamocortical model); i.e., connection strengths to and from the basal ganglia neuronal populations were set to zero. Third, neurons were driven by the full basal ganglia/thalamocortical model described above ("BG", the healthy basal ganglia model). Finally, neurons were driven by the full basal ganglia/thalamocortical model, using parameter values shown by Van Albada and Robinson (2009) to best match the electrophysiological changes associated with the degeneration of dopaminergic projections to the striatum ("PD", the Parkinson's disease model).

2.4. ANALYSIS

2.4.1. Fano factor

The Fano factor, a common measure of spiking variability (Churchland et al., 2010), is the ratio of the variance to the mean of the spike rate:

$$F = \frac{\sigma^2}{\mu}, \tag{5}$$

where σ is the standard deviation and μ is the mean of the time series of binned spiking activity across all neurons. To explore spiking variability on a range of different time scales, the time bin size was varied from 1 ms (resulting in 16,000 bins, with an average of roughly 10 spikes per bin) to 8 s (resulting in 2 bins, with roughly 80,000 spikes per bin).

2.4.2. Population burst probability

A population burst (Benayoun et al., 2010) was defined as ≥ 2 neurons firing within a given 10 ms time bin. The probability of a burst of size N was defined as the number of time bins with N cells firing divided by the total number of time bins. The relative burst probability was calculated by dividing the observed number of bursts of each size by the number of bursts of that size expected from uncorrelated activity, which in turn was determined via the observed firing rate (averaged over the entire simulation) and the binomial probability distribution.

2.4.3. Spectral granger causality

Information flow was quantified in terms of spectral Granger causality, also called the directed transfer function (Kaminski et al., 2001). Although many alternative tools for inferring causality exist, such as directed transfer entropy (Lizier et al., 2011), no others allow the spectral properties of the signals to be analyzed in detail.

As in standard Granger causality analysis, spectral Granger causality of $\alpha(f) \rightarrow \beta(f)$ is non-zero if prior knowledge of variable α at frequency f reduces error in the prediction of β at frequency f. The directionality of the causation arises from the fact that Granger causality quantifies how much the history of time series α can be used to predict the future of time series β: if α has a strong causal influence on β, then the prediction error will be reduced.

Spectral Granger causality is calculated by Fourier transforming the multivariate autoregressive model used in standard

Granger causality. Hence, the spectral Granger causality from time series $\alpha(t)$ to time series $\beta(t)$ is defined as (Cui et al., 2008)

$$G_{\alpha\to\beta}(f) = -\log\left(1 - \frac{\left(N_{\alpha\alpha} - \frac{N_{\beta\alpha}^2}{N_{\alpha\alpha}}\right)|H_{\beta,\alpha}(f)|^2}{S_{\beta,\beta}(f)}\right), \quad (6)$$

where N is the noise covariance, $H(f)$ is the transfer function, and $S(f)$ the spectral matrix, as derived from the bivariate autoregressive model of $\alpha(t)$ and $\beta(t)$. This analysis was performed in Matlab 2012a using code based on the BSMART toolbox, available via http://www.brain-smart.org.

3. RESULTS

The neural field model results were similar to those reported previously (Van Albada and Robinson, 2009; Van Albada et al., 2009), and are briefly presented here for completeness. We then present the overall dynamics of the spiking network model (Kerr et al., 2012), comparing its dynamics for each of the four drives (white noise, the thalamocortical model, the healthy basal ganglia model, and the PD model). Finally, we focus more closely on the alterations that occur in the PD-driven model and their implications. We have split the results into these sections in order to better accomplish our dual goals of (1) presenting the new composite model, and (2) applying this model to help understand the pathophysiology of PD.

3.1. FIELD MODEL DYNAMICS

Firing rates in each neuronal population were similar to those reported previously (Van Albada and Robinson, 2009; Van Albada et al., 2009). Because the drive from the field model to the network model was normalized to a range that provided realistic firing rates in the latter, tonic firing rates had negligible effect on the simulations.

Changes in coherence are a commonly reported finding in PD. In the PD model, coherence between the GPe and the GPi was lost, and high frequency power (>10 Hz) in the GPi was reduced (**Figure 4**). In the healthy state, activity in the GPe and GPi is strongly correlated ($r^2 = 0.9$). Following dopamine loss, this correlation is substantially reduced ($r^2 = 0.3$). This is because the GPe and GPi are both mostly influenced by the striatum in the healthy state, whereas the GPi is strongly driven by the STN in the parkinsonian state, resulting in strong coherence between the GPi and STN in the PD model. Increased STN-GPi coherence at frequencies up to about 35 Hz has indeed been found in PD off levodopa compared to the on-levodopa condition (Brown et al., 2001). Since the GPi is the only nucleus of the basal ganglia that projects to the thalamus or cortex (**Figure 1**), all changes observed in the network model in the healthy versus PD cases are due to the altered dynamics of the GPi.

To characterize the overall dynamics of the different field models, we looked at their power spectra. In the absence of the basal ganglia, cortical excitatory neurons had a strong alpha peak (10 Hz), and a weaker harmonic in the beta range (20 Hz), as shown in **Figure 4B**. Cortical inhibitory neurons were driven strongly by thalamocortical cells, evident both in the phase locking between the two populations (**Figure 4A**), and in the similarity of their power spectra below 70 Hz (**Figure 4B**). The addition of the basal ganglia (**Figure 4B**, middle panel) reduced the strength of the alpha peak in cortical excitatory neurons and reduced the slope of the power law spectral fall-off at high frequencies; in cortical excitatory neurons, this slope changed from $P(f) \propto f^{-5.3}$ to $P(f) \propto f^{-4.3}$. Reduced dopamine corresponding to PD reduced the power of higher frequencies (>10 Hz) relative to lower frequencies (<10 Hz) in the cortical, thalamic, and GPi spectra. For example, the GPi showed a 2% decrease in power at 10 Hz compared to a 76% decrease at 20 Hz. In contrast, reduced dopamine increased power in the STN at frequencies >10 Hz (e.g., 2.2 times larger at 20 Hz), a result also reported experimentally (Brown et al., 2001; Cassidy et al., 2002; Priori et al., 2004).

3.2. NETWORK MODEL DYNAMICS

The field drive into the network model strongly modulated its spiking activity (**Figure 5**). Firing rates varied from near zero during the troughs of input activity to >10 Hz during the peaks (**Figure 5A**). The temporal structure of the spiking activity depended strongly on the type of input drive used (**Figure 5B**). As a control, white noise produced no consistent temporal structure. The TC-driven model input produced some structure, with a characteristic time scale below 500 ms. The BG-driven model added some features on longer time scales (of order 1 s) to the activity produced by the TC-only field model. Variability in firing rate, as measured by the Fano factor, was lowest in the WN-driven model (**Figure 5D**)—as would be expected since the white noise had the lowest variability of the four inputs. On time scales <1 s, the PD-driven model had the greatest variability, while the BG-driven model had the greatest variability on scales >1 s.

The power spectra of the network model, shown in **Figure 6A**, were broadly similar to those of the input drives, but with several interesting differences. The basic filter properties of the network model are apparent from the shape of spectrum of the WN-driven model; to a first approximation, the network acts like a low-pass filter, with $P(f) \propto f^{-4.0}$ for $f > 20$ Hz. However, actual afferent activity in the brain is already low-pass filtered due to dendritic properties, so a more realistic input (the thalamocortical drive) results in even greater low-pass filtering. For example, the WN-driven model predicts 5.4 times more power at 10 Hz than the TC-driven model. Both BG- and PD-driven models differed markedly from the TC-driven model in the 20–30 Hz band, where many basal ganglia nuclei have their peak power. Interestingly, this peak was much sharper in the network model than in the input drive, demonstrating a resonance effect (compare **Figure 4A** with **Figure 6B**).

To quantify synchrony in the model on a population level, we used population burst size (Benayoun et al., 2010). All of the field-driven models showed substantially higher population bursting than the WN-driven model (**Figure 6B**). This is because the field drive applies a global modulatory signal to the network, which organizes the firing of its neurons into up and down states (as evident from the bands of spikes in **Figure 5A**); in contrast, the WN-driven model has a constant, intermediate level of activation.

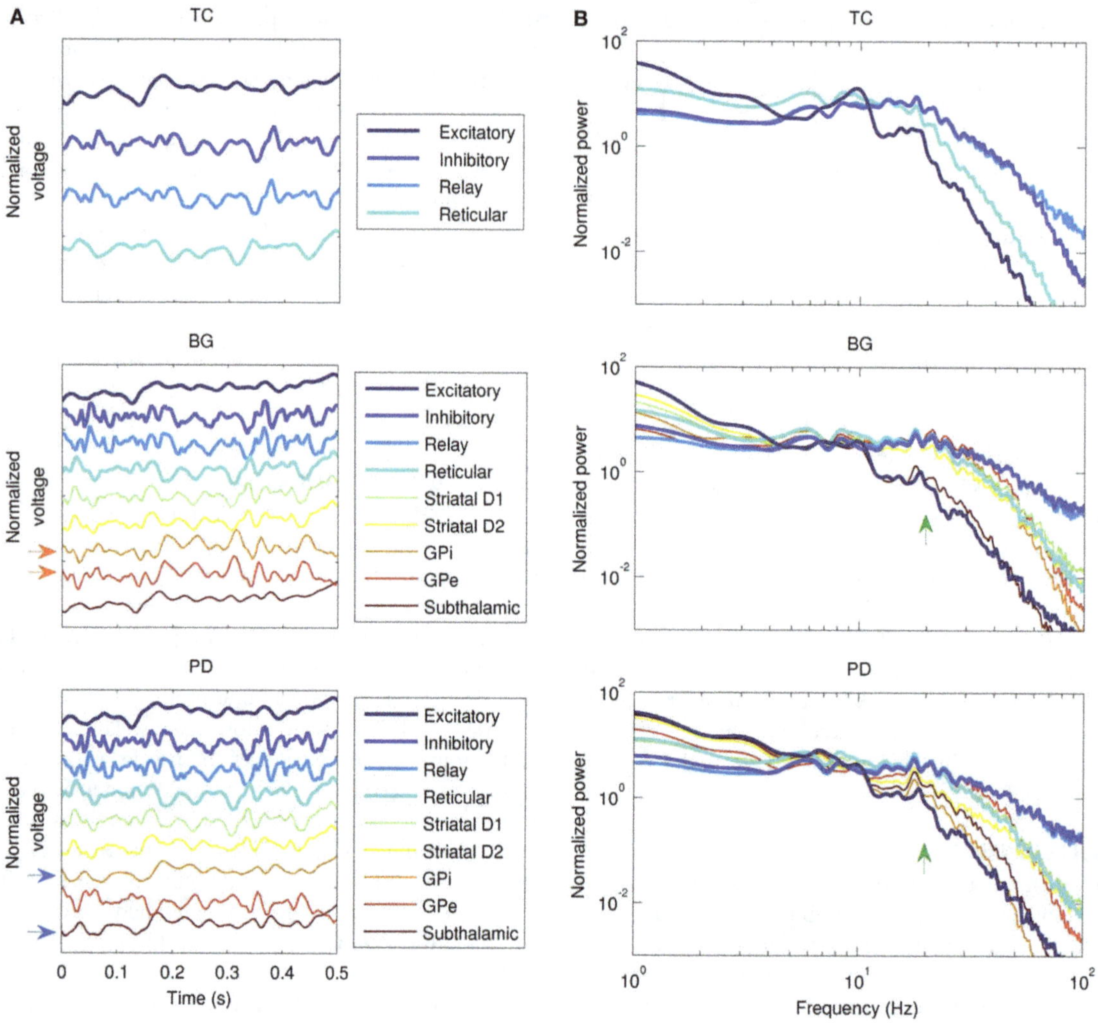

FIGURE 4 | Dynamics of the three field models (without the network model). TC, thalamocortical field model; BG, healthy basal ganglia model; PD, Parkinson's disease model; white noise model not shown. "Excitatory" and "inhibitory" refer to cortical subpopulations. **(A)** Local field potential (LFP) time series, showing phase relationships between populations. Activity in the globus pallidus internal (GPi) and external (GPe) segments is normally in phase (red arrows), but this relationship is lost in PD, since the GPi entrains to the subthalamic nucleus instead (blue arrows). **(B)** LFP spectra. Except for the subthalamic nucleus, healthy basal ganglia nuclei spectra are similar to the spectrum of the thalamic relay nuclei from 10–40 Hz. This is disrupted in PD (green arrows), especially in the GPi.

3.3. DYNAMICAL CHANGES IN THE PARKINSON'S DISEASE MODEL

The Parkinson's disease model (PD-driven model) showed a number of changes that suggest possible mechanisms underlying the clinical dysfunctions of the disease. Compared to the healthy control (BG-driven model), the PD-driven model showed a shift in the LFP spectrum toward lower frequencies, with higher delta power and a lower beta peak frequency (**Figure 6**), consistent with clinical findings (Stoffers et al., 2007). These changes were also readily apparent looking at the LFP time series, which showed a flattening of activity between the slow, high-amplitude features (**Figure 5B**). Soikkeli et al. (1991) noted such slowing in 10 out of 18 non-demented PD patients, as well as in all 18 demented PD patients studied [see Figure 1 in Soikkeli et al. (1991)].

The PD-driven model showed an $18 \pm 2\%$ decrease in firing rates compared to the healthy model (**Figure 5C**), consistent with changes in fMRI indicators of activity (Monchi et al., 2007). The PD-driven model also showed greater firing variability than the healthy model on most time scales. For example, with a bin size of 1 ms, the Fano factor was 41% higher in the PD-driven model (**Figure 5D**). However, it showed less variability on very long time scales: with a bin size of 8 s, the Fano factor was 2.4 times higher in the BG-driven model. The increased variability in the PD-driven model on all but the longest timescales is consistent with the enhanced oscillations and synchrony associated with PD (Goldberg et al., 2002). Note that maximal dynamical richness does not necessarily correspond to maximal variability in firing rates: for example, tonic firing will have low dynamical richness

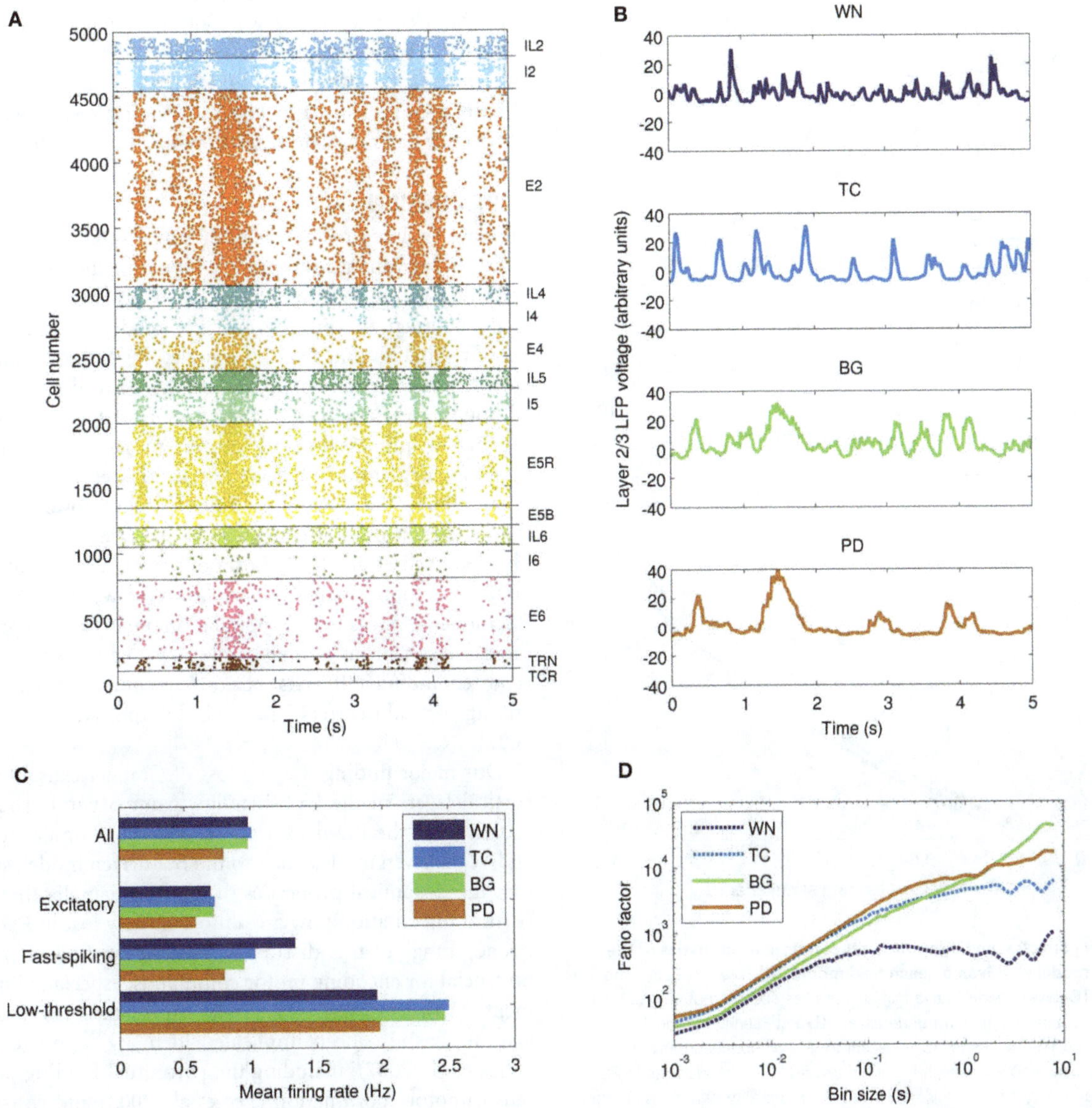

FIGURE 5 | Temporal dynamics of the network model with each type of input drive (WN, white noise; TC, thalamocortical; BG, healthy thalamocortical/basal ganglia; PD, Parkinson's disease). (A) Example spike raster from the BG-driven model. Low-frequency oscillations are clearly visible. **(B)** LFPs from layer 2/3 of each model. The BG case corresponds to the raster shown in **(A)**; peaks in voltage are correlated with peaks in spiking activity. **(C)** Mean firing rates by cell type (averaged over both cortical and thalamic populations). Overall, the PD-driven model had considerably lower firing rates, which result from excessive inhibition of the thalamic nuclei. **(D)** Variability in neuronal firing rates on different time scales. The PD- and BG-driven models (which receive the most highly structured input) show the most variability on short and long time scales, respectively; the WN-driven model (which receives the least structured input) shows the least variability on all scales.

and low variability on all time scales, while strong, seizure-like oscillations will also have low dynamical richness, despite very high variability (at least on the time scale of the oscillation).

The concentration of activity in large population bursts was a prominent feature of the PD-driven model. For example, bursts consisting of 40 neurons were 60% more common in the PD-driven model than in the healthy model, while 70-neuron bursts were three orders of magnitude more common. (Population bursts smaller than 30 neurons were more common in the healthy model, a result of its higher firing rate.) Although it is tempting to consider these large population events in the context of parkinsonian tremor, we did not note a clear periodicity in their occurrence.

A crucial question in PD is the mechanism by which information flow is disrupted from higher cortical areas (e.g., those involved in motor planning) to primary areas (e.g., those involved in motor execution). Although information flow between cortical layers is bidirectional, a dominant direction of information flow is suggested by both anatomical and functional studies (Bollimunta et al., 2008). This dominant information pathway is believed to

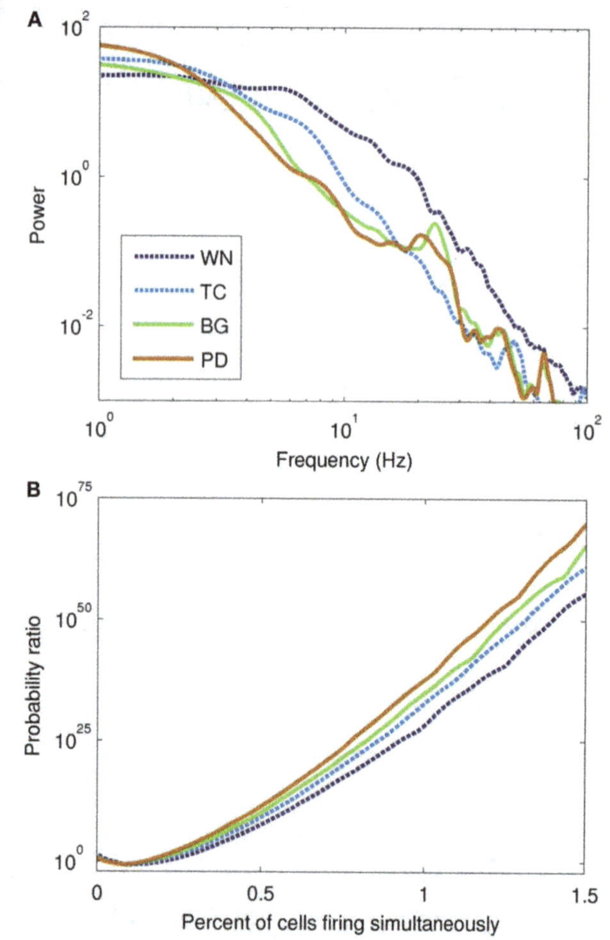

FIGURE 6 | Spectral and information-theoretic characteristics of the network model as driven by each field model. (A) Power spectra. The WN- and TC-driven models have fairly featureless spectra, but with different fall-off characteristics at high frequencies. BG- and PD-driven models are similar to the TC-driven spectrum, except for the pronounced peak at ~20 Hz. Spectral power is slightly shifted toward lower frequencies in PD. **(B)** Population burst frequency, defined as the probability of a given number of cells firing within a 10 ms time window, divided by the corresponding probability for uncorrelated processes. All models are many orders of magnitude more likely to show large bursts than would be predicted from uncorrelated activity; large population bursts are most likely in the PD-driven model.

stream from thalamic inputs to layer 4 (or upper layer 5 in agranular motor cortices), up to layer 2/3 for processing, and thence to layer 5, which in turn produces outputs to multiple sites including the thalamus, basal ganglia, and brainstem. We hypothesized that damage to this dominant pathway would represent a pathology with major functional consequences. We therefore used Granger causality to quantify information flow between the cortical layers that comprise this pathway.

Overall, interlaminar spectral Granger causality was highest in the BG-driven model, and lowest in the WN-driven model (**Figure 7**). Most notably, the BG-driven model showed a prominent peak in causality in the high-beta/low-gamma band (20–35 Hz). This peak was almost entirely absent in the PD-driven model; for example, peak causality from layer 4 to layer 5 in this frequency range was only half that of the BG-driven model (0.23 and 0.45 for PD- and BG-driven models, respectively), even though these models had similar spectral power (**Figure 6A**). As shown in **Figure 7**, similar results were seen in other layer pairs (e.g., 4 → 2/3, 2/3 → 5, and 6 → 2/3).

4. DISCUSSION

We have explored the effects of driving a spiking network model with several different types of input, including those corresponding to the healthy brain and to PD. Many of the differences between the healthy and PD models accord with prior experimental findings. For example, we found a modest but consistent reduction in firing rates of cortical neurons in PD. Although there are no direct studies of cortical firing rates during PD in humans, several indirect measures from functional imaging suggest such a decrease (Jenkins et al., 2004; Monchi et al., 2004, 2007). We also found a shift toward lower LFP frequencies, a finding consistent with PD electroencephalography (Soikkeli et al., 1991; Bosboom et al., 2006; Stoffers et al., 2007). We found increased synchrony between neurons in our PD model, as measured by population burst size and probability; increased synchrony among basal ganglia neurons is a commonly reported finding in PD (Raz et al., 1996), and increased synchrony among cortical neurons has also been reported (Goldberg et al., 2002).

Our major finding was the loss of Granger causality between cortical layers in the high-beta/low-gamma band. The Granger causality for the PD-driven model was more similar to the TC- and WN-driven models than to the BG-driven model, suggesting that the dynamical properties of the basal ganglia that facilitate cortical information flow are almost entirely lost in PD. The frequency range of this disrupted information flow is thought to be crucial for encoding motor commands, especially limb movements (Van Der Werf et al., 2008; Muthukumaraswamy, 2010). Gamma has also been implicated in many cognitive processes (Fries et al., 2007), including the perceptual binding underlying sensorimotor coordination (Lee et al., 2003) and consciousness (Llinas et al., 1998). Hence, our observation of disrupted causality might also partially account for some of the cognitive symptoms of PD, including bradyphrenia and planning deficits (Morris et al., 1988; Chaudhuri and Schapira, 2009).

The fact that Granger causality was disrupted in the PD-driven model (**Figure 7**) while the power spectrum was nearly unchanged in the same frequency band (**Figure 6A**) shows that the changed input drive has reorganized the dynamics of the network in complex ways. Since the GPi does not project directly to the cortex, these changes are entirely mediated by the thalamus; indeed, thalamic lesions alone are sufficient for producing parkinsonian symptoms in rats (Oehrn et al., 2007). Since the thalamus projects differentially to the different layers of the cortex, a major change in thalamic input is sufficient explanation for why the causality would shift so dramatically. Specifically, the thalamus normally projects strongly to layer 4; the peak in causality at 20–35 Hz is consistent with thalamic modulation by the GPi. In PD, inhibition to the thalamus is increased, which results in weaker drive to the cortex and thus a loss of information flow.

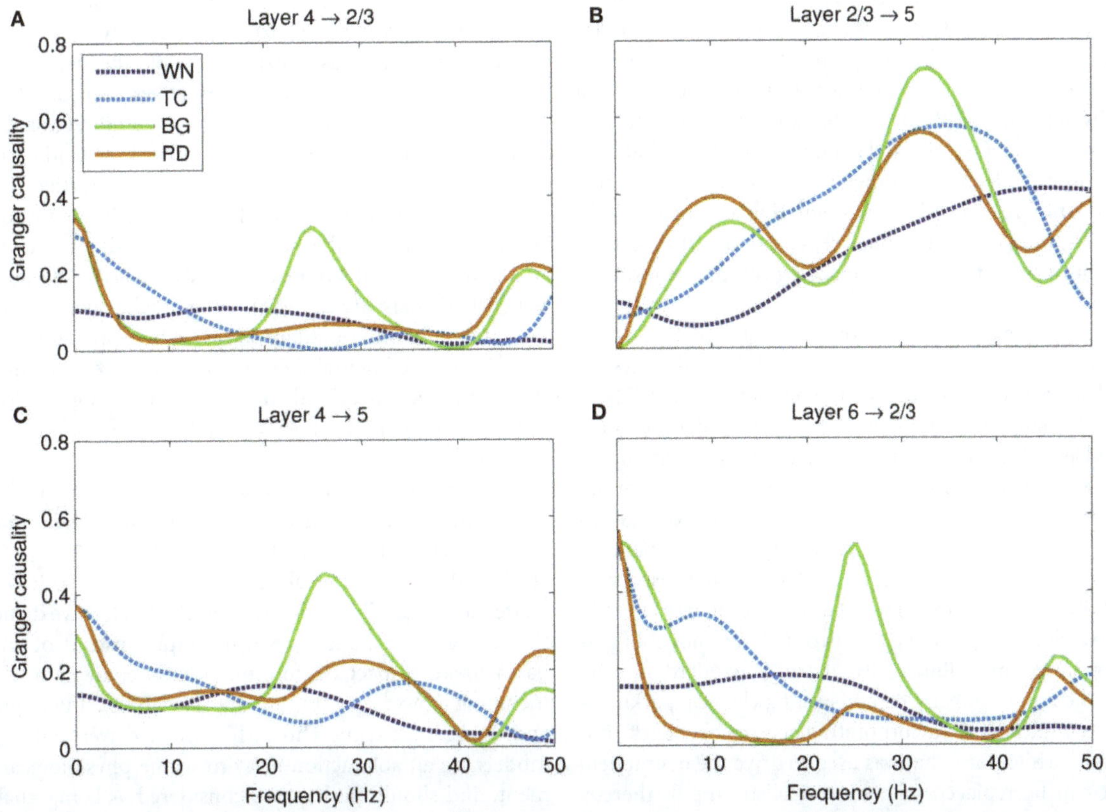

FIGURE 7 | Spectral Granger causality between cortical layers in each of the models. (A) The BG-driven model shows strong causality from layer 4 to 2/3 in the delta (<5 Hz) and high-beta/low-gamma (20–35 Hz) bands; causality in the latter band is almost entirely lost in Parkinson's disease. **(B)** The causality from layer 2/3 to layer 5 is slightly reduced in this band in Parkinson's disease. **(C)** These two effects combine to significantly reduce the total Granger causality from layer 4 to layer 5 in PD, especially in the high-beta/low-gamma band. **(D)** Similar reductions of Granger causality in this band were seen in other layer pairs, such as layer 6 to layer 2/3. In each case, the high-beta/low-gamma band Granger causality is significantly higher in the BG-driven model than in any of the other models.

Our findings suggest that therapeutic interventions, such as deep brain stimulation (Deuschl et al., 2006), may be more effective if they restore both the dynamics and the tonic level of activity of the GPi, rather than just the latter.

Several of our findings are qualitatively consistent with experimental results pointing to a loss of complexity in EEG time series from patients with a variety of cognitive disorders, including PD (Stam et al., 1994, 1995; Vaillancourt and Newell, 2002). For example, in the healthy model, the slope of the Fano factor increases roughly linearly on time scales from 1 ms to 10 s, indicating dynamical structure across a wide range of time scales (**Figure 5D**). This result can be seen qualitatively in the LFP time series of the healthy model, which appeared to show meaningful structure over a broader range of time scales than any of the other models (**Figure 5B**). We speculate that these properties may reflect the number of possible states that the network can assume, which may in turn be related to the number of different motor programs that can be implemented by the network. This principle is closely related to the concept of ϕ, defined as "the repertoire of causal states available to a system as a whole" (Balduzzi and Tononi, 2008). While ϕ cannot be easily computed for moderately large networks such as ours, we expect that it will be manifested in terms of the network's ability to perform real motor tasks—a topic we will explore in future work. Specifically, we predict that the BG-driven model will perform better on simulated reaching tasks than the WN-, TC-, or PD-driven models.

Beta-band activity (15–30 Hz) was predominantly generated by the thalamic and inhibitory cortical neuronal populations in our model (**Figure 4B**, top panel), in agreement with previous experimental and modeling studies (Brown and Williams, 2005; Hahn and McIntyre, 2010). Most empirical studies of beta activity in PD have focused on the basal ganglia nuclei, with increased power in the STN being a commonly reported finding (Brown and Williams, 2005; Kühn et al., 2005; Weinberger et al., 2006). In our model, we found that beta power in the STN was indeed enhanced in PD (**Figure 4B**, middle and bottom panels), which may reflect an idling or antikinetic state (Brown and Williams, 2005; Engel and Fries, 2010).

4.1. LIMITATIONS

Several experimentally observed features of PD, such as increased coherence among neurons in the STN, can only be explicitly represented using a neuronal network model of the basal ganglia

(Terman et al., 2002)—a major benefit of that modeling approach. However, it is not known whether these phenomena are causally linked to parkinsonian symptoms. Hence, in the present context, the benefits of using a neural field model for the basal ganglia outweigh the drawbacks of this approach. In future, a spiking network model of the basal ganglia would be desirable in order to account for these and other phenomena, such as reinforcement learning. An explicit representation of dopamine in such a mode—rather than the implicit representation used here—would also allow the effects of pharmacological interventions to be modeled directly.

Due to the eloquence of the motor system, movement disorders are the most obvious symptoms of PD. Yet the pathophysiology of the disease is widespread; even the retina is affected (Hajee et al., 2009). We stress that the spiking network model used here was designed as a model of association cortex, not primary motor cortex; for example, our model includes layer 4 cells, which are absent from the latter. However, since the thalamus and striatum have broad projections to the cortex, we expect the dynamical and information-theoretic changes in PD (such as increased synchrony and reduced complexity) to extend to motor areas as well. In the future, we will explore the effects of PD in a model of primary motor cortex controlling a virtual arm (Chadderdon et al., 2012), with the aim of directly demonstrating classical parkinsonian motor symptoms. By incorporating sensory feedback into this model, the white noise that was used to drive the neural field component can be replaced with more realistic input, thereby addressing another obvious limitation of the method used here.

4.2. MULTISCALE DYNAMICS IN A COMPOSITE MODEL

To our knowledge, this work represents the first composite spiking network/neural field model of the brain. This is a multiscale model that spans spatial scales from 10 μm to 30 cm and temporal scales from 1 ms to tens of seconds. The composite method provides a way of linking two types of models that provide access to different spatial scales—a network model than spans scales from individual neurons (10 μm) to a cortical column (600 μm), and a field model encompassing the whole diencephalon (30 cm). Temporally, both network and field models are valid over many orders of magnitude (approximately 10^{-3}–10^{4} s).

The mechanism used here to couple the field and network models is just one of several alternatives (Wilson et al., 2012). In the present case, the coupling was unidirectional; the network model did not affect the dynamics of the field model. While this can be easily justified in terms of the effective size of each model, an alternative approach generates the neural field based on the dynamics of the network model, using the new neuron-in-cell approach of Robinson and Kim (2012). Because spiking network models are still limited in their capacity to generate accurate dynamics on a large scale, this approach cannot yet be used in place of neural field models. However, this may change if scientific advances and improved computing facilities enable the development of larger and more realistic spiking network models.

Many spiking network models that are too small to show self-sustaining activity are driven by white noise (Hill and Tononi, 2005; Vogels and Abbott, 2005; Oswald et al., 2009; McDonnell et al., 2011; Volman et al., 2011; Kerr et al., 2012; Muller and Destexhe, 2012; Vijayan and Kopell, 2012). Here we demonstrated that using physiologically realistic input instead of white noise has a major impact on multiple measures of network activity, including power spectra, spiking variability, burst probability, and Granger causality. Thus, white-noise-driven spiking network models are an abstraction away from the physiological environment, and should perhaps be considered as being analogous to artificially driven slice preparations rather than *in vivo* activity.

ACKNOWLEDGMENTS

Cliff C. Kerr, Samuel A. Neymotin, George L. Chadderdon, and William W. Lytton were supported by DARPA grant N66001-10-C-2008; P. A. Robinson was supported by the Australian Research Council and the Westmead Millennium Institute; and Sacha J. van Albada was supported by EU FP7 Grant 269921 (BrainScaleS) and the Helmholtz Alliance on Systems Biology. The funders had no role in the study design, data collection and analysis, decision to publish, or preparation of the manuscript.

REFERENCES

Adesnik, H., and Scanziani, M. (2010). Lateral competition for cortical space by layer-specific horizontal circuits. *Nature* 464, 1155–1160.

Ananthanarayanan, R., Esser, S. K., Simon, H. D., and Modha, D. S. (2009). "The cat is out of the bag: cortical simulations with 10^9 neurons, 10^{13} synapses," in *Proceedings of the Conference on High Performance Computing Networking, Storage and Analysis*, SC '09 (New York, NY: ACM), 1–12.

Balduzzi, D., and Tononi, G. (2008). Integrated information in discrete dynamical systems: motivation and theoretical framework. *PLoS Comput. Biol.* 4:e1000091. doi: 10.1371/journal.pcbi.1000091

Benayoun, M., Cowan, J. D., Van Drongelen, W., and Wallace, E. (2010). Avalanches in a stochastic model of spiking neurons. *PLoS Comput. Biol.* 6:e1000846. doi: 10.1371/journal.pcbi.1000846

Binzegger, T., Douglas, R. J., and Martin, K. A. (2004). A quantitative map of the circuit of cat primary visual cortex. *J. Neurosci.* 24, 8441–8453.

Bolam, J. P., Hanley, J. J., Booth, P. A. C., and Bevan, M. D. (2002). Synaptic organisation of the basal ganglia. *J. Anat.* 196, 527–542.

Bollimunta, A., Chen, Y., Schroeder, C. E., and Ding, M. (2008). Neuronal mechanisms of cortical alpha oscillations in awake-behaving macaques. *J. Neurosci.* 28, 9976–9988.

Bosboom, J. L., Stoffers, D., Stam, C. J., Van Dijk, B. W., Verbunt, J., Berendse, H. W., et al. (2006). Resting state oscillatory brain dynamics in Parkinson's disease: an MEG study. *Clin. Neurophysiol.* 117, 2521–2531.

Bressloff, P. C. (2001). Traveling fronts and wave propagation failure in an inhomogeneous neural network. *Physica D* 155, 83–100.

Brown, P., Oliviero, A., Mazzone, P., Insola, A., Tonali, P., and Di Lazzaro, V. (2001). Dopamine dependency of oscillations between subthalamic nucleus and pallidum in Parkinson's disease. *J. Neurosci.* 21, 1033–1038.

Brown, P., and Williams, D. (2005). Basal ganglia local field potential activity: character and functional significance in the human. *Clin. Neurophysiol.* 116, 2510–2519.

Burns, B. D. (1951). Some properties of isolated cerebral cortex in the unanaesthetized cat. *J. Physiol.* 112, 156–175.

Carnevale, N. T., and Hines, M. L. (2006). *The NEURON Book*. Cambridge, UK: Cambridge University Press.

Cassidy, M., Mazzone, P., Oliviero, A., Insola, A., Tonali, P., Di Lazzaro, V., et al. (2002). Movement-related changes in synchronization in the human basal ganglia. *Brain* 125, 1235–1246.

Chadderdon, G. L., Neymotin, S. A., Kerr, C. C., and Lytton, W. W. (2012). Reinforcement learning of targeted movement in a spiking neuronal model of motor cortex. *PLoS ONE* 7:e47251. doi: 10.1371/journal.pone.0047251

Chaudhuri, K. R., and Schapira, A. H. (2009). Non-motor symptoms of Parkinson's disease: dopaminergic pathophysiology and treatment. *Lancet Neurol.* 8, 464–474.

Churchland, M. M., Byron, M. Y., Cunningham, J. P., Sugrue, L. P., Cohen, M. R., Corrado, G. S., et al. (2010). Stimulus onset quenches neural variability: a widespread cortical phenomenon. *Nat. Neurosci.* 13, 369–378.

Cools, R. (2006). Dopaminergic modulation of cognitive function-implications for L-DOPA treatment in Parkinson's disease. *Neurosci. Biobehav. Rev.* 30, 1–23.

Cui, J., Xu, L., Bressler, S. L., Ding, M., and Liang, H. (2008). BSMART: a Matlab/C toolbox for analysis of multichannel neural time series. *Neural Netw.* 21, 1094–1104.

Dayan, P., and Abbott, L. F. (2001). *Theoretical Neuroscience*, Vol. 31. Cambridge, MA: MIT Press.

Deco, G. and Jirsa, V. K. (2012). Ongoing cortical activity at rest: criticality, multistability, and ghost attractors. *J. Neurosci.* 32, 3366–3375.

Destexhe, A., and Sejnowski, T. J. (2009). The Wilson–Cowan model, 36 years later. *Biol. Cybern.* 101, 1–2.

Deuschl, G., Schade-Brittinger, C., Krack, P., Volkmann, J., Schäfer, H., Bötzel, K., et al. (2006). A randomized trial of deep-brain stimulation for parkinson's disease. *N. Engl. J. Med.* 355, 896–908.

Dovzhenok, A., Park, C., Worth, R. M., and Rubchinsky, L. L. (2013). Failure of delayed feedback deep brain stimulation for intermittent pathological synchronization in Parkinson's disease. *PLoS ONE* 8:e58264. doi: 10.1371/journal.pone.0058264

Engel, A. K., and Fries, P. (2010). Beta-band oscillations – signalling the status quo? *Curr. Opin. Neurobiol.* 20, 156–165.

Freeman, W. (1975). *Mass Action in the Nervous System*. New York, NY: Academic Press.

Fries, P., Nikolic, D., and Singer, W. (2007). The gamma cycle. *Trends Neurosci.* 30, 309–316.

Goldberg, J. A., Boraud, T., Maraton, S., Haber, S., Vaadia, E., and Bergman, H. (2002). Enhanced synchrony among primary motor cortex neurons in the 1-methyl-4-phenyl-1, 2, 3, 6-tetrahydropyridine primate model of Parkinson's disease. *J. Neurosci.* 22, 4639–4653.

Guo, Y., and Rubin, J. E. (2011). Multi-site stimulation of subthalamic nucleus diminishes thalamocortical relay errors in a biophysical network model. *Neural Netw.* 24, 602–616.

Hahn, P. J., and McIntyre, C. C. (2010). Modeling shifts in the rate and pattern of subthalamopallidal network activity during deep brain stimulation. *J. Comput. Neurosci.* 28, 425–441.

Hajee, M. E., March, W. F., Lazzaro, D. R., Wolintz, A. H., Shrier, E. M., Glazman, S., et al. (2009). Inner retinal layer thinning in Parkinson disease. *Arch. Ophthalmol.* 127, 737–741.

Hill, S., and Tononi, G. (2005). Modeling sleep and wakefulness in the thalamocortical system. *J. Neurophysiol.* 93, 1671–1698.

Hines, M. L., and Carnevale, N. T. (2001). NEURON: a tool for neuroscientists. *Neuroscientist* 7, 123–135.

Humphries, M. D., Stewart, R. D., and Gurney, K. N. (2006). A physiologically plausible model of action selection and oscillatory activity in the basal ganglia. *J. Neurosci.* 26, 12921–12942.

Izhikevich, E. M., and Edelman, G. M. (2008). Large-scale model of mammalian thalamocortical systems. *Proc. Natl. Acad. Sci. U.S.A.* 105, 3593–3598.

Jenkins, I. H., Fernandez, W., Playford, E. D., Lees, A. J., Frackowiak, R. S. J., Passingham, R. E., et al. (2004). Impaired activation of the supplementary motor area in Parkinson's disease is reversed when akinesia is treated with apomorphine. *Ann. Neurol.* 32, 749–757.

Jirsa, V. K., and Haken, H. (1996). Field theory of electromagnetic brain activity. *Phys. Rev. Lett.* 77, 960–963.

Kaminski, M., Ding, M., Truccolo, W. A., and Bressler, S. L. (2001). Evaluating causal relations in neural systems: Granger causality, directed transfer function and statistical assessment of significance. *Biol. Cybern.* 85, 145–157.

Kerr, C. C., Neymotin, S. A., Chadderdon, G. L., Fietkiewicz, C. T., Francis, J. T., and Lytton, W. W. (2012). Electrostimulation as a prosthesis for repair of information flow in a computer model of neocortex. *IEEE Trans. Neural. Syst. Rehabil. Eng.* 20, 153–160.

Kühn, A. A., Trottenberg, T., Kivi, A., Kupsch, A., Schneider, G.-H., and Brown, P. (2005). The relationship between local field potential and neuronal discharge in the subthalamic nucleus of patients with parkinson's disease. *Exp. Neurol.* 194, 212–220.

Leblois, A., Boraud, T., Meissner, W., Bergman, H., and Hansel, D. (2006). Competition between feedback loops underlies normal and pathological dynamics in the basal ganglia. *J. Neurosci.* 26, 3567–3583.

Lee, K. H., Williams, L. M., Breakspear, M., and Gordon, E. (2003). Synchronous gamma activity: a review and contribution to an integrative neuroscience model of schizophrenia. *Brain Res. Rev.* 41, 57–78.

Lefort, S., Tomm, C., Floyd Sarria, J.-C., and Peterson, C. C. H. (2009). The excitatory neuronal network of the C2 barrel column in mouse primary somatosensory cortex. *Neuron* 61, 301–316.

Lizier, J., Heinzle, J., Horstmann, A., Haynes, J.-D., and Prokopenko, M. (2011). Multivariate information-theoretic measures reveal directed information structure and task relevant changes in fMRI connectivity. *J. Comput. Neurosci.* 30, 85–107.

Llinas, R., Ribary, U., Contreras, D., and Pedroarena, C. (1998). The neuronal basis for consciousness. *Philos. Trans. R. Soc. Lond. B Biol. Sci.* 353, 1841–1849.

Lumer, E. D., Edelman, G. M., and Tononi, G. (1997). Neural dynamics in a model of the thalamocortical system. I. Layers, loops and the emergence of fast synchronous rhythms. *Cereb. Cortex* 7, 207–227.

Lytton, W. W., Neymotin, S. A., and Hines, M. L. (2008a). The virtual slice setup. *J. Neurosci. Methods* 171, 309–315.

Lytton, W. W., Omurtag, A., Neymotin, S. A., and Hines, M. L. (2008b). Just-in-time connectivity for large spiking networks. *Neural Comput.* 20, 2745–2756.

Lytton, W. W., and Omurtag, A. (2007). Tonic-clonic transitions in computer simulation. *J. Clin. Neurophysiol.* 24, 175–181.

Lytton, W. W., and Stewart, M. (2005). A rule-based firing model for neural networks. *Int. J. Bioelectromagnetism* 7, 47–50.

Lytton, W. W., and Stewart, M. (2006). Rule-based firing for network simulations. *Neurocomputing* 69, 1160–1164.

Mazzoni, A., Whittingstall, K., Brunel, N., Logothetis, N. K., and Panzeri, S. (2010). Understanding the relationships between spike rate and delta/gamma frequency bands of LFPs and EEGs using a local cortical network model. *Neuroimage* 52, 956–972.

McDonnell, M. D., Mohan, A., Stricker, C., and Ward, L. M. (2011). Input-rate modulation of gamma oscillations is sensitive to network topology, delays and short-term plasticity. *Brain Res.* 1434, 162–177.

Monchi, O., Petrides, M., Doyon, J., Postuma, R. B., Worsley, K., and Dagher, A. (2004). Neural bases of set-shifting deficits in Parkinson's disease. *J. Neurosci.* 24, 702–710.

Monchi, O., Petrides, M., Mejia-Constain, B., and Strafella, A. P. (2007). Cortical activity in Parkinson's disease during executive processing depends on striatal involvement. *Brain* 130, 233–244.

Morris, R. G., Downes, J. J., Sahakian, B. J., Evenden, J. L., Heald, A., and Robbins, T. W. (1988). Planning and spatial working memory in Parkinson's disease. *J. Neurol. Neurosurg. Psychiatry* 51, 757–766.

Muller, L., and Destexhe, A. (2012). Propagating waves in thalamus, cortex and the thalamocortical system: experiments and models. *J. Physiol. Paris* 106, 222–238.

Muthukumaraswamy, S. D. (2010). Functional properties of human primary motor cortex gamma oscillations. *J. Neurophysiol.* 104, 2873–2885.

Neymotin, S. A., Jacobs, K. M., Fenton, A. A., and Lytton, W. W. (2011a). Synaptic information transfer in computer models of neocortical columns. *J. Comput. Neurosci.* 30, 69–84.

Neymotin, S. A., Lee, H., Park, E., Fenton, A. A., and Lytton, W. W. (2011b). Emergence of physiological oscillation frequencies in a computer model of neocortex. *Front. Comput. Neurosci.* 5:19. doi: 10.3389/fncom.2011.00019

Niedermeyer, E., and Lopes da Silva., F. (1999). *Electroencephalography: Basic Principles, Clinical Applications, and Related Fields.* Baltimore, MD: Urban and Schwarzenberg.

Nunez, P. L. (1974). Wave-like properties of the alpha rhythm. *IEEE Trans. Biomed. Eng.* 21, 473–482.

Nunez, P. L. (1995). *Neocortical Dynamics and Human EEG Rhythms.* Oxford: Oxford University Press.

Oehrn, C., Allbutt, H., and Henderson, J. (2007). Effect of ventrolateral thalamic nucleus lesions in the unilateral 6-hydroxydopamine rat model. *Behav. Brain Res.* 183, 67–77.

Oswald, A. M. M., Doiron, B., Rinzel, J., and Reyes, A. D. (2009). Spatial profile and differential recruitment of $GABA_B$ modulate oscillatory activity in auditory cortex. *J. Neurosci.* 29, 10321–10334.

Park, C., Worth, R. M., and Rubchinsky, L. L. (2011). Neural dynamics in parkinsonian brain: the boundary between synchronized and nonsynchronized dynamics. *Phys. Rev. E* 83:042901. doi: 10.1103/PhysRevE.83.042901

Priori, A., Foffani, G., Pesenti, A., Tamma, F., Bianchi, A. M., Pellegrini, M., et al. (2004). Rhythm-specific pharmacological modulation of subthalamic activity in Parkinson's disease. *Exp. Neurol.* 189, 369–379.

Raz, A., Feingold, A., Zelanskaya, V., Vaadia, E., and Bergman, H. (1996). Neuronal synchronization of tonically active neurons in the striatum of normal and parkinsonian primates. *J. Neurophysiol.* 76, 2083–2088.

Rennie, C. J., Robinson, P. A., and Wright, J. J. (1999). Effects of local feedback on dispersion of electrical waves in the cerebral cortex. *Phys. Rev. E* 59, 3320–3329.

Rennie, C. J., Wright, J. J., and Robinson, P. A. (2000). Mechanisms of cortical electrical activity and emergence of gamma rhythm. *J. Theor. Biol.* 205, 17–35.

Robinson, P. A., Loxley, P. N., O'Connor, S. C., and Rennie, C. J. (2001). Modal analysis of corticothalamic dynamics, electroencephalographic spectra, and evoked potentials. *Phys. Rev. E* 63:041909. doi: 10.1103/PhysRevE.63.041909

Robinson, P. A., and Kim, J. W. (2012). Spike, rate, field, and hybrid methods for treating neuronal dynamics and interactions. *J. Neurosci. Methods* 205, 283–294.

Robinson, P. A., Rennie, C. J., and Rowe, D. L. (2002). Dynamics of large-scale brain activity in normal arousal states and epileptic seizures. *Phys. Rev. E* 65:041924. doi: 10.1103/PhysRevE.65.041924

Robinson, P. A., Rennie, C. J., Rowe, D. L., and O'Connor, S. C. (2004). Estimation of multiscale neurophysiologic parameters by electroencephalographic means. *Hum. Brain Mapp.* 23, 53–72.

Robinson, P. A., Rennie, C. J., Rowe, D. L., O'Connor, S. C., and Gordon, E. (2005). Multiscale brain modelling. *Philos. Trans. R. Soc. Lond. B Biol. Sci.* 360, 1043–1050.

Robinson, P. A., Rennie, C. J., and Wright, J. J. (1997). Propagation and stability of waves of electrical activity in the cerebral cortex. *Phys. Rev. E* 56, 826–840.

Rubchinsky, L. L., Kopell, N., and Sigvardt, K. A. (2003). Modeling facilitation and inhibition of competing motor programs in basal ganglia subthalamic nucleus–pallidal circuits. *Proc. Natl. Acad. Sci. U.S.A.* 100, 14427–14432.

Rubino, D., Robbins, K. A., and Hatsopoulos, N. G. (2006). Propagating waves mediate information transfer in the motor cortex. *Nat. Neurosci.* 9, 1549–1557.

Soikkeli, R., Partanen, J., Soininen, H., Pääkkönen, A., and Riekkinen, P. (1991). Slowing of EEG in Parkinson's disease. *Electroencephalogr. Clin. Neurophysiol.* 79, 159–165.

Song, S., Sjostrom, P., Reigl, M., Nelson, S., and Chklovskii, D. (2005). Highly nonrandom features of synaptic connectivity in local cortical circuits. *PLoS Biol.* 3:e68. doi: 10.1371/journal.pbio.0030068

Song, W., Kerr, C. C., Lytton, W. W., and Francis, J. T. (2013). Cortical plasticity induced by spike-triggered microstimulation in primate somatosensory cortex. *PLoS ONE* 8:e57453. doi: 10.1371/journal.pone.0057453

Stam, C. J., Jelles, B., Achtereekte, H. A. M., Rombouts, S., Slaets, J. P. J., and Keunen, R. W. M. (1995). Investigation of EEG non-linearity in dementia and Parkinson's disease. *Electroencephalogr. Clin. Neurophysiol.* 95, 309–317.

Stam, K. J., Tavy, D. L. J., Jelles, B., Achtereekte, H. A. M., Slaets, J. P. J., and Keunen, R. W. M. (1994). Nonlinear dynamical analysis of multichannel EEG: clinical applications in dementia and Parkinson's disease. *Brain Topogr.* 7, 141–150.

Steriade, M., Gloor, P., Llinás, R. R., Lopes da Silva, F. H., and Mesulam, M. M. (1990). Basic mechanisms of cerebral rhythmic activities. *Electroencephalogr. Clin. Neurophysiol.* 76, 481–508.

Stoffers, D., Bosboom, J. L. W., Deijen, J. B., Wolters, E. C., Berendse, H. W., and Stam, C. J. (2007). Slowing of oscillatory brain activity is a stable characteristic of Parkinson's disease without dementia. *Brain* 130, 1847–1860.

Terman, D., Rubin, J. E., Yew, A. C., and Wilson, C. J. (2002). Activity patterns in a model for the subthalamopallidal network of the basal ganglia. *J. Neurosci.* 22, 2963–2976.

Thomson, A., West, D., Wang, Y., and Bannister, A. (2002). Synaptic connections and small circuits involving excitatory and inhibitory neurons in layers 2–5 of adult rat and cat neocortex: triple intracellular recordings and biocytin labelling *in vitro*. *Cereb. Cortex* 12, 936–953.

Traub, R. D., Contreras, D., Cunningham, M. O., Murray, H., LeBeau, F. E., Roopun, A., et al. (2005). Single-column thalamocortical network model exhibiting gamma oscillations, sleep spindles, and epileptogenic bursts. *J. Neurophysiol* 93, 2194–2232.

Vaillancourt, D. E., and Newell, K. M. (2002). Changing complexity in human behavior and physiology through aging and disease. *Neurobiol. Aging* 23, 1–11.

Van Albada, S. J., Gray, R. T., Drysdale, P. M., and Robinson, P. A. (2009). Mean-field modeling of the basal ganglia-thalamocortical system. II. Dynamics of parkinsonian oscillations. *J. Theor. Biol.* 257, 664–688.

Van Albada, S. J., and Robinson, P. A. (2009). Mean-field modeling of the basal ganglia-thalamocortical system. I. Firing rates in healthy and parkinsonian states. *J. Theor. Biol.* 257, 642–663.

Van Der Werf, J., Jensen, O., Fries, P., and Medendorp, W. P. (2008). Gamma-band activity in human posterior parietal cortex encodes the motor goal during delayed prosaccades and antisaccades. *J. Neurosci.* 28, 8397–8405.

Vijayan, S., and Kopell, N. J. (2012). Thalamic model of awake alpha oscillations and implications for stimulus processing. *Proc. Natl. Acad. Sci. U.S.A.* 109, 18553–18558.

Vogels, T. P., and Abbott, L. F. (2005). Signal propagation and logic gating in networks of integrate-and-fire neurons. *J. Neurosci.* 25, 10786–10795.

Volman, V., Bazhenov, M., and Sejnowski, T. J. (2011). Pattern of trauma determines the threshold for epileptic activity in a model of cortical deafferentation. *Proc. Natl. Acad. Sci. U.S.A.* 108, 15402–15407.

Weinberger, M., Mahant, N., Hutchison, W. D., Lozano, A. M., Moro, E., Hodaie, M., et al. (2006). Beta oscillatory activity in the subthalamic nucleus and its relation to dopaminergic response in Parkinson's disease. *J. Neurophysiol.* 96, 3248–3256.

Wilson, H. R., and Cowan, J. D. (1973). A mathematical theory of the functional dynamics of cortical and thalamic nervous tissue. *Kybernetik* 13, 55–80.

Wilson, M. T., Robinson, P. A., O'Neill, B., and Steyn-Ross, D. A. (2012). Complementarity of spike-and rate-based dynamics of neural systems. *PLoS Comput. Biol.* 8:e1002560. doi: 10.1371/journal.pcbi.1002560

Wright, J. J., and Liley, D. T. J. (1995). Simulation of electrocortical waves. *Biol. Cybern.* 72, 347–356.

Wright, J. J., and Liley, D. T. J. (1996). Dynamics of the brain at global and microscopic scales: neural networks and the EEG. *Behav. Brain Sci.* 19, 285–294.

16

Implementing the cellular mechanisms of synaptic transmission in a neural mass model of the thalamo-cortical circuitry

Basabdatta S. Bhattacharya* *

Engineering Hub, School of Engineering, University of Lincoln, Lincoln, UK

Correspondence:
Basabdatta S. Bhattacharya, School of Engineering, University of Lincoln, Engineering Hub, Brayford Pool, Lincoln LN6 7TS, Lincolnshire, UK
e-mail: basab@ieee.org

A novel direction to existing neural mass modeling technique is proposed where the commonly used "alpha function" for representing synaptic transmission is replaced by a kinetic framework of neurotransmitter and receptor dynamics. The aim is to underpin neuro-transmission dynamics associated with abnormal brain rhythms commonly observed in neurological and psychiatric disorders. An existing thalamocortical neural mass model is modified by using the kinetic framework for modeling synaptic transmission mediated by glutamatergic and GABA (gamma-aminobutyric-acid)-ergic receptors. The model output is compared qualitatively with existing literature on *in vitro* experimental studies of ferret thalamic slices, as well as on single-neuron-level model based studies of neuro-receptor and transmitter dynamics in the thalamocortical tissue. The results are consistent with these studies: the activation of ligand-gated GABA receptors is essential for generation of spindle waves in the model, while blocking this pathway leads to low-frequency synchronized oscillations such as observed in slow-wave sleep; the frequency of spindle oscillations increase with increased levels of post-synaptic membrane conductance for AMPA (alpha-amino-3-hydroxy-5-methyl-4-isoxazolepropionic-acid) receptors, and blocking this pathway effects a quiescent model output. In terms of computational efficiency, the simulation time is improved by a factor of 10 compared to a similar neural mass model based on alpha functions. This implies a dramatic improvement in computational resources for large-scale network simulation using this model. Thus, the model provides a platform for correlating high-level brain oscillatory activity with low-level synaptic attributes, and makes a significant contribution toward advancements in current neural mass modeling paradigm as a potential computational tool to better the understanding of brain oscillations in sickness and in health.

Keywords: neural mass model, thalamocortical circuitry, kinetic framework, brain oscillations, AMPA, GABA

1. INTRODUCTION

Neural mass computational models mimicking synchronous behavior in populations of thalamocortical neurons are often used to study brain oscillations (David and Friston, 2003; Suffczyński et al., 2004; Breakspear et al., 2006; Sotero et al., 2007; Deco et al., 2008; Izhikevich and Edelman, 2008; Pons et al., 2010; Robinson et al., 2011; de Haan et al., 2012). The term "neural mass" was coined by Freeman (1975), while the neural mass modeling paradigm is based on the mathematical framework proposed by Wilson and Cowan (1973); each cell population in a neural mass model represents a neuronal "ensemble" of mesoscopic-scale (10^4–10^7), which are densely packed in space and work at the same temporal-scale, so that for all practical purposes, they can be mathematically treated as a single entity (Liljenström, 2012), whence "mass". In a seminal work, da Silva et al. (1974) used a neural mass model of a simple thalamocortical circuitry to simulate EEG (Electroencephalography) alpha rhythms (8–13 Hz). Subsequently, this model has been the basis of several research (Zetterberg et al., 1978; Stam et al., 1999; Suffczyński, 2000; Bhattacharya et al., 2011a), albeit with modifications and enhancements; of special mention is the modification introduced by Jansen and Rit (1995) where the model is expressed as a set of ordinary differential equations (ODE). This modification, in turn, has been the basis of many significant research (Wendling et al., 2002; Grimbert and Faugeras, 2006; Ursino et al., 2010). However, the computational basis of the models remain the same—the conversion from firing rate to membrane potential by excitatory and inhibitory neurotransmitters is simulated by convolution of the input from a pre-synaptic neuronal mass with an exponential function, commonly known as the "alpha function", proposed by Rall (1967). Although the alpha function is a fair estimate of the synaptic process (Bernard et al., 1994), it does not allow an insight into the underlying cellular mechanisms of synaptic transmission associated with abnormal brain oscillations—an aspect emphasized to be crucial as an aid to research in brain disorders (McCormick, 1992; Basar and Guntekin, 2008). The importance of understanding the neurotransmission mechanisms in slow wave synchronized as well as spindle oscillations is also discussed in several relevant experimental studies (Steriade et al., 1993; von Krosigk et al., 1993). Moreover, correlating synaptic kinetics with brain oscillatory activity has the potential to aid neuropharmacological advances in treating the diseased brain (Aradi and Erdi, 2006). Along these lines, Destexhe et al. (1998) argue that the alpha function is inappropriate for representing post synaptic events other than the originally proposed post-synaptic potential in spiking neural networks; they propose a kinetic framework as a more biologically plausible method of modeling synaptic transmission compared to the alpha function (Destexhe et al., 2002). The ability of such a modeling framework to capture the physiological properties of synaptic transmission was demonstrated by fitting the model outputs to experimental data from hippocampal slices. Moreover, kinetic modeling is reported to be computationally efficient (Destexhe et al., 1994), a vital prerequisite in large-scale computational models. Subsequently, the kinetic models of neurotransmission was used in several single-neuronal-level model-based studies—to investigate thalamic oscillations (Destexhe et al., 1996) and corticothalamic influence on brain oscillatory activity (Destexhe, 2008); to investigate network synchrony (Breakspear et al., 2003); to simulate synchronous behavior observed during *in vitro* experimental studies on ferret thalamic slice by Wang and Rinzel (1992), Golomb et al. (1994, 1996) and Wang et al. (1995).

A significant modification to current neural mass modeling framework was proposed by Suffczyński et al. (2004) by applying single-neuronal-level model based techniques. Toward this, they proposed an "ensemble" representation of the membrane conductance and post-synaptic current in a neuronal mass model of the thalamocortical circuitry; an integrator is used to generate the "ensemble" post-synaptic membrane potential. In the work presented here, a similar approach is adopted to implement the kinetic framework of synaptic transmission in neural mass models—each post-synaptic attribute is assumed to be an "ensemble" representation corresponding to a "neuronal mass". For brevity, only two-state ("open" and "closed") ion-channels (Destexhe et al., 1998) are considered, the desensitized state is ignored. While two-state models are a significant simplification of the very complex nature of ion channel dynamics in biology, they have shown a remarkable fit to biological data compared to more-than-two-state models (Destexhe et al., 1998, 2002). This work aims to interface an abstraction of the ion channel dynamics, such as the two-state ion channel kinetic models, with an abstraction of the population level neuronal behavior, such as neural mass models. The goal is to enable the correlation of higher-level brain dynamics observed in EEG with cellular-level dynamics.

The work is presented thus: first, the kinetic framework for modeling AMPA (α-amino-3-hydroxy-5-methyl-4-isoxazolepropionic-acid) and GABA (γ-amino-butyric-acid) receptor mediated synapses is introduced in an existing thalamocortical neural mass model (section 2); second, a qualitative comparison of the model behavior with experimental studies on ferret thalamocortical tissue reported in von Krosigk et al. (1993) as well as to single-neuronal-level model based observations reported in Golomb et al. (1996; section 3) is presented; the lack of a quantitative study is mainly to avoid erratic conclusions as difference in model structure and simulation techniques are bound to induce mismatch in numerical results. The model behavior is observed to be consistent with these studies (von Krosigk et al., 1993; Golomb et al., 1996)—The post synaptic membrane conductance in both the thalamocortical relay (TCR) and thalamic reticular nucleus (TRN) cell population plays a role in effecting a bifurcation in model behavior from spindling mode [oscillations with the characteristic waxing-and-waning pattern seen in early stages of sleep (Steriade et al., 1993; Hughes et al., 2004) as well as in alpha rhythmic oscillations during resting brain state (da Silva et al., 1973)] to a limit-cycle mode (synchronized oscillations as seen in later stages of sleep or during absence seizures). The post-synaptic membrane conductance for both AMPA and GABA in the TRN cell population is responsible for sustaining and modulating spindle oscillations in the model output. Blocking the GABA-ergic synapses in the self-inhibitory loop of the TRN cell population effects a low-frequency synchronized oscillation in the model; this is aided by the secondary-messenger-gated GABA synapses in the TCR cell population. In addition, the reverse rate of transmitter binding plays a role in increasing or decreasing the frequency of synchronized oscillations, besides functioning as a bifurcation parameter, an observation that has not been reported in experimental studies. A comparison of the simulation time of the model with previous research using neural mass models based on alpha functions show a factor of 10 improvement in simulation time. This is a dramatic improvement on computational efficiency and emphasizes the appropriateness of the model proposed herein toward building large-scale software models for investigating neuronal disorders. The observations from this study as well as issues related to the modeling approach are discussed in section 4.

2. MATERIALS AND METHODS

2.1. FROM ALPHA FUNCTION TO KINETIC MODEL: A BRIEF OUTLINE

A single neuronal mass structure as used commonly in neural mass models is shown in **Figure 1** and is defined in Equations (1–5):

$$h_{\bar{w}}(t) = \frac{H_{\bar{w}}}{\tau_{\bar{w}}} t\exp(-t/\tau_{\bar{w}}) \tag{1}$$

$$y_N(t) = \sum h_{\bar{w}}(t) \otimes E_{\bar{w}}^N(t) \tag{2}$$

$$\ddot{y}_N(t) = \frac{H_{\bar{w}}}{\tau_{\bar{w}}} E_{\bar{w}}^N(t) - \frac{2}{\tau_{\bar{w}}} \dot{y}_N(t) - \frac{1}{\tau_{\bar{w}}^2} y_N(t) \tag{3}$$

$$V_P(t) = \sum_{N \in \{1,2,3,\ldots n\}} C_N . y_N(t) \tag{4}$$

$$E_{\bar{w}}^P(t) = S(V_P) = \frac{2e_0}{1 + e^{\nu(s_0 - V_P)}} \tag{5}$$

where $\bar{w} \in \{e, i\}$ represents pre-synaptic neuronal populations which make excitatory *(e)* and inhibitory *(i)* synapses on a post-synaptic neuronal population; $\tau_{\bar{w}}$ is the time constant and

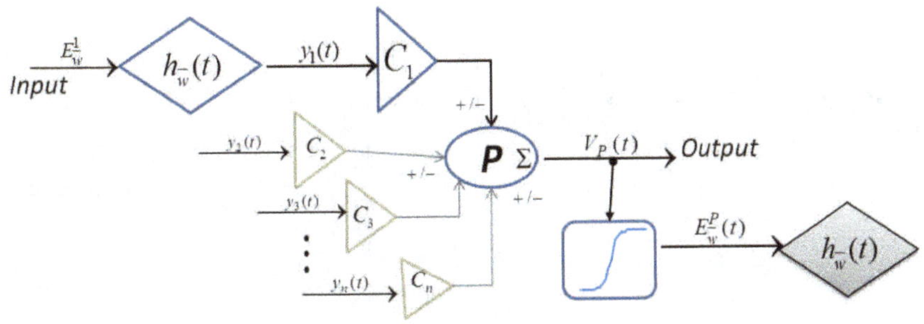

FIGURE 1 | Block diagram of a single "neuronal mass" in current state-of-the-art neural mass models.

$H_{\bar{w}}$ is the amplitude of the synapse; $E_{\bar{w}}^{N}(t),\ N \in \{1, 2 \ldots n\}$ is the firing frequency of an extrinsic or intrinsic cell population that is pre-synaptic to the population **P**; C_N is a percentage of the total number of synapses from all afferents to **P**; V_P is the "ensemble post-synaptic membrane potential"; $E_{\bar{w}}^{P}$ is the "ensemble firing rate" of **P** and is defined by a sigmoid function where $2e_0$ is the maximum firing rate of the population, s_0 is the threshold potential at which the neurons spike and ν is the sigmoid steepness parameter.

2.1.1. A modified neural mass representation

In a recent work, Suffczyński et al. (2004) modified the neural mass representation of a cell population and introduced post-synaptic current mediated by the ligand-gated glutamatergic receptors AMPA, and the ligand- and secondary-messenger-gated GABA-ergic receptors $GABA_A$ and $GABA_B$, respectively. The input $E_{\bar{\xi}}^{N}(t),\ \bar{\xi} \in \{\text{AMPA}, \text{GABA}_A, \text{GABA}_B\}$, is the firing rate of an excitatory (AMPA) or inhibitory ($GABA_A$ and $GABA_B$) pre-synaptic neuronal population $N \in \{1, 2 \ldots, n\}$. The model (**Figure 2A**) is defined in Equations (6–11):

$$h_{\bar{\xi}}(t) = H_{\bar{\xi}}\left(\exp\left(-t/\tau_{\bar{\xi}}^{a}\right) - exp\left(-t/\tau_{\bar{\xi}}^{b}\right)\right),\ \tau_{\bar{\xi}}^{b} > \tau_{\bar{\xi}}^{a} \quad (6)$$

$$g_{\bar{\xi}}^{N}(t) = \sum h_{\bar{\xi}}(t) \otimes E_{\bar{\xi}}^{N}(t) \quad (7)$$

$$\ddot{g}_{\bar{\xi}}^{N}(t) = \frac{1}{\tau_{\bar{\xi}}^{a}\tau_{\bar{\xi}}^{b}}\left[H_{\bar{\xi}}\left(\tau_{\bar{\xi}}^{a} - \tau_{\bar{\xi}}^{b}\right)E_{\bar{\xi}}^{N}(t) - \left(\tau_{\bar{\xi}}^{a} + \tau_{\bar{\xi}}^{b}\right)\dot{g}_{\bar{\xi}}^{N}(t) - g_{\bar{\xi}}^{N}(t)\right] \quad (8)$$

$$I_{\bar{\xi}}^{N}(t) = g_{\bar{\xi}}^{N}(t)\left(V^{P}(t) - V_{\bar{\xi}}\right) \quad (9)$$

$$\kappa_m \dot{V}^{P}(t) = -\sum_{N \in \{1,2,3,\ldots,n\}} C_N.I_{\bar{\xi}}^{N}(t) - I_{\lambda}(t) \quad (10)$$

$$I_{\lambda}(t) = g_{\lambda}\left(V^{P}(t) - V_{\lambda}\right) \quad (11)$$

where $h_{\bar{\xi}}(t)$ is the synaptic transmission function with $\tau_{\bar{\xi}}^{a}$ and $\tau_{\bar{\xi}}^{b}$ as the rise and decay times, respectively; $g_{\bar{\xi}}^{N}$ denote the post-synaptic "ensemble" membrane conductance; $V_{\bar{\xi}}$ is the reversal potential for the synapse mediated by $\bar{\xi}$; V^{P} is the ensemble post synaptic membrane potential of the population **P** due to PSC from all pre-synaptic cell populations $N \in \{1, 2 \ldots, n\}$; κ_m is the ensemble membrane capacitance; C_N is the synaptic connectivity parameter; I_{λ}, g_{λ} and V_{λ} are the ensemble leakage current, conductance and reversal potential, respectively for **P**. The ensemble firing rate $E_{\bar{\xi}}^{P}(t)$ is as defined in Equation (5) and is the pre-synaptic firing rate input to other neuronal populations.

2.1.2. Introducing kinetic model of synapses in a neural mass representation

The single neuronal mass structure presented in **Figures 1, 2A** is modified by replacing the alpha function with kinetic models of AMPA, $GABA_A$, and $GABA_B$ synapses; the enhanced representation (**Figure 2B**) is defined in Equations (12–19):

$$[T]_{\chi}(V_{\chi}) = \frac{T_{\max}}{1 + e^{-\frac{V_{\chi} - \theta_s}{\sigma_s}}} \quad (12)$$

$$\frac{dr_{\chi}^{\bar{\xi}_1}(t)}{dt} = \alpha^{\bar{\xi}_1}[T]_{\chi}\left(1 - r_{\chi}^{\bar{\xi}_1}(t)\right) - \beta^{\bar{\xi}_1} r_{\chi}^{\bar{\xi}_1}(t) \quad (13)$$

$$\frac{dR_{\chi}^{\bar{\xi}_2}(t)}{dt} = \alpha^{\bar{\xi}_2}[T]_{\chi}\left(1 - R_{\chi}^{\bar{\xi}_2}(t)\right) - \beta^{\bar{\xi}_2} R_{\chi}^{\bar{\xi}_2}(t) \quad (14)$$

$$\frac{d[X](t)}{dt} = \alpha^{\bar{\xi}_2} R_{\chi}^{\bar{\xi}_2}(t) - \beta^{\bar{\xi}_2}[X](t) \quad (15)$$

$$r_{\chi}^{\bar{\xi}_2}((t)) = \frac{[X]^{n}(t)}{[X]^{n}(t) + K_d} \quad (16)$$

$$I_{\chi}^{\bar{\xi}}(t) = g^{\bar{\xi}} r_{\chi}^{\bar{\xi}}(t)\left(V_P(t) - V^{\bar{\xi}}\right) \quad (17)$$

$$\kappa_m \frac{dV_P(t)}{dt} = -\sum_{\chi \in \{1,2\}} I_{\chi}^{\bar{\xi}}(t).C_{\chi} - I_P^{\lambda}(t) \quad (18)$$

$$I_P^{\lambda}(t) = g_P^{\lambda}\left(V_P(t) - V_P^{\lambda}\right) \quad (19)$$

Let $V_{\chi},\ \chi \in \{1, 2\}$ be the "ensemble" membrane potential of two pre-synaptic neuronal population that are afferent to the post-synaptic population **P** such that the synapses made by $\chi = 1$ is mediated by a ligand-gated receptor $\bar{\xi}_1 \in \{\text{AMPA}, \text{GABA}_A\}$ while that made by $\chi = 2$ is mediated by a secondary-messenger-gated receptor $\bar{\xi}_2 \in \{\text{GABA}_B\}$. The concentration of neurotransmitters

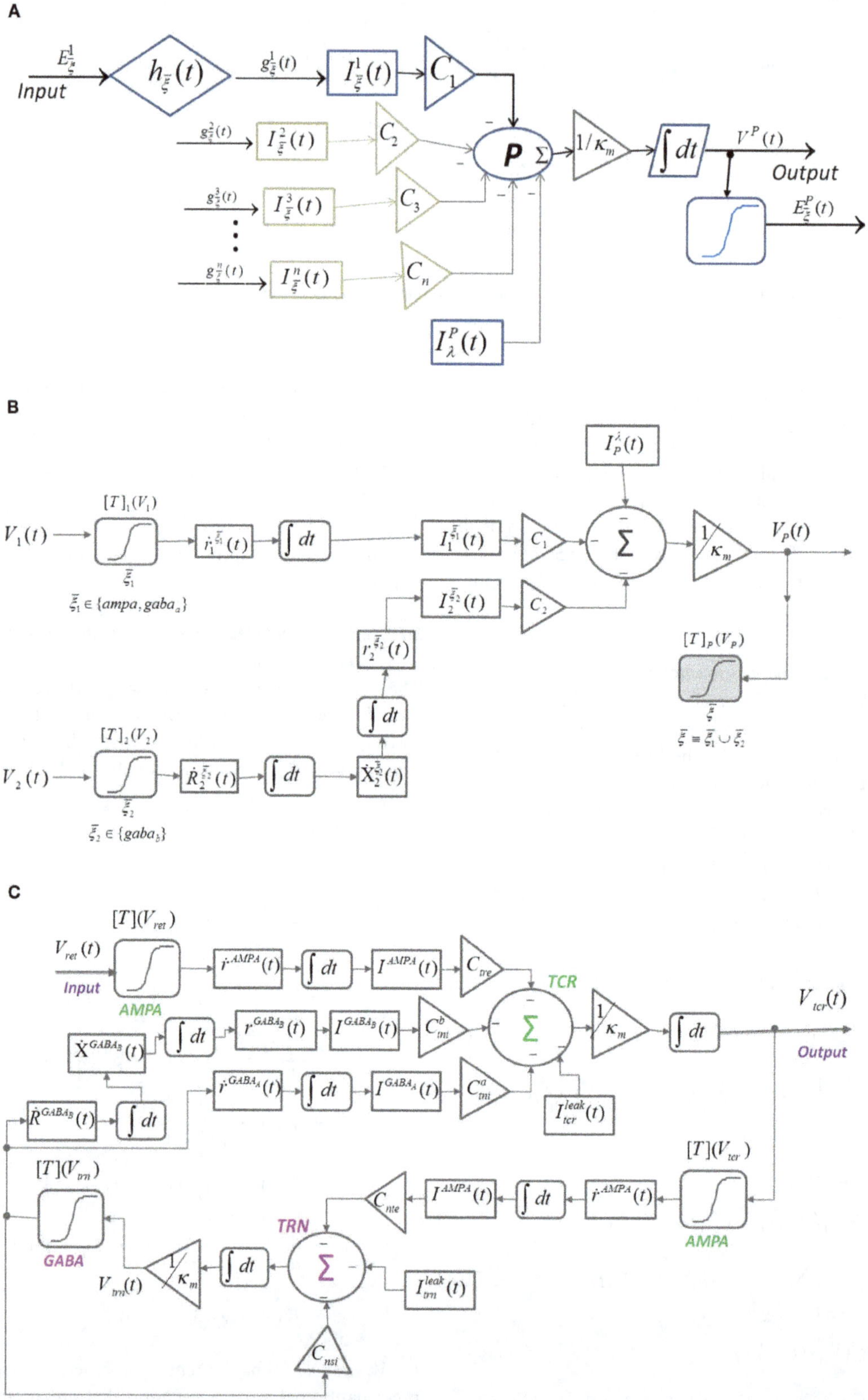

FIGURE 2 | Block diagram of (A) Suffczyński et al. (2004)'s modification of the structure in Figure 1 by introducing "ensemble" representation of post-synaptic membrane conductance and current. (B) Neuronal mass structure with the kinetic framework implemented for modeling synaptic transmission as an alternative to the alpha function ($h_{\bar{\psi}}(t)$ in **Figure 1**). A diagrammatic representation of the ion-channel kinetics during synaptic transmission is presented in **Figures 3A,B**. **(C)** A thalamocortical circuitry implementing the modified neuronal mass representation in **(B)**.

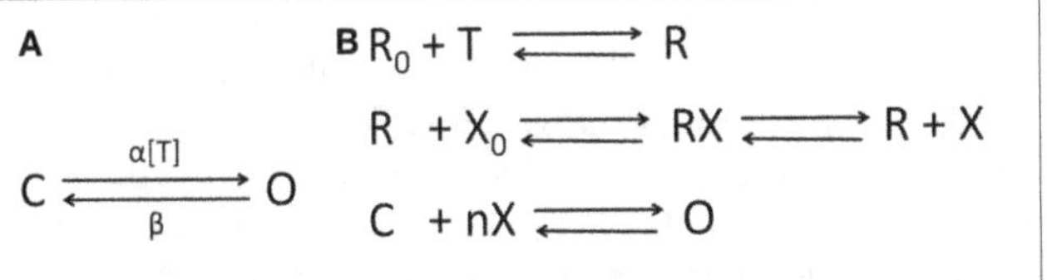

FIGURE 3 | The state transition diagrams for (A) AMPA and GABA$_A$ neuro-receptor dynamics defined in Equation (13); α and β are rate of transitions between the two states and α is a function of the transmitter concentration in the synaptic cleft [*T*] defined in Equation (12); (B) GABA$_B$ neuro-transmission as defined in Equations (14–16)—the neurotransmitter *T* binds to the inactivated receptor R_0; a fraction of activated receptors *R* act as a catalyst to transform the G-protein from an inactivated form X_0 to an activated form *X*, which binds at *n* independent sites to open a fraction of the ion channels. The desensitized state of the ion-channels are ignored in this work for brevity (see Destexhe et al., 1998 for a detailed comparison of kinetic models with more than two-states).

$[T]_\chi$ in the synaptic cleft is defined as a function of V_χ and is expressed by a sigmoid function (Equation 12) where T_{max} is the maximum neuronal concentration in the synaptic cleft and is well approximated by 1 mM (Destexhe et al., 1998), θ_s represents the threshold at which $[T] = 0.5T_{max}$ and σ_s denote the steepness of the sigmoid. The proportion of open ion-channels due to the bound receptors $\bar{\xi}_1$ on the ensemble membrane of the post-synaptic cell population corresponding to the synapse made by the population $\chi = 1$ is defined in Equation (13) where $\alpha^{\bar{\xi}_1}$ and $\beta^{\bar{\xi}_1}$ are the forward and backward rate constants, respectively for transmitter binding. The transition diagram is shown in **Figure 3A**. However, GABA$_B$ mediated synapses, unlike AMPA and GABA$_A$ synapses, activate G-proteins which in turn act as the "secondary messengers" and initiate the opening of ion channels. The process is defined in Equations (14–16) where $R^{\bar{\xi}_2}_\chi$ is the fraction of activated $\bar{\xi}_2$ receptors, which acts as a catalyst in activating the secondary-messenger G-protein (guanine nucleotideŰbinding proteins); [X] is the concentration of the activated G-protein; $r^{\bar{\xi}_2}_\chi$ is the fraction of open ion channels caused by binding of X with independent binding sites; $\alpha^{\bar{\xi}_2}$ and $\beta^{\bar{\xi}_2}$ are the binding rate constants; *n* is the number of bound receptor sites and K_d is the dissociation constant of binding of X with the ion channels. The transition diagram of this process is shown in **Figure 3B**. The resulting ensemble PSC mediated by the receptor $\bar{\xi} \equiv \bar{\xi}_1 \cup \bar{\xi}_2$ due to a synapse from the pre-synaptic population χ is defined in Equation (17) where $g^{\bar{\xi}}$ and $V^{\bar{\xi}}$ are the maximum conductance and reverse potential, respectively corresponding to $\bar{\xi}$ mediated synapse. V_P (Equation 18) is the ensemble post-synaptic potential (PSP) of **P**, where κ_m is the ensemble membrane capacitance of **P**, C_χ, $\chi \in \{1, 2\}$ is the synaptic connectivity parameter. I^λ_P (Equation 19) is the ensemble leak current of the post-synaptic membrane, where g^λ_P and V^λ_P are conductance and reverse potential, respectively, corresponding to "non-specific" leak (Golomb et al., 1996; Suffczyński et al., 2004) in the ensemble membrane of the post synaptic cell population. In the following section, we implement this framework in a neural mass model of the thalamocortical circuitry.

2.2. NEURAL MASS MODEL OF A THALAMOCORTICAL CIRCUITRY WITH KINETIC SYNAPSES

The thalamocortical circuitry is shown in **Figure 2C** and consists of the two thalamic cell populations that communicate with the cortex viz. the TCR and TRN. The third group of cells viz. the Interneurons (IN) participate in intra-thalamic communications and are ignored here for brevity. The synaptic structure and connectivity are informed from experimental data based on the dorsal thalamic Lateral Geniculate Nucleus (LGNd) (Horn et al., 2000). The input to the model is assumed to be the ensemble membrane potential of pre-synaptic retinal cells (V_{ret}) in a resting state with no sensory input and is simulated using a Gaussian white noise (da Silva et al., 1973). The TCR cells make AMPA receptor mediated glutamatergic synapses on the TRN cells (other types of glutamatergic receptors are ignored in this work for brevity); the TRN cells make GABA-ergic synapses on the TCR cells mediated by both the ligand-gated GABA$_A$ and the secondary-messenger-gated GABA$_B$ receptors. Furthermore, the TRN cells make GABA$_A$ receptor mediated synapses within the population. The model is defined in Equations (20–27); all variables and parameters in the model are assumed to be the ensemble representation corresponding to a neural mass:

$$[T]_{\bar\Psi}(V_{\bar\Psi}(t)) = \frac{T_{max}}{1 + exp\left(-\frac{V_{\bar\Psi}(t)-\theta_s}{\sigma_s}\right)} \quad (20)$$

$$\frac{dr^{\bar\eta_1}_{\bar\Psi}(t)}{dt} = \alpha^{\bar\eta_1}[T]_{\bar\Psi}\left(1 - r^{\bar\eta_1}_{\bar\Psi}(t)\right) - \beta^{\bar\eta_1} r^{\bar\eta_1}_{\bar\Psi}(t) \quad (21)$$

$$\frac{dR^{\bar\eta_2}_{\bar\Psi}(t)}{dt} = \alpha^{\bar\eta_2}_1[T]_{\bar\Psi}\left(1 - R^{\bar\eta_2}_{\bar\Psi}(t)\right) - \beta^{\bar\eta_2}_1 R^{\bar\eta_2}_{\bar\Psi}(t) \quad (22)$$

$$\frac{d[X](t)}{dt} = \alpha^{\bar\eta_2}_2 R^{\bar\eta_2}_{\bar\Psi}(t) - \beta^{\bar\eta_2}_2 [X](t) \quad (23)$$

$$r^{\bar\eta_2}_{\bar\Psi}((t)) = \frac{[X]^n(t)}{[X]^n(t) + K_d}, \quad (24)$$

$$I^{\bar\eta}_{\bar\Psi}(t) = g^{\bar\eta} r^{\bar\eta}_{\bar\Psi}(t)\left(V_{\bar\Upsilon}(t) - V^{\bar\eta}\right) \quad (25)$$

$$\kappa_m \frac{dV_{\bar\Upsilon}(t)}{dt} = -\sum_{\bar\Psi \in \{\text{ret, trn, trn}\}} I^{\bar\eta}_{\bar\Psi}(t).C_{\bar u\bar v\bar w} - I^\lambda_{\bar\Upsilon}(t), \quad (26)$$

$$I^\lambda_{\bar\Upsilon}(t) = g^\lambda_{\bar\Upsilon}(V_{\bar\Upsilon}(t) - V^\lambda_{\bar\Upsilon}), \quad (27)$$

where $\bar\Psi \in \{\text{ret, trn, trn}\}$ represent the afferent cell populations; $\bar\Upsilon = \{\text{trn, trn}\}$ represent the efferent cell populations; $\bar\eta_1 \in \{\text{AMPA, GABA}_A\}$, $\bar\eta_2 \in \{\text{GABA}_B\}$, $\bar\eta \equiv \bar\eta_1 \cup \bar\eta_2$; $C_{\bar u\bar v\bar w}$ are connectivity parameters where $\bar u \in \{t, n\}$ and $\bar v \in \{r, t, n, s\}$ denote the post-synaptic and pre-synaptic cell populations, respectively of the retina (*r*), TCR (*t*), TRN (*n*), while *s* denote an intra-population afferent; $\bar w \in \{e, i\}$ represent an excitatory (*e*) or an inhibitory (*i*) synapse. All other parameter nomenclatures are as defined in section 2.1. The initial parameter values are mentioned in **Table 1**.

Table 1 | Initial values of the parameters defined in Equations (21–27).

Neuroreceptors → Units↓	AMPA	GABA$_A$	GABA$_B$
(A) NEUROTRANSMISSION PARAMETERS			
mM.msec^{-1}	$\alpha^{\bar{\eta}_1} = 2$	$\alpha^{\bar{\eta}_1} = 2$	$\alpha_1^{\bar{\eta}_2} = 0.02$ $\alpha_2^{\bar{\eta}_2} = 0.03$
msec^{-1}	$\beta^{\bar{\eta}_1} = 0.1$	$\beta^{\bar{\eta}_1} = 0.08$	$\beta_1^{\bar{\eta}_2} = 0.05$ $\beta_2^{\bar{\eta}_2} = 0.01$
mS	$g^{\bar{\eta}} = 0.1$	$g^{\bar{\eta}}_{\text{TRN to TCR}} = 0.1$ $g^{\bar{\eta}}_{\text{TRN to TRN}} = 0.2$	$g^{\bar{\eta}} = 0.06$
mV	$V^{\bar{\eta}} = 0$	$V^{\bar{\eta}}_{\text{TRN to TCR}} = -85$ $V^{\bar{\eta}}_{\text{TRN to TRN}} = -75$	$V^{\bar{\eta}} = -100$
			$K_d = 100$ $n = 4$

(B) CELL MEMBRANE PARAMETERS

	TCR	TRN
$g^{\lambda}_{\bar{\Upsilon}}$ (mS)	0.01	0.01
$V^{\lambda}_{\bar{\Upsilon}}$ (mV)	−55	−72.5
V_{rest} (mV)	−61	−84

(C) CONNECTIVITY PARAMETERS

Efferents → / Afferents ↓	TCR	TRN: GABA$_A$	TRN: GABA$_B$	Retinal
TCR	X	C^a_{tni} $\frac{3}{4}$ of 30.9	C^b_{tni} $\frac{1}{4}$ of 30.9	C_{tre} 7.1
TRN	C_{nte} 35	C_{nsi} 20	X	X

Data in (A) and (B) are as in Golomb et al. (1996) and Suffczyński et al. (2004). In Equation (20), both θ_s and σ_s act as bifurcation parameters in the model (see Bhattacharya et al., 2012). However, the emphasis here is on post-synaptic membrane attributes as in von Krosigk et al. (1993) and Golomb et al. (1996). Thus these parameters ($\theta_s = -35$ and $\sigma_s = 2$) are set by trial and error at values just before the model undergoes bifurcation from a "point-attractor" mode to a "limit-cycle" mode, based on a recent study where we observed rich model dynamics and power spectral behavior around the bifurcation point (Bhattacharya et al., 2013); $T_{max} = 1\,mM$ (Destexhe et al., 1994). The input noise mean $\mu = -45\,mV$ and standard deviation $\varphi = 20\,mV^2$ are set by trial and error and represents the resting state membrane potential fluctuations in retinal cells. While the total number of GABA-ergic synaptic count on TCR cells is reported as 30.9%, specific data on GABA$_A$ and GABA$_B$ are not available in literature to the best of our knowledge. Thus, values for C^a_{tni}, C^b_{tni} and C_{nsi} in (C) are selected, within the reported biological range [see Bhattacharya et al. (2011b) for details], when the model output showed an increased frequency content within the theta (4–7 Hz) and alpha (8–13 Hz) bands. C_{tre} and C_{nte} are as in Bhattacharya et al. (2011b). All variables in the ODEs are initialized to an arbitrarily small value 0.0002.

3. RESULTS

The ODEs are solved using the 4th/5th order Runge-Kutta-Fehlberg method (RKF45) in Matlab for a total duration of 600 s (10 min) at a resolution of 1 ms. The output voltage time series is averaged over 20 simulations, each simulation run with different seed for the noisy input. For frequency analysis, an epoch from 100–599 s of the output signal is sampled every 4 ms (250 Hz) and bandpass filtered between 3.5–14 Hz with a Butterworth filter of order 10. Short Time Fourier Transform (STFT) is done with a Hamming window of duration 10 s and overlap of 50%.

The model displays a point-attractor mode behavior (initial transient oscillations before settling down to a low amplitude noisy output, which reflects the noisy input of the model) corresponding to initial parameter values (**Figure 4A**). There is a behavioral transition in the model to a limit cycle mode with increasing values of β^{ampa}, which correlates with a decrease in the fraction of open ion channels in the post-synaptic ensemble membrane (**Figures 4B,C**). Varying α^{ampa}, on the other hand, does not affect the model behaviour (**Figures 4D,E**). A transition from the limit cycle mode to a spindling mode is effected in the model by increasing g^{ampa}, the post-synaptic membrane conductance for AMPA mediated synapses in both TCR and TRN cell population, and shown in **Figures 4F,G**. STFT of the output time series indicates the non-stationary behavior of the model (**Figures 4H–K**). A decrease and increase, respectively of the theta and alpha band components imply an overall increase in frequency with increasing values of $g^{ampa} \equiv \{g^{ampa}_{TCR}, g^{ampa}_{TRN}\}$, where g^{ampa}_{TCR} and g^{ampa}_{TRN} correspond to the incoming signal from the retina (to the TCR) and TCR (to the TRN), respectively in the model. These observations are consistent with similar reports of a transition in the state of the model output with increasing values of g^{ampa} in Golomb et al. (1996; pp. 756–757), accompanied by an abrupt increase in the ratio of the frequency of oscillation of the TCR and the TRN cell populations; we have not studied the latter aspect in this work. A more detailed study on the model presented herein where g^{ampa}_{TCR} and g^{ampa}_{TRN} are varied separately specify the g^{ampa}_{TCR} as the control parameter that causes a bifurcation in the model output from a limit cycle mode to the spindling mode with an increase in its value. On the other hand, the g^{ampa}_{TRN} does not effect any behavioral change in the model output, rather, it is effective in increasing the inter-spindle frequency with an increase in its value when the model is in a spindling mode. This observation implies that a change in AMPA receptor related attributes in the TRN plays a role in modulating thalamocortical spindle oscillations, which finds strong support in the experimental study by von Krosigk et al. (1993), where "activation of AMPA-kainate receptors on the PGN" (Peri-geniculate nucleus—the part of the TRN associated with the LGNd) is described as "critical to the generation of spindle waves". Furthermore, this observation is in line with the TRN being widely implicated as being the key "ingredient" in the generation of thalamocortical spindle oscillations (McCormick, 1992; Steriade et al., 1993).

Varying the GABA-ergic synaptic attributes when the model is in a point-attractor mode does not show any change in model behavior. When the model is in a spindling mode (**Figure 5A**), increased synchronization within the limit cycle mode with increasing values of $g^{gaba_A}_{\text{TRN to TCR}}$ (**Figures 5B,C**) is observed. An increase in the parameter β^{gaba_A} affects the output only when the model is in a limit-cycle mode and counters the effect of increase in $g^{gaba_A}_{\text{TRN to TCR}}$ (**Figure 5D**). However, varying α^{gaba_A}

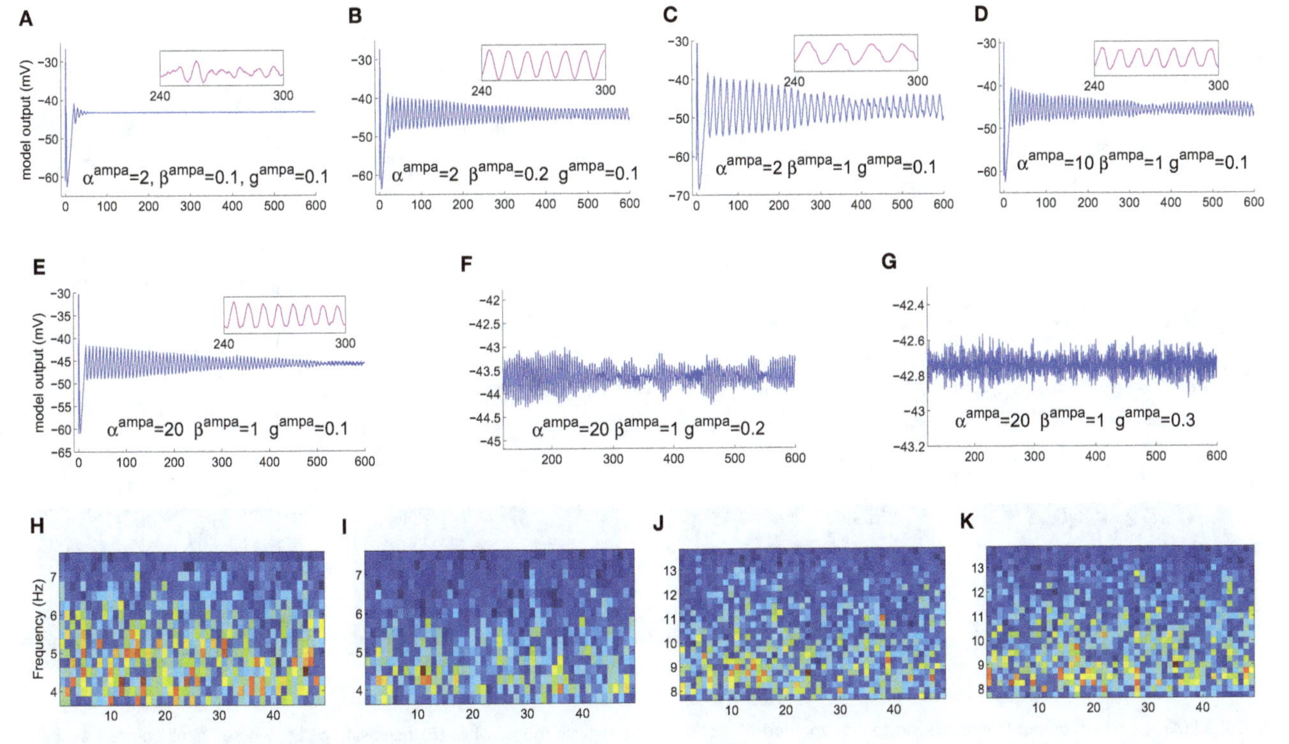

FIGURE 4 | The model output time series with (A) all parameters at their initial values as in Table 1. (B) The model displays a bifurcation in output behavior when β^{ampa} is increased to 0.2; **(C)** a further increase in the parameter shows sustained oscillations with increased magnitude and decreased frequency. The frequency behavior may be observed qualitatively in the embedded line plots displaying the respective time-series in each plot for an arbitrarily selected period of 60 s. **(D)** An increase in α^{ampa} has a reverse effect resulting in reduced magnitude and increased frequency in the limit-cycle mode; **(E)** further increase in the parameter do not show any significant effect on the magnitude or the limit-cycle behavior while there is a slight increase in frequency. **(F)** Maintaining these modified values of $\alpha^{ampa} = 20$ and $\beta^{ampa} = 1$, an increase in g^{ampa} brings a bifurcation in model behavior from a limit-cycle mode to a "spindling" mode. A "zoomed-in" plot from the 3rd minute to the 9th minute is shown; the initial transient oscillations are neglected. **(G)** The frequency of spindle oscillations increase with increasing values of g^{ampa}. This is indicated by a distinct **(H,I)** decrease (more blue pixels) in theta band components and **(J, K)** increase (more red, orange and yellow pixels) in alpha band components in the corresponding output time series plots. The abscissa in the figures denote (**A–G**) time (seconds) (**H–K**) time windows (seconds).

does not affect the model output. For $g^{gaba_A}_{\text{TRN to TCR}} \geqslant 0.5$, which is the approximate bifurcation point (**Figure 5B**), increasing $g^{gaba_A}_{\text{TRN to TRN}}$ causes the model to revert back to the spindling mode; the frequency of the inter-spindle oscillations increase with increasing values of the parameter (**Figures 5E,F**). This is also indicated by a decrease (**Figures 5H,I**) and increase (**Figures 5J,K**) of theta and alpha band components respectively in the STFT of the output time series. In other words, decreasing values of the parameter $g^{gaba_A}_{\text{TRN to TRN}}$ causes increased synchronization within the spindling mode behavior of the model along with a decrease in the inter-spindle frequency. However, blocking $g^{gaba_A}_{\text{TRN to TRN}}$ effects a switch in the model behavior to a very low-frequency oscillatory state (**Figure 5G**). These results are consistent with experimental findings (von Krosigk et al., 1993) where application of $GABA_A$ inhibitor either "abolished spindle waves or decreased within-spindle frequency," which correspond to the condition of either blocking or decreasing, respectively of $g^{gaba_A}_{\text{TRN to TRN}}$ in our model. Thus, the model implicate the intra-TRN synaptic activity to be a key factor in sustaining spindle oscillations in the thalamocortical circuitry, an observation which conforms to those made in Golomb et al. (1996; p. 755). Furthermore, a "frequency jump" with increasing g^{gaba_A}, and associated transition in model behavior is also reported in Golomb et al. (1996; see Figure 7) as a comparative study between the TCR and TRN cells. This is similar with the increase in frequency of the spindle oscillations corresponding to increasing $g^{gaba_A}_{\text{TRN to TRN}}$ in the present model, although we have not done a comparative study with the TRN cell population behavior. However, the current study implicate the increased post-synaptic conductance for $GABA_A$ receptors in the TCR cell population ($g^{gaba_A}_{\text{TRN to TCR}}$) to play a significant role in effecting state-transition between spindle and slow-wave oscillations, an observation that is yet to find support from experimental or model-based studies.

A quiescent state is observed corresponding to blocking either AMPA ($g^{ampa} = 0$) or both $GABA_A$ ($g^{gaba_A}_{\text{TRN to TCR}} = 0$) and $GABA_B$ ($g^{gaba_B}_{\text{TRN to TCR}} = 0$) mediated synapses in the TRN to TCR pathway (not shown). This is consistent with both experimental (von Krosigk et al., 1993) and model-based (Golomb et al., 1996) studies. The role of the synaptic parameters in the $GABA_B$ pathway in our model was minimal—to sustain a non-quiescent model behavior with blockage of $GABA_A$; to sustain a high amplitude of limit-cycle oscillations in the model. Again, this

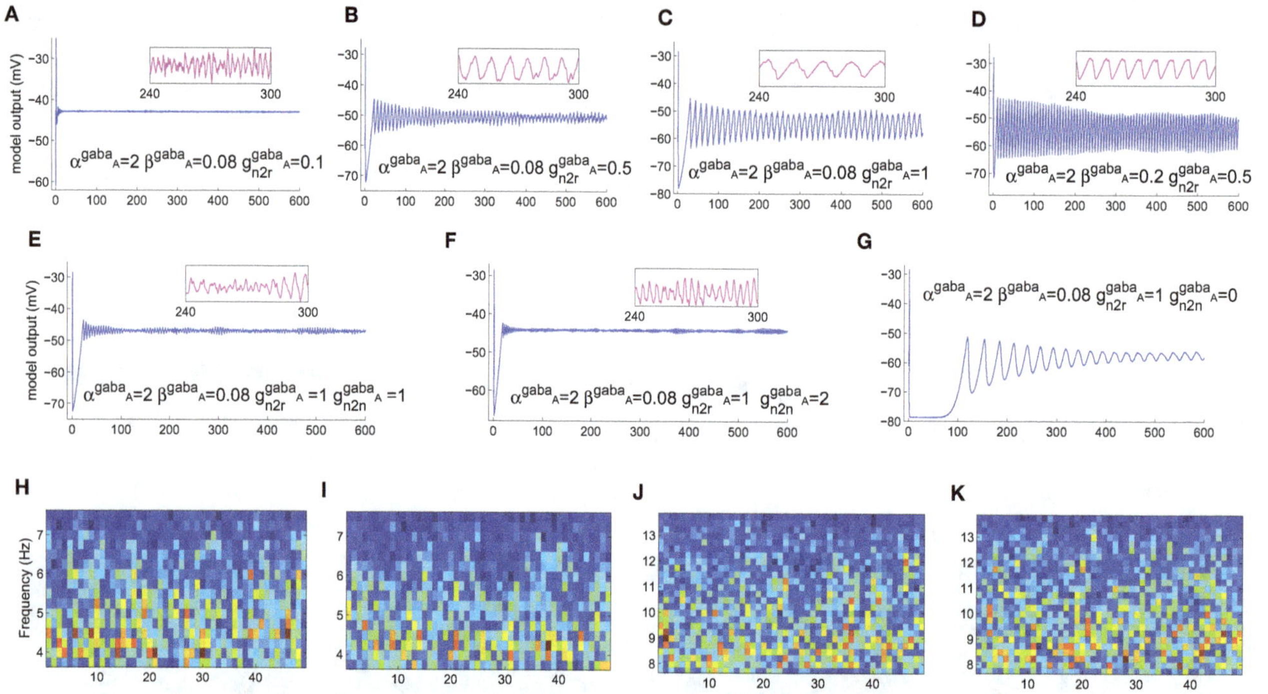

FIGURE 5 | (A) The model output (corresponding to the "zoomed-in" plot in **Figure 4G**) when $\alpha^{ampa} = 20$, $\beta^{ampa} = 1$, $g^{ampa} = 0.3$). Retaining these parameter values, **(B)** increasing $g_{n2r}^{gaba_A}$, where "*n2r*" denotes the TRN to TCR pathway, from its initial value effects a bifurcation in model behavior from a spindling mode to a limit-cycle mode, indicating highly synchronized oscillations in the thalamocortical circuitry. **(C)** Synchronization increases with increase in $g_{n2r}^{gaba_A}$, indicated by increased magnitude and decreased frequency of oscillation. For $g_{n2r}^{gaba_A} \geqslant 0.5$ [approximate point of bifurcation, shown in **(B)**], **(D)** increasing β^{gaba_A} effects an increase in frequency within the limit-cycle mode, while **(E)** increasing $g_{n2n}^{gaba_A}$, where "*n2n*" denotes the self inhibitory pathway of the TRN, effects a transition from the limit-cycle mode to the spindling mode. **(F)** Further increase in $g_{n2n}^{gaba_A}$ causes an increase in the frequency of the spindle oscillations, indicated by **(H,I)** a decrease (more blue pixels) in theta band components and **(J,K)** increase (more red, orange and yellow pixels) in alpha band components in the corresponding output time series plots. **(G)** Blocking of $g_{n2n}^{gaba_A}$ shows a very low-frequency (≈0.03 Hz) synchronized oscillation whose magnitude decreases with time. The abscissa in the figures denote **(A–G)** time (seconds) **(H–K)** time windows (seconds).

is in agreement with experimental studies (von Krosigk et al., 1993), where activation of $GABA_B$ receptors are reported as "not essential" for generating synchronized oscillations, while application of $GABA_B$ antagonist abolished "evoked or spontaneous slowed oscillations." The model in Golomb et al. (1996; see in Discussion p. 763) is also mentioned as being consistent with these experimental results.

In a recent work (Bhattacharya et al., 2012), a simple neural mass model implementing kinetic modeling for synaptic transmission is presented; the synaptic connectivity parameters in the model correlate directly to that of an alpha function based neural mass model [modified Alpha Rhythm model (modARm) from Bhattacharya et al. (2011a)]. The model behavior is studied corresponding to changes in the synaptic connectivity parameters as well as transmitter concentration related parameters, and a relevant comparison is made with the modARm. However, the model presented in this work has a larger set of synaptic connectivity parameters; model behavior corresponding to this parameter space and its usefulness in understanding neurological disorders will be the topic of a future work.

4. DISCUSSION

The work presented here explores a novel approach toward correlating current neural mass model based studies with underlying cellular mechanisms during synaptic transmission. The aim is to underpin the synaptic correlates of abnormal brain oscillations in neurological and psychiatric disorders such as observed in Electroencephalogram (EEG). A kinetic framework for modeling AMPA and GABA receptor mediated synapses is implemented in an existing thalamocortical neural mass model consisting of an excitatory and an inhibitory neural mass, representing cell populations of the thalamocortical relay (TCR) and the thalamic reticular nucleus (TRN), respectively. Parameters in the model are assumed to be "ensemble" representations of the corresponding attributes in a single neuron. A preliminary observation is made on the model behavior by varying the parameters corresponding to the post-synaptic membrane conductance of the cell populations as well as the forward and reverse rates of synaptic reaction; of specific interest is the transition of the model behavior between the spindle oscillatory mode and the limit-cycle mode, the latter resembling the slow-wave (high-amplitude, low-frequency) synchronized oscillations that are signatures of absence seizures as well as slow-wave sleep. Furthermore, only the alpha (8–13 Hz) and theta (4–7 Hz) frequency bands of the output power spectra are studied here, as EEG alpha and theta bands are believed to have a strong correlation with thalamocortical oscillations (Hughes et al., 2004).

The results indicate that: (1) The post synaptic membrane conductance for both AMPA and $GABA_A$ receptors in the TRN cell population play a role in sustaining spindle oscillations of the TCR cell population (the model output). (2) Blocking the $GABA_A$ mediated synapses in the self-inhibitory feedback pathway of the TRN cell population effects synchronized oscillations with high amplitude and increased time-period of oscillation ($\approx$0.03 Hz). (3) The post-synaptic membrane conductance for $GABA_B$ in the TCR cell population does not play any role in generating or sustaining spindle oscillations, but is responsible for sustaining the slow-wave oscillations in the model associated with blocking of the intra-TRN $GABA_A$ synapses. (4) Blocking both $GABA_A$ and $GABA_B$ or only the AMPA mediated synapses in the TCR cell population results in a quiescent model output. These findings are consistent with *in vitro* studies based on multiple unit recordings from ferret thalamic slices (von Krosigk et al., 1993) as well as single-neuron-level model based studies (Golomb et al., 1996). In addition, this study identifies—(a) the reverse rate of transmitter binding as an important attribute in effecting thalamocortical synchronized oscillations that can be induced in the model by increasing (decreasing) the fraction of open channels due to $GABA_A$ (AMPA) mediated synapses in the TCR (TRN) cell populations; (b) the post-synaptic membrane conductance for $GABA_A$ in the TCR cell population as a control parameter for effecting a behavioral transition in the model.

It may be noted that the above-mentioned observations are only a qualitative comparison with single-neuron-level model-based (Golomb et al., 1996) and experimental (von Krosigk et al., 1993) studies; a drawback of the current work is a lack of quantitative comparison with these studies. The neural mass model presented in this work is at a mesoscopic scale, representation of a population of $\approx 10^4 - 10^7$ neurons, unlike that in Golomb et al. (1996), which is at single-neuronal-level. Similarly, the multiple unit recording based study in von Krosigk et al. (1993) observes neuronal behavior of either a single neuron or a population of $<10^2$ neurons. In addition, the modeling and simulation methods in the current work and that in Golomb et al. (1996) are not similar. Thus, a quantitative comparison of the current work with these studies may lead to erroneous conclusions. However, model validation with experimental data is a crucial criteria when investigating brain disorders. Along these lines, an ongoing work is investigating ways to validate the model presented herein with EEG data, and will be the topic of a future study.

The model structure in the current work is a considerably simplified representation of the thalamocortical circuitry. The role of the thalamocortical circuitry in generating slow wave brain oscillations is discussed at length in Steriade et al. (1993), based on *in vivo* and *in vitro* studies. More recently, three parameters in the thalamo-cortico-thalamic loop viz. the cortico-thalamic, thalamo-cortical and intra-thalamic pathways are specified in Breakspear et al. (2006) for generating instabilities in the thalamocortical circuitry, leading to synchronized oscillations such as seen during absence seizures. Furthermore, a non-linear dynamical analysis of the model is shown to predict seizure onset by validating with patient EEG data. In a previous research (Bhattacharya et al., 2011b), we have proposed a more elaborate alpha-function based neural mass model that have considered these vital pathways in the thalamocorticothalamic loop. Also, we have performed a non-linear dynamical analysis of a simple thalamocortical model based on alpha functions in Bhattacharya et al. (2013) to understand EEG power spectra abnormalities associated with several neurological disorders. Such research directions will be considered as an extended work based on the model presented herein.

It is worth mentioning here that biologically plausible parameterizations has been a major constraint in neural mass modeling of brain dynamics. This is largely due to insufficient experimental data, published or otherwise, as well as to a lack of "homogeneity" of published data from different experimental laboratories. The trend thus far has been to use biologically plausible data if and when available; otherwise, i.e., for parameter values that cannot be availed from experimental data, the models are tuned to estimated parameter values which provide a desirable output in context to the objectives of the research [the reader may refer to Robinson et al. (2004) for a model parameterizations related work and discussion]. Thus, the model in Breakspear et al. (2006) was based on neurophysiological parameters obtained from Robinson et al. (2002), which in turn are based on inverse parameterizations during model validation with EEG data from patients of epileptic seizures. The parameterizations of the model presented in this work is largely based on neurophysiological parameters obtained from experimental studies: the cellular-level parameters, including those of the synaptic kinetics, are based on *in vitro* studies and model-based studies of thalamocortical tissue by von Krosigk et al. (1993) and Golomb et al. (1996), respectively; the model connectivity parameters are based on experimental studies of the cat and rat thalamus obtained from Horn et al. (2000); Sherman and Guillery (2001). On the other hand, the extrinsic (retinal) input and neuro-transmitter concentration parameter values are adjusted to maintain a "dynamically active" model behavior (this is as opposed to a continuous "quiescent" state of the model corresponding to certain parameter values, and does not conform to biology). However, technological advances in the field of neuro-imaging during the last decade such as functional Magnetic Resonance Imaging (fMRI), Diffusion Tensor Imaging (DTI) and Transcanial Magnetic Stimulation (TMS) are paving the way for biologically-realistic mapping of parameter values in computational models; for example as in Izhikevich and Edelman (2008).

The observations made herein support the motivation toward this preliminary work, which is to correlate higher-level brain dynamics with underlying cellular-level synaptic mechanisms. It may be noted that in all our previous works using alpha function based neural mass models, the emphasis has been on studying the model behavior with varying values of synaptic connectivity parameters toward a meaningful mapping to Alzheimer disease-related EEG anomalies. However, such "synaptic parameter variation only" studies are highly constrained and do not make much sense when trying to understand generic brain-state conditions e.g., the sleep-awake cycle, or several other neurological and psychiatric disorders e.g., absence seizures, which rely heavily on various aspects of cellular dynamics in the thalamocortical circuitry. Rather, the emphasis of this work is on laying the ground-work for a more elaborate, and yet computationally efficient scheme, whereby large-scale computational models may be simulated to mimic brain rhythms, which can then be correlated to model parameters emulating cellular dynamics. The synaptic transmission kinetics and subsequent post-synaptic membrane parameters are some of the key constituents of brain signaling, and are affected significantly in various brain diseases. Clearly, the alpha-function based neural mass models are inadequate in dealing with research directions where model parameters can be mapped in a biologically plausible manner to synaptic attributes. In terms of computational efficiency, the time for simulating 20 trials with the model presented in this work takes 60 s; this may be contrasted with 600 s for simulating a similar model [the modified Alpha Rhythm model in Bhattacharya et al. (2011a)] based on alpha functions. This is a dramatic improvement in computational efficiency and highlight the plausibility of using the kinetic-model based neural mass modeling framework in simulating large-scale computational models toward mimicking real-time EEG signals. This in turn will provide a powerful tool for specifying cellular pathways that need be targeted for symptomatic alleviation of anomalous brain rhythms as well as to inform effective neuropharmacological research directions.

REFERENCES

Aradi, I., and Erdi, P. (2006). Computational neuropharmacology: dynamical approaches in drug discovery. *Trends Pharmacol. Sci.* 27, 240–243. doi: 10.1016/j.tips.2006.03.004

Basar, E., and Guntekin, B. (2008). A review of brain oscillations in cognitive disorders and the role of neurotransmitters. *Brain Res. Rev.* 1235, 172–193. doi: 10.1016/j.brainres.2008.06.103

Bernard, C., Ge, Y., Stockley, E., Willis, J., and Wheal, H. (1994). Synaptic integration of NMDA and non-NMDA receptors in large neuronal network models solved by means of differential equations. *Biol. Cybern.* 70, 267–273. doi: 10.1007/BF00197607

Bhattacharya, B. S., Cakir, Y., Serap-Sengor, N., Maguire, L. P., and Coyle, D. (2013). Model-based bifurcation and power spectral analyses of thalamocortical alpha rhythm slowing in Alzheimer's disease. *Neurocomputing* 115, 11–22. doi: 10.1016/j.neucom.2012.10.023

Bhattacharya, B. S., Coyle, D., and Maguire, L. P. (2011a). "Alpha and theta rhythm abnormality in Alzheimer's disease: a study using a computational model," in *Advances in Experimental Medicine and Biology.* Vol. 718, eds C. Hernandez, J. Gomez, R. Sanz, I. Alexander, L. Smith, A. Hussain, et al. (New York, NY: Springer), 57–73.

Bhattacharya, B. S., Coyle, D., and Maguire, L. P. (2011b). A thalamo-cortico-thalamic neural mass model to study alpha rhythms in Alzheimer's disease. *Neural Netw.* 24, 631–645. doi: 10.1016/j.neunet.2011.02.009

Bhattacharya, B. S., Coyle, D., Maguire, L. P., and Stewart, J. (2012). "Kinetic modelling of synaptic functions in the alpha rhythm neural mass model," in *ICANN 2012 Part I, Lecture Notes in Computer Science 7552*, eds E. P. V. Alessandro, D. Wlodzislaw, E. Peter, M. Francesco, and P. Gunther (Berlin; Heidelberg: Springer Verlag), 645–652.

Breakspear, M., Roberts, J., Terry, J., Rodrigues, S., Mahant, N., and Robinson, P. A. (2006). A unifying explanation of primary generalized seizures through nonlinear brain modelling and bifurcation analysis. *Cereb. Cortex* 16, 1296–1313. doi: 10.1093/cercor/bhj072

Breakspear, M., Terry, J. R., and Friston, K. J. (2003). Modulation of excitatory synaptic coupling facilitates synchronization and complex dynamics in a nonlinear model of neuronal dynamics. *Neurocomputing* 52, 151–158. doi: 10.1016/S0925-2312(02)00740-3

da Silva, F. H. L., Hoeks, A., Smits, H., and Zetterberg, L. H. (1974). Model of brain rhythmic activity. *Kybernetic* 15, 27–37. doi: 10.1007/BF00270757

da Silva, F. H. L., van Lierop, T. H. M. T., Schrijer, C. F., and van Leeuwen, W. S. (1973). Essential differences between alpha rhythms and barbiturate spindles: spectra and thalamo-cortical coherences. *Electroencephalogr. Clin. Neurophysiol.* 35, 641–645. doi: 10.1016/0013-4694(73)90217-4

David, O., and Friston, K. J. (2003). A neural mass model for MEG/EEG: coupling and neuronal dynamics. *Neuroimage* 20, 1743–1755. doi: 10.1016/j.neuroimage.2003.07.015

de Haan, W., Mott, K., van Straaten, E. C. W., Scheltens, P., and Stam, C. J. (2012). Activity dependent degeneration explains hub vulnerability in Alzheimer's disease. *PLoS Comput. Biol.* 8:e1002582. doi: 10.1371/journal.pcbi.1002582

Deco, G., Jirsa, V. K., Robinson, P. A., Breakspear, M., and Friston, K. (2008). The dynamic brain: from spiking neurons to neural masses and cortical fields. *PLoS Comput. Biol.* 4:e1000092. doi: 10.1371/journal.pcbi.1000092

Destexhe, A. (2008). "Cortico-thalamic feedback: a key to explain absence seizures," in *Computational Neuroscience in Epilepsy*, eds I. Soltez and K. Staley (Amsterdam: Elsevier), 184–214. doi: 10.1016/B978-012373649-9.50016-8

Destexhe, A., Bal, T., McCormick, D., and Sejnowski, T. J. (1996). Ionic mechanisms underlying synchronised oscillations and propagating waves in a model of ferret thalamic slices. *J. Neurophysiol.* 76, 2049–2070.

Destexhe, A., Mainen, Z., and Sejnowski, T. (1994). An efficient method for computing synaptic conductances based on a kinetic model of receptor binding. *Neural Comput.* 6, 14–18. doi: 10.1162/neco.1994.6.1.14

Destexhe, A., Mainen, Z., and Sejnowski, T. (1998). "Kinetic models of synaptic transmission," in *Methods in Neuronal Modelling*, eds C. Koch and I. Segev (Cambridge, MA: MIT Press), 1–25.

Destexhe, A., Mainen, Z., and Sejnowski, T. (2002). "Kinetic models for synaptic interactions," in *The Handbook of Brain Theory and Neural Networks*, ed M. Arbib (Cambridge, MA: MIT Press), 1126–1130.

Freeman, W. J. (1975). *Mass Action in the Nervous System.* 1st Edn. New York, NY: Academic Press.

Golomb, D., Wang, X.-J., and Rinzel, J. (1994). Synchronization properties of spindle oscillations in a thalamic reticular nucleus model. *J. Neurophysiol.* 72, 1109–1126.

Golomb, D., Wang, X.-J., and Rinzel, J. (1996). Propagation of spindle waves in a thalamic slice model. *J. Neurophysiol.* 75, 750–769.

Grimbert, F., and Faugeras, O. (2006). Bifurcation analysis of Jansen's neural mass model. *Neural Comput.* 18, 3052–3068. doi: 10.1162/neco.2006.18.12.3052

Horn, S. C. V., Erisir, A., and Sherman, S. M. (2000). Relative distribution of synapses in the A-laminae of the lateral geniculate nucleus of the cat. *J. Compar. Neurol.* 416, 509–520. doi: 10.1002/(SICI)1096-9861(20000124)416:4<509::AID-CNE7>3.0.CO;2-H

Hughes, S. W., Lorincz, M., Cope, D. W., Blethyn, K. L., Kekesi, K. A., Parri, H. R., et al. (2004). Synchronised oscillations at α and θ frequencies in the lateral geniculate nucleus. *Neuron* 42, 253–268. doi: 10.1016/S0896-6273(04)00191-6

Izhikevich, E. M., and Edelman, G. M. (2008). Large-scale model of mammalian thalamocortical systems. *Proc. Natl. Acad. Sci. U.S.A.* 105, 3593–3598. doi: 10.1073/pnas.0712231105

Jansen, B. H., and Rit, V. G. (1995). Electroencephalogram and visual evoked potential generation in a mathematical model of coupled cortical columns. *Biol. Cybern.* 73, 357–366. doi: 10.1007/BF00199471

Liljenström, H. (2012). Mesoscopic brain dynamics. *Scholarpedia* 7:4601. doi: 10.4249/scholarpedia.4601

McCormick, D. A. (1992). Neurotransmitter actions in the thalamus and cerebral cortex and their role in neuromodulation of thalamocortical activity. *Progr. Neurobiol.* 39, 337–388. doi: 10.1016/0301-0082(92)90012-4

Pons, A. J., Cantero, J. L., Atienza, M., and Garcia-Ojalvo, J. (2010). Relating structural and functional anomalous connectivity in the ageing brain via neural mass modelling. *Neuroimage* 52, 848–861. doi: 10.1016/j.neuroimage.2009.12.105

Rall, W. (1967). Distinguishing theoretical synaptic potentials computed for different soma-dendritic distributions of synaptic inputs. *J. Neurophysiol.* 30, 1138–1168.

Robinson, P., Rennie, C., and Rowe, D. (2002). Dynamics of large-scale brain activity in normal arousal states and epileptic seizures.

Phys. Rev. E 65:041924. doi: 10.1103/PhysRevE.65.041924

Robinson, P., Rennie, C., Rowe, D., and Connor, S. O. (2004). Estimation of multiscale neurophysiologic parameters by electroencephalographic means. *Hum. Brain Mapp.* 23, 53–72. doi: 10.1002/hbm.20032

Robinson, P. A., Phillips, A. J. K., Fulcher, B. D., Puckeridge, M., and Roberts, J. A. (2011). Quantitative modelling of sleep dynamics. *Philos. Trans. R. Soc. A* 369, 3840–3854. doi: 10.1098/rsta.2011.0120

Sherman, S. M., and Guillery, R. W. (2001). *Exploring the Thalamus.* 1st Edn. New York, NY: Academic Press.

Sotero, R. C., Tujillo-Barreto, N. J., and Iturria-Medina, Y. (2007). Realistically coupled neural mass models can generate EEG rhythms. *Neural Comput.* 19, 479–512. doi: 10.1162/neco.2007.19.2.478

Stam, C. J., Pijn, J., Suffczyński, P., and da Silva, F. (1999). Dynamics of the human alpha rhythm: evidence for non-linearity? *Clin. Neurophysiol.* 110, 1801–1813. doi: 10.1016/S1388-2457(99)00099-1

Steriade, M., McCormick, D. A., and Sejnowski, T. J. (1993). Thalamocortical oscillations in the sleeping and aroused brain. *Science* 262, 679–685. doi: 10.1126/science.8235588

Suffczyński, P. (2000). *Neural Dynamics Underlying Brain Thalamic Oscillations Investigated with Computational Models.* Ph.D. Thesis, Institute of experimental physics, University of Warsaw.

Suffczyński, P., Kalitzin, S., and Silva, F. H. L. D. (2004). Dynamics of non-convulsive epileptic phenomena modelled by a bistable neuronal network. *Neuroscience* 126, 467–484. doi: 10.1016/j.neuroscience.2004.03.014

Ursino, M., Cona, F., and Zavaglia, M. (2010). The generation of rhythms within a cortical region: analysis of a neural mass model. *Neuroimage* 52, 1080–1094. doi: 10.1016/j.neuroimage.2009.12.084

von Krosigk, M., Bal, T., and McCormick, D. A. (1993). Cellular mechanisms of a synchronised oscillation in the thalamus. *Science* 261, 361–364. doi: 10.1126/science.8392750

Wang, X.-J., Golomb, D., and Rinzel, J. (1995). Emergent spindle oscillations and intermittent burst firing in a thalamic model: specific neuronal mechanisms. *Proc. Natl. Acad. Sci.* 92, 5577–5581. doi: 10.1073/pnas.92.12.5577

Wang, X.-J., and Rinzel, J. (1992). Alternating and synchronous rhythms in reciprocally inhibitory model neurons. *Neural Comput.* 4, 84–97. doi: 10.1162/neco.1992.4.1.84

Wendling, F., Bartolomei, F., Bellanger, J. J., and Chauvel, P. (2002). Epileptic fast activity can be explained by a model of impaired GABAergic dendritic inhibition. *Eur. J. Neurosci.* 15, 1499–1508. doi: 10.1046/j.1460-9568.2002.01985.x

Wilson, H. R., and Cowan, J. D. (1973). A mathematical theory of the functional dynamics of cortical and thalamic nervous tissue. *Kybernetik* 13, 55–80. doi: 10.1007/BF00288786

Zetterberg, L. H., Kristiansson, L., and Mossberg, K. (1978). Performance of a model for a local neuron population. *Biol. Cybern.* 31, 15–26. doi: 10.1007/BF00337367

Permissions

 Every chapter published in this book has been scrutinized by our experts. Their significance has been extensively debated. The topics covered herein carry significant findings which will fuel the growth of the discipline. They may even be implemented as practical applications or may be referred to as a beginning point for another development.

The contributors of this book come from diverse backgrounds, making this book a truly international effort. This book will bring forth new frontiers with its revolutionizing research information and detailed analysis of the nascent developments around the world.

We would like to thank all the contributing authors for lending their expertise to make the book truly unique. They have played a crucial role in the development of this book. Without their invaluable contributions this book wouldn't have been possible. They have made vital efforts to compile up to date information on the varied aspects of this subject to make this book a valuable addition to the collection of many professionals and students.

This book was conceptualized with the vision of imparting up-to-date information and advanced data in this field. To ensure the same, a matchless editorial board was set up. Every individual on the board went through rigorous rounds of assessment to prove their worth. After which they invested a large part of their time researching and compiling the most relevant data for our readers.

The editorial board has been involved in producing this book since its inception. They have spent rigorous hours researching and exploring the diverse topics which have resulted in the successful publishing of this book. They have passed on their knowledge of decades through this book. To expedite this challenging task, the publisher supported the team at every step. A small team of assistant editors was also appointed to further simplify the editing procedure and attain best results for the readers.

Apart from the editorial board, the designing team has also invested a significant amount of their time in understanding the subject and creating the most relevant covers. They scrutinized every image to scout for the most suitable representation of the subject and create an appropriate cover for the book.

The publishing team has been an ardent support to the editorial, designing and production team. Their endless efforts to recruit the best for this project, has resulted in the accomplishment of this book. They are a veteran in the field of academics and their pool of knowledge is as vast as their experience in printing. Their expertise and guidance has proved useful at every step. Their uncompromising quality standards have made this book an exceptional effort. Their encouragement from time to time has been an inspiration for everyone.

The publisher and the editorial board hope that this book will prove to be a valuable piece of knowledge for researchers, students, practitioners and scholars across the globe.

List of Contributors

Axel Hutt
INRIA CR Nancy - Grand Est, Team CORTEX, Villers-les-Nancy, France

Rosalyn Moran
Wellcome Trust Centre for Neuroimaging, Institute of Neurology, University College London, London, UK
Virginia Tech Carilion Research Institute, Virginia Tech, Roanoke, VA, USA
Bradley Department of Electrical and Computer Engineering, Virginia Tech, Blacksburg, VA, USA

Dimitris A. Pinotsis and Karl Friston
Wellcome Trust Centre for Neuroimaging, Institute of Neurology, University College London, London, UK

James Joseph Wright
Department of Psychological Medicine, Faculty of Medicine, The University of Auckland, Auckland, New Zealand
Liggins Institute, The University of Auckland, Auckland, New Zealand

Paul David Bourke
iVEC@UWA, University of Western Australia, Perth, WA, Australia

Paul C. Bressloff and Jeremy Wilkerson
Department of Mathematics, University of Utah, Salt Lake City, UT, USA

David T. J. Liley
Brain and Psychological Sciences Research Centre, Faculty of Life and Social Sciences, Swinburne University of Technology, Hawthorn, VIC, Australia
Cortical Dynamics Ltd., Hawthorn, VIC, Australia

Matthew Walsh
Brain and Psychological Sciences Research Centre, Faculty of Life and Social Sciences, Swinburne University of Technology, Hawthorn, VIC, Australia

Peter beim Graben
Bernstein Center for Computational Neuroscience Berlin, Berlin, Germany
Department of German Language and Linguistics, Humboldt-Universität zu Berlin, Berlin, Germany

Serafim Rodrigues
Centre for Robotics and Neural Systems, School of Computing and Mathematics, University of Plymouth, Plymouth, UK

Ingo Bojak
Centre for Computational Neuroscience and Cognitive Robotics, School of Psychology, University of Birmingham, Birmingham, UK
Donders Centre for Neuroscience, Donders Institute for Brain, Cognition and Behaviour, Radboud University Nijmegen Medical Centre, Nijmegen, Netherlands

Harry C. Day
Centre for Computational Neuroscience and Cognitive Robotics, School of Psychology, University of Birmingham, Birmingham, UK

Faten Mina, Pascal Benquet and Fabrice Wendling
INSERM, U1099, Universite de Rennes 1, Rennes, France
Laboratoire Traitement du Signal et de L'Image, Université de Rennes 1, Rennes, France

Anca Pasnicu
Unité d'Épileptologie, Service de Neurologie, CHU, Rennes, France

Arnaud Biraben
INSERM, U1099, Universite de Rennes 1, Rennes, France
Laboratoire Traitement du Signal et de L'Image, Université de Rennes 1, Rennes, France
Unité d'Épileptologie, Service de Neurologie, CHU, Rennes, France

Richard T. Gray
The Kirby Institute, The University of New South Wales, Sydney, NSW, Australia

Peter A. Robinson
School of Physics, University of Sydney, Sydney, NSW, Australia
Brain Dynamics Center, Sydney Medical School – Western, University of Sydney, Westmead, NSW, Australia

Moritz Augustin, Josef Ladenbauer and Klaus Obermayer
Department of Software Engineering and Theoretical Computer Science, Technische Universität Berlin, Berlin, Germany
Bernstein Center for Computational Neuroscience Berlin, Berlin, Germany

Stephen E. Robinson and Richard Coppola
MEG Core Facility, National Institute of Mental Health, National Institutes of Health, Bethesda, MD, USA

Arnold J. Mandell
Department of Psychiatry, University of California, San Diego, CA, USA

Dipanjan Roy
Theoretical Neuroscience Group, Faculté de Médecine, Institut de Neurosciences des Systèmes, Inserm UMR1106, Aix-Marseille Université, Marseille, France
Bernstein Center for Computational Neuroscience, Berlin, Germany
Department of Software Engineering and Theoretical Computer Science, Technische Universität Berlin, Berlin, Germany

Viktor Jirsa
Theoretical Neuroscience Group, Faculté de Médecine, Institut de Neurosciences des Systèmes, Inserm UMR1106, Aix-Marseille Université, Marseille, France

Ramesh Srinivasan
Department of Cognitive Sciences, University of California, Irvine, CA, USA
Department of Biomedical Engineering, University of California, Irvine, CA, USA
Institute for Mathematical Behavioral Sciences, University of California, Irvine, CA, USA

Samuel Thorpe
Institute for Mathematical Behavioral Sciences, University of California, Irvine, CA, USA

Paul L. Nunez
Cognitive Dissonance, LLC, San Diego, CA, USA

J. Modolo and A. W. Thomas
Human Threshold Research Group, Lawson Health Research Institute, London, ON, Canada
Department of Medical Biophysics, Western University, London, ON, Canada
Department of Medical Imaging, Western University, London, ON, Canada

A. Legros
Human Threshold Research Group, Lawson Health Research Institute, London, ON, Canada
Department of Medical Biophysics, Western University, London, ON, Canada
Department of Medical Imaging, Western University, London, ON, Canada
School of Kinesiology, Western University, London, ON, Canada

Cliff C. Kerr
Department of Physiology and Pharmacology, State University of New York Downstate Medical Center, Brooklyn, NY, USA
School of Physics, University of Sydney, NSW, Australia
Brain Dynamics Centre, Westmead Millennium Institute, Westmead, NSW, Australia

Sacha J. Van Albada
Institute of Neuroscience and Medicine (INM-6) and Institute for Advanced Simulation (IAS-6), Jülich Research Centre and JARA, Jülich, Germany

Samuel A. Neymotin
Department of Physiology and Pharmacology, State University of New York Downstate Medical Center, Brooklyn, NY, USA
Department of Neurobiology, Yale University, New Haven, CT, USA

George L. Chadderdon
Department of Physiology and Pharmacology, State University of New York Downstate Medical Center, Brooklyn, NY, USA

P. A. Robinson
School of Physics, University of Sydney, NSW, Australia
Brain Dynamics Centre, Westmead Millennium Institute, Westmead, NSW, Australia

William W. Lytton
Department of Physiology and Pharmacology, State University of New York Downstate Medical Center, Brooklyn, NY, USA
Department of Neurology, Kings County Hospital, Brooklyn, NY, USA

Basabdatta S. Bhattacharya
Engineering Hub, School of Engineering, University of Lincoln, Lincoln, UK

Index

O

P

R

S

T

W

www.ingramcontent.com/pod-product-compliance
Lightning Source LLC
LaVergne TN
LVHW082218200926
848484LV00008B/2273

31. Happé, F.; Frith, U. The Weak Coherence Account: Detail-focused Cognitive Style in Autism Spectrum Disorders. *J. Autism Dev. Disord.* **2006**, *36*, 5–25. [CrossRef]
32. Lang, K.; Lopez, C.; Stahl, D.; Tchanturia, K.; Treasure, J. Central coherence in eating disorders: An updated systematic review and meta-analysis. *World J. Biol. Psychiatry* **2014**, *15*, 586–598. [CrossRef] [PubMed]
33. Lang, K.; Roberts, M.; Harrison, A.; Lopez, C.; Goddard, E.; Khondoker, M.; Treasure, J.; Tchanturia, K. Central Coherence in Eating Disorders: A Synthesis of Studies Using the Rey Osterrieth Complex Figure Test. *PLoS ONE* **2016**, *11*, e0165467. [CrossRef] [PubMed]
34. Madsen, S.K.; Bohon, C.; Feusner, J.D. Visual processing in anorexia nervosa and body dysmorphic disorder: Similarities, differences, and future research directions. *J. Psychiatr. Res.* **2013**, *47*, 1483–1491. [CrossRef] [PubMed]
35. Freeman, R.; Touyz, S.; Sara, G.; Rennie, C.; Gordon, E.; Beumont, P. In the eye of the beholder: Processing body shape information in anorexic and bulimic patients. *Int. J. Eat. Disord.* **1991**, *10*, 709–714. [CrossRef]
36. Karlsson, L.; Rastam, M.; Wentz, E. The SWedish Eating Assessment for Autism spectrum disorders (SWEAA)-Validation of a self-report questionnaire targeting eating disturbances within the autism spectrum. *Res. Dev. Disabil.* **2013**, *34*, 2224–2233. [CrossRef]
37. NICE. Autism Spectrum Disorder in Adults: Diagnosis and Management, Clinical Guideline CG142. Available online: https://www.nice.org.uk/guidance/cg142 (accessed on 6 February 2020).
38. Ashwood, K.L.; Gillan, N.; Horder, J.; Hayward, H.; Woodhouse, E.; McEwen, F.S.; Findon, J.; Eklund, H.; Spain, D.; Wilson, C.E.; et al. Predicting the diagnosis of autism in adults using the Autism-Spectrum Quotient (AQ) questionnaire. *Psychol. Med.* **2016**, *46*, 2595–2604. [CrossRef]
39. Baron-Cohen, S.; Wheelwright, S.; Skinner, R.; Martin, J.; Clubley, E. The Autism-Spectrum Quotient (AQ): Evidence from Asperger syndrome/high-functioning autism, males and females, scientists and mathematicians. *J. Autism Dev. Disord.* **2001**, *31*, 5–17. [CrossRef]
40. Sizoo, B.B.; Horwitz, E.H.; Teunisse, J.P.; Kan, C.C.; Vissers, C.; Forceville, E.J.M.; Van Voorst, A.J.P.; Geurts, H.M. Predictive validity of self-report questionnaires in the assessment of autism spectrum disorders in adults. *Autism* **2015**, *19*, 842–849. [CrossRef]
41. Conner, C.M.; Cramer, R.D.; McGonigle, J.J. Examining the Diagnostic Validity of Autism Measures Among Adults in an Outpatient Clinic Sample. *Autism Adulthood* **2019**, *1*, 60–68. [CrossRef]
42. Sedgewick, F.; Kerr-Gaffney, J.; Leppanen, J.; Tchanturia, K. Anorexia Nervosa, Autism, and the ADOS: How Appropriate Is the New Algorithm in Identifying Cases? *Front. Psychiatry* **2019**, *10*, 507. [CrossRef]

2

The Effect of a Food Addiction Explanation Model for Weight Control and Obesity on Weight Stigma

Kerry S. O'Brien [1,*], Rebecca M. Puhl [2], Janet D. Latner [3], Dermot Lynott [4], Jessica D. Reid [1], Zarina Vakhitova [1], John A. Hunter [5], Damian Scarf [5], Ruth Jeanes [6], Ayoub Bouguettaya [1] and Adrian Carter [7]

1 School of Social Sciences, Faculty of Arts, Monash University, Melbourne 3800, Australia; jdorothea.reid@gmail.com (J.D.R.); zarina.vakhitova@monash.edu (Z.V.); ayoub.bouguettaya@monash.edu (A.B.)
2 Department of Human Development and Family Sciences, Rudd Center for Food Policy & Obesity, University of Connecticut, Storrs, CT 06269, USA; rebecca.puhl@uconn.edu
3 Department of Psychology, College of Social Sciences, University of Hawaii, Manoa, HI 96822, USA; jlatner@hawaii.edu
4 Department of Psychology, Faculty of Science and Technology University of Lancaster, Lancaster LA1 4YW, UK; d.lynott@lancaster.ac.uk
5 Division of Sciences, Department of Psychology, University of Otago, Dunedin 9016, New Zealand; jackie.hunter@otago.ac.nz (J.A.H.); damian@psy.otago.ac.nz (D.S.)
6 Curriculum & Pedagogy, Faculty of Education, Monash University, Melbourne 3800, Australia; ruth.jeanes@monash.edu
7 School of Psychology, Faculty of Medicine, Nursing, and Health Sciences, Monash University, Melbourne 3800, Australia; adrian.carter@monash.edu
* Correspondence: kerrykez@gmail.com

Abstract: There is increasing scientific and public support for the notion that some foods may be addictive, and that poor weight control and obesity may, for some people, stem from having a food addiction. However, it remains unclear how a food addiction model (FAM) explanation for obesity and weight control will affect weight stigma. In two experiments ($N = 530$ and $N = 690$), we tested the effect of a food addiction explanation for obesity and weight control on weight stigma. In Experiment 1, participants who received a FAM explanation for weight control and obesity reported lower weight stigma scores (e.g., less dislike of 'fat people', and lower personal willpower blame) than those receiving an explanation emphasizing diet and exercise ($F_{(4,525)} = 7.675$, $p = 0.006$; and $F_{(4,525)} = 5.393$, $p = 0.021$, respectively). In Experiment 2, there was a significant group difference for the dislike of 'fat people' stigma measure ($F_{(5,684)} = 5.157$, $p = 0.006$), but not for personal willpower weight stigma ($F_{(5,684)} = 0.217$, $p = 0.81$). Participants receiving the diet and exercise explanation had greater dislike of 'fat people' than those in the FAM explanation and control group (p values < 0.05), with no difference between the FAM and control groups ($p > 0.05$). The FAM explanation for weight control and obesity did not increase weight stigma and resulted in lower stigma than the diet and exercise explanation that attributes obesity to personal control. The results highlight the importance of health messaging about the causes of obesity and the need for communications that do not exacerbate weight stigma.

Keywords: stigma; obesity; food addiction; weight bias; weight stigma; obesity prejudice reduction

1. Introduction

Research on the extent, nature, and impact of weight stigma (also termed weight bias, obesity stigma) suggests that weight stigma has increased over time in adults [1] and children [2] and is associated with a host of negative social and health outcomes [3]. For example, research shows that women perceived to be overweight or obese encounter discrimination in education, health, and employment settings [4–6]. Similarly, experiences of weight stigma are associated with poorer psychological and physical outcomes arising from stigma-related stress, including increased depression and anxiety [7], emotional and stress-related eating [8], and avoidance of health care settings [9]. As such, there is a need for research that seeks to understand factors that contribute to and reinforce weight stigma.

Attribution theories, and specifically, the attribution-value model [10] suggests that antipathy toward a specific group or target is maintained by beliefs about the controllability of specific group behaviours. In the case of overweight and obesity, studies show that weight stigma is increased by attributions about controllability of weight and obesity [11,12]. That is, because people are exposed to public health and media messages that weight is under personal control, people conclude that obesity must be due to an individual's personal failures, which in turn leads to greater weight stigma [13,14]. Dominant public health messages on the cause of overweight and obesity remain focused, if simplistically, on individual control of diet and physical activity [15]. This individualistic public health narrative is increasingly criticised [16], as it ignores research on the myriad of uncontrollable factors contributing to weight control and obesity, such as neurophysiology, environment, and the interplay with genetics/epigenetics. Experimental evidence suggests that changing people's attributions about the causes of obesity away from individual blame, and to more biologically and environmentally pre-determined factors, can help to reduce weight stigma [11]. Accordingly, correcting public misattributions about weight has the potential not only to improve knowledge about the complex causes of obesity, but also the potential to reduce weight stigma and discrimination [17].

Recent research posits that some people may have a neurobiological addiction to certain foods, particularly ultra-processed hyper-palatable foods. This addiction may, in part, contribute to people's food choices and consumption behaviour, and in turn obesity rates [18,19]. Termed *food addiction*, neuropsychological and behavioural research on the addictive properties of food identifies considerable overlap in the food and drug reward and addiction-related centres and pathways of the brain; as a result, food can be as rewarding and addictive as other addictive substances such as drugs, which share overlapping brain reward pathways [20,21]. Large-scale studies suggest that a significant proportion (15%) of the general population [22], and a greater proportion of those with obesity (up to 30%) meet criteria for a diagnosis of food addiction [23]. Furthermore, between 28% and 52% of the general population perceive themselves to be addicted to food [24].

The food addiction model (FAM) for weight control and obesity raises questions about whether a FAM explanation could be helpful or harmful in efforts to reduce weight stigma. While it could be argued that a FAM explanation might increase weight stigma as a result of labelling individuals with obesity as having an addiction, it is possible that a FAM explanation could instead reduce stigma towards people perceived to have obesity by reducing attributions of individual controllability of weight [25]. Research examining these questions is scarce [26]. Some research suggests that the addition of the addiction label to obesity is associated with increased vulnerability to stigmatization [27], and experimental work suggests that the FAM explanation may increase stigma associated with obesity [28]. In contrast, experimental research by Latner and colleagues [25] found that a FAM explanation for weight control and obesity resulted in less stigma and less blame for targets at both lower and higher body weights. These mixed findings indicate the need for additional research to establish whether a FAM explanation increases or decreases weight stigma relative to current public health messaging that suggests diet and exercise as the primary drivers of weight and obesity [29,30].

The present study aimed to examine whether a food addiction explanation for weight control would exacerbate or ameliorate weight stigma relative to the dominant public health messaging emphasizing personal control of diet and exercise. We conducted two experiments to assess the impact of a food addiction explanation for obesity on expressions of weight stigma. In line with previous research with the attribution value model [10] for weight stigma, we predicted that the FAM explanation would result in less weight stigma towards people perceived to be obese or "fat".

2. Methods (Experiment 1 and 2)

2.1. Participants

Table 1 details the demographic characteristics of participants in Experiment 1 and 2. For Experiment 1, a sample of $N = 652$ university (college) students was invited to participate in the experiment in return for course credit. Most students (86%; $N = 561$) agreed to participate, with $N = 530$ (94%) of those agreeing to participate providing data on the outcome variables. For Experiment 2, university (college) students ($N = 717$) were invited to participate in the experiment in return for course credit. Most (96%; $N = 696$) agreed to participate, with $N = 690$ providing data on the outcome variables.

Table 1. Participant characteristics for Experiment 1 and Experiment 2.

Parameter	Value
Experiment 1 ($N = 530$)	
Age (years)	M = 19.7, SD = 1.8 (range: 18–35)
Gender (female/male)	73.8% ($n = 391$)/26.2% ($n = 139$)
Body Mass Index (BMI)	M = 22.5, SD = 4.1
Percentage underweight (BMI ≤ 18.5 kg/m^2)	10.9% ($n = 57$)
Percentage normal weight (BMI = 18.5 < 25.0)	69.4% ($n = 367$)
Percentage overweight or obese (BMI > 25+)	20% ($n = 106$)
Experiment 2 ($N = 690$)	
Age (years)	M = 19.7, SD = 2.51 (range: 18–52)
Gender (female/male)	72.2% ($n = 498$)/27.7% ($n = 191$)
Body Mass Index (BMI)	M = 22.4, SD = 4.1
Percentage underweight (BMI ≤ 18.5 kg/m^2)	11.1% ($n = 77$)
Percentage normal weight (BMI = 18.5 < 25.0)	68.0% ($n = 469$)
Percentage overweight or obese (BMI > 25+)	20.9% ($n = 144$)

A priori sample size calculations indicated a required minimum sample of $N = 142$ for Experiment 1 and $N = 216$ for Experiment 2 (72 per group) to detect a small to moderate effect size ($d = 0.30$) between experimental groups with desired power at 0.80 and α set at 0.05 (two-sided). The present sample sizes were sufficient for experimental designs and planned analyses.

2.2. Design (Experiments 1 and 2)

Experiment 1 used a between-subjects experimental design to test the effect of a food addiction explanation ($N = 263$) for weight control and obesity vs. the diet and exercise explanation ($N = 267$) on weight stigma (prejudice towards "fat" people). The host university's Qualtrics research platform randomisation function with a 1:1 ratio was used for randomisation to conditions. Participants received either a simulated news article from The Guardian on the food addiction explanation for weight control and obesity (food addiction condition) or an identically formatted news article positing the dominant public health message that weight control and obesity are due to poor dieting and/or exercise behaviour. Single-item post-manipulation measures were taken for all variables.

Experiment 2 ($N = 690$) was identical to Experiment 1, but introduced a control group that received no newspaper article. The randomisation ratio was set at 2:1:1 with the control condition ($N = 346$) having two participants for every one participant allocated to the food addiction ($N = 167$) and diet and exercise conditions ($N = 175$).

2.3. Manipulation (Food Addiction vs. Diet and Exercise News Articles, vs. Control/No News Article)

Two newspaper articles were constructed for the experiments. The two articles appeared authentic and were structurally identical, using The Guardian newspaper format, with identical author, date/time of publication, word length, and text/photo placement. Both articles contained identical text reporting on research from The Lancet suggesting that mortality from obesity-related diseases was high and, for the first time, greater than mortality from starvation. However, the articles differed considerably in the text regarding explanations for weight control and obesity.

The *food addiction* article described the concept of food addiction and explained how foods can be addictive through the involvement of the pleasure/reward centres of the brain, and the release of dopamine when eating some foods, which in turn leads to cravings and a vicious cycle of addiction. The article named the originator of the term food addiction, and stated that approximately 20% of the population may have a food addiction, particularly to highly processed or convenience foods. The article also suggested that food addiction was a key factor in weight control and overweight and obesity.

The *diet and exercise* news article made no reference to food addictions or cravings, but instead focused on people's lack of physical exercise, sedentary lifestyles, and overconsumption of unhealthy foods. The article stated that these personal behaviours were the cause of obesity. The article cited research from experts stating that more self-control was needed when choosing what foods to eat, and it concluded by stating that diet and exercise programs are our best chance at reducing the obesity epidemic and that people need to get moving more.

2.4. *Measures*

Along with demographic characteristics including age, sex, height in centimetres, weight in kilograms, and ethnicity, we assessed participant's weight stigma (i.e., anti-fat prejudice, weight bias). We also included simple measures to assess whether the manipulations affected beliefs about the causes of obesity and weight gain and loss and a food addiction condition manipulation check. All participants received all of the measures summarized below.

2.4.1. Weight Stigma

To measure weight stigma we used the Anti-Fat Attitudes Test (AFAT), a psychometrically sound measure that has been widely used in the field to measure weight bias [31]. The AFAT is a 13-item scale comprised of three subscales assessing dislike of "fat people" which assesses antipathy towards people perceived to be "fat" (Dislike: 7 items, e.g., "I really don't like fat people much"), fear of becoming fat (Fear of Fat: 3 items, e.g., "I worry about becoming fat"), and belief that excess weight is due to a lack personal willpower (Willpower: 3 items, e.g., "Some people are fat because they have no willpower"). Participants indicate their agreement to items using a scale ranging from 0 = *very strongly disagree* to 9 = *very strongly agree*. The mean of the subscale items is used for analyses. Previous work has identified that the 'fear of fat' subscale functions as a measure of personal body image rather than weight stigma toward others per se, with one of the items lacking face validity, so this subscale was not analysed in the present study [32]. Cronbach's alpha's for the dislike and willpower subscales were good in the present sample: $\alpha = 0.87$ and $\alpha = 0.79$, respectively.

2.4.2. Belief in the Food Addiction Explanation

The food addiction support index (FASI) [24] was used to assess participant beliefs in, and support for, the food addiction explanation for eating, obesity, and weight gain, following exposure to the food addiction vs. diet and exercise news articles (manipulation). Participants responded to the five-item FASI (e.g., "Obesity should be treated as an addiction"), using a five-point scale ranging from 0 = *strongly disagree* to 4 = *strongly agree* with items summed to form a scale total from 0 to 20. Cronbach's alpha's in the present experiment was $\alpha = 0.83$.

2.4.3. Belief in Diet and Exercise for Weight Control

Two items from the dieting beliefs scale [33] that directly capture beliefs about exercise and dieting for the control of weight were used to assess the following exposure to the food addiction vs. diet and exercise news article (manipulation). Specifically, participants were asked to indicate their agreement using a six-point scale ranging from 1 = *not at all descriptive of my beliefs* to 6 = *very descriptive of my beliefs* to the statements "By restricting what one eats, one can lose weight" and "By increasing the amount that one exercises, one can lose weight". The two items were combined to form a score ranging from 1 to 12, with higher scores indicating greater belief that diet and exercise are responsible for weight control and obesity.

2.5. *Food Addiction Manipulation Check*

To assess whether participants attended to the information in the food addition article, we asked a short question assessing recall for a specific piece of information in the food addiction article. Specifically, we asked participants to identify via a multi-choice recognition response (four answer options) "Who first introduced the term Food Addiction?" Participant responses were coded as either incorrect = 0 or correct = 1.

2.6. *Procedure*

Upon entering the experiment via a web-link to the host university's Qualtrics research platform, participants in both experiments were provided with the title and description of the study, and then were asked to provide consent to participate. To limit bias in sampling and responding, the study used deception in the advertising and description of the experiment. Participants were told that the experiment was interested in how cognitive information processing styles affect public opinion on a range of political, health, and social issues and that researchers were interested in how people deal with being saturated by the wide range of media messages they receive via TV, computer, and mobile devices.

Participants first answered demographic questions before being presented with one of the two news articles (FAM condition vs. diet/exercise condition) or no article for those in the control group for Experiment 2. To enhance the authenticity of the experiment guise, a large set of distractor questions taken from measures assessing experiential and analytical thinking styles [34] were interspersed in the outcome and manipulation measures. These measures asked participants whether they enjoy the process of thinking deeply about issues, and they have been used successfully elsewhere [35]. Finally, participants were presented with the outcome and manipulation measures. The experiment took approximately 22 min on average to complete. Ethical approval for the study was sought and provided by the host university's Human Research Ethics Committee (Project ID: 8912).

2.7. *Analysis*

Chi-squared (X^2) and t-tests were used to assess whether randomisation resulted in balanced groups based on gender, age, and body mass index (BMI). Because weight stigma scores were not normally distributed in either experiment, we adopted a two-step transformation to normalise the data [36]. Subsequent normality checks showed the data to have no issues with skewness or kurtosis. ANCOVAs accounting for age, sex, and BMI as covariates were used to test for significant mean group differences on the dislike and willpower weight stigma measures. A Chi-squared test assessed accurate recognition of the food addiction originator in a probe question (manipulation check). ANOVA was also used to examine whether there were any differences on the manipulation measures (i.e., FASI, dieting/exercise beliefs, and food addiction article attention; i.e., who was the originator of food addiction term). We report adjusted means (M) and standard deviations (SD) along with F and p-values (significance was set at 0.05) for all primary outcomes.

3. Results (Experiments 1 and 2)

3.1. Preliminary Analysis Experiment 1

Preliminary analyses (X^2 and *t*-tests) assessing whether randomisation resulted in balanced groups on demographic characteristics showed there were no significant differences between groups for sex, age, or BMI scores (all p values > 0.27). A higher proportion of participants in the food addiction condition (61%) correctly recalled the name of the originator of the term food addiction than did those in the diet and exercise condition (39%, $X^2 = 23.663$, $p < 0.0005$).

3.2. Experiment 1 Food Addiction vs. Diet and Exercise

ANCOVA found significant group difference for the 'dislike' weight stigma measure: $F_{(4,525)} = 7.675$, $p = 0.006$. Participants exposed to the FAM explanation had significantly lower dislike of "fat people" (M = 1.82, SD = 1.46) scores than did the participants in the diet and exercise condition (M = 2.13, SD = 1.70). Similarly, participants in the FAM group endorsed significantly lower willpower stigma scores (M = 4.29, SD = 205) than participants in the diet and exercise explanation group (M = 4.68, SD = 1.97; $F_{(4,525)} = 5.393$, $p = 0.021$), indicating that those in the FAM condition were less likely to attribute excess weight to a lack of personal willpower.

We examined whether there were differences between groups in the posited beliefs about the causes of weight control and obesity (i.e., FASI, dieting/exercise beliefs). There were statistically significant group difference on FASI scores. Participants receiving the FAM explanation for obesity and weight control had greater belief in the FAM explanation for obesity and weight control (FASI) (M = 14.57, SD = 3.78) than participants receiving the traditional diet and exercise explanation (M = 13.66, SD = 3.80; $F_{(4,525)} = 8.823$, $p = 0.003$). There was not a statistically significant group difference for the dieting and exercise beliefs measure (FAM, M = 8.60, SD = 2.04; diet and exercise M = 8.50, SD = 2.03; $F_{(4,525)} = 0.100$, $p = 0.75$).

3.3. Preliminary Analysis Experiment 2

Preliminary analyses (X^2 and *t*-tests) assessing whether randomisation resulted in balanced groups on demographic characteristics showed there were no significant differences between groups for sex, age, or BMI scores (all p values > 0.46). A higher proportion of participants in the food addiction condition (58%) correctly recalled the name of the originator of the term food addiction than did those in the diet and exercise condition (42%; $X^2 = 15.047$, $p < 0.0005$).

3.4. Experiment 2 Food Addiction vs. Diet and Exercise vs. Control/No News Article

ANCOVA found significant group difference for the dislike of 'fat people' weight stigma scores ($F_{(5,684)} = 5.157$, $p = 0.006$). Post-hoc tests showed that participants exposed to FAM explanation had significantly lower dislike of 'fat people' (M = 1.85, SD = 1.57) than participants in the diet and exercise condition (M = 2.23, SD = 1.76, $p < 0.001$). Participants in the diet and exercise condition also endorsed higher weight stigma scores than those in the control condition (M = 1.70, SD = 1.54). There was no significant difference in dislike of 'fat people' scores between the FAM condition and the control group ($p = 0.56$). There was also no significant group difference for willpower weight stigma scores ($F_{(5,684)} = 0.217$, $p = 0.81$), with the FAM, diet and exercise, and control groups having similar mean scores (M = 4.71, SD = 2.05, and M = 4.81, SD = 1.86, M = 4.62, SD = 2.16, respectively).

We examined whether there were differences between groups in the posited beliefs about the causes of weight control and obesity (i.e., dieting/exercise beliefs, FASI). There was no significant group difference for the dieting/exercise beliefs measure ($F_{(5,682)} = 2.055$, $p = 0.13$; diet and exercise condition M = 4.62, SD = 0.95, control condition M = 4.38, SD = 1.06, FAM group M = 4.43, SD = 1.03). We found no statistically significant group difference in FASI scores ($F_{(5,680)} = 1.764$, $p = 0.17$; control M = 14.54, SD = 4.17, FAM M = 15.01, SD = 3.29, diet and exercise M = 13.99, SD = 3.90).

4. Discussion

We examined whether the FAM explanation for weight control and obesity versus the traditional public health messaging around control of diet and exercise would affect weight stigma. Relative to the dominant public health narrative that obesity stems from lack of control over diet and exercise, the FAM explanation resulted in lower weight stigma. In Experiment 1, both dislike of 'fat people' and perceptions that excess weight is a result of lack of willpower were lower in people presented with the FAM explanation. In a second experiment, we introduced a control group that was not exposed to information about obesity or causal models for obesity. Similar to Experiment 1, participants in Experiment 2 who received the FAM explanation for weight control and obesity displayed less weight stigma (dislike of "fat people") than participants in the diet and exercise condition. Importantly, there was no difference between the FAM and control groups in levels of weight stigma. Contrary to Experiment 1, in Experiment 2 there was no significant group difference with respect to perceptions that excess weight is caused by a lack of willpower (blame). The results of these two experiments are consistent with work by Latner and colleagues [25] who reported less stigma following exposure to a food addiction explanation. The results do not appear to support the notion that attaching an addiction label to people with obesity would exacerbate weight stigma. Accordingly, a simple interpretation of the results of both experiments is that the dominant public health messaging around the diet and exercise explanation for weight control and obesity exacerbates weight stigma, but the FAM explanation does not.

We found mixed support for the attribution value model of weight stigma [10]. Analysis of the FASI scores in Experiment 1 suggest that the difference in weight stigma scores between the FAM and diet and exercise conditions was due to changes in participants' attributions about the causes of obesity. However, we found no significant group difference on FASI scores in Experiment 2. Similarly, there was no group differences in participant beliefs about personal control of diet and exercise as a primary cause for obesity and weight control in Experiment 1 or 2. This finding is unexpected, as it was reasonable to predict a decrease in attributions of dieting and exercise as a causal explanation among participants who received the FAM explanation. It is possible that the FAM explanation resulted in less stigma because of a greater understanding of, and/or empathy for, those facing the challenges of weight management when one is addicted to food. As we did not assess constructs related to empathy, it will be important for future work to assess the relationship between perceptions of food addiction and levels of empathy towards people with obesity. It is apparent that those in the FAM condition did not dismiss the notion of diet and exercise as contributors to weight control and obesity. Participants may already have firmly established beliefs about personal control of weight given pervasive societal messages emphasizing this message. However, this possible pre-existing belief did not interfere with participants' abilities to receive and incorporate a different message about the contributors to obesity emphasized in the FAM perspective.

The perception that weight is determined by the individual's personal control of choices regarding dieting and exercise behaviours is widespread and accepted in society [37]. Belief in this dominant public health model for overweight and obesity is thought to be linked to weight stigma because it infers and/or attributes overweight and obesity to personal responsibility, lack of discipline, and laziness. The FAM explanation for obesity and weight control is garnering attention in several research fields [19,38,39] and is gaining traction in popular culture [40]. Indeed, studies suggest that around 15% of people meet criteria for a food addiction and anywhere from 28–52% of people believe they may be addicted to a food [22–24]. The present findings support suggestions that popular societal messages of blame and personal responsibility for weight may be partly responsible for the prevalence and rise of weight bias [1]. In contrast, an alternative explanation for obesity, the FAM explanation, may have a positive effect of reducing weight stigma. As our studies did not assess attitudes over time, it will be important for future work to examine whether changes in participants' causal attributions for obesity can be maintained following brief interventions or information about alternative contributors to obesity. It is likely that repeated exposure to FAM information and messages would be needed to sustain shifts in people's perspectives over time, especially in the face of continued and prominent societal messages emphasizing personal behaviours as the primary cause of obesity. Nevertheless, findings from both of our studies suggest that it is possible to shift weight stigma attitudes with a brief intervention emphasizing a FAM narrative for obesity.

Several limitations of this research should be noted. First, study participants were mostly young and female, with a majority who did not have overweight or obesity. Future studies should examine the FAM explanation in a more representative population sample, including those with diverse body sizes. Baseline data on weight stigma variables were not collected, which could otherwise have been included as potential covariates in the analyses. However, the decision not to collect baseline data on these variables was balanced against the importance of maintaining the study's deception, to avoid tipping off participants to the nature of the study and cuing them in the direction of socially desirable responding. Still, future studies could employ within-participant designs to examine potential changes in weight stigma across subjects upon exposure to the FAM model of weight. In addition, future research should explore the longer-term outcomes of public health messages, particularly those delivered in real-world settings.

5. Conclusions

The present study found lower weight stigma after exposure to a food addiction model of weight and greater weight stigma after exposure to a diet and exercise model of weight. While several studies have attempted to reduce weight stigma, with varying success, far more work is needed to address this prevalent and harmful societal problem. The improvement found in weight stigma following an addiction explanation, and the worsening of weight stigma following a diet and exercise explanation, has implications for public health messages about body weight and obesity. The results support the growing popularity of the food addiction model for eating and associated body weight and obesity. Increasing public understanding of the role of a food addiction explanation for eating behaviour and weight may help to alleviate weight stigma, including, potentially, internalised weight bias/self-stigma. At the same time, our research suggests that the current dominant public health message that largely attributes weight control and obesity to lack of personal control of, and responsibility for, diet and exercise needs to be changed as it appears to be supporting weight stigma [41]. Future research is needed to explore ways to modify current public health messaging so that it is not exacerbating weight stigma. Such messaging could describe the interplay between biological (e.g., FAM, genes) and/or environmental factors (e.g., food security, access to healthy and affordable foods, exercise-facilitating living and work environments) contributing to weight, as well as the importance of healthy eating and physical activity for all individuals, regardless of body size.

Author Contributions: Conceptualization: K.S.OB., A.C., J.D.R., J.D.L. data curation: K.S.OB., J.D.R., A.B.; formal analysis: K.S.OB., J.D.R.; project administration: K.S.OB., A.C., J.D.R.; supervision: K.S.OB., A.C.; writing—original draft: K.S.OB., J.D.L., Z.V., R.M.P., A.B.; writing—review and editing: K.S.OB., A.B., R.J., J.A.H., Z.V., D.S., D.L. All authors have read and agreed to the published version of the manuscript.

References

1. Andreyeva, T.; Puhl, R.M.; Brownell, K.D. Changes in perceived weight discrimination among Americans, 1995–1996 through 2004–2006. *Obesity* **2008**, *16*, 1129–1134. [CrossRef]
2. Latner, J.D.; Stunkard, A.J. Getting worse: The stigmatization of obese children. *Obes. Res.* **2003**, *11*, 452–456. [CrossRef]
3. Puhl, R.M.; Heuer, C.A. The stigma of obesity: A review and update. *Obesity* **2009**, *17*, 941–964. [CrossRef]
4. Nutter, S.; Ireland, A.; Alberga, A.S.; Brun, I.; Lefebvre, D.; Hayden, K.A.; Russell-Mayhew, S. Weight bias in educational settings: A systematic review. *Curr. Obes. Rep.* **2019**, *8*, 185–200. [CrossRef] [PubMed]
5. Phelan, S.M.; Burgess, D.J.; Yeazel, M.W.; Hellerstedt, W.L.; Griffin, J.M.; van Ryn, M. Impact of weight bias and stigma on quality of care and outcomes for patients with obesity. *Obes. Rev.* **2015**, *16*, 319–326. [CrossRef] [PubMed]

6. O'Brien, K.S.; Latner, J.D.; Ebneter, D.; Hunter, J.A. Obesity discrimination: The role of physical appearance, personal ideology, and anti-fat prejudice. *Int. J. Obes.* **2013**, *37*, 455–460. [CrossRef] [PubMed]
7. Papadopoulos, S.; Brennan, L. Correlates of weight stigma in adults with overweight and obesity: A systematic literature review. *Obesity* **2015**, *23*, 1743–1760. [CrossRef]
8. O'Brien, K.S.; Latner, J.D.; Puhl, R.M.; Vartanian, L.R.; Giles, C.; Griva, K.; Carter, A. The relationship between weight stigma and eating behavior is explained by weight bias internalization and psychological distress. *Appetite* **2016**, *102*, 70–76. [CrossRef]
9. Mensinger, J.L.; Tylka, T.L.; Calamari, M.E. Mechanisms underlying weight status and healthcare avoidance in women: A study of weight stigma, body-related shame and guilt, and healthcare stress. *Body Image* **2019**, *25*, 139–147. [CrossRef]
10. Crandall, C.S.; D'Anello, S.; Sakalli, N.; Lazarus, E.; Wieczorkowska, G.; Feather, N.T. An attribution-value model of prejudice: Anti-fat attitudes in six nations. *Pers. Soc. Psychol. Bull.* **2001**, *27*, 30–37. [CrossRef]
11. O'Brien, K.S.; Puhl, R.M.; Latner, J.D.; Mir, A.S.; Hunter, J.A. Reducing anti-fat prejudice in preservice health students: A randomized trial. *Obesity* **2010**, *18*, 2138–2144. [CrossRef]
12. Pearl, R.L.; Lebowitz, M.S. Beyond personal responsibility: Effects of causal attributions for overweight and obesity on weight-related beliefs, stigma, and policy support. *Psychol. Health* **2014**, *29*, 1176–1191. [CrossRef]
13. Barry, C.L.; Brescoll, V.L.; Brownell, K.D.; Schlesinger, M. Obesity metaphors: How beliefs about the causes of obesity affect support for public policy. *Milbank Q.* **2009**, *87*, 7–47. [CrossRef] [PubMed]
14. Barry, C.L.; Jarlenski, M.; Grob, R.; Schlesinger, M.; Gollust, S.E. News media framing of childhood obesity in the United States from 2000 to 2009. *Pediatrics* **2011**, *128*, 132–145. [CrossRef] [PubMed]
15. World Health Organisation Fact Sheet. Available online: https://www.who.int/news-room/fact-sheets/detail/obesity-and-overweight#targetText=In%202016%2C%20more%20than%201.9,women)%20were%20obese%20in%202016 (accessed on 28 July 2019).
16. Kleinert, S.; Horton, R. Obesity needs to be put into a much wider context. *Lancet* **2019**, *393*, 724–726. [CrossRef]
17. Danielsdottir, S.; O'Brien, K.S.; Ciao, A. Anti-fat prejudice reduction: A review of published studies. *Obes. Facts* **2010**, *3*, 47–58. [CrossRef]
18. Gearhardt, A.N.; Davis, C.; Kuschner, R.; Brownell, K.D. The addiction potential of hyperpalatable foods. *Curr. Drug Res. Rev.* **2011**, *4*, 140–145. [CrossRef]
19. Adams, R.C.; Sedgmond, J.; Maizey, L.; Chambers, C.D.; Lawrence, N.S. Food addiction: Implications for the diagnosis and treatment of overeating. *Nutrients* **2019**, *11*, 2086. [CrossRef]
20. Alonso-Alonso, M.; Woods, S.C.; Pelchat, M.; Grigson, P.S.; Stice, E.; Farooqi, S.; Khoo, C.S.; Mattes, R.D.; Beauchamp, G.K. Food reward system: Current perspectives and future research needs. *Nutr. Rev.* **2015**, *73*, 296–307. [CrossRef]
21. Volkow, N.D.; Wise, R.A.; Baler, R. The dopamine motive system: Implications for drug and food addiction. *Nat. Rev. Neurosci.* **2017**, *18*, 741–752. [CrossRef]
22. Gearhardt, A.N.; Corbin, W.R.; Brownell, K.D. Development of the yale food addiction scale version 2.0. *Psychol. Addict. Behav.* **2016**, *30*, 113–121. [CrossRef] [PubMed]
23. Meadows, A.; Nolan, L.J.; Higgs, S. Self-perceived food addiction: Prevalence, predictors, and prognosis. *Appetite* **2017**, *114*, 282–298. [CrossRef] [PubMed]
24. Latner, J.D.; Puhl, R.M.; Murakami, J.M.; O'Brien, K.S. Food addiction as a causal model of obesity. Effects on stigma, blame, and perceived psychopathology. *Appetite* **2014**, *77*, 79–84. [CrossRef] [PubMed]
25. Reid, J.; O'Brien, K.S.; Puhl, R.; Hardman, C.A.; Carter, A. Food addiction and its potential links with weight stigma. *Curr. Addict. Rep.* **2018**, *5*, 192–201. [CrossRef]
26. DePierre, J.D.; Puhl, R.M.; Luedicke, J. Public perceptions of food addiction: A comparison with alcohol and tobacco. *J. Subst. Use* **2013**, *19*, 1–6. [CrossRef]
27. DePierre, J.A.; Puhl, R.M.; Luedicke, J. A new stigmatized identity? Comparisons of a 'Food Addict' label with other stigmatized health conditions. *Basic Appl. Soc. Psych.* **2013**, *35*, 10–21. [CrossRef]
28. Eller, D. Are You Addicted to Food? *Prevention magazine*. Available online: http://www.prevention.com/ (accessed on 30 November 2011).
29. Micco, N. Addicted to Food? 5 Tips to Control Your Cravings. *The Huffington Post*. Available online: http://www.huffingtonpost.com/eatingwell/could-you-be-addicted-to-_b_828270.html (accessed on 27 February 2011).

30. Crandall, C.S. Prejudice against fat people: Ideology and selfinterest. *J. Pers. Soc. Psychol.* **1994**, *66*, 882–894. [CrossRef]
31. O'Brien, K.S.; Hunter, J.A.; Banks, M. Implicit anti-fat bias in physical educators: Physical attributes, ideology, and socialisation. *Int. J. Obes.* **2007**, *31*, 308–314. [CrossRef]
32. Lee, N.M.; Lucke, J.; Hall, W.D.; Meurk, C.; Boyle, F.M.; Carter, A. Public views on food addiction and obesity: Implications for policy and treatment. *PLoS ONE* **2013**, *8*, e74836. [CrossRef]
33. Stotland, S.; Zuroff, D.C. A new measure of weight locus of control: The dieting beliefs scale. *J. Pers. Assess.* **1990**, *54*, 191–203. [CrossRef]
34. Epstein, S.; Pacini, R.; Denes-Raj, V.; Heier, H. Individual differences in intuitive experiential and analytical-rational thinking styles. *J. Pers. Soc. Psychol.* **1996**, *71*, 390–405. [CrossRef] [PubMed]
35. O'Brien, K.S.; Latner, J.D.; Halberstadt, J.; Hunter, J.A.; Anderson, J.; Caputi, P. Do antifat attitudes predict antifat behaviors? *Obesity* **2008**, *16*, S87–S92. [CrossRef] [PubMed]
36. Templeton, G.F. A two-step approach for transforming continuous variables to normal: Implications and recommendations for IS research. *Commun. Assoc. Inf. Syst.* **2011**, *28*, 41–58. [CrossRef]
37. Brownell, K.D.; Kersh, R.; Ludwig, D.S.; Post, R.C.; Puhl, R.M.; Schwartz, M.B.; Willett, W.C. Personal responsibility and obesity: A constructive approach to a controversial issue. *Health Aff.* **2010**, *29*, 379–387. [CrossRef]
38. Davis, C.; Curtis, C.; Levitan, R.D.; Carter, J.C.; Kaplan, A.S.; Kennedy, J.L. Evidence that 'food addiction'is a valid phenotype of obesity. *Appetite* **2011**, *57*, 711–717. [CrossRef]
39. Schulte, E.M.; Joyner, M.A.; Potenza, M.N.; Grilo, C.M.; Gearhardt, A.N. Current considerations regarding food addiction. *Curr. Psychiatry Rep.* **2015**, *17*, 19. [CrossRef]
40. Almendrala, A. Food Addiction vs. Eating Addiction: Why A Single Word Makes All The Difference [Internet]. *HuffPost Australia*. 2014. Available online: https://www.huffingtonpost.com.au/2014/09/23/food-addiction-eating-addiction_n_5844712.html?guccounter=1 (accessed on 23 November 2015).
41. Puhl, R.M.; Latner, J.D.; O'Brien, K.; Luedicke, J.; Forhan, M.; Danielsdottir, S. Cross-national perspectives about weight-based bullying in youth: Nature, extent and remedies. *Pediatr. Obes.* **2015**, *11*, 241–250. [CrossRef]

3

Outcomes of an Accelerated Inpatient Refeeding Protocol in 103 Extremely Underweight Adults with Anorexia Nervosa at a Specialized Clinic in Prien, Germany

Thorsten Koerner [1], Verena Haas [2], Julia Heese [1], Matislava Karacic [1], Elmar Ngo [1], Christoph U. Correll [2,3,4], Ulrich Voderholzer [1,5,*] and Ulrich Cuntz [1,6]

1 Schön Clinic Roseneck; Am Roseneck 6, 83209 Prien am Chiemsee, Germany; thkoerner@schoen-klinik.de (T.K.); jheese@schoen-klinik.de (J.H.); mkaracic@schoen-klinik.de (M.K.); engo@schoen-klinik.de (E.N.); UCuntz@schoen-klinik.de (U.C.)

2 Clinic for Psychiatry, Psychosomatics and Psychotherapy of childhood and adolescence, Charité – University Berlin, corporate member of Free University Berlin, Humboldt-University Berlin, and Berlin Institute of Health, 13353 Berlin, Germany; verena.haas@charite.de (V.H.); christoph.correll@charite.de (C.U.C.)

3 Department of Psychiatry and Molecular medicine, Donald and Barbara Zucker School of Medicine at Hofstra/Northwell, Hempstead, NY 11549, USA

4 Department of Psychiatry, the Zucker Hillside Hospital, Glen Oaks, NY 11004, USA

5 Department of Psychiatry and Psychotherapy, Ludwig-Maximilians-Universität München (LMU), 80336 München, Germany

6 Research program for the evaluation of psychotherapy in complex therapeutic settings, PMU Paracelsus Medical University Salzburg, 5020 Salzburg, Austria

* Correspondence: uvoderholzer@schoen-klinik.de

Abstract: Background: In mildly to moderately malnourished adolescent patients with anorexia nervosa (AN), accelerated refeeding protocols using higher initial calory supply coupled with phosphate supplements were not associated with a higher incidence of refeeding syndrome (RS). It is unclear whether this is also a feasible approach for extremely malnourished, adult AN patients. Methods: Outcomes of a clinical refeeding protocol involving a targeted initial intake of ≥2000 kcal/day, routine supplementation of phosphate and thiamine as well as close medical monitoring, were evaluated. A retrospective chart review including AN patients with a body mass index (BMI) <13 kg/m^2 was conducted, to describe changes in weight, BMI, and laboratory parameters (phosphate, creatine kinase, hematocrit, sodium, liver enzymes, and blood count) over four weeks. Results: In 103 female patients (age, mean ± standard deviation (SD) = 23.8 ± 5.3 years), BMI between admission and follow-up increased from 11.5 ± 0.9 to 13.1 ± 1.1 kg/m^2 and total weight gain within the first four weeks was 4.2 ± 2.0 kg (mean, SD). Laboratory parameter monitoring indicated no case of RS, but continuous normalization of blood parameters. Conclusions: Combined with close medical monitoring and electrolyte supplementation, accelerated refeeding may also be applied to achieve medical stabilization in extremely underweight adults with AN without increasing the risk of RS.

Keywords: anorexia nervosa; caloric intake; refeeding syndrome; refeeding protocol

---

1. Introduction: Refeeding and Refeeding Syndrome

Refeeding syndrome (RS) is a sudden, threatening deterioration in the general physical condition of a cachectic patient undergoing refeeding, especially in the first two to three weeks of refeeding following a prolonged period of hunger. RS has been scientifically described, among other conditions, in prisoners of war after the Second World War [1,2] and later in the refeeding of predominantly older underweight patients and patients with tumor cachexia [3,4]. Characteristic features of RS are fluid shifts and electrolyte fluctuations, which can occur as a result of endocrine and metabolic changes resulting from the onset of refeeding. At the center of RS are hypophosphatemia, hyponatremia, disturbed glucose metabolism, and insufficient thiamine supply [5]. Drastic malnutrition is associated with depleted intracellular phosphate stores. Initially, refeeding causes a change from a catabolic to anabolic metabolism, and concomitant hyperparathyroidism may contribute to the development of hypophosphatemia [6]. This process can lead to a critical drop in the intracellular concentration of adenosine triphosphate (ATP) and thus in the energy supply of the cells [7]. Clinical consequences range from severe organ dysfunction and rhabdomyolysis to seizures, delirium, coma, and death. The definition of RS is not clear-cut, and so there are no clear prevalence figures for RS in patients with anorexia nervosa (AN). In adult AN patients, the incidence of hypophosphatemia during refeeding is reported to range from 0%–80% [8,9]. Appropriate control of energy intake, as well as monitoring and adequate supplementation of electrolytes, are essential in the early stages of refeeding to avoid complications [10].

Due to the fear of serious medical complications related to RS, "start low, go slow" approaches (e.g., starting at 1200 kcal/d and increasing by 200 calories every other day) have been practiced for a long time in the refeeding of patients with AN. In practice, this approach leads initially to a hypocaloric diet and the maintenance of severe energy deficiency and to additional weight loss, which, in some cases, can lead to pronounced hypoglycemia with subsequent organ damage, as well as to longer hospital stays. In adolescent patients with AN, higher initial weight gain has been linked with a higher likelihood of remission by the end of treatment [11].

There is currently no consensus regarding the adequate initial energy supply during the refeeding of AN patients, which leads to inconsistent procedures. A scientific basis for the very restrictive dietary guidelines for the initial caloric intake in severely underweight adult patients is still missing, and presumably, the initial BMI [12] or the expression of cachexia is a predictor of RS [13]. Study protocols, in which an initially higher caloric intake was compared with a low-caloric diet [14] or with high energy intake in the first week and a gradual reduction of energy supply [15], showed no difference in the occurrence of components of RS, but larger and faster weight gain with the higher-caloric refeeding approach. In addition, a review of 22 studies by Garber et al. [16] showed that in mildly to moderately malnourished AN patients a low initial energy intake was too conservative and that higher initial energy levels were not associated with an increased risk of RS, as long as electrolytes, water balance, and cardiovascular parameters were closely monitored and controlled; however, most studies included in the review were conducted in adolescents. For extremely underweight adult patients, there are currently only a few studies examining higher caloric refeeding, and therefore no commonly accepted, reliable recommendations regarding the value and safety of accelerated refeeding strategies exist. In a recent study on 119 adults with AN, higher initial caloric refeeding (i.e., 1500 instead of 1000 kcal/d) was described to provide additional nourishment, to medically stabilize patients, and to prevent RS [17]. The authors concluded that future research is needed to examine whether higher-calorie intakes (i.e., 2000 kcal/d), similar to those studied in adolescent patients, may also be beneficial to treat adult patients.

This retrospective study aimed to describe (i) a clinical, high-caloric refeeding protocol established in a specialist ward of a psychosomatic clinic, targeting an initial intake of 2000 kcal/d and the accompanying essential medical measures; (ii) the outcomes of this approach regarding changes in weight and selected blood parameters to reflect physiological status and risk of RS.

2. Methods

2.1. Design and Population

The 24-bed ward featured in this study admitted patients with a diagnosis of anorexia nervosa who are at least 18 years old and who, due to their underweight, excessive exercising and/or vomiting and/or medical complications, require intensive medical and therapeutic surveillance.

For this retrospective chart review, patient data from all consecutive admissions were included if they fulfilled the following inclusion criteria:

- Age > 18 years; no upper age limit was defined as an inclusion criterion.
- Treated at a 24-bed unit for extremely underweight patients with 6 surveillance beds at Schön Klinik Roseneck, Rosenheim, Germany, between 1/1/2016 and 12/31/2018 (oral nutrition, no forced feeding or medication, no tube feeding, and all meals accompanied).
- Main diagnosis of AN (restrictive, active, and atypical AN).
- BMI ≤ 13 kg/m^2.
- Retention period of ≥28 days, as RS and related phenomena, are expected in this time window.
- Availability of laboratory data: five measurements from the time of admission until day 28.

Exclusion criteria were age <18 years, treatment at the institution outside of the time window, a BMI > 13 kg/m^2, and other eating disorder diagnoses, such as bulimia nervosa and binge eating disorders.

2.2. *Ethical Approval*

All procedures performed in studies involving human participants were in accordance with the ethical standards of the institutional review board of the Ludwig Maximilian Universität (LMU) Munich and with the 1964 Helsinki declaration and its later amendments or comparable ethical standards. According to the guidelines by the institutional review board of the LMU Munich, retrospective studies conducted on already available, anonymized data are exempt from requiring ethics approval.

2.3. *Routine, Clinical Management of Meals, and Refeeding*

All patients received three meals with an average total energy content of 2000 kcal per day from day 1 after admission to the ward, divided into three main meals with a choice between vegetarian and non-vegetarian menus. The caloric intake was adjusted and increased according to weight development to aim for an increase in body weight of 700–1000 g/week. The criterion for sufficient food intake was weight gain, which should be at least 100 g per day. If the agreed amount of food intake for weight gain could not be achieved, the portion size of one or more main meals was increased, and up to three snacks between meals were added. In addition, liquid food was offered to substitute for energy losses in case a part of the meals could not be eaten. All meals were therapeutically accompanied by a nurse or therapist in a 1:6 group supervision. Patient adherence to dietary intake was supported through daily therapeutic contacts and medical rounds. Patients ate their meals in a stable group setting and supported each other. Peer pressure may play an important role. In weekly eating protocol sessions, patients reviewed their progress and committed to new goals related to food avoidance, fears, and counteractive behavior. Patients did not receive nasogastric feeding since the normalization of eating behavior is a common therapeutic goal. All patients were prescribed 2000 kcal/d (three meals) starting from the day of admission. The average caloric value (data provided by the caterer and controlled in samples) for the non-vegetarian menu was 743, 717, and 704 (total 2164) kcal for breakfast, lunch, and dinner; and 743, 737, and 683 (total: 2162) for the vegetarian option. If patients did not finish their meal (50%–99% eaten) they were asked to drink 1 supplemental drink (400 kcal, Fresubin 200 mL with 2 kcal/mL). If patients ate less than 50% of their respective meal, they were asked to replace the missed-out calories by drinking 2 supplemental drinks (2 × 400 kcal). The group setting and the support from experienced therapists were considered essential for compliance with dietary adherence. Contingency measures were often necessary to regulate excessive exercising and slow weight gain. During the first 28 days, it was rare that patients required more than 2000 kcal/d but many patients received liquid food to replace unfinished meals. Patients reduced their calorie consumption by limiting their physical activity. Contingency contracts and video surveillance with 24/7 nursing staff presence as well as very moderate exercise therapy play an important role in normalizing movement behavior.

During the first 4 weeks, which was the observation period in this study, most patients gained sufficient weight with 2000 kcal/d spread over three meals. This was supported by restricting their physical activity and exercising. In individual cases, an energy intake of more than 4000 kcal was necessary to ensure sufficient weight gain. All patients participated in an intensive therapeutic program adapted to the special needs of the severely underweight women and suitable for therapeutically addressing the considerable anxieties and resistance associated with weight gain. This included daily individual cognitive behavioral therapy (CBT) sessions and medical rounds, accompanied meals, participation in group therapy (twice weekly problem-solving group, Cognitive Remediation Therapy (CRT), and art therapy, and daily morning and evening rounds with the nursing staff).

Daily documentation occurred for clinical and therapeutic observations and nursing contacts as well as weight measurement and comments on the accompanied meals. Physical examination including neurological assessment and vital signs was a standard procedure at admission and brief daily medical check during rounds. The SUSS (Sit up, squat, stand) test, as specified by the British Royal College of Psychiatrists MARSIPAN (Management of Really Sick Patients with AN) workgroup, assessed physical performance. It was used at admission and during rounds to follow up on physical performance. Patients used wheelchairs during the first weeks on the ward if their weight is below 13 kg/m^2. A normal result of the SUSS test plus a BMI of 13 kg/m^2 and above show that a wheelchair was no longer necessary.

As part of the routine refeeding protocol: weight was monitored daily in underwear (Scale: Seca Model Nr. 6357021004). Height was measured at admission. Blood work was performed at least once a week including blood count (without white blood cell differential), electrolytes (sodium, potassium, phosphate, and chloride), transaminases, gamma-glutamyl-transferase (γ-GT), creatine kinase, creatinine, and urea. Further investigations included continuous monitoring of vital signs (electrocardiogram (ECG), heart rate, and blood pressure), hematocrit (<25%) and weight progression, routine clinical examination including neurological assessment and vital signs, SUSS test, sonography, and bioelectrical impedance analysis to assess edema status. Phosphate (612 mg to 1224 mg/d) and thiamine (200 mg/d) were supplemented routinely for two weeks and phosphate thereafter if needed. In some patients, the administration of diuretics was necessary at times when either the severity of the edema was subjectively too stressful or the heart rate per minute exceeded the systolic blood pressure in mmHg.

2.4. Data Assessment

The American Society of Parental and Enteral Nutrition developed consensus guidelines for the following diagnostic criteria for RS [18]: (i) a decrease of serum phosphorus, potassium, and/or magnesium levels by 10%–20% (mild RS), 20%–30% (moderate RS), or >30% and/or organ dysfunction resulting from a decrease in any of these and/or due to thiamin deficiency (severe RS) (ii) and occurring within 5 days of reinitiating or substantially increasing energy provision. These ASPEN criteria did not appear suitable to us for assessing the risk of the patients we treat in our unit: phosphate and thiamine were routinely supplemented and it was therefore unlikely that such a deficiency will occur in the context of malnutrition. Potassium was controlled even more closely (possibly several times a day), because of the risk of cardiac arrhythmia. If a drop in serum potassium occurred, potassium, as well as magnesium, were supplemented. In this respect, we chose not to adhere to these guidelines, and to report on a broad range of blood parameters to cover as many of the risks associated with re-nutrition as it was possible using our retrospective data from routine treatment.

The following criteria were used to define a case of RS:

- Critical deterioration of the general condition (e.g., severe edema, pericardial effusion, and weakness).
- Critical drop of serum phosphate to values <0.75 mmol/L.
- Increase in creatine kinase to >1000 U/L.
- Decrease of hematocrit to <25%.

- Decrease of serum sodium to <125 mmol/L.
- For the assessment of the clinical condition, the following laboratory parameters were also used:
    - Aspartate aminotransferase (GOT) (>35 U/L) and alanine aminotransferase (GPT) (>35 U/L) for estimation of liver cell damage.
    - Leukocytes (<3.98 G/L), hemoglobin (<11.2 g/L), and thrombocytes (<182 G/L) for the assessment of bone marrow function.

The following data were collected on admission and weekly thereafter for 4 weeks in clinical care and are presented in this study: body weight, height, BMI, and blood work (creatin kinase, phosphate, sodium, GOT, GPT, leucocytes, hematocrit, hemoglobin, and thrombocytes).

The following cut-off values were used to define pathological blood values: creatin kinase, >170 U/L; phosphate, <0.75 mmol/L; sodium, <12 mmol/L; GOT, GPT >35 U/L; leucocytes, <3.98 G/L, hemoglobin, <25%; thrombocytes, <182 G/L.

2.5. Statistical Analysis

All data were examined with the Shapiro–Wilk test for normal distribution and presented as mean ± standard deviation (normally distributed data) or as median and 25th/75th percentile (non-normally distributed data). For the change of BMI, weight, laboratory values over time, a paired samples t-test (for normally distributed differences), or a non-parametric, related samples Wilcoxon test (difference not normally distributed) was chosen. To assess how pathological laboratory values developed over time, the change in the percentage of pathological values in the total sample was treated as a categorical variable (pathological: y/n) and examined at the beginning and after 4 weeks using the two-sided Fisher's Exact Test (https://www.graphpad.com/quickcalcs/contingency1.cfm). The Fisher's Exact Test (Fisher–Yates test, exact chi-square test) is a significant test for independence in contingency tables. In contrast to the Chi-square independence test, however, it does not impose any requirements on the sample size and provides reliable results even with a small number of observations per cell.

A two-sided p-value <0.05 was considered statistically significant. Statistical analyses were performed by using SPSS version 21.0 for Windows (IBM Corp., Armonk, NY, USA).

3. Results

Between 01/01/2016 and 12/31/2018, 335 patients were admitted to the 24-bed unit for extremely underweight patients at Schön Klinik Roseneck in Rosenheim, Germany within a 120-bed hospital for psychosomatic medicine and psychotherapy. Of these 335 patients, 181 had a main diagnosis of AN, and 161 had a BMI <13 kg/m^2 as well as a length of stay ≥28 days, with 43 of these (27.3%) discontinuing therapy in the first four weeks. None of these 43 patients had refeeding syndrome. A total of 103 patients with a BMI <13 kg/m^2, a stay of ≥4 weeks, and available laboratory data per the inclusion criteria were included in this study. These 103 patients had complete data sets, i.e., the laboratory values were available weekly (+− 2 days) for all measurement times. Most of the patients with incomplete data sets were discharged or transferred before the end of the 28 days, mostly due to lack of motivation—in none of these cases was a transfer necessary due to critical deterioration of the general condition. All participants were female and aged 23.8 ± 5.3 (range = 18–47) years. No males in the weight range <13 kg/m^2 were admitted in the observation period.

The weekly change in weight and BMI is shown in Table 1. The weight of the female patients increased during four weeks by an average of 1.0 ± 0.5 kg/week, and by a total of 4.2 ± 2.0 kg over four weeks (mean, SD). This weight change corresponds to a total increase of 1.6 ± 0.8 BMI units in four weeks (p = 0.001). None of the patients experienced a critical deterioration of their physical condition, and all patients improved their performance level with weight gain (sit up, squat, stand (SUSS) test score as specified by the MARSIPAN workgroup (32).

Table 1. Weekly change in weight and body mass index.

	Weight	BMI		Weight	BMI
Week 1	31.5 ± 3.6 (23.5–40.1)	11.5 ± 0.9 (9.5–13.0)	Week 1–2	1.3 (0.6/3.0) *** (−2.2–8.4)	0.5 (0.2/1.1) *** (−0.8–3.4)
Week 2	33.4 ± 3.7 (24.0–41.5)	12.3 ± 1.1 (9.7–15.2)	Week 2–3	0.8 ± 0.9 *** (−1.2–3.4)	0.3 (0.1/0.5) *** (−0.5–1.4)
Week 3	34.2 ± 3.6 (26.0–41.5)	12.6 ± 1.1 (9.8–15.9)	Week 3–4	0.7 ± 0.7 *** (−0.8–2.8)	0.2 (0.1/0.4) *** (−0.4–1.2)
Week 4	35.0 ± 3.5 (26.5–42.0)	12.8 ± 1.1 (10.0–16.1)	Week 4–5	0.8 (0.4/1.1) *** (−1.4–1.9)	0.3 (0.1/0.5) *** (−0.5–0.8)
Week 5	35.7 ± 3.4 (27.8–43.9)	13.1 ± 1.1 (10.0–16.9)	Week 1–5	4.0 (2.9 / 5.0) *** (−2.5–9.7)	1.4 (1.1/1.9) *** (−0.8–4.1)

***, $p < 0.001$; t-test for normally distributed data are presented as mean (SD), and for non-normally distributed data as median (25/75 percentile) using a Wilcoxon test. change; BMI: body mass index; data in parenthesis are ranges.

The weight gain was highest in the first week with an average of 1.9 ± 2.0 kg, leveling off to 0.7–0.8 kg/week in the following three weeks. The maximum increase observed in the first week was 8.4 kg, which was mostly due to rehydration (traceable by hematocrit decrease). In 20 patients (19%), the weekly weight gain in the first week was between 0.1 and 0.6 kg, in 13 (13%) between 0.7 and 1.0 kg, in 22 (21%) between 1.1 and 2.0 kg, in 24 (23%) between 2.1 and 4.0 kg, and in 13 (13%) >4.0 kg. In 11 patients (11%) a weight stagnation or weight loss was recorded in the first week, and this group had a mean weight loss of 0.7 kg (max. 2.2 kg to min. 0 kg).

All patients received 200 mg thiamine daily for the first four weeks and 612–1024 mg phosphate daily for the first two weeks. With this supplementation, serum phosphate levels increased during the observation period (Table 2, Figure 1). On admission, 7 (6.2%) of the 103 subjects had hypophosphatemia with values <0.75 mmol/L, and one subject had a critical value <0.5 mmol/L. After one week, only five patients had slightly decreased serum phosphate levels (<0.75 mmol/L) and after two weeks only three patients.

The decrease in the mean creatine kinase values during the observation period of the first four weeks of treatment clearly shows that the increase in energy intake and the consecutive significant weight gain right at the beginning of treatment was not associated with an increased risk of rhabdomyolysis (Table 2, Figure 1). Strongly elevated values for creatine kinase (>1000 U/L) were only observed in one patient at intake with 9941 U/L, which completely normalized within fourteen days with adequate nutrition and phosphate substitution.

While critical hyponatremia with values <125 mmol/L also occurred only on admission in one patient, the initially already low average value for hematocrit fell from 37% to 35% after fourteen days, and then slowly rose again to 36% after four weeks. Accordingly, up to three (different) patients with their hematocrit fell below the critical value of 25% at the first three measurement points. After four weeks, the values in two patients were still below the critical value. In parallel to the increase in weight, the transaminases, which were strongly elevated at admission, decreased significantly. Further, 54 (51.9%) of the patients had elevated GOT and 62 patients (59.6%) had elevated GPT > 35 U/L at admission, only 12 patients (11.5%) still had elevated values of GOT after four weeks, and the number of pathological values for GPT did not change on average during the four weeks being still $n = 61$ (59.2%).

Similarly, the rapid refeeding led to a highly significant increase in thrombocytes and leukocytes (Figure 1, Table 2), while the hemoglobin, in parallel to the hematocrit, dropped from an initial average of 12.5 ± 1.76 g/dL to 11.5 ± 1.69 g/dL in the third week, and stabilized at 11.6 ± 1.5 g/dL by week 4.

Table 2. Laboratory values at admission (T1) and after four weeks (T5), Mean and SD for 103 pt.

	CK	Phos	Sodium	GOT	GPT	Leuco	Haematocrit	Hb	Pla
cut off	>170 U/L	<0.75 mmol/L	<125 mmol/L	>35 U/L	>35 U/L	<3.98 G/L	<25 %	<11.2 g/L	<182 G/L
At admission	222 ± 974 (27–9941)	1.15 ± 0.29 (0.46–1.92)	138.7 ± 4.7 (112.0–152.0)	67.9 ± 117.8 (15.3–1078.0)	85.6 ± 121.9 (8.3–742.0)	4.1 ± 1.8 (1.1–14.0)	37.0 ± 5.0 (22.9–44.7)	12.5 ± 1.8 (7.5–15.6)	242 ± 81 (45–494)
After four weeks	75 ± 54 *** (22–374)	1.34 ± 0.18 *** (0.94–1.88)	141.3 ± 2.7 *** (133.0–148.0)	25.9 ± 8.0 *** (12.7–53.0)	42.3 ± 21.6 *** (10.7–133.0)	4.8 ± 1.8 *** (1.6–12.8)	36.1 4.2 ** (23.0–42.0)	11.6 ± 1.5 *** (6.6–14.3)	300 ± 92 *** (185–849)
pathologic at admission	19 (103) 18.4%	7 (103) 6.8%	7 (103) 6.8%	54 (103) 52.4%	62 (103) 60.2%	54 (103) 52.4%	23 (103) 22.3%	21 (103) 20.4%	21 (103) (20.4%)
pathologic after four weeks	6 (103) 5.8% *	0 (103) 0% *	0 (103) 0% *	12 (103) 11.7% ***	61 (103) 59.2%	37 (101) 36.6% *	22 (101) 21.8%	36 (101) 35.6% *	0 (101) (0%) ***

The T-test was used for normally distributed differences in blood values between two measurement points. A Wilcoxon test was used for non-normally distributed differences. For the percentage change in the proportion of pathological blood values, the two-sided Fischer's exact test was used * $p < 0.05$; ** $p < 0.01$;***. $p < 0.001$; data in parenthesis are ranges. Abbreviations: CK: creatine kinase; Phos: inorganic phosphate; GOT: aspartate aminotransferase; GPT: alanine aminotransferase; Leuco: leukocytes; Hb: hemoglobin; Pla: platelets; SD, standard deviation.

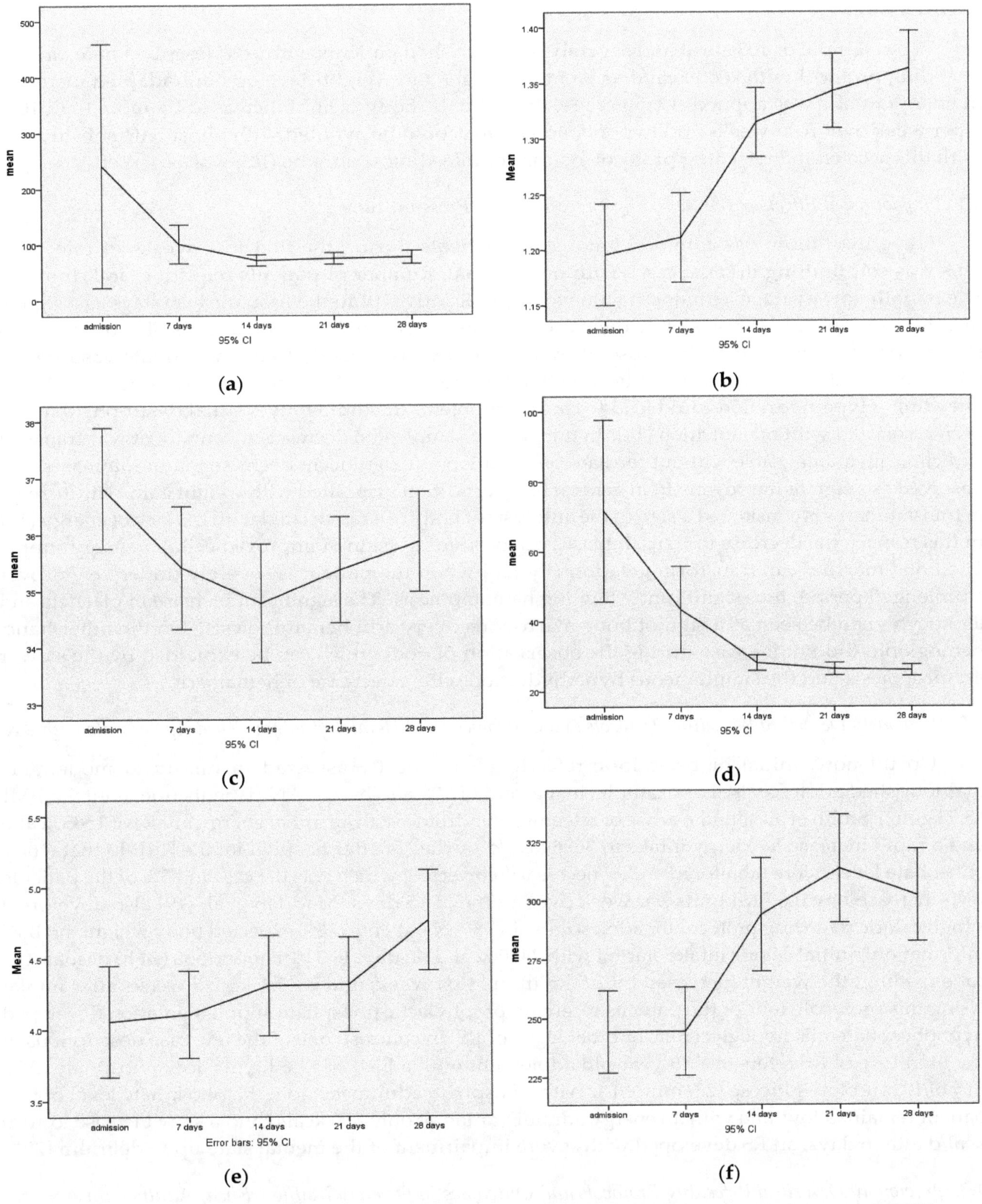

Figure 1. The course of creatine kinase (CK), inorganic phosphate (Phos) × 100, hematocrit (HK), and aspartate aminotransferase (GOT) leukocytes and platelets over four weeks with F-values of the measurement repeatability analysis. T1 to T5 (T1 intake, followed by weekly intervals of the laboratory survey). (**a**) Creatin kinase (F 2,3 df 4, *p* 0.056.); (**b**) Phosphate (F 23,9, df 4, *p* 0.000); (**c**) Hematocrit (F 12,3 df 4, *p* 0.000); (**d**) GOT (F 13,8 df 4, *p* 0.000); (**e**) Leucocytes (F 8,9, df 4, *p* 0.000); (**f**) Platelets (F 19,8, df 4 *p* 0.000.). T1, admission; T5, 28 days after admission.

4. Discussion

In the sample of 103 adult and severely malnourished patients with AN described here, an oral refeeding protocol with 2000 kcal/d as an initial target and weight-development-adapted increases in energy intake was applied. On average, the patients' body weight increased by more than 1040 g per week over four weeks and hypophosphatemia could be avoided with phosphate substitution. With this accelerated refeeding protocol, no case of refeeding syndrome (RS) was observed.

4.1. *Physiological Effects of the Refeeding Protocol in the Present Study*

Hyperhydration was common among the patients during the first four weeks of refeeding. This was self-limiting in most cases with only a small number of patients requiring oral diuretics. The initially low average hematocrit value fell significantly within the first fourteen days as a sign of hyperhydration, only to rise slowly thereafter; however, sodium levels remained stable or increased slightly on average, so that the cause of hyperhydration is unlikely to be inadequate vasopressin release or polydipsia. There is no indication that the drop in hematocrit could be avoided with slower refeeding. Hyperhydration could lead to cardiac problems, including myocardial dystrophy that has been associated with malnutrition [14]. In the present sample, the decrease in hematocrit was transient and clinically manageable without cardiac complications. A significant decrease in transaminases was observed as a sign of improvement in general body condition associated with weight gain. The increase in transaminases is considered a sign of the autolysis of body cells associated with the lack of energy [19]. In this respect, the decrease in transaminases can be seen as a sign of improved cellular energy supply. The bone marrow can transform gelatinously [20] when the patient is severely underweight over a prolonged period, thus significantly limiting hematopoiesis. The significant increase in platelets and leukocytes can be seen as a sign of bone marrow recovery and hematopoiesis. On the other hand, hemoglobin did not increase during the observation period, which can be explained by the slower erythropoiesis and the simultaneous hyperhydration with a decrease of hematocrit.

4.2. *Previously Described Refeeding Protocols and Outcomes in Moderately Malnourished Adolescents with AN*

Up till now, initial higher-caloric refeeding was mostly assessed in mildly to moderately malnourished adolescents. For example, in a group of 129 adolescent AN patients (mean intake BMI: 15.9 kg/m^2), Smith et al. found no case of refeeding syndrome with an initial energy intake of 1585 kcal/d and a rapid increase in energy intake to 3626 kcal/d by day 14 after hospital intake [14]. In that study, phosphate levels were monitored and, if necessary, corrected, which was the case in 75% of the patients. BMI increased by 0.6 BMI units per week over a time of 15 days. Madden et al. [19] also developed a high caloric refeeding protocol for adolescents: in 78 AN patients (78% expected body weight, no BMI information), initial caloric intake started with 2400 kcal/d on days 0–3 by continuous (24 h) nasogastric tube feeding, the weight increased by 2.5 kg in the first week, and by 5.1 kg 2.5 weeks after intake. Using this protocol, none of the patients receiving prophylactic phosphate supplementation developed hypophosphatemia, hypoglycemia, or other signs of RS. In contrast, one of the few case descriptions in the literature of RS refers to a 15-year-old adolescent with a BMI of 11.6 kg/m^2, low phosphate (0.78 mmol/L), and low glucose (2.6 mmol/L). With phosphate administration, the phosphate level of this patient remained low, and with an energy administration of only 800 kcal/d and a slow increase to 1000 kcal/d after 6 days, an RS developed with severe impairment of the mental state up to delirium [20].

4.3. *Previously Described Refeeding Protocols and Outcomes in Severely Malnourished, Adults with AN*

Gaudiani et al. [9] prescribed 990 kcal/d at the beginning with an increase to 2000 kcal/d after 19 days in 25 adults with AN (mean BMI at admission 13.1 kg/m^2), resulting in a BMI increase of 0.5 BMI units per week over a time of 19 days. Hypoglycemia occurred in 44% of patients, 76% showed abnormal liver function, 45% developed hypophosphatemia, and 92% developed hypothermia [9]. The observed complications by Gaudiani may have been due to initial low caloric intake (hypoglycemia and consecutive liver dysfunction) and less proactive phosphate substitution (hypophosphatemia). Hofer et al. [21] reported on 65 adults with AN (mean BMI at intake 13.7 kg/m^2) who were refed at 437 kcal/d with an initial increase to 1506 kcal/d, leading to an increase of 0.3 BMI units per week over a time of three weeks. This strategy was associated with severe hypokalemia in two patients, but no patient developed hypophosphatemia (due to phosphate supplementation). In 10.5% of patients, the following medical complications occurred: pretibial edema (n = 4), organ dysfunction as mild and transient pancreatitis, transient stage 2 renal failure, and urinary tract infection (n = 3). In two patients with already existing heart failure at admission with an echocardiographic ejection fraction of 40%, the malnutrition increased the severity of the existing disease. In a recent retrospective, observational study by Matthews et al. with 119 adult AN patients, higher caloric refeeding (group 1: baseline BMI of 17.2 kg/m^2 and intake of 1500 kcal/d vs. group 2: baseline BMI of 14.9 kg/m^2 and intake of 1000 kcal/d) along with close medical monitoring stabilized the patients and prevented RS. Our findings are in line with these results, and firstly, extend to an even more malnourished group of patients and second, to higher initial caloric intake.

4.4. Relevance of the Findings with Respect to Current Guideline Recommendations

Given these data, it is important to question the recommendations of the current guidelines for the management of AN. The German S3 guideline refers to the U.S.–American studies in adolescents, which recommend faster re-nutrition, but with the remark that at the time of the guideline update no comparable studies from the German-speaking countries and in adults were available. Other guidelines, however, seem to be based on older studies in which the paradigm shift towards faster refeeding had not yet become apparent. For example, the current guidelines for adults with AN (Table 3) recommend a consistently low energy intake, which does not allow for adequate weight gain.

Table 3. Current, national refeeding guidelines for malnourished patients with anorexia nervosa.

Guidelines	Age	Recommended Energy Intake
Australia and New Zealand	adult	1400 kcal/d [22]
Europe [23]	adult	start at 10, slowly increase to 15 kcal/kg/d (Day 1–3)
United Kingdom: Royal College of Psychiatrists [24]	adult	10–20 kcal/kg/d
United Kingdom: MARSIPAN [25]	adult	5–20 kcal/kg/d
American Psychiatric Association/American Dietetic Association [26]	adult	30–40 kcal/kg/d (1000–1600 kcal/d)
United Kingdom: Junior MARSIPAN [27]	<18 years	20 kcal/kg/d

Recent data implies that combined with close medical monitoring, a more accelerated approach appears to be safe, minimize complications, prevent mortality, and to reduce the length of stay in hospitals for patients with AN; however, as long as there is still not sufficient evidence-based data to support a new, general recommendation for severely malnourished, adult patients, nutritional rehabilitation must remain tailored to the individual patient.

There is still a need for systematic research to finally answer the question, which initial refeeding strategy for managing severe malnutrition should be the first-line treatment for AN patients. Further studies are needed that allow a detailed analysis of energy intake, weight change, and any associated complications. The approach presented in the current analysis appears promising and, to our knowledge, unique in this form in adults concerning faster and at the same time safe refeeding.

The strength of the present study is the large sample size and the uniform medical and therapeutic care under the largely standardized medication and diagnostics. One of the methodological limitations is that this is not a randomized patient selection, but a naturalistic setting in a single clinic. A randomized controlled trial (RCT) comparing "slow or regular" versus "fast" refeeding would be the next step to provide evidence for changing refeeding guidelines. We analyzed data from a consecutive cohort of extremely underweight patients. For such patients, inclusion in an RCT might be problematic for ethical reasons. With the chosen procedure, there was no evidence of critical deterioration of the physical condition, on the contrary, a consolidation of critical health status due to the rapid increase in weight was observed. Another limitation of the study is that the individual energy intake of the patients as well as adherence to the dietary recommendations and frequency of contingency measures were not objectively recorded and could only be given with a description of the general refeeding protocol that was as accurate as possible. On the other hand, an exact and objective recording of the energy intake of patients with AN is difficult to achieve, even under controlled conditions, and the comparatively high and rapid initial weight gain proves that correspondingly high energy intake must have taken place. Even though low blood glucose levels and thus hypoglycemia have been reported during refeeding in patients with AN, data on blood glucose levels is not included in the manuscript. To our experience hypoglycemia does not occur if the patients are sufficiently nourished, however, we cannot be sure that there were periods of hypoglycemia in the patient cohort described in our study.

Key messages:

(1) There are few evidence-based high caloric refeeding protocols for severely malnourished adult AN patients.
(2) In the present study, a rapid initial weight restoration strategy targeting oral energy intake of 2000 kcal/d from day one of treatment resulted in an average weight gain of 1040 g/week over four weeks. Combined with close medical monitoring and supplementation of phosphate and thiamine, this accelerated refeeding strategy was not associated with refeeding complications in severely malnourished adult AN patients.
(3) To derive safe and commonly accepted guidelines, further and prospective studies comparing different refeeding regimes are required.
(4) Following previous recommendations [18], the findings of the present study do not constitute medical advice. While the acknowledgment of the accelerated refeeding protocol presented in this study may assist in rethinking models of nutritional management of adult, severely malnourished AN patients, the judgment of the treating professional about the choice of an adequate refeeding strategy for an individual patient should prevail.

5. Conclusions

In summary, data from this naturalistic study indicate that the rapid refeeding strategy described here was effective and safe and that RS was not a consequence of more rapid refeeding. Future studies should further assess the efficacy and safety of rapid refeeding protocols in adults with AN who are severely underweight.

Author Contributions: Conceptualization: U.C., T.K., and U.V.; methodology: U.C. and V.H.; validation: V.H.; formal analysis, U.C., J.H., M.K.; Investigation, U.C., U.V., T.K., J.H., M.K., and E.N.; resources: U.C., and U.V.; data curation, U.C., J.H., and M.K.; writing—original draft preparation, T.K., U.C., V.H., and E.N.; writing—review and editing, U.V., V.H., C.U.C., and T.K.; visualization, U.C.; supervision, U.C. and U.V.; project administration: T.K. All authors have read and agreed to the published version of the manuscript.

References

1. Keys, A. Human starvation and its consequences. *J. Am. Diet. Assoc.* **1946**, *22*, 582–587. [PubMed]
2. Schnitker, M.A.; Mattman, P.E.; Bliss, T.L. A clinical study of malnutrition in Japanese prisoners of war. *Ann. Intern. Med.* **1951**, *35*, 69–96. [CrossRef] [PubMed]
3. Apovian, C.M.; McMahon, M.M.; Bistrian, B.R. Guidelines for refeeding the marasmic patient. *Crit. Care Med.* **1990**, *18*, 1030–1033. [CrossRef] [PubMed]
4. Vaszar, L.T.; Culpepper-Morgan, J.A.; Winter, S.M. Refeeding syndrome induced by cautious enteral alimentation of a moderately malnourished patient. *Gastroenterologist* **1998**, *6*, 79–81.
5. Solomon, S.M.; Kirby, D.F. The refeeding syndrome: A review. *JPEN J. Parenter Enter. Nutr.* **1990**, *14*, 90–97. [CrossRef]

6. Cumming, A.D.; Farquhar, J.R.; Bouchier, I.A.D. Refeeding Hypophosphatemia in Anorexia-Nervosa and Alcoholism. *Brit. Med. J.* **1987**, *295*, 490–491. [CrossRef]
7. Gourley, D.R.H. The Role of Adenosine Triphosphate in the Transport of Phosphate in the Human Erythrocyte. *Arch. Biochem. Biophys.* **1952**, *40*, 1–12. [CrossRef]
8. Friedli, N.; Stanga, Z.; Sobotka, L.; Culkin, A.; Kondrup, J.; Laviano, A.; Mueller, B.; Schuetz, P. Revisiting the refeeding syndrome: Results of a systematic review. *Nutrition* **2017**, *35*, 151–160. [CrossRef]
9. Gaudiani, J.L.; Sabel, A.L.; Mascolo, M.; Mehler, P.S. Severe anorexia nervosa: Outcomes from a medical stabilization unit. *Int. J. Eat. Disord.* **2012**, *45*, 85–92. [CrossRef]
10. Hilbert, A.; Hoek, H.W.; Schmidt, R. Evidence-based clinical guidelines for eating disorders: International comparison. *Curr. Opin. Psychiatry* **2017**, *30*, 423–437. [CrossRef]
11. Le Grange, D.; Accurso, E.C.; Lock, J.; Agras, S.; Bryson, S.W. Early weight gain predicts outcome in two treatments for adolescent anorexia nervosa. *Int. J. Eat. Disord.* **2014**, *47*, 124–129. [CrossRef] [PubMed]
12. Lund, B.C.; Hernandez, E.R.; Yates, W.R.; Mitchell, J.R.; McKee, P.A.; Johnson, C.L. Rate of Inpatient Weight Restoration Predicts Outcome in Anorexia Nervosa. *Int. J. Eat. Disord.* **2009**, *42*, 301–305. [CrossRef] [PubMed]
13. Redgrave, G.W.; Coughlin, J.W.; Schreyer, C.C.; Martin, L.M.; Leonpacher, A.K.; Seide, M.; Verdi, A.M.; Pletch, A.; Guarda, A.S. Refeeding and weight restoration outcomes in anorexia nervosa: Challenging current guidelines. *Int. J. Eat. Disord.* **2015**, *48*, 866–873. [CrossRef] [PubMed]
14. Smith, K.; Lesser, J.; Brandenburg, B.; Lesser, A.; Cici, J.; Juenneman, R.; Beadle, A.; Eckhardt, S.; Lantz, E.; Lock, J.; et al. Outcomes of an inpatient refeeding protocol in youth with Anorexia Nervosa and atypical Anorexia Nervosa at Children's Hospitals and Clinics of Minnesota. *J. Eat. Disord.* **2016**, *4*, 35. [CrossRef]
15. Pettersson, C.; Tubic, B.; Svedlund, A.; Magnusson, P.; Ellegard, L.; Swolin-Eide, D.; Forslund, H.B. Description of an intensive nutrition therapy in hospitalized adolescents with anorexia nervosa. *Eat. Behav.* **2016**, *21*, 172–178. [CrossRef]
16. Garber, A.K.; Sawyer, S.M.; Golden, N.H.; Guarda, A.S.; Katzman, D.K.; Kohn, M.R.; Le Grange, D.; Madden, S.; Whitelaw, M.; Redgrave, G.W. A systematic review of approaches to refeeding in patients with anorexia nervosa. *Int. J. Eat. Disord.* **2016**, *49*, 293–310. [CrossRef]
17. Matthews, K.; Hill, J.; Jeffrey, S.; Patterson, S.; Davis, A.; Ward, W.; Palmer, M.; Capra, S. A Higher-Calorie Refeeding Protocol Does Not Increase Adverse Outcomes in Adult Patients with Eating Disorders. *J. Acad. Nutr. Diet.* **2018**, *118*, 1450–1463. [CrossRef]
18. da Silva, J.S.V.; Seres, D.S.; Sabino, K.; Adams, S.C.; Berdahl, G.J.; Citty, S.W.; Cober, M.P.; Evans, D.C.; Greaves, J.R.; Gura, K.M.; et al. ASPEN Consensus Recommendations for Refeeding Syndrome. *Nutr. Clin. Pr.* **2020**, *35*, 178–195. [CrossRef]
19. Madden, S.; Miskovic-Wheatley, J.; Clarke, S.; Touyz, S.; Hay, P.; Kohn, M.R. Outcomes of a rapid refeeding protocol in Adolescent Anorexia Nervosa. *J. Eat. Disord.* **2015**, *3*, 8. [CrossRef]
20. Norris, M.L.; Pinhas, L.; Nadeau, P.O.; Katzman, D.K. Delirium and refeeding syndrome in anorexia nervosa. *Int. J. Eat. Disord.* **2012**, *45*, 439–442. [CrossRef]
21. Hofer, M.; Pozzi, A.; Joray, M.; Ott, R.; Hahni, F.; Leuenberger, M.; von Kanel, R.; Stanga, Z. Safe refeeding management of anorexia nervosa inpatients: An evidence-based protocol. *Nutrition* **2014**, *30*, 524–530. [CrossRef] [PubMed]
22. Hay, P.; Chinn, D.; Forbes, D.; Madden, S.; Newton, R.; Sugenor, L.; Touyz, S.; Ward, W.; Royal, A.; Royal Australian and New Zealand College of Psychiatrists. Royal Australian and New Zealand College of Psychiatrists clinical practice guidelines for the treatment of eating disorders. *Aust. N Z J Psychiatry* **2014**, *48*, 977–1008. [CrossRef] [PubMed]
23. Stanga, Z.; Brunner, A.; Leuenberger, M.; Grimble, R.F.; Shenkin, A.; Allison, S.P.; Lobo, D.N. Nutrition in clinical practice-the refeeding syndrome: Illustrative cases and guidelines for prevention and treatment. *Eur. J. Clin. Nutr.* **2008**, *62*, 687–694. [CrossRef] [PubMed]
24. Guidelines for the Nutritional Management of Anorexia Nervosa. Available online: https://cdn.ymaws.com/www.feast-ed.org/resource/resmgr/Docs/Meal_Plans/Guidelines_nutritional_AN_cr.pdf (accessed on 29 July 2019).
25. Robinson, P.; Jones, W.R. Management of really sick patients with anorexia nervosa. *Bjpsych Adv.* **2018**, *24*, 20–32. [CrossRef]

26. Practice Guideline for the Treatment of Patients with Eating Disorders Third edition. Available online: https://psychiatryonline.org/pb/assets/raw/sitewide/practice_guidelines/guidelines/eatingdisorders.pdf (accessed on 24 April 2020).
27. Junior MARSIPAN: Management of Really Sick Patients under 18 with Aanorexia Nervosa. Available online: https://www.rcpsych.ac.uk/docs/default-source/improving-care/better-mh-policy/college-reports/college-report-cr168.pdf (accessed on 31 July 2019).

4

Impulsivity, Emotional Dysregulation and Executive Function Deficits Could be Associated with Alcohol and Drug Abuse in Eating Disorders

María Lozano-Madrid [1,2,3], Danielle Clark Bryan [4], Roser Granero [3,5], Isabel Sánchez [1,2,3], Nadine Riesco [1,2,3], Núria Mallorquí-Bagué [3,6], Susana Jiménez-Murcia [1,2,3,7], Janet Treasure [4] and Fernando Fernández-Aranda [1,2,3,7,*]

1. Department of Psychiatry, Bellvitge University Hospital-IDIBELL, 08907 L'Hospitalet de Llobregat, Barcelona, Spain; maria.lozano@bellvitgehospital.cat (M.L.-M.); isasanchez@bellvitgehospital.cat (I.S.); nriesco@bellvitgehospital.cat (N.R.); sjimenez@bellvitgehospital.cat (S.J.-M.)
2. Psychiatry and Mental Health Group, Neuroscience Program, Institut d'Investigació Biomèdica de Bellvitge—IDIBELL, 08907 L'Hospitalet de Llobregat, Barcelona, Spain
3. Ciber Fisiopatologia Obesidad y Nutrición (CIBERobn), Instituto Salud Carlos III, 28029 Madrid, Spain; Roser.Granero@uab.cat (R.G.); nmallorqui@live.com (N.M.-B.)
4. Department of Psychological Medicine, Section of Eating Disorders, Institute of Psychiatry, Psychology and Neuroscience, King's College London, SE5 8AF London, UK; danielle.clarkbryan@kcl.ac.uk (D.C.B.); janet.treasure@kcl.ac.uk (J.T.)
5. Departament de Psicobiologia i Metodologia. Universitat Autònoma de Barcelona, 08035 Barcelona, Spain
6. Department of Psychiatry, Addictive Behavior Unit, Hospital de la Santa Creu i Sant Pau, Biomedical Research Institute Sant Pau, 08001 Barcelona, Spain
7. Department of Clinical Sciences, School of Medicine and Health Sciences, University of Barcelona, 08907 L'Hospitalet de Llobregat, Barcelona, Spain

* Correspondence: ffernandez@bellvitgehospital.cat

Abstract: Background: Empirical data suggests a high comorbid occurrence of eating disorders (EDs) and substance use disorders (SUDs), as well as neurological and psychological shared characteristics. However, no prior study has identified the neuropsychological features of this subgroup. This study examines the prevalence of alcohol and/or drug abuse (A/DA) symptoms in ED patients. It also compares the clinical features and neuropsychological performance of ED patients with and without A/DA symptoms. Methods: 145 participants (74.5% females) with various forms of diagnosed EDs underwent a comprehensive clinical (TCI-R, SCL-90-R and EDI-2) and neuropsychological assessment (Stroop, WCST and IGT). Results: Approximately 19% of ED patients (across ED subtypes) had A/DA symptoms. Those with A/DA symptoms showed more impulsive behaviours and higher levels of interoceptive awareness (EDI-2), somatisation (SCL-90-R) and novelty seeking (TCI-R). This group also had a lower score in the Stroop-words measure, made more perseverative errors in the WCST and showed a weaker learning trajectory in the IGT. Conclusions: ED patients with A/DA symptoms display a specific phenotype characterised by greater impulsive personality, emotional dysregulation and problems with executive control. Patients with these temperamental traits may be at high risk of developing a SUD.

Keywords: eating disorder; alcohol and/or drug abuse; substance use disorder; executive functions; impulsivity; emotional dysregulation

1. Introduction

Eating disorders (EDs) are mental illnesses characterized by abnormal eating behaviours, which normally lead to significant impairments in physical health and psychosocial functioning [1]. EDs often co-occur with other untreated mental conditions such as substance use disorders (SUDs) [2], summarised as the inability to control the usage or craving of substances despite problems related to their use [1]. A recent meta-analysis of 43 studies estimated that the lifetime prevalence of any SUD among adults with EDs is 25.4%, with tobacco, caffeine and alcohol most commonly abused [2]. The prevalence of substance abuse varies according to demographic factors (e.g., age, sex, ethnicity) and ED diagnostic subtype [2–4]. According to the above-mentioned meta-analysis [2], the lifetime prevalence of SUDs seems to be higher in female-sample studies (26%) compared to mixed studies (15%), in adult populations (26%) compared to young adults (19%) and in primarily Caucasian samples (24%) compared to Asian samples (7%). Similarly, several studies have reported a stronger association between substance abuse and bulimia nervosa (BN) compared to anorexia nervosa (AN) [3,4]. Overall, it seems that those ED patients with purging behaviours are at higher risk of developing a comorbid SUD [2,5].

This comorbidity might be due to shared biological and psychological endophenotypes [6]. Genetic studies reveal that EDs and SUDs share overlapping genetic risk factors, especially those ED subtypes characterized by binge-purge behaviours [7,8]. Personality traits such as impulsivity are also shared [9–11], as are the elevated rates of psychopathology (especially social anxiety, antisocial behaviour, and cluster B and C personality disorders) and emotional dysregulation [12–14]. Neuropsychological impairments are another common feature [15–27], especially in executive functions (i.e., high-level cognitive processes implicated in the formation of successful goal-directed behaviours [28]). Difficulties in decision-making, cognitive flexibility and inhibitory control have been reported in all ED subtypes [15–20], as well as in SUD patients [21–27]. However, no studies have explored neuropsychological performance in ED patients with substance abuse comorbidity.

Empirical data on the comorbidity of EDs and SUDs, as well as their biological and psychological shared characteristics are available. However, there are no prior studies which have assessed the neuropsychological profile in ED patients with substance abuse symptomatology. Identifying these neuropsychological features might help to develop specific treatments that target these deficits with the purpose of preventing the later evolution into a SUD. As such, the first aim of this study was to examine the prevalence of alcohol and/or drug abuse (A/DA) symptoms in a heterogeneous series of ED patients. Our hypothesis was that A/DA symptoms would be most common in those with binge-purge behaviours. A second aim was to compare clinical (i.e., eating symptomatology, general psychopathology and personality traits) and neuropsychological features (i.e., decision-making, cognitive flexibility and inhibitory control) of patients with or without A/DA symptoms. Our hypothesis was that ED patients with A/DA symptoms will display higher impulsivity and emotional dysregulation, along with poorer executive functions.

2. Materials and Methods

2.1. Participants

The total sample comprised of 145 participants (74.5% females) aged between 18 and 60 years old. All participants were diagnosed with an ED by experienced clinicians according to the DSM-5 diagnostic criteria [1]. The final sample included: AN-restrictive subtype [AN-R] (n = 57), AN-binge/purge subtype [AN-BP] (n = 26), BN (n = 28), binge eating disorder [BED] (n = 22) and other specified feeding or eating disorder [OSFED] (n = 12).

Participants were recruited at the *Eating Disorders Unit* within the Department of Psychiatry at Bellvitge University Hospital (Barcelona, Spain), where they were receiving outpatient treatment. All participants were informed about the research procedures and gave their informed consent in writing. Procedures were approved by the Ethical Committee of the above-mentioned institution in accordance with the Helsinki Declaration of 1975 as revised in 1983 (reference: PR146/14). Exclusion criteria were the following: (1) history of chronic medical illness or neurological condition that might affect cognitive function; (2) head trauma with loss of consciousness for more than 2 min, learning disability or intellectual disability; (3) use of psycho-active medications or drugs; (4) age under 18 or over 60 (to discard neuropsychological deficits associated with the age).

2.2. Procedure and Assessment

As part of the protocol, all patients who arrived at the *Eating Disorders Unit* seeking treatment for an ED were assessed by experienced clinicians using a semi-structured clinical interview based on the DSM-5 diagnostic criteria [1]. All patients consecutively diagnosed with an ED were screened for the inclusion criteria of the study. Those who met the criteria and voluntarily accepted to be part of the study underwent a comprehensive neuropsychological and clinical assessment within the first week of their outpatient treatment. Weight and Body Mass Index (BMI) were measured for all subjects on the day of assessment. Additional sociodemographic information was also taken. The neuropsychological tests were selected to cover various aspects of executive functions including decision-making, response inhibition, strategic planning and cognitive flexibility and were administered by a trained psychologist in a single session and in a randomised order. Finally, information regarding the presence or absence of impulsive behaviours (including alcohol abuse, drugs abuse, binge episodes, theft, kleptomania and compulsive buying) was taken from the semi-structured clinical interview. The presence of A/DA symptoms was defined as the confirmation of current or lifetime behaviours of alcohol abuse, illicit drug abuse or both, causing significant distress or impairments in daily functioning.

2.2.1. Psychopathological/Personality Measures

Semi-structured clinical interview: This interview is based on the ED module of the Structured Clinical Interview for DSM-5 (SCID-5 [29]) and is used to ascertain the presence of a current ED according to the DSM-5 criteria. It provides specific information regarding the symptomatology and course of the ED. It also includes other questions in relation to the impulsive behaviours frequently found in ED patients, such us alcohol abuse, drug abuse, theft, compulsive buying, etc.

The *Temperament and Character Inventory-Revised* (TCI-R [30]; Spanish validation [31]) is a reliable and valid 240-item questionnaire that measures seven personality dimensions: four temperament dimensions (novelty seeking, harm avoidance, reward dependence and persistence) and three about character (self-directedness, cooperativeness and self-transcendence). The scales in the revised version showed a mean internal consistency of 0.87 (α coefficient).

The *Symptom Checklist-90 Revised* (SCL-90-R [32]; Spanish validation [33]) is a 90-item questionnaire which evaluates psychopathological symptoms; these are grouped as follows: somatization, obsessive-compulsive, interpersonal sensitive, depression, anxiety, hostility, phobic anxiety, paranoia and psychotic. It also includes a global severity index (GSI), designed to measure overall psychological distress. This instrument has demonstrated satisfactory psychometric properties in the Spanish version, obtaining a mean internal consistency of 0.75 (α coefficient).

The *Eating Disorders Inventory-2* (EDI-2 [34]; Spanish validation [35]) is a 91-item self-report questionnaire that assesses the following ED factors: drive for thinness, bulimia, body dissatisfaction, ineffectiveness, perfectionism, interpersonal distrust, interoceptive awareness, maturity fears, asceticism, impulse regulation and social insecurity. This instrument was validated in a Spanish population with a mean internal consistency of 0.63 (α coefficient).

2.2.2. Neuropsychological Measures

The Stroop Colour and Word Test (SCWT [36]; Spanish version [37]) is an extensively used neuropsychological test to assess inhibitory control (including response inhibition and interference control). It consists of three different lists: a word list containing the names of colours printed in black ink, a colour list that comprises letter Xs printed in colour and a colour-word list comprised of names of colours in a colour ink that does not match the written name. Three final scores are obtained based on the number of items that the participant is able to read on each of the three lists in a time window of 45 s. An interference score is computed from all three lists. A higher score is interpreted as better inhibitory control.

The Wisconsin Card Sorting Test (WCST [38]) is a computerized set-shifting task for assessing cognitive flexibility. It includes 128 cards that vary according to three attributes: number (N), colour (C) and shape (S). The participant has to pile the cards beneath four reference cards that also vary along these same dimensions, and in order to succeed, they have to settle upon a predetermined sorting rule. The only feedback given to the participant is the word "right" or "wrong" after each sorting. Initially, C is the correct sorting category, and positive feedback is given only if the card is placed in the pile with the same colour. After 10 consecutive correct sorts, the rule changes. Thus, the positive feedback is only given when the sorting matches the new category. By trial and error, the participant must learn to change the sorting categories according to the given feedback. There are up to six attempts to derive a rule, providing rule shifts in the following category sequence: C-S-N-C-S-N. Participants are not informed of the correct sorting principle and that the sorting principle shifts during the test. The test is completed when all 128 cards are sorted or after the six full categories are completed. The number of completed categories, the percentage of perseverative errors (i.e., failures to change sorting strategy after negative feedback) and the percentage of non-perseverative errors are recorded.

The Iowa Gambling Task (IGT [39]) is a computerized task to evaluate decision-making, which has also been proposed as a measure of choice impulsivity [40]. It involves a total of 100 turns distributed across four decks of cards (A, B, C and D), and each time the participant selects a deck, a specified amount of play money is awarded. The interspersed rewards among these decks are probabilistic punishments (monetary losses with different amounts). Participants are instructed that the final aim of the task is to win as much money as possible and to avoid losing as much money as possible. Moreover, they may choose cards from any deck, and switch decks at any time. This test is scored by subtracting the number of cards selected from decks A and B from the number of cards selected from decks C and D. Decks A and B are not advantageous as the final loss is higher than the final gain; however, decks C and D are advantageous since the punishments are smaller. Higher scores indicate better performance on the task.

2.3. Statistical Analyses

Statistical analysis was carried out with Stata16 for Windows [41]. The comparisons between the groups with and without A/DA symptoms were based on T-TEST procedures for quantitative variables and chi-square tests (χ^2) for categorical variables. The effect size of the mean differences in the clinical variables was estimated with Cohen's-*d* coefficient, considering null effect for $|d| < 0.20$, low-poor for $|d| > 0.20$, moderate-medium for $|d| > 0.5$ and large-high for $|d| > 0.8$ [42]. The significance tests were complemented with other standardised measures of the effect size: partial eta-squared coefficients (η^2), which measures the proportion of the total variance in a criterion associated with the membership of the different groups, defined by the independent variable once the potential effects of other predictors and interactions are partialled out (in one way ANOVA, eta-squared and partial eta-squared come out the same, but in multivariate ANOVA, their values differ). The comparisons between the proportions were based on the Cohen's-*h* coefficient, a standardised measure of the distance between the proportions obtained in two groups; it is estimated as the difference of the arcsine transformation for the two probabilities [43]. In addition, and due the multiple statistical comparisons performed on the clinical and neuropsychological variables, Finner-correction was used to control the increase in the Type-I error [44]. Finner-method uses a stepwise multiple comparisons procedure, which solves the monotonicity of the critical values by means of an inequality for the distribution function of the statistic range, using the principle of family-wise Type I correction. The post-hoc power calculation was also conducted for each observed effect based on the sample size and the parameter estimates, defining an alpha value $\alpha = 0.05$.

A 2×5 mixed analysis of variance was obtained to analyse the learning curve in the IGT test. For this analysis, the group was defined as the between-subjects factor (2 levels: with versus without

A/DA) and the IGT-block as the within-subjects factor (5 levels: blocks 1 to 5). Tests of within-subjects included polynomial contrasts for assessing the presence of trends in the mean estimates (linear, quadratic, cubic and order-4). Effect size of the parameter estimates were assessed with eta-squared values (η^2).

3. Results

3.1. Characteristics of the Sample

Most participants were women (108, 74.5%), born in Spain (130, 89.7%) and single (105, 72.4%). Mean chronological age was 30.3 years (SD = 10.3), age of ED onset was 22.7 years (SD = 9.1) and duration of the ED symptoms 7.7 years (SD = 7.4). The prevalence of impulsive behaviours was 43.1% for binges episodes, 18.6% for theft, 3.4% for kleptomania and 11.0% for compulsive buying. No participants reported instances of problematic gambling behaviours.

Table 1 shows the comparison between the groups with and without A/DA symptoms. Statistical differences were found for the presence of impulsive behaviours (higher prevalence among patients with A/DA).

Table 1. Descriptive of the sample.

		Without A/DA		With A/DA		
		n = 118		*n* = 27		*p*
		n	%	*n*	%	
Sex	Women	88	74.6%	20	74.1%	0.957
	Men	30	25.4%	7	25.9%	
ED subtype	Anorexia restrictive	49	41.5%	8	29.6%	0.751
	Anorexia binge/purge	20	16.9%	6	22.2%	
	Bulimia	21	17.8%	7	25.9%	
	Binge eating disorder	18	15.3%	4	14.8%	
	Other specified feeding eating dis.	10	8.5%	2	7.4%	
Education	Primary	30	25.4%	10	37.0%	0.438
	Secondary	52	44.1%	11	40.7%	
	University	36	30.5%	6	22.2%	
		Mean	SD	Mean	SD	*p*
	Age (years-old)	30.30	10.13	30.56	11.22	0.907
	Onset of the ED (years-old)	22.94	8.99	21.59	9.83	0.491
	Duration of the ED (years)	7.36	7.58	8.96	6.72	0.312
	BMI (kg/m^2)	21.70	8.47	22.50	8.87	0.663
	Other impulsive behaviours	*n*	%	*n*	%	*p*
	Binges episodes	46	39.3%	16	59.3%	0.049 *
	Theft	18	15.3%	9	33.3%	0.029 *
	Kleptomania	2	1.7%	3	11.1%	0.045 *
	Compulsive buying	10	8.5%	6	22.2%	0.040 *

A/DA: alcohol and/or drugs abuse symptoms. ED: eating disorder. BMI: body mass index. SD: standard deviation. *: significant comparison (0.05 level).

3.2. Prevalence of A/DA in ED Patients

The number of patients with A/DA symptoms was 27 (prevalence = 18.6%). Table 2 compares prevalence estimates between ED subtypes and gender. No differences by gender (women (18.5%) and men (18.9%) ($\chi^2 = 0.01$, $df = 1$, $p = 0.957$)) or subtype (14.0% for AN-R, 23.1% for AN-BP, 25.0% for BN, 18.2% for BED and 16.7% for OSFED ($\chi^2 = 1.92$, $df = 4$, $p = 0.751$)) were found. The highest effect size for the comparison between AN-R and BN was a Cohen's-h into the low range $|h| = 0.28$.

Table 2. Prevalence estimate of A/DA depending on ED subtype and gender.

Total		AN-R		AN-BP		BN		BED		OSFED		Women		Men	
$n = 145$		$n = 57$		$n = 26$		$n = 28$		$n = 22$		$n = 12$		$n = 108$		$n = 37$	
n	%	n	%	n	%	n	%	n	%	n	%	n	%	n	%
27	18.6%	8	14.0%	6	23.1%	7	25.0%	4	18.2%	2	16.7%	20	18.5%	7	18.9%
	χ^2	1.92	($df = 4$)									0.01	($df = 1$)		
	p	0.751										0.957			

AN-R: anorexia restrictive. AN-BP: anorexia binge/purge. BN: bulimia. BED: binge eating disorder. OSFED: other specified feeding eating disorder. df: degrees of freedom.

3.3. Comparison of the Clinical and Neuropsychological Profile of Patients with and without A/DA

Table 3 compares the clinical measures of patients with and without A/DA symptoms. Those with A/DA had higher levels of interoceptive awareness (EDI-2), somatisation (SCL-90-R) and novelty seeking (TCI-R). Internal consistency in the sample of the study was between good to excellent for all the psychometrical scales (Cronbach's alpha values).

Table 3. Comparison of the clinical profile between groups with and without A/DA.

	α	Without A/DA $n = 118$		With A/DA $n = 27$		p	$\lvert d \rvert$	η^2	Power
		Mean	SD	Mean	SD				
EDI Drive for thinness	0.846	11.24	6.65	12.10	6.50	0.544	0.13	0.003	0.093
EDI Body dissatisfaction	0.922	13.35	8.86	15.66	7.70	0.213	0.28	0.011	0.237
EDI Interoceptive awareness	0.868	8.98	7.13	12.10	5.95	0.036 *	0.52 †	0.030	0.556
EDI Bulimia	0.791	4.92	5.20	6.51	4.83	0.148	0.32	0.015	0.303
EDI Interpersonal distrust	0.824	5.59	4.84	5.92	4.47	0.752	0.07	0.001	0.061
EDI Ineffectiveness	0.905	8.61	6.89	10.78	6.91	0.142	0.32	0.015	0.312
EDI Maturity fears	0.841	7.54	5.08	7.58	5.89	0.975	0.01	0.001	0.050
EDI Perfectionism	0.842	5.31	4.40	5.16	4.54	0.878	0.03	0.001	0.053
EDI Impulse regulation	0.850	5.43	5.85	5.60	4.43	0.886	0.03	0.001	0.052
EDI Ascetic	0.703	5.99	4.37	6.92	3.76	0.307	0.23	0.007	0.175
EDI Social insecurity	0.825	6.37	5.17	7.28	5.72	0.417	0.17	0.005	0.127
EDI Total score	0.974	83.33	48.73	95.62	42.19	0.228	0.27	0.010	0.225
SCL-90R Somatization	0.857	1.45	0.90	1.82	0.77	0.049 *	0.44	0.026	0.497
SCL-90-R Obsessive-compulsive	0.909	1.57	0.98	1.78	0.89	0.308	0.22	0.007	0.174
SCL-90-R Interpersonal sensitive	0.912	1.76	1.04	1.94	0.91	0.416	0.18	0.005	0.128
SCL-90-R Depression	0.946	2.00	1.05	2.21	0.82	0.329	0.22	0.007	0.164
SCL-90-R Anxiety	0.911	1.38	0.95	1.66	0.74	0.145	0.34	0.015	0.307
SCL-90-R Hostility	0.774	1.17	0.88	1.25	0.97	0.672	0.09	0.001	0.071
SCL-90-R Phobic anxiety	0.854	0.78	0.87	0.86	0.73	0.667	0.10	0.001	0.072
SCL-90-R Paranoia	0.875	1.27	0.89	1.32	0.81	0.821	0.05	0.001	0.056
SCL-90-R Psychotic	0.893	1.17	0.77	1.28	0.67	0.529	0.14	0.003	0.096
SCL-90-R GSI	0.980	1.50	0.82	1.69	0.68	0.257	0.26	0.009	0.204
SCL-90-R PST	0.980	56.61	19.91	63.15	17.64	0.119	0.35	0.017	0.345
SCL-90-R PSDI	0.980	2.20	0.66	2.32	0.42	0.383	0.21	0.005	0.140
TCI-R Novelty seeking	0.797	94.68	13.80	103.37	13.83	0.004 *	0.63 †	0.057	0.834
TCI-R Harm avoidance	0.925	112.31	20.84	116.07	21.50	0.402	0.18	0.005	0.133
TCI-R Reward dependence	0.700	101.21	15.47	102.56	17.33	0.691	0.08	0.001	0.068
TCI-R Persistence	0.860	114.12	20.30	107.33	24.13	0.133	0.30	0.016	0.323
TCI-R Self-directedness	0.908	125.72	21.84	119.33	24.19	0.181	0.28	0.012	0.266
TCI-R Cooperativeness	0.831	136.66	17.28	135.89	15.97	0.832	0.05	0.001	0.055
TCI-R Self-transcendence	0.893	63.16	15.28	63.37	18.91	0.951	0.01	0.001	0.050

SD: standard deviation. Cronbach's alpha in the sample. *: significant comparison (0.05 level). †: effect size into the moderate ($\lvert d \rvert > 0.50$) to high range ($\lvert d \rvert > 0.80$). p-values with Finner-correction.

Table 4 shows the comparison of the neuropsychological profile. Higher scores in perseverative errors (WCST) and in the first block of the IGT and lower scores in the Stroop-words measure were found.

Table 4. Comparison of the neuropsychological profile between groups with and without A/DA.

	Without A/DA		With A/DA					
	$n = 118$		$n = 27$		p	$\lvert d\rvert$	η^2	Power
	Mean	SD	Mean	SD				
Stroop Words	104.43	19.39	95.61	24.53	0.045 *	0.40	0.028	0.521
Stroop Colour	75.84	16.06	80.24	19.74	0.221	0.24	0.010	0.231
Stroop Words-colour	48.27	11.75	46.50	9.33	0.467	0.17	0.004	0.112
Stroop Interference	5.09	8.99	4.42	7.92	0.725	0.08	0.001	0.064
WCST Total trials	94.42	20.72	100.55	20.70	0.168	0.30	0.013	0.280
WCST Correct	67.83	10.87	68.06	14.02	0.924	0.02	0.001	0.051
WCST Perseverative errors	12.40	10.33	18.54	19.41	0.023 *	0.39	0.036	0.629
WCST Non-perseverative errors	14.20	15.25	14.22	11.91	0.993	0.01	0.001	0.050
WCST Conceptual	60.64	16.54	59.18	19.97	0.692	0.08	0.001	0.068
WCST Categories completed	5.10	1.80	4.88	1.98	0.577	0.12	0.002	0.086
WCST Trials completed 1st categ.	20.36	24.17	26.73	31.78	0.248	0.23	0.009	0.210
IGT Block 1	−2.59	4.21	−0.62	2.84	0.023 *	0.55 †	0.036	0.629
IGT Block 2	−1.11	4.91	0.32	4.41	0.165	0.31	0.013	0.284
IGT Block 3	0.29	5.80	−1.39	3.55	0.152	0.35	0.014	0.298
IGT Block 4	0.38	6.69	0.68	6.67	0.834	0.04	0.001	0.055
IGT Block 5	0.51	7.78	0.06	5.42	0.777	0.07	0.001	0.059
IGT Total	−2.52	20.79	−0.95	11.51	0.704	0.09	0.001	0.067

SD: standard deviation. *: significant comparison (0.05 level). †: effect size into the moderate ($\lvert d\rvert > 0.50$) to high range ($\lvert d\rvert > 0.80$). p-values with Finner-correction.

The results of the mixed ANOVA obtained to analyse the learning curve in the IGT showed a quasi-significant interaction parameter IGT-by-Group ($F_{(3.42;488.5)} = 2.02$, $p = 0.091$, $\eta^2 = 0.014$; Greenhouse–Geisser adjusted) as well as a main effect of the IGT-block ($F_{(3.42;488.5)} = 2.65$, $p = 0.041$, $\eta^2 = 0.018$). Figure 1 shows the adjusted mean net scores in the blocks, showing a learning trajectory only for patients without A/DA symptoms: Among this group, polynomial contrasts for the IGT-block showed a significant linear trend ($F_{(1;117)} = 18.3$, $p < 0.001$, $\eta^2 = 0.135$) and a significant quadratic trend ($F_{(1;117)} = 6.97$, $p = 0.009$, $\eta^2 = 0.056$), while non-significant results were found for the cubic ($F_{(1;117)} = 0.01$, $p = 0.931$ $\eta^2 = 0.001$) and order 4 ($F_{(1;117)} = 0.59$, $p = 0.442$, $\eta^2 = 0.005$) trends. In patients without A/DA symptoms, post-hoc pairwise comparisons defining the difference-type contrasts (based on comparing each block with the previous) showed statistical differences between blocks 2 versus block 1 ($p = 0.008$) and block 3 versus block 2 ($p = 0.011$), while no statistical differences were found between blocks 4 versus block 3 ($p = 0.886$) and block 5 versus block 4 ($p = 0.832$). However, patients with A/DA symptoms did not have significant results (linear: $F_{(1;26)} = 0.27$, $p = 0.607$, $\eta^2 = 0.010$; quadratic: $F_{(1;26)} = 0.06$, $p = 0.815$, $\eta^2 = 0.002$; cubic: $F_{(1;26)} = 0.01$, $p = 0.988$, $\eta^2 = 0.001$; order 4: $F_{(1;26)} = 2.30$, $p = 0.141$, $\eta^2 = 0.081$). No statistical differences were found in the post-hoc pairwise comparisons comparing the IGT blocks among patients who reported the presence of A/DA.

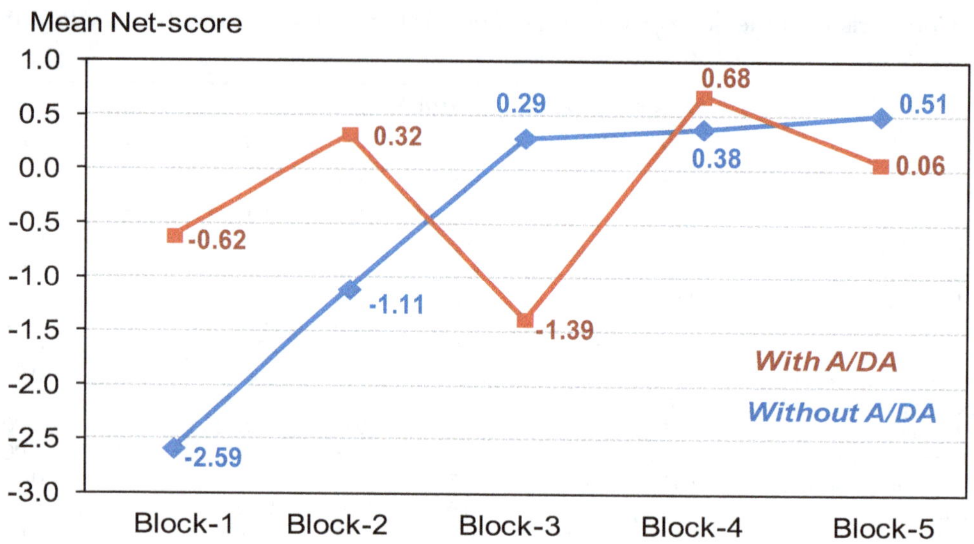

Figure 1. Learning curve in the IGT measure. Note. A/DA: alcohol and/or drug abuse. Sample size: $n = 145$.

4. Discussion

The first aim of this study was to assess the prevalence of A/DA symptoms in a sample of patients across the range of ED diagnoses. The lifetime A/DA prevalence was similar to that found previously in ED patients [2], although slightly lower. This small difference could be explained by the fact that we only assessed symptoms of alcohol and illicit drugs abuse, whereas previous studies considered other substances such as tobacco and caffeine [2]. Although this study had insufficient power to detect differences between subtypes, the trends were in the same direction as previous studies, with BN patients showing the highest prevalence [2–5] and those with AN-BP higher than those with AN-R [45], confirming our first hypothesis based on previous studies. We failed to find the gender difference in prevalence observed in a previous systematic review [2]; however, this might be a question of low power and methodology. While our study compares female and male patients within the same sample, Bahji et al. [2] compared the prevalence observed in female sample studies to mixed studies.

When comparing the clinical profile, the A/DA group scored higher on interoceptive awareness subscale (EDI-2), which indicates a poorer ability to recognise and differentiate between hunger and satiety and emotional states [34]. In ED patients, emotional dysregulation is associated with difficulties in controlling impulsive behaviours (e.g., compulsive binging, purging and overeating) in both negative and positive states [46,47], and this may lead to abuse of alcohol and drugs [13,14]. Indeed, the weaker interoceptive awareness previously found in individuals with BN [48] may explain their higher vulnerability to develop comorbid A/DA symptoms [3,4].

Moreover, the A/DA group had higher levels of somatisation (SCL-90-R), the experience of psychological distress in the presence of unexplained physical symptoms [49]. It is suggested that patients experiencing high levels of somatising symptoms use substances to numb uncomfortable experiences [49]. Furthermore, somatising symptoms are closely associated with symptoms of substance intoxication or withdrawal, but whether they are a cause or effect of substance abuse remains unclear [50]. In any case, our results seem to reflect this association between somatising and substance abuse symptoms, yet longitudinal studies would be needed to clarify the direction of these interactions.

The group with A/DA symptoms had higher scores for the novelty seeking trait (TCI-R), mainly related to impulsivity [30]. Our findings align with other neurobehavioural research, which suggests that novelty seeking is associated with vulnerability to substance abuse [10,11] and with the finding of a higher prevalence of binge episodes, theft, kleptomania and compulsive buying in this subgroup. Strong associations among all the impulsive behaviours mentioned above are documented in the literature. For instance, ED patients who engage in binge-purge behaviours frequently display high prevalence of SUD [2–5,45] and compulsive buying [51,52]. Similarly, several studies have reported high rates of SUDs in individuals with kleptomania and compulsive buying [53,54].

The neuropsychological assessment results revealed that ED patients with A/DA symptoms display significantly lower scores in the Stroop-words measure, demonstrating a poorer reading ability in terms of speed and accuracy [36]. Contrary to expectations, no differences between groups were found in the Stroop-interference measure, meaning no differences in inhibitory control [36]. Impairments in inhibitory control are found to be a core deficit among binge/purge-type EDs [15,16] and SUDs [21,23], especially when examining stimuli related to each disorder (e.g., food, body shape, use of substances, etc.) [15,55,56]. Since inhibitory deficits seem to represent a risk factor for the development of both disorders separately, we expected to find greater inhibitory control impairments when both disorders co-occur. The fact that we failed to find this result might be explained because of the limited statistical power of this study. Further studies with larger samples are needed to clarify this issue.

In addition, patients with A/DA symptoms made more perseverative errors (WCST). Previous research demonstrated that individuals with EDs perform worse on set-shifting tasks than healthy individuals, which translates to poorer cognitive flexibility and higher rigidity [17,18]. Reduced cognitive flexibility has also been observed in individuals with SUDs, which may negatively impact on their problem-solving strategies [24,25]. In summary, poor cognitive flexibility is shown to be a common feature in EDs and SUDs, and our results point out that it might be highlighted when both disorders are present at the same time. However, due to the relatively small sample size of one of the groups and the low statistical power, our results should be interpreted with caution until more evidence is available.

Lastly, even though no differences between groups were found on the IGT total score, both groups displayed an impaired decision-making performance in comparison to healthy population [18,57,58]. However, when comparing the learning curve of both groups, patients with A/DA symptoms showed a weaker learning trajectory and greater difficulties to learn the reward/punishment contingencies of their choices [59]. Our results point out that decision-making problems seem to be present in ED patients [18–20], particularly in those with comorbid substance abuse symptomatology. Once again, future studies are needed to confirm this finding.

The results of this study should be interpreted in the context of some limitations. First, although our sample size is relatively large, the subgroups vary in size, and one of them is relatively small, leading to a low statistical power. Studies with small samples are severely underpowered, which might represent a concern if the "null hypothesis" cannot be rejected. For this reason, the significance tests were complemented with other standardized measure of the effect size. In any case, the results of this study should be interpreted with caution and considering this limitation. Furthermore, because the design is cross-sectional, claims regarding causality cannot be made. Future longitudinal studies should examine the extent to which psychopathology and cognitive function improve after treatment. Another limitation was the lack of a formal diagnosis of SUD in our sample. Finally, our sample was largely made up of young adults, and it would be of clinical interest to explore whether similar impairments in neuropsychological functioning are present in older samples.

5. Conclusions

To conclude, although previous studies have explored comorbidity between EDs and SUDs, this is the first study to explore gender differences. Moreover, it is the first to assess the neuropsychological profile in ED patients with A/DA symptoms. We found that this subgroup displays a specific phenotype characterised by greater impulsivity (i.e., high novelty seeking and difficulties to control impulsive behaviours), noticeable emotional dysregulation (i.e., decreased interoceptive awareness) and more impaired executive control (i.e., low cognitive flexibility and poor decision-making). Of future benefit would be the consolidation of our findings in larger samples and clarifying if these deficits are involved in the development and maintenance of substance abuse comorbidity. As such, this subgroup of ED patients might benefit from augmented treatment that targets these problems, such as inhibitory control training [60], emotion regulation training [61] or cognitive remediation therapy [62]. This may reduce the present substance abuse symptomatology and prevent later evolution into a SUD, as previous studies have reported that ED patients who do not receive any adjunctive treatment for substance abuse are at high risk for switching from one problematic behaviour to the other, especially during the recovery process [2].

Author Contributions: Conceptualization, M.L.-M., F.F.-A., S.J.-M. and J.T.; methodology, M.L.-M. and F.F.-A.; formal analysis, R.G.; data curation, M.L.-M. and N.M.-B.; investigation, I.S. and N.R.; writing—original draft preparation, M.L.-M. and D.C.B.; writing—review and editing, M.L.-M., D.C.B., F.F.-A. and J.T.; funding acquisition, F.F.-A., M.L.-M. and J.T. All authors have read and agreed to the published version of the manuscript.

References

1. American Psychiatric Association. *Diagnostic and Statistical Manual of Mental Disorders*, 5th ed.; American Psychiatric Association: Washington, DC, USA, 2013.
2. Bahji, A.; Mazhar, M.N.; Hudson, C.C.; Nadkarni, P.; MacNeil, B.A.; Hawken, E. Prevalence of substance use disorder comorbidity among individuals with eating disorders: A systematic review and meta-analysis. *Psychiatry Res.* **2019**, *273*, 58–66. [CrossRef] [PubMed]
3. Hudson, J.I.; Hiripi, E.; Pope, H.G.; Kessler, R.C. The Prevalence and Correlates of Eating Disorders in the National Comorbidity Survey Replication. *Biol. Psychiatry* **2007**, *61*, 348–358. [CrossRef] [PubMed]
4. Fouladi, F.; Mitchell, J.E.; Crosby, R.D.; Engel, S.G.; Crow, S.; Hill, L.; Le Grange, D.; Powers, P.; Steffen, K.J. Prevalence of Alcohol and Other Substance Use in Patients with Eating Disorders. *Eur. Eat. Disord. Rev.* **2015**, *23*, 531–536. [CrossRef] [PubMed]
5. Dennis, A.B.; Pryor, T. The Complex Relationship between Eating Disorders and Substance Use Disorders. In *Clinical Handbook of Complex and Atypical Eating Disorders*; Anderson, L.K., Murray, S.B., Kaye, W.H., Eds.; Oxford University Press: New York, NY, USA, 2017; pp. 60–78.
6. Harrop, E.N.; Marlatt, G.A. The comorbidity of substance use disorders and eating disorders in women: Prevalence, etiology, and treatment. *Addict. Behav.* **2010**, *35*, 392–398. [CrossRef] [PubMed]
7. Munn-Chernoff, M.A.; Baker, J.H. A Primer on the Genetics of Comorbid Eating Disorders and Substance Use Disorders. *Eur. Eat. Disord. Rev.* **2016**, *24*, 91–100. [CrossRef] [PubMed]
8. Munn-Chernoff, M.A.; Johnson, E.C.; Chou, Y.L.; Coleman, J.R.I.; Thornton, L.M.; Walters, R.K.; Yilmaz, Z.; Baker, J.H.; Hübel, C.; Gordon, S.; et al. Shared genetic risk between eating disorder- and substance-use-related phenotypes: Evidence from genome-wide association studies. *Addict. Biol.* **2020**. [CrossRef]
9. Krug, I.; Pinheiro, A.P.; Bulik, C.; Jiménez-Murcia, S.; Granero, R.; Penelo, E.; Masuet, C.; Agüera, Z.; Fernández-Aranda, F. Lifetime substance abuse, family history of alcohol abuse/dependence and novelty seeking in eating disorders: Comparison study of eating disorder subgroups. *Psychiatry Clin. Neurosci.* **2009**, *63*, 82–87. [CrossRef]
10. Fernández-Mondragón, S.; Adan, A. Personality in male patients with substance use disorder and/or severe mental illness. *Psychiatry Res.* **2015**, *228*, 488–494. [CrossRef]
11. Wingo, T.; Nesil, T.; Choi, J.S.; Li, M.D. Novelty Seeking and Drug Addiction in Humans and Animals: From Behavior to Molecules. *J. Neuroimmune Pharmcol.* **2016**, *11*, 456–470. [CrossRef]
12. Lilenfeld, L.R.; Kaye, W.H.; Greeno, C.G.; Merikangas, K.R.; Plotnicov, K.; Pollice, C.; Rao, R.; Strober, M.; Bulik, C.M.; Nagy, L. Psychiatric disorders in women with bulimia nervosa and their first-degree relatives: Effects of comorbid substance dependence. *Int. J. Eat. Disord.* **1997**, *22*, 253–264. [CrossRef]
13. Sloan, E.; Hall, K.; Moulding, R.; Bryce, S.; Mildred, H.; Staiger, P.K. Emotion regulation as a transdiagnostic treatment construct across anxiety, depression, substance, eating and borderline personality disorders: A systematic review. *Clin. Psychol. Rev.* **2017**, *57*, 141–163. [CrossRef]
14. Aldao, A.; Nolen-Hoeksema, S. Specificity of cognitive emotion regulation strategies: A transdiagnostic examination. *Behav. Res. Ther.* **2010**, *48*, 974–983. [CrossRef]
15. Wu, M.; Hartmann, M.; Skunde, M.; Herzog, W.; Friederich, H.-C. Inhibitory Control in Bulimic-Type Eating Disorders: A Systematic Review and Meta-Analysis. *PLoS ONE* **2013**, *8*, e83412. [CrossRef]
16. Lavagnino, L.; Arnone, D.; Cao, B.; Soares, J.C.; Selvaraj, S. Inhibitory control in obesity and binge eating disorder: A systematic review and meta-analysis of neurocognitive and neuroimaging studies. *Neurosci. Biobehav. Rev.* **2016**, *68*, 714–726. [CrossRef]

17. Roberts, M.E.; Tchanturia, K.; Treasure, J.L. Overlapping neurocognitive inefficiencies in anorexia nervosa: A preliminary investigation of women with both poor set-shifting and weak central coherence. *Eat. Weight Disord. Stud. Anorex. Bulim. Obes.* **2016**, *21*, 725–729. [CrossRef]
18. Aloi, M.; Rania, M.; Caroleo, M.; Bruni, A.; Palmieri, A.; Cauteruccio, M.A.; De Fazio, P.; Segura-García, C. Decision making, central coherence and set-shifting: A comparison between Binge Eating Disorder, Anorexia Nervosa and Healthy Controls. *BMC Psychiatry* **2015**, *15*, 1–10. [CrossRef]
19. Fagundo, A.B.; de la Torre, R.; Jiménez-Murcia, S.; Agüera, Z.; Granero, R.; Tárrega, S.; Botella, C.; Baños, R.; Fernández-Real, J.M.; Rodríguez, R.; et al. Executive Functions Profile in Extreme Eating/Weight Conditions: From Anorexia Nervosa to Obesity. *PLoS ONE* **2012**, *7*, e43382. [CrossRef]
20. Guillaume, S.; Gorwood, P.; Jollant, F.; Van den Eynde, F.; Courtet, P.; Richard-Devantoy, S. Impaired decision-making in symptomatic anorexia and bulimia nervosa patients: A meta-analysis. *Psychol. Med.* **2015**, *45*, 3377–3391. [CrossRef]
21. Luijten, M.; Machielsen, M.W.J.; Veltman, D.J.; Hester, R.; de Haan, L.; Franken, I.H.A. Systematic review of ERP and fMRI studies investigating inhibitory control and error processing in people with substance dependence and behavioural addictions. *J. Psychiatry Neurosci.* **2014**, *39*, 149–169. [CrossRef]
22. Allen, D.N.; Woods, S.P. *Neuropsychological Aspects of Substance Use Disorders: Evidence-Based Perspectives*; Oxford University Press: New York, NY, USA, 2014; ISBN 9780199930838.
23. Ersche, K.D.; Turton, A.J.; Chamberlain, S.R.; Müller, U.; Bullmore, E.T.; Robbins, T.W. Cognitive dysfunction and anxious-impulsive personality traits are endophenotypes for drug dependence. *Am. J. Psychiatry* **2012**, *169*, 926–936. [CrossRef]
24. Fernández-Serrano, M.J.; Pérez-García, M.; Verdejo-García, A. What are the specific vs. generalized effects of drugs of abuse on neuropsychological performance? *Neurosci. Biobehav. Rev.* **2011**, *35*, 377–406. [CrossRef]
25. Henry, B.L.; Minassian, A.; Perry, W. Effect of methamphetamine dependence on everyday functional ability. *Addict. Behav.* **2010**, *35*, 593–598. [CrossRef]
26. Ersche, K.D.; Sahakian, B.J. The neuropsychology of amphetamine and opiate dependence: Implications for treatment. *Neuropsychol. Rev.* **2007**, *17*, 317–336. [CrossRef] [PubMed]
27. Fernández-Serrano, M.J.; Perales, J.C.; Moreno-López, L.; Pérez-García, M.; Verdejo-García, A. Neuropsychological profiling of impulsivity and compulsivity in cocaine dependent individuals. *Psychopharmacology* **2012**, *219*, 673–683. [CrossRef]
28. Lezak, M.D.; Howieson, D.B.; Bigler, E.D.; Tranel, D. *Neuropsychological Assessment*, 5th ed.; Oxford University Press: New York, NY, USA, 2012; ISBN 9780195395525.
29. First, M.; Williams, J.; Karg, R.; Spitzer, R. *Structured Clinical Interview for DSM-5 Disorders, Clinician Version (SCID-5-CV)*; American Psychiatric Association: Arlington, VA, USA, 2016.
30. Cloninger, C.R.; Przybeck, T.R.; Svrakic, D.M.; Wetzel, R.D. *The Temperament and Character Inventory (TCI): A Guide to Its Development and Use*; Center for Psychobiology of Personality, Washington University: St. Louis, MO, USA, 1994; ISBN 0-9642917-03.
31. Gutiérrez-Zotes, J.A.; Bayón, C.; Montserrat, C.; Valero, J.; Labad, A.; Cloninger, C.; Fernández-Aranda, F. Temperament and Character Inventory-Revised (TCI-R). Standardization and normative data in a general population sample. *Actas Esp Psiquiatr* **2004**, *32*, 8–15.
32. Derogatis, L.R. *Symptom Checklist-90-R (SCL-90-R): Administration, scoring, and procedures manual*, 3rd ed.; NCS Pearson: Minneapolis, MN, USA, 1994; ISBN 2090-6684 (Print) 2090-6692.
33. González de Rivera, J.L.; de las Cuevas, C.; Rodríguez-Abuín, M.; y Rodríguez-Pulido, F. *SCL-90-R. Cuestionario de 90 Síntomas. Manual*; TEA Ediciones: Madrid, Spain, 2002.
34. Garner, D.M. *Eating Disorder Inventory-2*; Psychological Assessment Resources: Odessa, Ukraine, 1991.
35. Garner, D.M. *Inventario de Trastornos de la Conducta Alimentaria (EDI-2)-Manual*; TEA: Madrid, Spain, 1998.
36. Golden, C.J. Stroop colour and word test. *Age* **1978**, *15*, 90.
37. Golden, C.J. *Stroop: Test de Colores y Palabras: Manual*; TEA Ediciones: Madrid, Spain, 2001.
38. Heaton, R.K. *PAR Staff Wisconsin Card Sorting TestTM: Computer Version 4, Research Edition*; Psychological Assessment Resources: Lutz, FL, USA, 2003.
39. Bechara, A.; Damasio, A.R.; Damasio, H.; Anderson, S.W. Insensitivity to future consequences following damage to human prefrontal cortex. *Cognition* **1994**, *50*, 7–15. [CrossRef]
40. Eisinger, A.; Magi, A.; Gyurkovics, M.; Szabo, E.; Demetrovics, Z.; Kokonyei, G. Iowa Gambling Task: Illustration of a behavioral measurement. *Neuropsychopharmacol. Hung.* **2016**, *18*, 45–55.

41. *StataCorp Stata Statistical Software: Release 16*; StataCorp LLC.: College Station, TX, USA, 2019.
42. Kelley, K.; Preacher, K.J. On effect size. *Psychol. Methods* **2012**, *17*, 137–152. [CrossRef]
43. Cohen, J. *Statistical Power Analysis for Behavioural Sciences*; Lawrence Earlbaum Associates: Hillsdale, NJ, USA, 1998; ISBN 0805802835.
44. Finner, H. On a Monotonicity Problem in Step-Down Multiple Test Procedures. *J. Am. Stat. Assoc.* **1993**, *88*, 920. [CrossRef]
45. Root, T.L.; Pinheiro, A.P.; Thornton, L.; Strober, M.; Fernandez-Aranda, F.; Brandt, H.; Crawford, S.; Fichter, M.M.; Halmi, K.A.; Johnson, C.; et al. Substance use disorders in women with anorexia nervosa. *Int. J. Eat. Disord.* **2010**, *43*, 14–21. [CrossRef] [PubMed]
46. Bongers, P.; Jansen, A.; Houben, K.; Roefs, A. Happy eating: The single target implicit association test predicts overeating after positive emotions. *Eat. Behav.* **2013**, *14*, 348–355. [CrossRef] [PubMed]
47. Leehr, E.J.; Krohmer, K.; Schag, K.; Dresler, T.; Zipfel, S.; Giel, K.E. Emotion regulation model in binge eating disorder and obesity-a systematic review. *Neurosci. Biobehav. Rev.* **2015**, *49*, 125–134. [CrossRef] [PubMed]
48. Fassino, S.; Pierò, A.; Gramaglia, C.; Abbate-Daga, G. Clinical, psychopathological and personality correlates of interoceptive awareness in anorexia nervosa, bulimia nervosa and obesity. *Psychopathology* **2004**, *37*, 168–174. [CrossRef]
49. Hasin, D.; Katz, H. Somatoform and substance use disorders. *Psychosom. Med.* **2007**, *69*, 870–875. [CrossRef]
50. Kanner, R. Substance Abuse, Somatization, and Personality Disorders. In *Emergency Neurology*; Roos, K.L., Ed.; Elseiver: Boston, MA, USA, 2012; pp. 375–384. ISBN 9780387885858.
51. Fernández-Aranda, F.; Jiménez-Murcia, S.; Álvarez-Moya, E.M.; Granero, R.; Vallejo, J.; Bulik, C.M. Impulse control disorders in eating disorders: Clinical and therapeutic implications. *Compr. Psychiatry* **2006**, *47*, 482–488. [CrossRef]
52. Jiménez-Murcia, S.; Granero, R.; Moragas, L.; Steiger, H.; Israel, M.; Aymamí, N.; Gómez-Peña, M.; Sauchelli, S.; Agüera, Z.; Sánchez, I.; et al. Differences and similarities between bulimia nervosa, compulsive buying and gambling disorder. *Eur. Eat. Disord. Rev.* **2015**, *23*, 126–132. [CrossRef]
53. Grant, J.E. Impulse control disorders, a clinician's guide to understanding and treating behavi oral addictions. *Psicoter. Cogn. E Comport.* **2011**, *17*, 130–131. [CrossRef]
54. Schreiber, L.; Odlaug, B.L.; Grant, J.E. Impulse control disorders: Updated review of clinical characteristics and pharmacological management. *Front. Psychiatry* **2011**, *2*. [CrossRef]
55. Schag, K.; Schönleber, J.; Teufel, M.; Zipfel, S.; Giel, K.E. Food-related impulsivity in obesity and Binge Eating Disorder-a systematic review. *Obes. Rev.* **2013**, *14*, 477–495. [CrossRef]
56. Wrege, J.; Schmidt, A.; Walter, A.; Smieskova, R.; Bendfeldt, K.; Radue, E.-W.; Lang, U.; Borgwardt, S. Effects of Cannabis on Impulsivity: A Systematic Review of Neuroimaging Findings. *Curr. Pharm. Des.* **2014**, *20*, 2126–2137. [CrossRef] [PubMed]
57. Verdejo-Garcia, A.; Benbrook, A.; Funderburk, F.; David, P.; Cadet, J.L.; Bolla, K.I. The differential relationship between cocaine use and marijuana use on decision-making performance over repeat testing with the Iowa Gambling Task. *Drug Alcohol Depend.* **2007**, *90*, 2–11. [CrossRef] [PubMed]
58. Bechara, A.; Tranel, D.; Damasio, H. Characterization of the decision-making deficit of patients with ventromedial prefrontal cortex lesions. *Brain* **2000**, *123*, 2189–2202. [CrossRef] [PubMed]
59. Bechara, A.; Damasio, H.; Damasio, A.R.; Lee, G.P. Different contributions of the human amygdala and ventromedial prefrontal cortex to decision-making. *J. Neurosci.* **1999**, *19*, 5473–5481. [CrossRef] [PubMed]
60. Turton, R.; Nazar, B.P.; Burgess, E.E.; Lawrence, N.S.; Cardi, V.; Treasure, J.; Hirsch, C.R. To Go or Not to Go: A Proof of Concept Study Testing Food-Specific Inhibition Training for Women with Eating and Weight Disorders. *Eur. Eat. Disord. Rev.* **2018**, *26*, 11–21. [CrossRef] [PubMed]
61. Claudat, K.; Brown, T.A.; Anderson, L.; Bongiorno, G.; Berner, L.A.; Reilly, E.; Luo, T.; Orloff, N.; Kaye, W.H. Correlates of co-occurring eating disorders and substance use disorders: A case for dialectical behavior therapy. *Eat. Disord.* **2020**, *28*, 142–156. [CrossRef]
62. Hagan, K.E.; Christensen, K.A.; Forbush, K.T. A preliminary systematic review and meta-analysis of randomized-controlled trials of cognitive remediation therapy for anorexia nervosa. *Eat. Behav.* **2020**, *37*. [CrossRef]

5

Does ADHD Symptomatology Influence Treatment Outcome and Dropout Risk in Eating Disorders?

Giulia Testa [1,2,†], Isabel Baenas [1,2,†], Cristina Vintró-Alcaraz [1,2], Roser Granero [1,3], Zaida Agüera [1,2,4], Isabel Sánchez [1,2], Nadine Riesco [1,2], Susana Jiménez-Murcia [1,2,5] and Fernando Fernández-Aranda [1,2,5,*]

1 Ciber Physiopathology, Obesity and Nutrition (CIBERObn), Instituto de Salud Carlos III, 08907 Barcelona, Spain; gtesta@idibell.cat (G.T.); ibaenas@bellvitgehospital.cat (I.B.); cvintro@bellvitgehospital.cat (C.V.-A.); Roser.Granero@uab.cat (R.G.); zaguera@bellvitgehospital.cat (Z.A.); isasanchez@bellvitgehospital.cat (I.S.); nriesco@bellvitgehospital.cat (N.R.); sjimenez@bellvitgehospital.cat (S.J.-M.)

2 Department of Psychiatry, Bellvitge University Hospital-IDIBELL, 08907 Barcelona, Spain

3 Department of Psychobiology and Methodology of Health Sciences, Universitat Autònoma de Barcelona, 08193 Barcelona, Spain

4 Department of Public Health, Mental Health and Maternal-Child Nursing, School of Nursing, University of Barcelona, 08907 Barcelona, Spain

5 Department of Clinical Sciences, School of Medicine, University of Barcelona, 08907 Barcelona, Spain

* Correspondence: ffernandez@bellvitgehospital.cat

† Share first authorship.

Abstract: Attention-deficit/hyperactivity disorder (ADHD) and its symptoms have been shown to be present in patients with eating disorders (EDs) and are associated with increased psychopathology and more dysfunctional personality traits. This study aimed to assess if the presence of ADHD symptoms in patients with EDs affects their short and long-term therapy outcome. A total of 136 consecutively treated ED patients were considered in this study. Baseline pre-treatment evaluation included the Adult ADHD Self-Report Scale (ASRS v1.1) for ADHD symptoms and the assessment of eating symptomatology using the Eating Disorders Inventory (EDI-2). Treatment outcome was evaluated in terms of ED symptoms after cognitive behavioral therapy (CBT) and dropout rate during treatment. Furthermore, we evaluated ED symptoms in treatment completers after a follow-up of 8 years on average. Path analyses assessed the potential mediational role of the EDI-2 total score in the relationship between ADHD and treatment outcome. Results showed that baseline symptoms of ADHD indirectly affected treatment outcome after CBT; the ASRS positive screening was related to higher eating symptomatology (standardized coefficient $B = 0.41$, $p = 0.001$, 95% CI: 0.26 to 0.55), and the presence of high ED levels contributed to the increase of dropout ($B = 0.15$, $p = 0.041$, 95% CI: 0.03 to 0.33) and a worse treatment outcome ($B = 0.18$, $p = 0.041$, 95% CI: 0.01 to 0.35). No direct effect was found between the ASRS positive screening with the risk of dropout ($B = -0.08$, $p = 0.375$) and worse treatment outcome ($B = -0.07$, $p = 0.414$). These results suggest the relevance of identifying specific treatment approaches for patients with ADHD symptoms and severe eating symptomatology.

Keywords: attention-deficit/hyperactivity disorder; ADHD; eating disorders; longitudinal; treatment outcome; dropout

1. Introduction

Attention-deficit/hyperactivity disorder (ADHD), which is characterized by symptoms of impulsivity, hyperactivity and inattention, has been described in relation to several psychiatric disorders including eating disorders (EDs) [1–4]. Accordingly, a higher prevalence of ADHD symptoms in EDs has been reported in many studies, in comparison with the general population [4–10]. Likewise, ADHD has been related with increased risk of disordered eating in childhood and adulthood [11–14], obesity [15] and behavioral addictions [16,17].

From a neurobiological perspective, a recent study examined the genetic factors common to both disorders and observed a stronger genetic association between ADHD and binge-eating behaviors [18]. From a clinical view, ADHD symptoms in ED were associated with higher ED symptomatology [19], specifically binge ED subtypes, with greater psychopathology [19–21], and increased levels of motor and cognitive impulsivity [22,23], as well as impulsive personality traits [24,25].

Despite the evidence linking ADHD and EDs, there is a lack of studies investigating whether ADHD symptoms may impact treatment response in patients with EDs, both in terms of treatment adherence (i.e., dropout rate) and outcome. To the best of our knowledge, there is only one previous study in female patients with EDs reporting higher ADHD symptoms at baseline as a predictor of non-recovery from eating-related symptomatology one year after treatment, especially for patients with loss of control overeating, bingeing and purging [26]. However, a high dropout rate (61%) was shown in that study, highlighting the need for future studies examining the impact of ADHD symptoms over dropout rate in EDs treatment.

The first aim of the present study was to evaluate if the initial presence of ADHD symptomatology impacts the therapy outcome after a cognitive behavioral therapy (CBT) treatment for EDs and dropout rate during treatment. The second aim was to analyze whether the baseline ADHD symptomatology had an impact on long-term therapy outcome (after eight years on average). Furthermore, we assessed the influence of EDs severity over the relationship between ADHD symptoms and treatment results.

2. Materials and Methods

2.1. Participants

The initial sample was comprised of 191 adult women diagnosed with an ED and presented for treatment to the Eating Disorder Unit within the Department of Psychiatry at Bellvitge University Hospital (HUB) (Barcelona, Spain) from 16 April 2009 to 31 January 2011. The baseline data of the initial sample was previously reported by Fernández-Aranda et al. (2013). Patients were diagnosed according to the DSM-IV-TR criteria [27], and diagnoses were reanalyzed and recodified post hoc using the DSM-5 criteria [28]. In the present study, we analyzed this sample of patients following a CBT treatment and after a longer follow-up (mean = 8.81 years; SD = 1.5). To that end, clinical records and an online shared medical network were analyzed retrospectively throughout the region of Catalonia (Spain). Thirty-three patients who did not start treatment were excluded from the original sample ($n = 191$); however, neither online nor paper clinical records were available for 22 out of 158 patients who started treatment. Thus, a final sample of 136 patients was included in the principal analysis. There were no baseline differences between patients who were included in this study and those who were not. Sixty-four participants included in the final sample did not complete treatment sessions (dropout) whereas 72 patients out of 136 completed the treatment (see flowchart; Figure 1).

2.2. Assessment

Adult ADHD Self-Report Scale (ASRS-v1.1) [29]: The ASRS-v1.1 is a self-administered scale designed to screen ADHD in the adult population (aged 18 years and older). It comprises 6 items that are consistent with the DSM-IV-TR [27] criteria and address the manifestation of ADHD in adults; the first 4 questions examine the inattention component of ADHD, and the final 2, the hyperactivity component. Each item is assessed using a 5-point Likert scale (0–4). The total score ranges between 0 and 24, with the cut-off being set at 12. The Spanish validation reported good psychometric properties [30]. Internal consistency in the sample analyzed in this work was good (Cronbach's alpha $\alpha = 0.77$).

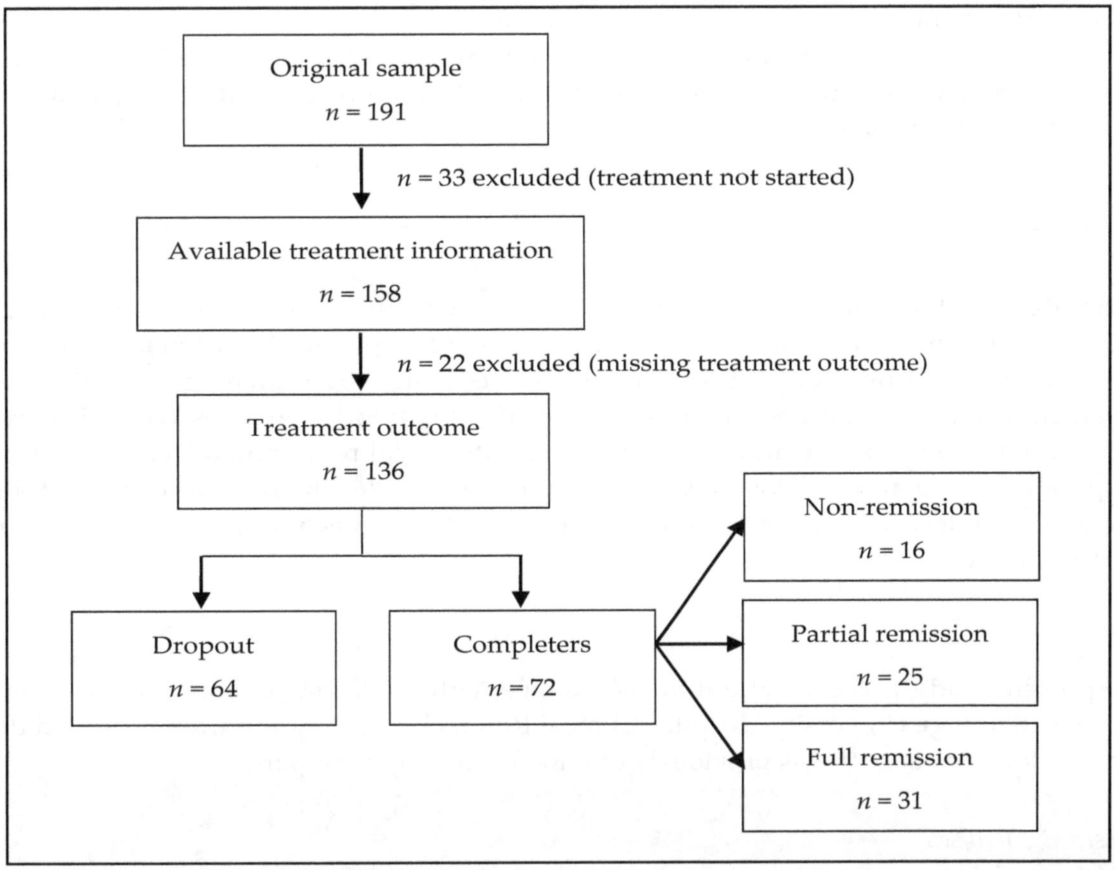

Figure 1. Flow chart for the sampling procedure.

Eating Disorders Inventory-2 (EDI-2) [31]: This self-report questionnaire consists of 91 items, answered on a 6-point Likert scale, that assess different cognitive and behavioral characteristics related to ED. The EDI-2 provides standardized subscale scores as well as a global measure of ED severity, which can be obtained based on the sum of all the items. A Spanish version of this questionnaire [32] has been validated and it obtained excellent psychometrical properties as an external global measure of ED severity. Internal consistency for the total score in this study was good (Cronbach's alpha $\alpha = 0.85$).

2.3. Treatment

As described elsewhere [33,34], all patients received cognitive behavioral therapy (CBT) at HUB, which was carried out by clinical psychology experts in the field. The CBT group therapy intervention for bulimia nervosa (BN), binge eating disorder (BED) and other specified feeding or eating disorders (OSFED) consisted of 16 weekly outpatient sessions lasting 90 minutes each and a follow-up period of about two years' duration that was carried out in a group format. Patients with BN first received six sessions of psychoeducational brief group therapy to offer information and psychoeducation about the negative consequences of BN. Patients diagnosed with anorexia nervosa (AN) completed a day hospital treatment program, which included two daily group CBT sessions during an average of 3 months. If they were severely underweight (IMC < 15 kg/m^2), they were offered an in-patient treatment with a maximum duration of three months. Patients with AN also had a two-year follow-up period with individual/group sessions. The goals of the treatment were to train patients to implement CBT strategies to reduce eating symptoms and to enable patients to acquire good healthy habits.

Patients were re-evaluated at discharge and categorized into the following three categories: full remission, partial remission and non-remission. According to DSM-5 criteria [28], the definition of full remission is a total absence of symptoms meeting diagnostic criteria for at least 4 consecutive weeks; partial remission is defined as a substantial symptomatic improvement but with residual symptoms; and patients who present poor outcomes are defined as non-remission. These categories were previously used to assess treatment outcome in threshold ED in other published studies [33,34]. Voluntary treatment discontinuation was categorized as dropout (i.e., not attending treatment for at least three consecutive sessions).

2.4. Follow-Up

A longitudinal follow-up of the patients was collected during an average period of 8.8 years (SD = 1.5), from the end of the first contact made in our unit to April 2020. This first contact coincided with the assessment using the ASRS screening questionnaire. By searching through centralized Catalonian clinical records and an online shared medical network, we assessed clinical evolution of all ED patients over the time, in terms of symptomatological remission (categorized as positive follow-up) or clinical non-remission of eating symptomatology (categorized as negative follow-up). From the total sample, clinical records were available for 123 patients, while 13 patients were missing (10.5% attrition rate).

2.5. Ethics

The present study was carried out in accordance with the latest version of the Declaration of Helsinki. The Bellvitge University Hospital Clinical Research Ethics Committee approved the study and signed informed consent was previously obtained from all participants.

2.6. Statistical Analyses

Stata16 for Windows was used to carry out statistical analyses [35]. A comparison between the groups defined by the risk of dropout during the CBT (yes/no) and the classification of the therapy outcome (full/partial remission versus dropout/non-remission) was done with a chi-square test (χ^2).

Survival function (Kaplan–Meier product-limit estimator) modeled the rate of dropout during the therapy. This procedure is usually used to describe the probability of the patients "living/surviving" for a certain amount of time after one concrete intervention [36]. In this study, "surviving" was defined for patients without dropout after the beginning of the CBT.

Path analyses assessed the potential mediational role of the ED severity level (EDI-2 total score) in the relationship between ADHD and treatment outcome (i.e., therapy outcome after a CBT treatment and dropout rate during treatment). This procedure was defined in this work as a case of structural equation modeling (SEM), with the maximum-likelihood estimation method of parameter estimation, adjusting by the covariates participants' age and the duration of the ED. The goodness-of-fit was evaluated using a standard statistical test, and it was considered adequate fitting for [37]: non-significant result ($p > 0.05$) in the χ^2 test, root mean square error of approximation (RMSEA) < 0.08, Bentler's comparative fit index (CFI) > 0.90, Tucker–Lewis Index (TLI) > 0.90 and standardized root mean square residual (SRMR) < 0.10. In this study, the relatively low sample size and the high correlations between the EDI-2 scores did not allow the SEM to be included in all the EDI-2 subscales registered for the participants (goodness-of-fit was not achieved).

3. Results

3.1. Characteristics of the Sample

No statistical differences between participants selected for the study and those excluded were found for marital status ($\chi^2 = 0.07, p = 0.982$), education level ($\chi^2 = 1.03, p = 0.317$), socioeconomic status ($\chi^2 = 2.67, p = 0.446$), age ($T = 1.04, p = 0.300$), duration of the eating problems ($T = 0.62, p = 0.535$), onset of the ED ($T = 0.70, p = 0.487$), ED-symptom levels ($T = 0.52, p = 0.603$) and ADHD-symptom levels ($T = 0.74, p = 0.462$).

Table 1 shows the descriptive for the sociodemographic and clinical variables of the final sample included in the study. All participants were women, with a mean age of 28.7 years (SD = 9.6), most were single (66.9%) and had achieved a secondary education level (61.0%). The number of patients within the ASRS positive screening group was n = 46 (point prevalence estimate equal to 33.8%). Regarding CBT outcomes, the dropout rate in the total sample was 47.0%, non-remission was registered for 11.8%, partial remission for 18.4% and full remission for 22.8%. Within the completers subsample (n = 72), non-remission was registered for 22.2% of the participants, partial remission for 34.7% and full remission for 43.1%.

Table 1. Descriptive for the sample (n = 136).

Sociodemographic		n	%	Therapy Outcomes	n	%
Marital	Single	91	66.9%	Total sample (n = 136)		
	Married/Partner	34	25.0%	Dropout	64	47.0%
	Divorced/Separated	11	8.1%	Non-remission	16	11.8%
Education	Primary	32	23.5%	Partial remission	25	18.4%
	Secondary	83	61.0%	Full remission	31	22.8%
	University	21	15.5%	Completers subsample (n = 72)		
Age and ED severity level		Mean	SD	Non-remission	16	22.2%
Chronological age (years)		28.74	9.59	Partial remission	25	34.7%
EDI-2 total score		97.91	44.52	Full remission	31	43.1%
ADHD (ASRS screening)		n	%			
Positive screening		46	33.8%			
Negative screening		90	66.2%			

Note. SD: standard deviation.

Table 2 includes the correlation matrix (Pearson correlation coefficients, R) between the ADHD level (measured through the ASRS scales) with the ED symptom level (EDI-2 scales). Due the strong relationship between the significance test for the correlation model and the sample size (high coefficients estimated in low samples sizes tend to show non-significance, while low coefficients tend to show significance obtained in samples with a large number of participants), Table 2 shows in bold the coefficients with an effect size that is in the moderate-mild ($|R| > 0.24$) to high-large range ($|R| > 0.37$). While moderate to high correlations were found between most EDI-2 scales, low correlation was found between ASRS inattention with hyperactive scores (R = 0.166). ASRS inattention positively correlated with all the EDI-2 scales, except for maturity fears, perfectionism and impulse regulation. ASRS hyperactivity also positively correlated with drive for thinness, body dissatisfaction, interoceptive awareness, impulse regulation and total. ASRS total correlated with all the EDI-2 scales (except for perfectionism), achieving the highest R-coefficient with the EDI-2 total (R = 0.497).

Table 2. Correlation matrix for the Adult ADHD Self-Report Scale (ASRS) and Eating Disorders Inventory (EDI-2) scores (n = 136).

		2	3	4	5	6	7	8	9	10	11	12	13	14	15
1.	ASRS: inattention	0.166	**0.882** †	**0.252** †	**0.356** †	**0.384** †	**0.287** †	**0.287** †	**0.425** †	0.183	0.033	0.220	**0.312** †	**0.419** †	**0.420** †
2.	ASRS: hyperactive	—	**0.609** †	**0.372** †	**0.282** †	**0.341** †	0.226	0.086	0.207	0.214	0.116	**0.336** †	0.210	0.149	**0.342** †
3.	ASRS: total		—	**0.379** †	**0.419** †	**0.474** †	**0.337** †	**0.267**	**0.438** †	**0.246** †	0.078	**0.337** †	**0.346** †	**0.402** †	**0.497** †
4.	EDI-2: Drive.thinness			—	**0.622** †	**0.582** †	**0.367** †	**0.341**	**0.483** †	**0.297** †	**0.339** †	**0.364** †	**0.628** †	**0.440** †	**0.720** †
5.	EDI-2: Body.dissatisf.				—	**0.503** †	**0.483** †	**0.383**	**0.596** †	**0.283** †	0.211	**0.429** †	**0.506** †	**0.457** †	**0.751** †
6.	EDI-2: Interoc.awar.					—	**0.508** †	**0.500**	**0.700** †	**0.371** †	**0.305** †	**0.604** †	**0.666** †	**0.637** †	**0.838** †
7.	EDI-2: Bulimia						—	0.238	**0.430** †	0.032	0.056	**0.385** †	**0.486** †	**0.262** †	**0.562** †
8.	EDI-2: Interp.distrust							—	**0.561** †	**0.306** †	0.168	**0.347** †	**0.385** †	**0.697** †	**0.626** †
9.	EDI-2: Ineffectiveness								—	**0.503** †	**0.296** †	**0.568** †	**0.650** †	**0.749** †	**0.865** †
10.	EDI-2: Maturity fears									—	**0.277** †	**0.366** †	**0.279** †	**0.496** †	**0.549** †
11.	EDI-2: Perfectionism										—	**0.331** †	**0.314** †	**0.299** †	**0.438** †
12.	EDI-2: Impulse.regul.											—	**0.541** †	**0.576** †	**0.717** †
13.	EDI-2: Ascetic												—	**0.503** †	**0.768** †
14.	EDI-2: Social.insec.													—	**0.790** †
15.	EDI-2: Total score														—

Note. † Correlation with effect size in the moderate-mild (|R| > 0.24) to high-large range (|R| > 0.37).

The ADHD level was not directly related to the short-term therapy outcomes in the study; the prevalence of the ASRS positive screening score was statistically equal for completers and dropouts, as well as for participants with partial remission and full remission versus those with dropout and non-remission (Table 3). No association was found even when stratified by the diagnostic subtype (Supplementary Table S1). Regarding data registered after the follow-up, neither was there any statistical association found between the ASRS positive screening with therapy outcome.

Table 3. Description of ADHD measures within the groups defined by the short term therapy outcomes (n = 136) and the follow-up (n = 123).

Treatment Outcome	Completers (n = 72)		Dropout (n = 64)		p
ADHD screening (+); n-%	25	34.7%	21	32.8%	0.814
Short-term therapy outcome	Full/partial remission (n = 56)		Dropout/non-remission (n = 80)		p
ADHD screening (+); n-%	21	37.5%	25	31.3%	0.448
Outcome at follow-up	Remission (n = 87)		Non-remission (n = 36)		p
ADHD screening (+); n-%	29	33.3%	12	33.3%	1.00

Figure 2 includes the cumulate survival function for the time to dropout. The higher proportion of dropouts was registered during the two weeks after the beginning of the treatment (12.1% for the total sample), followed by the next two weeks (at the end of the first month 24.1% had followed). No statistical contribution was found between ASRS score with the rate to dropout (log rank test = 0.01, p = 0.995).

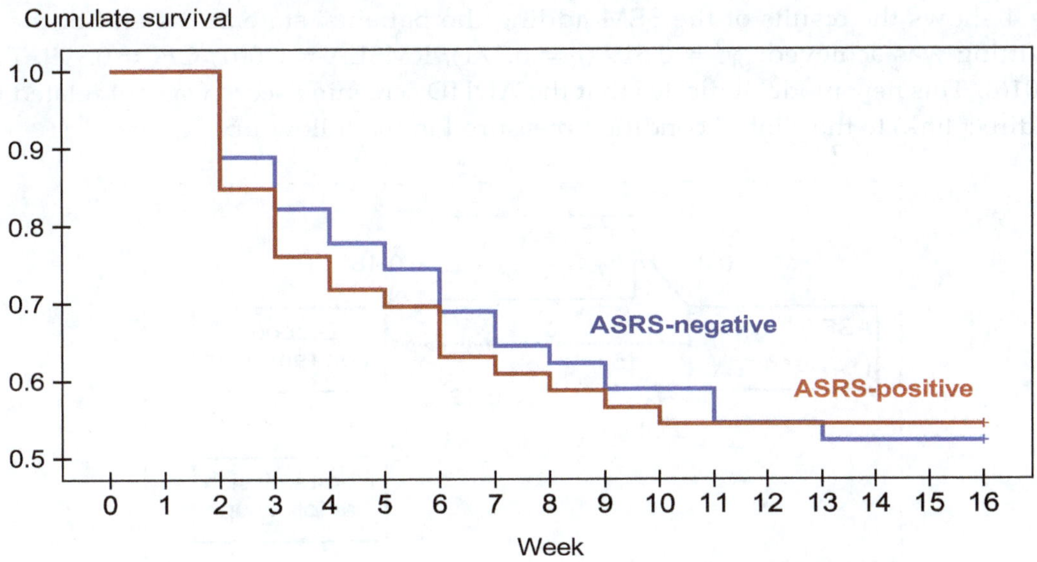

Figure 2. Survival function for dropout (n = 136).

Supplementary Table S2 includes the associations between the ADHD levels (registered in the ASRS inattention, hyperactivity and total score) and the ED symptom levels (registered in the EDI-2 scores) with the treatment outcomes (during therapy, at short-term and in the follow-up). No statistical differences were found comparing the mean scores in the ASRS and the EDI-2 between the groups of the study.

3.2. Path Analysis

Figure 3 shows the results of the SEM assessing the mediational link of the ED severity into the relationship between ADHD and the CBT outcomes. Goodness of fit was achieved for both models (risk of dropout: χ^2 = 0.807 (p = 0.848), RMSEA = 0.001, CFI = 0.999, TLI = 0.998, SRMR = 0.015;

better CBT outcome: $\chi^2 = 0.029$ ($p = 0.864$), RMSEA = 0.001, CFI = 0.999, TLI = 0.998, SRMR = 0.004). These results confirmed the indirect effect of ADHD on the therapy outcome; being in the ASRS positive screening group is related to higher ED severity (higher EDI-2 total), and this worse ED level contributed to the increase in the risk of dropout and a worse treatment outcome.

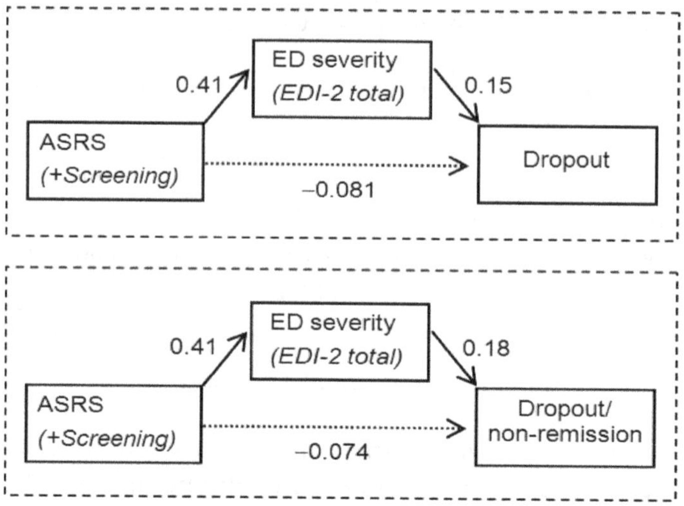

Figure 3. Path-diagrams: standardized coefficients in the SEM for the short-term therapy outcome ($n = 136$). Continuous line: significant coefficient. Dash line: non-significant coefficient. Results adjusted by age and duration of the ED.

Figure 4 shows the results of the SEM adding the patients' state at the end of the follow-up (adequate fitting was achieved: $\chi^2 = 0.519$ ($p = 0.771$), RMSEA = 0.001, CFI = 0.999, TLI = 0.998, SRMR = 0.016). This new model indicates that the ADHD screening score was not related (through a direct or indirect link) to the clinical condition measured in the follow-up.

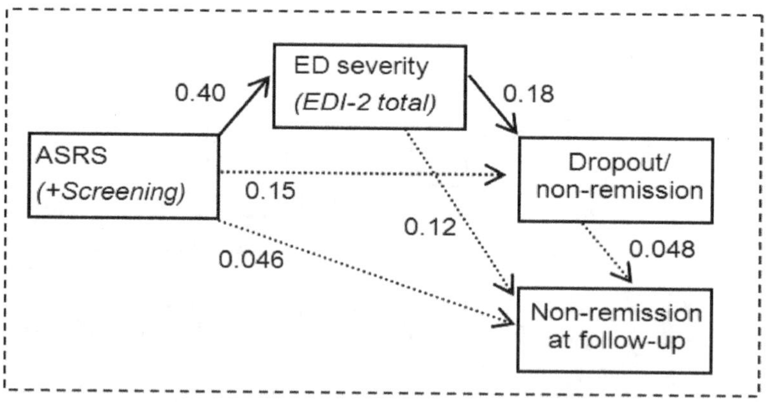

Figure 4. Path-diagrams: standardized coefficients in the SEM for the follow-up ($n = 123$). Continuous line: significant coefficient. Dash line: non-significant coefficient. Results adjusted by age and duration of the ED.

4. Discussion

This study investigated whether the presence of ADHD symptoms in patients with EDs may impact treatment outcome and dropout for EDs. The second aim was to examine the influence of EDs severity on the relationship between ADHD symptoms and treatment outcome/dropout rate. Finally, a long-term follow-up was included to assess the effect of ADHD symptoms at baseline on the clinical evolution of EDs.

ADHD screening at baseline did not directly predict treatment outcome or dropout rate in patients attending a CBT for EDs. However, our results highlighted that the severity of eating symptomatology mediates the relation between ADHD and treatment outcome/dropout rate. Specifically, positive screening for ADHD symptoms was directly associated with the severity of EDI-2, which in turn is related to a higher dropout rate and a worse treatment outcome, in terms of dropout during treatment and non-remission of ED symptomatology.

The only previous study investigating the effect of ADHD over treatment for ED suggested that patients with higher ADHD symptoms presented a higher risk of poor post-treatment outcome, although the impact of ED severity on this relation was not assessed [26]. Interestingly, a high dropout from treatment was also reported in that study (61%), further suggesting the importance of taking into account dropout as a negative outcome of ED treatment. Considering that patients with ADHD tend to act impulsively, they may be more likely to abandon treatment, although limited information has been reported linking the effect of ADHD symptomatology in the treatment of comorbid psychopathology, in terms of dropout. These studies were mostly focused on substance use disorder (SUD), such as tobacco [38] or cocaine [39–41]. When SUD and ADHD are co-morbid, some factors seem to increase the risk of dropout, including: disruptive behaviors related to ADHD [40], cognitive deficit (e.g., executive dysfunctions) and the type of substance of abuse [41]. Concerning EDs, this is the first study suggesting that higher severity of EDs and co-occurring ADHD symptoms increase the risk of dropout.

In spite of the higher proportion of dropouts registered within the first two weeks of treatment, the ASRS score does not differ between early or later dropout, suggesting that ADHD symptoms may increase the dropout rate at different stages of treatment. Furthermore, we included a longer follow-up of the majority of the patients, showing that positive screening for ADHD symptoms at baseline did not affect the longer terms evolution of EDs. This is the first retrospective study which allows the evaluation of the impact of ADHD symptoms on EDs with a longitudinal follow-up of roughly 8 years.

This study must be interpreted in light of its limitations. First, a self-reporting instrument was used to measure the frequency of adult ADHD symptoms, which may lead to an overestimation of this symptomatology. Therefore, future studies should focus on EDs patients with comorbidity with ADHD, not only taking into account ADHD symptomatology. Furthermore, comorbidity with others psychiatric disorders often associated with EDs (e.g., anxiety, depression) should be addressed by future studies in larger samples. Second, only female EDs patients were included in this study, so further studies would benefit from including male population as men report a higher prevalence of ADHD in adult life [42]. Third, it would have been advisable to have objective measures available after the follow-up. Finally, the retrospective nature of the design should be considered.

In conclusion, the present findings suggest a higher risk for dropout of treatment (i.e., CBT for EDs) and worse treatment outcomes in patients with more severe ED-symptoms, and an indirect effect of ADHD symptomatology on the treatment outcomes mediated by the ED severity levels. This was the first study to examine the effect of ADHD over the risk of dropout in patients treated for EDs, suggesting the relevance of identifying specific treatment approaches for patients with greater degrees of ADHD symptoms and severe EDs.

Author Contributions: G.T., I.B. and C.V.-A. contributed to the conceptualization and writing of the present study; S.J.-M. and F.F.-A. supervised the study; R.G. performed the formal analysis; Z.A., I.B., I.S. and N.R. aided with data collection and also with the interpretation of data; G.T. and I.B. shared first authorship. All authors have read and agreed to the published version of the manuscript.

Acknowledgments: We thank the CERCA Programme/Generalitat de Catalunya for institutional support.

References

1. Bleck, J.; DeBate, R.D. Exploring the co-morbidity of attention-deficit/hyperactivity disorder with eating disorders and disordered eating behaviors in a nationally representative community-based sample. *Eat. Behav.* **2013**, *14*, 390–393. [CrossRef] [PubMed]

2. Mikami, A.Y.; Hinshaw, S.P.; Patterson, K.A.; Lee, J.C. Eating Pathology Among Adolescent Girls With Attention-Deficit/Hyperactivity Disorder. *J. Abnorm. Psychol.* **2008**, *117*, 225–235. [CrossRef]
3. Mikami, A.Y.; Hinshaw, S.P.; Arnold, L.E.; Hoza, B.; Hechtman, L.; Newcorn, J.H.; Abikoff, H.B. Bulimia nervosa symptoms in the multimodal treatment study of children with ADHD. *Int. J. Eat. Disord.* **2010**, *43*, 248–259. [CrossRef]
4. Nazar, B.P.; Pinna, C.M.D.S.; Coutinho, G.; Segenreich, D.; Duchesne, M.; Appolinario, J.C.; Mattos, P. Review of literature of attention-deficit/hyperactivity disorder with comorbid eating disorders. *Rev. Bras. Psiquiatr.* **2008**, *30*, 384–389. [CrossRef]
5. Blinder, B.J.; Cumella, E.J.; Sanathara, V.A. Psychiatric comorbidities of female inpatients with eating disorders. *Psychosom. Med.* **2006**, *68*, 454–462. [CrossRef]
6. Farber, S.K. The Comorbidity of Eating Disorders and Attention-Deficit Hyperactivity Disorder. *Eat. Disord.* **2009**, *18*, 81–89. [CrossRef] [PubMed]
7. Stulz, N.; Hepp, U.; Gächter, C.; Martin-Soelch, C.; Spindler, A.; Milos, G. The severity of ADHD and eating disorder symptoms: A correlational study. *BMC Psychiatry* **2013**, *13*, 44. [CrossRef] [PubMed]
8. Svedlund, N.E.; Norring, C.; Ginsberg, Y.; von Hausswolff-Juhlin, Y. Symptoms of Attention Deficit Hyperactivity Disorder (ADHD) among adult eating disorder patients. *BMC Psychiatry* **2017**, *17*, 19. [CrossRef]
9. Wentz, E.; Lacey, J.H.; Waller, G.; Råstam, M.; Turk, J.; Gillberg, C. Childhood onset neuropsychiatric disorders in adult eating disorder patients. *Eur. Child. Adolesc. Psychiatry* **2005**, *14*, 431–437. [CrossRef]
10. Yates, W.R.; Lund, B.C.; Johnson, C.; Mitchell, J.; McKee, P. Attention-deficit hyperactivity symptoms and disorder in eating disorder inpatients. *Int. J. Eat. Disord.* **2009**, *42*, 375–378. [CrossRef]
11. Reinblatt, S.P.; Leoutsakos, J.-M.S.; Mahone, E.M.; Forrester, S.; Wilcox, H.C.; Riddle, M.A. Association between binge eating and attention-deficit/hyperactivity disorder in two pediatric community mental health clinics. *Int. J. Eat. Disord.* **2015**, *48*, 505–511. [CrossRef] [PubMed]
12. Levin, R.L.; Rawana, J.S. Attention-deficit/hyperactivity disorder and eating disorders across the lifespan: A systematic review of the literature. *Clin. Psychol. Rev.* **2016**, *50*, 22–36. [CrossRef] [PubMed]
13. Sonneville, K.R.; Calzo, J.P.; Horton, N.J.; Field, A.E.; Crosby, R.D.; Solmi, F.; Micali, N. Childhood hyperactivity/inattention and eating disturbances predict binge eating in adolescence. *Psychol. Med.* **2015**, *45*, 2511–2520. [CrossRef] [PubMed]
14. Nazar, B.P.; de Sousa Pinna, C.M.; Suwwan, R.; Duchesne, M.; Freitas, S.R.; Sergeant, J.; Mattos, P. ADHD Rate in Obese Women With Binge Eating and Bulimic Behaviors From a Weight-Loss Clinic. *J. Atten. Disord.* **2016**, *20*, 610–616. [CrossRef]
15. Sepúlveda, A.R.; Solano, S.; Blanco, M.; Lacruz, T.; Veiga, O. Feasibility, acceptability, and effectiveness of a multidisciplinary intervention in childhood obesity from primary care: Nutrition, physical activity, emotional regulation, and family. *Eur. Eat. Disord. Rev.* **2020**, *28*, 184–198. [CrossRef]
16. Mestre-Bach, G.; Steward, T.; Potenza, M.N.; Granero, R.; Fernández-Aranda, F.; Mena-Moreno, T.; Magaña, P.; Vintró-Alcaraz, C.; del Pino-Gutiérrez, A.; Menchón, J.M.; et al. The Role of ADHD Symptomatology and Emotion Dysregulation in Gambling Disorder. *J. Atten. Disord.* **2019**, 108705471989437. [CrossRef]
17. Aymamí, N.; Jiménez-Murcia, S.; Granero, R.; Ramos-Quiroga, J.A.; Fernández-Aranda, F.; Claes, L.; Sauvaget, A.; Grall-Bronnec, M.; Gómez-Peña, M.; Savvidou, L.G.; et al. Clinical, Psychopathological, and Personality Characteristics Associated with ADHD among Individuals Seeking Treatment for Gambling Disorder. *Res. Artic. Clin.* **2015**. [CrossRef]
18. Yao, S.; Kuja-Halkola, R.; Martin, J.; Lu, Y.; Lichtenstein, P.; Hübel, C.; Almqvist, C.; Magnusson, P.K.; Bulik, C.M.; Larsson, H.; et al. Associations Between Attention-Deficit/Hyperactivity Disorder and Various Eating Disorders: A Swedish Nationwide Population Study Using Multiple Genetically Informative Approaches. *Biol. Psychiatry* **2019**, *86*, 577–586. [CrossRef]
19. Fernández-Aranda, F.; Agüera, Z.; Castro, R.; Jiménez-Murcia, S.; Ramos-Quiroga, J.A.; Bosch, R.; Fagundo, A.B.; Granero, R.; Penelo, E.; Claes, L.; et al. ADHD symptomatology in eating disorders: A secondary psychopathological measure of severity? *BMC Psychiatry* **2013**, *13*, 166. [CrossRef]
20. Barkley, R.A.; Murphy, K.; Kwasnik, D. Psychological adjustment and adaptive impairments in young adults with ADHD. *J. Atten. Disord.* **1996**, *1*, 41–54. [CrossRef]
21. Schredl, M.; Alm, B.; Sobanski, E. Sleep quality in adult patients with attention deficit hyperactivity disorder (ADHD). *Eur. Arch. Psychiatry Clin. Neurosci.* **2007**, *257*, 164–168. [CrossRef]

22. Malloy-Diniz, L.; Fuentes, D.; Leite, W.B.; Correa, H.; Bechara, A. Impulsive behavior in adults with attention deficit/hyperactivity disorder: Characterization of attentional, motor and cognitive impulsiveness. *J. Int. Neuropsychol. Soc. JINS* **2007**. [CrossRef]
23. Scheres, A.; Lee, A.; Sumiya, M. Temporal reward discounting and ADHD: Task and symptom specific effects. *J. Neural. Transm.* **2008**, *115*, 221–226. [CrossRef] [PubMed]
24. Donfrancesco, R.; Di Trani, M.; Porfirio, M.C.; Giana, G.; Miano, S.; Andriola, E. Might the temperament be a bias in clinical study on attention-deficit hyperactivity disorder (ADHD)?: Novelty Seeking dimension as a core feature of ADHD. *Psychiatry Res.* **2015**, *227*, 333–338. [CrossRef] [PubMed]
25. Valko, L.; Doehnert, M.; Müller, U.C.; Schneider, G.; Albrecht, B.; Drechsler, R.; Maechler, M.; Steinhausen, H.C.; Brandeis, D. Differences in neurophysiological markers of inhibitory and temporal processing deficits in children and adults with ADHD. *J. Psychophysiol.* **2009**, *23*, 235–246. [CrossRef]
26. Svedlund, N.E.; Norring, C.; Ginsberg, Y.; von Hausswolff-Juhlin, Y. Are treatment results for eating disorders affected by ADHD symptoms? A one-year follow-up of adult females. *Eur. Eat. Disord. Rev.* **2018**, *26*, 337–345. [CrossRef]
27. American Psychiatric Association. *Diagnostic and Statistical Manual of Mental Disorders*, 4th ed.; American Psychiatric Association: Washington, DC, USA, 2000.
28. APA American Psychiatric Association. *Diagnostic and Statistical Manual of Mental Disorders*, 5th ed.; American Psychiatric Association: Washington, DC, USA, 2013.
29. Kessler, R.C.; Adler, L.; Ames, M.; Demler, O.; Faraone, S.; Hiripi, E.; Howes, M.J.; Jin, R.; Secnik, K.; Spencer, T.; et al. The World Health Organization adult ADHD self-report scale (ASRS): A short screening scale for use in the general population. *Psychol. Med.* **2005**, *35*, 245–256. [CrossRef] [PubMed]
30. Ramos-Quiroga, J.A.; Daigre, C.; Valero, S.; Bosch, R.; Gómez-Barros, N.; Nogueira, M.; Palomar, G.; Roncero, C.; Casas, M. Validation of the Spanish version of the attention deficit hyperactivity disorder adult screening scale (ASRS v. 1.1): A novel scoring strategy. *Rev. Neurol.* **2009**, *48*, 449–452. [CrossRef] [PubMed]
31. Garner, D.M. *Inventario de Trastornos de la Conducta Alimentaria (EDI-2)-Manual*; TEA: Madrid, Spain, 1998.
32. Corral, S.; González, M.; Pereña, J.; Seisdedos, N. *Adaptación española del Inventario de trastornos de la conducta alimentaria, Inventario de Trastornos de la Conducta Alimentaria*; TEA: Madrid, Spain, 1998.
33. Agüera, Z.; Sánchez, I.; Granero, R.; Riesco, N.; Steward, T.; Martín-Romera, V.; Jiménez-Murcia, S.; Romero, X.; Caroleo, M.; Segura-García, C.; et al. Short-Term Treatment Outcomes and Dropout Risk in Men and Women with Eating Disorders. *Eur. Eat. Disord. Rev.* **2017**, *25*, 293–301. [CrossRef] [PubMed]
34. Riesco, N.; Agüera, Z.; Granero, R.; Jiménez-Murcia, S.; Menchón, J.M.; Fernández-Aranda, F. Other Specified Feeding or Eating Disorders (OSFED): Clinical heterogeneity and cognitive-behavioral therapy outcome. *Eur. Psychiatry* **2018**, *54*, 109–116. [CrossRef]
35. *StataCorp Stata Statistical Software*, Release 16; StataCorp LLC: College Station, TX, USA, 2019.
36. Singer, J.D.; Willett, J.B.; Willett, J.B. *Applied Longitudinal Data Analysis: Modeling Change and Event Occurrence*; Oxford University Press: New York, NY, USA, 2003.
37. Barrett, P. Structural equation modelling: Adjudging model fit. *Pers. Individ. Dif.* **2007**, *42*, 815–824. [CrossRef]
38. Bidwell, L.C.; Karoly, H.C.; Hutchison, K.E.; Bryan, A.D. ADHD symptoms impact smoking outcomes and withdrawal in response to Varenicline treatment for smoking cessation. *Drug Alcohol Depend.* **2017**, *179*, 18–24. [CrossRef] [PubMed]
39. Carroll, K.M.; Rounsaville, B.J. History and significance of childhood attention deficit disorder in treatment-seeking cocaine abusers. *Compr. Psychiatry* **1993**, *34*, 75–82. [CrossRef]
40. Sullivan, M.A.; Rudnik-Levin, F. Attention Deficit/Hyperactivity Disorder and Substance Abuse. *Ann. N. Y. Acad. Sci.* **2006**, *931*, 251–270. [CrossRef]
41. Van Emmerik-van Oortmerssen, K.; Blankers, M.; Vedel, E.; Kramer, F.; Goudriaan, A.E.; van den Brink, W.; Schoevers, R.A. Prediction of drop-out and outcome in integrated cognitive behavioral therapy for ADHD and SUD: Results from a randomized clinical trial. *Addict. Behav.* **2020**, *103*, 106228. [CrossRef] [PubMed]
42. Faraone, S.V.; Biederman, J. What is the prevalence of adult ADHD? Results of a population screen of 966 adults. *J. Atten. Disord.* **2005**, *9*, 384–391. [CrossRef] [PubMed]

6

Emotion Recognition Abilities in Adults with Anorexia Nervosa are Associated with Autistic Traits

Jess Kerr-Gaffney [1], Luke Mason [2], Emily Jones [2], Hannah Hayward [3], Jumana Ahmad [4], Amy Harrison [5,6], Eva Loth [3], Declan Murphy [3] and Kate Tchanturia [1,6,7,*]

1 Department of Psychological Medicine, Institute of Psychiatry, Psychology and Neuroscience, King's College London, London SE5 8AB, UK; jess.kerr-gaffney@kcl.ac.uk
2 Centre for Brain & Cognitive Development, Birkbeck, University of London, London WC1E 7JL, UK
3 Department of Forensic & Neurodevelopmental Sciences, Institute of Psychiatry, Psychology and Neuroscience, King's College London, London SE5 8AB, UK
4 School of Human Sciences, University of Greenwich, London SE10 9LS, UK
5 Department of Psychology and Human Development, University College London, London WC1H 0AA, UK
6 South London and Maudsley NHS Trust, National Eating Disorders Service, Psychological Medicine Clinical Academic Group, London SE5 8AZ, UK
7 Department of Psychology, Ilia State University, Tbilisi 0162, Georgia
* Correspondence: kate.tchanturia@kcl.ac.uk

Abstract: Difficulties in socio-emotional functioning are proposed to contribute to the development and maintenance of anorexia nervosa (AN). This study aimed to examine emotion recognition abilities in individuals in the acute and recovered stages of AN compared to healthy controls (HCs). A second aim was to examine whether attention to faces and comorbid psychopathology predicted emotion recognition abilities. The films expressions task was administered to 148 participants (46 AN, 51 recovered AN, 51 HC) to assess emotion recognition, during which attention to faces was recorded using eye-tracking. Comorbid psychopathology was assessed using self-report questionnaires and the Autism Diagnostic Observation Schedule–2nd edition (ADOS-2). No significant differences in emotion recognition abilities or attention to faces were found between groups. However, individuals with a lifetime history of AN who scored above the clinical cut-off on the ADOS-2 displayed poorer emotion recognition performance than those scoring below cut-off and HCs. ADOS-2 scores significantly predicted emotion recognition abilities while controlling for group membership and intelligence. Difficulties in emotion recognition appear to be associated with high autism spectrum disorder (ASD) traits, rather than a feature of AN. Whether individuals with AN and high ASD traits may require different treatment strategies or adaptations is a question for future research.

Keywords: anorexia nervosa; ASD; comorbidity; emotion recognition; attention

---

1. Introduction

Anorexia nervosa (AN) is a severe psychiatric disorder characterised by an intense fear of weight gain, persistent behaviour to restrict energy intake, and a disturbance in the way one's body weight or shape are experienced [1]. Difficulties in social functioning have been identified as key factors in the development and maintenance of AN [2]. For example, before illness onset, individuals with AN report more social difficulties, fewer childhood friends, and engage in more solitary activities than healthy controls (HCs) [3–6]. During the illness, a variety of difficulties are seen, including high social anxiety, poorer social skills and social problem-solving abilities, loss of interest in social activities, and reduced social networks [7–14]. Given that interpersonal difficulties are associated with poorer outcomes in those with AN [15–17], it is important to understand potential underlying socio-cognitive mechanisms.

One area that has received considerable attention is emotion recognition. Given that up to two-thirds of human communication occurs through non-verbal means, recognising emotions from faces is considered key to successful social interaction [18]. Findings from studies in individuals with AN are mixed, with some reporting those with AN are significantly less accurate at inferring emotions from faces than HCs [19–22], and others reporting no differences [23–26]. A meta-analysis of 10 studies found that individuals with AN were significantly poorer at recognising basic and complex emotions relative to HCs, with small-to-medium and large effect sizes, respectively [27]. Given the effects of starvation on higher level cognitive processes, it is important to establish whether these effects may be a result of the ill state in AN. However, very few studies have examined emotion recognition performance in those recovered from AN, and results are equally mixed. While some report performance similar to that of HCs [28], others have reported poorer emotion recognition abilities, similar to those who are acutely unwell [20,29]. It is therefore not known whether potential differences in emotion recognition abilities are a result of the ill state in AN. However, one study found that emotion recognition difficulties were also present in unaffected twins of those with AN, suggesting that difficulties in this domain might represent an endophenotype for the disorder [30].

Clinical presentation of AN is associated with high levels of depression [31], anxiety [32], alexithymia [7], and autism spectrum disorder (ASD) traits [33], factors which by themselves may alter social-cognitive abilities. It is therefore possible that comorbid psychopathology might moderate emotion recognition abilities in those with AN. Although few studies have directly investigated this issue, a few have examined the impact of alexithymia. Alexithymia is a sub-clinical trait also present within the general population, describing an inability to recognise or describe one's own emotions. When matched for levels of alexithymia, individuals with AN or bulimia nervosa (BN) have been found to show similar emotion recognition abilities to HCs [34,35], suggesting that emotion recognition difficulties may be attributable to alexithymia rather than the eating disorder (ED) per se. However, the use of mixed ED groups and small sample sizes limit interpretation of the results for AN specifically. Given the profound effects of ASD on social cognitive abilities, it is perhaps surprising that very few studies have examined the impact of ASD traits on emotion recognition in individuals with AN. Dinkler and colleagues [28] reported that individuals recovered from AN with comorbid ASD were more accurate at recognising low intensity emotional expressions than those without ASD, who did not differ from HCs. However, due to the very small sample size in the AN+ASD group ($n = 6$), analyses were treated as exploratory only. Nonetheless, these findings support the proposition that AN with or without comorbid ASD may be two qualitatively different forms of the illness [36].

Another variable that has received little attention in emotion recognition research in AN is social attention. Attending to nonverbal social cues provided by others, such as eye gaze, gestures, and facial expressions, is a necessary precursor to higher-order social cognitive abilities such as emotion recognition [37]. In typical human development, social information in the environment is highly salient, and stimuli such as faces and eyes hold particular importance [38]. This attentional bias towards social information is demonstrated from infancy, and reductions in this capacity are among one of the first signs of socio-communicative disorders such as ASD [39]. There is also emerging evidence to suggest that individuals with AN show reduced attention to faces [40] and eyes [41]. Reduced attention to facial features has been found to predict the degree of emotion recognition impairment and lower social competence in individuals with ASD [37,42,43], however only a few studies have measured attention during emotion recognition in individuals with AN. Phillipou and colleagues [44] demonstrated that while individuals with AN and HCs did not differ in their ability to recognise basic emotions, AN displayed more fixations of shorter duration to faces, indicating a "hyperscanning" strategy. Unfortunately, this study did not examine whether eye movements were associated with emotion recognition performance. In a mixed ED sample (AN or BN), Fujiwara and colleagues [35] found that difficulties in emotion recognition were predicted by less visual attention to faces in those with an ED, but not in HCs. This raises the possibility that difficulties in emotion recognition sometimes associated with EDs are a result of differences in spontaneous social attention, rather than misinterpretation of emotional displays. Finally, Dinkler et al. [28] found no differences in eye movements between those recovered from AN and HCs, and accuracy was not associated with attention to facial features. Together, these findings suggest there may be differences in the relationship between emotion recognition and attention in the acute stage of AN compared to the recovered stage or those who have never had an ED. However, studies including an acute AN group (rather than AN and BN together) are required to test this hypothesis.

The current study aimed to examine emotion recognition performance in adults in the acute and recovered stages of AN compared to HCs. It has been suggested that difficulties in this area in those with AN may be more subtle and less detectable using basic emotions [27], therefore a paradigm allowing for assessment of both basic and complex emotion recognition was selected. In order to understand why individuals with AN might display emotion recognition deficits, a secondary aim was to examine whether visual attention to faces predicted emotion recognition performance. Relatedly, a third aim was to examine whether levels of comorbid psychopathology were associated with emotion recognition performance. As well as including measures of alexithymia and ASD traits, we included depression, anxiety, and social anxiety due to their high co-occurrence with AN [8,32,45] and potential effects on social cognition [46–51]. We hypothesised that individuals with AN would be less accurate at recognising complex emotions compared to HCs, and that those recovered from AN would show intermediate levels of performance. No significant differences in basic emotion recognition were predicted. Finally, we predicted that more attention to faces, as well as lower alexithymia and ASD traits would be associated with better emotion recognition performance.

2. Methods

Ethical approval was obtained from the National Health Service (NHS) Research Ethics Committee (Camberwell St Giles, 17/LO/1960).

2.1. Participants

All participants were required to be between 18 and 55 years old and fluent in English. Exclusion criteria were a history of brain trauma or learning disability. HC participants were recruited through a King's College London email circular and posters around campuses. Before taking part, HC participants were screened using the Structured Clinical Interview for DSM-5 Disorders, research version (SCID-5-RV) [52], to ensure they did not meet criteria for any psychiatric disorders. HCs were required to have a body mass index (BMI) between 19 and 27.

In addition to the university advertisements, participants with a lifetime history of AN were recruited through online advertisements (B-eat, call for participants, MQ Mental Health), and through two specialist NHS ED services in London. Participants were screened using the SCID-5-RV to confirm a current or past diagnosis of AN. Participants with AN were required to have a BMI ≤ 18.5 and recovered participants needed to have a BMI between 19 and 27.

2.2. Materials

The Films Expressions Task (FET) [53] is a facial emotion recognition task, modified to enable concurrent recording of eye movements. In each trial, participants are first presented with an emotion word on-screen. Three images are then presented for 500 ms each, one after another (with a 500 ms blank screen between images; see Figure 1). The height of each image was 15.7° at a viewing distance of 60 cm from the screen. The widths of each image were adjusted to ensure a correct aspect ratio and ranged from 12.4° to 21.4°. Images within each trial present the same actor displaying different emotional expressions (see Figure 2 for an example). Participants were then asked to indicate, as quickly and as accurately as they could, which of the images displayed the emotion word by pressing the corresponding key (1, 2, or 3). There were 53 trials in total (preceded by 3 practice trials). Prior to the task, participants were presented with a sheet listing the target emotion words and their definitions to ensure they were familiar with the words. A full list of the target emotion words is presented in the

Supplementary Materials. Images were from films made in non-English speaking countries to reduce the probability that participants would recognise the actors.

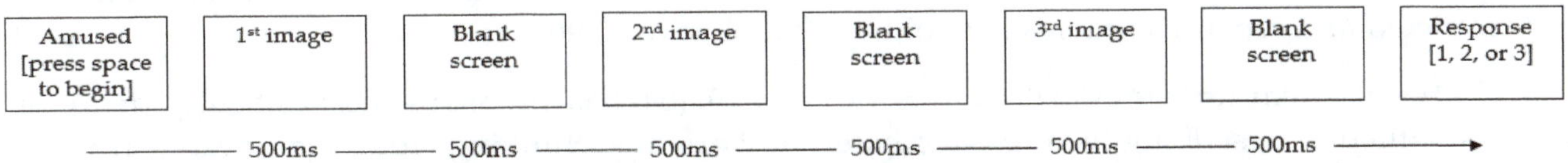

Figure 1. Sequence of events for an example trial of the films expression task.

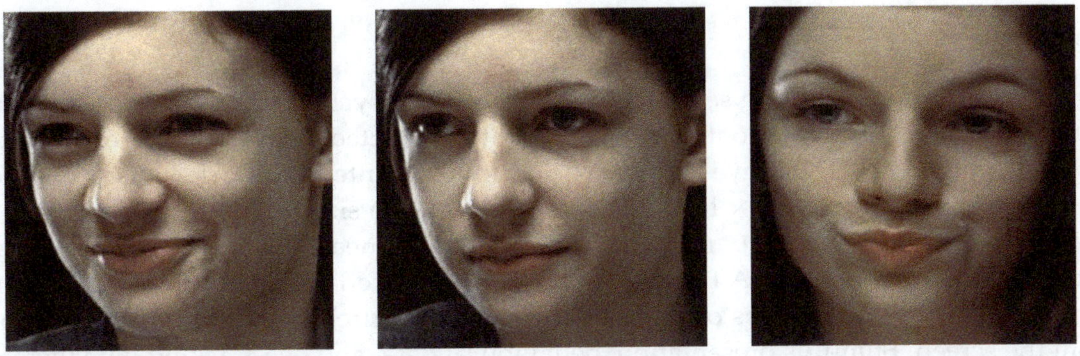

Figure 2. Images from an example trial [amused] of the films expression task.

The FET was chosen due to its depiction of naturalistic facial expressions; its inclusion of a range of both basic and complex emotions; and relatively brief presentation times. Basic and complex emotion trials were presented interleaved in a fixed random order. Foil emotional expressions were selected to be similar to the target emotion in terms of intensity of the expression and perceptual features. Development and validation of the test stimuli is presented in [53]. Dependent measures were: Accuracy (% of trials correct), mean RTs, and time spent looking at the stimuli (as a proportion of presentation time).

The Wechsler Abbreviated Scale of Intelligence, Second Edition (WASI-II) [54] measures verbal intelligence and perceptual reasoning, as well as full-scale IQ. The two subtest version was used (vocabulary and matrix reasoning).

The Autism Diagnostic Observation Schedule–2nd edition (ADOS-2), Module 4 [55] is a standardised semi-structured interview recommended for the assessment of ASD [56]. It includes a range of questions and activities designed to evoke behaviours and cognitions associated with ASD. Interviews were administered by the first author who received ADOS-2 training and met requirements for research reliability for module 4 and also attended reliability meetings throughout the study period. The revised algorithm, which was designed to more closely reflect the DSM-5 criteria for ASD was used for scoring [57]. The algorithm has two subscales: social affect and restrictive and repetitive behaviours, and total scores of 8 or more indicate possible ASD. The ADOS-2 was used in this study to identify participants with low or high ASD traits.

2.3. Questionnaires

The Eating Disorder Examination Questionnaire (EDE-Q) [58] measures severity of ED psychopathology. Global scores are calculated by averaging responses across items, with higher scores indicating more severe symptoms (max 6). HCs with a score of >2.7 were excluded from analyses to ensure those with possible sub-threshold ED symptoms were not included [59]. Cronbach's alpha was 0.93.

The Hospital Anxiety and Depression Scale (HADS) [60] is a 14-item scale with two subscales: anxiety and depression. Subscale scores are interpreted as: normal (0–7), mild (8–10), moderate (11–14), and severe (15–21). Cronbach's alpha was 0.93.

The Liebowitz Social Anxiety Scale (LSAS) [61] has two subscales: fear and avoidance of social situations. A score of 60 has been established as a cut-off indicative of social anxiety disorder (SAD) [62]. Cronbach's alpha was 0.97.

The Social Responsiveness Scale-2nd Edition, adult self-report form (SRS-2) [63] measures symptoms associated with ASD, with higher scores (max 195) indicating more autistic symptoms. There are 5 sub-scales: social awareness, social cognition, social communication, social motivation, and restricted and repetitive interests. Cronbach's alpha was 0.96.

The twenty-item Toronto Alexithymia Scale (TAS-20) [64] has three subscales: difficulty identifying feelings, difficulty describing feelings, and externally oriented thinking. Total scores range from 0 to 100, and cut-offs are as follows: ≤51 = no alexithymia; 52–60 = borderline alexithymia; and ≥61 = alexithymia [65]. Cronbach's alpha was 0.90.

2.4. Procedure

Participants attended a testing session at the Institute of Psychiatry, Psychology & Neuroscience. After written informed consent was obtained, participants completed the FET while their eye movements were recorded using a Tobii TX300 eye-tracker. The desktop mounted eye-tracker has a sampling rate of 300 Hz, a screen resolution of 1920 × 1080, and a diagonal screen size of 23". During tracking, infrared diodes generate reflections on the participant's retinas and corneas. From this reflection the angular rotation of each eye is estimated. A five-point calibration procedure relates this angular rotation to corresponding x and y coordinates on the screen surface. Participants were seated approximately 60 cm from the screen. Stimulus presentation, behavioural data, and eye-tracking data were managed and recorded using custom-written MATLAB software [66].

After the FET, the first author administered the WASI-II and the ADOS-2, and the participant completed the questionnaires. Weight and height measurements were taken to calculate BMI (weight/height^2). Participants were reimbursed £20 for their time.

2.5. Analysis

Histograms and Q-Q plots were inspected to check for normal distributions. Where variables were positively skewed, as was the case for RT and age data, a logarithmic transformation was applied. Homogeneity was assessed using Levene's test. Group differences in psychopathology and demographic information were assessed using one-way ANOVAs and Tukey's post-hoc tests, or Welch's ANOVA with Games-Howell post-hoc tests where the assumption of homogeneity was violated.

Group differences in FET accuracy and RT were assessed with two-way mixed ANOVAs, with the within-subjects factor emotion complexity (basic or complex) and the between-subjects factor group (AN, recovered AN (REC), HC). Although analyses were conducted on log-transformed RT values, medians and interquartile range for the untransformed variable are reported for ease of interpretation, as these are similar to the geometric means. Proportion of time spent looking at faces violated the assumptions of an ANOVA (non-normal distribution, strongly negatively skewed). Therefore, group differences were assessed using the nonparametric Kruskall-Wallis test, and the effects of emotion complexity were analysed using Wilcoxon signed rank tests, with the significance level adjusted for multiple comparisons (p <0.01). Effects of medication on FET outcome measures were examined using independent samples t-tests (or a Mann-Whitney U test in the case of the non-normally distributed time spent looking at faces), comparing those with past or current AN who were on medication to those who were not.

Spearman's correlations were run to examine relationships between emotion recognition performance (the primary outcome measure), demographic variables (age, IQ, BMI), psychopathology scores (EDE-Q, HADS anxiety and depression, LSAS, SRS-2, and TAS-20, ADOS-2 total), and proportion of time spent looking at faces. Variables that showed statistically significant relationships with emotion recognition performance were entered into a hierarchical regression analysis to determine which, if any, explained variance in the outcome measure.

3. Results

3.1. Demographics

In total, 148 participants were recruited (46 AN, 51 REC, 51 HC). Five HCs were subsequently excluded based on their EDE-Q scores and one REC participant was excluded due to a BMI > 27. Due to equipment failure on the day of testing, one AN and one REC participant could not complete the FET and were therefore excluded. Thus, data from 45 participants with AN, 49 REC, and 46 HC were analysed. Eye-tracking data from three HC and one REC participant was of low quality (excessive eye blinks) and was therefore excluded from analyses, however all other data (including FET accuracy and RT) from these participants was retained.

Demographic information and psychopathology scores are presented in Table 1. There were no significant group differences in age, IQ, years of education, or sex.

Table 1. Mean (SD) demographic information and psychopathology scores.

	AN (n = 45)	REC (n = 49)	HC (n = 46)	Test Statistics	p-Value	$\eta p^2/d$
Age (years) †	27.04 (8.92)	26.00 (8.10)	23.87 (4.52)	F (2, 85.23) = 2.16	0.12	0.02
% female	93.5	98.0	91.1	Fisher's exact test = 2.17	0.31	
BMI	15.75 (1.41) ^{a}	21.14 (1.91) ^{b}	21.69 (1.88) ^{b}	F (2, 136) = 159.75	**<0.001**	0.70
Years of education	16.06 (3.07)	16.52 (2.62)	16.63 (2.45)	F (2, 136) = 0.54	0.58	0.01
IQ	110.86 (12.29)	110.16 (10.38)	113.78 (7.25)	F (2, 85.30) = 2.18	0.12	0.02
Age diagnosed †	19.84 (7.39) ^{a}	16.41 (3.53) ^{b}	-	t (73.24) = 2.92	**0.01**	0.59
Illness length (years)	7.19 (7.88)	5.40 (5.65)	-	t (79.67) = 1.24	0.22	0.26
% on psychiatric medication	53.3 ^{a}	32.7 ^{b}	-	χ^2 = 4.10	**0.04**	
EDE-Q	3.86 (1.25) ^{a}	1.81 (1.52) ^{b}	0.61 (0.58) ^{c}	F (2, 75.81) = 125.35	**<0.001**	0.56
HADS-A	13.56 (4.51) ^{a}	10.84 (5.11) ^{b}	5.02 (3.09) ^{c}	F (2, 87.46) = 61.90	**<0.001**	0.40
HADS-D	9.87 (4.40) ^{a}	5.04 (4.02) ^{b}	1.54 (1.68) ^{c}	F (2, 76.50) = 77.66	**<0.001**	0.48
LSAS	68.95 (30.78) ^{a}	57.08 (29.98) ^{a}	27.91 (18.32) ^{b}	F (2, 84.80) = 36.34	**<0.001**	0.29
SRS-2	82.43 (31.99) ^{a}	70.04 (31.97) ^{a}	39.23 (20.18) ^{b}	F (2, 85.60) = 34.67	**<0.001**	0.28
TAS-20	58.16 (13.50) ^{a}	49.81 (15.08) ^{b}	37.47 (11.26) ^{c}	F (2, 136) = 26.86	**<0.001**	0.29
ADOS-2						
Total	4.67 (3.94) ^{a}	4.16 (4.50) ^{ab}	2.70 (2.52) ^{b}	F (2, 85.99) = 4.79	**0.01**	0.05
SA	4.02 (3.61) ^{a}	3.71 (3.96) ^{ab}	2.50 (2.38) ^{b}	F (2, 86.95) = 3.48	**0.04**	0.04
RRB	0.64 (1.00) ^{a}	0.45 (0.89) ^{ab}	0.20 (0.58) ^{b}	F (2, 86.10) = 3.82	**0.03**	0.05
% above clinical cut-off	17.8 ^{a,b}	24.5 ^{a}	4.3 ^{b}	χ^2 = 7.48	**0.02**	

ADOS-2: autism diagnostic observation schedule–2nd edition; AN: anorexia nervosa; BMI: body mass index; EDE-Q: eating disorder examination questionnaire; HADS-A: hospital anxiety and depression scale, anxiety subscale; HADS-D: hospital anxiety and depression scale, depression subscale; HC: healthy control; IQ: intelligence quotient; LSAS: Liebowitz social anxiety scale; REC: recovered anorexia nervosa; RRB: restrictive and repetitive behaviors; SA: social affect; SD: standard deviation; SRS-2: social responsiveness scale–2nd edition; TAS-20: twenty-item Toronto alexithymia scale. Different superscripts indicate significant differences between groups, significant p-values are highlighted in bold. † Variable was log transformed for analyses, original values are displayed.

3.2. Films Expression Task

Mean emotion recognition accuracy, RTs, and proportion of time spent looking at faces across groups are displayed in Table 2. A 3 (group: AN, REC, HC) × 2 (emotion complexity: basic, complex) mixed ANOVA was computed to examine group differences in emotion recognition accuracy (% correct) for basic and complex emotions. The interaction effect was not significant, though it did reach trend level, F (2, 137) = 2.43, p = 0.09, ηp^2 = 0.03. The main effect of emotion complexity was significant, F (1, 137) = 26.65, p <0.001, ηp^2 = 0.16, indicating accuracy was significantly higher for basic emotions (M = 89.34%, SD = 10.92%) than complex ones (M = 85.44%, SD = 10.19). The main effect of group was not significant, F (2, 132) = 1.10, p = 0.34, ηp^2 = 0.02. Accuracy (all faces) did not differ between medicated and unmedicated participants t (92) = 0.42, p = 0.67.

Table 2. Mean (SD) performance and attention during the films expression task.

	AN (n = 45)	REC (n = 49)	HC (n = 46)
Accuracy (% correct)			
Basic emotions	88.25 (11.61)	89.80 (12.88)	89.91 (7.62)
Complex emotions	84.10 (10.79)	84.09 (11.65)	88.18 (7.14)
Reaction time (ms) †			
Basic emotions	786.86 (546.32)	668.86 (415.61)	556.61 (352.43)
Complex emotions	875.69 (597.10)	703.59 (518.45)	662.13 (376.79)
Time spent looking at faces (%)			
Basic emotions	95.79 (5.85)	97.60 (2.79)	94.60 (8.23)
Complex emotions	96.54 (5.26)	97.81 (2.64)	94.37 (8.64)

AN: anorexia nervosa; HC: healthy control; REC: recovered anorexia nervosa; SD: standard deviation. † Variable was log transformed for analyses, median and IQR (of the untransformed variable) are displayed.

A 3 (group: AN, REC, HC) × 2 (emotion complexity: basic, complex) mixed ANOVA was computed to examine group differences in RTs for basic and complex emotions. The interaction effect was not significant, F (2, 132) = 0.86, p = 0.43, ηp^2 = 0.01. The main effect of emotion complexity was significant, F (1, 137) = 60.72, p <0.001, ηp^2 = 0.31, indicating RTs were significantly shorter for basic emotions (median = 654.14 ms, IQR = 464.68 ms) than complex ones (median = 718.29 ms, IQR = 474.55 ms). The main effect of group was not significant, F (2, 137) = 2.06, p = 0.13, ηp^2 = 0.03. RTs (all trials) did not differ between medicated and unmedicated participants, t (92) = −1.03, p = 0.31.

Kruskall-Wallis tests indicated there were no significant differences between groups in the proportion of time spent looking at faces displaying basic emotions, χ^2 (2) = 4.75, p = 0.09, or complex ones, χ^2 (2) = 4.61, p = 0.10. Wilcoxon signed-ranks tests indicated that time spent looking at basic versus complex emotions did not significantly differ within either of the three groups (all p >0.01, adjusted significance level for multiple comparisons). Proportion of time spent looking at faces (overall) did not differ between medicated and unmedicated participants, U = 980.00, p = 0.57.

3.3. Predicting Emotion Recognition Performance

In the whole sample, emotion recognition accuracy was significantly positively associated with the proportion of time spent looking at faces (r = 0.17, p = 0.04) and IQ (r = 0.23, p = 0.01), and negatively correlated with TAS-20 (r = −0.18, p = 0.04) and ADOS-2 scores (r = −0.17, p = 0.04) (see Supplementary Materials for full table of correlations). To establish whether the relationship between accuracy and attention to faces differed across groups, correlations were run for each of the three groups separately. Proportion of time spent looking at faces significantly correlated with emotion recognition accuracy in the AN group only (r = 0.34, p = 0.02). However, a linear regression showed that proportion of time spent looking at faces did not significantly predict emotion recognition abilities in those with AN, although the association did reach trend level, F (1, 42) = 3.36, p = 0.07, adjusted R^2 = 0.05. In the whole sample, a hierarchical multiple regression was run to determine if the addition of attention to faces, TAS-20, and ADOS-2 scores would improve the prediction of emotion recognition performance over group membership and IQ. The full model was significant, R^2 = 0.22, F (6, 126) = 5.95, p <0.001, adjusted R^2 = 0.18. Details of each regression model are shown in Table 3. The addition of ADOS-2 scores (model 3) led to a significant increase in R^2 of 0.11, F (1, 127) = 17.54, p <0.001. The addition of proportion of time spent looking at faces (model 2) and TAS-20 scores (model 4) did not significantly add to the prediction.

Table 3. Hierarchical regression analysis predicting emotion recognition accuracy from associated demographic variables and psychopathology scores.

	Model 1	Model 2	Model 3	Model 4
IQ	0.22 *	0.23 **	0.17 *	0.15
% of time spent looking at faces		0.17	0.10	0.11
ADOS-2			−0.35 ***	−0.31 ***
TAS-20				−0.14
R^2	0.07	0.10	0.21	0.22

ADOS-2: autism diagnostic observation schedule–2nd edition; IQ: intelligence quotient; TAS-20: twenty-item Toronto Alexithymia Scale. Figures shown are standardized coefficients. Group membership was entered in model 1 but was not significant and not displayed here. * $p < 0.05$; ** $p < 0.01$; *** $p < 0.001$.

3.4. ASD, Emotion Recognition Performance, and Attention to Faces

To further explore the relationship between ASD symptoms and emotion recognition performance, individuals with past or current AN were grouped according to whether they met the clinical cut-off for ASD on the ADOS-2 and compared with HCs. The two HCs who scored above cut-off on the ADOS-2 were excluded, due to their being too few cases to assess group differences. Thus, 44 HC, 20 lifetime AN scoring above the ADOS-2 cut-off (AN + ASD), and 74 lifetime AN scoring below the ADOS-2 cut-off (AN − ASD) were included in analyses.

A 3 (group: AN + ASD, AN − ASD, HC) × 2 (emotion complexity: basic, complex) mixed ANOVA was computed to examine group differences in emotion recognition accuracy (Figure 3). The interaction effect was not significant, though it did reach trend level, F (2, 135) = 2.70, $p = 0.07$, $\eta p^2 = 0.04$. The main effect of emotion complexity was significant, F (1, 135) = 23.13, $p < 0.001$, $\eta p^2 = 0.15$, indicating accuracy was significantly higher for basic emotions (M = 89.34%, SD = 10.99%) than complex ones (M = 85.49%, SD = 10.22). The main effect of group was also significant, F (2, 135) = 10.51, $p < 0.001$, $\eta p^2 = 0.14$, indicating AN + ASD (M = 77.36%, SD = 16.54%) were significantly less accurate at recognising emotions than AN − ASD (M = 87.58, SD = 7.36), and HCs (M = 88.85%, SD = 6.10%), who did not differ from one another. Kruskall-Wallis tests indicated there were no significant differences across groups in the proportion of time spent looking at faces displaying basic emotions χ^2 (2) = 2.06, $p = 0.36$, or complex ones, χ^2 (2) = 2.92, $p = 0.23$.

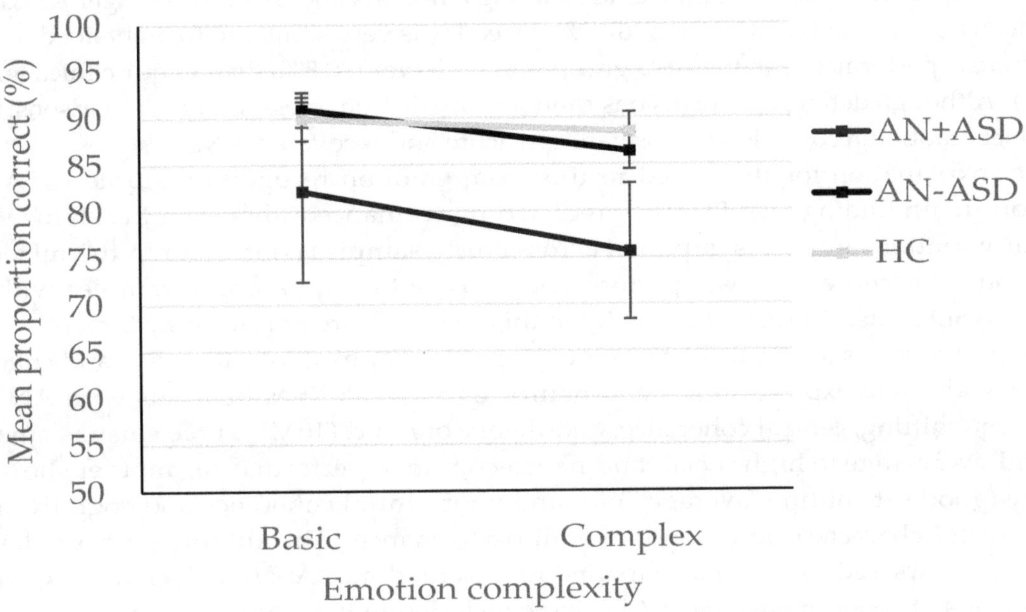

Figure 3. Mean proportion of correct trials on the films expression task. Error bars represent 95% confidence intervals. HC = healthy controls; AN + ASD = lifetime AN, above cut-off on the ADOS-2; AN − ASD = lifetime AN, below cut-off on the ADOS-2.

4. Discussion

The current study aimed to examine emotion recognition abilities in those with acute AN, REC, and HCs. Contrary to our hypotheses, there were no significant differences between groups in basic or complex emotion recognition. Our prediction that emotion recognition abilities would be associated with attention to faces, as well as alexithymia and ASD traits, was partially supported. Emotion recognition accuracy was significantly positively correlated with proportion of time spent looking at faces, and negatively correlated with alexithymia (TAS-20) and autistic features (ADOS-2 scores). However, in regression analyses, only ADOS-2 scores remained a significant predictor of emotion recognition performance while controlling for IQ and group membership. A subsequent analysis demonstrated that considering acute and recovered AN together, those who scored above the clinical cut-off for ASD on the ADOS-2 were significantly less accurate at recognising emotions than those who scored below the ADOS-2 cut off and HCs. These groups did not differ in the proportion of time spent looking at faces, suggesting differences in emotion recognition abilities were not due to differences in attention. Thus, in our sample of adults with a lifetime diagnosis of AN, difficulties in emotion recognition abilities appear to be associated with high ASD traits, rather than a feature of AN.

Our findings suggest that difficulties in emotion recognition are not a feature of the socio-emotional profile hypothesised to contribute to the maintenance of AN [2]. Although our results contrast with studies showing facial emotion recognition difficulties in acute and recovered AN [19,20,29,67], several studies have failed to detect significant differences between groups [23–25,68,69]. It is possible that the different emotion recognition tasks used across studies contribute to the mixed results. The FET was chosen for its relative difficulty; faces are presented for 500 ms only, stimuli are naturalistic facial expressions, and a wide range of complex emotions are included in addition to the six basic emotions. Nonetheless, given that accuracy was relatively high across groups, it may be the case that there were ceiling effects in our sample. This might be due to educational levels or IQ; participants were generally highly educated and mean IQ scores across groups were higher than the population average. Indeed, in the original pilot studies of the FET, distractors were only chosen if they were misidentified as the target emotion less than 30% of the time [53], possibly resulting in the high level of accuracy seen in our sample. It should be noted that the FET has not yet been validated in a normative sample, limiting comparisons with previous literature. However, a recent study using the FET found that individuals with ASD were significantly less accurate at identifying emotions and displayed longer RTs compared to HCs [70]. Mean accuracy in the HC group (87.5% correct) was very similar to that obtained in our sample (88.64%), whereas performance in the ASD group was far lower (70.8%) than in our clinical group (acute AN = 85.2%). Although definitive conclusions cannot be made from cross-study comparisons, this pattern supports intact emotion recognition performance in acute and recovered AN.

Another explanation for the mixed results from emotion recognition studies in AN concern another of our main findings: ASD traits predicted performance rather than ED status. It could be the case that variations in ASD symptoms across study samples contribute to the mixed findings, such that group differences in mean performance may not be apparent in samples with relatively low levels of ASD traits. To further investigate this issue, future studies may benefit from looking beyond group differences in social-cognitive performance. For example, Renwick and colleagues [36] used cluster analysis to explore social- and neuro-cognitive abilities in adults with AN, including measures of set-shifting, central coherence, and theory of mind (ToM). Three clusters emerged: One characterised by average to high social- and neuro-cognitive performance; another showing mixed performance (good set-shifting, average ToM, and poor central coherence and cognitive flexibility); and a final cluster characterised by poor overall performance. The authors propose that the third cluster, which comprised 17% of participants, represented an "ASD-like" cluster. Unfortunately, no diagnostic or self-report measures of ASD were included in the study, so is in not known whether these participants met diagnostic criteria for ASD. Nonetheless, this study demonstrates that distinct sub-groups within the overall diagnosis of AN may exist, potentially with different aetiologies and developmental pathways.

Although our cross-sectional design prevents conclusions regarding the differing developmental pathways that may characterise participants in the current study, recent research presents some interesting hypotheses. For example, individuals with ASD report sensory sensitivities and a limited range of acceptable foods, often from childhood [71,72]. Further, women with ASD report high levels of eating disturbances compared to both men with ASD and neurotypical women, particularly in regards to eating rituals, sensory sensitivity to the taste, smell, and texture of food, and difficulties around eating with others [73]. These difficulties may reinforce food restriction, resulting in energy deficits and a potential trigger for the development of a clinical ED in some individuals with ASD [74]. Another possible pathway through which EDs and ASD may co-occur is via interacting influences of body dissatisfaction and gender identity. There is emerging evidence to suggest that having ASD increases one's chances of experiencing gender dysphoria [75] and rejecting a binary gender identity [76]. In addition, qualitative reports from women with ASD often report conflict between expected feminine roles and their autistic identities [77]. At the same time, transgender individuals are at increased risk of body dissatisfaction and clinical EDs [78,79]. Specifically, restrictive eating and exercise can be a means of achieving a body congruent with one's gender identity [80]. These differing aetiological pathways and maintenance factors for EDs are likely to have important implications for treatment.

The findings from the current study have important clinical implications. In our sample, 17.8% of acute AN and 24.5% of REC scored above the clinical cut-off on the ADOS-2, compared to 4.3% of HCs. Similar findings have been reported previously [69,81]. Interestingly, total scores on the ADOS-2 were significantly higher in acute AN than HCs, while scores in the REC group lay between the two. This pattern of results suggests that although a small proportion of ASD symptoms may be a result of starvation in acute AN, the ADOS-2 algorithm might be robust against picking up false positives. The findings from our recovered group suggest that ASD symptoms may be a stable trait, present before and after the illness in individuals with AN. Consequently, a more personalised approach to treatment in individuals with AN might be required. Treatment modules designed to improve social cognition may not be suitable for the majority of individuals with AN, however, they could prove useful in those with high ASD traits and accompanying emotion recognition difficulties. Interventions such as social skills training groups may be effective in adults and adolescents with ASD, with several studies reporting improvements in social cognition measures, social skills knowledge, and friendship quality [82–86]. In addition, some studies have shown improvements in mental health outcomes, suggesting a relationship between social functioning and wider mental health [87,88]. Whether such interventions might be useful for those with AN and ASD comorbidity is yet to be addressed. Thus far, interventions in AN that have incorporated emotion or social skills training, such as Cognitive Remediation and Emotion Skills Training (CREST) [89] have more heavily emphasised identifying and managing one's own emotions rather than identifying emotions in others. Future treatment protocols may benefit from the inclusion of more extensive social cognition training specifically for those with AN and comorbid ASD.

The current study has a number of strengths. The sample size is one of the largest among eye-tracking studies in individuals with EDs (for a review, see [90]), and it is the first study to measure attention during emotion recognition in both acute and recovered AN. The inclusion of both basic and complex emotions, as well as the use of realistic photo stimuli allowed for a more ecologically valid assessment of emotion recognition abilities. However, several limitations should also be discussed. Most notably, given the short stimuli presentation times (500 ms), our paradigm only provided an assessment of early attentional engagement during emotion recognition. It may be that individuals with AN show differences in attention at later processing stages where attention is under conscious control [91]. This may explain why although attention to faces significantly correlated with emotion recognition accuracy, it did not explain a significant amount of the variance in accuracy in regression analyses. Although our quick presentation times might have replicated the fleeting facial expressions encountered in real life, future studies would benefit from measuring attention over longer periods in order to gain a better understanding of attentional processes in individuals with AN. Further, given the inclusion of both basic and complex emotion words in the FET, it is likely that verbal comprehension abilities explain significant variance in accuracy. Although we assessed associations between full-scale IQ and emotion recognition accuracy, our analyses may have benefited from including verbal IQ instead. Nonetheless, our findings show that individuals with AN have the capacity to process emotions rapidly to the same extent as HCs.

Relatedly, the short stimuli presentation times in the FET prevented a more fine-grained analysis of scan paths across the facial features. Reduced attention to the eyes has been demonstrated in acute AN during free viewing of face images, as well as during real-life social interactions [40,41]. Thus, it could be the case that our measure of overall looking times to faces was too blunt to detect group differences. Another limitation of the current study is the cross-sectional design. It cannot be ruled out that differences in socio-cognitive functioning or psychological resources contributed to the recovery of the recovered AN group. To our knowledge, no study has tested emotion recognition abilities and/or social attention over time in the same group of individuals with AN before and after recovery. Further, it must be noted that although the ADOS-2 is recommended as part of an ASD diagnostic assessment, it does not provide enough information on its own to confer a diagnosis of ASD [56]. Research using developmental measures in addition to assessing current symptoms would be informative in further defining social cognition in the AN+ASD sub-group.

To conclude, the findings of the current study suggest that emotion recognition difficulties are not a feature of the socio-emotional phenotype proposed to characterise AN. Instead, difficulties in emotion recognition appear to only be present in those with high ASD traits, independent of illness state. While it is not known whether this subgroup of individuals meets full diagnostic criteria for ASD, our findings support the notion that AN with and without high ASD traits might be two qualitatively different conditions. Whether these individuals may require different treatment strategies or adaptations to accommodate different communicative styles is a question for future research. Our results also suggest individuals in the acute and recovered stages of AN do not show any differences in attention to faces compared to HCs. However, given the limitations of our study design and the lack of research in this area, future studies should examine attention to individual facial features to expand on our findings.

Author Contributions: Conceptualization, J.K.-G. and K.T.; formal analysis, J.K.-G. and E.J.; funding acquisition, J.K.-G.; investigation, J.K.-G.; methodology, E.L. and J.A.; resources, H.H. and D.M.; software, L.M.; supervision, A.H., D.M. and K.T.; writing—original draft, J.K.-G.; writing—review & editing, L.M., E.J., H.H., A.H., E.L., J.A. and K.T. All authors have read and agreed to the published version of the manuscript.

Acknowledgments: The authors would like to thank the participants who took part in the research for their time.

References

1. American Psychiatric Association. *Diagnostic and Statistical Manual of Mental Disorders*, 5th ed.; American Psychiatric Publishing: Arlington, TX, USA, 2013.
2. Treasure, J.; Schmidt, U. The Cognitive-Interpersonal Maintenance Model of Anorexia Nervosa Revisited: A Summary of the Evidence for Cognitive, Socio-Emotional and Interpersonal Predisposing and Perpetuating Factors. *J. Eat. Disord.* **2013**, *1*, 13. [CrossRef] [PubMed]
3. Lie, S.Ø.; Rø, Ø.; Bang, L. Is Bullying and Teasing Associated with Eating Disorders? A Systematic Review and Meta-Analysis. *Int. J. Eat. Disord.* **2019**, *52*, 497–514. [CrossRef] [PubMed]
4. Cardi, V.; Mallorqui-Bague, N.; Albano, G.; Monteleone, A.M.; Fernandez-Aranda, F.; Treasure, J. Social Difficulties as Risk and Maintaining Factors in Anorexia Nervosa: A Mixed-Method Investigation. *Front. Psychiatry* **2018**, *9*, 12. [CrossRef] [PubMed]
5. Fairburn, C.G.; Cooper, Z.; Doll, H.A.; Welch, S.L. Risk Factors for Anorexia Nervosa: Three Integrated Case-Control Comparisons. *Arch. Gen. Psychiatry* **1999**, *56*, 468–476. [CrossRef]
6. Krug, I.; Penelo, E.; Fernandez-Aranda, F.; Anderluh, M.; Bellodi, L.; Cellini, E.; di Bernardo, M.; Granero, R.; Karwautz, A.; Nacmias, B.; et al. Low Social Interactions in Eating Disorder Patients in Childhood and Adulthood: A Multi-Centre European Case Control Study. *J. Health Psychol.* **2012**, *18*, 26–37. [CrossRef]

7. Westwood, H.; Kerr-Gaffney, J.; Stahl, D.; Tchanturia, K. Alexithymia in Eating Disorders: Systematic Review and Meta-Analyses of Studies Using the Toronto Alexithymia Scale. *J. Psychosom. Res.* **2017**, *99*, 66–81. [CrossRef]
8. Kerr-Gaffney, J.; Harrison, A.; Tchanturia, K. Social Anxiety in the Eating Disorders: A Systematic Review and Meta-Analysis. *Psychol. Med.* **2018**, *48*, 2477–2491. [CrossRef]
9. Rhind, C.; Bonfioli, E.; Hibbs, R.; Goddard, E.; Macdonald, P.; Gowers, S.; Schmidt, U.; Tchanturia, K.; Micali, N.; Treasure, J. An Examination of Autism Spectrum Traits in Adolescents with Anorexia Nervosa and Their Parents. *Mol. Autism* **2014**, *5*, 56. [CrossRef]
10. Winecoff, A.A.; Ngo, L.; Moskovich, A.; Merwin, R.; Zucker, N. The Functional Significance of Shyness in Anorexia Nervosa. *Eur. Eat. Disord. Rev.* **2015**, *23*, 327–332. [CrossRef]
11. Tiller, J.M.; Sloane, G.; Schmidt, U.; Troop, N.; Power, M.; Treasure, J.L. Social Support in Patients with Anorexia Nervosa and Bulimia Nervosa. *Int. J. Eat. Disord.* **1997**, *21*, 31–38. [CrossRef]
12. Patel, K.; Tchanturia, K.; Harrison, A. An Exploration of Social Functioning in Young People with Eating Disorders: A Qualitative Study. *PLoS ONE* **2016**, *11*, e0159910. [CrossRef] [PubMed]
13. Westwood, H.; Lawrence, V.; Fleming, C.; Tchanturia, K. Exploration of Friendship Experiences, before and after Illness Onset in Females with Anorexia Nervosa: A Qualitative Study. *PLoS ONE* **2016**, *11*, e0163528. [CrossRef] [PubMed]
14. Harrison, A.; Mountford, V.A.; Tchanturia, K. Social Anhedonia and Work and Social Functioning in the Acute and Recovered Phases of Eating Disorders. *Psychiatry Res.* **2014**, *218*, 187–194. [CrossRef] [PubMed]
15. Jones, A.; Lindekilde, N.; Lübeck, M.; Clausen, L. The Association between Interpersonal Problems and Treatment Outcome in the Eating Disorders: A Systematic Review. *Nord. J. Psychiatry* **2015**, *9488*, 1–11. [CrossRef] [PubMed]
16. Zipfel, S.; Löwe, B.; Reas, D.L.; Deter, H.-C.; Herzog, W. Long-Term Prognosis in Anorexia Nervosa: Lessons from a 21-Year Follow-up Study. *Lancet* **2000**, *355*, 721–722. [CrossRef]
17. Franko, D.L.; Keshaviah, A.; Eddy, K.T.; Krishna, M.; Davis, M.C.; Keel, P.K.; Herzog, D.B. A Longitudinal Investigation of Mortality in Anorexia Nervosa and Bulimia Nervosa. *Am. J. Psychiatry* **2013**, *170*, 917–925. [CrossRef]
18. Ko, B.C. A Brief Review of Facial Emotion Recognition Based on Visual Information. *Sensors* **2018**, *18*, 401. [CrossRef]
19. Kucharska-Pietura, K.; Nikolaou, V.; Masiak, M.; Treasure, J. The Recognition of Emotion in the Faces and Voice of Anorexia Nervosa. *Int. J. Eat. Disord.* **2004**, *35*, 42–47. [CrossRef]
20. Harrison, A.; Tchanturia, K.; Treasure, J. Attentional Bias, Emotion Recognition, and Emotion Regulation in Anorexia: State or Trait? *Biol. Psychiatry* **2010**, *68*, 755–761. [CrossRef]
21. Jänsch, C.; Harmer, C.; Cooper, M.J. Emotional Processing in Women with Anorexia Nervosa and in Healthy Volunteers. *Eat. Behav.* **2009**, *10*, 184–191. [CrossRef]
22. Russell, T.A.; Schmidt, U.; Doherty, L.; Young, V.; Tchanturia, K. Aspects of Social Cognition in Anorexia Nervosa: Affective and Cognitive Theory of Mind. *Psychiatry Res.* **2009**, *168*, 181–185. [CrossRef] [PubMed]
23. Kessler, H.; Schwarze, M.; Filipic, S.; Traue, H.C.; von Wietersheim, J. Alexithymia and Facial Emotion Recognition in Patients with Eating Disorders. *Int. J. Eat. Disord.* **2006**, *39*, 245–251. [CrossRef] [PubMed]
24. Kim, Y.R.; Eom, J.S.; Yang, J.W.; Kang, J.; Treasure, J. The Impact of Oxytocin on Food Intake and Emotion Recognition in Patients with Eating Disorders: A Double Blind Single Dose within-Subject Cross-over Design. *PLoS ONE* **2015**, *10*, e0137514. [CrossRef]
25. Kucharska, K.; Jeschke, J.; Mafi, R. Intact Social Cognitive Processes in Outpatients with Anorexia Nervosa: A Pilot Study. *Ann. Gen. Psychiatry* **2016**, *15*, 1–6. [CrossRef] [PubMed]
26. Mendlewicz, L.; Linkowski, P.; Bazelmans, C.; Philippot, P. Decoding Emotional Facial Expressions in Depressed and Anorexic Patients. *J. Affect. Disord.* **2005**, *89*, 195–199. [CrossRef] [PubMed]
27. Oldershaw, A.; Hambrook, D.; Stahl, D.; Tchanturia, K.; Treasure, J.; Schmidt, U. The Socio-Emotional Processing Stream in Anorexia Nervosa. *Neurosci. Biobehav. Rev.* **2011**, *35*, 970–988. [CrossRef]
28. Dinkler, L.; Rydberg Dobrescu, S.; Råstam, M.; Gillberg, I.C.; Gillberg, C.; Wentz, E.; Hadjikhani, N. Visual Scanning during Emotion Recognition in Long-Term Recovered Anorexia Nervosa: An Eye-Tracking Study. *Int. J. Eat. Disord.* **2019**, *52*, 691–700. [CrossRef]

29. Oldershaw, A.; Hambrook, D.; Tchanturia, K.; Treasure, J.; Schmidt, U. Emotional Theory of Mind and Emotional Awareness in Recovered Anorexia Nervosa Patients. *Psychosom. Med.* **2010**, *72*, 73–79. [CrossRef]
30. Kanakam, N.; Krug, I.; Raoult, C.; Collier, D.; Treasure, J. Social and Emotional Processing as a Behavioural Endophenotype in Eating Disorders: A Pilot Investigation in Twins. *Eur. Eat. Disord. Rev.* **2013**, *21*, 294–307. [CrossRef]
31. Godart, N.; Radon, L.; Curt, F.; Duclos, J.; Perdereau, F.; Lang, F.; Venisse, J.L.; Halfon, O.; Bizouard, P.; Loas, G.; et al. Mood Disorders in Eating Disorder Patients: Prevalence and Chronology of ONSET. *J. Affect. Disord.* **2015**, *185*, 115–122. [CrossRef]
32. Swinbourne, J.; Touyz, S. The Co-Morbidity of Eating Disorders and Anxiety Disorders: A Review. *Eur. Eat. Disord. Rev.* **2007**, *15*, 215–221. [CrossRef] [PubMed]
33. Westwood, H.; Tchanturia, K. Autism Spectrum Disorder in Anorexia Nervosa: An Updated Literature Review. *Curr. Psychiatry Rep.* **2017**, *19*, 41. [CrossRef] [PubMed]
34. Brewer, R.; Cook, R.; Cardi, V.; Treasure, J.; Bird, G. Emotion Recognition Deficits in Eating Disorders Are Explained by Co-Occurring Alexithymia. *R. Soc. Open Sci.* **2015**, *2*, 140382. [CrossRef] [PubMed]
35. Fujiwara, E.; Kube, V.L.; Rochman, D.; Macrae-Korobkov, A.K.; Peynenburg, V. Visual Attention to Ambiguous Emotional Faces in Eating Disorders: Role of Alexithymia. *Eur. Eat. Disord. Rev.* **2017**, *25*, 451–460. [CrossRef]
36. Renwick, B.; Musiat, P.; Lose, A.; Dejong, H.; Broadbent, H.; Kenyon, M.; Loomes, R.; Watson, C.; Ghelani, S.; Serpell, L.; et al. Neuro- and Social-Cognitive Clustering Highlights Distinct Profiles in Adults with Anorexia Nervosa. *Int. J. Eat. Disord.* **2015**, *48*, 26–34. [CrossRef] [PubMed]
37. Klin, A.; Jones, W.; Schultz, R.; Volkmar, F.; Cohen, D. Visual Fixation Patterns During Viewing of Naturalistic Social Situations as Predictors of Social Competence in Individuals With Autism. *Arch. Gen. Psychiatry* **2002**, *59*, 809. [CrossRef]
38. Klein, J.T.; Shepherd, S.V.; Platt, M.L. Social Attention and the Brain. *Curr. Biol.* **2009**, *19*, R958–R962. [CrossRef]
39. Jones, E.J.H.; Gliga, T.; Bedford, R.; Charman, T.; Johnson, M.H. Developmental Pathways to Autism: A Review of Prospective Studies of Infants at Risk. *Neurosci. Biobehav. Rev.* **2014**, *39*, 1–33. [CrossRef]
40. Watson, K.K.; Werling, D.M.; Zucker, N.L.; Platt, M.L. Altered Social Reward and Attention in Anorexia Nervosa. *Front. Psychol.* **2010**, *1*, 36. [CrossRef]
41. Harrison, A.; Watterson, S.V.; Bennett, S.D. An Experimental Investigation into the Use of Eye-Contact in Social Interactions in Women in the Acute and Recovered Stages of Anorexia Nervosa. *Int. J. Eat. Disord.* **2019**, *52*, 61–70. [CrossRef]
42. Corden, B.; Chilvers, R.; Skuse, D. Avoidance of Emotionally Arousing Stimuli Predicts Social–Perceptual Impairment in Asperger's Syndrome. *Neuropsychologia* **2008**, *46*, 137–147. [CrossRef] [PubMed]
43. Müller, N.; Baumeister, S.; Dziobek, I.; Banaschewski, T.; Poustka, L. Validation of the Movie for the Assessment of Social Cognition in Adolescents with ASD: Fixation Duration and Pupil Dilation as Predictors of Performance. *J. Autism Dev. Disord.* **2016**, *46*, 2831–2844. [CrossRef] [PubMed]
44. Phillipou, A.; Abel, L.A.; Castle, D.J.; Hughes, M.E.; Gurvich, C.; Nibbs, R.G.; Rossell, S.L. Self Perception and Facial Emotion Perception of Others in Anorexia Nervosa. *Front. Psychol.* **2015**, *6*, 1–9. [CrossRef] [PubMed]
45. Pollice, C.; Kaye, W.H.; Greeno, C.G.; Weltzin, T.E. Relationship of Depression, Anxiety, and Obsessionality to State of Illness in Anorexia Nervosa. *Int. J. Eat. Disord.* **1997**, *21*, 367–376. [CrossRef]
46. Attwood, A.S.; Easey, K.E.; Dalili, M.N.; Skinner, A.L.; Woods, A.; Crick, L.; Ilett, E.; Penton-Voak, I.S.; Munafò, M.R. State Anxiety and Emotional Face Recognition in Healthy Volunteers. *R. Soc. Open Sci.* **2017**, *4*, 160855. [CrossRef] [PubMed]
47. Bourke, C.; Douglas, K.; Porter, R. Processing of Facial Emotion Expression in Major Depression: A Review. *Aust. N. Z. J. Psychiatry* **2010**, *44*, 681–696. [CrossRef]
48. Demenescu, L.R.; Kortekaas, R.; den Boer, J.A.; Aleman, A. Impaired Attribution of Emotion to Facial Expressions in Anxiety and Major Depression. *PLoS ONE* **2010**, *5*, e15058. [CrossRef]
49. Hezel, D.M.; McNally, R.J. Theory of Mind Impairments in Social Anxiety Disorder. *Behav. Ther.* **2014**, *45*, 530–540. [CrossRef]
50. Schreiter, S.; Pijnenborg, G.H.M.; Aan Het Rot, M. Empathy in Adults with Clinical or Subclinical Depressive Symptoms. *J. Affect. Disord.* **2013**, *150*, 1–16. [CrossRef]

51. Washburn, D.; Wilson, G.; Roes, M.; Rnic, K.; Harkness, K.L. Theory of Mind in Social Anxiety Disorder, Depression, and Comorbid Conditions. *J. Anxiety Disord.* **2016**, *37*, 71–77. [CrossRef]
52. First, M.B.; Williams, J.B.; Karg, R.S.; Spitzer, R.L. *Structured Clinical Interview for DSM-5 Disorders, Research Version*; American Psychiatric Association: Arlington, TX, USA, 2015.
53. Garrido, L.; Furl, N.; Draganski, B.; Weiskopf, N.; Stevens, J.; Tan, G.C.Y.; Driver, J.; Dolan, R.J.; Duchaine, B. Voxel-Based Morphometry Reveals Reduced Grey Matter Volume in the Temporal Cortex of Developmental Prosopagnosics. *Brain* **2009**, *132*, 3443–3455. [CrossRef] [PubMed]
54. Wechsler, D. *Wechsler Abbreviated Scale of Intelligence, Second Edition (WASI-II)*; NCS Pearson: San Antonio, TX, USA, 2011.
55. Lord, C.; Rutter, M.; Dilavore, P.; Risi, S.; Gotham, K.; Bishop, S. *Autism Diagnostic Observation Schedule, Second Edition (ADOS-2) Modules 1-4*; Western Psychological Services: Los Angeles, CA, USA, 2012.
56. National Institute for Health and Clinical Excellence. *Autism: Recognition, Referral, Diagnosis and Management of Adults on the Autism Spectrum (CG142)*; NICE: London, UK, 2012.
57. Hus, V.; Lord, C. The Autism Diagnostic Observation Schedule, Module 4: Revised Algorithm and Standardized Severity Scores. *J. Autism Dev. Disord.* **2014**, *44*, 1996–2012. [CrossRef] [PubMed]
58. Fairburn, C.G.; Beglin, S.J. Assessment of Eating Disorders: Interview or Self-Report Questionnaire? *Int. J. Eat. Disord.* **1994**, *16*, 363–370. [CrossRef] [PubMed]
59. Lang, K.; Larsson, E.; Mavromara, L.; Simic, M.; Treasure, J.; Tchanturia, K. Diminished Facial Emotion Expression and Associated Clinical Characteristics in Anorexia Nervosa. *Psychiatry Res.* **2016**, *236*, 165–172. [CrossRef] [PubMed]
60. Zigmond, A.S.; Snaith, R.P. The Hospital Anxiety and Depression Scale. *Acta Psychiatr. Scand.* **1983**, *67*, 361–370. [CrossRef] [PubMed]
61. Liebowitz, M.R. Social Phobia. *Mod. Probl. Pharmacopsychiatry* **1987**, *22*, 141–173.
62. Rytwinski, N.K.; Fresco, D.M.; Heimberg, R.G.; Coles, M.E.; Liebowitz, M.R.; Cissell, S.; Stein, M.B.; Hofmann, S.G. Screening for Social Anxiety Disorder with the Self-Report Version of the Liebowitz Social Anxiety Scale. *Depress. Anxiety* **2009**, *26*, 34–38. [CrossRef]
63. Constantino, J.N.; Gruber, C.P. *Social Responsiveness Scale-Second Edition (SRS-2)*; Western Psychological Services: Torrance, CA, USA, 2012.
64. Bagby, R.M.; Parker, J.D.A.; Taylor, G.J. The Twenty-Item Toronto Alexithymia Scale—I. Item Selection and Cross-Validation of the Factor Structure. *J. Psychosom. Res.* **1994**, *38*, 23–32. [CrossRef]
65. Parker, J.D.A.; Taylor, G.J.; Bagby, R.M. Alexithymia and the Processing of Emotional Stimuli: An Experimental Study. *New Trends Exp. Clin. Psychiatry* **1993**, *9*, 9–14.
66. Task Engine. Available online: https://sites.google.com/site/taskenginedoc/ (accessed on 13 February 2020).
67. Tapajõz Pereira De Sampaio, F.; Soneira, S.; Aulicino, A.; Allegri, R.F. Theory of Mind in Eating Disorders and Their Relationship to Clinical Profile. *Eur. Eat. Disord. Rev.* **2013**, *21*, 479–487. [CrossRef]
68. Adenzato, M.; Todisco, P.; Ardito, R.B. Social Cognition in Anorexia Nervosa: Evidence of Preserved Theory of Mind and Impaired Emotional Functioning. *PLoS ONE* **2012**, *7*, e44414. [CrossRef] [PubMed]
69. Bentz, M.; Jepsen, J.R.M.; Pedersen, T.; Bulik, C.M.; Pedersen, L.; Pagsberg, A.K.; Plessen, K.J. Impairment of Social Function in Young Females with Recent-Onset Anorexia Nervosa and Recovered Individuals. *J. Adolesc. Heal.* **2017**, *60*, 23–32. [CrossRef] [PubMed]
70. Loth, E.; Garrido, L.; Ahmad, J.; Watson, E.; Duff, A.; Duchaine, B. Facial Expression Recognition as a Candidate Marker for Autism Spectrum Disorder: How Frequent and Severe Are Deficits? *Mol. Autism* **2018**, *9*, 7. [CrossRef] [PubMed]
71. Marí-Bauset, S.; Zazpe, I.; Mari-Sanchis, A.; Llopis-González, A.; Morales-Suárez-Varela, M. Food Selectivity in Autism Spectrum Disorders. *J. Child Neurol.* **2014**, *29*, 1554–1561. [CrossRef] [PubMed]
72. Sharp, W.G.; Berry, R.C.; McCracken, C.; Nuhu, N.N.; Marvel, E.; Saulnier, C.A.; Klin, A.; Jones, W.; Jaquess, D.L. Feeding Problems and Nutrient Intake in Children with Autism Spectrum Disorders: A Meta-Analysis and Comprehensive Review of the Literature. *J. Autism Dev. Disord.* **2013**, *43*, 2159–2173. [CrossRef]
73. Spek, A.A.; van Rijnsoever, W.; van Laarhoven, L.; Kiep, M. Eating Problems in Men and Women with an Autism Spectrum Disorder. *J. Autism Dev. Disord.* **2019**, 1–8. [CrossRef]

74. Kinnaird, E.; Norton, C.; Stewart, C.; Tchanturia, K. Same Behaviours, Different Reasons: What Do Patients with Co-Occurring Anorexia and Autism Want from Treatment? *Int. Rev. Psychiatry* **2019**, *31*, 308–317. [CrossRef]
75. Strang, J.F.; Kenworthy, L.; Dominska, A.; Sokoloff, J.; Kenealy, L.E.; Berl, M.; Walsh, K.; Menvielle, E.; Slesaransky-Poe, G.; Kim, K.E.; et al. Increased Gender Variance in Autism Spectrum Disorders and Attention Deficit Hyperactivity Disorder. *Arch. Sex. Behav.* **2014**, *43*, 1525–1533. [CrossRef]
76. Kristensen, Z.E.; Broome, M.R. Autistic Traits in an Internet Sample of Gender Variant UK Adults. *Int. J. Transgenderism* **2015**, *16*, 234–245. [CrossRef]
77. Bargiela, S.; Steward, R.; Mandy, W. The Experiences of Late-Diagnosed Women with Autism Spectrum Conditions: An Investigation of the Female Autism Phenotype. *J. Autism Dev. Disord.* **2016**, *46*, 3281–3294. [CrossRef]
78. Diemer, E.W.; Grant, J.D.; Munn-Chernoff, M.A.; Patterson, D.A.; Duncan, A.E. Gender Identity, Sexual Orientation, and Eating-Related Pathology in a National Sample of College Students. *J. Adolesc. Heal.* **2015**, *57*, 144–149. [CrossRef] [PubMed]
79. Jones, B.A.; Haycraft, E.; Bouman, W.P.; Brewin, N.; Claes, L.; Arcelus, J. Risk Factors for Eating Disorder Psychopathology within the Treatment Seeking Transgender Population: The Role of Cross-Sex Hormone Treatment. *Eur. Eat. Disord. Rev.* **2018**, *26*, 120–128. [CrossRef] [PubMed]
80. Couturier, J.; Pindiprolu, B.; Findlay, S.; Johnson, N. Anorexia Nervosa and Gender Dysphoria in Two Adolescents. *Int. J. Eat. Disord.* **2015**, *48*, 151–155. [CrossRef] [PubMed]
81. Sedgewick, F.; Kerr-Gaffney, J.; Leppanen, J.; Tchanturia, K. Anorexia Nervosa, Autism, and the ADOS: How Appropriate Is the New Algorithm in Identifying Cases? *Front. Psychiatry* **2019**, *10*, 1–7. [CrossRef]
82. Hillier, A.; Fish, T.; Cloppert, P.; Beversdorf, D.Q. Outcomes of a Social and Vocational Skills Support Group for Adolescents and Young Adults on the Autism Spectrum. *Focus Autism Other Dev. Disabl.* **2007**, *22*, 107–115. [CrossRef]
83. Kandalaft, M.R.; Didehbani, N.; Krawczyk, D.C.; Allen, T.T.; Chapman, S.B. Virtual Reality Social Cognition Training for Young Adults with High-Functioning Autism. *J. Autism Dev. Disord.* **2013**, *43*, 34–44. [CrossRef]
84. Turner-Brown, L.M.; Perry, T.D.; Dichter, G.S.; Bodfish, J.W.; Penn, D.L. Brief Report: Feasibility of Social Cognition and Interaction Training for Adults with High Functioning Autism. *J. Autism Dev. Disord.* **2008**, *38*, 1777–1784. [CrossRef]
85. Laugeson, E.A.; Frankel, F.; Mogil, C.; Dillon, A.R. Parent-Assisted Social Skills Training to Improve Friendships in Teens with Autism Spectrum Disorders. *J. Autism Dev. Disord.* **2009**, *39*, 596–606. [CrossRef]
86. Schohl, K.A.; Van Hecke, A.V.; Carson, A.M.; Dolan, B.; Karst, J.; Stevens, S. A Replication and Extension of the PEERS Intervention: Examining Effects on Social Skills and Social Anxiety in Adolescents with Autism Spectrum Disorders. *J. Autism Dev. Disord.* **2014**, *44*, 532–545. [CrossRef]
87. Hillier, A.J.; Fish, T.; Siegel, J.H.; Beversdorf, D.Q. Social and Vocational Skills Training Reduces Self-Reported Anxiety and Depression Among Young Adults on the Autism Spectrum. *J. Dev. Phys. Disabil.* **2011**, *23*, 267–276. [CrossRef]
88. Yoo, H.-J.; Bahn, G.; Cho, I.-H.; Kim, E.-K.; Kim, J.-H.; Min, J.-W.; Lee, W.-H.; Seo, J.-S.; Jun, S.-S.; Bong, G.; et al. A Randomized Controlled Trial of the Korean Version of the PEERS Parent-Assisted Social Skills Training Program for Teens With ASD. *Autism Res.* **2014**, *7*, 145–161. [CrossRef] [PubMed]
89. Davies, H.; Fox, J.; Naumann, U.; Treasure, J.; Schmidt, U.; Tchanturia, K. Cognitive Remediation and Emotion Skills Training for Anorexia Nervosa: An Observational Study Using Neuropsychological Outcomes. *Eur. Eat. Disord. Rev.* **2012**, *20*, 211–217. [CrossRef] [PubMed]
90. Kerr-Gaffney, J.; Harrison, A.; Tchanturia, K. Eye-Tracking Research in Eating Disorders: A Systematic Review. *Int. J. Eat. Disord.* **2018**, 3–27. [CrossRef] [PubMed]
91. Bauer, A.; Schneider, S.; Waldorf, M.; Cordes, M.; Huber, T.J.; Braks, K.; Vocks, S. Visual Processing of One's Own Body over the Course of Time: Evidence for the Vigilance-Avoidance Theory in Adolescents with Anorexia Nervosa? *Int. J. Eat. Disord.* **2017**, *50*, 1205–1213. [CrossRef]

7

Cognitive Interpersonal Model for Anorexia Nervosa Revisited: The Perpetuating Factors that Contribute to the Development of the Severe and Enduring Illness

Janet Treasure [1,†], Daniel Willmott [1,†,*], Suman Ambwani [2], Valentina Cardi [1], Danielle Clark Bryan [1], Katie Rowlands [1] and Ulrike Schmidt [1]

1. Section of Eating Disorders, Department of Psychological Medicine, Institute of Psychiatry, Psychology and Neuroscience, King's College London, SE5 8AF London, UK; janet.treasure@kcl.ac.uk (J.T.); valentina.cardi@kcl.ac.uk (V.C.); danielle.clarkbryan@kcl.ac.uk (D.C.B.); katie.rowlands@kcl.ac.uk (K.R.); ulrike.schmidt@kcl.ac.uk (U.S.)
2. Department of Psychology, Dickinson College, Carlisle, PA17013, USA; ambwanis@dickinson.edu

* Correspondence: daniel.p.willmott@kcl.ac.uk

† These authors equally contributed to this work.

Abstract: The cognitive interpersonal model was outlined initially in 2006 in a paper describing the valued and visible aspects of anorexia nervosa (Schmidt and Treasure, 2006). In 2013, we summarised many of the cognitive and emotional traits underpinning the model (Treasure and Schmidt, 2013). In this paper, we describe in more detail the perpetuating aspects of the model, which include the inter- and intrapersonal related consequences of isolation, depression, and chronic stress that accumulate in the severe and enduring stage of the illness. Since we developed the model, we have been using it to frame research and development at the Maudsley. We have developed and tested interventions for both patients and close others, refining the model through iterative cycles of model/intervention development in line with the Medical Research Council (MRC) framework for complex interventions. For example, we have defined the consequences of living with the illness on close others (including medical professionals) and characterised the intense emotional reactions and behaviours that follow. For the individual with an eating disorder, these counter-reactions can allow the eating disorder to become entrenched. In addition, the consequent chronic stress from starvation and social pain set in motion processes such as depression, neuroprogression, and neuroadaptation. Thus, anorexia nervosa develops a life of its own that is resistant to treatment. In this paper, we describe the underpinnings of the model and how this can be targeted into treatment.

Keywords: anorexia nervosa; cognitive interpersonal model; severe enduring

1. Introduction

The Medical Research Council has described a framework for the process of development of complex interventions [1]. This involves a procedure in which treatments targeting risk or maintaining factors for an illness are fine-tuned following feedback from proof of concept, feasibility, and pilot studies, including both quantitative and qualitative outcomes. Furthermore, within UK health care research conducted in the National Health Service (NHS), a strong emphasis is placed upon the involvement of patients, carers, and the public to co-design interventions and services. We have used this combined approach to design interventions and services for people with anorexia nervosa (AN).

The first iteration of the cognitive interpersonal model for AN outlined core valued and visible maintaining factors of the illness (Figure 1) [2]; the visible aspects of the disorder elicit deep concern from close others, which is in stark contrast to the egosyntonic nature of the illness, where the sufferer values certain aspects of the illness and does not identify themselves as 'sick'. In the next iteration of the model, we outlined the underpinning neuroscience, the interaction between vulnerability traits and eating disorder behaviours, and how this serves to strengthen the hold of the disorder, allowing it over time to develop a life of its own [3]. Indeed, individuals with a persistent form of the illness often state that they want to change but cannot do so. Examples of interactions between vulnerability traits and eating disorder behaviours include personality traits such as conscientiousness and introversion [4], which can predispose to disordered eating [5] and allow eating disorder habits to become fixed. Furthermore, recent genetic findings reported on correlations between polygenic risk scores, not only with other "brain" disorders, but also with "metabolic" traits related to growth, size, lipids, and insulin sensitivity [6]. Thus, a possible hypothesis is that homeostatic forces maintaining energy balance might be weaker in terms of increasing appetite and stronger in terms of a foraging or over active response to "food shortage". This argument has been developed in more detail in an evolutionary-based model of AN and might benefit from further exploration [7].

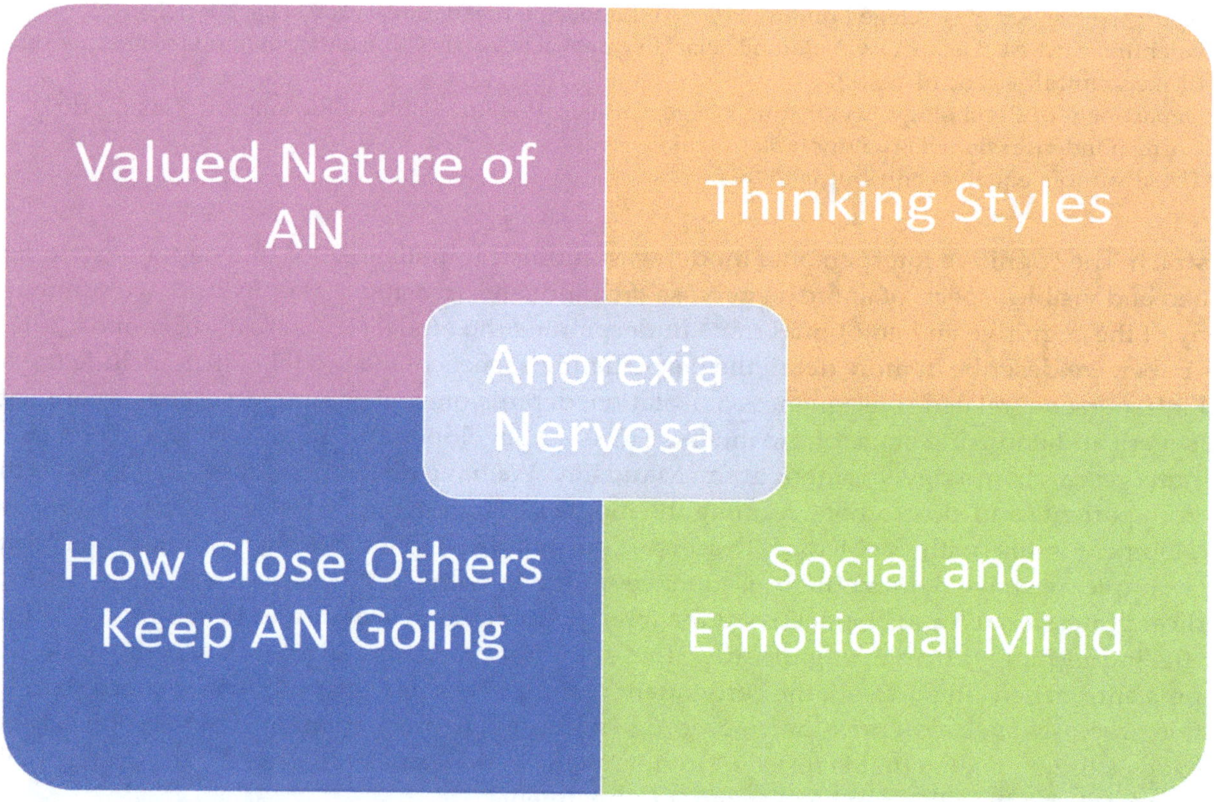

Figure 1. The cognitive–interpersonal maintenance model of anorexia nervosa.

2. Staging Models of Anorexia Nervosa: the Enhanced Cognitive Interpersonal Maintenance Model

This next iteration of the model describes in more detail the development of the severe and enduring form of AN [8]. Current diagnostic procedures do not account for clinical features such as illness trajectory, severity, and co-morbidity, which may impact on the effectiveness of current treatments. The maintenance model of severe and enduring AN consists of three components (Figure 2). The first domain includes the interpersonal consequences of AN. These arise in part because of the impact of chronic starvation on social cognition and the reaction of others to the illness. The next domain relates to the behavioural consequences of AN. Neuroadaptation and habits develop as a consequence of repeated behaviours. Moreover, feeding experiences can increase aversive learning towards food. The third domain relates to the chronic stress response, which may relate to a genetic predisposition to susceptibility, early adversity, or be a secondary response to chronic starvation.

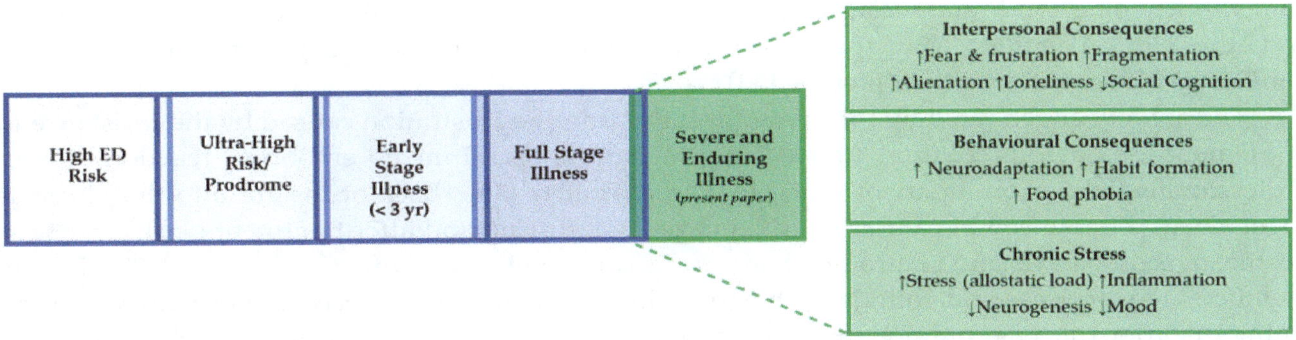

Figure 2. Severe and enduring anorexia nervosa: a maintenance model.

In this paper, we consider in more depth these three domains that contribute to the development of the severe enduring form of illness.

3. Social Risk and Maintaining Factors

Difficulties with interpersonal relationships predispose to the development of AN and are also secondary consequences of the disorder, contributing to the perseverance of the illness.

Social anxiety is a common precursor of eating disorders [9]. In some cases, this is part of the autistic spectrum profile of symptoms that has been observed [10,11], and problems with social cognition may form part of the genetic liability. For example, the offspring of mothers with a history of an eating disorder had anomalies in social cognition during childhood [12]. This familial association suggests that problems in social cognition may be an endophenotype that increases the risk of developing an ED. In addition, adverse social experiences during development such as childhood maltreatment [13], insecure attachment [14], or teasing, bullying, or social exclusion [15] can shape interpersonal relationships and disrupt normal identity development, potentially by increasing the salience of competitive patterns of interaction that can fuel striving for perfection and greater internalisation of beauty ideals as a standard to define the self [16].

Furthermore, people with AN are more likely to report early maladaptive schema (pervasive negative themes regarding the self and one's relationship with others [17]) and difficulties in emotion regulation, with a greater use of dysfunctional interpersonal emotion regulation strategies [18,19]. Problems in emotion regulation may play a key role in maintaining the symptoms of AN [20]. Thus, an interaction between social vulnerability traits, risks within the interpersonal environment, and dysfunctional emotion processing can predispose to the development of AN, a "social–emotional disorder" [21].

Problems in social cognition also can arise as secondary consequences of starvation. Anomalies in social cognition are most pronounced in the acute phase of illness and are less marked after recovery [22]. The anomalies include deficits in nonverbal emotional expression [23,24], an inability to provide a spontaneous social narrative and to identify the social salience of stimuli [25], a sensitivity to threat [26], to social comparison [27], misalignments in social reciprocity [28], and the avoidance or suppression of emotions, particularly to avoid conflict [19]. Impairments in nonverbal communication and a lack of reciprocation of warmth elicits the "uncanny valley" aversive response in others [29–31]. This can lead to social exclusion and isolation, which is a defining facet of the illness [32].

3.1. Interpersonal Reactions to Living with Anorexia Nervosa

A mental health professional with lived experience of AN used one word to epitomize the illness: "isolation" [32]. However, family members are usually closely involved in the evolution of AN, which commonly has its onset in early adolescence. Close others can encourage help seeking in the early phase of the illness, which in turn may have a favourable effect on the prognosis. Nevertheless, the individual's resistance to the need for treatment can make negotiating this transition difficult. The disruption of family functioning, work, and social adjustment varies accordingly with the developmental age, mood, and other clinical features. Many patients with a chronic form of illness remain dependent on their families or the state during their lifetime [33].

The anxiety engendered by the overt "ill state" and the frustration caused by the resistance to implement the obvious solution "to eat" fuels a profound and mixed emotional reaction in both professionals (nurses on inpatient units) [34] and families [35]. Lack of insight into the illness is particularly pronounced in restrictive AN and persists during and after treatment [36,37]. Critical, hostile, overprotective, and controlling behaviours can develop as counter reactions [38,39]. Family members may appease and collude with eating disorder behaviours, becoming organised around eating disorder rules (accommodating to the illness) and ignoring or covering up for the negative consequences of the behaviours (inadvertently enabling the illness) [40].

These diverse reactions can cause divisions amongst family members. Some family members shoulder an overly high burden, whilst others become disempowered and disengaged. Aspects of the caregiving experience are summarised in systematic reviews [35]. High perceived burden and low caregiving efficacy are common and are associated with clinical levels of depression and anxiety. In addition, the societal reaction to the illness (including interactions with services) can be problematic.

Carers' own practical and emotional reactions to the illness can cause harm to the family unit as relationship ruptures occur in response to accommodating and enabling behaviours [41] or divergent forms of reactive expressed emotion develop. Siblings can be drawn into caregiving, develop their own problems, or leave home prematurely as their needs may be neglected [42,43]. Thus, a vicious circle of escalating interpersonal stress can develop.

The protracted course of the illness and the entanglement between eating and social function means that close others have the potential to remediate these difficulties. Therefore, it is important that carers and close others are involved across the lifespan and not excluded from the treatment process. Clinicians explain this exclusion through concerns around confidentiality, but this is considered a misinterpretation of the law [44].

3.2. Targeting Stressful Interpersonal Reactions

A hypothesis that follows from the cognitive interpersonal model is that the toxic consequences that accrue from the isolation and loneliness of an eating disorder can be ameliorated by skills training for family members or close others across the lifespan [45]. Improving the interpersonal environment often begins at home. Close others are highly motivated to help but are often uncertain of what they can do. Materials coproduced with carers and patients have been developed to illustrate these problems [39] and provide a curriculum for workshops to help carers provide effective support.

These materials explain how the patients' primary and secondary difficulties in social cognition make relationships difficult. For example, the reduced facial expressivity of eating disorder patients [23,24] makes it hard for others to appreciate their level of terror or show appreciation of the carers' distress. AN patients appear to be impervious to the impact of their behaviours on other people. This lack of concern for others appears in the domain of caregiving when others are distressed at their lack of insight and unwillingness to accept the sick role. It also can be evident in treatment facilities where overt demonstration and discussion of eating disorder behaviours can trigger distress in their peers.

The three basic elements of carer skill-sharing interventions include:

(1) Psychoeducation about the illness and framing patient presentation within the cognitive–interpersonal model, highlighting predisposing, precipitating, and perpetuating factors.

(2) Information about how carers might be able to moderate and mould the energy and insight from their own emotional reactions to foster a calm, compassionate, and collaborative context (a life skill that they can role model to the person with the eating disorder).

(3) Introduction to effective support and behaviour change skills such as motivational interviewing, the use of risk-taking experiments, and exposure to fear [46].

Interventions based on this model have been delivered in a range of different formats including workshops and guided self-help interventions with individual or group support. An improved understanding about the illness reduces carer distress and burden [35,45,47,48]. Several studies have found that augmenting treatment with these resources for carers reduces both carer and service burden [49–51]. Often this has involved a 'train the trainer' approach whereby carers and patients deliver these interventions. Pépin and King [52] tested the workshops in a pilot study in Australia, finding participation led to reductions in carer distress and burden and helped them to modify their emotional reactions to the illness. Psychoeducational carer workshops reduce carer psychological distress and burden, yet when collaborative carer skills are taught as well, there are secondary effects on alleviating patients' anxiety and depression [53].

Treatment for individuals with AN based on the cognitive interpersonal model, the Maudsley Model of Anorexia Treatment for Adults (MANTRA) [54,55], also includes a section for carers. Carers are encouraged to cultivate their own emotional and social intelligence by examining the relevant modules for patients so that they can role model these skills to their loved ones. It is helpful if both parties externalise the illness and understand how the AN voice can trap everyone into spirals of confusion. A compassionate, mutually supportive family environment is essential as it is inevitable that miscues and mistakes will happen, but these can be reframed as being valuable opportunities of learning.

4. Behavioural Consequences of Anorexia Nervosa

The repeated patterns of behaviour that underpin the development of AN, such as avoiding high caloric, highly palatable foods, becomes habitual. Initially, these behaviours are initiated to achieve a specific goal and are reinforced as they are positively rewarding. With daily repetition, the actions become automatic and entrenched until they are activated with no conscious effort in response to a stimulus or cue [56]. A recent cognitive neuroscience model of AN proposes that habitual behaviours are mediated within dorsal frontostriatal circuits [57–59]. In line with this, techniques from habit reversal therapy with inpatients led to significant reductions in eating disorder symptoms and self-reported habit strengths [60]. These preliminary findings could be used to augment or guide developments in treatment for those with severe and enduring difficulties.

In addition, fear and/or disgust responses to food represents a key challenge to weight restoration [61]. People with AN show reduced extinction of fear learning but increased fear generalisation and reinstatement, which may contribute to the strength of these fear learning networks [62]. These fears may originate from adverse experiences relating to food and body shape during sensitive periods of development [63]. Furthermore, these could be iatrogenically aggravated by coercive treatment experiences such as nasogastric feeding under restraint. A qualitative study with nurses identified that power battles over 'punitive' feeding causes patients great anguish and can rupture the therapeutic alliance [64]. These interactions may be overlooked as a complicating feature within family-based treatment [65]. Interestingly, in adolescence, reduced extinction of fears appears to be more pronounced with co-morbid depression [66].

Exposure is the standard treatment for fear learning. The underlying mechanism involves developing new learning to the threatening stimulus (as opposed to habituation to anxiety) and updating the fear pathways in the brain [67,68]. There are some caveats in applying this treatment to AN. First, one of the feared consequences, weight gain, is an expected and necessary consequence of refeeding. Furthermore, with fluid fluxes and other aspects of metabolic instability during this phase, a "lack of control of weight" can maintain AN cognitions. Moreover, it is probable that neurogenesis is reduced as a sequelae of the chronic stress of AN, reducing the effectiveness of exposure. A variety of techniques have been used to facilitate this learning. These include positive mood induction [69], the addition of cycloserine to consolidate learning [70,71], and virtual reality [72].

Other training approaches developed to target risk factors show some promise in proof-of-concept studies. These include cognitive remediation approaches that focus on cultivating a flexible, big picture style of thinking [73], cognitive skills training for social avoidance [74], and go/no-go inhibition training [75], which may be of value for the binge–purge form of the illness. Food-related attention bias modification training is also being investigated as an add-on intervention for AN, following directions from anxiety disorder research [76,77].

5. Chronic Stress Response: Co-Morbidity with Depression and Anxiety

Another maintaining factor in the model is the impact of chronic starvation leading to anhedonia and accentuating existing co-morbidities. Emotional distress is common as both a predisposition and a secondary consequence that perpetuates the illness [20,78,79]. This emotional distress may occur due to a shared genetic predisposition [6]; developmental trauma [80], with emotional abuse (e.g., bullying) playing a central role [81]; or as a feature of starvation [82].

Depressive symptomatology may follow a persistent trajectory over the lifetime, independently from eating disorder symptoms [83,84]. Approximately 50% of patients with AN report a minimum of one episode of a mood disorder during their lifetime [85,86]. Depression, anxiety, and interpersonal sensitivity are central nodes in a network analysis of symptoms [87] with key bridging roles [81]. The symptom profile differs somewhat from that of unipolar depression in that somatic features such as loss of energy and reduced activation are less pronounced, whereas cognitive features such as negative views of the self are higher [88]. Indeed, the chance of recovery is reduced in people who developed AN after they had experienced depression [89]. In addition, the long-term outcomes of patients with AN complicated with mood comorbidity were reduced [90]. Consequently, psychological well-being, positive supportive relationships, hope, identity, meaning, and purpose are important markers of recovery [91,92].

Anxiety traits are also linked to eating disorders. Obsessive–compulsive personality traits, obsessive–compulsive disorders, and anxiety [9,93,94] often present in childhood prior to the onset of AN. In addition, there is a strong familial association with these traits [95,96]. The strongest polygenic risk correlations from genome wide association studies (GWAS) of AN is shared with OCD [97], whereas correlations with neuroticism, depression, and anxiety are half the size [6]. In a network analysis of eating disorder and anxiety traits, avoidance of social eating was the strongest bridge node, with eating symptoms and low self-confidence being the strongest bridge node with anxiety traits [98].

In a longitudinal study, the neural correlates of disordered eating and obsessive–compulsive disorder at age 14 included an increase in grey matter volume in the orbitofrontal cortex, the right dorsolateral prefrontal cortex, and the ventral striatum [99]. However, people with a chronic illness had a decrease in grey matter in the cerebellum and the mesencephalon, specifically the substantia nigra and ventral tegmental area [100]. Hippocampal volume is particularly reduced [101–103] which is associated with anxiety and depression [102] and correlated with raised cortisol [104]. Patients in the later stage of AN have increased ventral striatal activation to body image cues than patients in the early stage of illness [105,106].

The chronic stress profile associated with enduring AN [107] is similar to that found in treatment resistant depression [108] and with the 'ecophenotype' associated with childhood maltreatment [109]. This chronic stress response includes hyperactivity of the hypothalamic pituitary adrenal (HPA) axis [101,110–112], activation of the immune system [113,114], and anomalies in the microbiome [115,116]. There is a widespread reduction in brain volume, which is possibly secondary to reduced neurogenesis [117], which may be the most marked in the hippocampus [118] and associated with raised cortisol levels [104]. This broad stress response reduces resilience [119] and may be accompanied by reduced mesolimbic dopamine function, anhedonia, and lack of motivation [120]. Thus, a sizeable proportion of patients could be classified as fulfilling the criteria of treatment-resistant depression.

Treatment-Resistant Depression and other Co-Morbidities as Maintaining Factors: Implications for Treatment

Treatments targeting nutritional recovery are less effective for improving mood [49,50,79,121–123]. Therefore, it is possible that strategies used for treatment-resistant depression might be of benefit for people with severe enduring AN. Proof-of-concept studies of neuromodulation such as deep brain stimulation [124] and repetitive transcranial magnetic stimulation have shown potential [125–127]. Interestingly, the trajectory of symptom change following these neuromodulation techniques shows differences to that found with more traditional eating disorder treatment, in that an improvement in mood is the main initial effect, whereas improvements in eating disorder psychopathology follow later [125,126,128].

Interest in pharmacological approaches is starting to increase, as summarised in a recent review [129]. There is mixed evidence for the use of antipsychotic medications to treat AN [130], although a recent multicenter outpatient study of olanzapine found small positive effects on agitation and weight gain (albeit with no difference in rates of hospitalisation) [131]. The field may need to consider using drugs that have been shown to have benefit in OCD. For example, high doses of Selective Serotonin Reuptake Inhibitors (SSRIs), exposure, and response treatment are effective for people in the later stages of OCD [132], which has also been recently conceptualized within a staging framework [133]. In addition, there is interest in pharmacological approaches that are being used for treatment-resistant depression, such as ketamine and psilocybin [134]. Interestingly, ketamine showed some promise in a small series of studies in the 1990s [135]. A pilot study of the effects of ketamine on mood and eating disorder cognitions in people with severe and enduring AN is registered on the Australia New Zealand Clinical Trial Registry (anzctr.org.au, ACTRN12618001393246p) and additionally, a psilocybin trial for AN is currently registered (ClinicalTrials.gov, NCT04052568). Therefore, we echo the call by Franko and colleagues [90] to consider using a combined approach to target both mood and eating disorder symptoms, with clear characterization of the patient group.

Although not the topic of this paper, given the similarities between staging models for other psychiatric disorders [8], it may be of interest to look at the other end of the trajectory, the ultra-high risk (UHR) group, and consider whether there might be interventions that could be matched to this stage and provide primary or secondary prevention approaches. The first step is to define the UHR phenotype, which may include traits such as behavioural inhibition, perfectionism, early symptoms of OCD, or social–emotional difficulties.

6. Conclusions

In this latest iteration of the cognitive interpersonal model, we have described treatments targeting modifiable elements. Increasing social connection through encouraging a collaborative inclusive approach towards recovery, by increasing the knowledge and skills of family members, decreases the need for high-intensity care (day or inpatient) and reduces carer burden and patient isolation [49–51,136]. Treatment using MANTRA focuses on both inter and intrapersonal model elements [55,56]. Augmenting treatment through digital technology is showing potential [137]. Finally, we are borrowing approaches that show promise in other domains of psychiatry in which a chronic stress response has led to the illness having a life of its own. Neuromodulation techniques are encouraging, and new pharmacological approaches are in progress. Services may need to implement broader clinical assessment skills to more accurately stage the illness to personalise treatments to match patient's needs and preferences.

However, it is too early for this model to be ossified. The field of eating disorders has been starved of resources for research, and so the evidence is limited. Nevertheless, we think that by using this framework in order to identify targets and by using high-quality randomised controlled trials, we will be able to develop more effective treatments through an iterative process.

Author Contributions: Conceptualization, J.T.; writing—original draft preparation, J.T. and D.W.; writing and editing, J.T. and D.W.; reviewing manuscript, S.A., D.C.B., V.C., K.R. and U.S. All authors have read and agreed to the published version of the manuscript.

Acknowledgments: VC, JT and US acknowledge financial support from the National Institute for Health Research (NIHR) Specialist Biomedical Research Centre for Mental Health award to the South London and Maudsley NHS

Foundation Trust and the Institute of Psychiatry, King's College London. US is supported by an NIHR Senior Investigator Award.

References

1. Craig, P.; Dieppe, P.; Macintyre, S.; Michie, S.; Nazareth, I.; Petticrew, M. Developing and evaluating complex interventions: The new Medical Research Council guidance. *BMJ* **2008**, *337*, a1655. [CrossRef] [PubMed]
2. Schmidt, U.; Treasure, J. Anorexia nervosa: Valued and visible. A cognitive-interpersonal maintenance model and its implications for research and practice. *Br. J. Clin. Psychol.* **2006**, *45*, 343–366. [CrossRef] [PubMed]
3. Treasure, J.; Schmidt, U. The cognitive-interpersonal maintenance model of anorexia nervosa revisited: A summary of the evidence for cognitive, socio-emotional and interpersonal predisposing and perpetuating factors. *J. Eat. Disord.* **2013**, *1*, 13. [CrossRef]
4. Farstad, S.M.; McGeown, L.M.; von Ranson, K.M. Eating disorders and personality, 2004–2016: A systematic review and meta-analysis. *Clin. Psychol. Rev.* **2016**, *46*, 91–105. [CrossRef]
5. Miller, J.L.; Schmidt, L.A.; Vaillancourt, T.; McDougall, P.; Laliberte, M. Neuroticism and introversion: A risky combination for disordered eating among a non-clinical sample of undergraduate women. *Eat. Behav.* **2006**, *7*, 69–78. [CrossRef]
6. Watson, H.J.; Yilmaz, Z.; Thornton, L.M.; Hübel, C.; Coleman, J.R.; Gaspar, H.A.; Medland, S.E. Genome-wide association study identifies eight risk loci and implicates metabo-psychiatric origins for anorexia nervosa. *Nat. Genet.* **2019**, *51*, 1207–1214. [CrossRef]
7. Guisinger, S. Adapted to flee famine: Adding an evolutionary perspective on anorexia nervosa. *Psychol. Rev.* **2003**, *110*, 745. [CrossRef]
8. Treasure, J.; Stein, D.; Maguire, S. Has the time come for a staging model to map the course of eating disorders from high risk to severe enduring illness? An examination of the evidence. *Early Interv. Psychiatry* **2015**, *9*, 173–184. [CrossRef]
9. Goddard, E.; Treasure, J. Anxiety and social-emotional processing in eating disorders: Examination of family trios. *Cogn. Ther. Res.* **2013**, *37*, 890–904. [CrossRef]
10. Rhind, C.; Bonfioli, E.; Hibbs, R.; Goddard, E.; Macdonald, P.; Gowers, S.; Treasure, J. An examination of autism spectrum traits in adolescents with anorexia nervosa and their parents. *Mol. Autism* **2014**, *5*, 56. [CrossRef]
11. Nielsen, S.; Anckarsäter, H.; Gillberg, C.; Gillberg, C.; Råstam, M.; Wentz, E. Effects of autism spectrum disorders on outcome in teenage-onset anorexia nervosa evaluated by the Morgan-Russell outcome assessment schedule: A controlled community-based study. *Mol. Autism* **2015**, *6*, 14. [CrossRef] [PubMed]
12. Kothari, R.; Barona, M.; Treasure, J.O.; Micali, N. Social cognition in children at familial high-risk of developing an eating disorder. *Front. Behav. Neurosc.* **2015**, *9*, 208. [CrossRef] [PubMed]
13. Johnson, J.G.; Cohen, P.; Kasen, S.; Brook, J.S. Childhood adversities associated with risk for eating disorders or weight problems during adolescence or early adulthood. *Am. J. Psychiatry* **2002**, *159*, 394–400. [CrossRef] [PubMed]
14. Jewell, T.; Collyer, H.; Gardner, T.; Tchanturia, K.; Simic, M.; Fonagy, P.; Eisler, I. Attachment and mentalization and their association with child and adolescent eating pathology: A systematic review. *Int. J. Eat. Disord.* **2016**, *49*, 354–373. [CrossRef]
15. Cardi, V.; Tchanturia, K.; Treasure, J. Premorbid and illness-related social difficulties in eating disorders: An overview of the literature and treatment developments. *Curr. Neuropharmacol.* **2018**, *16*, 1122–1130. [CrossRef]
16. Vartanian, L.R.; Hayward, L.E.; Smyth, J.M.; Paxton, S.J.; Touyz, S.W. Risk and resiliency factors related to body dissatisfaction and disordered eating: The identity disruption model. *Int. J. Eat. Disord.* **2018**, *51*, 322–330. [CrossRef]
17. Young, J.E.; Klosko, J.S.; Weishaar, M.E. *Schema Therapy: A Practitioner's Guide*; Guilford Press: New York, NY, USA, 2003.
18. Arcelus, J.; Haslam, M.; Farrow, C.; Meyer, C. The role of interpersonal functioning in the maintenance of eating psychopathology: A systematic review and testable model. *Clin. Psychol. Rev.* **2013**, *33*, 156–167. [CrossRef]

19. Oldershaw, A.; Lavender, T.; Sallis, H.; Stahl, D.; Schmidt, U. Emotion generation and regulation in anorexia nervosa: A systematic review and meta-analysis of self-report data. *Clin. Psychol. Rev.* **2015**, *39*, 83–95. [CrossRef]
20. Engel, S.G.; Wonderlich, S.A.; Crosby, R.D.; Mitchell, J.E.; Crow, S.; Peterson, C.B.; Gordon, K.H. The role of affect in the maintenance of anorexia nervosa: Evidence from a naturalistic assessment of momentary behaviors and emotion. *J. Abnorm. Psychol.* **2013**, *122*, 709. [CrossRef]
21. Rapee, R.M.; Oar, E.L.; Johnco, C.J.; Forbes, M.K.; Fardouly, J.; Magson, N.R.; Richardson, C.E. Adolescent development and risk for the onset of social-emotional disorders: A review and conceptual model. *Behav. Res. Ther.* **2019**, *123*, 103501. [CrossRef]
22. Caglar-Nazali, H.P.; Corfield, F.; Cardi, V.; Ambwani, S.; Leppanen, J.; Olabintan, O.; Micali, N. A systematic review and meta-analysis of 'Systems for Social Processes' in eating disorders. *Neurosci. Biobehav. Rev.* **2014**, *42*, 55–92. [CrossRef] [PubMed]
23. Cardi, V.; Corfield, F.; Leppanen, J.; Rhind, C.; Deriziotis, S.; Hadjimichalis, A.; Treasure, J. Emotional processing, recognition, empathy and evoked facial expression in eating disorders: An experimental study to map deficits in social cognition. *PLoS ONE* **2015**, *10*, e0133827. [CrossRef] [PubMed]
24. Davies, H.; Wolz, I.; Leppanen, J.; Fernandez-Aranda, F.; Schmidt, U.; Tchanturia, K. Facial expression to emotional stimuli in non-psychotic disorders: A systematic review and meta-analysis. *Neurosci. Biobehav. Rev.* **2016**, *64*, 252–271. [CrossRef] [PubMed]
25. Oldershaw, A.; DeJong, H.; Hambrook, D.; Schmidt, U. Social attribution in anorexia nervosa. *Eur. Eat. Disord. Rev.* **2018**, *26*, 197–206. [CrossRef]
26. Cardi, V.; Di Matteo, R.; Corfield, F.; Treasure, J. Social reward and rejection sensitivity in eating disorders: An investigation of attentional bias and early experiences. *World J. Biol. Psychiatry* **2013**, *14*, 622–633. [CrossRef]
27. Cardi, V.; Di Matteo, R.; Gilbert, P.; Treasure, J. Rank perception and self-evaluation in eating disorders. *Int. J. Eat. Disord.* **2014**, *47*, 543–552. [CrossRef]
28. Ambwani, S.; Berenson, K.R.; Simms, L.; Li, A.; Corfield, F.; Treasure, J. Seeing things differently: An experimental investigation of social cognition and interpersonal behavior in anorexia nervosa. *Int. J. Eat. Disord.* **2016**, *49*, 499–506. [CrossRef]
29. Szczurek, L.; Monin, B.; Gross, J.J. The Stranger Effect: The Rejection of Affective Deviants. *Psychol. Sci.* **2012**, *23*, 1105–1111. [CrossRef]
30. Hess, U.; Fischer, A. Emotional Mimicry as Social Regulation. *Personal. Soc. Psychol. Rev.* **2013**, *17*, 142–157. [CrossRef]
31. Schneider, K.G.; Hempel, R.J.; Lynch, T.R. That "poker face" just might lose you the game! the impact of expressive suppression and mimicry on sensitivity to facial expressions of emotion. *Emotion* **2013**, *13*, 852–866. [CrossRef]
32. McKnight, R.; Boughton, N. Anorexia Nervosa. *Br. Med. J.* **2014**, *22*, 1–9. [CrossRef] [PubMed]
33. Hjern, A.; Lindberg, L.; Lindblad, F. Outcome and prognostic factors for adolescent female in-patients with anorexia nervosa: 9-to 4-year follow-up. *Br. J. Psychiatry* **2006**, *189*, 428–432. [CrossRef] [PubMed]
34. Treasure, J.; Crane, A.; McKnight, R.; Buchanan, E.; Wolfe, M. First do no harm: Iatrogenic maintaining factors in anorexia nervosa. *Eur. Eat. Disord. Rev.* **2011**, *19*, 296–302. [CrossRef] [PubMed]
35. Anastasiadou, D.; Medina-Pradas, C.; Sepulveda, A.R.; Treasure, J. A systematic review of family caregiving in eating disorders. *Eat. Behav.* **2014**, *15*, 464–477. [CrossRef]
36. Konstantakopoulos, G.; Tchanturia, K.; Surguladze, S.A.; David, A.S. Insight in eating disorders: Clinical and cognitive correlates. *Psychol. Med.* **2011**, *41*, 1951–1961. [CrossRef]
37. Gorwood, P.; Duriez, P.; Lengvenyte, A.; Guillaume, S.; Criquillion, S. Clinical insight in anorexia nervosa: Associated and predictive factors. *Psychiatry Res.* **2019**, *281*, 112561. [CrossRef]
38. Treasure, J.; Schmidt, U.; Macdonald, P. (Eds.) *The Clinician's Guide to Collaborative Caring in Eating Disorders: The New Maudsley Method*; Routledge: London, UK, 2009.
39. Treasure, J.; Smith, G.; Crane, A. *Skills-Based Caring for a Loved One With an Eating Disorder: The New Maudsley Method*; Routledge: London, UK, 2016.
40. Sepulveda, A.R.; Kyriacou, O.; Treasure, J. Development and validation of the accommodation and enabling scale for eating disorders (AESED) for caregivers in eating disorders. *BMC Health Serv. Res.* **2009**, *9*, 171. [CrossRef]

41. Salerno, L.; Rhind, C.; Hibbs, R.; Micali, N.; Schmidt, U.; Gowers, S.; Treasure, J. An examination of the impact of care giving styles (accommodation and skilful communication and support) on the one year outcome of adolescent anorexia nervosa: Testing the assumptions of the cognitive interpersonal model in anorexia nervosa. *J. Affect. Disord.* **2016**, *191*, 230–236. [CrossRef]
42. Dimitropoulos, G.; Klopfer, K.; Lazar, L.; Schacter, R. Caring for a sibling with anorexia nervosa: A qualitative study. *Eur. Eat. Disord. Rev. Prof. J. Eat. Disord. Assoc.* **2009**, *17*, 350–365. [CrossRef]
43. Dimitropoulos, G.; Freeman, V.E.; Bellai, K.; Olmsted, M. Inpatients with severe anorexia nervosa and their siblings: Non-shared experiences and family functioning. *Eur. Eat. Disord. Rev.* **2013**, *21*, 284–293. [CrossRef]
44. House of Commons Health Committee. *Suicide Prevention: Interim Report. Fourth Report of Session*; House of Commons: London, UK, 2016.
45. Treasure, J.; Nazar, B.P. Interventions for the carers of patients with eating disorders. *Curr. Psychiatry Rep.* **2016**, *18*, 16. [CrossRef] [PubMed]
46. Langley, J.; Treasure, J.; Todd, G. *Caring for a Loved One with an Eating Disorder: The New Maudsley Skills-Based Training Manual*; Routledge: London, UK, 2018.
47. Treasure, J.; Murphy, T.; Szmukler, T.; Todd, G.; Gavan, K.; Joyce, J. The experience of caregiving for severe mental illness: A comparison between anorexia nervosa and psychosis. *Soc. Psychiatry Psychiatr. Epidemiol.* **2001**, *36*, 343–347. [CrossRef]
48. Magill, N.; Rhind, C.; Hibbs, R.; Goddard, E.; Macdonald, P.; Arcelus, J.; Treasure, J. Two-year follow-up of a pragmatic randomised controlled trial examining the effect of adding a carer's skill training intervention in inpatients with anorexia nervosa. *Eur. Eat. Disord. Rev.* **2016**, *24*, 122–130. [CrossRef] [PubMed]
49. Hibbs, R.; Magill, N.; Goddard, E.; Rhind, C.; Raenker, S.; Macdonald, P.; Schmidt, U. Clinical effectiveness of a skills training intervention for caregivers in improving patient and caregiver health following in-patient treatment for severe anorexia nervosa: Pragmatic randomised controlled trial. *BJPsych Open* **2015**, *1*, 56–66. [CrossRef] [PubMed]
50. Hodsoll, J.; Rhind, C.; Micali, N.; Hibbs, R.; Goddard, E.; Nazar, B.P.; Landau, S. A pilot, multicentre pragmatic randomised trial to explore the impact of carer skills training on carer and patient behaviours: Testing the cognitive interpersonal model in adolescent anorexia nervosa. *Eur. Eat. Disord. Rev.* **2017**, *25*, 551–561. [CrossRef]
51. Adamson, J.; Cardi, V.; Kan, C.; Harrison, A.; Macdonald, P.; Treasure, J. Evaluation of a novel transition support intervention in an adult eating disorders service: ECHOMANTRA. *Int. Rev. Psychiatry* **2019**, *31*, 382–390. [CrossRef]
52. Pépin, G.; King, R. Collaborative care skills training workshops: Helping carers cope with eating disorders from the UK to Australia. *Soc. Psychiatry Psychiatr. Epidemiol.* **2013**, *48*, 805–812. [CrossRef]
53. Quiles, M.Y.; Quiles, S.M.; Escolano, H.M.; Sanmartín, R.; Treasure, J. Testing carer skill training programs in Spanish carers of patients with eating disorders. *Psicothema* **2018**, *30*, 295.
54. Schmidt, U.; Wade, T.D.; Treasure, J. The Maudsley Model of Anorexia Nervosa Treatment for Adults (MANTRA): Development, key features, and preliminary evidence. *J. Cog. Psychother.* **2014**, *28*, 48–71. [CrossRef]
55. Schmidt, U.; Startup, H.; Treasure, J. *A Cognitive-Interpersonal Therapy Workbook for Treating Anorexia Nervosa: The Maudsley Model*; Routledge: London, UK, 2018.
56. Walsh, B.T. The enigmatic persistence of anorexia nervosa. *Am. J. Psychiatry* **2013**, *170*, 477–484. [CrossRef]
57. Steinglass, J.E.; Walsh, B.T. Neurobiological model of the persistence of anorexia nervosa. *J. Eat. Disord.* **2016**, *4*, 19. [CrossRef] [PubMed]
58. Uniacke, B.; Walsh, B.T.; Foerde, K.; Steinglass, J. The role of habits in anorexia nervosa: Where we are and where to go from here? *Curr. Psychiatry Rep.* **2018**, *20*, 61. [CrossRef] [PubMed]
59. Steinglass, J.E.; Berner, L.A.; Attia, E. Cognitive neuroscience of eating disorders. *Psychiatr. Clin.* **2019**, *42*, 75–91. [CrossRef] [PubMed]
60. Steinglass, J.E.; Glasofer, D.R.; Walsh, E.; Guzman, G.; Peterson, C.B.; Walsh, B.T.; Wonderlich, S.A. Targeting habits in anorexia nervosa: A proof-of-concept randomized trial. *Psychol. Med.* **2018**, *48*, 2584–2591. [CrossRef]

61. Levinson, C.A.; Brosof, L.C.; Ma, J.; Fewell, L.; Lenze, E.J. Fear of food prospectively predicts drive for thinness in an eating disorder sample recently discharged from intensive treatment. *Eat. Behav.* **2017**, *27*, 45–51. [CrossRef]
62. Lambert, E.; Purves, K.; McGregor, T.; Treasure, J.; Cardi, V. Fear conditioning in women with a lifetime diagnosis of anorexia nervosa and healthy controls. In Preparation.
63. Cardi, V.; Leppanen, J.; Mataix-Cols, D.; Campbell, I.C.; Treasure, J. A case series to investigate food-related fear learning and extinction using in vivo food exposure in anorexia nervosa: A clinical application of the inhibitory learning framework. *Eur. Eat. Disord. Rev.* **2019**, *27*, 173–181. [CrossRef]
64. Ramjan, L.M. Nurses and the 'therapeutic relationship': Caring for adolescents with anorexia nervosa. *J. Adv. Nurs.* **2004**, *45*, 495–503. [CrossRef]
65. Kimber, M.; McTavish, J.R.; Couturier, J.; Le Grange, D.; Lock, J.; MacMillan, H.L. Identifying and responding to child maltreatment when delivering family-based treatment—A qualitative study. *Int. J. Eat. Disord.* **2019**, *52*, 292–298. [CrossRef]
66. Den, M.L.; Graham, B.M.; Newall, C.; Richardson, R. Teens that fear screams: A comparison of fear conditioning, extinction, and reinstatement in adolescents and adults. *Dev. Psychobiol.* **2015**, *57*, 818–832. [CrossRef]
67. Koskina, A.; Campbell, I.C.; Schmidt, U. Exposure therapy in eating disorders revisited. *Neurosci. Biobehav. Rev.* **2013**, *37*, 193–208. [CrossRef]
68. Murray, S.B.; Treanor, M.; Liao, B.; Loeb, K.L.; Griffiths, S.; Le Grange, D. Extinction theory & anorexia nervosa: Deepening therapeutic mechanisms. *Behav. Res. Ther.* **2016**, *87*, 1–10. [PubMed]
69. Cardi, V.; Esposito, M.; Clarke, A.; Schifano, S.; Treasure, J. The impact of induced positive mood on symptomatic behaviour in eating disorders. An experimental, AB/BA crossover design testing a multimodal presentation during a test-meal. *Appetite* **2015**, *87*, 192–198. [CrossRef] [PubMed]
70. Steinglass, J.; Sysko, R.; Schebendach, J.; Broft, A.; Strober, M.; Walsh, B.T. The application of exposure therapy and D-cycloserine to the treatment of anorexia nervosa: A preliminary trial. *J. Psychiatr. Pract.* **2007**, *13*, 238. [CrossRef]
71. Levinson, C.A.; Rodebaugh, T.L.; Fewell, L.; Kass, A.E.; Riley, E.N.; Stark, L.; Lenze, E.J. D-Cycloserine facilitation of exposure therapy improves weight regain in patients with anorexia nervosa: A pilot randomized controlled trial. *J. Clin. Psychiatry* **2015**, *76*, e787. [CrossRef]
72. Cardi, V.; Krug, I.; Perpiñá, C.; Mataix-Cols, D.; Roncero, M.; Treasure, J. The use of a nonimmersive virtual reality programme in anorexia nervosa: A single case-report. *Eur. Eat. Disord. Rev.* **2012**, *20*, 240–245. [CrossRef]
73. Tchanturia, K.; Davies, H.; Reeder, C.; Wykes, T. Cognitive Remediation Therapy for AN Therapist Manual. 2010. Available online: http://www.katetchanturia.com/publications/c1y51 (accessed on 26 February 2020).
74. Cardi, V.; Esposito, M.; Bird, G.; Rhind, C.; Yiend, J.; Schifano, S.; Treasure, J. A preliminary investigation of a novel training to target cognitive biases towards negative social stimuli in Anorexia Nervosa. *J. Affect. Disord.* **2015**, *188*, 188–193. [CrossRef]
75. Turton, R.; Nazar, B.P.; Burgess, E.E.; Lawrence, N.S.; Cardi, V.; Treasure, J.; Hirsch, C.R. To go or not to go: A proof of concept study testing food-specific inhibition training for women with eating and weight disorders. *Eur. Eat. Disord. Rev.* **2018**, *26*, 11–21. [CrossRef]
76. Werthmann, J.; Simic, M.; Konstantellou, A.; Mansfield, P.; Mercado, D.; van Ens, W.; Schmidt, U. Same, same but different: Attention bias for food cues in adults and adolescents with anorexia nervosa. *Int. J. Eat. Disord.* **2019**, *52*, 681–690. [CrossRef]
77. Mercado, D.; Schmidt, U.; O'Daly, O.; Campbell, I.; Werthmann, J. Food related attention bias modification training for anorexia nervosa and its potential underpinning mechanisms. *J. Eat. Disord.* **2020**, *8*, 1. [CrossRef]
78. Wildes, J.E.; Marcus, M.D.; Bright, A.C.; Dapelo, M.M. Emotion and eating disorder symptoms in patients with anorexia nervosa: An experimental study. *Int. J. Eat. Disord.* **2012**, *45*, 876–882. [CrossRef]
79. Rodgers, R.F.; Paxton, S.J. The impact of indicated prevention and early intervention on co-morbid eating disorder and depressive symptoms: A systematic review. *J. Eat. Disord.* **2014**, *2*, 30. [CrossRef] [PubMed]
80. Molendijk, M.L.; Hoek, H.W.; Brewerton, T.D.; Elzinga, B.M. Childhood maltreatment and eating disorder pathology: A systematic review and dose-response meta-analysis. *Psychol. Med.* **2017**, *47*, 1402–1416. [CrossRef] [PubMed]

81. Monteleone, A.M.; Mereu, A.; Cascino, G.; Criscuolo, M.; Castiglioni, M.C.; Pellegrino, F.; Zanna, V. Re-conceptualization of anorexia nervosa psychopathology: A network analysis study in adolescents with short duration of the illness. *Int. J. Eat. Disord.* **2019**, *52*, 1263–1273. [CrossRef] [PubMed]
82. Sauro, C.L.; Ravaldi, C.; Cabras, P.L.; Faravelli, C.; Ricca, V. Stress, hypothalamic-pituitary-adrenal axis and eating disorders. *Neuropsychobiology* **2008**, *57*, 95–115. [CrossRef] [PubMed]
83. Chua, Y.W.; Lewis, G.; Easter, A.; Lewis, G.; Solmi, F. Eighteen-year trajectories of depressive symptoms in mothers with a lifetime eating disorder: Findings from the ALSPAC cohort. *Br. J. Psychiatry* **2019**, *14*, 1–7. [CrossRef]
84. Tomba, E.; Tecuta, L.; Crocetti, E.; Squarcio, F.; Tomei, G. Residual eating disorder symptoms and clinical features in remitted and recovered eating disorder patients: A systematic review with meta-analysis. *Int. J. Eat. Disord.* **2019**, *52*, 759–776. [CrossRef]
85. Godart, N.; Radon, L.; Curt, F.; Duclos, J.; Perdereau, F.; Lang, F.; Corcos, M. Mood disorders in eating disorder patients: Prevalence and chronology of ONSET. *J. Affect. Disord.* **2015**, *185*, 115–122. [CrossRef]
86. Dobrescu, S.R.; Dinkler, L.; Gillberg, C.; Råstam, M.; Gillberg, C.; Wentz, E. Anorexia nervosa: 30-year outcome. *Br. J. Psychiatry* **2019**, *22*, 1–8. [CrossRef]
87. Solmi, M.; Collantoni, E.; Meneguzzo, P.; Tenconi, E.; Favaro, A. Network analysis of specific psychopathology and psychiatric symptoms in patients with anorexia nervosa. *Eur. Eat. Disord. Rev.* **2019**, *27*, 24–33. [CrossRef]
88. Voderholzer, U.; Hessler-Kaufmann, J.B.; Lustig, L.; Läge, D. Comparing severity and qualitative facets of depression between eating disorders and depressive disorders: Analysis of routine data. *J. Affect. Disord.* **2019**, *257*, 758–764. [CrossRef]
89. Keski-Rahkonen, A.; Raevuori, A.; Bulik, C.M.; Hoek, H.W.; Rissanen, A.; Kaprio, J. Factors associated with recovery from anorexia nervosa: A population-based study. *Int. J. Eat. Disord.* **2014**, *47*, 117–123. [CrossRef] [PubMed]
90. Franko, D.L.; Tabri, N.; Keshaviah, A.; Murray, H.B.; Herzog, D.B.; Thomas, J.J.; Eddy, K.T. Predictors of long-term recovery in anorexia nervosa and bulimia nervosa: Data from a 22-year longitudinal study. *J. Psychiatr. Res.* **2018**, *96*, 183–188. [CrossRef] [PubMed]
91. Duncan, T.K.; Sebar, B.; Lee, J. Reclamation of power and self: A meta-synthesis exploring the process of recovery from anorexia nervosa. *Adv. Eat. Disord. Theory Res. Pract.* **2015**, *3*, 177–190. [CrossRef]
92. de Vos, J.A.; LaMarre, A.; Radstaak, M.; Bijkerk, C.A.; Bohlmeijer, E.T.; Westerhof, G.J. Identifying fundamental criteria for eating disorder recovery: A systematic review and qualitative meta-analysis. *J. Eat. Disord.* **2017**, *5*, 34. [CrossRef]
93. Measelle, J.R.; Stice, E.; Hogansen, J.M. Developmental trajectories of co-occurring depressive, eating, antisocial, and substance abuse problems in female adolescents. *J. Abnorm. Psychol.* **2006**, *115*, 524. [CrossRef]
94. Degortes, D.; Zanetti, T.; Tenconi, E.; Santonastaso, P.; Favaro, A. Childhood obsessive–compulsive traits in anorexia nervosa patients, their unaffected sisters and healthy controls: A retrospective study. *Eur. Eat. Disord. Rev.* **2014**, *22*, 237–242. [CrossRef]
95. Lilenfeld, L.R.; Kaye, W.H.; Greeno, C.G.; Merikangas, K.R.; Plotnicov, K.; Pollice, C.; Nagy, L. A controlled family study of anorexia nervosa and bulimia nervosa: Psychiatric disorders in first-degree relatives and effects of proband comorbidity. *Arch. Gen. Psychiatry* **1998**, *55*, 603–610. [CrossRef]
96. Cederlöf, M.; Thornton, L.M.; Baker, J.; Lichtenstein, P.; Larsson, H.; Rück, C.; Mataix-Cols, D. Etiological overlap between obsessive-compulsive disorder and anorexia nervosa: A longitudinal cohort, multigenerational family and twin study. *World Psychiatry* **2015**, *14*, 333–338. [CrossRef]
97. Yilmaz, Z.; Halvorsen, M.; Bryois, J.; Yu, D.; Thornton, L.M.; Zerwas, S.; Erdman, L. Examination of the shared genetic basis of anorexia nervosa and obsessive–compulsive disorder. *Mol. Psychiatry* **2018**. [CrossRef]
98. Forrest, L.N.; Jones, P.J.; Ortiz, S.N.; Smith, A.R. Core psychopathology in anorexia nervosa and bulimia nervosa: A network analysis. *Int. J. Eat. Disord.* **2018**, *51*, 668–679. [CrossRef]
99. Montigny, C.; Castellanos-Ryan, N.; Whelan, R.; Banaschewski, T.; Barker, G.J.; Büchel, C.; Nees, F. A phenotypic structure and neural correlates of compulsive behaviors in adolescents. *PLoS ONE* **2013**, *8*, e80151. [CrossRef] [PubMed]
100. Fonville, L.; Giampietro, V.; Williams, S.C.R.; Simmons, A.; Tchanturia, K. Alterations in brain structure in adults with anorexia nervosa and the impact of illness duration. *Psychol. Med.* **2014**, *44*, 1965–1975. [CrossRef]

101. Connan, F.; Treasure, J. Stress, eating and neurobiology. In *Neurobiology in the Treatment of Eating Disorders*; Wiley: Chichester, UK, 1998; pp. 211–236.
102. Myrvang, A.D.; Vangberg, T.R.; Stedal, K.; Rø, Ø.; Endestad, T.; Rosenvinge, J.H.; Aslaksen, P.M. Hippocampal subfields in adolescent anorexia nervosa. *Psychiatry Res. Neuroimaging* **2018**, *282*, 24–30. [CrossRef] [PubMed]
103. Nickel, K.; Joos, A.; Tebartz van Elst, L.; Matthis, J.; Holovics, L.; Endres, D.; Maier, S. Recovery of cortical volume and thickness after remission from acute anorexia nervosa. *Int. J. Eat. Disord.* **2018**, *51*, 1056–1069. [CrossRef]
104. Chui, H.T.; Christensen, B.K.; Zipursky, R.B.; Richards, B.A.; Hanratty, M.K.; Kabani, N.J.; Katzman, D.K. Cognitive function and brain structure in females with a history of adolescent-onset anorexia nervosa. *Paediatrics* **2008**, *122*, e426–e437. [CrossRef] [PubMed]
105. Fladung, A.K.; Grön, G.; Grammer, K.; Herrnberger, B.; Schilly, E.; Grasteit, S.; von Wietersheim, J. A neural signature of anorexia nervosa in the ventral striatal reward system. *Am. J. Psychiatry* **2009**, *167*, 206–212. [CrossRef]
106. Fladung, A.K.; Schulze, U.M.E.; Schöll, F.; Bauer, K.; Grön, G. Role of the ventral striatum in developing anorexia nervosa. *Transl. Psychiatry* **2013**, *3*, e315. [CrossRef]
107. Chami, R.; Treasure, J. *The Neurobiology of Trauma and Eating Disorders. Trauma-Informed Approaches to Eating Disorders*; Springer Publishing Company: New York, NY, USA, 2018.
108. Akil, H.; Gordon, J.; Hen, R.; Javitch, J.; Mayberg, H.; McEwen, B.; Nestler, E.J. Treatment resistant depression: A multi-scale, systems biology approach. *Neurosci. Biobehav. Rev.* **2018**, *84*, 272–288. [CrossRef]
109. Teicher, M.H.; Samson, J.A. Childhood maltreatment and psychopathology: A case for ecophenotypic variants as clinically and neurobiologically distinct subtypes. *Am. J. Psychiatry* **2013**, *170*, 1114–1133. [CrossRef]
110. Putignano, P.; Dubini, A.; Toja, P.; Invitti, C.; Bonfanti, S.; Redaelli, G.; Cavagnini, F. Salivary cortisol measurement in normal-weight, obese and anorexic women: Comparison with plasma cortisol. *Eur. J. Endocrinol.* **2001**, *145*, 165–171. [CrossRef]
111. Misra, M.; Klibanski, A. Endocrine consequences of anorexia nervosa. *Lancet Diabetes Endocrinol.* **2014**, *2*, 581–592. [CrossRef]
112. Chami, R.; Monteleone, A.M.; Treasure, J.; Monteleone, P. Stress hormones and eating disorders. *Mol. Cell. Endocrinol.* **2018**, *497*, 110349. [CrossRef] [PubMed]
113. Dalton, B.; Campbell, I.; Chung, R.; Breen, G.; Schmidt, U.; Himmerich, H. Inflammatory Markers in Anorexia Nervosa: An Exploratory Study. *Nutrients* **2018**, *10*, 1573. [CrossRef]
114. Dalton, B.; Leppanen, J.; Campbell, I.C.; Chung, R.; Breen, G.; Schmidt, U.; Himmerich, H. A longitudinal analysis of cytokines in anorexia nervosa. *Brain Behav. Immun.* **2019**. [CrossRef]
115. Herpertz-Dahlmann, B.; Seitz, J.; Baines, J. Food matters: How the microbiome and gut–brain interaction might impact the development and course of anorexia nervosa. *Eur. Child Adolesc. Psychiatry* **2017**, *26*, 1031–1041. [CrossRef]
116. Seitz, J.; Trinh, S.; Herpertz-Dahlmann, B. The microbiome and eating disorders. *Psychiatr. Clin.* **2019**, *42*, 93–103. [CrossRef]
117. Barona, M.; Brown, M.; Clark, C.; Frangou, S.; White, T.; Micali, N. White matter alterations in anorexia nervosa: Evidence from a voxel-based meta-analysis. *Neurosc. Biobehav. Rev.* **2019**, *100*, 285–295. [CrossRef]
118. Connan, F.; Murphy, F.; Connor, S.E.; Rich, P.; Murphy, T.; Bara-Carill, N.; Morris, R.G. Hippocampal volume and cognitive function in anorexia nervosa. *Psychiatry Res. Neuroimaging* **2006**, *146*, 117–125. [CrossRef]
119. Cathomas, F.; Murrough, J.W.; Nestler, E.J.; Han, M.H.; Russo, S.J. Neurobiology of resilience: Interface between mind and body. *Biol. Psychiatry* **2019**, *86*, 410–420. [CrossRef]
120. Collo, G.; Pich, E.M. A human translational model based on neuroplasticity for pharmacological agents potentially effective in Treatment-Resistant Depression: Focus on dopaminergic system. *Neural Regen. Res.* **2020**, *15*, 1027. [CrossRef]
121. Schmidt, U.; Oldershaw, A.; Jichi, F.; Sternheim, L.; Startup, H.; McIntosh, V.; Landau, S. Out-patient psychological therapies for adults with anorexia nervosa: Randomised controlled trial. *Br. J. Psychiatry* **2012**, *201*, 392–399. [CrossRef]
122. Albano, G.; Hodsoll, J.; Kan, C.; Lo Coco, G.; Cardi, V. Task-sharing interventions for patients with anorexia nervosa or their carers: A systematic evaluation of the literature and meta-analysis of outcomes. *Int. Rev. Psychiatry* **2019**, *31*, 367–381. [CrossRef] [PubMed]

123. Schmidt, U.; Magill, N.; Renwick, B.; Keyes, A.; Kenyon, M.; Dejong, H.; Watson, C. The Maudsley Outpatient Study of Treatments for Anorexia Nervosa and Related Conditions (MOSAIC): Comparison of the Maudsley Model of Anorexia Nervosa Treatment for Adults (MANTRA) with specialist supportive clinical management (SSCM) in outpatients with broadly defined anorexia nervosa: A randomized controlled trial. *J. Consult. Clin. Psychol.* **2015**, *83*, 796. [PubMed]
124. Lipsman, N.; Woodside, D.B.; Giacobbe, P.; Hamani, C.; Carter, J.C.; Norwood, S.J.; Smith, G.S. Subcallosal cingulate deep brain stimulation for treatment-refractory anorexia nervosa: A phase 1 pilot trial. *Lancet* **2013**, *381*, 1361–1370. [CrossRef]
125. McClelland, J.; Kekic, M.; Bozhilova, N.; Nestler, S.; Dew, T.; Van den Eynde, F.; Schmidt, U. A randomised controlled trial of neuronavigated repetitive transcranial magnetic stimulation (rTMS) in anorexia nervosa. *PLoS ONE* **2016**, *11*, e0148606. [CrossRef]
126. Dalton, B.; Bartholdy, S.; McClelland, J.; Kekic, M.; Rennalls, S.J.; Werthmann, J.; Glennon, D. Randomised controlled feasibility trial of real versus sham repetitive transcranial magnetic stimulation treatment in adults with severe and enduring anorexia nervosa: The TIARA study. *BMJ Open* **2018**, *8*, e021531. [CrossRef]
127. Knyahnytska, Y.O.; Blumberger, D.M.; Daskalakis, Z.J.; Zomorrodi, R.; Kaplan, A.S. Insula H-coil deep transcranial magnetic stimulation in severe and enduring anorexia nervosa (SE-AN): A pilot study. *Neuropsychiatr. Dis. Treat.* **2019**, *15*, 2247. [CrossRef]
128. Lipsman, N.; Lam, E.; Volpini, M.; Sutandar, K.; Twose, R.; Giacobbe, P.; Lozano, A.M. Deep brain stimulation of the subcallosal cingulate for treatment-refractory anorexia nervosa: 1 year follow-up of an open-label trial. *Lancet Psychiatry* **2017**, *4*, 285–294. [CrossRef]
129. Himmerich, H.; Treasure, J. Psychopharmacological advances in eating disorders. *Expert Rev. Clin. Pharmacol.* **2018**, *11*, 95–108. [CrossRef]
130. Dold, M.; Aigner, M.; Klabunde, M.; Treasure, J.; Kasper, S. Second-generation antipsychotic drugs in anorexia nervosa: A meta-analysis of randomized controlled trials. *Psychother. Psychosom.* **2015**, *84*, 110–116. [CrossRef]
131. Attia, E.; Steinglass, J.E.; Walsh, B.T.; Wang, Y.; Wu, P.; Schreyer, C.; Marcus, M.D. Olanzapine versus placebo in adult outpatients with anorexia nervosa: A randomized clinical trial. *Am. J. Psychiatry* **2019**, *176*, 449–456. [CrossRef] [PubMed]
132. Hirschtritt, M.E.; Bloch, M.H.; Mathews, C.A. Obsessive-compulsive disorder: Advances in diagnosis and treatment. *JAMA* **2017**, *317*, 1358–1367. [CrossRef] [PubMed]
133. Fontenelle, L.F.; Yücel, M. A Clinical Staging Model for Obsessive–Compulsive Disorder: Is It Ready for Prime Time? *EClinicalMedicine* **2019**, *7*, 65–72. [CrossRef] [PubMed]
134. Rucker, J.J.; Iliff, J.; Nutt, D.J. Psychiatry & the psychedelic drugs. Past, present & future. *Neuropharmacology* **2018**, *142*, 200–218. [PubMed]
135. Mills, I.H.; Park, G.R.; Manara, A.R.; Merriman, R.J. Treatment of compulsive behaviour in eating disorders with intermittent ketamine infusions. *QJM Mon. J. Assoc. Physicians* **1998**, *91*, 493–503. [CrossRef]
136. Cardi, V.; Albano, G.; Ambwani, S.; Cao, L.; Crosby, R.D.; Macdonald, P.; Treasure, J. A randomised clinical trial to evaluate the acceptability and efficacy of an early phase, online, guided augmentation of outpatient care for adults with anorexia nervosa. *Psychol. Med.* **2019**, *16*, 1–12. [CrossRef]
137. Cardi, V.; Ambwani, S.; Robinson, E.; Albano, G.; MacDonald, P.; Aya, V.; Arcelus, J. Transition care in anorexia nervosa through guidance online from peer and carer expertise (TRIANGLE): Study protocol for a randomised controlled trial. *Eur. Eat. Disord. Rev.* **2017**, *25*, 512–523. [CrossRef]

8

Brain Stimulation in Eating Disorders: State of the Art and Future Perspectives

Philibert Duriez [1,2,†], Rami Bou Khalil [3,4,†], Yara Chamoun [3], Redwan Maatoug [5], Robertas Strumila [6], Maude Seneque [4,7], Philip Gorwood [1,2], Philippe Courtet [4,7] and Sébastien Guillaume [4,7,*]

1 GHU Paris Psychiatry and Neuroscience, Clinique des Maladies Mentales et de l'Encéphale (CMME), Sainte-Anne Hospital, 75014 Paris, France; phduriez@gmail.com (P.D.); P.GORWOOD@ghu-paris.fr (P.G.)
2 Institute of Psychiatry and Neurosciences of Paris (IPNP), UMR_S1266, INSERM, Université de Paris, 102-108 rue de la Santé, 75014 Paris, France
3 Department of Psychiatry, Hotel Dieu de France- Saint Joseph University, 166830 Beirut, Lebanon; ramiboukhalil@hotmail.com (R.B.K.); yara.chamoun@hotmail.com (Y.C.)
4 Neuropsychiatry: Epidemiological and Clinical Research, Université Montpellier, INSERM, CHU de Montpellier, 34295 Montpellier, France; maude.seneque@gmail.com (M.S.); p-courtet@chu-montpellier.fr (P.C.)
5 Sorbonne Université, AP-HP, Service de Psychiatrie Adulte de la Pitié-Salpêtrière, Institut du Cerveau, ICM, 75013 Paris, France; redwanmaatoug@gmail.com
6 Faculty of Medicine, Institute of Clinical Medicine, Psychiatric Clinic, Vilnius University, 03101 Vilnius, Lithuania; robertas.strumila@gmail.com
7 Department of Emergency Psychiatry and Post-Acute Care, CHRU Montpellier, 34295 Montpellier, France
* Correspondence: s-guillaume@chu-montpellier.fr
† These authors contributed equally to this work.

Abstract: The management of eating disorders (EDs) is still difficult and few treatments are effective. Recently, several studies have described the important contribution of non-invasive brain stimulation (repetitive transcranial magnetic stimulation, transcranial direct current stimulation, and electroconvulsive therapy) and invasive brain stimulation (deep brain stimulation and vagal nerve stimulation) for ED management. This review summarizes the available evidence supporting the use of brain stimulation in ED. All published studies on brain stimulation in ED as well as ongoing trials registered at clinicaltrials.gov were examined. Articles on neuromodulation research and perspective articles were also included. This analysis indicates that brain stimulation in EDs is still in its infancy. Literature data consist mainly of case reports, cases series, open studies, and only a few randomized controlled trials. Consequently, the evidence supporting the use of brain stimulation in EDs remains weak. Finally, this review discusses future directions in this research domain (e.g., sites of modulation, how to enhance neuromodulation efficacy, personalized protocols).

Keywords: rTMS; deep brain stimulation; treatment; anorexia; bulimia; binge eating disorders

1. Introduction

Eating disorders (EDs) are serious psychiatric disorders characterized by abnormal eating or weight-control behaviors [1]. These disorders are most often chronic and relapsing, and this has a heavy impact on the patients' physical and mental health and life expectancy. Anorexia nervosa (AN) is a multifactorial ED characterized by significantly low body weight for the individual's height, age, and developmental stage, intense fear of gaining weight despite obvious thinness, and extreme behaviors designed to lose weight, such as food restriction with or without induced vomiting, or use of laxatives. The consequence is massive weight loss and/or pathological thinness. Binge eating disorder (BED) and bulimia nervosa (BN) are EDs characterized by recurrent episodes of binge eating and loss of personal control during binging. Individuals with BN counteract binge eating with compensatory behaviors to prevent weight gain, whereas individuals with BED do not exhibit recurrent compensatory behaviors. BED and BN are characterized by compulsive overeating, and shared neural alterations and neurobiological mechanisms underlie these EDs. EDs impair the quality of life of both patients and their families [2]. Among individuals with EDs, mortality and morbidity are increased and health service use is particularly high, resulting in elevated healthcare costs [3].

To date, ED management is still difficult, and few treatments have demonstrated their efficacy. In accordance with most guidelines, management programs are generally multidisciplinary. In AN, the available treatment recommendations aim at restoring normal weight, adapting and relaxing eating behaviors, improving social and interpersonal relationships, and improving the patient's self-image. Psychotherapy is the main therapeutic approach. However, data to guide the psychotherapy choice are limited and controversial [4]. Medication trials have been disappointing [5]. Overall, about one-third of patients will not recover, and the standardized mortality rate is 5.9 [6]. In patients with BN or BED, the best validated and most frequently used treatment is ED-specific cognitive behavioral therapy [7]. Nevertheless, a meta-analysis found that core BN symptoms are still present in more than 60% of patients, even after receiving the best available treatments [8]. Other psychotherapies have been proposed. Moreover, serotonergic antidepressants, the most frequently used pharmacological option, improve the medium-term symptomatology to some degree, but do not allow full remission. In this context, the development of alternative therapeutic strategies is crucial.

Brain stimulation is a therapeutic modality in which the activity of a specific neural circuit is modified by applying an electric current with predefined frequency, amplitude, and pulse width to restore the functional state without any tissue damage [9]. Brain stimulation is obtained by invasive and non-invasive interventions that stimulate or block the action potentials in the nervous system [9,10]. The ultimate aim of brain stimulation is to reverse maladaptive neurocircuitry changes in neural tissue and improve inter-neuronal connectivity [9–11]. These changes implicate synaptic potentiation or depression via regulation of neurotransmitters and ion channels and modification of the expression of intracellular second messengers [12,13]. In direct electrical stimulation, electrodes are used to apply a potential gradient across a neuron that induces intracellular ionic current flow, localized depolarization and hyperpolarization of the cell membrane, resulting in neural stimulation or inhibition [9]. The mechanism for magnetic stimulation is similar, except that the potential gradients are induced in the tissue by a rapidly changing strong magnetic field that is implemented transcutaneously [9]. Non-invasive brain stimulation (NIBS) techniques include electroconvulsive therapy (ECT), repetitive transcranial magnetic stimulation (rTMS), and transcranial direct current stimulation (tDCS). In ECT, seizures are induced by a direct current passing through the brain under general anesthesia [14]. In rTMS, excitability is induced by delivering magnetic stimulation pulses with a wire coil placed externally on the scalp above specific cortical regions [15]. In tDCS, direct current is delivered through electrodes implanted on the scalp, without seizure induction, with the aim of exciting (anodal stimulation) or inhibiting (cathodal stimulation) the activity in specific brain regions [16,17]. Invasive neuromodulation includes deep brain stimulation (DBS) and vagal nerve stimulation (VNS). In DBS, a pulse generator usually implanted in the subclavicular region delivers electrical current to the brain parenchyma through implanted electrodes. On the other hand, in VNS the left cervical vagal nerve is stimulated through a device implanted in the left chest wall [18].

The number of studies on brain stimulation in EDs and/or in dimensions associated with EDs is progressively increasing. In this review, we present the available data, issues, and future directions concerning the use of brain stimulation in EDs.

2. Methods

This is a non-systematic review of the literature on brain stimulation techniques used in patients with EDs. Nevertheless, a systematic research of the available literature was performed in the PubMed database by combining the search terms "eating disorders", "anorexia nervosa", "bulimia nervosa", "binge eating disorders" with the terms "neuromodulation", "rTMS", "tDCS", "DBS", "ECT", "VNS". All papers in English or French published up to June 2020 were retrieved. All original articles on brain stimulation in patients with EDs were included. Studies in high risk populations without EDs (e.g., patients with obesity or healthy subjects with high levels of food craving) were not included. This search was then supplemented by internet searches and manual search of the reference lists of potentially relevant articles and reviews, and by examining pertinent trials registered at clinicaltrial.gov. Among the 121 manuscripts identified, after duplicate removal, 72 were screened. All manuscripts are not cited because when a recent systematic review was available, it was included and prioritized in the synthesis of results. Additional studies on neuromodulation mechanisms, ED treatment, potential ED biomarkers, and mechanistic models of circuitries involved in EDs were also added. The search was performed independently by three researchers (P.D., R.B.K., Y.C.). Disagreements were resolved by consensus among all authors.

3. Results

3.1. rTMS in Eating Disorders

3.1.1. Anorexia Nervosa

As shown in Table 1

, In 2008, the first published case on rTMS concerned a patient with AN and comorbid depression. The study reported weight gain and amelioration of the depressive symptoms after 41 sessions of rTMS over the left dorsolateral prefrontal cortex (DLPFC) [19]. This was followed by other case reports and case series on left DLPFC rTMS in patients with AN, often with comorbid depression [20–22]. The first case series on five patients with AN and without a clinically manifest comorbidity reported AN symptom improvement at 6 months but no longer at 12 months after 20 sessions of rTMS delivered over the left DLPFC [23]. A pilot study in which one session of high-frequency rTMS (10 Hz) was delivered to the left DLPFC in 10 patients showed that the procedure was well tolerated, leading to a reduction in the sensation of feeling full, fat, and anxious as well as in the urge to exercise after exposure to visual and real food stimuli [24]. These studies were followed by double-blind, controlled clinical trials [25–27]. In one of these trials, one rTMS session was delivered to the left DLPFC in 49 patients with AN, but the effect on AN core symptoms was not significant [25] compared with the sham session group. However, in the group analysis, AN core symptoms improved in the rTMS arm compared with baseline (before rTMS), and the results persisted at 24 h of follow-up [25]. Several studies suggest that a higher number of rTMS sessions give better clinical results [26,27]. An ancillary analysis of the sample of a randomized controlled feasibility trial on rTMS [26], using a food choice task, found a decrease in self-controlled food choices, suggesting than rTMS may promote more flexibility in relation to food choices [28]. Finally, the feasibility and safety of rTMS of DLPFC in patients with AN have been confirmed by these randomized controlled trials [25–27].

Table 1. Repetitive transcranial magnetic stimulation (rTMS) in eating disorders.

Reference	Type of Study	Participants	Modulation Target	Treatment Characteristics	Main Results
			Anorexia Nervosa		
Kamolz et al., 2008 [19]	Case report	24-year-old female with AN	Left DLPFC Manual targeting	41 sessions 100 × 2 s trains/10 s inter-train interval at 10 Hz = 2000 pulses per session, 110 % MT	Full remission
Van den Eynde et al., 2013 [24]	Case series (pilot study)	10 patients with AN	Left DLPFC Manual targeting	1 session, 20 × 5 s trains/55 s inter-train interval, 10 Hz, intensity of 110% MT, 1000 pulses over 20 min	Reduced levels of feeling full, feeling fat, and feeling anxious
McClelland et al., 2013 [20]	Case report	23-year-old and 52-year-old women with AN [1]	Left DLPFC Neuronavigation	20 and 19 sessions 20 × 5 s trains/55 s inter-train interval, 10 Hz, intensity of 110% MT, 1000 pulses over 20 min within each session	Significant improvement
McClelland et al., 2016 [23]	Case series	5 women with AN [1]	Left DLPFC Neuronavigation	~20 sessions, 20 × 5 s trains/55 s inter-train interval, 10 Hz, intensity of 110% MT, 1000 pulses over 20 min within each session	Significant improvement of ED and affective symptoms after 6 months, but positive results waned at 12 months follow-up
McClelland et al., 2016 [25]	RCT	49 patients with AN [1]	Left DLPFC Neuronavigation	1 session 5 s trains/55 s inter-train interval, 10 Hz, intensity of 110% MT, 1000 pulses over 20 min	No significant effect on core symptoms of ED compared to sham rTMS, but improvement in individuals who received real rTMS when compared before and after the session and the results persisted at 24 h of follow-up
Choudhary et al., 2017 [21]	Case report	23-year-old female with AN	Left DLPFC Manual targeting	21 sessions High-frequency rTMS (10 Hz) at 110% of resting MT, 1000 pulses	Significant improvement
Jaššová et al., 2018 [22]	Case report	25-year-old female with AN	Left DLPFC Targeting method not available	10 sessions, 10 Hz, 15 trains/day, 100 pulses/train, intertrain interval 107 s	No improvement of ED, anxiety, or depression
Woodside et al., 2017 [29]	Case series	Fourteen subjects with eating disorders (6 AN, 5 BN, and 3 ednos) and comorbid PTSD	DMPFC Neuronavigation	20–30 sessions 120% resting MT, at 10 Hz, 5 s on, 10 s off, 3000 pulses/hemisphere, with left then right lateralized coil orientation	Improvement in emotional regulation and PTSD symptoms
Dalton et al., 2018 [26]	RCT	30 patients (16 real, 14 sham) with AN [2]	Left DLPF CNeuronavigation	20 sessions, 20 × 5 s trains/55 s inter-train interval, 10 Hz, intensity of 110% MT, 1000 pulses over 20 min within each session	Between-group effect sizes of change scores (baseline to follow-up) were small for BMI (d = 0.2, 95% CI −0.49 to 0.90) and eating disorder symptoms (d = 0.1, 95% CI −0.60 to 0.79), medium for quality of life and moderate to large (d = 0.61 to 1.0) for mood outcomes, all favoring rTMS over sham

Table 1. *Cont.*

Reference	Type of Study	Participants	Modulation Target	Treatment Characteristics	Main Results
Knyahnytska et al., 2019 [30]	Case series (pilot study)	8 women with AN	Insula Manual targeting	42 sessions, H-coil dTMS 18 Hz, 2 s on, 20 s off, number of pulses 36, number of trains 80, over 20 min	Reduction in AN-related obsessions and compulsions, as well as depression and anxiety scores
Dalton et al., 2020 [28]	RCT	34 anorexic female patients (17 real, 17 sham) vs. 30 healthy controls [2]	Left DLPFC Neuronavigation	20 sessions 20 × 5 s trains/55 s inter-train interval, 10 Hz, intensity of 110% MT, 1000 pulses over 20 min within each session	No significant effect of rTMS nor time on food choices related to fat content. Among AN participants who received real rTMS, there was a decrease in self-controlled food choices at post-treatment
Bulimic Disorders (Bulimia and/or Binge Eating Disorders)					
Hausmann et al., 2004 [31]	Case report	One woman with BN and depression	Left DLPFC Neuronavigation	10 sessions, 20 × 5 s trains/55 s inter-train interval, 10 Hz, intensity of 110% MT	Significant improvement in BN symptoms
Walpoth et al., 2008 [32]	RCT	14 females with BN	Left DLPFC Manual targeting	15 sessions, 10 × 10 s trains/60 s inter-train interval at 20 Hz, = 2000 pulses; 120% MT	No difference between real and sham group
Van den Eynde et al., 2010 [33]	RCT	38 females with BN [3]	Left DLPFC Manual targeting	1 session, 20 × 5 s trains/55 s inter-train interval, 10 Hz, intensity of 110% MT, 1000 pulses over 20 min	Real rTMS associated with a decrease in self-reported urge to eat and binge eating
Van den Eynde et al., 2011 [34]	RCT	33 females with BN [3]	Left DLPFC Manual targeting	1 session, 20 × 5 s trains/55 s inter-train interval, 10 Hz, intensity of 110% MT, 1000 pulses over 20 min	No differences between the real and sham groups on stroop task
Van den Eynde et al., 2011 [35]	RCT	38 females with BN [3]	Left DLPFC Manual targeting	1 session, 20 × 5 s trains/55 s inter-train interval, 10 Hz, intensity of 110% MT, 1000 pulses over 20 min	TMS did not alter blood pressure or heart rate
Claudino et al., 2011 [36]	RCT	22 patients (11 real, 11 sham) with BN [3]	Left DLPFC Manual targeting	1 session, 20 × 5 s trains/55 s inter-train interval, 10 Hz, intensity of 110% MT, 1000 pulses over 20 min	Decreased salivary cortisol concentrations compared with sham rTMS
Van den Eynde et al., 2012 [37]	Case series	7 left-handed females with BN	Left DLPFCM anual targeting	1 session, 20 × 5 s trains/55 s inter-train interval, 10 Hz, intensity of 110% MT, 1000 pulses over 20 min	Different effects in left- and right-handed people
Downar et al., 2012 [38]	Case report	One woman with severe refractory BN and depression	DMPFC Neuronavigation	2 × 20 sessions 60 trains of 10 Hz stimulation at 120% of resting motor threshold in 5 s trains with a 10-s inter-train interval	Significant improvement in BN symptoms
Baczynski et al., 2014 [39]	Case report	One woman with BED and comorbid depression	Left DLPFC Manual targeting	20 sessions 20 × 4 s trains/26 s inter-train interval, 10 Hz, intensity of 110% MT	Improvement in binge eating scale

Table 1. *Cont.*

Reference	Type of Study	Participants	Modulation Target	Treatment Characteristics	Main Results
Dunlop, 2015 [40]	Case series	28 subjects with anorexia nervosa, binge-purge subtype or bulimia nervosa	DMPFC Neuronavigation	20–30 sessions 120% resting MT, at 10 Hz, 5 s on, 10 s off, 3000 pulses/hemisphere, with left then right lateralized coil orientation	Enhanced frontostriatal connectivity was associated with responders to DMPFC-rTMS for binge/purge behavior
Sutoh et al., 2016 [41]	Case series (pilot study)	8 women with BN	Left DLPFC Manual targeting	1 session, 15 × 5 s trains/55 s inter-train interval, 10 Hz, intensity of 110% MT, 1000 pulses over 20 min within each session	Significant reduction of food craving and decrease in cerebral oxygenation of the left DLPFC
Gay et al., 2016 [42]	RCT	47 women (23 real, 24 sham) with BN [4]	Left DLPFC Manual targeting	10 sessions, 20 × 5 s trains/55 s inter-train interval, 10 Hz intensity of 110% MT, 1000 pulses over 20 min within each session	No significant improvement of bingeing or purging
Guillaume et al., 2018 [43]	RCT	39 patients (22 real, 17 sham) with BN [4]	Left DLPFC Manual targeting	10 sessions, 20 × 5 s trains/55 s inter-train interval, 10 Hz, intensity of 110% MT	Improvement of inhibitory control and decision-making

Note: All studies are cited in bibliography, because when a recent systematic review was available, it was included and prioritized in the synthesis of results. [1,2,3,4]: Partial or total overlap on sample.

Besides DLPFC, one study on rTMS of the inferior parietal cortex was stopped for safety reasons (NCT01717079). The study promoter informed us that the study was halted following two suicide attempts after the first inclusions. Another pilot case series ($n = 8$ patients with long-lasting AN) used deep rTMS to target the insula and found that this approach was safe and well-tolerated. At the end of the 42 sessions, AN-related obsessions and compulsions were reduced, as were the depression and anxiety scores [30].

3.1.2. Bulimia Nervosa and Binge-Eating Disorder

In a recent review of the literature, Dalton et al. identified eight studies on rTMS for BN. The areas stimulated were mainly the left DLPFC, and the dorsomedial prefrontal cortex (DMPFC). The results showed a decrease in food craving, and in some studies a reduction in food binging or purging behavior (for review see Dalton et al. [44]). DLPFC stimulation may also improve the inhibitory control and decision making in patients with BN [43]. A study on the correlation between salivary cortisol and rTMS on the left DLPFC in BN showed that salivary cortisol concentrations were significantly lower in the rTMS arm compared with the sham rTMS arm. This suggests that stimulation of this area modifies the hypothalamic–pituitary–adrenal axis activity in people with BN [36]. Moreover, frontal lobe oxygenation is decreased after one rTMS session [41]. On the other hand, one randomized controlled trial showed no improvement of binge/purge behavior after 10 sessions of high-frequency rTMS on the left DLPFC [42]. A groundbreaking research study demonstrated that self-reported food craving during exposure to experimental foods remained stable before and after stimulation of the left DLPFC compared with the sham group in which craving increased [45].

Another interesting finding is the relationship between frontostriatal connectivity and response to 20 sessions of rTMS in patients with refractory binge/purge behavior. In this case series, enhanced frontostriatal connectivity was associated with binge/purge behavior improvement after DMPFC-rTMS. Conversely, in non-responders, who showed high connectivity on the resting-state fMRI, rTMS caused paradoxical suppression of frontostriatal connectivity [40]. Finally, in an open-label case series that included patients with various EDs (mainly binge form) and comorbid post-traumatic stress disorder, post-traumatic stress symptoms were improved after 20 to 30 sessions of high-frequency rTMS on the DMPFC [29].

Hence, rTMS is an important tool to explore the neurobiology of craving and binge eating (BE). An ongoing study is investigating rTMS tolerability and safety and its effects on food craving and BE behavior, and also on ED-related psychopathology (including depression, anxiety, and stress symptoms), anthropometric measures, cognition, brain structure and function, hormones, and inflammatory biomarkers [46].

3.1.3. rTMS and Site of Modulation

As shown in Table 1, most of the published studies targeted the left DLPFC with excitatory modulation. Nevertheless, other neuroanatomical targets should be investigated. The first is the DMPFC, which plays an important role in self-control, including self-inhibition of movements, self-cessation of loss-chasing in pathological gamblers, self-suppression of emotional responses, and impulse control. It has been hypothesized that DMPFC stimulation may alter the DMPFC top-down executive control of the striatal regions associated with the urge to binge, thereby improving binge symptoms. The available open label studies using 10 Hz stimulation [40] emphasize the interest of this target particularly in BN and BED, although more work is needed to allow definitive conclusions.

The insula has also been considered in one pilot study. The insula is involved in the process of imagination of food images and food intake, in the perception of taste during food intake and of satiety, and in the feeling of disgust after eating. The insular lobe plays a role in the disturbed body image perception in patients with AN and is implicated in the brain response to stress through its close connection with the hypothalamus–pituitary–adrenal axis [12]. This brain area is reduced in patients with AN [47]. Moreover, Kaye et al. demonstrated a functional disconnection between the insula and ventral caudal putamen in patients with AN in a hungry state [48]. All these findings suggest that insula is a potential target in AN.

The corticostriatal circuits through the orbitofrontal cortex (OFC) might also represent a valuable target. They play key roles in complex human behaviors, such as evaluation, affect regulation, and reward-based decision making, and have been implicated in all ED types [49]. A functional hyperconnectivity between NAcc and the orbitofrontal cortex has been shown in AN [50]. Few studies have targeted this area with NIBS, and to our knowledge, it has not been done in patients with ED. Nevertheless, the good response to inhibitory (1 Hz) rTMS in patients with obsessive-compulsive disorder (OCD) who share some features with ED (e.g., functional hyperconnectivity between NAcc and OFC) [51] supports testing this target in ED.

Finally, other targets have also been explored in patients with addictions with promising results, particularly high-frequency stimulation of the superior frontal gyrus [52] and inhibition of the medial prefrontal cortex in patients with cocaine use disorder [53]. All these areas might constitute interesting targets in bulimic disorders, but it is challenging to decide which region to stimulate to obtain the best results.

3.2. tDCS and Eating Disorders

As shown in Table 2, in AN, tDCS approaches on the right and left DLPFC have been tested [54]. In an open-label single-arm study, seven patients with AN underwent left DLPFC anodal tDCS for 25 min daily for 10 days. In three patients, the levels of eating and depressive symptoms improved immediately after the sessions, and the response was maintained at 1 month in one patient [55]. Of note, only patients concomitantly treated with selective serotonin reuptake inhibitors (SSRI) improved. In another open-label study, nine patients with AN received 20 sessions of tDCS (the anode over the left DLPFC and the cathode over the right DLPFC). The treatment was effective on several AN dimensions and the comorbid depression at 1 month of follow-up [56]. Finally, a pilot study is currently testing the efficacy and safety of high-definition tDCS over the left inferior parietal lobe [57].

Table 2. Transcranial direct current stimulation (tDCS) and eating disorders.

Reference	Type of Study	Participants	Modulation Target	Treatment Characteristics	Main Results
Khedr et al., 2014 [55]	Open-label, single arm study (pilot study)	7 patients with AN	Left DLPFC	10 sessions Anodal tDCS for 25 min at 2 mA (15 s ramp in and 15 s ramp out)	Immediate improvement in 3 patients after the sessions on eating and depressive symptoms, with one patient maintaining the response at 1 month
Burgess et al., 2016 [58]	RCT (proof-of-concept study)	30 participants with BED	Right DLPFC	1 session, 2 mA, 20 min	Decreased craving for sweets, savory proteins, and an all-foods category, with strongest reductions in men
Kekic et al., 2017 [59]	RCT	39 patients (2 male) with BN	Right and left DLPFC (3 montages: AR/CL; AL/CR; sham)	1 session 20 min, 2 mA, 10 s ramp on/off	Reduction in ED cognitions with AR/CL tDCS Suppression of urge to binge-eat and increased self-regulatory control with both active montages Improvement of mood with AR/CL
Sreeraj et al., 2018 [60]	Case report	37 year old female with schizophrenia and binge-eating	Right DLPFC	10 sessions, 2 mA, 30 min	Improvement in subjective reporting on cognitive restraint and control over eating as well as feeling of satiation and ability to eat after exposure to cues 3 kg weight loss by the end of the treatment, 7 kg at 10-month follow-up
Strumila et al., 2019 [56]	Open-label study	10 females with AN	Anode over left DLPFC and cathode over right DLPFC	20 sessions of anodal 2 mA stimulation during a period of two weeks	Improvement of anorexic and depressive symptoms

In BN and BED, suppression of the urge to binge eat and increased self-regulatory control were reported by the only double-blind sham-controlled proof-of-principle trial on the effects of bilateral tDCS over the DLPFC in 39 adults with BN [59]. Two electrode montages were tested: anode on the right and cathode on the left (AR/CL) and the reverse (AL/CR). One session of AR/CL led to bulimic cognition reduction and mood improvement, compared with the AL/CR and sham conditions [59]. A case report [60] and the study by Burgess et al. (n = 30 participants with BED) showed that compared with the sham arm, tDCS on the right DLPFC decreased cravings for sweets, savory proteins, and an all-food category with stronger reductions in men. A possible explanation of this finding is that stimulation of the right DLPFC enhances cognitive control and/or decreases the need for reward [58].

3.3. *ECT in Eating Disorders*

3.3.1. Anorexia Nervosa

As shown in Table 3, only case reports and case series have evaluated ECT in AN (n = 50 patients in total) [61]. In most cases, ECT was proposed to treat a comorbid major depressive disorder (MDD), especially treatment-refractory MDD or associated with suicide attempts or obsessive-compulsive disorder (OCD). Indeed, due to the high suicide rate in patients with EDs, intensive treatments, like ECT, are often proposed. The recent and largest case series on patients with AN treated by ECT concerned 30 adolescents with comorbid depression [62]. All were severely depressed and suicidal upon admission and resistant to antidepressants. Improvement in depressive and ED symptoms was observed after ECT with minimal adverse effects. Several years after discharge, 46.6% of patients had no evidence of depression, suicidality, and ED symptomatology, and 23% had only ED symptomatology. Due to the simultaneous improvement of AN symptoms, body weight, and depression, a specific effect on ED cannot be easily identified. Finally, two recent case reports show contradictory results of ECT in patients with AN without psychiatric comorbidity [63,64]. Specifically, Naguy et al. demonstrated a strong improvement of eating behaviors in a 16-year-old girl after only six ECT sessions. However, the absence of comorbid depression or OCD was not clearly stated, and high-dose antidepressant treatment was introduced during the ECT course. Duriez et al. reported that 10 sessions of ECT had a negative outcome and rapid relapse after discharge in patients with careful evaluation of depression, anxiety, and ED dimensions before and after ECT.

Table 3. Electroconvulsive therapy (ECT) and eating disorders.

Reference	Type of Study	Participants	Modulation Target	Treatment Characteristics	Main Results
		Anorexia Nervosa			
Davis et al., 1961 [65]	Case report	12-year-old girl with AN-R	-	12 sessions (bilateral)	Weight gain and discharge
Bernstein et al., 1964 [66]	Case report	20-year-old female with AN-R and personality disorder	-	21 sessions followed by maintenance ECT	Weight gain and mood improvement
Bernstein et al., 1972 [67]	Case report	94-year-old female with AN-R and psychotic disorder	-	5 sessions	Short term weight gain
Ferguson et al., 1993 [68]	Case series	3 patients with AN and MDD	-	11, 8 and 16 sessions (bilateral)	Transient improvement on weight and symptomatology for 2/3 patients
Bek et al., 1996 [69]	Case series	8 females with AN, one had psychosis and five had personality disorders	-	11 sessions	Modest weight gain
Hill et al., 2001 [70]	Case report	77-year-old female with AN-R and MDD	-	9 sessions	Modest weight gain and mood improvement
Poutanen et al., 2009 [71]	Case report	21-year-old female with AN-B/P and MDD	-	45 sessions in three courses (bilateral)	Modest thymic and eating amelioration. Cognitive impairment.

Table 3. *Cont.*

Reference	Type of Study	Participants	Modulation Target	Treatment Characteristics	Main Results
Andrews et al., 2014 [72]	Case report	17-year-old with AN-B/P, MDD, and NSSI	-	10 unilateral and 21 bilateral sessions/13 weeks	Mood improvement
Andersen et al., 2017 [73]	Case report	14-year-old girl with AN-R, MDD, and GAD	-	22 sessions (bilateral)	Weight gain
Saglam et al., 2018 [74]	Case report	24-year-old male with AN-B/P, OCD, and MDD	-	12 sessions (bitemporal)	Weight restoration and OCD improvement, stopped diuretic and laxative abuse.
Pacillio et al., 2019 [61]	Case report	30-year-old female patient with AN and MDD	-	11 sessions (unilateral)	Modest increase of eating disorder, mood improvement
Naguy et al., 2019 [63]	Case report	16-year-old female with AN and personality disorder	-	6 sessions (bitemporal)	Weight gain and improvement in eating behavior
Duriez et al., 2020 [75]	Case report	19-year-old female with AN	-	10 sessions	No improvement of AN symptoms
Shilton et al., 2020 [62]	Case series	30 female adolescents with AN and MDD	-	-	Mood improvement, treatment well tolerated, no specific improvement for eating disorder symptoms
		Bulimic Disorders (Bulimia and/or Binge Eating Disorders)			
Rapinesi et al., 2013 [76]	Case report	41-year-old male with BED and bipolar disorder. Personal history of AN	-	8 sessions (bitemporal)	Important weight loss and decrease of psychotic symptoms

AN: anorexia nervosa; AN-R: anorexia nervosa restricting subtype; AN-B/P: anorexia nervosa binge/purge subtype; BED: binge eating disorder; OCD: obsessive-compulsive disorder; MDD: major depressive disorder; NSSI: non-suicidal self-injury.

To our knowledge, no controlled trial is currently testing ECT efficacy in AN. Furthermore, as only case series have been published, no standardized evaluation has been provided, thus preventing the precise comparison of patients with different AN profiles. Moreover, we hypothesize a strong publication bias towards ECT in severe and enduring AN without comorbid psychiatric disorders.

Nevertheless, the available results suggest that ECT is safe in this population and might improve AN symptomatology in addition to its positive effects on comorbid mood disorders. ECT appears to be well tolerated in this population, and it is even used in late-onset AN in older adults [67,70].

3.3.2. Bulimia Nervosa and Binge Eating Disorder

MDD is more frequent in patients with BN than in AN [77]. According to a recent systematic review [61], only one case report described ECT use in BED and none in BN. In this patient with a psychiatric comorbidity, ECT was safe and effective on bulimic symptoms.

3.4. VNS in Eating Disorders

To date, no study assessed VNS effects in patients with EDs [78]. However, a growing body of evidence suggests the relevance of VNS in patients with ED. Some studies in animal models showed an association between VNS and reduction in food intake and/or weight loss, suggesting that vagal stimulation might mediate satiety signals (for review see McClelland 2013 [79]). Several fMRI studies have also shown that VNS modulates the activity in brain regions related to the processing of afferent vagal signals and interoception, such as the thalamus, precentral gyrus, and insular cortex [80–82]. A recent study demonstrated that transcutaneous VNS improves interoceptive accuracy [83]. This is a very valuable point given the central role of interoception in ED [84–86].

3.5. Deep Brain Stimulation in Eating Disorders

3.5.1. Deep Brain Stimulation in Anorexia Nervosa

In a recent review, Sobstyl et al. described all trials on DBS in patients with AN [87]. Ten years ago, the first description of DBS in a patient with severe and treatment-resistant MDD and comorbid AN opened the way to a new therapeutic modality [88]. To date, 58 case reports on DBS in AN have been published (Table 4). The first studies concerned well known targets in MDD or OCD, mostly in the limbic system linked to the anxiety and emotion pathways. Barbier et al. [89] described AN remission and complete weight recovery in a patients with comorbid OCD/AN after treatment first by bilateral stimulation of the anterior limb of the internal capsule and then of the bed nucleus of the stria terminalis. In 2012, McLaughlin et al. reported the improvement of severe OCD in a patient with comorbid AN treated by DBS of the ventral capsule and ventral striatum [90]. Moreover, they observed a small weight gain, but less distress about caloric intake. Blomstedt et al. [91] showed that bilateral stimulation of the medial forebrain bundle (MFB) and then of the bed nucleus of the stria terminalis (BNST) improved MDD and AN. However, it should be noted that this 60-year-old woman lost weight during the procedure. The first case series came from an open-label trial involving 16 patients with AN, among whom 14 had comorbid depression or other major psychiatric comorbidities [92]. The primary outcomes were acceptability and safety of DBS applied to the subgenual cingulate cortex (SCC), a validated target for the treatment of resistant depression [93]. After 1 year, patients exhibited weight gain and improvement in depressive and anxious symptoms. In 2013, AN remission was observed in four patients after implanting electrodes bilaterally in the nucleus accumbens (NAcc) [94]. Wang et al. [95] used the same method in two patients with AN and a comorbid psychiatric disorder (OCD, generalized anxiety disorder, or MDD). These two trials also demonstrated glucose metabolism changes after DBS in the NAcc and SCC by positron emission tomography [96,97]. Recently, the Shanghai group published the largest series on DBS in AN involving 28 patients with refractory AN who were followed for at least 2 years after electrode implantation in the NAcc [98]. All patients had a major psychiatric comorbidity at inclusion (n = 9 OCD, n = 7 severe anxiety, and n = 12 MDD). Post-hoc analysis suggests that NAcc DBS is less effective for weight restoration in the binge/purge AN subtype than in the restrictive subtype [98]. Another recent preliminary study proposes for the first time two targets in the same trial chosen according to the main psychiatric comorbidities associated with AN: SCC for affective disorder (n = 4) and NAcc for anxiety disorder (n = 4) (Martinez et al., 2020). Four patients considered as responders after 6 months will be randomized in two arms (ON/OFF or OFF/ON) for a double-blind controlled cross over trial.

Regarding tolerance and safety, DBS is a reversible procedure, and the device can be removed if requested by the patient [93,96]. The clinical situation of malnutrition is a key issue for surgical procedures, like DBS [92]. The existing studies did not report any permanent neurological deficit after the procedure. In one patient, the device was removed due to infection (new implantation 6 months later). Moreover, Lipsman et al. observed excessive pain at the incision site in five patients, treatment withdrawal by two patients (device off or removal) without any precise reason, and seizures in two patients. Liu et al. reported device removal in one patient (3%) at 18 months due to rejection. It has been suggested that the surgical risk is higher in patients with severe AN and BMI lower than 14 kg/m^2 due to malnutrition. These first findings are encouraging, but more investigations and controlled trials are needed. Nevertheless, the high mortality and morbidity in severe and enduring AN and the increasing knowledge of AN functional neuroanatomy give strong ethical support for this procedure.

Table 4. Deep brain stimulation (DBS) in eating disorders.

Reference	Type of Study	Participants	Modulation Target	Treatment Characteristics *	Main Results
			Anorexia Nervosa		
Israël et al., 2010 [88]	Case report	56-year-old female with AN and severe depression	SCC (bilateral)	Intermittent stimulation 2 min on/1 min off 5 mA/91 µs/130 Hz	Maintenance of normal BMI (average 19.1 kg/m^2) at 3 years, normal scores in restraint and weight and shape concerns
Barbier et al., 2011 [89]	Case report	39-year-old female with AN and severe OCD	ALIC and BNST (bilateral)	Unknown	Full recovery of AN and strong improvement of OCD
McLaughlin et al., 2012 [90]	Case report	52-year-old female with refractory OCD and AN	Ventral capsule and ventral striatum (bilateral)	Left unilateral, monopolar 7.5 V/120 µs/120 Hz	Significant weight improvement, reduction in AN-related obsession and patient can go out to eat
Wu et al., 2013 and Sun et al., 2012 [94,99]	Case series	4 females with AN (3 OCD, 1 GAD) [1]	NAcc (bilateral)	Unknown	Full remission of AN, restoration of menstrual cycle and return to school for 3 patients
Wang et al., 2013 [95]	Case series	2 females with AN, depression, and OCD	NAcc (bilateral)	2.5–3.8 V/120–210 µs/135–185 Hz	Significant weight gain and affective improvement
Lipsman et al., 2013 [96]	Open label clinical trial	6 females with AN, 5 with psychiatric comorbidities (MDD, OCD, SUD, PTSD) [2]	SCC (bilateral)	5–7 V/90 µs/130 Hz	Weight gain in 3 patients, changes in brain metabolism
Hayes et al., 2015 [100]	Ancillary Study	8 females with AN, 7 with psychiatric comorbidities (MDD, OCD, GAD, PTSD, BPD) [2]	SCC (bilateral)	Unknown	Weight loss in 3 patients, weight gain in 5 patients
Lipsman et al., 2017 [93]	Open label clinical trial	16 females with AN, 14 with psychiatric comorbidities (MDD, OCD, SUD, PTSD, GAD, BPD) [2]	SCC (bilateral)	5–6.5 V/90 µs/130 Hz	Significant weight gain for 8 patients Adverse effects: 1 surgical-site infection, 2 devices explanted at patient request, 1 seizure
Blomstedt et al., 2017 [91]	Case report	60-year-old female with AN and depression	MFB (bilateral) and subsequent BNST (bilateral)	Bipolar MFB stimulation 3 V/60 µs/130 Hz two years later: monopolar BNST stimulation 4.3 V/120 µs/130 Hz	Improvement of affective symptoms Weight stabilization Target change due to blurred vision
Manuelli et al., 2019 [101]	Case report	37-year-old female with AN-BP	BNST (bilateral)	4 V/60 µs/130 Hz	Full weight restoration after 4 months
Wei Liu et al., 2020 [98]	Open label clinical trial	29 females with AN, 28 with psychiatric comorbidities (12 MDD, 9 OCD, 7 GAD)	NAcc (bilateral)	2.5–4 V/120–150 µs/160–180 Hz	12 patients obtained full weight restoration and 5 significant weight increase after 2 years of follow up Less effective with AN-BP than AN-R
Martinez et al., 2020 [102]	Open label clinical trial [3]	7 female and 1 male with AN, 4 with affective disorder and 4 with anxiety disorder as main psychiatric comorbidities	SCC (bilateral) or NAcc (bilateral)	7–8 mA/90 µs/130 Hz	No weight gain. Subjective improvement of quality of life

Table 4. *Cont.*

Reference	Type of Study	Participants	Modulation Target	Treatment Characteristics *	Main Results
Bulimic Disorders (Bulimia and/or Binge Eating Disorders)					
Whiting et al., 2013 [103]	Case series	3 patients with BED	LHA (bilateral)	Monopolar unknown V/90 µs/185 Hz	1/3 significantly improvement in binge eating Significant weight loss in 2/3
Tronnier et al., 2018 [104]	Case report	47-year-old female with BED and severe depression	NAcc (bilateral)	Bipolar 3 V/90 µs/130 Hz	Weight loss (2.8 kg/month), affective improvement and decrease of binge eating behaviors

AN: anorexia nervosa; AN-R: anorexia nervosa restricting subtype; AN-BP: anorexia nervosa binge/purge subtype; BED: binge eating disorder; OCD: obsessive-compulsive disorder; MDD: major depressive disorder; GAD: generalized anxiety disorder; SUD: substance use disorder; PTSD: post traumatic stress disorder; BMI: body mass index; BNST: bed nucleus of the stria terminalis; SCC: subgenual cingulate cortex; NAcc: nucleus accumbens; MFB: medial forebrain bundle; ALIC: anterior limb of internal capsule; LHA: lateral hypothalamus; PET: positron emission tomography. * We retained the main stimulation parameter after adjustments: amplitude/pulse width/frequency. [1,2]: Partial overlap on sample; [3]: in a second phase, patients will be included in a randomized trial with two arms (ON/OFF or OFF/ON).

3.5.2. Deep Brain Stimulation in Bulimia Nervosa and Binge Eating Disorder

As shown in Table 4, several patients have been treated by DBS of the hypothalamus or NAcc for severe obesity [105]. In some cases, binge eating behaviors were mentioned, but without a clear ED diagnosis. A pilot study with a 2-year follow-up assessed DBS of the lateral hypothalamic area in three patients with refractory obesity [103]. Only one patient reported binge eating reduction. Tronier et al. observed a reduction of binge eating behaviors after bilateral DBS of NAcc in one patient with treatment-resistant depression and severe obesity previously treated by gastric bypass [104].

3.5.3. Neuroanatomical Targets in DBS

SCC was the first DBS target tested in AN by Andres Lozano's group after their extensive experience with DBS in depression. This region is an affective regulatory center [106]. Substantial evidence indicates the main role of dysregulated emotional processing in AN pathogenesis [107]. SCC stimulation in AN also benefits from the experience in refractory MDD, and is an extensively interconnected component of the limbic system.

Other limbic regions have also been targeted. The BNST is a center of integration for limbic information and valence monitoring [108]. The MFB is a key structure of the reward-seeking circuitry and is highly connected to the limbic system [109]. Preclinical data supports the interest of NAcc modulation in EDs and the stimulation of the ventral striatum. NAcc stimulation increased food intake and weight gain in a rodent model of food restriction and hyperactivity [110,111]. Abnormalities in goal-directed behavior and the establishment of a compulsive/restrictive behavior might be the consequences of dysregulation of neurocircuits that control positive/negative valence as well as reward and decision-making behaviors [112]. A recent study highlighted the role of the mesolimbic reward circuitry in a rodent model of AN [113].

It is important to stress that when choosing targets for brain stimulation, the dysfunctional networks in EDs must be taken into account, as illustrated by recent studies on DBS. Lipsman et al. and Zhang et al. observed broad changes in glucose metabolism in many brain regions after DBS of the SCC and NAcc, respectively. Specifically, SCC stimulation increases activity in the insula and glucose metabolism in parietal and temporal regions, and decreases cingulate activity [93]. NAcc stimulation decreases activity in the frontal lobe, lentiform nucleus (putamen), and hippocampus [97]. More studies are needed to investigate the influence of ventral striatum (NAcc) stimulation and dorsal striatum (caudate nucleus and putamen) on habit formation. The DBS mechanism of action on neuronal pathways is only partially understood, but the target choice is the focus of the current research because a highly focal intervention can have a very broad effect.

4. Discussion

4.1. Current Evidence and Issues

Altogether, the evidence for the use of brain stimulation in EDs is promising, but more studies are needed before it will be considered an effective intervention. Indeed, the literature consists mainly of case reports, cases series, and open studies, and only a few randomized controlled trials. Most studies had small samples and focused mainly on the immediate effects on craving or neurocognition, without follow-up data. Moreover, methodologies were very heterogeneous among studies. For instance, some studies on rTMS effects on craving did not use cues to induce craving, while others used them only during stimulation or for pre-stimulation craving induction, but not for post-stimulation craving assessment. Some studies assessed craving using a visual analogic scale, whereas other used questionnaires. Moreover, only a few studies assessed the (immediate and long-term) clinical effects of brain stimulation. Yet, a crucial question is whether brain stimulation can induce lasting changes in a well-established behavior. Studies using ECT are limited to case reports. Nevertheless, there have been more studies on ECT in AN in the past two years than in the previous thirty years. This is probably due to a global increase of interest in ECT after years of stigma and the recent demonstration of neurogenesis induction by ECT [114]. Although the level of evidence is low, ECT may be useful and safe for the management of severe and treatment-resistant MDD in patients with AN. Its wider accessibility compared to other brain stimulation techniques should facilitate the organization of a prospective trial, particularly in patients with severe comorbid MDD, given the lower efficacy of SSRI in AN [5]. The cognitive and memory effects of ECT are a challenging aspect. They are the strongest limiting factors of ECT use in MDD and should be thoroughly evaluated in the specific metabolic context of AN. DBS is the most recent and promising brain stimulation technique for severe and enduring AN (due to the ethical issues linked to an invasive procedure). Although the lack of consensus on the best neuroanatomical target strongly limits the level of evidence, there are already prospective studies and a few randomized trials currently recruiting. Park et al. proposed a double-blind cross-over study that includes a sham-stimulation phase [92]. Perez et al. are currently recruiting for a cross-over trial in Spain (NCT03168893) [102].

The main issue of the reviewed studies is that many of them were underpowered. Therefore, their findings must interpreted with caution due to the high risk of type II error and inflated effect sizes. Future studies should include larger samples, and the number of patients needed for a robust statistical analysis should be calculated in advance. In rTMS, most studies used manual methods rather than MRI-based methods to locate the target, particularly those on rTMS of the DLPFC. As the location of the intended target region varied across individuals, this might have affected the results and resulted in low effect-size. Moreover, the standard figure-8-shaped rTMS coil, used in most studies, allows a relatively limited and shallow stimulation area that does not induce direct stimulation of deep cortical areas [115]. Stimulation of deeper areas using an H coil might be more effective, leading to enduring benefits. With the exception of Dalton et al. [28,44], the randomized controlled studies only proposed a limited number of pulses and 1 to 10 sessions (i.e., about 10,000 pulses maximum). It is likely that more sessions are needed to modify neural programs and their associated behaviors. Future studies should determine the optimal dose of neuromodulation and duration (for example by comparing different rTMS durations or by investigating in ancillary studies non-responders to a specific program).

Psychiatric comorbidities are the norm in people with eating disorders (>70%) [1]. Binge disorders are often comorbid with a substance use disorders [1]. Binge eating is also frequently compared to addictions, based on the evidence that they share common characteristics, such as escalating frequency of the behavior, ambivalence towards treatments, and frequent relapses [116,117]. In addition, brain stimulation is a successful strategy in MDD. ECT is recommended in most guideline and rTMS in some of them [118]. Given the high rate of these comorbid disorders in patients with EDs, some of the published studies were built on this background. Protocols targeting DMPFC in BN were adapted from substance use disorders studies, ECT studies on severe MDD have been one of the main drivers to begin ECT in patients with MDD and AN. In DBS, AN comorbid with MDD and OCD was one of the reasons to target the SCC. In their study targeting two areas in the same trial for the first time, the targets were chosen based on two of the major psychiatric comorbidities associated with AN: SCC for affective disorder ($n = 4$) and NAcc for anxiety disorder ($n = 4$) [102]. Indeed, most studies reported positive effects on depressive symptoms with rTMS [26], tDCS [56], ECT [62], and DBS [93]. Future studies in EDs might benefit from this knowledge in brain target selection (Figure 1), in studies design (add-on with another modalities of treatment, inclusion and exclusion criteria, etc.), or in the stimulation parameters: number of sessions, type of coil or electrode, stimulation duration, etc.

Nevertheless, regarding the mood component, there is a crucial methodological problem: because of the simultaneous improvement of ED weight and mood features, a specific effect on ED cannot be identified. Systematic measurement of depressive symptoms associated with subgroup analyses of patients without depression will make it possible to address this problem.

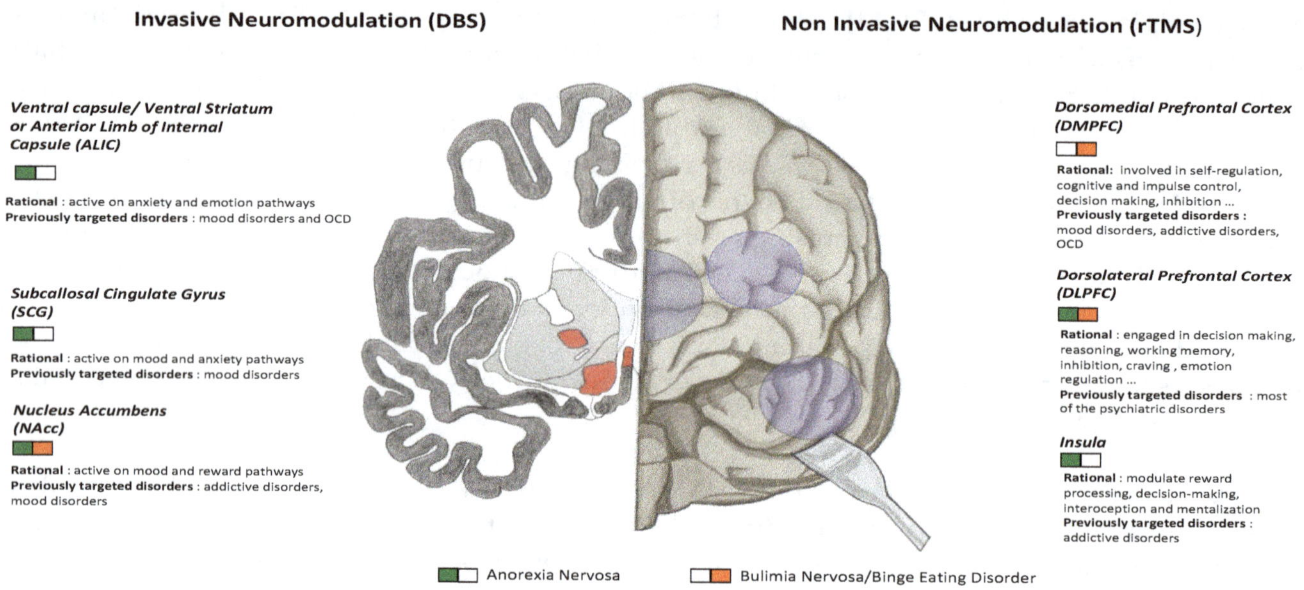

Figure 1. Overview of main neuromodulation targets in eating disorders. Schematic coronal section of right brain and front view of left brain. DBS: deep brain stimulation; rTMS: repetitive transcranial magnetic stimulation; tDCS: transcranial direct current stimulation; OCD: obsessive-compulsive disorder.

Another factor that should be considered is the variability in brain activity related to the metabolic state. The nutritional state in patients with ED might affect brain functions more than in any other psychiatric disorder. Starvation and nutritional status affect behavior, cognition, and disease symptoms. The nutritional status also influences the treatment response, especially to antidepressants that are less effective in acutely ill and underweight patients [5]. To the best of our knowledge, no study has determined whether the nutritional status affects the resting brain state and the neuromodulatory response. Nevertheless, it is possible that the nutritional status influences the response/non-response to a treatment and acts as a confounding factor on brain stimulation efficiency. Better metabolic monitoring could be useful to limit some central deficit that might affect the stimulation response, as reported for folate deficiency in people with comorbid depression [119] and for kynurenic pathway defects [120]. This should be investigated in view of personalized treatment programs.

Finally, in most of the studies reviewed here, samples only included adults and mainly patients with severe, chronic ED. However, due to the good safety and acceptability profile of NIBS, it would be interesting to assess their effects in patients with less severe ED forms, as is usually done in studies on SSRI efficiency in bulimia [121].

4.2. Perspectives

4.2.1. Improving Brain Stimulation Efficiency

A promising strategy consists in stimulating a specific disorder-related circuitry involved in ED using NIBS and in functionally engaging the targeted circuit through cognitive tasks or therapies. This is particularly relevant for neurocognition.

Behavioral abnormalities driven by cognitive processes are a prominent ED feature. For instance, studies in adults with AN suggest poor set-shifting [122], weak central coherence [123], and impaired decision making [124]. Similarly, in BN and BED, decision making and cognitive inhibition seem to be impaired [94,124]. Cognitive remediation programs that target specifically some of these functions have been developed, and some have proved their effectiveness, notably in AN [125]. NIBS also may modulate some of these cognitive functions [126]. It would be interesting to determine whether concomitant brain stimulation might enhance cognitive remediation training. This is especially true for tDCS, which is easier to administer and does not interfere with the psychotherapy sessions. Some proof of concept studies are currently testing them in EDs [127]. Moreover, studies on other disorders showed that when a patient experiences salient cues before modulation with TMS, the benefits increase significantly compared with patients who receive no provocation task [128]. An optimized provocation task before or during brain stimulation is one of the future challenges. In this context, the widespread availability of virtual reality gaming environments that could be customized and adapted to EDs (for example with cues related to food or body shape) might be an opportunity.

In DBS, the stimulation parameters also may be critical. This includes frequency, voltage, pulse width, and also number of contacts and number of directions depending on the electrode model. The choice of parameters remains challenging [129] because symptom improvement cannot be immediately monitored, in contrast to movement disorders. None of the reviewed studies on DBS evaluated the stimulation parameters, although this is a crucial issue. Awake surgery, proposed by Lipsman to increase the procedure safety, could be used also to optimize the target location by testing during implantation [93]. Alternatively, deep electroencephalography during a neurocognitive task immediately before electrode positioning may help to precisely choose the target. In addition, in the currently used open-loop DBS, the medical team can modify the stimulation parameters at different times based on clinical changes. In closed-loop DBS, the stimulation parameters are programmed automatically based on the measured biomarker. Closed-loop devices could adapt the stimulation as a function of the eating behaviors during food consumption or food deprivation. External interventions can modulate some therapeutic strategies to model behaviors like exposition work during specific cognitive behavioral therapy. Finally, the current brain stimulation strategies have little access to important therapeutic targets, deep within the brain. Recent NIBS studies [130,131] in rodent models suggest that deep-brain areas could be targeted in a non-invasive manner, potentially enlarging the number of patients who might benefit from deep-brain stimulation due to the reduction of risk and the perspective of mapping deep-brain targets. Currently, this promising technique has only shown its effectiveness on rodent brains. Its relevance and spatial resolution in human brains, which are much larger, are unknown. Resolution might be increased also using optogenetic techniques, but these methods raise ethical questions linked to their translation from animals to humans [132,133].

4.2.2. Toward More Personalized Protocols

As EDs and each subtype are highly heterogeneous and have many overlapping features, finding a single "optimal" protocol is highly unlikely. Moreover, it has been suggested that there are distinct neural endophenotypes, not readily apparent when using standard diagnostic criteria, but with differential neural and clinical responses to interventions.

Targeting specific subgroups is a valuable option. For instance, many findings support a specific disease trajectory, and preliminary evidence suggests that interventions should be matched to the disease stage [134]. Interventions tailored according to ED stage or to the developmental trajectory were tested in a recent pilot study [30]. Some clinical features could also be considered because they are associated with a specific disease form or poorer prognosis, such as ED subtype (restrictive versus binge), age, gender, associated personality traits, psychiatric comorbidities, or history of childhood abuse. Latent class and profile analyses have been performed and could be a starting point for patient stratification.

Another possible solution is to move from a categorical to a dimensional approach and to target relevant dimensions associated with the disorders rather than with the specific diagnosis. This might be particularly relevant within the research domain criteria (RDoC) research framework. This project seeks to characterize the fundamental domains of cognitive, perceptual, and social processing with the aim of identifying novel targets for mental health disorder treatment. It integrates many levels of information (from genomics and circuits to behavior and self-reports) to assess basic dimensions of functioning that span the full range of human behavior from normal to abnormal. These basic dimensions, independent of DSM diagnoses, are then used to describe the pathological behaviors of psychiatric disorders. Many dimensions associated with EDs can be studied within the RDoC matrix, such as delay discounting, sensitivity to reward/punishment, compulsive behavior, and cognitive functions [135,136]. Brain stimulation is a tremendously interesting approach to modulate the cerebral circuits involved in these dimensions and to assess the impact of this modulation in an integrative way from the molecular level to behavior.

The effects of a given protocol can vary widely across individuals. Some patients will drastically improve, whereas others will not improve, or will even worsen. ED heterogeneity and the potential confounding factors might play a major role, and therefore it is crucial to identify predictors and correlates of the response to a treatment. The perfect illustration of this is the study by Dunlop et al. [40] where enhanced frontostriatal connectivity was associated with response to DMPFC rTMS for binge/purge behavior. rTMS caused paradoxical suppression of frontostriatal connectivity in non-responders who had a high connectivity on resting-state fMRI. Thus, resting-state fMRI could be a key tool to optimize the stimulation parameters. Moreover, in a study on cocaine users treated by continuous theta-burst stimulation of the medial prefrontal cortex, the effects on the neural circuitry of cravings were not uniform and may depend on the individual baseline frontal-striatal reactivity to cues [137]. Hayes et al. also demonstrate that presurgical fornix and anterior limb of internal capsule (ALIC) connectivity are correlated with DBS response [100]. If these results are replicated, this feature might be useful in selecting potential responders. These examples indicate that future studies should include as secondary objectives the profiles of responders/non-responders. It also illustrates the relevance of fMRI neuromodulation studies for patient selection and for investigating the neuromodulatory mechanism. Martinez et al. adapted the DBS target depending on the main comorbidity in patients with severe and resistant AN: SCC for affective disorder or NAcc for anxiety disorder [102]. Finally, all DBS studies defined a minimal illness duration (from 7 to 10 years) as eligibility criterion. Better evidence for choosing the criteria of ED severity, based on neurocognitive tasks, neuroimaging, neuronal metabolism, genetic, or other metabolic patterns, is needed to allow evaluating DBS in patients with shorter illness duration [138]. More precise neurocognitive analyses correlated with neurophysiological measures are also needed.

5. Conclusions

Brain stimulation techniques in EDs are still in their infancy. Different potential targets have been considered (Figure 1), but the literature includes mainly open studies with only a few randomized controlled trials, and many issues remain to be addressed. At this time, the evidence for using brain stimulation as a routine treatment in ED management is weak. However, several ongoing studies should bring new information on optimal stimulation protocols and targets. This is a major source of hope for EDs where the development of alternative treatments is crucial.

Author Contributions: Conceptualization, P.D., R.B.K., S.G.; methodology P.D., R.B.K., P.G., P.C., S.G.; validation P.G., P.C., S.G.; investigation, P.D., R.B.K., Y.C., R.S., M.S., R.M., S.G.; resources, R.S., M.S., R.M.; writing—original draft preparation P.D., R.B.K., S.G.; writing—review and editing, all co-authors; supervision P.C., S.G.; project administration, M.S.; All authors have read and agreed to the published version of the manuscript.

References

1. Treasure, J.; Duarte, T.A.; Schmidt, U. Eating disorders. *Lancet* **2020**, *395*, 899–911. [CrossRef]
2. Zabala, M.J.; Macdonald, P.; Treasure, J. Appraisal of caregiving burden, expressed emotion and psychological distress in families of people with eating disorders: A systematic review. *Eur. Eat. Disord. Rev. Prof. J. Eat. Disord. Assoc.* **2009**, *17*, 338–349. [CrossRef] [PubMed]
3. Striegel-Moore, R.H.; DeBar, L.; Wilson, G.T.; Dickerson, J.; Rosselli, F.; Perrin, N.; Lynch, F.; Kraemer, H.C. Health services use in eating disorders. *Psychol. Med.* **2008**, *38*, 1465–1474. [CrossRef] [PubMed]
4. Mitchell, J.E.; Peterson, C.B. Anorexia Nervosa. *N. Engl. J. Med.* **2020**, *382*, 1343–1351. [CrossRef] [PubMed]

5. Blanchet, C.; Guillaume, S.; Bat-Pitault, F.; Carles, M.E.; Clarke, J.; Dodin, V.; Duriez, P.; Gerardin, P.; Hanachi-Guidoum, M.; Iceta, S.; et al. Medication in AN: A Multidisciplinary Overview of Meta-Analyses and Systematic Reviews. *J. Clin. Med.* **2019**, *8*, 278. [CrossRef]
6. Treasure, J.; Claudino, A.M.; Zucker, N. Eating disorders. *Lancet* **2015**, *375*, 375–583. [CrossRef]
7. Eating Disorders: Recognition and Treatment (NICE Guideline 69). Available online: https://www.nice.org.uk/guidance/ng69 (accessed on 8 June 2020).
8. Slade, E.; Keeney, E.; Mavranezouli, I.; Dias, S.; Fou, L.; Stockton, S.; Saxon, L.; Waller, G.; Turner, H.; Serpell, L.; et al. Treatments for bulimia nervosa: A network meta-analysis. *Psychol. Med.* **2018**, *48*, 2629–2636. [CrossRef]
9. Luan, S.; Williams, I.; Nikolic, K.; Constandinou, T.G. Neuromodulation: Present and emerging methods. *Front. Neuroeng.* **2014**, *7*, 27. [CrossRef]
10. De Pitta, M.; Brunel, N.; Volterra, A. Astrocytes: Orchestrating synaptic plasticity? *Neuroscience* **2016**, *323*, 43–61. [CrossRef]
11. Gomez-Fernandez, L. Cortical plasticity and restoration of neurologic functions: An update on this topic. *Rev. Neurol.* **2000**, *31*, 749–756.
12. Pascual-Leone, A.; Tormos-Munoz, J.M. Transcranial magnetic stimulation: The foundation and potential of modulating specific neuronal networks. *Rev. Neurol.* **2008**, *46* (Suppl. 1), S3–S10. [PubMed]
13. Lopez-Rojas, J.; Almaguer-Melian, W.; Bergado-Rosado, J.A. Synaptic tagging and memory trace. *Rev. Neurol.* **2007**, *45*, 607–614. [PubMed]
14. Read, J.; Bentall, R. The effectiveness of electroconvulsive therapy: A literature review. *Epidemiol. Psichiatr. Soc.* **2010**, *19*, 333–347. [CrossRef] [PubMed]
15. Klomjai, W.; Katz, R.; Lackmy-Vallee, A. Basic principles of transcranial magnetic stimulation (TMS) and repetitive TMS (rTMS). *Ann. Phys. Rehabil. Med.* **2015**, *58*, 208–213. [CrossRef]
16. Impey, D.; de la Salle, S.; Knott, V. Assessment of anodal and cathodal transcranial direct current stimulation (tDCS) on MMN-indexed auditory sensory processing. *Brain Cogn.* **2016**, *105*, 46–54. [CrossRef]
17. Uher, R.; Murphy, T.; Brammer, M.J.; Dalgleish, T.; Phillips, M.L.; Ng, V.W.; Andrew, C.M.; Williams, S.C.; Campbell, I.C.; Treasure, J. Medial prefrontal cortex activity associated with symptom provocation in eating disorders. *Am. J. Psychiatry* **2004**, *161*, 1238–1246. [CrossRef]
18. Marangell, L.B.; Martinez, M.; Jurdi, R.A.; Zboyan, H. Neurostimulation therapies in depression: A review of new modalities. *Acta Psychiatr. Scand.* **2007**, *116*, 174–181. [CrossRef]
19. Kamolz, S.; Richter, M.M.; Schmidtke, A.; Fallgatter, A.J. Transcranial magnetic stimulation for comorbid depression in anorexia. *Nervenarzt* **2008**, *79*, 1071–1073. [CrossRef]
20. McClelland, J.; Bozhilova, N.; Nestler, S.; Campbell, I.C.; Jacob, S.; Johnson-Sabine, E.; Schmidt, U. Improvements in symptoms following neuronavigated repetitive transcranial magnetic stimulation (rTMS) in severe and enduring anorexia nervosa: Findings from two case studies. *Eur. Eat. Disord. Rev.* **2013**, *21*, 500–506. [CrossRef]
21. Choudhary, P.; Roy, P.; Kumar Kar, S. Improvement of weight and attitude towards eating behaviour with high frequency rTMS augmentation in anorexia nervosa. *Asian J. Psychiatr* **2017**, *28*, 160. [CrossRef]
22. Jassova, K.; Albrecht, J.; Papezova, H.; Anders, M. Repetitive Transcranial Magnetic Stimulation (rTMS) Treatment of Depression and Anxiety in a Patient with Anorexia Nervosa. *Med. Sci. Monit.* **2018**, *24*, 5279–5281. [CrossRef] [PubMed]
23. McClelland, J.; Kekic, M.; Campbell, I.C.; Schmidt, U. Repetitive Transcranial Magnetic Stimulation (rTMS) Treatment in Enduring Anorexia Nervosa: A Case Series. *Eur. Eat. Disord. Rev.* **2016**, *24*, 157–163. [CrossRef] [PubMed]
24. Van den Eynde, F.; Guillaume, S.; Broadbent, H.; Campbell, I.C.; Schmidt, U. Repetitive transcranial magnetic stimulation in anorexia nervosa: A pilot study. *Eur Psychiatry* **2013**, *28*, 98–101. [CrossRef] [PubMed]
25. McClelland, J.; Kekic, M.; Bozhilova, N.; Nestler, S.; Dew, T.; Van den Eynde, F.; David, A.S.; Rubia, K.; Campbell, I.C.; Schmidt, U. A Randomised Controlled Trial of Neuronavigated Repetitive Transcranial Magnetic Stimulation (rTMS) in Anorexia Nervosa. *PLoS ONE* **2016**, *11*, e0148606. [CrossRef] [PubMed]
26. Dalton, B.; Bartholdy, S.; McClelland, J.; Kekic, M.; Rennalls, S.J.; Werthmann, J.; Carter, B.; O'Daly, O.G.; Campbell, I.C.; David, A.S.; et al. Randomised controlled feasibility trial of real versus sham repetitive transcranial magnetic stimulation treatment in adults with severe and enduring anorexia nervosa: The TIARA study. *BMJ Open* **2018**, *8*, e021531. [CrossRef]

27. Bartholdy, S.; McClelland, J.; Kekic, M.; O'Daly, O.G.; Campbell, I.C.; Werthmann, J.; Rennalls, S.J.; Rubia, K.; David, A.S.; Glennon, D.; et al. Clinical outcomes and neural correlates of 20 sessions of repetitive transcranial magnetic stimulation in severe and enduring anorexia nervosa (the TIARA study): Study protocol for a randomised controlled feasibility trial. *Trials* **2015**, *16*, 548. [CrossRef]
28. Dalton, B.; Foerde, K.; Bartholdy, S.; McClelland, J.; Kekic, M.; Grycuk, L.; Campbell, I.C.; Schmidt, U.; Steinglass, J.E. The effect of repetitive transcranial magnetic stimulation on food choice-related self-control in patients with severe, enduring anorexia nervosa. *Int. J. Eat. Disord.* **2020**, 1–11. [CrossRef]
29. Woodside, D.B.; Colton, P.; Lam, E.; Dunlop, K.; Rzeszutek, J.; Downar, J. Dorsomedial prefrontal cortex repetitive transcranial magnetic stimulation treatment of posttraumatic stress disorder in eating disorders: An open-label case series. *Int. J. Eat. Disord.* **2017**, *50*, 1231–1234. [CrossRef]
30. Knyahnytska, Y.O.; Blumberger, D.M.; Daskalakis, Z.J.; Zomorrodi, R.; Kaplan, A.S. Insula H-coil deep transcranial magnetic stimulation in severe and enduring anorexia nervosa (SE-AN): A pilot study. *Neuropsychiatr. Dis. Treat.* **2019**, *15*, 2247–2256. [CrossRef]
31. Hausmann, A.; Mangweth, B.; Walpoth, M.; Hoertnagel, C.; Kramer-Reinstadler, K.; Rupp, C.I.; Hinterhuber, H. Repetitive transcranial magnetic stimulation (rTMS) in the double-blind treatment of a depressed patient suffering from bulimia nervosa: A case report. *Int. J. Neuropsychopharmacol.* **2004**, *7*, 371–373. [CrossRef]
32. Walpoth, M.; Hoertnagl, C.; Mangweth-Matzek, B.; Kemmler, G.; Hinterholzl, J.; Conca, A.; Hausmann, A. Repetitive transcranial magnetic stimulation in bulimia nervosa: Preliminary results of a single-centre, randomised, double-blind, sham-controlled trial in female outpatients. *Psychother. Psychosom.* **2008**, *77*, 57–60. [CrossRef] [PubMed]
33. Van den Eynde, F.; Claudino, A.M.; Mogg, A.; Horrell, L.; Stahl, D.; Ribeiro, W.; Uher, R.; Campbell, I.; Schmidt, U. Repetitive transcranial magnetic stimulation reduces cue-induced food craving in bulimic disorders. *Biol. Psychiatry* **2010**, *67*, 793–795. [CrossRef]
34. Van den Eynde, F.; Samarawickrema, N.; Kenyon, M.; DeJong, H.; Lavender, A.; Startup, H.; Schmidt, U. A study of neurocognition in bulimia nervosa and eating disorder not otherwise specified-bulimia type. *J. Clin. Exp. Neuropsychol.* **2012**, *34*, 67–77. [CrossRef] [PubMed]
35. Van den Eynde, F.; Claudino, A.M.; Campbell, I.; Horrell, L.; Andiappan, M.; Stahl, D.; Schmidt, U. Cardiac safety of repetitive transcranial magnetic stimulation in bulimic eating disorders. *Brain Stimul.* **2011**, *4*, 112–114. [CrossRef] [PubMed]
36. Claudino, A.M.; Van den Eynde, F.; Stahl, D.; Dew, T.; Andiappan, M.; Kalthoff, J.; Schmidt, U.; Campbell, I.C. Repetitive transcranial magnetic stimulation reduces cortisol concentrations in bulimic disorders. *Psychol. Med.* **2011**, *41*, 1329–1336. [CrossRef] [PubMed]
37. Van den Eynde, F.; Broadbent, H.; Guillaume, S.; Claudino, A.; Campbell, I.C.; Schmidt, U. Handedness, repetitive transcranial magnetic stimulation and bulimic disorders. *Eur. Psychiatry* **2012**, *27*, 290–293. [CrossRef]
38. Downar, J.; Sankar, A.; Giacobbe, P.; Woodside, B.; Colton, P. Unanticipated Rapid Remission of Refractory Bulimia Nervosa, during High-Dose Repetitive Transcranial Magnetic Stimulation of the Dorsomedial Prefrontal Cortex: A Case Report. *Front. Psychiatry* **2012**, *3*, 30. [CrossRef]
39. Baczynski, T.P.; de Aquino Chaim, C.H.; Nazar, B.P.; Carta, M.G.; Arias-Carrion, O.; Silva, A.C.; Machado, S.; Nardi, A.E. High-frequency rTMS to treat refractory binge eating disorder and comorbid depression: A case report. *CNS Neurol. Disord. Drug Targets* **2014**, *13*, 771–775. [CrossRef]
40. Dunlop, K.; Woodside, B.; Lam, E.; Olmsted, M.; Colton, P.; Giacobbe, P.; Downar, J. Increases in frontostriatal connectivity are associated with response to dorsomedial repetitive transcranial magnetic stimulation in refractory binge/purge behaviors. *Neuroimage Clin.* **2015**, *8*, 611–618. [CrossRef]
41. Sutoh, C.; Koga, Y.; Kimura, H.; Kanahara, N.; Numata, N.; Hirano, Y.; Matsuzawa, D.; Iyo, M.; Nakazato, M.; Shimizu, E. Repetitive Transcranial Magnetic Stimulation Changes Cerebral Oxygenation on the Left Dorsolateral Prefrontal Cortex in Bulimia Nervosa: A Near-Infrared Spectroscopy Pilot Study. *Eur. Eat. Disord. Rev.* **2016**, *24*, 83–88. [CrossRef]
42. Gay, A.; Jaussent, I.; Sigaud, T.; Billard, S.; Attal, J.; Seneque, M.; Galusca, B.; Van Den Eynde, F.; Massoubre, C.; Courtet, P.; et al. A Lack of Clinical Effect of High-frequency rTMS to Dorsolateral Prefrontal Cortex on Bulimic Symptoms: A Randomised, Double-blind Trial. *Eur. Eat. Disord. Rev.* **2016**, *24*, 474–481. [CrossRef] [PubMed]

43. Guillaume, S.; Gay, A.; Jaussent, I.; Sigaud, T.; Billard, S.; Attal, J.; Seneque, M.; Galusca, B.; Thiebaut, S.; Massoubre, C.; et al. Improving decision-making and cognitive impulse control in bulimia nervosa by rTMS: An ancillary randomized controlled study. *Int. J. Eat. Disord.* **2018**, *51*, 1103–1106. [CrossRef] [PubMed]
44. Dalton, B.; Bartholdy, S.; Campbell, I.C.; Schmidt, U. Neurostimulation in Clinical and Sub-clinical Eating Disorders: A Systematic Update of the Literature. *Curr. Neuropharmacol.* **2018**, *16*, 1174–1192. [CrossRef] [PubMed]
45. Uher, R.; Yoganathan, D.; Mogg, A.; Eranti, S.V.; Treasure, J.; Campbell, I.C.; McLoughlin, D.M.; Schmidt, U. Effect of left prefrontal repetitive transcranial magnetic stimulation on food craving. *Biol. Psychiatry* **2005**, *58*, 840–842. [CrossRef]
46. Maranhao, M.F.; Estella, N.M.; Cury, M.E.; Amigo, V.L.; Picasso, C.M.; Berberian, A.; Campbell, I.; Schmidt, U.; Claudino, A.M. The effects of repetitive transcranial magnetic stimulation in obese females with binge eating disorder: A protocol for a double-blinded, randomized, sham-controlled trial. *BMC Psychiatry* **2015**, *15*, 194. [CrossRef]
47. Titova, O.E.; Hjorth, O.C.; Schioth, H.B.; Brooks, S.J. Anorexia nervosa is linked to reduced brain structure in reward and somatosensory regions: A meta-analysis of VBM studies. *BMC Psychiatry* **2013**, *13*, 110. [CrossRef]
48. Kaye, W.H.; Wierenga, C.E.; Bischoff-Grethe, A.; Berner, L.A.; Ely, A.V.; Bailer, U.F.; Paulus, M.P.; Fudge, J.L. Neural Insensitivity to the Effects of Hunger in Women Remitted From Anorexia Nervosa. *Am. J. Psychiatry* **2020**. [CrossRef]
49. Steward, T.; Menchon, J.M.; Jimenez-Murcia, S.; Soriano-Mas, C.; Fernandez-Aranda, F. Neural Network Alterations Across Eating Disorders: A Narrative Review of fMRI Studies. *Curr. Neuropharmacol.* **2018**, *16*, 1150–1163. [CrossRef]
50. Cha, J.; Ide, J.S.; Bowman, F.D.; Simpson, H.B.; Posner, J.; Steinglass, J.E. Abnormal reward circuitry in anorexia nervosa: A longitudinal, multimodal MRI study. *Hum. Brain Mapp.* **2016**, *37*, 3835–3846. [CrossRef]
51. Ruffini, C.; Locatelli, M.; Lucca, A.; Benedetti, F.; Insacco, C.; Smeraldi, E. Augmentation effect of repetitive transcranial magnetic stimulation over the orbitofrontal cortex in drug-resistant obsessive-compulsive disorder patients: A controlled investigation. *Prim. Care Companion J. Clin. Psychiatry* **2009**, *11*, 226–230. [CrossRef]
52. Rose, J.E.; McClernon, F.J.; Froeliger, B.; Behm, F.M.; Preud'homme, X.; Krystal, A.D. Repetitive transcranial magnetic stimulation of the superior frontal gyrus modulates craving for cigarettes. *Biol. Psychiatry* **2011**, *70*, 794–799. [CrossRef] [PubMed]
53. Hanlon, C.A.; Dowdle, L.T.; Austelle, C.W.; DeVries, W.; Mithoefer, O.; Badran, B.W.; George, M.S. What goes up, can come down: Novel brain stimulation paradigms may attenuate craving and craving-related neural circuitry in substance dependent individuals. *Brain Res.* **2015**, *1628*, 199–209. [CrossRef] [PubMed]
54. Hecht, D. Transcranial direct current stimulation in the treatment of anorexia. *Med. Hypotheses* **2010**, *74*, 1044–1047. [CrossRef]
55. Khedr, E.M.; Elfetoh, N.A.; Ali, A.M.; Noamany, M. Anodal transcranial direct current stimulation over the dorsolateral prefrontal cortex improves anorexia nervosa: A pilot study. *Restor. Neurol. Neurosci.* **2014**, *32*, 789–797. [CrossRef] [PubMed]
56. Strumila, R.; Thiebaut, S.; Jaussent, I.; Seneque, M.; Attal, J.; Courtet, P.; Guillaume, S. Safety and efficacy of transcranial direct current stimulation (tDCS) in the treatment of Anorexia Nervosa. The open-label STAR study. *Brain Stimul.* **2019**, *12*, 1325–1327. [CrossRef]
57. Phillipou, A.; Kirkovski, M.; Castle, D.J.; Gurvich, C.; Abel, L.A.; Miles, S.; Rossell, S.L. High-definition transcranial direct current stimulation in anorexia nervosa: A pilot study. *Int. J. Eat. Disord.* **2019**, *52*, 1274–1280. [CrossRef]
58. Burgess, E.E.; Sylvester, M.D.; Morse, K.E.; Amthor, F.R.; Mrug, S.; Lokken, K.L.; Osborn, M.K.; Soleymani, T.; Boggiano, M.M. Effects of transcranial direct current stimulation (tDCS) on binge eating disorder. *Int. J. Eat. Disord.* **2016**, *49*, 930–936. [CrossRef]
59. Kekic, M.; McClelland, J.; Bartholdy, S.; Boysen, E.; Musiat, P.; Dalton, B.; Tiza, M.; David, A.S.; Campbell, I.C.; Schmidt, U. Single-Session Transcranial Direct Current Stimulation Temporarily Improves Symptoms, Mood, and Self-Regulatory Control in Bulimia Nervosa: A Randomised Controlled Trial. *PLoS ONE* **2017**, *12*, e0167606. [CrossRef]

60. Sreeraj, V.S.; Masali, M.; Shivakumar, V.; Bose, A.; Venkatasubramanian, G. Clinical Utility of Add-On Transcranial Direct Current Stimulation for Binge Eating Disorder with Obesity in Schizophrenia. *Indian J. Psychol. Med.* **2018**, *40*, 487–490. [CrossRef]
61. Pacilio, R.M.; Livingston, R.K.; Gordon, M.R. The Use of Electroconvulsive Therapy in Eating Disorders: A Systematic Literature Review and Case Report. *J. ECT* **2019**, *35*, 272–278. [CrossRef]
62. Shilton, T.; Enoch-Levy, A.; Giron, Y.; Yaroslavsky, A.; Amiaz, R.; Gothelf, D.; Weizman, A.; Stein, D. A retrospective case series of electroconvulsive therapy in the management of comorbid depression and anorexia nervosa. *Int. J. Eat. Disord.* **2020**, *53*, 210–218. [CrossRef] [PubMed]
63. Naguy, A.; Al-Tajali, A.; Alamiri, B. An Adolescent Case of Treatment-Refractory Anorexia Nervosa Favorably Responded to Electroconvulsive Therapy. *J. ECT* **2019**, *35*, 217–218. [CrossRef] [PubMed]
64. Duriez, P.; Ramoz, N.; Gorwood, P.; Viltart, O.; Tolle, V. A Metabolic Perspective on Reward Abnormalities in Anorexia Nervosa. *Trends Endocrinol. Metab.* **2019**, *30*, 915–928. [CrossRef] [PubMed]
65. Davis, H.K. Anorexia nervosa: Treatment with hypnosis and ECT. *Dis. Nerv. Syst.* **1961**, *22*, 627–631. [PubMed]
66. Bernstein, I.C. Anorexia Nervosa Treated Successfully with Electroshock Therapy and Subsequently Followed by Pregnancy. *Am. J. Psychiatry* **1964**, *120*, 1023–1024. [CrossRef]
67. Bernstein, I.C. Anorexia nervosa, 94-year-old woman treated with electroshock. *Minn. Med.* **1972**, *55*, 552–553.
68. Ferguson, J.M. The use of electroconvulsive therapy in patients with intractable anorexia nervosa. *Int. J. Eat. Disord.* **1993**, *13*, 195–201. [CrossRef]
69. Bek, R.; Hotujak, L. Clinical characteristics of female patients suffering from anorexia nervosa. *Soc. Psihijat.* **1996**, *24*, 159–161.
70. Hill, R.; Haslett, C.; Kumar, S. Anorexia nervosa in an elderly woman. *Aust. N. Z. J. Psychiatry* **2001**, *35*, 246–248. [CrossRef]
71. Poutanen, O.; Huuhka, K.; Perko, K. Severe anorexia nervosa, co-occurring major depressive disorder and electroconvulsive therapy as maintenance treatment: A case report. *Cases J.* **2009**, *2*, 9362. [CrossRef]
72. Andrews, J.T.; Seide, M.; Guarda, A.S.; Redgrave, G.W.; Coffey, D.B. Electroconvulsive therapy in an adolescent with severe major depression and anorexia nervosa. *J. Child. Adolesc. Psychopharmacol.* **2014**, *24*, 94–98. [CrossRef] [PubMed]
73. Andersen, L.; LaRosa, C.; Gih, D.E. Reexamining the Role of Electroconvulsive Therapy in Anorexia Nervosa in Adolescents. *J. ECT* **2017**, *33*, 294–296. [CrossRef] [PubMed]
74. Saglam, T.; Aksoy Poyraz, C.; Poyraz, B.C.; Tosun, M. Successful use of electroconvulsive therapy in a patient with anorexia nervosa and severe acute-onset obsessive-compulsive disorder. *Int. J. Eat. Disord.* **2018**, *51*, 1026–1028. [CrossRef] [PubMed]
75. Duriez, P.; Maatoug, R.; Verbe, J. Failure of Electroconvulsive Therapy to Improve Anorexia Nervosa in the Absence of Other Psychiatric Comorbidities: A Case Report. *J. ECT* **2020**. [CrossRef] [PubMed]
76. Rapinesi, C.; Del Casale, A.; Serata, D.; Caccia, F.; Di Pietro, S.; Scatena, P.; Carbonetti, P.; Fensore, C.; Angeletti, G.; Tatarelli, R.; et al. Electroconvulsive therapy in a man with comorbid severe obesity, binge eating disorder, and bipolar disorder. *J. ECT* **2013**, *29*, 142–144. [CrossRef] [PubMed]
77. Jaite, C.; Hoffmann, F.; Glaeske, G.; Bachmann, C.J. Prevalence, comorbidities and outpatient treatment of anorexia and bulimia nervosa in German children and adolescents. *Eat. Weight Disord.* **2013**, *18*, 157–165. [CrossRef]
78. Val-Laillet, D.; Aarts, E.; Weber, B.; Ferrari, M.; Quaresima, V.; Stoeckel, L.E.; Alonso-Alonso, M.; Audette, M.; Malbert, C.H.; Stice, E. Neuroimaging and neuromodulation approaches to study eating behavior and prevent and treat eating disorders and obesity. *Neuroimage Clin.* **2015**, *8*, 1–31. [CrossRef]
79. McClelland, J.; Bozhilova, N.; Campbell, I.; Schmidt, U. A systematic review of the effects of neuromodulation on eating and body weight: Evidence from human and animal studies. *Eur. Eat. Disord. Rev.* **2013**, *21*, 436–455. [CrossRef]
80. Badran, B.W.; Dowdle, L.T.; Mithoefer, O.J.; LaBate, N.T.; Coatsworth, J.; Brown, J.C.; DeVries, W.H.; Austelle, C.W.; McTeague, L.M.; George, M.S. Neurophysiologic effects of transcutaneous auricular vagus nerve stimulation (taVNS) via electrical stimulation of the tragus: A concurrent taVNS/fMRI study and review. *Brain Stimul.* **2018**, *11*, 492–500. [CrossRef]

81. Dietrich, S.; Smith, J.; Scherzinger, C.; Hofmann-Preiss, K.; Freitag, T.; Eisenkolb, A.; Ringler, R. A novel transcutaneous vagus nerve stimulation leads to brainstem and cerebral activations measured by functional MRI. *Biomed. Tech.* **2008**, *53*, 104–111. [CrossRef]
82. Yakunina, N.; Kim, S.S.; Nam, E.C. Optimization of Transcutaneous Vagus Nerve Stimulation Using Functional MRI. *Neuromodulation* **2017**, *20*, 290–300. [CrossRef] [PubMed]
83. Villani, V.; Tsakiris, M.; Azevedo, R.T. Transcutaneous vagus nerve stimulation improves interoceptive accuracy. *Neuropsychologia* **2019**, *134*, 107201. [CrossRef] [PubMed]
84. Kaye, W.H.; Wagner, A.; Fudge, J.L.; Paulus, M. Neurocircuity of eating disorders. *Curr. Top. Behav. Neurosci.* **2011**, *6*, 37–57. [CrossRef] [PubMed]
85. Khalsa, S.S.; Adolphs, R.; Cameron, O.G.; Critchley, H.D.; Davenport, P.W.; Feinstein, J.S.; Feusner, J.D.; Garfinkel, S.N.; Lane, R.D.; Mehling, W.E.; et al. Interoception and Mental Health: A Roadmap. *Biol Psychiatry Cogn. Neurosci. Neuroimaging* **2018**, *3*, 501–513. [CrossRef] [PubMed]
86. Berner, L.A.; Simmons, A.N.; Wierenga, C.E.; Bischoff-Grethe, A.; Paulus, M.P.; Bailer, U.F.; Kaye, W.H. Altered anticipation and processing of aversive interoceptive experience among women remitted from bulimia nervosa. *Neuropsychopharmacology* **2019**, *44*, 1265–1273. [CrossRef]
87. Sobstyl, M.; Stapinska-Syniec, A.; Sokol-Szawlowska, M.; Kupryjaniuk, A. Deep brain stimulation for the treatment of severe intractable anorexia nervosa. *Br. J. Neurosurg.* **2019**, *33*, 601–607. [CrossRef] [PubMed]
88. Israel, M.; Steiger, H.; Kolivakis, T.; McGregor, L.; Sadikot, A.F. Deep brain stimulation in the subgenual cingulate cortex for an intractable eating disorder. *Biol. Psychiatry* **2010**, *67*, e53–e54. [CrossRef]
89. Barbier, J.; Gabriels, L.; van Laere, K.; Nuttin, B. Successful anterior capsulotomy in comorbid anorexia nervosa and obsessive-compulsive disorder: Case report. *Neurosurgery* **2011**, *69*, E745–E751, discussion E751. [CrossRef]
90. McLaughlin, N.C.; Didie, E.R.; Machado, A.G.; Haber, S.N.; Eskandar, E.N.; Greenberg, B.D. Improvements in anorexia symptoms after deep brain stimulation for intractable obsessive-compulsive disorder. *Biol. Psychiatry* **2013**, *73*, e29–e31. [CrossRef]
91. Blomstedt, P.; Naesstrom, M.; Bodlund, O. Deep brain stimulation in the bed nucleus of the stria terminalis and medial forebrain bundle in a patient with major depressive disorder and anorexia nervosa. *Clin. Case Rep.* **2017**, *5*, 679–684. [CrossRef]
92. Park, R.J.; Singh, I.; Pike, A.C.; Tan, J.O. Deep Brain Stimulation in Anorexia Nervosa: Hope for the Hopeless or Exploitation of the Vulnerable? The Oxford Neuroethics Gold Standard Framework. *Front. Psychiatry* **2017**, *8*, 44. [CrossRef] [PubMed]
93. Lipsman, N.; Lam, E.; Volpini, M.; Sutandar, K.; Twose, R.; Giacobbe, P.; Sodums, D.J.; Smith, G.S.; Woodside, D.B.; Lozano, A.M. Deep brain stimulation of the subcallosal cingulate for treatment-refractory anorexia nervosa: 1 year follow-up of an open-label trial. *Lancet Psychiatry* **2017**, *4*, 285–294. [CrossRef]
94. Wu, H.; Van Dyck-Lippens, P.J.; Santegoeds, R.; van Kuyck, K.; Gabriels, L.; Lin, G.; Pan, G.; Li, Y.; Li, D.; Zhan, S.; et al. Deep-brain stimulation for anorexia nervosa. *World Neurosurg.* **2013**, *80*, S29.e1–S29.e10. [CrossRef] [PubMed]
95. Wang, J.; Chang, C.; Geng, N.; Wang, X.; Gao, G. Treatment of intractable anorexia nervosa with inactivation of the nucleus accumbens using stereotactic surgery. *Stereotact. Funct. Neurosurg.* **2013**, *91*, 364–372. [CrossRef]
96. Lipsman, N.; Woodside, D.B.; Giacobbe, P.; Lozano, A.M. Neurosurgical treatment of anorexia nervosa: Review of the literature from leucotomy to deep brain stimulation. *Eur. Eat. Disord. Rev.* **2013**, *21*, 428–435. [CrossRef]
97. Zhang, H.W.; Li, D.Y.; Zhao, J.; Guan, Y.H.; Sun, B.M.; Zuo, C.T. Metabolic imaging of deep brain stimulation in anorexia nervosa: A 18F-FDG PET/CT study. *Clin. Nucl. Med.* **2013**, *38*, 943–948. [CrossRef]
98. Liu, W.; Zhan, S.; Li, D.; Lin, Z.; Zhang, C.; Wang, T.; Pan, S.; Zhang, J.; Cao, C.; Jin, H.; et al. Deep brain stimulation of the nucleus accumbens for treatment-refractory anorexia nervosa: A long-term follow-up study. *Brain Stimul.* **2020**, *13*, 643–649. [CrossRef]
99. Sun, B.; Liu, W. Stereotactic surgery for eating disorders. *Surg. Neurol. Int.* **2013**, *4*, S164–S169. [CrossRef]
100. Hayes, D.J.; Lipsman, N.; Chen, D.Q.; Woodside, D.B.; Davis, K.D.; Lozano, A.M.; Hodaie, M. Subcallosal Cingulate Connectivity in Anorexia Nervosa Patients Differs From Healthy Controls: A Multi-tensor Tractography Study. *Brain Stimul.* **2015**, *8*, 758–768. [CrossRef]

101. Manuelli, M.; Franzini, A.; Galentino, R.; Bidone, R.; Dell'Osso, B.; Porta, M.; Servello, D.; Cena, H. Changes in eating behavior after deep brain stimulation for anorexia nervosa. A case study. *Eat. Weight Disord.* **2019**. [CrossRef]
102. Villalba Martinez, G.; Justicia, A.; Salgado, P.; Gines, J.M.; Guardiola, R.; Cedron, C.; Polo, M.; Delgado-Martinez, I.; Medrano, S.; Manero, R.M.; et al. A Randomized Trial of Deep Brain Stimulation to the Subcallosal Cingulate and Nucleus Accumbens in Patients with Treatment-Refractory, Chronic, and Severe Anorexia Nervosa: Initial Results at 6 Months of Follow Up. *J. Clin. Med.* **2020**, *9*, 1946. [CrossRef] [PubMed]
103. Whiting, D.M.; Tomycz, N.D.; Bailes, J.; de Jonge, L.; Lecoultre, V.; Wilent, B.; Alcindor, D.; Prostko, E.R.; Cheng, B.C.; Angle, C.; et al. Lateral hypothalamic area deep brain stimulation for refractory obesity: A pilot study with preliminary data on safety, body weight, and energy metabolism. *J. Neurosurg.* **2013**, *119*, 56–63. [CrossRef] [PubMed]
104. Tronnier, V.M.; Rasche, D.; Thorns, V.; Alvarez-Fischer, D.; Munte, T.F.; Zurowski, B. Massive weight loss following deep brain stimulation of the nucleus accumbens in a depressed woman. *Neurocase* **2018**, *24*, 49–53. [CrossRef] [PubMed]
105. Formolo, D.A.; Gaspar, J.M.; Melo, H.M.; Eichwald, T.; Zepeda, R.J.; Latini, A.; Okun, M.S.; Walz, R. Deep Brain Stimulation for Obesity: A Review and Future Directions. *Front. Neurosci.* **2019**, *13*, 323. [CrossRef] [PubMed]
106. Mayberg, H.S.; Liotti, M.; Brannan, S.K.; McGinnis, S.; Mahurin, R.K.; Jerabek, P.A.; Silva, J.A.; Tekell, J.L.; Martin, C.C.; Lancaster, J.L.; et al. Reciprocal limbic-cortical function and negative mood: Converging PET findings in depression and normal sadness. *Am. J. Psychiatry* **1999**, *156*, 675–682. [CrossRef]
107. Lipsman, N.; Woodside, D.B.; Lozano, A.M. Neurocircuitry of limbic dysfunction in anorexia nervosa. *Cortex* **2015**, *62*, 109–118. [CrossRef]
108. Lebow, M.A.; Chen, A. Overshadowed by the amygdala: The bed nucleus of the stria terminalis emerges as key to psychiatric disorders. *Mol. Psychiatry* **2016**, *21*, 450–463. [CrossRef]
109. Coenen, V.A.; Panksepp, J.; Hurwitz, T.A.; Urbach, H.; Madler, B. Human medial forebrain bundle (MFB) and anterior thalamic radiation (ATR): Imaging of two major subcortical pathways and the dynamic balance of opposite affects in understanding depression. *J. Neuropsychiatry Clin. Neurosci.* **2012**, *24*, 223–236. [CrossRef]
110. van der Plasse, G.; Schrama, R.; van Seters, S.P.; Vanderschuren, L.J.; Westenberg, H.G. Deep brain stimulation reveals a dissociation of consummatory and motivated behaviour in the medial and lateral nucleus accumbens shell of the rat. *PLoS ONE* **2012**, *7*, e33455. [CrossRef]
111. Guercio, L.A.; Schmidt, H.D.; Pierce, R.C. Deep brain stimulation of the nucleus accumbens shell attenuates cue-induced reinstatement of both cocaine and sucrose seeking in rats. *Behav. Brain Res.* **2015**, *281*, 125–130. [CrossRef]
112. Steding, J.; Boehm, I.; King, J.A.; Geisler, D.; Ritschel, F.; Seidel, M.; Doose, A.; Jaite, C.; Roessner, V.; Smolka, M.N.; et al. Goal-directed vs. habitual instrumental behavior during reward processing in anorexia nervosa: An fMRI study. *Sci. Rep.* **2019**, *9*, 13529. [CrossRef] [PubMed]
113. Foldi, C.J.; Milton, L.K.; Oldfield, B.J. The Role of Mesolimbic Reward Neurocircuitry in Prevention and Rescue of the Activity-Based Anorexia (ABA) Phenotype in Rats. *Neuropsychopharmacology* **2017**, *42*, 2292–2300. [CrossRef]
114. Joshi, S.H.; Espinoza, R.T.; Pirnia, T.; Shi, J.; Wang, Y.; Ayers, B.; Leaver, A.; Woods, R.P.; Narr, K.L. Structural Plasticity of the Hippocampus and Amygdala Induced by Electroconvulsive Therapy in Major Depression. *Biol. Psychiatry* **2016**, *79*, 282–292. [CrossRef] [PubMed]
115. Zangen, A.; Roth, Y.; Voller, B.; Hallett, M. Transcranial magnetic stimulation of deep brain regions: Evidence for efficacy of the H-coil. *Clin. Neurophysiol.* **2005**, *116*, 775–779. [CrossRef] [PubMed]
116. Gearhardt, A.N.; White, M.A.; Potenza, M.N. Binge eating disorder and food addiction. *Curr. Drug Abuse Rev.* **2011**, *4*, 201–207. [CrossRef] [PubMed]
117. Volkow, N.D.; Wang, G.J.; Fowler, J.S.; Tomasi, D.; Baler, R. Food and drug reward: Overlapping circuits in human obesity and addiction. *Curr. Top. Behav. Neurosci.* **2012**, *11*, 1–24. [CrossRef] [PubMed]
118. Bayes, A.J.; Parker, G.B. Comparison of guidelines for the treatment of unipolar depression: A focus on pharmacotherapy and neurostimulation. *Acta Psychiatr. Scand.* **2018**, *137*, 459–471. [CrossRef]
119. Pan, L.A.; Martin, P.; Zimmer, T.; Segreti, A.M.; Kassiff, S.; McKain, B.W.; Baca, C.A.; Rengasamy, M.; Hyland, K.; Walano, N.; et al. Neurometabolic Disorders: Potentially Treatable Abnormalities in Patients With Treatment-Refractory Depression and Suicidal Behavior. *Am. J. Psychiatry* **2017**, *174*, 42–50. [CrossRef]

120. Schwieler, L.; Samuelsson, M.; Frye, M.A.; Bhat, M.; Schuppe-Koistinen, I.; Jungholm, O.; Johansson, A.G.; Landen, M.; Sellgren, C.M.; Erhardt, S. Electroconvulsive therapy suppresses the neurotoxic branch of the kynurenine pathway in treatment-resistant depressed patients. *J. Neuroinflamm.* **2016**, *13*, 51. [CrossRef]
121. Romano, S.J.; Halmi, K.A.; Sarkar, N.P.; Koke, S.C.; Lee, J.S. A placebo-controlled study of fluoxetine in continued treatment of bulimia nervosa after successful acute fluoxetine treatment. *Am. J. Psychiatry* **2002**, *159*, 96–102. [CrossRef]
122. Roberts, M.E.; Tchanturia, K.; Stahl, D.; Southgate, L.; Treasure, J. A systematic review and meta-analysis of set-shifting ability in eating disorders. *Psychol. Med.* **2007**, *37*, 1075–1084. [CrossRef] [PubMed]
123. Lang, K.; Lopez, C.; Stahl, D.; Tchanturia, K.; Treasure, J. Central coherence in eating disorders: An updated systematic review and meta-analysis. *World J. Biol. Psychiatry* **2014**, *15*, 586–598. [CrossRef] [PubMed]
124. Guillaume, S.; Gorwood, P.; Jollant, F.; Van den Eynde, F.; Courtet, P.; Richard-Devantoy, S. Impaired decision-making in symptomatic anorexia and bulimia nervosa patients: A meta-analysis. *Psychol. Med.* **2015**, *45*, 3377–3391. [CrossRef] [PubMed]
125. Leppanen, J.; Adamson, J.; Tchanturia, K. Impact of Cognitive Remediation Therapy on Neurocognitive Processing in Anorexia Nervosa. *Front. Psychiatry* **2018**, *9*, 96. [CrossRef] [PubMed]
126. Brevet-Aeby, C.; Brunelin, J.; Iceta, S.; Padovan, C.; Poulet, E. Prefrontal cortex and impulsivity: Interest of noninvasive brain stimulation. *Neurosci. Biobehav. Rev.* **2016**, *71*, 112–134. [CrossRef]
127. Gordon, G.; Brockmeyer, T.; Schmidt, U.; Campbell, I.C. Combining cognitive bias modification training (CBM) and transcranial direct current stimulation (tDCS) to treat binge eating disorder: Study protocol of a randomised controlled feasibility trial. *BMJ Open* **2019**, *9*, e030023. [CrossRef]
128. Dinur-Klein, L.; Dannon, P.; Hadar, A.; Rosenberg, O.; Roth, Y.; Kotler, M.; Zangen, A. Smoking cessation induced by deep repetitive transcranial magnetic stimulation of the prefrontal and insular cortices: A prospective, randomized controlled trial. *Biol. Psychiatry* **2014**, *76*, 742–749. [CrossRef]
129. Karas, P.J.; Lee, S.; Jimenez-Shahed, J.; Goodman, W.K.; Viswanathan, A.; Sheth, S.A. Deep Brain Stimulation for Obsessive Compulsive Disorder: Evolution of Surgical Stimulation Target Parallels Changing Model of Dysfunctional Brain Circuits. *Front. Neurosci.* **2018**, *12*, 998. [CrossRef]
130. Grossman, N.; Bono, D.; Dedic, N.; Kodandaramaiah, S.B.; Rudenko, A.; Suk, H.J.; Cassara, A.M.; Neufeld, E.; Kuster, N.; Tsai, L.H.; et al. Noninvasive Deep Brain Stimulation via Temporally Interfering Electric Fields. *Cell* **2017**, *169*, 1029–1041. [CrossRef]
131. Lozano, A.M. Waving Hello to Noninvasive Deep-Brain Stimulation. *N. Engl. J. Med.* **2017**, *377*, 1096–1098. [CrossRef]
132. Delbeke, J.; Hoffman, L.; Mols, K.; Braeken, D.; Prodanov, D. And Then There Was Light: Perspectives of Optogenetics for Deep Brain Stimulation and Neuromodulation. *Front. Neurosci.* **2017**, *11*, 663. [CrossRef]
133. Gradinaru, V.; Mogri, M.; Thompson, K.R.; Henderson, J.M.; Deisseroth, K. Optical deconstruction of parkinsonian neural circuitry. *Science* **2009**, *324*, 354–359. [CrossRef] [PubMed]
134. Treasure, J.; Stein, D.; Maguire, S. Has the time come for a staging model to map the course of eating disorders from high risk to severe enduring illness? An examination of the evidence. *Early Interv. Psychiatry* **2015**, *9*, 173–184. [CrossRef] [PubMed]
135. Dunlop, K.A.; Woodside, B.; Downar, J. Targeting Neural Endophenotypes of Eating Disorders with Non-invasive Brain Stimulation. *Front. Neurosci.* **2016**, *10*, 30. [CrossRef] [PubMed]
136. Wildes, J.E.; Marcus, M.D. Application of the Research Domain Criteria (RDoC) framework to eating disorders: Emerging concepts and research. *Curr. Psychiatry Rep.* **2015**, *17*, 30. [CrossRef] [PubMed]
137. Kearney-Ramos, T.E.; Dowdle, L.T.; Mithoefer, O.J.; Devries, W.; George, M.S.; Hanlon, C.A. State-Dependent Effects of Ventromedial Prefrontal Cortex Continuous Thetaburst Stimulation on Cocaine Cue Reactivity in Chronic Cocaine Users. *Front. Psychiatry* **2019**, *10*, 317. [CrossRef]
138. Wonderlich, S.A.; Bulik, C.M.; Schmidt, U.; Steiger, H.; Hoek, H.W. Severe and enduring anorexia nervosa: Update and observations about the current clinical reality. *Int. J. Eat. Disord.* **2020**. [CrossRef]

9

Clinical and Neurophysiological Correlates of Emotion and Food Craving Regulation in Patients with Anorexia Nervosa

Nuria Mallorquí-Bagué [1,2,3,*,†], María Lozano-Madrid [1,2,†], Giulia Testa [1,2], Cristina Vintró-Alcaraz [1,2], Isabel Sánchez [1], Nadine Riesco [1], José César Perales [4], Juan Francisco Navas [5,6], Ignacio Martínez-Zalacaín [1,7], Alberto Megías [4], Roser Granero [2,8], Misericordia Veciana De Las Heras [9], Rayane Chami [10], Susana Jiménez-Murcia [1,2,7], José Antonio Fernández-Formoso [2], Janet Treasure [10] and Fernando Fernández-Aranda [1,2,7,*]

1 Department of Psychiatry, University Hospital of Bellvitge-IDIBELL, 08907 Barcelona, Spain; maria.lozano@bellvitgehospital.cat (M.L.-M.); gtesta@idibell.cat (G.T.); cvintro@bellvitgehospital.cat (C.V.-A.); isasanchez@bellvitgehospital.cat (I.S.); nriesco@bellvitgehospital.cat (N.R.); imartinezz@outlook.es (I.M.-Z.); sjimenez@bellvitgehospital.cat (S.J.-M.)

2 CIBER Fisiopatologia Obesidad y Nutrición (CIBERobn), Instituto de Salud Carlos III, 28029 Madrid, Spain; Roser.Granero@uab.cat (R.G.); tono.fernandez@ciberisciii.es (J.A.F.-F.)

3 Addictive Behavior Unit, Department of Psychiatry, Hospital de la Santa Creu i Sant Pau, 08001 Barcelona, Spain

4 Department of Experimental Psychology, Mind, Brain, and Behavior Research Centre, University of Granada, 18071 Granada, Spain; jcesar@ugr.es (J.C.P.); megiasrobles@gmail.com (A.M.)

5 Department of Basic Psychology, Autonomous University of Madrid, 28049 Madrid, Spain; juan.fco.navas@gmail.com

6 Universitat Oberta de Catalunya, 08018 Barcelona, Spain

7 Clinical Sciences Department, School of Medicine, University of Barcelona, 08907 Barcelona, Spain

8 Department of Psychobiology and Methodology, Autonomous University of Barcelona, 08035 Barcelona, Spain

9 Neurophysiology Unit, Neurology Department, Hospital Universitari de Bellvitge, 08907 Barcelona, Spain; mveciana@bellvitgehospital.cat

10 Section of Eating Disorders, Institute of Psychiatry, Psychology & Neuroscience (IoPPN), King's College London, London SE5 8AF, UK; rayane.chami@kcl.ac.uk (R.C.); janet.treasure@kcl.ac.uk (J.T.)

* Correspondence: nmallorqui@santpau.cat (N.M.-B.); ffernandez@bellvitgehospital.cat (F.F.-A.)

† Shared First authorship: Nuria Mallorquí-Bagué and María Lozano-Madrid.

Abstract: Background: Difficulties in emotion regulation and craving regulation have been linked to eating symptomatology in patients with anorexia nervosa (AN), contributing to the maintenance of their eating disorder. Methods: To investigate clinical and electrophysiological correlates of these processes, 20 patients with AN and 20 healthy controls (HC) completed a computerized task during EEG recording, where they were instructed to down-regulate negative emotions or food craving. Participants also completed self-report measures of emotional regulation and food addiction. The P300 and Late Positive Potential (LPP) ERPs were analysed. Results: LPP amplitudes were significantly smaller during down-regulation of food craving among both groups. Independent of task condition, individuals with AN showed smaller P300 amplitudes compared to HC. Among HC, the self-reported use of re-appraisal strategies positively correlated with LPP amplitudes during emotional regulation task, while suppressive strategies negatively correlated with LPP amplitudes. The AN group, in comparison to the HC group, exhibited greater food addiction, greater use of maladaptive strategies, and emotional dysregulation. Conclusions: Despite the enhanced self-reported psychopathology among AN, both groups indicated neurophysiological evidence of food craving regulation as evidenced by blunted LPP amplitudes in the relevant task condition. Further research is required to delineate the mechanisms associated with reduced overall P300 amplitudes among individuals with AN.

Keywords: food craving; food addiction; emotion regulation; eating disorders; anorexia nervosa; event related potentials; EEG; neurophysiology; psychopathology

---

1. Introduction

Anorexia nervosa (AN) is recognized as a severe mental disorder characterized by restrained eating, dysfunctional thoughts, preoccupation concerning food and body image disturbance [1,2]. In addition to maladaptive cognitions and behaviours, difficulties in emotion regulation and food craving regulation have been linked to disordered eating symptomatology (i.e., binging, purging, or restriction), which are considered to be contributing factors to the maintenance of eating disorders [3–5].

Emotion regulation is understood as the process by which individuals are able to modulate the way they experience and express their emotions [6]. Two strategies have been of special interest when studying emotion regulation: suppression and reappraisal. Suppression consists of inhibiting the behavioural expression of an emotional response to a stressor, while reappraisal implicates reinterpreting the meaning of an emotional event [7]. Although the former is considered to be a maladaptive response, the latter is considered to be an adaptive strategy used to reduce the impact of negative emotional states evoked during stressful situations. In this sense, reappraisal appears to be particularly effective because it implies less physiological and cognitive costs, as well as less negative impact on memory compared to suppression [8].

It is hardly surprising that dysfunctional emotion regulation is considered to be a key mechanism underpinning numerous psychopathologies [9–12], among which we can find the whole spectrum of eating disorders [13–15]. Several studies suggest that, due to emotion regulation being adopted as a means of regulating negative emotions, difficulties in this area could be involved in the development and maintenance of problematic eating disorder-related behaviours [16,17]. Accordingly, emotion dysregulation has been exhibited as a trait among patients with AN, and also as a key element of their therapy [18,19].

Interestingly, food craving (i.e., intense desire for specific food), which is considered a hallmark of food addiction, has been recently proposed as an affective state involving behavioural and physiological changes [20]. Food craving is not necessary followed by increasing eating [21] and can be regulated like other affective states as suggested in recent studies in the non-clinical population [22–24]. In the eating disorder population, food craving and the related food addiction have been frequently reported [25], with a few studies suggesting the presence of these features even in patients with AN, especially those with binging/purging symptoms [26,27]. However, to our best knowledge, there is a lack of studies investigating food craving regulation in eating disorders, including AN.

Event-related potentials (ERPs) are electrical changes in electroencephalographic (EEG) recordings that are time-locked to sensory or cognitive events. Given the excellent time resolution, the event-related potential (ERP) technique has been adopted to investigate the time course of emotion regulation and craving regulation [28]. During late processing, the P300 component has been relevant to attention research as it increases with stimulus salience. Following it, the late positive potential (LPP) is thought to reflect motivated attention [7,29].

Previous ERP studies in the non-clinical population showed that the amplitude of the P300 and LPP components can be modulated by different emotion regulation strategies [30–38]. Due to the clinical relevance of emotions in daily life, numerous EEG studies have focused on down-regulation of P300 and LPP amplitudes in response to negative and positive emotions [30–38]. Although most studies point to a reduction of LPP amplitudes when participants try to down-regulate their negative emotions [30–33,39,40], other research studies have found no significant modulation of this component [35,38], or even a modulation in the opposite direction [41]. Focusing on the eating disorders field, several ERP studies have shown emotion regulation difficulties among individuals with comorbidities, such as anxiety disorders and alexithymia [42,43]. Nevertheless, no studies to date have examined ERP modulations by emotion regulation in specific eating disorder populations such as AN.

On the other hand, several ERP studies have strived to demonstrate the efficacy of different emotion regulation techniques in modulating food craving in healthy individuals. For instance, using reappraisal in order to change the emotional meaning of food increased LPP amplitude when participants tried to focus on the long-term consequences of eating high-caloric food [44]. Reappraisal was also employed in another study in which participants were instructed to increase or decrease the appetitive value of food. Results showed that P300 and LPP amplitudes to food cues were larger when participants tried to increase the appetitive value of food in comparison to the condition of decreasing or just watching the images [45]. Moreover, research instructing restrained eaters to either reappraise cravings, suppress cravings, or watch food during a food task found that engaging in cognitive reappraisal or suppression significantly reduced ERP amplitudes compared to the food watch condition [46]. Although research has demonstrated the efficacy of emotion regulation techniques in normal-weight healthy individuals, up to date there is a lack of ERP research assessing regulation of food craving in AN patients [47]. Elucidating neurophysiological mechanisms of food craving regulation could pave the way for new treatment approaches for anorexia nervosa, in which emotion regulation techniques might be employed to alter the motivational value of certain foods.

The primary aims of the study were to explore clinical and electrophysiological features of emotion regulation and food craving regulation among patients with AN. As for the clinical profile, we hypothesized that individuals with AN would present higher self-reported emotion dysregulation and food addiction compared to a group of healthy control (HC). Regarding electrophysiological data, we hypothesize that there will be a significant reduction in LPP amplitudes during conditions requiring participants to down-regulate negative emotions or food craving, as opposed to neutral conditions. Based on previous clinical research reporting emotion and food craving regulation difficulties in AN, we also aim to explore between-group differences in ERP during down-regulation of emotion or food craving. Finally, we explored to which extent self-reported emotion regulation strategies (adaptive or maladaptive) correlates with ERP (i.e., P300, LPP) during down-regulation of food craving or negative emotions. Maladaptive strategies are expected to be predominant in AN and possibly correlate with brain response during down-regulation of emotions/food craving.

2. Materials and Methods

2.1. Participants

The present study involved two different groups: a clinical group of patients with anorexia nervosa (AN) and a healthy control group (HC). The AN clinical group was comprised of 20 female treatment-seeking patients diagnosed with AN (60% AN restrictive subtype, 40% AN binge/purging subtype) according to DSM-5 criteria (Body Mass Index (BMI) < 18.5) [48]. Recruitment was conducted at the Eating Disorders Unit within the Department of Psychiatry at Bellvitge University Hospital, a public health hospital certified as a tertiary care centre with a highly specialised unit for the treatment of eating disorders in Barcelona (Spain). The HC group consisted of 21 female participants who had no history of an eating disorder. Participant groups were matched by age and education level. All participants were recruited between June 2016 and July 2018.

Data from one healthy control participant had to be excluded due to poor EEG data quality. The final sample size consisted of 40 participants, of whom 20 were patients with AN (mean age = 22.7 years, SD = 6.51, age range 18 to 43, mean BMI = 16.6 kg/m^2, SD = 1.1), and 20 were HC (mean age = 21.0 years, SD = 5.12, age range 18 to 39; mean BMI = 20.7 kg/m^2, SD = 1.78). Among AN group, 9 patients (45%) reported psychotropic treatment (antidepressants: n = 4, 20%; anxiolytics: n = 1 5%; both: n =

4, 20%). Exclusion criterion for all participants were: (a) being male, (b) younger than 18 years, (c) current or life-time history of chronic illness or neurological condition (abnormal EEG activity), which could influence electrophysiology and/or the neuropsychological assessment, (c) lifetime diagnosis of a severe mental health condition (bipolar disorder, lifetime diagnosis of psychotic disorder), (d) current substance dependence or any other mental disorder that could interfere cortical activity or the assessment. Additionally, in the HC group, an exclusion criteria was a lifetime diagnosis of any eating disorder, assessed by means of the Mini International Neuropsychiatric Interview (MINI) [49], being overweight/obese (Body Mass Index (BMI) ≥ 25), or underweight (BMI < 18.5).

Written informed consent was obtained before participation in the study, which was approved by the Ethics Committee of University Hospital of Bellvitge in accordance with the Helsinki Declaration of 1975 as revised in 1983. Participants received no compensation for taking part in the study.

2.2. Procedure

Patients who sought treatment for AN as their primary health concern were assessed by an experienced clinical psychologist as part of the Eating Disorders Unit protocol, which is based on DSM-5 criteria and includes height and weight measurements. All patients consecutively diagnosed with AN were screened for the inclusion criteria of the study and gave informed consent for voluntarily accepting to be part of the study. HC participants were recruited within a university campus and, if they were interested in taking part in the study, an eligibility screening was conducted prior to the initial face-to-face assessment session.

The variables explored in the present study were assessed in two separate sessions of approximately 90 minutes each. Firstly, participants were evaluated with the MINI to exclude those patients with any severe psychiatric condition. Afterwards, they completed a battery of self-reported questionnaires (DERS, ERQ, SCL-90-R, YFAS-2). Next, participants performed the experimental tasks (food craving and emotion regulation) during EEG acquisition. Participants were instructed to have a 'normal' meal 90 minutes before the session and then to refrain from eating or drinking coffee. Additional information was collected on the day of the experimental session, in order to control for a set of variables (i.e., food consumed on the day of the session, menstrual cycle, and alcohol or drugs consumption in the last 24h). In a second session, participants completed a different set of experimental neurophysiological tests (data will be reported in separate manuscript).

2.3. Clinical Assessment

The *Mini-International Neuropsychiatric Interview* (MINI) [49] is a short structured diagnostic interview for the major psychiatric disorders in DSM-III-R [50], DSM-IV [51] and DSM-5 [16] and ICD-10 [52]. Validation and reliability studies have been done comparing the MINI to the Structured Clinical Interview (SCID-P) [53] based on DSM-III-R [50] and the Composite International Diagnostic Interview (CIDI) [54], which is a structured interview developed by the World Health Organization. These studies showed that the MINI has similar reliability and validity properties to both instruments. With an administration time of approximately 15 minutes, it was designed to meet the needs for a short, yet accurate, structured psychiatric interview for multicentre clinical trials and epidemiology studies and to be used as a first step in outcome tracking in non-research clinical settings. The standard MINI assesses the 17 most common disorders in mental health. The disorders were selected based on current prevalence rates of 0.5% or higher in the general population in epidemiology studies. In the interest of brevity, it uses branching tree logic.

Difficulties in Emotion Regulation Scale (DERS; Spanish validation) [15,55,56] is a 36-item self-report scale that assesses relevant difficulties in emotion regulation on six subscales: non-acceptance of emotional responses, difficulties engaging in goal directed behaviour, impulse control difficulties, lack of emotional awareness, limited access to emotion regulation strategies and lack of emotional clarity. The measure yields a total score as well as scores on the six subscales. Higher scores indicate greater problems with emotion regulation. Cronbach's α for the total score in the present study was 0.91.

Emotion Regulation Questionnaire, Spanish version (ERQ) [57] is a 10-item questionnaire to assess the respondents' tendency to implement two emotion regulation strategies: reappraisal and emotional suppression. For the present study it shows a Cronbach's α of 0.76 for the suppression scale, and 0.85 for the reappraisal scale.

Symptom Checklist-90 Revised (SCL-90; Spanish validation) [58,59] is a 90-item questionnaire which evaluates psychopathological symptoms. It also includes a global severity index (GSI), designed to measure overall psychological distress. Internal consistency for GSI scale in the present study sample was 0.98.

The Yale Food Addiction Scale Version 2.0 (YFAS-2) [25] is a 25 item self-report questionnaire to measure addictive food behaviours. It consists of seven scales which refer to the criteria for substance dependence: (1) tolerance, (2) withdrawal, (3) substance taken in larger amount/period of time than intended, (4) persistent desire/unsuccessful efforts to cut down, (5) great deal of time spent to obtain substance, (6) important activities given up to obtain substance, (7) use continued despite psychological/physical problems. The Cronbach's α value for the present study was 0.97.

2.4. Electrophysiological Assessment

Participants completed an emotion regulation task and a food craving regulation task during continuous EEG recording.

Emotion regulation task: The task stimuli consisted of 180 images, of which 120 were negative images distributed in two blocks of 60 images each and 60 were neutral images grouped in a third block. Stimuli were presented for 3000 ms, with an inter-trial interval ranging from 3500 ms to 4500 ms. Negative images and neutral images were matched on contrast, brightness, resolution and complexity. Images were taken from the International Affective Picture System (IAPS) [60] and each image was presented only once during the task. Stimulus presentation was carried out by Presentation®software (Version 16.0) [61]. Participants were seated approximately 60 cm in front of a computer screen and the images were shown serially and occupied 35.1° of visual angle horizontally and 28.1° vertically.

For negative images, participants were instructed to either view each picture and allow themselves to feel any emotional response it might elicit (from now on referred to as Observe Negative) or to view each picture and try to reduce the emotional response that it might elicit (from now on referred to as Regulate Negative). For neutral images, participants were instructed to view each picture and allow themselves to feel any emotional response it might elicit (from now on referred to as Observe Neutral) while viewing the images and feeling the elicited emotion.

Food craving regulation task: Task stimuli consisted of 180 images, of which 120 were highly palatable food images distributed in two blocks of 60 images each and 60 were neutral images (i.e., office items) grouped in a third block. Stimuli were presented for 3000 ms, with an inter-trial interval ranging from 3500 ms to 4500 ms. Food images and neutral images were matched on contrast, brightness, resolution and complexity. Images were taken from Food Pics [62] and each image was presented only once during the task. Stimulus presentation was carried out by Presentation®software (Version 16.0) [61]. Participants were seated approximately 60 cm in front of a computer screen. The images were shown serially and occupied 18.9° of visual angle horizontally and 17.1° vertically.

For food images, participants were instructed to either view each picture and allow themselves to feel any emotional response it might elicit (from now on referred to as Observe Negative) or to view each picture and try to reduce the emotional response that it might elicit (from now on referred to as Regulate Negative). For neutral images, participants were instructed to view each picture and allow themselves to feel any emotional response it might elicit (from now on referred to as Observe Neutral).

2.5. *Electrophysiological Recording and Analysis*

The electroencephalogram (EEG) was recorded continuously throughout the experimental task using PyCorder (BrainVision). 60 active Ag/AgCI electrodes were inserted into an EEG recording cap (EASYCAP GmbH), distributed after the 10–20 system; additional three electrodes were adopted for recording vertical and horizontal electrooculogram (EOG) and Cz was used as online reference. Impedances were kept below 20 KOhm using the SuperVisc high-viscosity electrolyte gel for active electrodes. Signals from all channels were digitized with a sampling rate of 500 Hz and 24 bit/channel resolution and online filtered between 0.1 and 100 Hz.

Offline EEG analyses were performed with Brain Vision Analyzer (Version 2.2.0) [63] consisting of the following steps: high pass filtering 0.1 Hz, low pass filtering at 30 Hz (Butterworth zero phase filter; 24 dB/octave slope) and notch filter at 50 Hz; raw data inspection for manual detection of artefact and screening for bad channels, semi-automatic eye-blink correction using independent component analysis (ICA); artefact rejection of trials with an amplitude exciding ±80 μV; and baseline correction adopting the pre-stimulus interval between −200 and 2000 ms. EEG data were segmented into 2200 ms epochs from 200 ms before to 2000 ms after stimulus onset. Data were baseline corrected against the mean voltage during the −200 pre stimulus period. Artefact free epochs were separately averaged for each subject in each experimental condition for each paradigm.

ERP analyses were based on visual inspection of the grand average waveforms and the existing literature [45,46]. ERP components were analysed in a central-parietal cluster (CP1, CP5, P3, P7, CP2, CP6, P4, P8). P300 mean amplitude (μV) was computed in the time-window between 280 and 400 ms; LPP mean amplitude (μV) was measured within two time-windows: at 500-1000 ms (LPP1) and 1000-1500 ms (LPP2) [64–66].

2.6. *Statistical Analysis*

Statistical analysis was carried out with Stata Statistical Software: Release 15 for Windows [67]. The variables of the study (ERQ, YFAS, DERS and SCL-90-R) were compared between groups using t-tests for quantitative measures and chi square (χ^2) tests for categorical measures. Comparisons were considered significant with $p < 0.05$ after Bonferroni-Finner correction to avoid Type-I errors (Finner, 1993). The effect size for the mean differences/proportions was measured through Cohen's-*d* coefficient (low/small effect size was considered for $|d| > 0.2$, moderate for $|d| > 0.5$ and large/high for $|d| > 0.8$; Kelly and Preacher, 2012). In this study, different dimensional and categorical measures for the YFAS 2.0 were analysed: firstly, the YFAS 2.0 dimensional symptom count, which measures the 11 DSM-5 SRAD criteria (raw scores are in the range of 0–11); and secondly, the categorical classification based on the dimensional symptom count, a threshold for food addiction (presents for individuals with at least two symptoms plus self-reported clinically significant impairment or distress, and absent for participants who did not meet these criteria). The capacity of the dimensional YFAS 2.0 symptom count to discriminate between the groups was tested through two sample T-test, and the capacity of the YFAS 2.0 categorical classifications to discriminate between the diagnostic sub-types was tested through chi-square tests (χ^2).

The mean amplitudes (μV) of the emotion regulation and food craving regulation tasks were analysed for each ERP component (P300, LPP1, LPP2) with independent 3×2 mixed design analyses of variance (ANOVA), with condition as the within-subject variable (Regulate Negative/Food, Observe Negative/Food, Observe Neutral) and group as the between subject variable (HC versus AN). Pairwise comparisons were used to follow up main effects (for non-significant interaction condition-by-group) and single effects (for significant interaction condition-by-group).

Pearson's correlations were calculated for each group to estimate correlations between ERPs in the "regulation" condition of the emotion/food craving regulation tasks and ERQ subscales (ERQ-suppression; ERQ-reappraisal). Due to the strong association between this model and the sample size, practical relevance was based on the own coefficient measure (effect size was considered low/poor for $|R| > 0.10$, moderate for $|R| > 0.24$ and large/high for $|R| > 0.37$) [66].

3. Results

3.1. Comparison of Clinical Profiles

There were no significant between-group differences in age (p = 0.364, $|d|$ = 0.29). As expected, the HC group had significantly greater BMIs ($p < 0.001$, $|d| = 2.79$), lower mean scores on psychopathological self-report measures (i.e., the SCL-90-R GSI, DERS and YFAS), and higher mean scores on ERQ-Reappraisal. The prevalence of participants with food addiction positive screening score was also higher in the AN group (70% vs. 0%, $p < 0.001$, $|d| = 2.16$) (See Table 1). When comparing food addiction between AN sub-types, significant higher scores were displayed by the AN-BP subtype on the YFAS total score ($p = 0.031$, $|d| = 1.00$) and in all the YFAS criteria with exception of "withdrawal symptoms" (See Table 2).

Table 1. Comparison of the clinical profile between groups.

	HC (n = 20)		**AN (n = 20)**		*T-stat*	*p*	$\|d\|$
	Mean	*(SD)*	*Mean*	*(SD)*			
Age (years-old)	21.00	(5.12)	22.70	(6.51)	0.92	0.364	0.29
BMI (current, kg/m^2)	20.72	(1.78)	16.63	(1.06)	8.82	**<0.001** *	**2.79** †
SCL-90-R: GSI score	0.65	(0.45)	1.59	(0.70)	5.10	**<0.001** *	**1.61** †
DERS: Total score	73.30	(16.12)	114.25	(23.36)	6.45	**<0.001** *	**2.04** †
ERQ: Reappraisal	33.50	(5.94)	24.25	(6.69)	4.62	**<0.001** *	**1.46** †
ERQ: Suppression	13.45	(5.71)	15.75	(4.64)	1.40	0.170	**0.51** †
YFAS2 total score	0.75	(1.12)	4.35	(3.73)	4.13	**<0.001** *	**1.31** †
	n	(%)	*n*	(%)	χ^2	*p*	$\|d\|$
FA positive screening (YFAS-2)	0	(0.0%)	14	(70.0%)	21.54	**<0.001** *	**2.16** †

Note. SD: standard deviation. HC: healthy control. AN: anorexia. FA: food addiction. * Bold: significant parameter (.05 level). † Bold: effect size into the mild/moderate ($|d|$ > 0.80) to large/good range ($|d|$ > 0.80).

Table 2. Comparison of the FA measures between AN sub-types.

	AN-R (n = 12)		**AN-BP (n = 8)**		χ^2	*p*	$\|d\|$
	n	(%)	*n*	(%)			
Substance taken in larger amount	4	33.3%	4	50.0%	0.56	0.456	0.34
Persistent desire	3	25.0%	4	50.0%	1.32	0.251	**0.53** †
Much time-activity to obtain, use, recover	5	41.7%	6	75.0%	2.15	0.142	**0.72** †
Social or occupational affectation	7	58.3%	7	87.5%	1.94	0.163	**0.69** †
Use continues despite consequences	4	33.3%	5	62.5%	1.65	0.199	**0.61** †
Tolerance	0	0.0%	5	62.5%	10.00	**0.002** *	**1.83** †
Withdrawal symptoms	5	41.7%	5	62.5%	0.83	0.361	0.43
Continued use despite social problems	1	8.3%	4	50.0%	4.44	**0.035** *	**1.03** †
Failure to fulfil major rule obligations	1	8.3%	4	50.0%	4.44	**0.035** *	**1.03** †
Use in physically hazardous situations	3	25.0%	4	50.0%	1.32	0.251	**0.53** †
Craving, or a strong desire or urge to use	2	16.7%	4	50.0%	2.54	0.111	**0.76** †
Clinically significant impairment-distress	8	66.7%	7	87.5%	1.11	0.292	**0.51** †
FA positive screening score	8	66.7%	6	75.0%	0.16	0.690	0.18
	Mean	*(SD)*	*Mean*	*(SD)*	*T-stat*	*P*	$\|d\|$
FA dimensional (YFAS2 total)	2.92	2.39	6.50	4.47	2.34	**0.031** *	**1.00** †

Note. AN-R: anorexia restrictive subtype. AN-BP: anorexia bulimic-purgative subtype. FA: food addiction. SD: standard deviation. * Bold: significant parameter (.05 level). † Bold: effect size into the mild/moderate ($|d|$ > 0.80) to large/good range ($|d|$ > 0.80).

3.2. ERP Results: Emotion Regulation Task

P300. The mixed design ANOVA yielded a significant main effect of condition (Regulate Negative, Observe Negative, Observe Neutral; F:27.7, df = 2/38, $p < 0.001$; $\eta^2 = 0.421$) and a significant main effect of group (HC versus AN; F = 10.9, df = 1/38, $p = 0.002$; $\eta^2 = 0.223$). No significant group x condition interaction was detected (F = 1.51, df = 2/37, $p = 0.229$; $\eta^2 = 0.038$). Post-hoc t-tests revealed that the main effect of condition was due to higher P300 mean amplitude in Observe Negative and in Regulate Negative conditions compared to the neutral one (Observe Negative vs. Observe Neutral $p < 0.001$; Regulate vs. Observe Neutral $p < 0.001$). With regards to the main effect of group, the AN group showed significantly smaller mean P300 amplitudes compared to HC group ($p = 0.002$).

LPP1. The mixed design ANOVA showed a significant main effect of condition (F = 51.7, df = 2/38, $p < 0.001$; $\eta^2 = 0.577$), but no significant main effect for group (F = 3.04, df = 1/38 $p = 0.089$; $\eta^2 = 0.074$) or group x condition interaction (F = 1.01, df = 2/37, $p = 0.369$; $\eta^2 = 0.026$). Post hoc t-tests for the main effect of condition showed higher LPP1 amplitudes in the Observe Negative and Regulate Negative conditions, compared to Neutral condition (Observe Negative vs. Observe Neutral $p < 0.001$; Regulate vs. Observe Neutral $p < 0.001$).

LPP2. The mixed design ANOVA showed a significant main effect of condition (F = 13.1, df = 2/38, $p < 0.001$; $\eta^2 = 0.256$), but no main significant effect of group (F = 0.22, df = 1/38, $p = 0.643$; $\eta^2 = 0.006$) or group x condition interaction (F = 0.05, df = 2/37, $p = 0.954$; $\eta^2 = 0.001$). Post-hoc t-tests revealed that the effect of condition was due to higher mean LPP2 amplitudes in both the Observe Negative and Regulate Negative conditions, compared to the neutral one (Observe Negative vs. Observe Neutral $p = 0.002$; Regulate Negative vs. Observe Neutral $p < 0.001$).

Means and standard deviations of the ERP amplitudes (μV) for each component (P300, LPP1, LPP2) are reported in Table 3 (see also Figure 1).

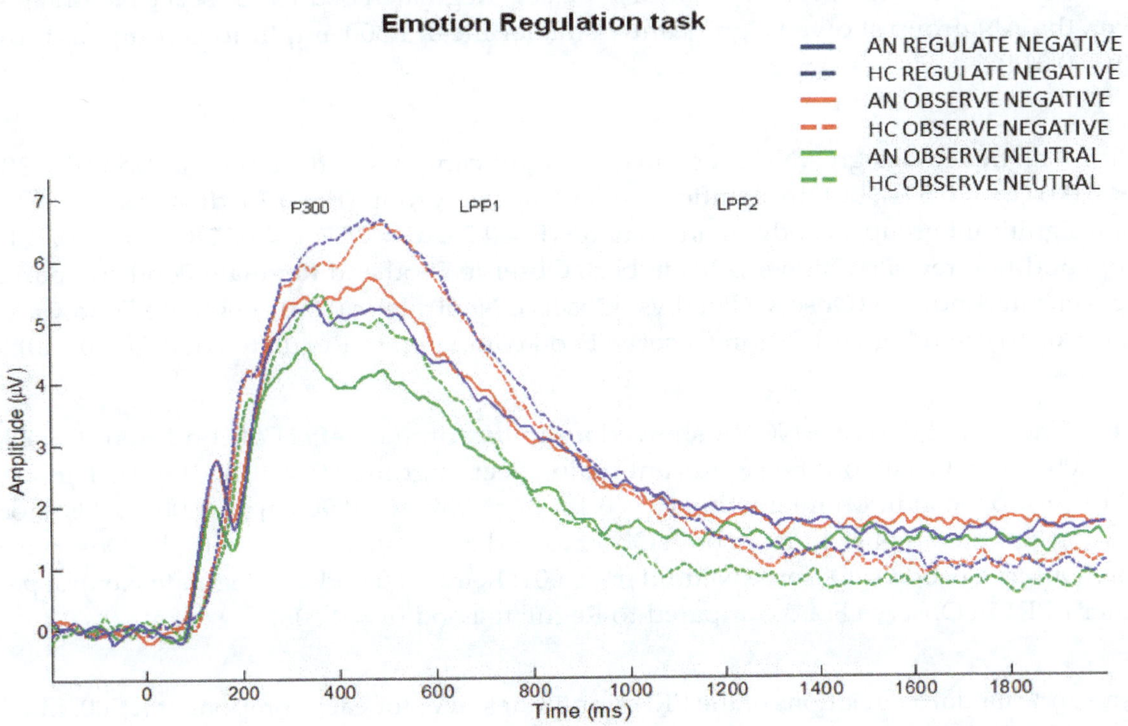

Figure 1. Grand average waveforms of the ER task, for each experimental condition (Regulate Negative, Observe Negative, Observe Neutral) and group (HC, AN), in the centro-parietal cluster of electrodes.

Table 3. Mean (SD) amplitudes (μV) of P300, LPP1 and LPP2 during the emotion regulation task.

	HC (n = 20)		AN (n = 20)	
	Mean	**(SD)**	**Mean**	**(SD)**
P300:				
observe negative	6.53	(2.72)	4.85	(1.97)
regulate negative	6.96	(2.93)	4.44	(1.84)
observe neutral	5.17	(1.86)	3.10	(1.44)
LPP1:				
observe negative	4.71	(2.59)	3.69	(1.63)
regulate negative	4.81	(2.27)	3.65	(1.49)
observe neutral	2.34	(1.53)	1.83	(1.20)
LPP2:				
observe negative	1.77	(2.16)	2.03	(1.48)
regulate negative	2.04	(2.04)	2.16	(1.11)
observe neutral	0.86	(1.47)	1.08	(1.10)

Note. HC: healthy control. AN: anorexia. SD: standard deviation.

3.3. ERP Results: Food Craving Regulation Task

P300. The mixed design ANOVA showed a significant main effect of condition (Regulate Food, Observe Food, Observe Neutral; F = 47.2, df = 2/38, $p < 0.001$; $\eta^2 = 0.560$) and a significant main effect of group (HC versus AN; F = 6.72, df = 1/38, $p = 0.014$; $\eta^2 = 0.154$), but no significant group x condition interaction (F = 1.40, df = 2/37, $p = 0.252$; $\eta^2 = 0.037$). Post-hoc t-tests for the main effect of condition showed higher amplitude in Observe Food and Regulate Food compared to the Observe Neutral condition (Observe Food vs. Observe Neutral $p < 0.001$; Regulate Food vs. Observe Neutral $p < 0.001$). Moreover, the AN group showed significantly smaller mean P300 amplitudes compared to the HC group ($p = 0.014$).

LPP1. The mixed design ANOVA showed a significant main effect of condition (F = 38.5, df = 2/38, $p < 0.001$; $\eta^2 = 0.504$), but no significant main effect of group (F = 0.73, df = 1/38, $p = 0.397$, $\eta^2 = 0.019$) or a significant group x condition interaction (F = 0.25, df = 2/37, $p = 0.778$; $\eta^2 = 0.007$). Post-hoc t-tests for condition revealed higher LPP1 in both Observe Food and Regulate Food compared to the Observe Neutral condition (Observe Food vs. Observe Neutral $p < 0.001$; Regulate Food vs. Observe Neutral $p < 0.001$), and higher LPP1 in Observe Food compared to Regulate Food ($p = 0.040$).

LPP2. The mixed design ANOVA showed a significant main effect of condition (F = 23.3, df = 2/38, $p < 0.001$; $\eta^2 = 0.380$), but no significant main effect of group (F = 0.13, df = 1/38, $p = 0.911$, $\eta^2 = 0.001$) or group x condition interaction (F = 0.10, df = 2/37, $p = 0.906$, $\eta^2 = 0.003$). Post-hoc t-tests for condition revealed higher LPP1 in both Observe and Regulate compared to the Observe Neutral condition (Observe Food vs. Observe Neutral $p < 0.001$; Regulate Food vs. Regulate Neutral $p < 0.001$), and higher LPP1 in Observe Food compared to Regulate Food ($p = 0.008$).

Mean and standard deviations of the ERP amplitudes (μV) for each component (P300, LPP1, LPP2) are reported in Table 4 (see also Figure 2).

Table 4. Mean (SD) amplitudes (μV) of P300, LPP1 and LPP2 during the food craving regulation task.

	HC (n = 20)		AN (n = 20)	
	Mean	**(SD)**	**Mean**	**(SD)**
P300:				
observe food	5.23	(2.39)	3.82	(1.47)
regulate food	5.60	(2.64)	3.67	(1.52)
observe neutral	3.68	(2.46)	2.32	(1.13)
LPP1:				
observe food	3.20	(1.91)	2.73	(1.38)
regulate food	2.86	(2.14)	2.38	(1.38)
observe neutral	1.49	(1.59)	1.25	(0.97)
LPP2:				
observe food	1.71	(1.45)	1.75	(1.19)
regulate food	1.26	(1.62)	1.21	(1.07)
observe neutral	0.42	(1.24)	0.54	(0.83)

Note. HC: healthy control. AN: anorexia. SD: standard deviation.

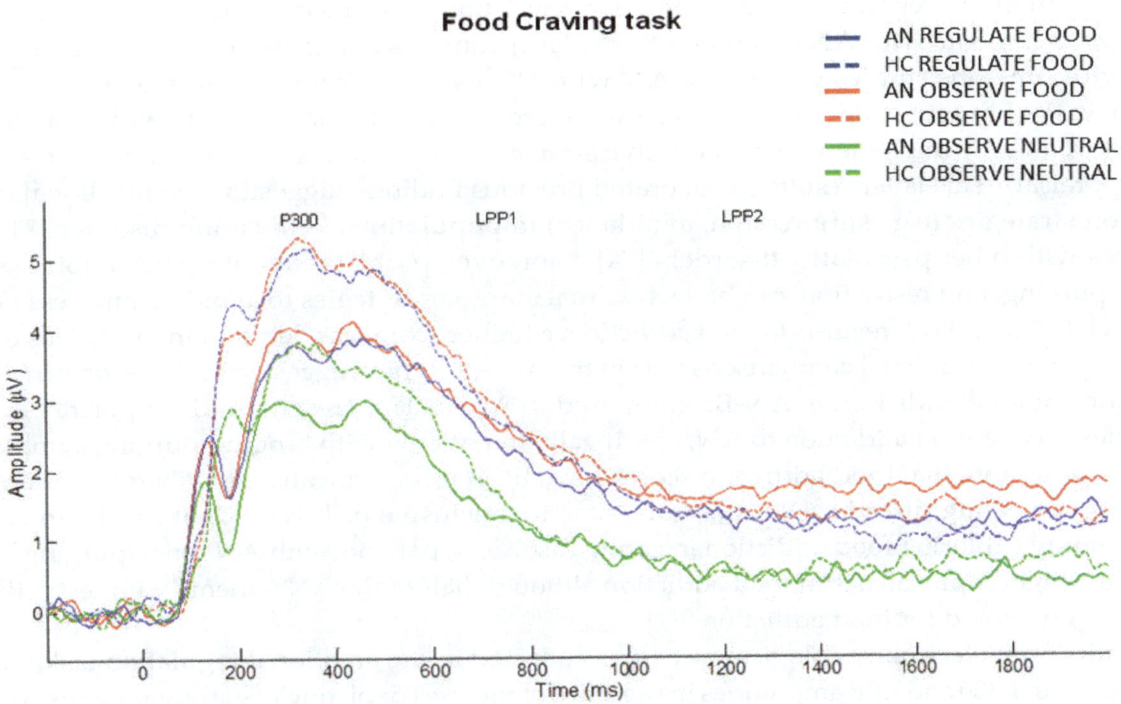

Figure 2. Grand average waveforms of the FRC task, for each experimental condition (Regulate Food, Observe Food, Observe Neutral) and group (HC, AN), in the centro-parietal cluster of electrodes.

3.4. Correlations between ERPs and Self-reported Emotional Regulation Strategies

Emotion Regulation Task and ERQ. In the HC group, reappraisal, as measured using the ERQ, was positively correlated with mean LPP1 amplitudes, while suppression was negatively correlated with mean LPP2 amplitudes. No significant correlations were found in the AN group.

Food Craving Regulation Task and ERQ. ERQ-reappraisal was positively correlated with mean LPP2 in the HC group, but not in the AN group. ERQ-suppression was negatively correlated with mean LPP1 and LPP2 amplitudes among patients with AN, but not in the HC group.

Table 5 shows the correlation matrix measuring the correlation between self-report measures of emotion regulation strategies (ERQ-suppression; ERQ-reappraisal) and ERPs amplitudes during emotion regulation (Regulate Negative) and food craving regulation (Regulate Food).

Table 5. Pearson's correlation between the amplitudes (μV) of the P300, LPP1, LPP2 during the "regulate" condition of the emotion regulation and the food craving regulation tasks.

	Emotion Regulation Task				Food Craving Regulation Task			
	HC (n = 20)		AN (n = 20)		HC (n = 20)		AN (n = 20)	
	ERQ reappr.	ERQ suppr.	ERQ reappr.	ERQ suppr.	ERQ reappr.	ERQ suppr.	ERQ reappr.	ERQ suppr.
P300	0.003	−0.195	0.119	−0.051	0.201	−0.187	0.101	0.018
LPP1	**0.247** †	−0.205	0.130	−0.103	0.144	−0.207	0.204	**−0.258** †
LPP2	0.196	**−0.281** †	0.173	−0.058	**0.396**†	−0.129	0.215	**−0.370** †

Note. HC: healthy control. AN: anorexia. † Bold: effect size into the mild/moderate (|R| > 0.24) to large/good range (|R| > 0.37). Sample size: Healthy control = 20; Anorexia = 20.

4. Discussion

In the present study, clinical and electrophysiological features of emotion regulation and food craving regulation among patients with AN were investigated by means of self-report and ERP measures.

Results from self-report measures of emotion regulation, confirmed greater difficulties in emotion regulation in patients with AN compared to the HC group (as suggested by DERS scores). This is in line with previous studies comparing AN with HC using the same questionnaire [5,68–70]. In addition, in the ERQ subscales, differences between groups were found, suggesting that patients with AN most frequently implemented maladaptive strategies (i.e., suppression) than adaptive strategies (i.e., reappraisal). This latter results corroborated previous findings suggesting dysfunctional emotion regulation strategies (e.g. suppression, avoidance) in populations with eating disorder [71–73], as is the case with other psychiatric disorders [74]. Moreover, problematic eating behaviours, such as binging, purging, and restriction, can be seen as maladaptive strategies to avoid or suppress negative emotions [68,75,76]. With regards to food addiction, a higher score was detected in the AN, as opposed to the HC group. Additional comparisons within the AN sub-types suggested higher scores in multiple dimensions of food addiction in AN-BP compared to AN-R. The present findings portray evidence of the relevance of food addiction to AN, specifically in patients with binging/purging symptoms. It is important to note that food addiction scores have been more typically described in patients with binge-subtype eating disorder [77–80], with some inconclusive or less evident results in AN. In a previous study exploring food addiction in eating disorders, patients with AN binge/purging subtype showed the highest prevalence of food addiction although half of the AN patients with restrictive type also positively scored for food addiction [27].

Results from electrophysiological measures collected in the emotional regulation task indicated enhanced mean P300 and LPP amplitudes in presence of pictures depicting negative emotions compared to neutral pictures in both AN and HC groups. This suggested enhanced processing of emotional stimuli, potentially due to their evolutionary salience, in accordance with previous ERP literature on 'healthy' populations [7,81–85]. Based on our results, we can suggest that, similarly to HC, patients with AN display a facilitated processing of stimuli with negative emotional valence. Although a previous ERP study reported altered processing of emotional stimuli in patients with AN [86], these controversial findings could be explained by the use of different types of stimuli and task (i.e., recognition of emotional faces).

Despite of the reported ERP indices of emotional processing, the instruction to down-regulate negative emotions did not elicit significant differences in mean P300 and LPP amplitudes when compared to passive viewing of negatively valenced emotional stimuli in any group. Since a reduction in LPP amplitude has been previously shown during emotion down-regulation in healthy population [30–33,39,40], the lack of this effect can be explained by a failure in emotion down-regulation that occurred in both AN patients and controls. This can be due to the fact that participants were not instructed to adopt a specific regulation strategy (e.g. reappraisal; suppression), which makes it more difficult to successfully achieve emotion regulation. However, adopting visual analogue scales to measure self-reported down-regulation is necessary to avoid premature conclusions.

During the food craving regulation task, pictures of food elicited greater mean P300 and LPP amplitudes compared to neutral non-food pictures in both AN and HC groups. This can be interpreted as motivated attention, meaning a higher amount of attentional resources allocated to process food stimuli [87]. However, we did not find higher motivated attention toward food in patients with AN when compared to HC, suggesting similar allocation of attentional resources toward food-stimuli, at latest stages of attentional processing. This is in accordance with a previous study in which patients with AN did not display enhanced P300/LPP toward high-caloric food, but only for low-caloric food pictures when compared with HC [88]. Since we were interested in investigating regulation of food craving, which is generally experienced in response to "forbidden foods" (i.e., high caloric), low-caloric food was not included in our study.

Interestingly, smaller LPP amplitudes were detected during down-regulation of craving compared to passing viewing food pictures, possibly suggesting successful down-regulation of food craving in both groups. This result is in line with a previous study in non-clinical 'restrained' eaters, showing that P300 and LPP amplitudes were reduced during down-regulation of food craving compared to the passive viewing of food-related pictures [46]. As the first ERP study which explores food craving regulation in patients with AN, we could observe that, despite AN reported greater "food addiction" symptomatology, these subjects were able to regulate food craving, as depicted at a neurophysiological level. Nevertheless, differential ERP response during food craving regulation may be expected between AN-BP and AN-R. Thus, further research in larger sample sized including different AN sub-types is needed to deeply understand the neurophysiological mechanisms underpinning this craving modulation in AN.

Finally, differences in ERP between patients and controls were depicted by smaller P300 amplitudes in the AN group. This overall reduction in mean P300 amplitudes was consistent in both tasks and regardless of experimental condition. Reduced neurophysiological response in AN could reflect neurocognitive alterations, possibly as a secondary effect of malnutrition which consequently affect cognitive functioning [89]. Accordingly, cognitive difficulties have been suggested in patients with AN, especially in memory, attention and executive functions (i.e. decision-making, set-shifting [90–92]. Similarly to our findings, previous ERP studies adopting different tasks showed reduced P300 in AN compared to controls, regardless of the emotional relevance of the stimuli [93,94].

Exploratory correlations in each group were performed in order to explore how emotion regulation strategies modulate both emotion and food craving regulation at a neurophysiological level. As for the emotion regulation task, our findings suggest that, only among HC, the tendency to suppress emotions correlated with larger LPP amplitudes, while the tendency to reappraise emotions correlated with lower LPP amplitudes. This may suggest that the tendency to adopt different emotion regulation strategies (i.e. reappraisal or suppression) is related with different modulation of the LPP amplitude while regulating emotions, at least in healthy individuals. Since the modulation of LPP amplitude has been linked to reappraisal of negative emotions in HC [30–33,39,40], the present results may further suggest a link between neurophysiological markers of emotion regulation and the tendency to adopt reappraisal as cognitive strategy to down-regulate negative emotions in the non-clinical population. By contrast, LPP response did not significantly correlate with emotion regulation strategies among patients with AN.

Similarly to the emotion regulation task, the LPP amplitude during down-regulation of food craving was positively related to ERQ-reappraisal in HC. By contrast, LPP amplitudes negatively correlated with ERQ-suppression in patients with AN. These latter results could suggest that neurophysiological response during down-regulation of food craving is related to different emotion regulation strategies in patients as compared to controls, which is in line with the differences observed in ERQ scores among groups. Interestingly, significant correlations with suppression in AN were specifically present in the food craving regulation task, and this can be linked to the fact that patients tend to adopt dysfunctional eating behaviours (e.g. bingeing/purging, restriction) as maladaptive strategies to regulate negative emotions, as showed by higher scores in ERQ-suppression.

It is important to consider some limitations when interpreting the results of the present study. Firstly, our sample size is rather low, which might have decreased the likelihood of detecting a significant difference if it existed [95]. Further studies with larger samples would be required to confirm our findings. Moreover, the small size of the sample did not allow us to distinguish and compare restrictive and purging AN sub-types. Given that different AN sub-types may exhibit different neurobiological correlates [96], future studies with larger samples should explore neural correlates of emotion regulation and food craving in different AN sub-types. In addition, our sample only consisted of female participants, which limits the generalizability of the results to a wider population. Additionally, we did not expose individuals to real food stimuli, which would have mimicked real-life situations and perhaps elicited stronger emotional and physiological reactions than food pictures [97]. Given the nature of the paradigms, another limitation of the study is the lack of eye-tracking and the lack of arousal tracing. Additional studies should further control eye-movements and attention focus during the image presentation. Furthermore, a proportion of patients with AN were under psychopharmacological medication (i.e., antidepressants, neuroleptic drugs, and benzodiazepines) and our sample did not allow us to control for medication. Finally, the present study design is cross-sectional in nature and claims regarding causality cannot be made. Future longitudinal studies are required to examine the extent to which the repetitive use of emotion regulation and food craving regulation techniques might modify the long-term neurophysiological responses in AN patients.

5. Conclusions

To conclude, previous ERP findings did not appear to mirror clarifying findings regarding eating disorders' aetiology and functioning. Therefore, to this date, they might not be used as accurate parameters or biomarkers that could be directly employed in the diagnosis or treatment of eating disorders [98]. To our knowledge, this is the first study which has examined the electrophysiological features of emotion and food craving regulation among patients with AN. Interestingly, ERP results suggest a successful down-regulation of food craving in AN, despite the fact that AN reported greater food addiction symptomatology. Nevertheless, further research including different AN sub-types is needed to deeply understand the neurophysiological mechanisms underpinning this craving modulation in AN.

Furthermore, although ERP did not depict differential response between AN and HC while down-regulating emotions or food craving, reduced P300 mean amplitudes were detected in AN when compared to HC. This result might reflect a general alteration in the neurophysiological responses of AN patients, which is possibly related to their prolonged state of malnutrition [99]. In this regard, this study provides an objective parameter of those impairments which long-lasting malnutrition might be occasioning in the neural systems of AN patients. Previous research has also found neurophysiological dysfunctions in AN, which do not always seem to be normalised after weight gain [98]. In that respect, it would be of great interest that future studies explore not only if neurophysiological alterations remain or, on the contrary, are ameliorated after patients' recovery, but also investigate the factors which might contribute to normalise neural responses in AN (e.g., weight gain, pharmacological treatments, specific psychological interventions, etc.).

On the other hand, clinical measures showed that patients with AN were characterized by food addiction symptoms and difficulties in emotion regulation with the tendency to use maladaptive techniques (i.e., suppression) to manage negative emotions. Moreover, this is the first study which relates the use of suppression strategies to smaller ERP amplitudes during food craving regulation in AN patients. This possibly reflects their tendency to adopt dysfunctional eating behaviours as maladaptive strategies to regulate negative emotions. Future interventions should focus on implementing more effective emotion regulation techniques such as reappraisal, which act through a reinterpretation of emotional situation in order to reduce its emotional impact. Reappraisal has shown a better capacity to decrease negative emotional experience, consequently reducing distress [100].

Further research with larger samples and considering AN sub-types is needed to deeply understand the neurophysiological mechanisms underpinning emotion and food craving modulation in AN.

Author Contributions: N.M.-B., J.C.P., S.J.-M. and F.F.-A. conceived and designed the study; N.M.-B., M.L.-M. and G.T. curated the data; G.T. and R.G. analysed the data; F.F.-A. acquired the fundings; N.M.-B., M.L.M., C.V.-A., I.S., N.R. and J.F.N. collected the data; J.C.P., S.J.-M., J.T. and F.F.-A. supervised this study; N.M.-B., M.L.M., G.T. and R.G. wrote the original draft; N.M.-B., M.L.M., G.T., J.C.P., J.F.N., I.M.-Z., A.M., M.V.D.L.H., R.C., S.J.-M., J.A.F.-F., J.T. and F.F.-A. reviewed and edited the manuscript. All authors have read and agreed to the published version of the manuscript.

References

1. Schaumberg, K.; Welch, E.; Breithaupt, L.; Hübel, C.; Baker, J.H.; Munn-Chernoff, M.A.; Yilmaz, Z.; Ehrlich, S.; Mustelin, L.; Ghaderi, A.; et al. The Science Behind the Academy for Eating Disorders' Nine Truths About Eating Disorders. *Eur. Eat. Disord. Rev.* **2017**, *25*, 432–450. [CrossRef]
2. Glashouwer, K.A.; van der Veer, R.M.L.; Adipatria, F.; de Jong, P.J.; Vocks, S. The role of body image disturbance in the onset, maintenance, and relapse of anorexia nervosa: A systematic review. *Clin. Psychol. Rev.* **2019**, *74*. [CrossRef]
3. Giel, K.E.; Teufel, M.; Friederich, H.-C.; Hautzinger, M.; Enck, P.; Zipfel, S. Processing of pictorial food stimuli in patients with eating disorders-A systematic review. *Int. J. Eat. Disord.* **2010**, *44*, 105–117. [CrossRef]
4. Aviram-Friedman, R.; Astbury, N.; Ochner, C.N.; Contento, I.; Geliebter, A. Neurobiological evidence for attention bias to food, emotional dysregulation, disinhibition and deficient somatosensory awareness in obesity with binge eating disorder. *Physiol. Behav.* **2018**, *184*, 122–128. [CrossRef]
5. Harrison, A.; Sullivan, S.; Tchanturia, K.; Treasure, J. Emotional functioning in eating disorders: Attentional bias, emotion recognition and emotion regulation. *Psychol. Med.* **2010**, *40*, 1887–1897. [CrossRef]
6. Gross, J.J. The emerging field of emotion regulation: An integrative review. *Rev. Gen. Psychol.* **1998**, *2*, 271–299. [CrossRef]
7. Hajcak, G.; MacNamara, A.; Olvet, D.M. Event-Related Potentials, Emotion, and Emotion Regulation: An Integrative Review. *Dev. Neuropsychol.* **2010**, *35*, 129–155. [CrossRef]
8. Richards, J.M.; Gross, J.J. Emotion regulation and memory: The cognitive costs of keeping one's cool. *J. Pers. Soc. Psychol.* **2000**, *79*, 410–424. [CrossRef]
9. Daros, A.R.; Rodrigo, A.H.; Norouzian, N.; Darboh, B.S.; McRae, K.; Ruocco, A.C. Cognitive Reappraisal of Negative Emotional Images in Borderline Personality Disorder: Content Analysis, Perceived Effectiveness, and Diagnostic Specificity. *J. Pers. Disord.* **2018**, 1–17. [CrossRef]
10. Tenenbaum, R.B.; Musser, E.D.; Morris, S.; Ward, A.R.; Raiker, J.S.; Coles, E.K.; Pelham, W.E. Response Inhibition, Response Execution, and Emotion Regulation among Children with Attention-Deficit/Hyperactivity Disorder. *J. Abnorm. Child Psychol.* **2018**. [CrossRef]
11. Joormann, J.; Quinn, M.E. Cognitive processes and emotion regulation in depression. *Depress. Anxiety* **2014**, *31*, 308–315. [CrossRef] [PubMed]
12. Malik, S.; Wells, A.; Wittkowski, A. Emotion regulation as a mediator in the relationship between attachment and depressive symptomatology: A systematic review. *J. Affect. Disord.* **2015**, *172*, 428–444. [CrossRef] [PubMed]
13. Mallorquí-Bagué, N.; Vintró-Alcaraz, C.; Sánchez, I.; Riesco, N.; Agüera, Z.; Granero, R.; Jiménez-Murcia, S.; Menchón, J.M.; Treasure, J.; Fernández-Aranda, F.; et al. Emotion Regulation as a Transdiagnostic Feature Among Eating Disorders: Cross-sectional and Longitudinal Approach. *Eur. Eat. Disord. Rev.* **2018**, *26*, 53–61. [CrossRef] [PubMed]
14. Monell, E.; Clinton, D.; Birgegård, A. Emotion dysregulation and eating disorders-Associations with diagnostic presentation and key symptoms. *Int. J. Eat. Disord.* **2018**. [CrossRef]
15. Wolz, I.; Agüera, Z.; Granero, R.; Jiménez-Murcia, S.; Gratz, K.L.; Menchón, J.M.; Fernández-Aranda, F. Emotion regulation in disordered eating: Psychometric properties of the Difficulties in Emotion Regulation Scale among Spanish adults and its interrelations with personality and clinical severity. *Front. Psychol.* **2015**, *6*, 907. [CrossRef]

16. Engel, S.G.; Wonderlich, S.A.; Crosby, R.D.; Mitchell, J.E.; Crow, S.; Peterson, C.B.; Le Grange, D.; Simonich, H.K.; Cao, L.; Lavender, J.M.; et al. The role of affect in the maintenance of anorexia nervosa: Evidence from a naturalistic assessment of momentary behaviors and emotion. *J. Abnorm. Psychol.* **2013**, *122*, 709–719. [CrossRef]
17. Haynos, A.F.; Roberto, C.A.; Martinez, M.A.; Attia, E.; Fruzzetti, A.E. Emotion regulation difficulties in anorexia nervosa before and after inpatient weight restoration. *Int. J. Eat. Disord.* **2014**, *47*, 888–891. [CrossRef]
18. Adamson, J.; Leppanen, J.; Murin, M.; Tchanturia, K. Effectiveness of emotional skills training for patients with anorexia nervosa with autistic symptoms in group and individual format. *Eur. Eat. Disord. Rev.* **2018**, *26*, 367–375. [CrossRef]
19. Oldershaw, A.; Lavender, T.; Schmidt, U. Are socio-emotional and neurocognitive functioning predictors of therapeutic outcomes for adults with anorexia nervosa? *Eur. Eat. Disord. Rev.* **2018**, *26*, 346–359. [CrossRef]
20. Giuliani, N.R.; Berkman, E.T. Craving Is an Affective State and Its Regulation Can Be Understood in Terms of the Extended Process Model of Emotion Regulation. *Psychol. Inq.* **2015**, *26*, 48–53. [CrossRef]
21. Hill, A.J. Symposium on "molecular mechanisms and psychology of food intake"—The psychology of food craving. *Proc. Nutr. Soc.* **2007**, *66*, 277–285. [CrossRef]
22. Giuliani, N.R.; Calcott, R.D.; Berkman, E.T. Piece of cake. Cognitive reappraisal of food craving. *Appetite* **2013**, *64*, 56–61. [CrossRef]
23. Giuliani, N.R.; Mann, T.; Tomiyama, A.J.; Berkman, E.T. Neural Systems Underlying the Reappraisal of Personally Craved Foods. *J. Cogn. Neurosci.* **2014**, *26*, 1390–1402. [CrossRef]
24. Siep, N.; Roefs, A.; Roebroeck, A.; Havermans, R.; Bonte, M.; Jansen, A. Fighting food temptations: The modulating effects of short-term cognitive reappraisal, suppression and up-regulation on mesocorticolimbic activity related to appetitive motivation. *Neuroimage* **2012**, *60*, 213–220. [CrossRef]
25. Granero, R.; Jiménez-Murcia, S.; Gerhardt, A.N.; Agüera, Z.; Aymamí, N.; Gómez-Peña, M.; Lozano-Madrid, M.; Mallorquí-Bagué, N.; Mestre-Bach, G.; Neto-Antao, M.I.; et al. Validation of the Spanish version of the Yale Food Addiction Scale 2.0 (YFAS 2.0) and clinical correlates in a sample of eating disorder, gambling disorder, and healthy control participants. *Front. Psychiatry* **2018**, *9*, 1–11. [CrossRef]
26. Gendall, K.A.; Sullivan, P.F.; Joyce, P.R.; Bulik, C.M. Food cravings in women with a history of anorexia nervosa. *Int. J. Eat. Disord.* **1997**, *22*, 403–409. [CrossRef]
27. Granero, R.; Hilker, I.; Agüera, Z.; Jiménez-Murcia, S.; Sauchelli, S.; Islam, M.A.; Fagundo, A.B.; Sánchez, I.; Riesco, N.; Dieguez, C.; et al. Food Addiction in a Spanish Sample of Eating Disorders: DSM-5 Diagnostic Subtype Differentiation and Validation Data. *Eur. Eat. Disord. Rev.* **2014**, *22*, 389–396. [CrossRef]
28. Blackwood, D.H.; Muir, W.J. Cognitive brain potentials and their application. *Br. J. Psychiatry. Suppl.* **1990**, 96–101. [CrossRef]
29. Wolz, I.; Sauvaget, A.; Granero, R.; Mestre-Bach, G.; Baño, M.; Martín-Romera, V.; Veciana de las Heras, M.; Jiménez-Murcia, S.; Jansen, A.; Roefs, A.; et al. Subjective craving and event-related brain response to olfactory and visual chocolate cues in binge-eating and healthy individuals. *Sci. Rep.* **2017**, *7*, 41736. [CrossRef]
30. Moser, J.S.; Hajcak, G.; Bukay, E.; Simons, R.F. Intentional modulation of emotional responding to unpleasant pictures: An ERP study. *Psychophysiology* **2006**, *43*, 292–296. [CrossRef]
31. Hajcak, G.; Nieuwenhuis, S. Reappraisal modulates the electrocortical response to unpleasant pictures. *Cogn. Affect. Behav. Neurosci.* **2006**, *6*, 291–297. [CrossRef]
32. Blechert, J.; Sheppes, G.; Di Tella, C.; Williams, H.; Gross, J.J. See What You Think. *Psychol. Sci.* **2012**, *23*, 346–353. [CrossRef]
33. Moser, J.S.; Krompinger, J.W.; Dietz, J.; Simons, R.F. Electrophysiological correlates of decreasing and increasing emotional responses to unpleasant pictures. *Psychophysiology* **2009**, *46*, 17–27. [CrossRef]
34. Baur, R.; Conzelmann, A.; Wieser, M.J.; Pauli, P. Spontaneous emotion regulation: Differential effects on evoked brain potentials and facial muscle activity. *Int. J. Psychophysiol.* **2015**, *96*, 38–48. [CrossRef]
35. Gardener, E.K.T.; Carr, A.R.; Macgregor, A.; Felmingham, K.L. Sex differences and emotion regulation: An event-related potential study. *PLoS ONE* **2013**, *8*, e73475. [CrossRef]

36. Yang, Q.; Gu, R.; Tang, P.; Luo, Y.-J. How does cognitive reappraisal affect the response to gains and losses? *Psychophysiology* **2013**, *50*, 1094–1103. [CrossRef]
37. Shafir, R.; Zucker, L.; Sheppes, G. Turning off hot feelings: Down-regulation of sexual desire using distraction and situation-focused reappraisal. *Biol. Psychol.* **2018**, *137*, 116–124. [CrossRef]
38. Langeslag, S.J.E.; van Strien, J.W. Cognitive reappraisal of snake and spider pictures: An event-related potentials study. *Int. J. Psychophysiol.* **2018**, *130*, 1–8. [CrossRef]
39. Yang, B.; Cao, J.; Zhou, T.; Dong, L.; Zou, L.; Xiang, J. Exploration of Neural Activity under Cognitive Reappraisal Using Simultaneous EEG-fMRI Data and Kernel Canonical Correlation Analysis. *Comput. Math. Methods Med.* **2018**, *2018*, 1–11. [CrossRef]
40. Reva, N.V.; Pavlov, S.V.; Korenek, V.V.; Loktev, K.V.; Tumialis, A.V.; Brak, I.V.; Aftanas, L.I. The regulation of negative and positive emotions during picture viewing: An ERP study. *Ross. Fiziol. zhurnal Im. I.M. Sechenova* **2015**, *101*, 114–122.
41. Langeslag, S.J.E.; Surti, K. The effect of arousal on regulation of negative emotions using cognitive reappraisal: An ERP study. *Int. J. Psychophysiol.* **2017**, *118*, 18–26. [CrossRef]
42. Han, H.Y.; Gan, T.; Li, P.; Li, Z.J.; Guo, M.; Yao, S.M. Attentional bias modulation by reappraisal in patients with generalized anxiety disorder: An event-related potential study. *Brazilian J. Med. Biol. Res. = Rev. Bras. Pesqui. medicas e Biol.* **2014**, *47*, 576–583. [CrossRef]
43. Pollatos, O.; Gramann, K. Attenuated modulation of brain activity accompanies emotion regulation deficits in alexithymia. *Psychophysiology* **2012**, *49*, 651–658. [CrossRef]
44. Meule, A.; Kübler, A.; Blechert, J. Time course of electrocortical food-cue responses during cognitive regulation of craving. *Front. Psychol.* **2013**, *4*. [CrossRef]
45. Sarlo, M.; Übel, S.; Leutgeb, V.; Schienle, A. Cognitive reappraisal fails when attempting to reduce the appetitive value of food: An ERP study. *Biol. Psychol.* **2013**, *94*, 507–512. [CrossRef]
46. Svaldi, J.; Tuschen-Caffier, B.; Biehl, S.C.; Gschwendtner, K.; Wolz, I.; Naumann, E. Effects of two cognitive regulation strategies on the processing of food cues in high restrained eaters. An event-related potential study. *Appetite* **2015**, *92*, 269–277. [CrossRef]
47. Wolz, I.; Fagundo, A.B.; Treasure, J.; Fernández-Aranda, F. The processing of food stimuli in abnormal eating: A systematic review of electrophysiology. *Eur. Eat. Disord. Rev.* **2015**, *23*, 251–261. [CrossRef]
48. APA. *Diagnostic and Statistical Manual of Mental Disorders*, 5th ed.; American Journal of Psychiatry: Washington, DC, USA, 2013; ISBN 9780890425541.
49. Sheehan, D.V.; Lecrubier, Y.; Sheehan, K.H.; Amorim, P.; Janavs, J.; Weiller, E.; Hergueta, T.; Baker, R.; Dunbar, G.C. The Mini-International Neuropsychiatric Interview (M.I.N.I.): The development and validation of a structured diagnostic psychiatric interview for DSM-IV and ICD-10. *J. Clin. Psychiatry* **1998**, *59* (Suppl. 2), 22–33; quiz 34-57.
50. APA. *DSM-III-R: Diagnostic and Statistical Manual of Mental Disorders (Rev.)*; APA: Washington, DC, USA, 1987.
51. APA. *American Psychiatric Association, Diagnostic and Statistical Manual of Mental Disorders*, 4th ed.; American Psychiatric Association: Washington, DC, USA, 1994.
52. World Health Organization. *International Statistical Classification of disease and related health problems, Tenth Revision (ICD-10)*; World Health Organization: Geneva, Switzerland, 1992.
53. Spitzer, R.L.; Williams, J.B.W.; Gibbon, M.; First, M.B. The Structured Clinical Interview for DSM-III-R (SCID). *Arch. Gen. Psychiatry* **1992**, *49*, 624. [CrossRef]
54. World Health Organization. *Composite international diagnostic interview (CIDI)*; World Health Organization: Geneva, Switzerland, 1993.
55. Gratz, K.L.; Roemer, L. Multidimensional Assessment of Emotion Regulation and Dysregulation: Development, Factor Structure, and Initial Validation of the Difficulties in Emotion Regulation Scale. *J. Psychopathol. Behav. Assess.* **2004**, *26*, 41–54. [CrossRef]
56. Hervás, G.; Jódar, R. Adaptación al castellano de la Escala de Dificultades en la Regulación Emocional The spanish version of the Difficulties in Emotion Regulation Scale. *Clínica y Salud* **2008**, *19*, 139–156.
57. Cabello, R.; Salguero, J.M.; Fernández-Berrocal, P.; Gross, J.J. A Spanish Adaptation of the Emotion Regulation Questionnaire. *Eur. J. Psychol. Assess.* **2013**, *29*, 234–240. [CrossRef]

58. Derogatis, L. *SCL-90-R. Cuestionario de 90 síntomas. [SCL-90-R. 90-Symptoms Questionnaire]*; TEA Ediciones: Madrid, Spain, 1994.
59. González de Rivera, J.L.; de las Cuevas, C.; Rodríguez Abuín, M.; y Rodríguez Pulido, F. *SCL-90-R. Cuestionario de 90 síntomas. Manual*; TEA Ediciones: Madrid, Spain, 2002.
60. Lang, P.J. *International Affective Picture System (IAPS): Affective Ratings of Pictures and Instruction Manual*; University of Florida: Gainesville, FL, USA, 2005.
61. *Presentation®Software (Version 16.0)*, Neurobehavioral Systems, Inc.: Berkeley, CA, USA.
62. Blechert, J.; Meule, A.; Busch, N.A.; Ohla, K. Food-pics: An image database for experimental research on eating and appetite. *Front. Psychol.* **2014**, *5*, 617. [CrossRef]
63. *Brain Vision Analyzer (Version 2.2.0) [Computer Software]*, Brain Products GmbH: Gilching, Germany, 2019.
64. Finner, H. On a Monotonicity Problem in Step-Down Multiple Test Procedures. *J. Am. Stat. Assoc.* **1993**, *88*, 920–923. [CrossRef]
65. Kelley, K.; Preacher, K.J. On effect size. *Psychol. Methods* **2012**, *17*, 137–152. [CrossRef]
66. Rosnow, R.L.; Rosenthal, R. Computing contrasts, effect sizes, and counternulls on other people's published data: General procedures for research consumers. *Psychol. Methods* **1996**, *1*, 331–340. [CrossRef]
67. StataCorp. *Stata Statistical Software: Release 15*; StataCorp LLC: College Station, TX, USA, 2017.
68. Harrison, A.; Sullivan, S.; Tchanturia, K.; Treasure, J. Emotion recognition and regulation in anorexia nervosa. *Clin. Psychol. Psychother.* **2009**, *16*, 348–356. [CrossRef]
69. Rowsell, M.; Macdonald, D.E.; Carter, J.C. Emotion regulation difficulties in anorexia nervosa: Associations with improvements in eating psychopathology. *J. Eat. Disord.* **2016**. [CrossRef]
70. Oldershaw, A.; Lavender, T.; Sallis, H.; Stahl, D.; Schmidt, U. Emotion generation and regulation in anorexia nervosa: A systematic review and meta-analysis of self-report data. *Clin. Psychol. Rev.* **2015**, *39*, 83–95. [CrossRef]
71. Svaldi, J.; Griepenstroh, J.; Tuschen-Caffier, B.; Ehring, T. Emotion regulation deficits in eating disorders: A marker of eating pathology or general psychopathology? *Psychiatry Res.* **2012**, *197*, 103–111. [CrossRef]
72. Aldao, A.; Nolen-Hoeksema, S.; Schweizer, S. Emotion-regulation strategies across psychopathology: A meta-analytic review. *Clin. Psychol. Rev.* **2010**, *30*, 217–237. [CrossRef] [PubMed]
73. Meule, A.; Richard, A.; Schnepper, R.; Reichenberger, J.; Georgii, C.; Naab, S.; Voderholzer, U.; Blechert, J. Emotion regulation and emotional eating in anorexia nervosa and bulimia nervosa. *Eat. Disord.* **2019**, 1–17. [CrossRef] [PubMed]
74. Sloan, E.; Hall, K.; Moulding, R.; Bryce, S.; Mildred, H.; Staiger, P.K. Emotion regulation as a transdiagnostic treatment construct across anxiety, depression, substance, eating and borderline personality disorders: A systematic review. *Clin. Psychol. Rev.* **2017**, *57*, 141–163. [CrossRef]
75. Brockmeyer, T.; Skunde, M.; Wu, M.; Bresslein, E.; Rudofsky, G.; Herzog, W.; Friederich, H.-C. Difficulties in emotion regulation across the spectrum of eating disorders. *Compr. Psychiatry* **2014**, *55*, 565–571. [CrossRef]
76. Lavender, J.M.; Wonderlich, S.A.; Peterson, C.B.; Crosby, R.D.; Engel, S.G.; Mitchell, J.E.; Crow, S.J.; Smith, T.L.; Klein, M.H.; Goldschmidt, A.B.; et al. Dimensions of Emotion Dysregulation in Bulimia Nervosa. *Eur. Eat. Disord. Rev.* **2014**, *22*, 212–216. [CrossRef]
77. Cassin, S.E.; von Ranson, K.M. Is binge eating experienced as an addiction? *Appetite* **2007**, *49*, 687–690. [CrossRef]
78. Gearhardt, A.N.; White, M.A.; Masheb, R.M.; Morgan, P.T.; Crosby, R.D.; Grilo, C.M. An examination of the food addiction construct in obese patients with binge eating disorder. *Int. J. Eat. Disord.* **2012**, *45*, 657–663. [CrossRef]
79. Meule, A.; von Rezori, V.; Blechert, J. Food Addiction and Bulimia Nervosa. *Eur. Eat. Disord. Rev.* **2014**, *22*, 331–337. [CrossRef]
80. Gearhardt, A.N.; White, M.A.; Masheb, R.M.; Grilo, C.M. An examination of food addiction in a racially diverse sample of obese patients with binge eating disorder in primary care settings. *Compr. Psychiatry* **2013**, *54*, 500–505. [CrossRef]
81. Lang, P.J.; Bradley, M.M.; Cuthbert, B.N. Motivated attention: Affect, activation, and action. In *Attention and Orienting: Sensory and Motivational Processes*; Psychology Press: East Sussex, UK, 1997; pp. 97–135. ISBN 9781135808273.

82. Schupp, H.T.; Markus, J.; Weike, A.I.; Hamm, A.O. Emotional Facilitation of Sensory Processing in the Visual Cortex. *Psychol. Sci.* **2003**, *14*, 7–13. [CrossRef]
83. Schupp, H.T.; Flaisch, T.; Stockburger, J.; Junghöfer, M. Emotion and attention: Event-related brain potential studies. *Prog. Brain Res.* **2006**, *156*, 31–51.
84. Cuthbert, B.N.; Schupp, H.T.; Bradley, M.M.; Birbaumer, N.; Lang, P.J. Brain potentials in affective picture processing: Covariation with autonomic arousal and affective report. *Biol. Psychol.* **2000**, *52*, 95–111. [CrossRef]
85. Amrhein, C.; Mühlberger, A.; Pauli, P.; Wiedemann, G. Modulation of event-related brain potentials during affective picture processing: A complement to startle reflex and skin conductance response? *Int. J. Psychophysiol.* **2004**, *54*, 231–240. [CrossRef]
86. Pollatos, O.; Herbert, B.M.; Schandry, R.; Gramann, K. Impaired Central Processing of Emotional Faces in Anorexia Nervosa. *Psychosom. Med.* **2008**, *70*, 701–708. [CrossRef]
87. Bradley, M.M.; Sabatinelli, D.; Lang, P.J.; Fitzsimmons, J.R.; King, W.; Desai, P. Activation of the visual cortex in motivated attention. *Behav. Neurosci.* **2003**, *117*, 369–380. [CrossRef]
88. Novosel, A.; Lackner, N.; Unterrainer, H.F.; Dunitz-Scheer, M.; Scheer, P.J.Z.; Wallner-Liebmann, S.J.; Neuper, C. Motivational processing of food cues in anorexia nervosa: A pilot study. *Eat. Weight Disord.* **2014**, *19*, 169–175. [CrossRef]
89. Micali, N.; Kothari, R.; Nam, K.W.; Gioroukou, E.; Walshe, M.; Allin, M.; Rifkin, L.; Murray, R.M.; Nosarti, C. Eating Disorder Psychopathology, Brain Structure, Neuropsychological Correlates and Risk Mechanisms in Very Preterm Young Adults. *Eur. Eat. Disord. Rev.* **2015**, *23*, 147–155. [CrossRef]
90. Fagundo, A.B.; de la Torre, R.; Jiménez-Murcia, S.; Agüera, Z.; Granero, R.; Tárrega, S.; Botella, C.; Baños, R.; Fernández-Real, J.M.; Rodríguez, R.; et al. Executive Functions Profile in Extreme Eating/Weight Conditions: From Anorexia Nervosa to Obesity. *PLoS ONE* **2012**, *7*, e43382. [CrossRef]
91. Tchanturia, K.; Liao, P.-C.; Forcano, L.; Fernández-Aranda, F.; Uher, R.; Treasure, J.; Schmidt, U.; Penelo, E.; Granero, R.; Jiménez-Murcia, S.; et al. Poor Decision Making in Male Patients with Anorexia Nervosa. *Eur. Eat. Disord. Rev.* **2012**, *20*, 169–173. [CrossRef]
92. Tchanturia, K.; Campbell, I.C.; Morris, R.; Treasure, J. Neuropsychological studies in anorexia nervosa. *Int. J. Eat. Disord.* **2005**, *37*, S72–S76. [CrossRef]
93. Nikendei, C.; Friederich, H.C.; Weisbrod, M.; Walther, S.; Sharma, A.; Herzog, W.; Zipfel, S.; Bender, S. Event-related potentials during recognition of semantic and pictorial food stimuli in patients with anorexia nervosa and healthy controls with varying internal states of hunger. *Psychosom. Med.* **2012**, *74*, 136–145. [CrossRef] [PubMed]
94. Hatch, A.; Madden, S.; Kohn, M.R.; Clarke, S.; Touyz, S.; Gordon, E.; Williams, L.M. Emotion brain alterations in anorexia nervosa: A candidate biological marker and implications for treatment. *J. Psychiatry Neurosci.* **2010**, *35*, 267–274. [CrossRef] [PubMed]
95. Ellis, P.D. *The Essential Guide to Effect Sizes: Statistical Power, Meta-analysis, and the Interpretation of Research Results*; Cambridge University Press: Cambridge, MA, USA, 2010; ISBN 0521142466.
96. Van Autreve, S.; De Baene, W.; Baeken, C.; van Heeringen, C.; Vervaet, M. Do Restrictive and Bingeing/Purging Subtypes of Anorexia Nervosa Differ on Central Coherence and Set Shifting? *Eur. Eat. Disord. Rev.* **2013**, *21*, 308–314. [CrossRef] [PubMed]
97. Gorini, A.; Griez, E.; Petrova, A.; Riva, G. Assessment of the emotional responses produced by exposure to real food, virtual food and photographs of food in patients affected by eating disorders. *Ann. Gen. Psychiatry* **2010**, *9*, 30. [CrossRef] [PubMed]
98. Jáuregui-Lobera, I. Electroencephalography in eating disorders. *Neuropsychiatr. Dis. Treat.* **2012**, *8*, 1–11. [CrossRef]
99. Tóth, E.; Kondákor, I.; Túry, F.; Gáti, Á.; Weisz, J.; Molnár, M. Nonlinear and linear EEG complexity changes caused by gustatory stimuli in anorexia nervosa. *Int. J. Psychophysiol.* **2004**, *51*, 253–260. [CrossRef]
100. Wang, Y.; Yang, L.; Wang, Y. Suppression (but Not Reappraisal) Impairs Subsequent Error Detection: An ERP Study of Emotion Regulation's Resource-Depleting Effect. *PLoS ONE* **2014**, *9*, e96339. [CrossRef]

10

Reduction of High Expressed Emotion and Treatment Outcomes in Anorexia Nervosa—Caregivers' and Adolescents' Perspective

Julia Philipp [1], Stefanie Truttmann [1], Michael Zeiler [1], Claudia Franta [1], Tanja Wittek [1], Gabriele Schöfbeck [1], Michaela Mitterer [1], Dunja Mairhofer [1], Annika Zanko [2], Hartmut Imgart [2], Ellen Auer-Welsbach [3], Janet Treasure [4], Gudrun Wagner [1] and Andreas F. K. Karwautz [1,*]

1 Eating Disorders Unit, Department of Child and Adolescent Psychiatry, Medical University of Vienna, 1090 Vienna, Austria; julia.philipp@meduniwien.ac.at (J.P.); stefanie.truttmann@meduniwien.ac.at (S.T.); michael.zeiler@meduniwien.ac.at (M.Z.); claudiaparfuss@gmx.at (C.F.); tanja.wittek@meduniwien.ac.at (T.W.); gabriele.schoefbeck@meduniwien.ac.at (G.S.); michaela.mitterer@meduniwien.ac.at (M.M.); dunja.mairhofer@meduniwien.ac.at (D.M.); gudrun.wagner@meduniwien.ac.at (G.W.)

2 Parkland Clinic, Clinic for Psychosomatic Medicine and Psychotherapy, 34537 Bad Wildungen, Germany; annika.zanko@parkland-klinik.de (A.Z.); hartmut.imgart@parkland-klinik.de (H.I.)

3 Department for Neurology and Child and Adolescent Psychiatry, 9020 Klagenfurt am Wörthersee, Austria; Ellen.Auer-Welsbach@kabeg.at

4 Section of Eating Disorders, Department of Psychological Medicine, Institute of Psychiatry, Psychology & Neuroscience, King's College London, London WC2R 2LS, UK; janet.treasure@kcl.ac.uk

* Correspondence: andreas.karwautz@meduniwien.ac.at

Abstract: High expressed emotion (EE) is common in caregivers of patients with anorexia nervosa (AN) and associated with poorer outcome for patients. In this study, we examined the prevalence of high EE in caregivers of adolescents with AN and analyzed predictors for EE using multivariate linear regression models. We further analyzed whether EE is reduced by the "Supporting Carers of Children and Adolescents with Eating Disorders in Austria" (SUCCEAT) intervention using general linear mixed models and whether a reduction of EE predicts patients' outcomes. Caregivers were randomly allocated to the SUCCEAT workshop ($N = 50$) or online intervention ($N = 50$) and compared to a comparison group ($N = 49$). EE and patients' outcomes were assessed at the baseline, post-intervention, and at the 12-month follow-up. Up to 47% of caregivers showed high EE. Lower caregiver skills, higher AN symptom impact, higher levels of depression and motivation to change in caregivers were significant predictors for high EE. EE significantly decreased in the SUCCEAT groups and the comparison group according to the caregivers', but not the patients' perspective. The level of reduction could partially predict subjective improvement and improvement in clinically assessed AN symptoms and body mass index of patients. Implementing interventions for caregivers addressing EE in the treatment of adolescents with AN is strongly recommended.

Keywords: anorexia nervosa; high expressed emotion; children and adolescents; intervention; caregivers

1. Introduction

Expressed emotion (EE) is a concept that describes a set of attitudes and behaviors (e.g., criticism, hostility, warmth, emotional involvement) of relatives towards an ill person. Specifically, the components of EE that have been mainly investigated so far are critical comments/criticism (CC) and emotional overinvolvement (EOI) [1,2]. High EE may represent a maladaptive response to an illness and may contribute to an exacerbation of psychiatric symptoms [2]. EE has been extensively studied in schizophrenia and has been confirmed to be a robust and significant predictor of relapse [3]. High levels of EE have further consistently been associated with treatment outcome, relapse, and treatment dropout in several other psychiatric disorders, including depression, bipolar disorder, anxiety disorders, and also eating disorders (EDs) [1–3].

In the field of EDs, caring for someone with an ED is known to be associated with high EE [1,4,5]. Caregivers often show extreme patterns of emotional reactions [6]. They might respond too intensely and too emotional, be too directive, negative and hostile, and blame the patient (CC), or they can be overprotective, overinvolved, and take over control (EOI). In a systematic review, up to 73.2% of caregivers showed high levels of CC and 89.3% showed high levels of EOI [5]. High EE has been found to be associated with caring for older patients and longer illness duration [4], higher anxiety and depression in caregivers [7], more contact time with the patient [8], higher caregivers' distress [8,9], and less caregiver skills [9]. Other studies revealed no clear association of high EE with the patients' weight or ED psychopathology [1,10], time spent caregiving, and ED severity [9]. Only few studies investigated the ED patients' point of view of EE within the family. Perceived EE in the family assessed by ED patients was reported to be higher than in healthy controls [11]. Patients reported higher EOI for their mothers, but no difference between mothers and fathers for CC [9]. The level of perceived EE from the patients' point of view was independent from age, contact time, and duration of treatment [11]. However, it has consistently been shown that high levels of EE in caregivers, especially in mothers, seem to negatively affect engagement, outcome, and effectiveness of ED treatment [1–3,10,12,13]. Thus, considering EE of caregivers in the patients' treatment seems to be highly relevant.

The key role of interpersonal relationships, particularly, communication and high EE within the family has also been highlighted in the interpersonal maintenance model of anorexia nervosa (AN) [14–16]. EE was related to caregivers' distress. Caregivers' distress was related to patients' distress, which predicted eating disorder symptoms [8]. Interventions based on this model were developed to reduce high EE [17] in order to improve the psychological wellbeing in caregivers and support recovery from the ED in patients [4]. These interventions address misperceptions of EDs and unhelpful reactions to the illness [18] and aim to improve communication skills, reduce negative emotion and build a warm and compassionate family atmosphere [19]. Caregivers learn to use reflective listening and motivational interviewing techniques, reduce confrontation, and be warm, calm, and compassionate.

A meta-analysis showed a moderate-sized reduction of EE in caregivers after participating in such interventions, including workshop-based, online, and self-help interventions [18]. Other recent studies also reported a reduction of high EE following interventions for caregivers [20–22]. However, having investigated the effects of such interventions, the previous literature almost exclusively focused on the parents' perception, while not considering the perception of the patients, although including the patients' perception is recommended and valued to gain additional insight in the family climate of ED patients [1]. One study that included the patients' perspective found that patients did not perceive a change in their caregivers' level of EE after caregivers participated in a specialized intervention [23], while in another study, qualitative improvement in caregivers' EE was mentioned by patients [24].

So far, only few studies have investigated whether a reduction in EE can also improve the patients' treatment outcomes. Two studies reported that an improvement of maternal EE was associated with better ED symptoms at the end of the treatment [10,25]. However, whether the level of reduction in parental EE is associated with the level of reduction in ED symptoms has not been investigated up to now.

SUCCEAT (Supporting Carers of Children and Adolescents with Eating Disorders in Austria) is an intervention for caregivers of adolescents with AN based on the interpersonal maintenance model [14–16] that has already been shown to effectively reduce caregiving burden and increase caregiver skills [26]. This paper presents secondary analyses of the SUCCEAT study, focusing on various aspects of high EE. Firstly, we aimed to examine the prevalence of high EE in a sample of caregivers and whether the level of EE assessed in parents is associated with the level of EE assessed in patients. Secondly, we explored whether different characteristics of caregivers and patients can predict the level of EE. Thirdly, this study aims to investigate whether EE can be reduced by participating in the SUCCEAT intervention and whether a change in assessed parental EE is also perceived by patients. Finally, we aimed to investigate whether a reduction in high EE is associated with patients' outcomes (AN symptoms, body mass index (BMI)).

2. Methods

2.1. Study Design

The SUCCEAT study is a two-arm parallel-group quasi-randomized controlled efficacy trial comparing two types of the SUCCEAT intervention (workshop and online) to a non-randomized control group. This study was conducted between 2014 and 2019. Caregivers of children and adolescents (10–19 years) with typical or atypical AN who received regular inpatient or outpatient treatment according to the National Institute for Health and Care Excellence (NICE) guidelines [27] were included. Caregivers and patients who were not fluent in German or suffered from severe comorbidities (e.g., psychosis) were excluded. For detailed information on the study protocol, see Franta et al. [28]. Written informed consent was obtained from all the participants prior to data collection. The SUCCEAT study protocol and all the informed consent forms were approved by the Ethics Committee of the Medical University of Vienna (#1840/2013). The SUCCEAT study was registered at ClinicalTrials.gov (Identifier: NCT02480907).

2.2. Recruitment and Randomisation

Caregivers of the SUCCEAT intervention group were recruited at the Eating Disorder Unit of the Department of Child and Adolescent Psychiatry at the Medical University of Vienna. If willing to participate, caregivers completed the baseline assessment and were allocated to one of the two intervention arms: workshop (SUCCEAT–WS) or online (SUCCEAT–ONL). The start dates of the groups had been previously fixed. The first block of participants was allocated to the SUCCEAT–WS group, the following block—to the SUCCEAT–ONL group, and so forth. Block sizes of eight participants were planned, however, sizes actually varied due to varying numbers of incoming participants prior to the upcoming group (median group size = 7). Caregivers were informed about the group allocation after they had completed the baseline assessments. Those who declined to participate in the allocated intervention arm were excluded from the study. The procedure slightly differed from the originally planned randomization [28] due to practical reasons, now corresponding to the definition of quasi-randomization [29]. However, there were no systematic differences between the WS and ONL groups at the baseline. Details on the randomization procedure are reported elsewhere [26].

2.3. Interventions

SUCCEAT is an intervention for caregivers of children and adolescents with AN based on the cognitive interpersonal model of maintaining factors for EDs [14–16] with the aim to reduce EE and burden in caregivers and improve caregiver skills. Dysfunctional communication, unhelpful reactions and emotions were addressed to increase communication skills, skills to handle difficult behavior, and strategies to encourage autonomy in patients in order to reduce EE. Additionally, caregivers' burden, wellbeing, and self-care were addressed as burden and psychopathology had been highly correlated with EE. The program was delivered in eight weekly modules as a WS or ONL, designed with the same content and structure and guided by two professional clinicians. Caregivers received weekly handouts, a manual to read more about the topics addressed [30], and a DVD [31] with case examples of unhelpful and helpful communication. A detailed description of the interventions is provided by Franta et al. [28] and Truttmann, Philipp et al. [26].

2.4. Comparison Group

The SUCCEAT groups were compared to a non-randomized comparison group (COMP) of caregivers who received other forms of family treatment within the same time frame at two other facilities: the Department for Neurology and Child and Adolescent Psychiatry, Klagenfurt, Austria (four double sessions of systemic family therapy [32]), and the Parkland Clinic, Clinic for Psychosomatic Medicine and Psychotherapy, Bad Wildungen, Germany (two-day workshop on multi-family therapy based on the Maudsley model of multi-family therapy for AN [33]). Several other inpatient and outpatient units that offer treatment as usual with and without any specialized intervention for caregivers were invited to participate as the control group declined the offer. Therefore, only the two named facilities that already implemented well-established family treatment agreed to participate and served as the COMP group.

2.5. Assessment Measures

Caregivers and patients completed self-report questionnaires at baseline (T0), at post-intervention (T1, approximately 3 months after T0), and at 12-month follow-up (FU) (T2), including the assessment of EE described below.

The Family Questionnaire (FQ [34]) is a self-report questionnaire for caregivers to detect the emotional climate and EE within the family. The 20 questions were answered using a four-point Likert scale providing two subscales of EE in caregivers: "Emotional overinvolvement" (EOI) and "Criticism" (CC). We used the established cut-off values (CC score $\geq$ 23, EOI score $\geq$ 27) to define high EE.

The Family Emotional Involvement and Criticism Scale (FEICS [35]) is a self-report questionnaire for children and adolescents to assess perceived EE within the family. Two subscales were calculated ("Emotional Involvement" and "Criticism") using 14 questions that were answered using a four-point Likert scale. For the FEICS scores, no established cut-off values are available.

In addition, self-assessments for caregivers were used to explore predictors of high EE and associations with perceived changes as described below (for details, see Franta et al. [28]).

The General Health Questionnaire (GHQ [36]) was fulfilled by caregivers and used to assess the level of psychological morbidity and distress in caregivers; a higher score indicates higher psychological distress.

The Eating Disorder Symptom Impact Scale (EDSIS [37]) assessed specific caregiving difficulties in caregivers associated with the ED of a child, such as difficulties related to "nutrition", "dysregulated behavior", "guilt", and "social isolation." A higher global score represents higher AN symptom impact in the family reported by caregivers.

The Beck Depression Inventory (BDI-II [38]) measured depression in caregivers; higher scores indicate higher levels of depression.

The State and Trait Anxiety Inventory (STAI [39]) assessed anxiety in caregivers; higher scores indicate higher levels of anxiety.

The Caregiver Skills (CASK) Scale [17] was used to measure self-assessed skills in caregivers (e.g., "insight and acceptance", "emotional intelligence", "frustration tolerance"). A higher total score means more caregiver skills.

The University of Rhode Island Change Assessment Scale (URICA [40]) was used to measure motivation to change in caregivers regarding their own behavior, revealing three scales: "precontemplation", "contemplation", and "action." A lower score on the precontemplation scale and higher scores on the contemplation and action scales represent higher motivation to change in caregivers.

Finally, two more assessments for patients were used as described below.

The Eating Disorder Examination (EDE [41]) is a semi-structured interview with patients reflecting the clinical assessment of ED psychopathology ("restraint", "eating concerns", "weight concerns", "shape concerns"). A higher global score indicates higher ED psychopathology.

The Eating Disorder Inventory-2 (EDI-2 [42]) was completed by the patients and assessed subjective ED symptoms from the patients' perspective (e.g., "drive for thinness", "perfection", "dissatisfaction with the body", etc.). A higher total score indicates more subjective ED symptoms.

Sociodemographic and clinical characteristics of caregivers (sex, age, marital status, highest educational degree, time spent caregiving) and patients (sex, age, AN subtype, BMI percentile, illness duration, type of current treatment) were obtained.

2.6. Statistical Analysis

The statistical analyses were performed using IBM SPSS Statistics 25.0 and R. We first calculated descriptive statistics and compared key sociodemographic and clinical characteristics between caregivers and patients of the SUCCEAT–WS, SUCCEAT–ONL, and the COMP group. We used Chi^2 tests for categorical and ANOVA tests for continuous variables, respectively, and Kruskal–Wallis tests for variables with skewed distribution. We calculated *t*-tests to analyze differences in CC and EOI scores between a mother and a father and Pearson correlation coefficients to explore associations between CC and EOI obtained from the parents and patients. To analyze predictors for assessed parental and patients' CC and EOI scores at the baseline, we first carried out a series of univariate linear regressions. The following predictors were considered: sex and age of the parent, parental psychological distress and psychopathology (including the GHQ, BDI, and STAI scores), AN symptom impact on the family (EDSIS score), self-reported caregiver skills (CASK score), parental motivation to change (URICA scores), the average time spent caregiving per day (<3 h vs. ≥3 h), the patient's age, treatment type (inpatient vs. outpatient), ED duration in months, BMI percentile (≤1st percentile vs. >1st percentile) and ED symptomatology (EDE and EDI-2 total scores). Variables reaching significance in univariate regressions ($p < 0.05$) were then considered for multivariate regression models using the forward selection method where variables were added to the model of ascending *p*-values.

In order to analyze the efficacy of the SUCCEAT intervention on EE, we calculated general linear mixed models using the FQ/FEICS scores (CC and EOI) obtained at the baseline, post-intervention, and at 12-month FU as the within factor and the group as the between factor. Firstly, we contrasted the SUCCEAT–WS group to the SUCCEAT–ONL intervention group. Secondly, we tested whether the SUCCEAT intervention (including all WS and ONL participants) differ from participants of the COMP group. Additionally, we performed sensitivity analyses by calculating paired sample *t*-tests for each group to explore the baseline-to-post-intervention and the baseline-to-12-month FU effect sizes (Cohen's dz). Furthermore, we explored the moderating effect of the patient's treatment type (inpatient vs. outpatient) on the EE outcome by adding a time x treatment type interaction term to the mixed design model.

Further, we explored whether a pre–post change in assessed parental CC and EOI scores corresponds to a change in CC and EOI assessed in the patients by calculating Pearson correlation coefficients.

Finally, we used linear regression analyses to analyze whether the degree of reduction in CC and EOI can predict improvements in ED symptomatology of the patients by using the EDE and EDI-2 change scores as well as the change in the BMI percentile as outcome variables and CC/EOI change scores as predictor variables.

3. Results

3.1. Sample

In total, 149 caregivers (83% mothers, 17% fathers; mean age (SD): 47.2 (4.74) years) provided informed consent and were included in the study. Forty-five percent had a university degree and 77% were married or lived in a partnership. According to their self-reports, the average amount of time spent with their child diagnosed with AN during weekdays was distributed as follows: 0–1 h (10%), 1–3 h (19%), 3–4 h (35%), > 4 h (35%). A total of 50 caregivers were allocated to the SUCCEAT–WS intervention, another 50 caregivers—to the SUCCEAT–ONL intervention, and 49 caregivers were included in the COMP group.

Of the 149 caregivers participating, we obtained data from 144 related patients with AN. The patients were predominantly female (83%) with a mean age of 15.1 years (SD: 1.7). According to ICD-10, most patients were diagnosed with AN restrictive subtype (89%), followed by AN binge/purging subtype (9%) and atypical AN (2%). At the baseline, the median sex-and age-specific BMI percentile was 1%, the average ED duration was 16.6 months (SD: 13.8), 59% received inpatient treatment, and 41% received outpatient treatment of their ED.

Baseline sample characteristics by intervention arm are shown in Table 1. There was a significantly lower proportion of caregivers with university degree in the COMP and patients of caregivers in the COMP had a significantly longer ED duration and higher subjective ED symptomatology scores as measured with EDI-2 and received inpatient treatment more often compared to SUCCEAT groups.

Table 1. Sample characteristics at the baseline (caregivers and eating disorder patients).

	SUCCEAT–WS (N = 50)	SUCCEAT–ONL (N = 50)	COMP (N = 49)	p
Caregivers' characteristics				
Mothers (%)	84.0%	88.0%	75.5%	0.248 [1]
Age (Mean, SD)	46.64 (5.43)	47.72 (4.25)	47.27 (4.48)	0.523 [2]
University degree (%)	60.0%	46.0%	27.7%	0.006 [1]
Married or living in partnership (%)	84.0%	75.0%	70.2%	0.264 [1]
Time spent with the patient during weekdays (%)				
0–1 h/day	6.1%	10.2%	15.2%	0.386 [1]
1–2 h/day	18.4%	22.4%	15.2%	
3–4 h/day	32.7%	42.9%	30.4%	
>4 h/day	42.9%	24.5%	39.1%	
FQ–CC score (Mean, SD)	20.76 (5.96)	21.78 (5.47)	21.82 (5.54)	0.559 [2]
FQ–EOI score (Mean, SD)	26.10 (5.17)	25.44 (4.98)	27.22 (5.05)	0.222 [2]
Patients' characteristics				
Females (%)	90.0%	96.0%	100%	0.061 [1]
Age (Mean, SD)	14.66 (1.91)	15.12 (1.80)	15.43 (1.08)	0.068 [2]
ED diagnosis (%)				
AN restrictive	90.0%	90.0%	87.8%	0.995 [1]
AN binge/purging	8.0%	8.0%	10.2%	
Atypical AN	2.0%	2.0%	2.0%	
ED duration (Mean, SD)	10.41 (7.10)	16.03 (16.05)	23.77 (12.93)	<0.001 [1]
BMI percentile (Median)	1.16	2.74	0.45	0.091 [3]
Inpatient treatment (%)	48.0%	48.0%	81.6%	<0.001 [1]
EDE score (Mean, SD)	3.27 (1.62)	3.32 (1.39)	3.22 (1.36)	0.945 [2]
EDI-2 score (Mean, SD)	67.32 (39.55)	69.62 (38.79)	91.57 (47.35)	0.009 [2]
FEICS–CC score (Mean, SD)	12.15 (4.17)	12.52 (4.44)	13.51 (4.08)	0.272 [2]
FEICS–EOI score (Mean, SD)	23.92 (4.43)	23.53 (4.17)	22.91 (3.94)	0.503 [2]

[1] Chi^2 test; [2] ANOVA test; [3] Kruskal–Wallis test. Abbreviations: AN, anorexia nervosa; CC, criticism; COMP, comparison group; ED, eating disorder; EDE, Eating Disorder Examination Interview, EDI-2, Eating Disorder Inventory-2; EOI, emotional overinvolvement; FEICS, Family Emotional Involvement and Criticism Scale; FQ, Family Questionnaire; ONL, online; SUCCEAT, Supporting Carers of Children and Adolescents with Eating Disorders in Austria; WS, workshop.

Dropout of caregivers in terms of non-completion at one of the FU assessments was 14.8% at the post-intervention assessment (SUCCEAT–WS: 4.0%, SUCCEAT–ONL: 6.0%, COMP: 34.7%) and 29.6% at the 12-month FU assessment (SUCCEAT–WS: 14.0%, SUCCEAT–ONL: 28.0%, COMP: 46.9%). Dropout of patients was 13.9% at the post-intervention assessment (SUCCEAT–WS: 8.3%, SUCCEAT–ONL: 6.1%, COMP: 27.7%) and 35.4% at the 12-month FU assessment (SUCCEAT–WS: 31.2%, SUCCEAT–ONL: 32.7%, COMP: 42.6%). Caregivers and patients who dropped out did not significantly differ from those who completed the study regarding the baseline EE scores (all p-values > 0.200).

3.2. *Baseline EE Characteristics*

Among the total sample, high CC defined as scores above the pre-defined cut-off in the FQ were observed in 39.2% (95% CI: 31.3; 47.1) and high EOI—in 46.6% (95% CI: 38.5; 54.7) of caregivers. Mean baseline CC and EOI scores obtained from the parents and patients are shown in Table 1. Mothers had slightly higher CC (mean: 21.79, SD: 5.52) and EOI scores (mean: 26.56, SD: 5.18) compared to fathers (CC: mean: 18.87, SD: 5.48; EOI: mean: 24.74, SD: 4.43); however, these differences did not reach statistical significance (CC: $t = 1.613$, $p = 0.109$; EOI: $t = 1.672$, $p = 0.097$).

3.3. *Bivariate Correlations between Parents' and Patients' EE Scores*

At the baseline, the parental EE scores were not significantly associated with the EE scores obtained from the patients' perspective neither for CC ($r = 0.078$, $p = 0.356$) nor for EOI ($r = 0.115$, $p = 0.171$). This correlation slightly increased at post-intervention (CC: $r = 0.142$, $p = 0.126$; EOI: $r = 0.117$, $p = 0.206$) and 12-month FU (CC: $r = 0.216$, $p = 0.042$; EOI: $r = 0.269$, $p = 0.011$). Considering mothers and fathers separately, we found a strong association between CC scores of fathers and patients at the baseline ($r = 0.509$, $p = 0.009$), while there was no association between CC scores of mothers and patients ($r = 0.006$, $p = 0.946$). No difference between mothers and fathers were found for EOI scores.

3.4. *Predictors for EE Scores at the Baseline*

Firstly, we explored whether different characteristics of parents and patients are predictive of the EE scores obtained from the parents. In the univariate regression analyses (Table S1 in the electronic Supplementary Materials), we found that the level of parental psychological distress, AN symptom impact, depression, anxiety, caregiver skills, parental motivation to change, and the current treatment setting (inpatient vs. outpatient) of the child were significantly associated with either the CC or EOI score or both. In the multivariate regression model (Table 2), lower caregiver skills, higher level of AN symptom impact, and an outpatient treatment setting were significant predictors for CC with the final model explaining 46.2% of the variance. The parental EOI score was significantly predicted by higher levels of AN symptom impact, higher distress, depression, as well as higher motivation to change and lower caregiving skills with the final model explaining 63.5% of the variance.

We repeated this analysis using the EE scores obtained from the patients' perspective as the outcome variable. In the univariate regression analyses (Table S2 in the electronic Supplementary Materials), ED duration and ED symptomatology as measured with EDE and EDI-2 were significantly associated with CC and parental motivation to change and BMI were significantly associated with EOI. In the multivariate regression model (Table 3), only higher ED symptomatology (EDI-2 score) significantly predicted CC explaining 14.2% of the variance. The EOI score was significantly predicted by lower BMI (<1st BMI percentile) and lower parental motivation to change. However, the final model only explained 8.1% of the variance.

Table 2. Multivariate regression (forward selection method) predicting criticism and emotional overinvolvement (FQ, parents).

Predictor	b(SE)	*t* (df)	*p*	R^2	ΔR^2
		Outcome: FQ, criticism			
Model 1				0.351	
CASK, total score	−0.240 (0.029)	−8.165 (1,123)	<0.001		
Model 2				0.435	0.084
CASK, total score	−0.171 (0.032)	−5.378	<0.001		
EDSIS, total score	0.127 (0.030)	4.253 (2,122)	<0.001		
Model 3				0.462	0.27
CASK, total score	−0.160 (0.032)	−5.079	<0.001		
EDSIS, total score	0.137 (0.030)	4.624	<0.001		
Treatment type [1]	1.849 (0.755)	2.450 (1,121)	0.016		
		Outcome: FQ, emotional overinvolvement			
Model 1				0.500	
EDSIS, total score	0.253 (0.023)	11.035 (1,122)	<0.001		
Model 2				0.567	0.068
EDSIS, total score	0.195 (0.025)	7.741	<0.001		
BDI, total score	0.203 (0.047)	4.354 (2,121)	<0.001		
Model 3				0.601	0.033
EDSIS, total score	0.173 (0.025)	6.863	<0.001		
BDI, total score	0.195 (0.045)	4.320	<0.001		
URICA, contemp.	0.173 (0.055)	3.170 (3,120)	0.002		
Model 4				0.620	0.020
EDSIS, total score	0.154 (0.026)	5.956	<0.001		
BDI, total score	0.160 (0.046)	3.437	0.001		
URICA, contemp.	0.169 (0.054)	3.164	0.002		
CASK, total score	−0.064 (0.026)	−0.2486 (4,119)	0.014		
Model 5				0.635	0.015
EDSIS, total score	0.137 (0.027)	5.119	<0.001		
BDI, total score	0.101 (0.053)	1.916	0.058		
URICA, contemp.	0.162 (0.053)	3.074	0.003		
CASK, total score	−0.061 (0.025)	−2.398	0.018		
GHQ, total score	0.248 (0.113)	2.185 (5,118)	0.031		

[1] 1 = inpatient, 2 = outpatient. Abbreviations: BDI, Beck Depression Inventory; CASK, Caregiver Skills Scale; contemp., contemplation; EDSIS, Eating Disorder Impact Scale; FQ, Family Questionnaire; GHQ, General Health Questionnaire; URICA, University of Rhode Island Change Assessment.

Table 3. Multivariate regression (forward selection method) predicting criticism and emotional overinvolvement (FEICS, patients).

Predictor	b(SE)	*t* (df)	*p*	R^2	ΔR^2
		Outcome: FEICS, criticism			
Model 1 (final)				0.145	
EDI-2, total score	0.040 (0.009)	4.555 (1,122)	<0.001		
		Outcome: FEICS, emotional overinvolvement			
Model 1				0.041	
BMI percentile [1]	−1.681 (0.701)	−2.399 (1,136)	0.018		
Model 2				0.085	0.044
BMI percentile [1]	−2.025 (0.701)	−2.894	0.004		
URICA, precon.	−0.191 (0.074)	−2.563 (2,135)	0.011		

[1] Categorized as follows: 1 ≤ 1st percentile, 2 > 1st percentile. Abbreviations: EDI-2, Eating Disorder Inventory-2; FEICS, Family Emotional Involvement and Criticism Scale; precon., precontemplation; URICA, University of Rhode Island Change Assessment.

3.5. Intervention Outcomes on EE

The change in EE scores by group from the baseline to the post-intervention and the 12-month FU assessment is shown in Figure 1. We first tested whether the SUCCEAT–WS group differs from SUCCEAT–ONL group. We found that the assessed parental CC ($F = 7.391$, $p = 0.001$) and EOI scores ($F = 45.704$, $p < 0.001$) significantly decreased over time across both groups, but there was no significant time × group interaction effect (CC: $F = 0.437$, $p = 0.782$; EOI: $F = 0.953$, $p = 0.435$). Considering the patients' perspective, there was no significant main effect of time and group difference neither for CC nor for EOI.

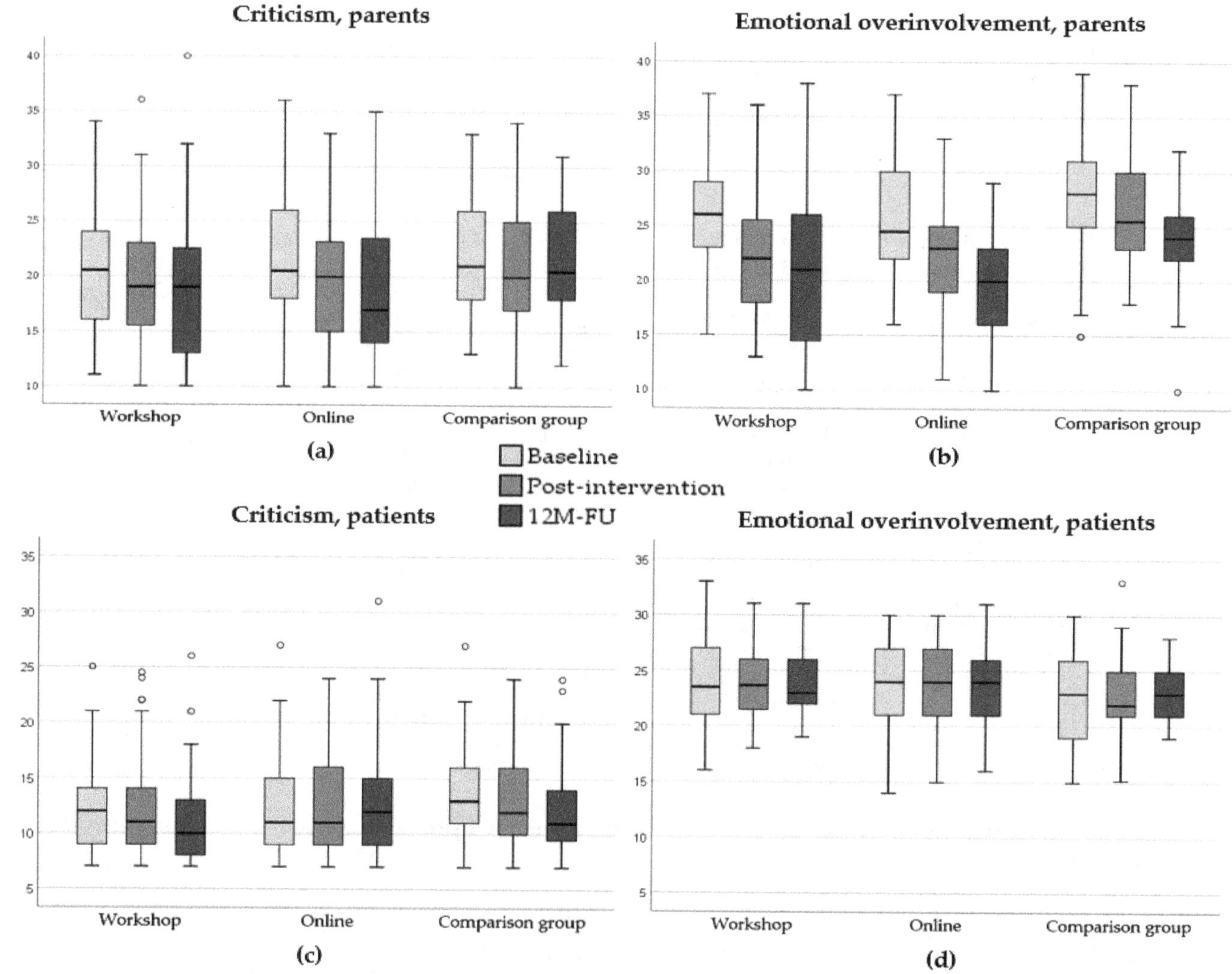

Figure 1. Change of high expressed emotion scores in the SUCCEAT workshop, online, and comparison groups from the baseline (light-grey box) to the post-intervention (mid-grey box) and the 12-month follow-up (dark-grey box) assessment: (**a**) Criticism score (parent perspective), (**b**) Emotional Overinvolvement score (parent perspective), (**c**) Criticism score (patient perspective), (**d**) Emotional Overinvolvement score (patient perspective). The size of the box represents the interquartile range (IQR); the whiskers indicate the minimum/maximum values in case no outliers were observed. Outliers (defined as values > 1.5 x IQR from the 25th quantile and 75th quantile) are depicted as circles. Abbreviations: 12M-FU, 12-month follow-up.

When contrasting the SUCCEAT groups to the COMP group, we found the same pattern of results. The assessed parental CC ($F = 5.400$, $p = 0.005$) and EOI scores ($F = 36.112$, $p < 0.001$) significantly decreased over time across the groups, but this change was the same for the SUCCEAT and COMP groups (CC: F = 0.089, $p = 0.914$; EOI: F = 1.612, $p = 0.202$). Again, no significant effects of time and time x group interaction effects were observed when considering the patients' perspective.

Sensitivity analyses using *t*-tests revealed that for the assessed parental CC, baseline-to-post-intervention reductions were highest for the SUCCEAT–ONL group (dz = 0.44, $t = 3.788$, $p < 0.001$) compared to the SUCCEAT–WS (dz = 0.20, $t = 1.806$, $p = 0.077$) and COMP groups (dz = 0.32, $t = 2.172$, $p = 0.038$). These effects remained stable to the 12-month FU for the SUCCEAT groups (WS: dz = 0.24; ONL: dz = 0.54) and slightly decreased in the COMP group (dz = 0.20). For the assessed parental EOI, baseline-to-post reductions were slightly higher for the SUCCEAT groups (WS: dz = 0.68, $t = 5.739$, $p < 0.001$; ONL: dz: 0.76, $t = 5.927$, $p < 0.001$) compared to the COMP group (dz = 0.36; $t = 2.061$, $p = 0.048$). The effect sizes further increased at the 12-month FU in all the groups (WS: dz = 0.76, ONL: dz = 1.11, COMP: dz = 0.89). Considering the patients' perspective, all effect sizes were close to zero in all the groups.

Further analyses revealed that the type of patients' treatment (inpatient vs. outpatient) was a significant moderator of the intervention outcome. Caregivers of outpatients reported a significantly higher reduction in CC scores than caregivers of inpatients (time x treatment type interaction: F = 4.076, $p = 0.018$). Regarding EOI, reductions of EOI scores were reported to be faster (from the baseline to post-intervention) in caregivers of outpatients, whereas the reduction was delayed (post-intervention to the 12-month FU) in caregivers of inpatients (time x treatment type interaction: F = 5.011, $p = 0.008$). This moderator effect was independent of the group.

Figure 2 presents the bivariate correlations between the baseline-to-post-intervention change of parental and patients' CC and EOI scores. In the SUCCEAT group, parental change of CC was moderately associated with the change of CC in patients ($r = 0.230$, $p = 0.031$). In the COMP group, this association was not significant ($r = 0.209$, $p = 0.285$). For EOI, no significant associations in the change scores were observed (SUCCEAT: $r = 0.160$, $p = 0.137$; COMP: $r = -0.088$, $p = 0.655$).

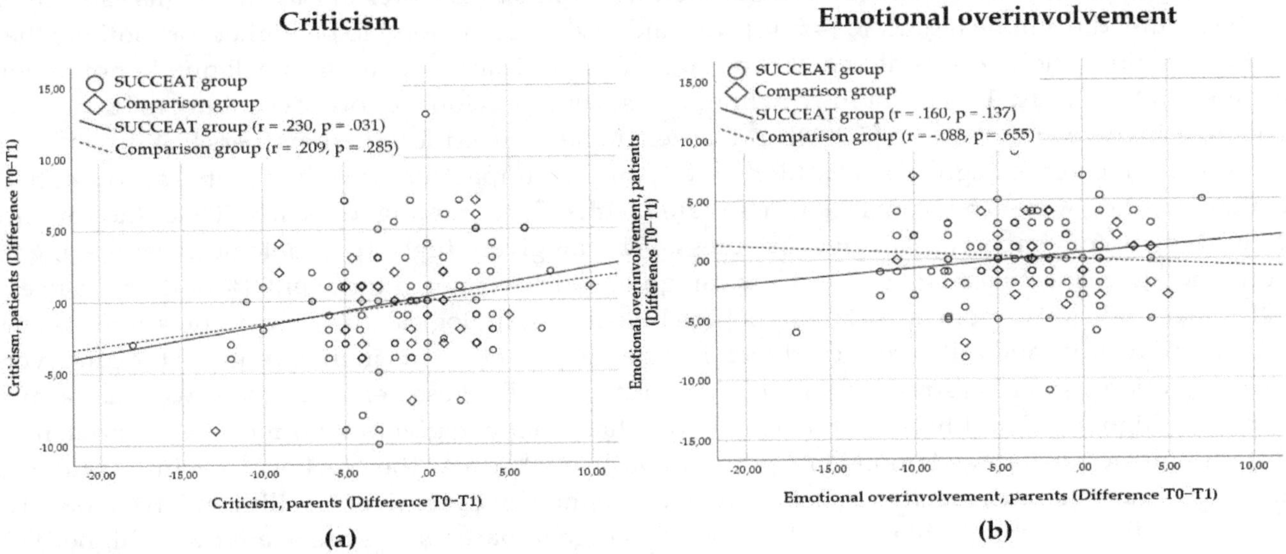

(a) (b)

Figure 2. The scatterplot depicting the association (Pearson correlation coefficients) between high expressed emotion change scores (baseline to post-intervention) of parents and patients: (**a**) Criticism change scores; (**b**) Emotional overinvolvement change scores. A significant positive correlation indicates that higher levels of change based on the parents' perspective are associated with higher levels of change based on the perspective of patients.

3.6. Impact of EE Change on the Patient's ED Symptomatology

Table 4 shows whether a reduction in parental or patients' EE scores significantly predicted improvements in ED symptoms (EDE and EDI-2 scores, BMI percentile) for the total sample and separately for inpatients and outpatients. We found that for the total sample, improvements in CC were significantly associated with improvements in ED symptomatology and BMI. On the contrary, reductions in EOI did not significantly predict improvements in ED symptoms.

Table 4. Results of linear regression analyses predicting the change in patient's eating disorder symptoms by the change in high expressed emotion.

	EDE Change Score		EDI-2 Change Score		BMI Perc. Change	
	T0–T1	T0–T2	T0–T1	T0–T2	T0–T1	T0–T2
Change in CC (FQ)	$p = 0.731$	$p = 0.239$	$p = 0.040$	$p = 0.073$	$p = 0.995$	$p = 0.099$
Change in EOI (FQ)	$p = 0.515$	$p = 0.148$	$p = 0.113$	$p = 0.050$	$p = 0.969$	$p = 0.066$
Change in CC (FEICS)	$p = 0.040$	$p = 0.087$	$p = 0.005$	$p < 0.001$	$p = 0.006$	$p = 0.561$
Change in EOI FEICS)	$p = 0.096$	$p = 0.438$	$p = 0.580$	$p = 0.867$	$p = 0.982$	$p = 0.307$

Abbreviations: CC, criticism, EOI, emotional overinvolvement, EDE, Eating Disorder Examination Interview, EDI-2, Eating Disorder Inventory-2, FQ, Family Questionnaire, FEICS, Family Emotional Involvement and Criticism Scale; T0–T1, difference between the baseline and post-intervention scores; T0-T2, difference between the baseline and 12-month FU scores.

4. Discussion

This study explored EE in caregivers and adolescents with AN at the baseline and following a skills training for caregivers, including a long-term FU. In addition, we aimed to investigate whether changes in EE affect patients' outcomes.

Firstly, the caregivers' perspective of EE was analyzed. One third of caregivers showed elevated CC scores and nearly half of the caregivers reported high EOI scores. These prevalence figures are somewhat lower compared to previous studies using the same questionnaire [5,7]. This may be due to older patients (mostly adults) and a longer illness duration in these reports (mostly far longer than one year) compared to our participants (approximately one year). Even though we only observed a tendency that longer illness duration is associated with higher EE scores in this study, this association can be assumed from the literature [4,5,10]. CC and EOI scores tended to be higher for mothers than for fathers, albeit these results did not reach statistical significance due to the small number of fathers included in this study. This is not fully in line with several previous reports describing mothers to be more overinvolved than fathers [5,9,43] and fathers to be more critical than mothers [5,43].

Low perceived caregiver skills, high AN symptom impact on caregivers, and an outpatient treatment setting were significant factors associated with CC, accounting for nearly 50% of the variance. High AN symptom impact on caregivers, depression in caregivers, higher psychological distress, higher motivation to change in caregivers, and less caregiver skills accounted for over 60% of the variance of EOI. Other studies also found associations of high EE with psychological distress or depression [1,43,44]. Caregivers' distress and self-care should therefore be the core elements in interventions for caregivers, beside emotion regulation strategies and communication skills. Less perceived skills were associated with both higher CC and higher EOI. This may reflect that caregivers who feel less competent to deal with ED in the family demonstrate high EE, probably because they feel overwhelmed with this situation. Consequently, one might also assume that enhancing caregivers' skills can have a positive impact on EE. Interestingly, higher motivation to change in parents was associated with higher EOI. This sounds paradoxical. However, caregivers who experience frustration and helplessness when confronted with ED symptoms or associated conflicts more often, which may consequently enhance EE, might also be highly motivated to change their own behavior or aspects of the actual situation. Therefore, it may be of benefit to target motivation to change in interventions for caregivers. Further research is needed to investigate the role of motivation to change in caregivers regarding high EE. Caregivers of outpatients reported higher scores for CC than caregivers of inpatients. It might be assumed that parents of outpatients feel more responsible for an improvement of symptoms compared to inpatients, whereas the responsibility for symptom improvement is delegated to the ED treatment team. This may lead to higher distress and burden in parents of outpatients which may promote more critical comments. Besides, an outpatient treatment setting might induce more situations where high

EE can occur compared to an inpatient setting. In contrast to the literature [43], there was no association with illness severity (patients with lower BMI or higher ED psychopathology). No associations were also found for age of caregivers and age of patients, with only a tendency for caregivers of older patients to report higher EOI scores, in contrast to other studies reporting significantly higher EE in caregivers of older patients [4,5]. This may be because the mean age of patients within those studies was higher than in our sample. As the patient's age and duration of illness often correlate, we assume that including adult patients in the study may lead to a similar result. The time spent caregiving did not play a role in our study regarding EE levels either, in contrast to another study [8]. This study included adult patients and concluded that caring for patients that live in the same household involves more time and leads to higher EE. However, as we only included adolescents, the great majority of whom still lived at home, the time spent caregiving may not play such an important role.

We also explored predictors of high EE based on the patients' perspective. Regarding the patients' point of view on EE, high ED psychopathology was solely associated with CC, whereas a lower BMI and higher motivation to change in caregivers were associated with EOI. Therefore, a somewhat more severe illness (lower BMI and higher ED psychopathology) was correlated with high EE in the family. Moreover, when parents were more motivated to change, the perceived EOI was higher, which is similar to the findings for parents described above. However, our model only accounted for 4% (CC) and 8% (EOI) of the variance. Hence, other factors associated with the patients' perception of EE in the family should be investigated in future research.

Another aim of the study was to explore whether parental and patients' perceptions of EE are correlated. Regarding the total group, there were no significant correlations at the baseline, while the correlations between caregivers and patients slightly increased with time and reached significance at the 12-month FU. It is unclear why parents and patients' perceptions are stronger associated with time, even though the patients' perception of high EE within the family did not decrease like the caregivers' perception did. We assume that either the patients' or the parents' ability to precisely assess the real family climate improves with time, probably due to successful weight restitution or less severe symptoms at T2 or because patients gain valuable insights on family dynamics during their ongoing psychotherapy. However, the low correlations indicate that the parent's and patient's perceptions of EE diverge, which can be targeted in family-based interventions. Interestingly, we found a significant high correlation between the fathers' and patients' perceptions of CC at the baseline and at post-intervention which has to be interpreted with caution due to the low number of fathers included in this study.

We further investigated the efficacy of the SUCCEAT intervention on EE in caregivers. A significant reduction of EE was observed in the SUCCEAT group for the short-term and the long-term FU. This is in line with the literature, showing that EE in caregivers can be reduced after participating in an intervention for caregivers including psychoeducation and skills training [18,20,21,45]. EE was also reduced in the COMP group with no significant difference to the SUCCEAT intervention. That might be because the facilities that recruited participants for the COMP group already implemented specialized family interventions (multi-family therapy [33] or systemic family therapy [32]) also including expressing emotions, conflict management, and communication within the family as the core elements. To note, there were no differences between the three study arms with regard to the majority of caregivers' and patients' sociodemographic and clinical characteristics at the baseline. However, the groups differed with respect to the highest educational degree, ED duration, treatment setting, and subjective ED symptoms with the caregivers of the SUCCEAT group having higher educational levels and the COMP patients having a longer illness duration, higher subjective ED psychopathology, and having been treated in an inpatient setting more often. This should be considered when interpreting the results regarding group differences. Yet, there was no difference for EE scores at the baseline between the three arms. The sensitivity analyses showed that reductions in EOI were generally higher than in CC and that intervention effects remained stable or increased further up to the 12-month FU except for CC in the COMP group where we found a small rebound effect indicating that parents of the COMP group were a bit more critical at the 12-month FU again. Indeed, the current literature suggests that CC is more susceptible to increase again in the long term [43]. Interestingly, the improvement of CC and EOI was stronger in caregivers of outpatients than of inpatients and EOI also improved faster. This might be due to the fact that caregivers of outpatients may have more time and more opportunities to use and practice the communication skills trained in the interventions than caregivers of inpatients.

Unfortunately, no improvements were found when considering the patients' perception of EE within the family. Thus, the patients did not perceive EE to be significantly reduced over time neither in the SUCCEAT nor in the COMP groups. This could be due to several reasons. Firstly, we used questionnaires that measure the same construct, but did not include exactly the same item contents, impeding direct comparisons. The FQ measures subjective CC and EOI towards the patient, whereas the FEICS assesses CC and EOI within the whole family from the patient's point of view, but not specifically towards the parent who completed the FQ. Secondly, in most cases, only one parent (either mother or father) participated in the intervention. It might be the case that the caregivers who did not participate did not change regarding their EE compared to the ones that participated and therefore they may still contribute to a highly negative emotional climate. Thus, if possible, both parents should be encouraged to participate in a caregiver's skills training and be included in further research. Another possible explanation is that parents feel a reduction of EE more intensely, whereas patients do not experience small changes. Rienecke [1] assumed patients with AN to be acutely sensitive to parental EE, so they may have difficulties to experience a change even if the frequency of EE has reduced. In that case, children and adolescents might need more information on EE themselves in order to be more sensitive to notice a change in the family climate [46]. It might be possible to encourage patients themselves to read some chapters of the manual or to watch some parts of the DVD used in the intervention. Another possibility is to arrange one family meeting where this topic can be discussed together or to implement this issue in the patients' therapy.

Although there was no reduction in EE from the patients' point of view, we found a significant association between the perceived change in CC in parents and the perceived change in CC in patients from the baseline to post-intervention in the SUCCEAT group only. However, this correlation was marginal. No such association was observed for EOI. These results were similar to another study [23] that reported a significant reduction of EE in caregivers, no perceived reduction in patients, but a positive correlation between changes in perceived EE between caregivers and patients. Furthermore, patients might experience qualitative improvements in EE as indicated by Goddard et al. [24] which might not have been covered with the questionnaire used in this study.

Finally, we investigated whether reductions in parental or perceived EE affect the outcome of ED pathology and BMI in AN patients. Indeed, improvement in the assessed parental CC was associated with greater changes in subjective ED symptoms. Similarly, greater improvement in CC assessed in patients was associated with greater changes in subjective ED symptoms, clinically assessed ED psychopathology, and BMI. For EOI, no clear association was observed. These results contribute to the literature indicating that a reduction in parental EE is associated with patients' outcomes [10,25]. Although our analyses were explorative, these results indicate that reducing EE through a caregiver skills training can positively affect the ED psychopathology and BMI in patients. These results highlight the benefit and need in a caregiver training in the routine ED treatment.

This study has a couple of strengths. It is the first study investigating whether a change in EE can predict a change in ED psychopathology and BMI in adolescent patients. A long-term outcome was included. Both SUCCEAT groups were uniformly designed and guided by the same two professional clinicians. The study has some limitations, too. The number of fathers included in this study was low. Therefore, the role of fathers and the correlation between patients and both parents as well as between mothers and fathers require further investigation. Furthermore, as ED duration and treatment setting (outpatient or inpatient setting) differ significantly between the three groups at the baseline, results regarding group differences should be interpreted with some caution.

5. Conclusions

Our study confirms that high EE is common in caregivers of adolescent patients with AN. It further highlights that EE can be reduced after interventions for caregivers and that this reduction positively influences patients' outcomes. Our results therefore underline the importance of including a focus on parental EE into the treatment of adolescents with AN. Parental EE was high and was associated with higher distress, higher depression, and a lack of skills. We found that parental EE was significantly reduced after participating in the SUCCEAT intervention or a specialized family intervention and that this reduction remained in the long term. Although the patients' perceptions did not match well with the caregivers' perceptions of EE, there was some evidence that reductions in EE positively affect the patient's treatment course. Altogether, we can strongly recommend to include interventions for caregivers, such as SUCCEAT, into the treatment of adolescents with AN in order to improve the outcome for caregivers and for patients. Patients might further benefit from a conjoint meeting with parents to discuss family climate and to get sensitive to perceive possible changes.

Author Contributions: Conceptualization, A.F.K.K., J.T., J.P., and G.W.; methodology, C.F., J.P., and M.Z.; formal analysis, M.Z.; investigation, J.P., S.T., A.Z., C.F., and T.W.; resources, H.I., E.A.-W., G.S., M.M., D.M., A.F.K.K., and G.W.; data curation, M.Z.; writing—original draft preparation, J.P.; writing—review and editing, M.Z., A.F.K.K., G.W., and J.P.; visualization, M.Z.; supervision, A.F.K.K. and G.W.; project administration, J.P., S.T., C.F., and T.W.; funding acquisition, A.F.K.K. and G.W. All authors have read and agreed to the published version of the manuscript.

Acknowledgments: We thank all the patients and caregivers who participated, as well as all the staff members that helped to conduct the study.

References

1. Rienecke, R. Expressed Emotion and Eating Disorders: An Updated Review. *Curr. Psychiatry Rev.* **2018**, *14*, 84–98. [CrossRef]
2. Peris, T.S.; Miklowitz, D.J. Parental Expressed Emotion and Youth Psychopathology: New Directions for an Old Construct. *Child Psychiatry Hum. Dev.* **2015**, *46*, 863–873. [CrossRef] [PubMed]
3. Butzlaff, R.L.; Hooley, J.M. Expressed emotion and psychiatric relapse: A meta-analysis. *Arch. Gen. Psychiatry* **1998**, *55*, 547–552. [CrossRef]
4. Zabala, M.J.; Macdonald, P.; Treasure, J. Appraisal of caregiving burden, expressed emotion and psychological distress in families of people with eating disorders: A systematic review. *Eur. Eat. Disord. Rev.* **2009**, *17*, 338–349. [CrossRef]
5. Anastasiadou, D.; Medina-Pradas, C.; Sepulveda, A.R.; Treasure, J. A systematic review of family caregiving in eating disorders. *Eat. Behav.* **2014**, *15*, 464–477. [CrossRef]
6. Treasure, J.; Sepulveda, A.R.; Whitaker, W.; Todd, G.; Lopez, C.; Whitney, J. Collaborative care between professionals and non-professionals in the management of eating disorders: A description of workshops focussed on interpersonal maintaining factors. *Eur. Eat. Disord. Rev.* **2007**, *15*, 24–34. [CrossRef]
7. Kyriacou, O.; Treasure, J.; Schmidt, U. Expressed emotion in eating disorders assessed via self-report: An examination of factors associated with expressed emotion in carers of people with anorexia nervosa in comparison to control families. *Int. J. Eat. Disord.* **2008**, *41*, 37–46. [CrossRef]
8. Goddard, E.; Salerno, L.; Hibbs, R.; Raenker, S.; Naumann, U.; Arcelus, J.; Ayton, A.; Boughton, N.; Connan, F.; Goss, K.; et al. Empirical examination of the interpersonal maintenance model of anorexia nervosa. *Int. J. Eat. Disord.* **2013**, *46*, 867–874. [CrossRef] [PubMed]
9. Rhind, C.; Salerno, L.; Hibbs, R.; Micali, N.; Schmidt, U.; Gowers, S.; Macdonald, P.; Goddard, E.; Todd, G.; Tchanturia, K.; et al. The Objective and Subjective Caregiving Burden and Caregiving Behaviours of Parents of Adolescents with Anorexia Nervosa. *Eur. Eat. Disord. Rev.* **2016**, *24*, 310–319. [CrossRef] [PubMed]
10. Allan, E.; Le Grange, D.; Sawyer, S.M.; McLean, L.A.; Hughes, E.K. Parental Expressed Emotion During Two Forms of Family-Based Treatment for Adolescent Anorexia Nervosa. *Eur. Eat. Disord. Rev.* **2018**, *26*, 46–52. [CrossRef] [PubMed]
11. Di Paola, F.; Faravelli, C.; Ricca, V. Perceived expressed emotion in anorexia nervosa, bulimia nervosa, and binge-eating disorder. *Compr. Psychiatry* **2010**, *51*, 401–405. [CrossRef]

12. Eisler, I.; Simic, M.; Russell, G.F.M.; Dare, C. A randomised controlled treatment trial of two forms of family therapy in adolescent anorexia nervosa: A five-year follow-up. *J. Child Psychol. Psychiatry* **2007**, *48*, 552–560. [CrossRef] [PubMed]
13. Berona, J.; Richmond, R.; Rienecke, R.D. Heterogeneous weight restoration trajectories during partial hospitalization treatment for anorexia nervosa. *Int. J. Eat. Disord.* **2018**, *51*, 914–920. [CrossRef] [PubMed]
14. Schmidt, U.; Treasure, J. Anorexia nervosa: Valued and visible. A cognitive-interpersonal maintenance model and its implications for research and practice. *Br. J. Clin. Psychol.* **2006**, *45*, 343–366. [CrossRef]
15. Treasure, J.; Schmidt, U. The cognitive-interpersonal maintenance model of anorexia nervosa revisited: A summary of the evidence for cognitive, socio-emotional and interpersonal predisposing and perpetuating factors. *J. Eat. Disord.* **2013**, *1*, 13. [CrossRef] [PubMed]
16. Treasure, J.; Willmott, D.; Ambwani, S.; Cardi, V.; Clark Bryan, D.; Rowlands, K.; Schmidt, U. Cognitive Interpersonal Model for Anorexia Nervosa Revisited: The Perpetuating Factors that Contribute to the Development of the Severe and Enduring Illness. *J. Clin. Med.* **2020**, *9*, 630. [CrossRef] [PubMed]
17. Hibbs, R.; Rhind, C.; Salerno, L.; Coco, G.L.; Goddard, E.; Schmidt, U.; Micali, N.; Gowers, S.; Beecham, J.; Macdonald, P.; et al. Development and validation of a scale to measure caregiver skills in eating disorders. *Int. J. Eat. Disord.* **2015**, *48*, 290–297. [CrossRef] [PubMed]
18. Hibbs, R.; Rhind, C.; Leppanen, J.; Treasure, J. Interventions for caregivers of someone with an eating disorder: A meta-analysis. *Int. J. Eat. Disord.* **2015**, *48*, 349–361. [CrossRef] [PubMed]
19. Treasure, J.; Whitaker, W.; Todd, G.; Whitney, J. A description of multiple family workshops for carers of people with anorexia nervosa. *Eur. Eat. Disord. Rev.* **2012**, *20*, e17–e22. [CrossRef]
20. Dimitropoulos, G.; Landers, A.; Freeman, V.; Novick, J.; Schmidt, U.; Olmsted, M. A feasibility study comparing a web-based intervention to a workshop intervention for caregivers of adults with eating disorders. *Eur. Eat. Disord. Rev.* **2019**, *27*, 641–654. [CrossRef]
21. Magill, N.; Rhind, C.; Hibbs, R.; Goddard, E.; Macdonald, P.; Arcelus, J.; Morgan, J.; Beecham, J.; Schmidt, U.; Landau, S.; et al. Two-year Follow-up of a Pragmatic Randomised Controlled Trial Examining the Effect of Adding a Carer's Skill Training Intervention in Inpatients with Anorexia Nervosa. *Eur. Eat. Disord. Rev.* **2015**, *24*. [CrossRef]
22. McEvoy, P.M.; Targowski, K.; McGrath, D.; Carter, O.; Fursland, A.; Fitzgerald, M.; Raykos, B. Efficacy of a brief group intervention for carers of individuals with eating disorders: A randomized control trial. *Int. J. Eat. Disord.* **2019**, *52*, 987–995. [CrossRef] [PubMed]
23. Hoyle, D.; Slater, J.; Williams, C.; Schmidt, U.; Wade, T.D. Evaluation of a web-based skills intervention for carers of people with anorexia nervosa: A randomized controlled trial. *Int. J. Eat. Disord.* **2013**, *46*, 634–638. [CrossRef] [PubMed]
24. Goddard, E.; Macdonald, P.; Treasure, J. An examination of the impact of the Maudsley Collaborative Care skills training workshops on patients with anorexia nervosa: A qualitative study. *Eur. Eat. Disord. Rev.* **2011**, *19*, 150–161. [CrossRef] [PubMed]
25. Moskovich, A.A.; Timko, C.A.; Honeycutt, L.K.; Zucker, N.L.; Merwin, R.M. Change in expressed emotion and treatment outcome in adolescent anorexia nervosa. *Eat. Disord.* **2017**, *25*, 80–91. [CrossRef] [PubMed]
26. Truttmann, S.; Philipp, J.; Zeiler, M.; Franta, C.; Wittek, T.; Merl, E.; Schöfbeck, G.; Koubek, D.; Laczkovics, C.; Imgart, H.; et al. Long-term Efficacy of the Workshop- vs. Online-SUCCEAT (Supporting Carers of Children and Adolescents with Eating Disorders) intervention: A quasi-randomised feasibility trial. *J. Clin. Med.* **2020**, *9*, 1912. [CrossRef]
27. National Guideline Alliance (UK). *Eating Disorders: Recognition and Treatment*; National Institute for Health and Care Excellence: Clinical Guidelines; National Institute for Health and Care Excellence: London, UK, 2017.
28. Franta, C.; Philipp, J.; Waldherr, K.; Truttmann, S.; Merl, E.; Schöfbeck, G.; Koubek, D.; Laczkovics, C.; Imgart, H.; Zanko, A.; et al. Supporting Carers of Children and Adolescents with Eating Disorders in Austria (SUCCEAT): Study protocol for a randomised controlled trial. *Eur. Eat. Disord. Rev.* **2018**, *26*, 447–461. [CrossRef]
29. Higgins, J.; Green, S. Cochrane Handbook for Systematic Reviews of Interventions. Available online: https://handbook-5-1.cochrane.org/ (accessed on 22 May 2020).
30. Treasure, J.; Smith, G.; Crane, A. *Skills-Based Learning for Caring for a Loved One with an Eating Disorder: The New Maudsley Method*; Routledge: London, UK, 2007.
31. The Succeed Foundation. *How to Care for Someone with an Eating Disorder [DVD]*; The Succeed Foundation: London, UK, 2011.

32. Reich, G. Familienbeziehungen und Familientherapie bei Essstörungen. *Prax. Kinderpsychol. Kinderpsychiatr.* **2005**, *54*, 318–336.
33. Imgart, H.; Plassmann, R. Effective factors in multifamily therapy in patients with eating disorders: Critical appraisal and implications for practice. *Neuropsychiatr* **2020**. [CrossRef]
34. Wiedemann, G.; Rayki, O.; Feinstein, E.; Hahlweg, K. The Family Questionnaire: Development and validation of a new self-report scale for assessing expressed emotion. *Psychiatry Res.* **2002**, *109*, 265–279. [CrossRef]
35. Kronmüller, K.-T.; Krummheuer, C.; Topp, F.; Zipfel, S.; Herzog, W.; Hartmann, M. Der Fragebogen zur familiären emotionalen Involviertheit und wahrgenommenen Kritik (FEIWK). *Psychother. Psychosom. Med. Psychol.* **2001**, *51*, 377–383. [CrossRef] [PubMed]
36. Linden, M.; Maier, W.; Achberger, M.; Herr, R.; Helmchen, H.; Benkert, O. Psychological disorders and their treatment in general practice in Germany: Results of a WHO study. *Nervenarzt* **1996**, *67*, 205–215. [PubMed]
37. Sepulveda, A.R.; Whitney, J.; Hankins, M.; Treasure, J. Development and validation of an Eating Disorders Symptom Impact Scale (EDSIS) for carers of people with eating disorders. *Health Qual. Life Outcomes* **2008**, *6*, 28. [CrossRef] [PubMed]
38. Hautzinger, M.; Keller, F.; Kühner, C. *Das Beck Depressionsinventar II*; Harcourt Test Services: Frankfurt, Germany, 2006.
39. Laux, L.; Glanzmann, P.; Schaffner, P.; Spielsberger, C.D. *Das State-Trait-Angstinventar*; Beltz: Weinheim, Germany, 1981.
40. Hasler, G.; Klaghofer, R.; Buddeberg, C. The University of Rhode Island Change Assessment Scale (URICA) psychometric testing of a German version. *PPmP* **2003**, *53*, 406–411. [CrossRef] [PubMed]
41. Hilbert, A.; Tuschen-Caffier, B. *Eating Disorder Examination*; Verlag für Psychotherapie: Münster, Germany, 2006.
42. Rathner, G.; Waldherr, K. Eating Disorder Inventory-2: A German language validation with norms for female and male adolescents. *Z. Klin. Psychol. Psychiatr. Psychother.* **1997**, *45*, 157–182.
43. Schwarte, R.; Timmesfeld, N.; Dempfle, A.; Krei, M.; Egberts, K.; Jaite, C.; Fleischhaker, C.; Wewetzer, C.; Herpertz-Dahlmann, B.; Seitz, J.; et al. Expressed Emotions and Depressive Symptoms in Caregivers of Adolescents with First-Onset Anorexia Nervosa-A Long-Term Investigation over 2.5 Years. *Eur. Eat. Disord. Rev.* **2017**, *25*, 44–51. [CrossRef]
44. Sepulveda, A.R.; Todd, G.; Whitaker, W.; Grover, M.; Stahl, D.; Treasure, J. Expressed emotion in relatives of patients with eating disorders following skills training program. *Int. J. Eat. Disord.* **2010**, *43*, 603–610. [CrossRef]
45. Marcos, Y.; Quiles, M.; Herrera, M.; Sanmartín, R.; Treasure, J. Testing carer skill training programs in Spanish carers of patients with eating disorders. *Psicothema* **2018**, *30*, 295–303. [CrossRef]
46. Giombini, L.; Nesbitt, S.; Kusosa, R.; Fabian, C.; Easter, A.; Tchanturia, K. Adapted emotion skills training group for young people with anorexia nervosa. *Neuropsychiatr* **2020**. [CrossRef]

11

Does Eating Addiction Favor a More Varied Diet or Contribute to Obesity?—The Case of Polish Adults

Marzena Jezewska-Zychowicz, Aleksandra Małachowska * and Marta Plichta

Institute of Human Nutrition Sciences, Warsaw University of Life Sciences (SGGW-WULS), 159C Nowoursynowska Street, 02-787 Warsaw, Poland; marzena_jezewska_zychowicz@sggw.edu.pl (M.J.-Z.); marta_plichta@sggw.edu.pl (M.P.)

* Correspondence: aleksandra_malachowska@sggw.edu.pl

Abstract: The rapidly increasing prevalence of overweight and obesity indicates a need to search for their main causes. Addictive-like eating and associated eating patterns might result in overconsumption, leading to weight gain. The aim of the study was to identify the main determinants of food intake variety (FIV) within eating addiction (EA), other lifestyle components, and sociodemographic characteristics. The data for the study were collected from a sample of 898 Polish adults through a cross-sectional survey in 2019. The questionnaire used in the study included Food Intake Variety Questionnaire (FIVeQ), Eating Preoccupation Scale (EPS), and questions regarding lifestyle and sociodemographic factors. High eating addiction was found in more than half of the people with obesity (54.2%). In the study sample, physical activity at leisure time explained FIV in the greatest manner, followed by the EPS factor: eating to provide pleasure and mood improvement. In the group of people with obesity, the score for this EPS factor was the best predictor of FIV, in that a higher score was conducive to a greater variety of food intake. Sociodemographic characteristics differentiated FIV only within groups with normal body weight (age) and with overweight (education). In conclusion, food intake variety (FIV) was associated with physical activity at leisure time, and then with EPS factor "Eating to provide pleasure and mood improvement", whereas sociodemographic characteristics were predictors of FIV only within groups identified by body mass index (BMI). Nevertheless, our observations regarding the eating to provide pleasure and mood improvement factor and its associations with food intake variety indicate a need for further research in this area. Future studies should also use other tools to explicitly explain this correlation.

Keywords: overweight; obesity; food addiction; eating addiction; food intake variety; eating behavior; overeating

---

1. Introduction

In spite of the growing prevalence of overweight and obesity, determining their main risk factors is still a challenge. Body weight and body mass index (BMI) are greatly influenced by energy intake and its adequacy [1]. However, the link between diet and those anthropometric parameters cannot be solely assessed on the basis of calorie intake, but should also include other elements of dietary patterns (eating frequency, diet quality, food variety, or proportions between different food groups) [2]. Lifestyle-related factors, such as unhealthy dietary patterns but also low physical activity, inadequate sleep hygiene, poor stress management, and tobacco smoking, can majorly alter energy intake and expenditure, and thus induce a positive energy balance [3]. Research shows that lifestyle factors are correlated with each other. Low physical activity is associated with the consumption of unhealthy foods [4,5]. In turn, less stress or negative as well as highly positive effects are associated with engagement in healthy behaviors, especially in physical activity [6]. Physical activity can reduce stress as well as negative emotions and, at the same time, enhance positive emotions. By contrast, human emotional functioning is associated with food, including emotional eating [7]. Physically active emotional eaters may want to eat when under emotional distress; however, they also choose more healthy foods to cope with this distress [8]. These interrelationships between selected lifestyle components, but also within human psychological functioning, implicate the necessity of including such parameters while exploring eating behaviors characteristics.

Some dietary patterns, such as uncontrolled excessive consumption, may resemble addictive behavior, and some foods may have addictive potential [9]. Gearhardt et al. [10] developed the first tool to assess FA, the Yale Food Addiction Scale (YFAS), as well as the follow-up, YFAS 2.0 [11]. These tools enable identification of addictive-like eating behaviors particularly towards highly processed and palatable foods. Elevated YFAS and YFAS 2.0 scores are both positively associated with body mass index (BMI), binge eating symptoms, and weight-cycling [11]. Research suggests that people diagnosed as food addicts consume more calories [12–16], especially derived from processed, energy-dense foods like confectionary, fast-food, and salty snacks, and their diet is higher in fat [12,14,16] than non-food-addicted individuals. Several studies have revealed that food addiction can be correlated with lower consumption of fruit, vegetables, and other core products [13,15].

Overeating might be associated with one of the following eating styles: restrained, emotional, or external. In restrained eating, when someone is following a strict dietary regimen, eating something forbidden may induce an "all-or-nothing" reaction leading to overconsumption [17]. Negative, positive, or neutral emotional states (e.g., sadness, anxiety, joy, boredom) might also increase food intake (emotional eating). Lastly, environmental factors, such as availability of food or presence of others eating, might also affect the consumption in so-called external eating [18]. Studies have found that emotional eating might favor undesirable food behaviors, including higher intake of snacks [19,20], "fast-food" [19], and sweet foods [21,22], whereas external eating may increase total calorie intake [19] as well as predispose to higher consumption of snacks [19,23]. Although dietary restraint can be conducive to lower intake of sweets [19] and total energy intake [19,24,25], it may simultaneously serve as a risk factor for excessive body weight [19,24,25]. The possible explanation of this phenomenon might be related to the possibility that people following strict dietary rules may be more susceptible to external and emotional eating, which can lead to weight gain [26]. Food-related thoughts are believed to be another crucial factor in the etiology of excessive food consumption as they can induce a specific food craving. When the urge to fulfill this craving arises, it can be difficult to resist overeating. Food preoccupation might therefore take the form of obsession [27].

In previous studies, also those using YFAS or YFAS 2.0, dietary assessment did not take into account food intake variety (FIV), which reflects the number of food products consumed by the individual. For many years, FIV was being promoted as a vital component of dietary guidelines. It was believed that a wider range of products will improve intake of macro- and micronutrients and provide adequate nutritional status [28]. Although a systematic review of 26 studies has shown that it is still unclear how total FIV affects body weight and measures of body adiposity [28], this parameter is of special concern to medical scientists and health professionals due to the growing obesity epidemic [29]. Results from the studies assessing the relationship between FIV and diet quality or eating habits remain inconsistent. Some research suggests a negative impact [30,31], whereas several studies have found that FIV might favor healthy eating habits, such as adequate intake of fruit and vegetables [32,33], or predispose to greater diet quality [34,35]. The existing research results suggest that sociodemographic characteristics, such as gender and age, can differentiate assessed variables and their correlations [30,33,34].

We assume that differences in food intake variety (FIV) can be explained by eating addiction assessed using the Eating Preoccupation Scale (EPS). However, we hypothesize that EPS explains the differences in FIV to a lesser extent than some components of lifestyle (i.e., physical activity, following a diet, smoking) but the importance of these factors may vary depending on BMI. Thus, the aim of the study is to assess eating addiction in a group of Polish adults, and to then answer the following questions: (1) Does eating addiction show a relationship with food intake variety? (2) Do such lifestyle components as following a diet, smoking, and physical activity differentiate the food intake variety more than the eating addiction? (3) Do the relationships between the examined variables differ after taking BMI into account?

2. Materials and Methods

2.1. Study Design and Sample Collection

The data were collected from February to March 2019 through a cross-sectional quantitative survey. The study was approved by the Ethics Committee of the Faculty of Human Nutrition and Consumer Science, Warsaw University of Life Sciences, in Poland on the 29 October 2018 (Resolution No. 22/2018). Informed consent to participate in the study was collected from participants.

According to the study design, recruitment and data collection were conducted by a research agency—ARC Market and Opinion. Adults aged 18–65 were recruited from the panel (epanel.pl) of approximately 64,000 adults. After sending an invitation to participate in the study, 2025 people gave their consent to participate in the study. Quota selection using gender, age, place of residence, and education was used to ensure the representativeness of the Polish population. During the recruitment, 78 people stopped filling out the questionnaire during the interview, and 932 people did not qualify due to filling the quota, while eight people were removed from the database at the collection control stage because of errors indicating the lack of credibility of their answers. As a result, the study consisted of 1007 participants. The computer-assisted web interviewing (CAWI) technique was used to collect all data. During the data check, 71 participants were excluded from the sample due to missing data, i.e., body mass and height, which did not allow calculation of the BMI. Then, during the data analysis, one more criterion of exclusion was used, namely being underweight (body mass index (BMI) < 18.5 kg/m^2). Thirty-eight participants were excluded from the analyses due to BMI lower than 18.5 kg/m^2. The total sample consisted of 898 people.

2.2. Food Intake Variety

Food intake variety was assessed using the food consumption frequency method, applying Food Intake Variety Questionnaire (FIVeQ) [36]. Information on the consumption of 63 food product groups over the last 7 days was collected using the FIVeQ questionnaire [36]. Quantity was specified for each product: seven slices for cereal products, seven cups for dairy and beverages with the exception of wine (quantity defined as 1 glass of wine—100 mL) and spirits (one shot of liquor—50 mL), amount sufficient for one slice of bread well covered (approx. 20 g) for cold cuts and sausages, 10 cubes for chocolate, and two tablespoons for the rest of the food products (e.g., groats, nuts, fish, and butter). The participant declared the consumption of such quantity of each product within the last 7 days (Yes/No). Food intake variety is expressed in the food intake variety index (FIVeI). FIVeI was calculated as the number of product groups eaten weekly (maximum 60 products/week) after excluding 3 groups of alcoholic beverages (beer, wine, vodka, and other strong alcohols). According to the methodology and assessment criteria developed by the authors of the questionnaire [35], the following four groups of people with a varied food intake (FIV) were distinguished:

Inadequate FIV (<20 food products weekly)
Sufficient FIV (20–29 food products weekly)
Good FIV (30–39 food products weekly)
Very good FIV (≥40 food products weekly)

2.3. Eating Addiction

Eating Preoccupation Scale (EPS) was used to assess eating addiction [37]. EPS consists of 18 statements, to which the respondent answers on a scale of 1—hardly/never; 2—rarely; 3—sometimes; 4—often; up to 5—almost/always (Table 1). This scale allows measuring an overall score of eating addiction and three EPS factors, which include focusing on eating activities; eating to provide pleasure and mood improvement; and compulsion to eat and loss of control over food. The overall score (range from 18 to 90 points), which was the sum of all ratings, allows evaluating a person's behavioral characteristics for eating addiction (EA) included in EPS. A score above 48 points indicates a high EA, 40–48 points an average EA, and below 40 points a low EA [37].

Table 1. The Eating Preoccupation Scale (EPS).

Statements from the Eating Preoccupation Scale (EPS)	**Mean Score ± Standard Deviation ***
EPS factor: Focusing on eating activities	
2. I think about eating and about my body weight	3.0 ± 1.2
6. I believe that my relationship with food is terrible	2.3 ± 1.1
8. I feel embarrassed about the amount of food I eat	2.2 ± 1.1
9. I plan ahead for situations when I will be able to eat alone	1.9 ± 1.0
10. I am worried about being unable to control the amount of food consumed	2.3 ± 1.1
16. I have a low self-esteem because of my uncontrolled eating	2.1 ± 1.1
EPS factor: Eating to provide pleasure and mood improvement	
1. Eating is a very important part of my life	3.4 ± 1.1
11. Eating greatly enhances my mood	3.2 ± 1.0
12. Eating is a great pleasure of mine	3.6 ± 1.0
13. I make myself "food feasts" for no clear reason	2.2 ± 1.1
17. I feel great satisfaction after an abundant meal	2.8 ± 1.1
18. I am willing to sacrifice other pleasures for eating	2.3 ± 1.0
EPS factor: Compulsion to eat and loss of control over food	
3. I eat vast amounts of high-calorie foods in a short period of time	2. 6 ± 1.0
4. I snack throughout the day	2.9± 1.0
5. I eat even when I am not feeling hunger	2.4 ± 1.0
7. I eat more than I had planned	2.7 ± 1.0
14. I wake up to eat at night	1.8 ± 1.0
15. I clear up my plate even when I am not feeling hungry anymore	2.9 ± 1.2

* 5-point scale: 1—hardly/never; 2—rarely, 3—sometimes, 4—often, 5—almost/always.

The internal compliance of the questionnaire was assessed using Cronbach's coefficient, which was 0.89. Internal stability, measured using a correlation coefficient in studies conducted after 6 weeks on a group of 30 women, was 0.72. Validity of the Eating Preoccupation Scale was tested by assessing the correlation of its results with the results of the Eating Related Behaviors Questionnaire [37], which measures the tendency toward habitual and emotional overeating, but also following dietary restrictions.

2.4. Physical Activity and Other Lifestyle Factors

Self-reported physical activity was recorded in the questionnaire on a 3-point scale: 1—"low", 2—"moderate", and 3—"high" [38]. The description of the scale was presented separately for physical activity during leisure and work/school time. For leisure time, "low" was described as "sedentary lifestyle, watching TV, reading the press, books, light housework, taking a walk for 1–2 h a week"; "moderate"—"walks, cycling, gymnastics, gardening or other light physical activity performed for 2–3 h a week ", and "high"—"cycling, running, working on a plot or garden, and other sports activities requiring physical effort, taking up more than 3 h a week". "Low" activity at work/school time was described as "over 70% of the time in a sitting position", "moderate" as "approximately 50% of the time in a sitting position and about 50% of time moving", and "high" as "about 70% of the time in motion or doing physical work associated with a lot of effort" [38].

Two questions were used to assess smoking: *"Do you smoke cigarettes?"* (Yes/No) and *"If you smoke, how many cigarettes a day do you smoke?"* (I smoke occasionally; up to 10 a day, 10–20 a day, more than 20 a day). In addition, respondents answered the question *"Have you followed a special diet in the last 3 months?"* (Yes/No).

2.5. Sociodemographic Characteristics

The questionnaire collected information about sociodemographic characteristics of the study sample, i.e., gender, age, education, and place of residence. Body mass index (BMI) was calculated using self-reported body weight and height and categorized according to International Obesity Task Force (IOTF) standards [39]. During the data analysis, three categories of respondents were identified, i.e., people with normal weight (BMI between 18.5 and 24.99 kg/m^2), overweight (BMI between 25.0 and 29.99 kg/m^2), and obesity (BMI $\geq$ 30 kg/m^2).

2.6. Statistical Analysis

Descriptive statistics were performed. The chi-square test and the one-way analysis of variance ANOVA test were used to compare variables, and $p < 0.05$ was considered significant.

The classification tree was used to determine independent variables explaining differences in food intake variety. This method was used because it allows computing both numerical and categorical data. Moreover, it offers clear graphic data presentation and is easy to interpret [40]. Separate classification trees were made in the study sample, and then in a group of people with normal body weight, overweight, and obesity. The method CHAID (chi-squared automatic interaction detector) was used to build the tree. The first node (node 0) is always the distribution of the dependent variable (FIV). The next nodes can include sociodemographic variables (gender, age, education, place of residence), variables describing eating addiction (eating addiction—overall score, three factors of eating addiction: focusing on eating activities, eating to provide pleasure and mood improvement, compulsion to eat and loss of control over food) and lifestyle variables (following a diet, smoking, physical activity during leisure time, and work/school time).

Statistical analysis was conducted using IBM SPSS Statistics for Windows, version 24.0 (IBM Corp, Armonk, NY, USA).

3. Results

3.1. Characteristics of the Study Sample

The sample consisted of 898 participants (433 women and 465 men) aged 18 to 65 years. Some details concerning sociodemographic characteristics of the study sample are displayed in Table 1.

More men than women were overweight or obese. Among people with normal weight the majority were people of the age of 18–34, while among overweight and people with obesity respondents aged 45–65 were the most numerous in this group. The average age of people with overweight and obesity did not differ, but was significantly higher compared to people with normal body weight. Education and place of residence did not differentiate groups identified according to BMI (Table 2).

3.2. Food Intake Variety and Other Lifestyle Factors

About 60% of the study sample displayed good or very good food intake variety (36.8% and 23.7%, respectively). FIV did not differ in BMI groups (Table 3).

Slightly more than 10% of participants declared following a diet. Almost two-thirds of the study participants (64.0%) declared they did not smoke. In the study sample, there were less heavy smokers (10 or more cigarettes a day) than light smokers (16.6% and 19.4%, respectively). About two-fifths of the study sample (38.3%) described their physical activity at work/school as low, and the same numbers of people evaluated their leisure activities in the same way. More than one-half of people with BMI $\geq$ 30 kg/m^2 (57.6%) declared low physical activity in leisure time. More people with overweight than ones with normal body weight indicated low activity in leisure time (37.7% and 32.8%, respectively) (Table 3).

3.3. Eating Addiction

Over two-fifths of study sample (42.1%) displayed a high eating addiction (EA) on the EPS. The mean value of the overall score from the EPS was 46.4 points, which indicates the average EA. Only differences in the overall score of EPS between people with normal weight and people with obesity were shown. The mean value of the overall score in the obese group exceeded 48 points and, therefore, meant a high EA. Low EA was displayed by 33.7% of people with normal body weight and by almost three times less of those with obesity (13.1%). However, a high EA was found in more than half of the people with obesity (54.2%) and in more than one-third of people with normal body weight (37.7%). Compulsive eating and loss of control of food consumption characterized eating behaviors of people with obesity to a higher extent compared to people with normal body weight. There were differences in the mean score for the "Focusing on eating activities" factor in the BMI groups. The larger the BMI, the more people were focused on eating behaviors were (Table 4).

3.4. Relationship between Food Intake Variety and Eating Addiction

Food intake variety (FIV) has shown differences only due to EPS factor "Eating to provide pleasure and mood improvement" (Figure 1). In the group of people with high or moderate physical activity at leisure time and at work/school time, a higher score for the EPS factor "Eating to provide pleasure and mood improvement" (above 18 points) favored an increase in FIV (nodes 7 and 8). Almost two-fifths of people with a score above 18 had very good FIV. Similarly, in the group of people with low physical activity at leisure time (nodes 5 and 6), a higher score for this EPS factor (above 16 points) was conducive to a greater variety of food intake (Figure 1).

In the group of people with obesity, the score of EPS factor "Eating to provide pleasure and mood improvement" was the most powerful predictor for FIV (nodes 1 and 2). A higher score for this EPS factor (above 16 points) was conducive to a greater variety of food intake. Almost three times more people with a score above 16 (29.5%) than with a score of 16 and below (10.3%) had a very good FIV (Figure 2).

3.5. Relationship between Food Intake Variety and Lifestyle and Sociodemographic Variables

In the study group, FIV has shown differences due to physical activity at leisure time (nodes 1 and 2) and physical activity at work/school (nodes 3 and 4), —as seen in Figure 1. Higher FIV was demonstrated in people with moderate and high physical activity at leisure time ($p < 0.001$). Over one-quarter of people (27.6%) with moderate or high physical activity and 17.7% of those with low physical activity at leisure time were characterized by very good FIV. Twice as many people with low physical activity in their leisure time were characterized by inadequate FIV compared to other people. Twice as many people with high and moderate physical activity in leisure time and the same physical activity at work/school showed very good FIV (32.5%) compared to people with low physical activity at work/school (15.5%) (nodes 3 and 4) (Figure 1).

In the group of people with overweight (nodes 1 and 2), more people with secondary education than the other categories had good FIV (46.8%, 34.9%, respectively) and very good FIV (29.4%, 22.2%, respectively (Figure 3).

In people with normal body weight, FIV differed among age groups (nodes 1, 2, and 3). The number of people aged 18–24 was the least when it came to showing very good FIV (8.3%), while most people aged 55–65 (31.8%). More than two-thirds of people aged 18–24 had inadequate FIV (11.1%) or sufficient FIV (56.9%). By contrast, more than three-quarters of people aged 25–54 years were characterized by good (40.9%) or very good FIV (25.5%). In this age group (nodes 4 and 5) more people with moderate or high physical activity in leisure time than others had good (44.4%, 34.3%, respectively) and very good (29.9%, 17.2%, respectively) FIV (Figure 4).

Table 2. Characteristics of the study sample.

Variables		Total (N = 898)		18.5 kg/m² ≤ BMI < 25 kg/m² (N = 424)		25.0 kg/m² ≤ BMI < 30 kg/m² (N = 321)		BMI ≥ 30 kg/m² (N = 153)	
		N	%	N	%	N	%	N	%
Gender *	Female	433	48.2	234	55.2	131	40.8	68	44.4
	Male	465	51.8	190	44.8	190	59.2	85	55.6
Education	Lower than secondary	348	38.8	153	36.1	123	38.3	72	47.1
	Secondary	309	34.4	153	36.1	109	34.0	47	30.7
	Higher	241	26.8	118	27.8	89	27.7	34	22.2
Place of residence	Rural area	329	36.6	159	37.5	113	35.2	57	37.3
	City ≤ 100,000 residents	291	32.4	140	33.0	106	33.0	45	29.4
	City > 100,000 residents	278	31.0	125	29.5	102	31.8	51	33.3
Age *	18–24 years	97	10.8	72	17.0	18	5.6	7	4.6
	25–34 years	205	22.8	117	27.6	62	19.3	26	17.0
	35–44 years	209	23.3	105	24.8	67	20.9	37	24.2
	45–54 years	168	18.7	64	15.1	70	21.8	34	22.2
	55–65 years	219	24.4	66	15.5	104	32.4	49	32.0
Age (years)	Mean; standard deviation	42.0; 13.7		38.0^{a}; 13.3		45.6^{b}; 13.1		45.5^{b}; 12.9	
Height (cm)	Mean; standard deviation	171.4; 9.5		170.8^{a}; 9.1		172.4^{a}; 9.6		170.8^{a}; 9.9	
Weight (kg)	Mean; standard deviation	76.6; 15.8		65.7^{a}; 9.2		81.0^{b}; 10.2		97.6^{c}; 13.8	
BMI (kg/m²)	Mean; standard deviation	26.0; 4.5		22.4^{a}; 1.8		27.2^{b}; 1.4		33.4^{c}; 3.6	

N—number of participants; * Significant at $p < 0.001$ between BMI groups (chi-square test); ^{a,b,c} Different letters in each line indicate significant differences at $p < 0.05$ between BMI groups (ANOVA test).

Table 3. Food intake variety and other lifestyle characteristics of the study sample.

Variables		Total Sample (N = 898)		18.5 kg/m^2 ≤ BMI < 25 kg/m^2 (N = 424)		25.0 kg/m^2 ≤ BMI < 30 kg/m^2 (N = 321)		BMI ≥ 30 kg/m^2 (N = 153)	
		N	%	N	%	N	%	N	%
Food intake variety—FIV	inadequate	79	8.8	38	9.0	25	7.8	16	10.5
	sufficient	276	30.7	139	32.7	92	28.7	45	29.4
	good	330	36.8	147	34.7	125	38.9	58	37.9
	very good	213	23.7	100	23.6	79	24.6	34	22.2
Following a diet	yes	97	10.9	42	10.0	37	11.6	18	12.0
Number of cigarettes smoked **	no smoking	575	64.0	266	62.7	223	69.5	86	56.2
	less than 10 cigarettes a day	174	19.4	91	21.5	56	17.4	27	17.6
	10 or more cigarettes a day	149	16.6	67	15.8	42	13.1	40	26.2
Physical activity during work/school time	low	329	38.3	137	34.3	123	39.4	69	47.3
	moderate	329	38.3	158	39.5	120	38.5	51	34.9
	high	200	23.4	105	26.2	69	22.1	26	17.8
Physical activity during leisure time ***	low	344	38.8	137	32.8	120	37.7	87	57.6
	moderate	415	46.8	208	49.8	153	48.1	54	35.8
	high	128	14.4	73	17.4	45	14.2	10	6.6
Food intake variety—FIV (number of products)	Mean; standard deviation	32.6; 10.7		32.4 [a]; 10.6		33.0 [a]; 10.5		32.6 [a]; 11.3	

N—number of participants; ** Significant at $p < 0.01$; *** Significant at $p < 0.001$ between BMI groups (chi-square test). [a] Having the same letter means no significant differences at $p < 0.05$ between groups (ANOVA test).

Table 4. Eating addiction in the study sample.

Variables		Total Sample (N = 898)		18.5 kg/m^2 ≤ BMI < 25 kg/m^2 (N = 424)		25.0 kg/m^2 ≤ BMI < 30 kg/m^2 (N = 321)		BMI ≥ 30 kg/m^2 (N = 153)	
		N	%	N	%	N	%	N	%
Eating Preoccupation Scale (EPS)—total score ***	low	237	26.4	143	33.7	74	23.1	20	13.1
	average	283	31.5	121	28.6	112	34.8	50	32.7
	high	378	42.1	160	37.7	135	42.1	83	54.2
Eating Preoccupation Scale (EPS)—total score	Mean; standard deviation	46.4; 11.0		45.2 [a]; 11.6		46.7 [a,b]; 10.6		49.1 [b]; 9.9	
EPS factor: Focus on eating activities	Mean; standard deviation	13.7; 4.8		12.9 [a]; 5.0		13.8 [b]; 4.6		15.5 [c]; 4.1	
EPS factor: Eating to provide pleasure and mood improvement	Mean; standard deviation	17.5; 4.4		17.5 [a]; 4.5		17.6 [a]; 4.2		17.5 [a]; 4.3	
EPS factor: Compulsion to eat and loss of control over food	Mean; standard deviation	15.2; 4.2		14.8 [a]; 4.4		15.3 [a,b]; 4.1		16.1 [b]; 3.9	

N—number of participants; *** Significant at $p < 0.001$ between BMI groups (chi-square test). [a,b,c] Different letters in each line mean significant differences at $p < 0.05$ between groups (ANOVA test).

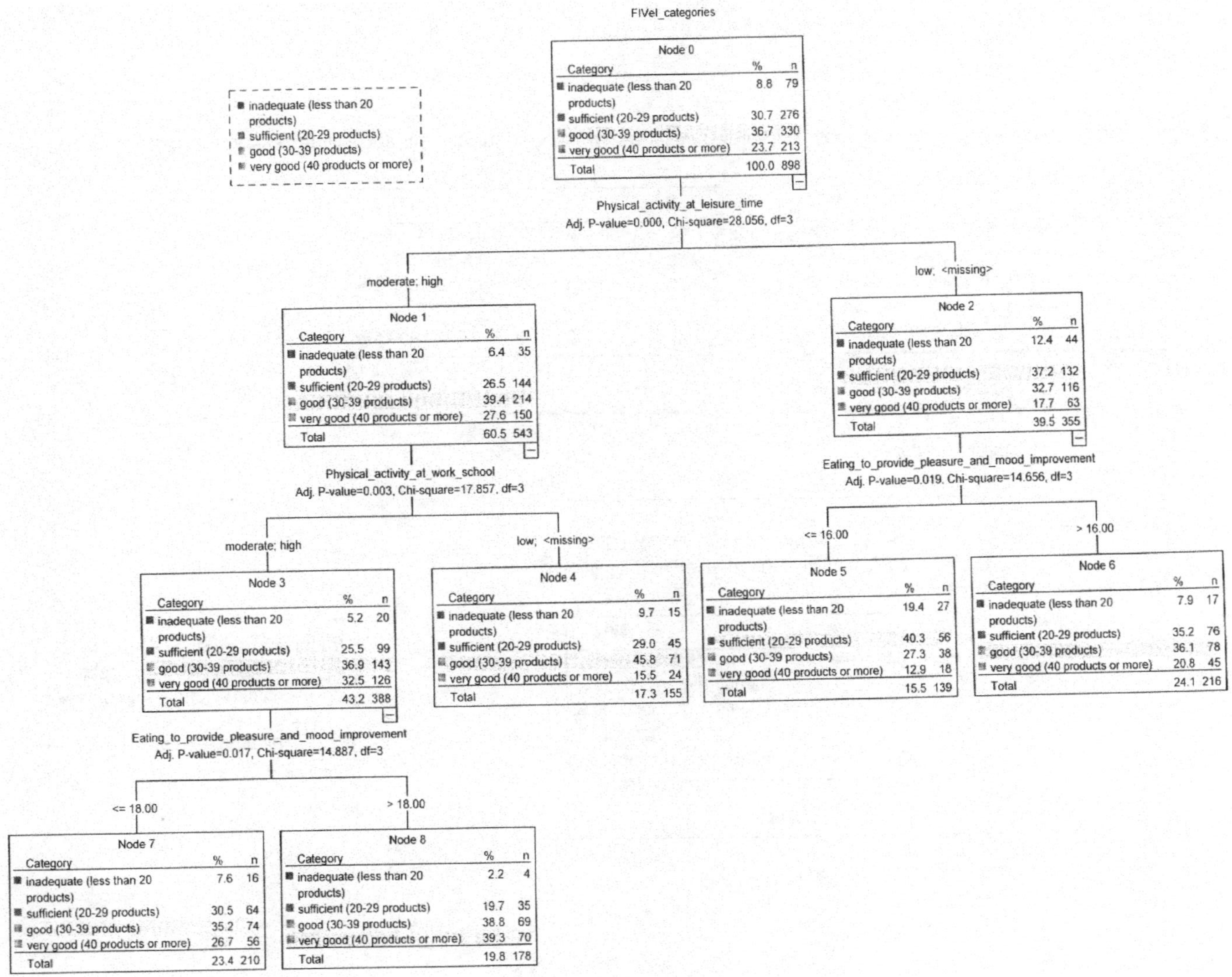

Figure 1. Relationship between food intake variety, eating addiction, selected lifestyles variables and sociodemographic characteristics in the study sample.

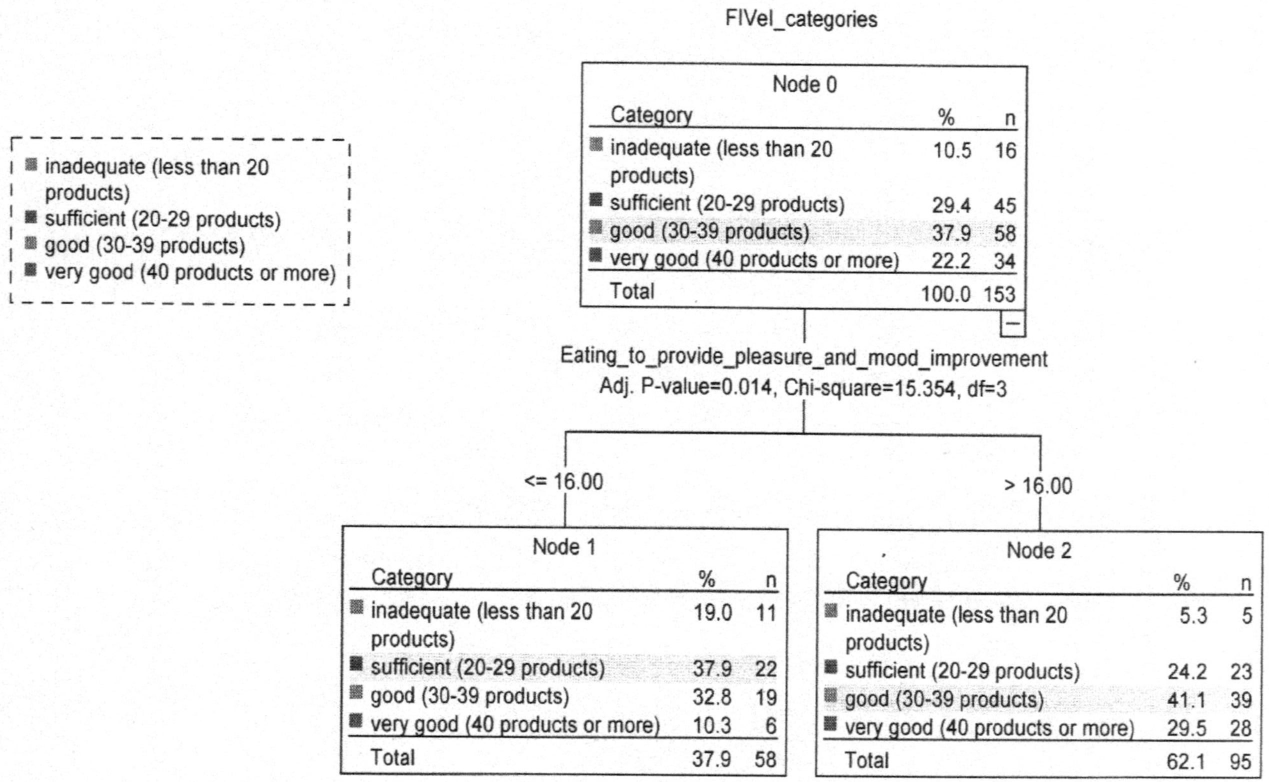

Figure 2. Relationship between food intake variety, eating addiction, selected lifestyles variables and sociodemographic characteristics in the group with obesity.

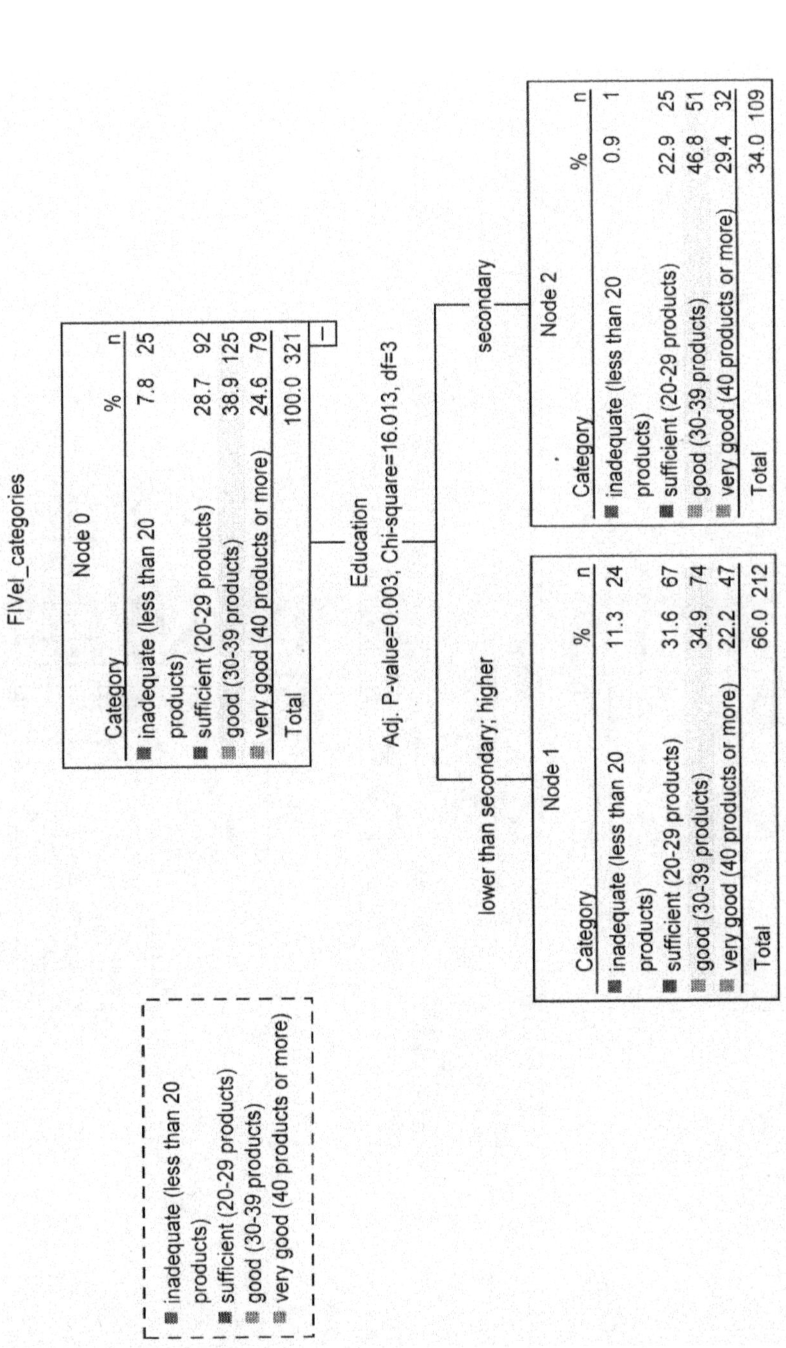

Figure 3. Relationship between food intake variety, eating addiction, selected lifestyles variables and sociodemographic characteristics in the group with overweight.

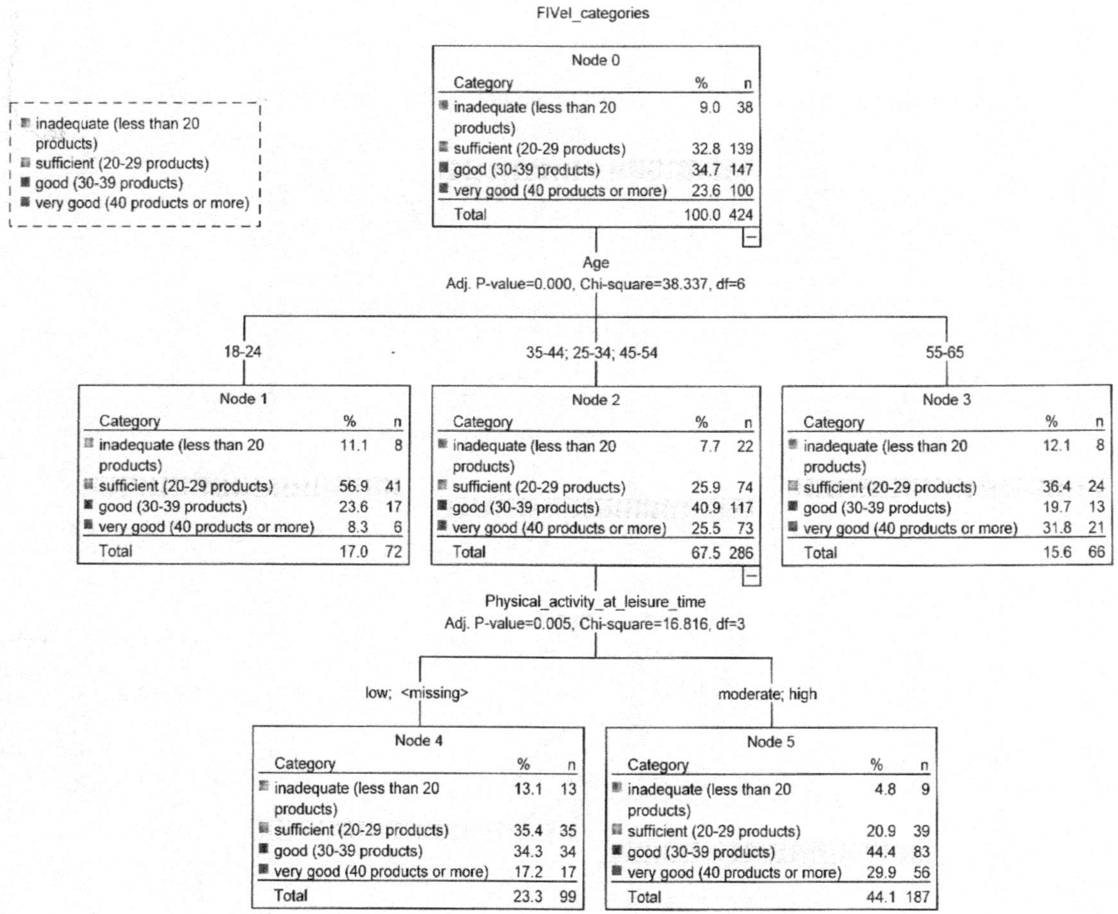

Figure 4. Relationship between food intake variety, eating addiction, selected lifestyles variables, and sociodemographic characteristics in the group with normal body weight.

4. Discussion

The study provided some support for our hypotheses that differences in food intake variety (FIV) can be explained by eating addiction assessed using the Eating Preoccupation Scale (EPS). The results concerning associations between FIV and EPS indicate that only one of the EPS factors, "Eating to provide pleasure and mood improvement", was related to FIV. Moreover, this indicator did not serve as the most important predictor of FIV, as physical activity during leisure time explained this parameter in a greater manner. Other EPS factors and total EPS did not differentiate FIV. In view of the previous research, it can be assumed that "Eating to provide pleasure and mood improvement" as a factor correlated with FIV might favor both overall dietary variety and dietary variety within particular food groups only. Few available studies, which attempted to explain differences in food intake variety, indicate that this parameter might be linked to the amount of food consumed with regard to selected foods [13,41]. People with overeating tendencies usually opt for a wide range of food products, yet it only applies to products considered as palatable. Thus, a wide range of palatable foods might be a factor involved in the development of addictive-like eating behaviors [42]. Other authors also point out that not all foods seem to be equally related to addictive-like eating behaviors. Foods rich in refined carbohydrates and added fat are more likely to be consumed in an addictive manner than low-processed foods [43,44]. High-fat and high-sugar foods were consumed more frequently among individuals who met the criteria of the Yale Food Addiction Scale for food addiction [13]. These foods also appear to trigger behavioral responses that are consistent with addictive-like eating behavior, for example such foods are frequently consumed during binge episodes [45]. Moreover, foods high in fat and sugar are more likely to be intensely craved [41,46,47] and consumed in greater quantities in response to negative affect [48,49]. The results of these studies are consistent with those obtained in our research among people with obesity. Within this group, the EPS factor "Eating to provide pleasure and mood improvement" was the most important factor in explaining FIV. Almost three times more people with a higher score of this EPS factor were characterized by higher FIV in comparison to people scoring lower on this subscale. It might be considered as a cause of overconsumption though longitudinal research is required to determine the direction of causality.

Our hypothesis was also supported, that EPS explains the differences in FIV to a lesser extent than some components of lifestyle (i.e., physical activity, following a diet, smoking) but the importance of these factors may vary depending on BMI. Physical activity at leisure time was the most important predictor of FIV in the study sample, while in the groups distinguished by BMI, differences in FIV predictors were observed. Greater food intake variety (FIV) correlated with moderate or high physical activity during leisure time, which may be the result of higher awareness of healthy lifestyle, healthier food choices, and greater adherence to dietary rules among physically active people [50,51]. Similarly as for the whole study group, the association between food intake variety (FIV) and physical activity in leisure time was supported among individuals with normal body weight aged 25–54, and greater FIV was observed in those more physically active within this age group. According to our best knowledge, an association between FIV and physical activity has not been the subject of previous research. Nevertheless, some studies have shown that physical activity favors healthier food choices among adults [52–54]. However, a few studies have revealed that being physically active might not always determine healthy eating nor prevent unfavorable eating behaviors [55]. On the premise that FIV might be linked to both health benefits and the higher intake of unhealthy foods, our results indicating that greater FIV is observed among physically active people is supported by previous studies.

Higher levels of physical activity observed in individuals presenting eating addiction symptoms might be caused by an attempt to make up for the excessive amount of calories consumed through exercise [56]. Physically active people are able to self-regulate food intake more precisely due to the effect of working out in lowering the reactivity of the brain reward system to food stimuli [57]. Moreover, among individuals in the group of moderate or high physical activity, both in leisure or school/work time, a positive correlation was seen for the result of "Eating to provide pleasure and mood improvement" subscale and FIV, which can be linked to self-contentment associated with satisfaction from living a healthy lifestyle, beneficial for health and wellbeing. A similar correlation was noted in the group with low physical activity in leisure time. It seems that low physical activity can induce food cravings in a manner resembling an addiction mechanism [58]. In those individuals, food can serve as a major source of pleasure, since sedentary behaviors favor food consumption. This association was not seen for the eating addiction total score in our study, and these results are supported by Li et al. [56].

Sociodemographic features as predictors of FIV were noticed only in groups separated due to BMI. Food intake variety in individuals with normal body weight was associated with age, which can be confirmed by previous research. Due to involutional processes along with environmental and psychological factors, older people tend to change their eating habits, which leads to lower calorie as well as macro- and micronutrient intake. Inadequate intake of nutrients increases the risk of malnutrition [59,60]. Greater FIV among older adults in our study, including having the largest number of very good FIV and, at the same time, the largest number of inadequate FIV, indicates that the recommendations on dietary diversity in older people [35,60] are being partly fulfilled. Higher FIV in older people was also noted by Drewnowski et al. [61].

The age was not associated with food intake variety in individuals with overweight and obesity. However, people with overweight with secondary education had greater FIV than the others. The impact of education on FIV in people with overweight may be explained in different ways. Environment, awareness of physical activity, dietary knowledge, and health literacy as well as social roles and cultural norms related to health and nutrition seem to be significant factors affecting this correlation [62]. Among people with lower educational status, a less varied diet might be linked to their living environment with limited access to more diverse and affordable fresh foods, but also to other components of a healthy lifestyle, including safe places for physical activity. On the other hand, alcohol, tobacco, and fast-food might be more accessible, which are conducive to a high-calorie diet combined with sedentary behaviors [63]. By contrast, people with higher education are expected to have more opportunities for being physically active, but also greater access to diverse food products. Educational status might be considerably associated with salary, and thus influence food choices and food variety [64,65]. Moreover, higher educated people should be more predisposed to favoring new or unfamiliar foods [66]. Nonetheless, the above possible explanations and mechanisms involving dietary knowledge and health literacy [67,68] cannot explain the results revealed in our study indicating that among those in the overweight group, people with higher education had lower FIV than individuals with secondary education. Despite having greater nutrition knowledge, more highly educated individuals might conform more to cultural norms, e.g., the thin ideal, which is often perceived as a condition of success [69]. Some authors suggested that body weight dissatisfaction might serve as a driver for unhealthy dieting behaviors [70,71]. It can be assumed that in our study sample, overweight people with higher education could have been particularly susceptible to social norms which, in turn, led to following a strict dietary regimen, thus resulting in lower FIV [70,71].

Strengths and Limitations

The strength of our study is its relatively large sample, representative of the Polish population in terms of the region of residence, gender, education, and age. Although our findings are specific to the Polish population and should not be generalized to populations of other cultural backgrounds, the observations could be of potential use in designing research and interventions. The analysis of relationships between eating addiction and lifestyle elements of great importance for health, i.e., diet (dietary variety and following a diet), and physical activity brought a wider perspective on adequate diet. To the best of our knowledge, this paper is the first to study the association between eating addiction and food intake variety. The use of the hitherto unknown Eating Preoccupation Scale can be considered as both a strength and a weakness. On the one hand, it may be noticed by other researchers and recognized as a tool that deserves further use. On the other hand, the use of this scale is a limitation of our study. The measure of eating addiction used in the present study (EPS) has not been extensively used and there is a need for additional research on its psychometric properties and its association with measures of related constructs such as food addiction, emotional eating, and binge eating. Additionally, this cross-sectional study design does not provide an opportunity to find a causal relationship between food intake variety and other variables. Some limitations are related to the potential biases that may occur when self-reported data are analyzed [72]. People tend to underreport their weight and overreport their body height [73], which may have led to underestimation of individuals with excessive body weight according to the BMI categories in our research. Self-reported indicators of lifestyle can be considered not quite satisfying, however, and using other measurement indicators confirms the results from the analysis of self-reported data [74].

5. Conclusions

The study found that food intake variety (FIV) was associated with physical activity at leisure time, and then with the EPS factor "Eating to provide pleasure and mood improvement", whereas sociodemographic characteristics were predictors of FIV only within groups determined by BMI. In the study sample, physical activity both at leisure and at work/school time proved to be a stronger predictor than the EPS factor related to pleasure and mood. However, the EPS factor "Eating to provide pleasure and mood improvement" was the only predictor of FIV among people with obesity. Sociodemographic characteristics differentiated FIV only within the group with normal body weight (age) and with overweight (education). Based on the findings of this study, it is possible to better understand the relationships between food intake variety and some components of lifestyle, including addictive behaviors. Moreover, additional focus on the groups identified by BMI and the performed analysis will allow the results to be used in dietary practice. However, there is still a need for further research involving the use of tools that can identify the "eating addiction" construct. Symptoms of eating addiction might serve as a marker of disordered eating, while early diagnosis can significantly affect both prevention and treatment of overweight and obesity. Further research attempting to clarify the association between FIV and EA should use also other tools to explicitly explain this correlation.

Author Contributions: M.P. and M.J.-Z. made substantial contributions to the study conception and design; M.P. was involved in the data acquisition; M.J.-Z. analyzed the data; M.J.-Z. and A.M. interpreted the data and wrote the manuscript; M.J.-Z., M.P., and A.M. were involved in critically revising the manuscript, and have given their approval to the manuscript submitted. All authors have read and agreed to the published version of the manuscript.

Acknowledgments: We wish to thank all our study participants for their participation.

References

1. Elmadfa, I.; Meyer, A. Developing Suitable Methods of Nutritional Status Assessment: A Continuous Challenge. *Adv. Nutr.* **2014**, *5*, 5905–5985. [CrossRef] [PubMed]
2. Schulze, M.; Martínez-González, M.; Fung, T.; Lichtenstein, A.; Forouhi, N. Food based dietary patterns and chronic disease prevention. *BMJ* **2018**, *361*, k2396. [CrossRef] [PubMed]
3. Blair, S.N.; Hand, G.A.; Hill, J.O. Energy balance: A crucial issue for exercise and sports medicine. *Br. J. Sports Med.* **2015**, *49*, 970–971. [CrossRef] [PubMed]
4. Hobbs, M.; Pearson, N.; Foster, P.J.; Biddle, S.J. Sedentary behaviour and diet across the lifespan: An updated systematic review. *Br. J. Sports Med.* **2014**, *49*, 1179–1188. [CrossRef]
5. Compernolle, S.; De Cocker, K.; Teixeira, P.J.; Oppert, J.-M.; Roda, C.; Mackenbach, J.D.; Lakerveld, J.; McKee, M.; Glonti, K.; Rutter, H.; et al. The associations between domain-specific sedentary behaviours and dietary habits in European adults: A cross-sectional analysis of the SPOTLIGHT survey. *BMC Public Health* **2016**, *16*, 1057. [CrossRef]
6. Schultchen, D.; Reichenberger, J.; Mittl, T.; Weh, T.R.M.; Smyth, J.M.; Blechert, J.; Pollatos, O. Bidirectional relationship of stress and affect with physical activity and healthy eating. *Br. J. Health Psychol.* **2019**, *24*, 315–333. [CrossRef]
7. Devonport, T.J.; Nicholls, W.; Fullerton, C. A systematic review of the association between emotions and eating behaviour in normal and overweight adult populations. *J. Health Psychol.* **2019**, *24*, 3–24. [CrossRef]

8. Dohle, S.; Hartmann, C.; Keller, C. Physical activity as a moderator of the association between emotional eating and BMI: Evidence from the Swiss Food Panel. *Psychol. Health* **2014**, *29*, 1062–1080. [CrossRef]
9. Gearhardt, A.N.; Corbin, W.R.; Brownell, K.D. Food addiction: An examination of the diagnostic criteria for dependence. *J. Addict. Med.* **2009**, *3*, 1–7. [CrossRef]
10. Gearhardt, A.N.; Corbin, W.R.; Brownell, K.D. Preliminary validation of the Yale Food Addiction Scale. *Appetite* **2009**, *52*, 430–436. [CrossRef]
11. Gearhardt, A.N.; Corbin, W.R.; Brownell, K.D. Development of the Yale Food Addiction Scale Version 2.0. *Psychol Addict. Behav.* **2016**, *30*, 113–121. [CrossRef] [PubMed]
12. Ayaz, A.; Nergiz-Unal, R.; Dedebayraktar, D.; AkyoL, A.; Pekcan, A.G.; Besler, H.T.; Buyuktuncer, Z. How does food addiction influence dietary intake profile? *PLoS ONE* **2018**, *13*, e0195541. [CrossRef] [PubMed]
13. Pursey, K.; Collins, C.; Stanwell, P.; Burrows, T. Foods and dietary profiles associated with 'food addiction' in young adults. *Addict. Behav. Rep.* **2015**, *2*, 41–48. [CrossRef] [PubMed]
14. Pedram, P.; Sun, G. Hormonal and dietary characteristics in obese human subjects with and without food addiction. *Nutrients* **2014**, *7*, 223–238. [CrossRef]
15. Burrows, T.; Hides, L.; Brown, R.; Dayas, C.V.; Kay-Lambkin, F. Differences in Dietary Preferences, Personality and Mental Health in Australian Adults with and without Food Addiction. *Nutrients* **2017**, *9*, 285. [CrossRef]
16. Küçükerdönmez, Ö.; Urhan, M.; Altın, M.; Hacıraifoğlu, Ö.; Yıldız, B. Assessment of the relationship between food addiction and nutritional status in schizophrenic patients. *Nutr. Neurosci.* **2019**, *22*, 392–400. [CrossRef]
17. Linardon, J. The relationship between dietary restraint and binge eating: Examining eating-related self-efficacy as a moderator. *Appetite* **2018**, *127*, 126–129. [CrossRef]
18. Denny, K.N.; Loth, K.; Eisenberg, M.E.; Neumark-Sztainer, D. Intuitive eating in young adults. Who is doing it, and how is it related to disordered eating behaviors? *Appetite* **2013**, *60*, 13–19. [CrossRef]
19. Paans, N.; Gibson-Smith, D.; Bot, M.; van Strien, T.; Brouwer, I.; Visser, M.; Penninx, B. Depression and eating styles are independently associated with dietary intake. *Appetite* **2019**, *134*, 103–110. [CrossRef]
20. Camilleri, G.; Méjean, C.; Kesse-Guyot, E.; Andreeva, V.; Bellisle, F.; Hercberg, S.; Péneau, S. The Associations between Emotional Eating and Consumption of Energy-Dense Snack Foods Are Modified by Sex and Depressive Symptomatology. *J. Nutr.* **2014**, *144*, 1264–1273. [CrossRef]
21. Konttinen, H.; Männistö, S.; Sarlio-Lähteenkorva, S.; Silventoinen, K.; Haukkala, A. Emotional eating, depressive symptoms and self-reported food consumption. A population-based study. *Appetite* **2010**, *54*, 473–479. [CrossRef] [PubMed]
22. van Strien, T.; Cebolla, A.; Etchemendy, E.; Gutiérrez-Maldonado, J.; Ferrer-García, M.; Botella, C.; Baños, R. Emotional eating and food intake after sadness and joy. *Appetite* **2013**, *66*, 20–25. [CrossRef] [PubMed]
23. Cleobury, L.; Tapper, K. Reasons for eating 'unhealthy' snacks in overweight and obese males and females. *J. Hum. Nutr. Diet.* **2013**, *27*, 333–341. [CrossRef] [PubMed]
24. Lluch, A.; Herbeth, B.; Méjean, L.; Siest, G. Dietary intakes, eating style and overweight in the Stanislas Family Study. *Int. J. Obes.* **2000**, *24*, 1493–1499. [CrossRef] [PubMed]
25. Klesges, R.C.; Isbell, T.R.; Klesges, L.M. Relationship between dietary restraint, energy intake, physical activity, and body weight: A prospective analysis. *J. Abnorm. Psychol.* **1992**, *101*, 668–674. [CrossRef]
26. van Strien, T.; Konttinen, H.; Ouwens, M.; van de Laar, F.; Winkens, L. Mediation of emotional and external eating between dieting and food intake or BMI gain in women. *Appetite* **2020**, *145*, 104493. [CrossRef]
27. Houben, K.; Jansen, A. When food becomes an obsession: Overweight is related to food-related obsessive-compulsive behavior. *J. Health Psychol.* **2019**, *24*, 1145–1152. [CrossRef]
28. Vadiveloo, M.; Dixon, L.B.; Parekh, N. Associations between dietary variety and measures of body adiposity: A systematic review of epidemiological studies. *Br. J. Nutr.* **2013**, *109*, 1557–1572. [CrossRef]
29. Hruby, A.; Hu, F.B. The Epidemiology of Obesity: A Big Picture. *Pharmacoeconomics* **2015**, *33*, 673–689. [CrossRef]
30. Bezerra, I.N.; Sichieri, R. Household food diversity and nutritional status among adults in Brazil. *Int. J. Behav. Nutr. Phys. Act.* **2011**, *8*, 22. [CrossRef]
31. Zhang, Q.; Chen, X.; Liu, Z.; Varma, D.S.; Wan, R.; Zhao, S. Diet diversity and nutritional status among adults in southwest China. *PLoS ONE* **2017**, *12*, e0172406. [CrossRef] [PubMed]
32. Keim, N.L.; Forester, S.M.; Lyly, M.; Aaron, G.J.; Townsend, M.S. Vegetable variety is a key to improved diet quality in low-income women in California. *J. Acad. Nutr. Diet.* **2014**, *114*, 430–435. [CrossRef] [PubMed]

33. Azadbakht, L.; Esmaillzadeh, A. Dietary diversity score is related to obesity and abdominal adiposity among Iranian female youth. *Public Health Nutr.* **2011**, *14*, 62–69. [CrossRef] [PubMed]
34. Murphy, S.P.; Foote, J.A.; Wilkens, L.R.; Basiotis, P.P.; Carlson, A.; White, K.K.; Yonemori, K.M. Simple measures of dietary variety are associated with improved dietary quality. *J. Am. Diet. Assoc.* **2006**, *106*, 425–429. [CrossRef]
35. Bernstein, M.A.; Tucker, K.L.; Ryan, N.D.; O'Neill, E.F.; Clements, K.M.; Nelson, M.E.; Evans, W.J.; Fiatarone Singh, M.A. Higher dietary variety is associated with better nutritional status in frail elderly people. *J. Am. Diet. Assoc.* **2002**, *102*, 1096–1104. [CrossRef]
36. Niedzwiedzka, E.; Wadolowska, L. Accuracy Analysis of the Food Intake Variety Questionnaire (FIVeQ). Reproducibility Assessment among Older People. *Pakistan J. Nutr.* **2008**, *7*, 426–435. [CrossRef]
37. Ogińska-Bulik, N. *Osobowość Typu D: Teoria i Badania; Type D Personality*; Theory and Research; Wyd.WSHE: Łódź, Poland, 2009.
38. Beliefs and Eating Habits Questionnaire. Behavioral Conditions of Nutrition Team, Committee of Human Nutrition Science. Polish Academy of Science. Warsaw 2014. Available online: http://www.knozc.pan.pl/ (accessed on 15 October 2018).
39. Cole, T.J.; Lobstein, T. Extended international (IOTF) body mass index cut-offs for thinness, overweight and obesity. *Pediatr. Obes.* **2012**, *7*, 284–294. [CrossRef]
40. James, G.; Witten, D.; Hastie, T.; Tibshirani, R. *An Introduction to Statistical Learning*; Springer: New York, NY, USA, 2015; ISBN 978-1-4614-7137-0.
41. Gilhooly, C.H.; Das, S.K.; Golden, J.K.; McCrory, M.A.; Dallal, G.E.; Saltzman, E.; Kramer, F.M.; Robert, S.B. Food cravings and energy regulation: The characteristics of craved foods and their relationship with eating behaviors and weight change during 6 months of dietary energy restriction. *Int. J. Obes.* **2007**, *31*, 1849–1858. [CrossRef]
42. Hebebrand, J.; Albayrak, Ö.; Adan, R.; Antel, J.; Dieguez, C.; de Jong, J.; Leng, G.; Menzies, J.; Mercer, J.G.; Murphy, M.; et al. "Eating addiction", rather than "food addiction", better captures addictive-like eating behavior. *Neurosci. Biobehav. Rev.* **2014**, *47*, 295–306. [CrossRef]
43. Curtis, C.; Davis, C. A qualitative study of binge eating and obesity from an addiction perspective. *Eat. Disord.* **2014**, *22*, 19–32. [CrossRef]
44. Schulte, E.M.; Avena, N.M.; Gearhardt, A.N. Which foods may Be Addictive? The roles of processing, fat content, and glycemic load. *PLoS ONE* **2015**, *10*, e0117959. [CrossRef] [PubMed]
45. Vanderlinden, J.; Dalle Grave, R.; Vandereycken, W.; Noorduin, C. Which factors do provoke binge-eating? An exploratory study in female students. *Eat. Behav.* **2001**, *2*, 79–83. [CrossRef]
46. Ifland, J.R.; Preuss, H.G.; Marcus, M.T.; Rourke, K.M.; Taylor, W.; Theresa Wright, H. Clearing the confusion around processed food addiction. *J. Am. Coll. Nutr.* **2015**, *34*, 240–243. [CrossRef] [PubMed]
47. White, M.A.; Grilo, C.M. Psychometric properties of the Food Craving Inventory among obese patients with binge eating disorder. *Eat. Behav.* **2005**, *6*, 239–245. [CrossRef]
48. Epel, E.; Lapidus, R.; McEwen, B.; Brownell, K. Stress may add bite to appetite in women: A laboratory study of stress-induced cortisol and eating behavior. *Psychoneuroendocrinology* **2001**, *26*, 37–49. [CrossRef]
49. Zellner, D.A.; Loaiza, S.; Gonzalez, Z.; Pita, J.; Morales, J.; Pecora, D.; Wolf, A. Food selection changes under stress. *Physiol. Behav.* **2006**, *87*, 789–793. [CrossRef]
50. Loprinzi, P.; Smit, E.; Mahoney, S. Physical Activity and Dietary Behavior in US Adults and Their Combined Influence on Health. *Mayo Clin. Proc.* **2014**, *89*, 190–198. [CrossRef]
51. Wadolowska, L.; Kowalkowska, J.; Lonnie, M.; Czarnocinska, J.; Jezewska-Zychowicz, M.; Babicz-Zielinska, E. Associations between physical activity patterns and dietary patterns in a representative sample of Polish girls aged 13–21 years: A cross-sectional study (GEBaHealth Project). *BMC Public Health* **2016**, *16*, 698. [CrossRef]
52. Wammes, B.; French, S.; Brug, J. What young Dutch adults say they do to keep from gaining weight: Self-reported prevalence of overeating, compensatory behaviours and specific weight control behaviours. *Public Health Nutr.* **2007**, *10*, 790–798. [CrossRef]
53. Lee, I.; Djoussé, L.; Sesso, H.D.; Wang, L.; Buring, J.E. Physical activity and weight gain prevention. *JAMA* **2010**, *303*, 1173–1179. [CrossRef]
54. Charreire, H.; Kesse-Guyot, E.; Bertrai, S.; Simon, C.; Chaix, B.; Weber, C.; Touvier, M.; Galan, P.; Hercberg, S.; Oppert, J.-M. Associations between dietary patterns, physical activity (leisure-time and occupational) and television viewing in middle-aged French adults. *Br. J. Nutr.* **2011**, *105*, 902–910. [CrossRef] [PubMed]

55. Kesse-Guyot, E.; Bertrais, S.; Peneau, S.; Estaquio, C.; Dauchet, L.; Vergnaud, A.-C.; Czernichow, S.; Galan, P.; Hercberg, S.; Bellisle, F. Dietary patterns and their sociodemographic and behavioural correlates in French middle-aged adults from the SU.VI.MAX cohort. *Eur. J. Clin. Nutr.* **2009**, *63*, 521–528. [CrossRef] [PubMed]
56. Li, J.T.E.; Pursey, K.M.; Duncan, M.J.; Burrows, T. Addictive Eating and Its Relation to Physical Activity and Sleep Behavior. *Nutrients* **2018**, *10*, 1428. [CrossRef]
57. Luo, S.; O'Connor, S.G.; Belcher, B.R.; Page, K.A. Effects of Physical Activity and Sedentary Behavior on Brain Response to High-Calorie Food Cues in Young Adults. *Obesity* **2018**, *26*, 540–546. [CrossRef] [PubMed]
58. Shook, R.; Hand, G.; Drenowatz, C.; Hebert, J.R.; Paluch, A.E.; Blundell, J.E.; Hill, J.O.; Katzmarzyk, P.T.; Church, T.S.; Blair, S.N. Low levels of physical activity are associated with dysregulation of energy intake and fat mass gain over 1 year. *Am. J. Clin. Nutr.* **2015**, *102*, 1332–1338. [CrossRef] [PubMed]
59. Yannakoulia, M.; Mamalaki, E.; Anastasiou, C.; Mourtzi, N.; Lambrinoudaki, I.; Scarmeas, N. Eating habits and behaviors of older people: Where are we now and where should we go? *Maturitas* **2018**, *114*, 14–21. [CrossRef]
60. Tsujim, T.; Yamamoto, K.; Yamasaki, K.; Hayashi, F.; Momoki, C.; Yasui, Y.; Ohfuji, S.; Fukushima, W.; Habu, D. Lower dietary variety is a relevant factor for malnutrition in older Japanese home-care recipients: A cross-sectional study. *BMC Geriatr.* **2019**, *19*, 197. [CrossRef]
61. Drewnowski, A.; Henderson, S.A.; Driscoll, A.; Rolls, B.J. The Dietary Variety Score: Assessing diet quality in healthy young and older adults. *J. Am. Diet. Assoc.* **1997**, *97*, 266–271. [CrossRef]
62. Morozink Boylan, J.; Cundiff, J.M.; Jakubowski, K.P.; Pardini, D.A.; Matthews, K.A. Pathways Linking Childhood SES and Adult Health Behaviors and Psychological Resources in Black and White Men. *Ann. Behav. Med.* **2018**, *52*, 1023–1035. [CrossRef]
63. Adler, N.E.; Stewart, J. Health disparities across the lifespan: Meaning, methods, and mechanisms. *Ann. NY Acad. Sci.* **2010**, *1186*, 5–23. [CrossRef]
64. Pechey, R.; Monsivais, P. Socioeconomic inequalities in the healthiness of food choices: Exploring the contributions of food expenditures. *Prev. Med.* **2016**, *88*, 203–209. [CrossRef] [PubMed]
65. Worsley, A.; Blaschea, R.; Ball, K.; Crawford, D. The relationship between education and food consumption in the 1995 Australian National Nutrition Survey. *Public Health Nutr.* **2004**, *7*, 649–663. [CrossRef] [PubMed]
66. Eertmans, A.; Baeyens, F.; Van den Bergh, O. Food likes and their relative importance in human eating behavior. Review and preliminary suggestions for health promotion. *Health Educ. Res.* **2001**, *16*, 443–456. [CrossRef] [PubMed]
67. Lumbers, M.; Raats, M. Food choices in later life. In *The Psychology of Food Choice*; Frontiers in Nutritional Sciences; Shepherd, R., Raats, M., Eds.; CABI Publishing: Wallingford, UK, 2006; Volume 3, pp. 280–310.
68. Conklin, A.; Forouhi, N.; Suhrcke, M.; Surtees, P.; Wareham, N.; Monsivais, P. Variety More Than Quantity of Fruit And Vegetable Intake Varies By Socioeconomic Status And Financial Hardship. Findings From Older Adults In The EPIC Cohort. *Appetite* **2014**, *83*, 248–255. [CrossRef]
69. Glass, C.; Haas, S.; Reither, E. The Skinny On Success: Body Mass, Gender And Occupational Standing Across The Life Course. *Social Forces* **2010**, *88*, 1777–1806. [CrossRef]
70. Duncan, D.; Wolin, K.; Scharoun-Lee, M.; Ding, E.; Warner, E.; Bennett, G. Does Perception Equal Reality? Weight Misperception in Relation to Weight-Related Attitudes and Behaviors among Overweight and Obese US Adults. *Int. J. Behav. Nutr. Phys. Act.* **2011**, *8*, 20. [CrossRef]
71. Millstein, R.A.; Carlson, S.A.; Fulton, J.E.; Galuska, D.A.; Zhang, J.; Blanck, H.M.; Ainsworth, B.E. Relationships between body size satisfaction and weight control practices among US adults. *Medscape J. Med.* **2008**, *10*, 119.
72. Burton, N.W.; Brown, W.; Dobson, A. Accuracy of body mass index estimated from self-reported height and weight in mid-aged Australian women. *Aust. N. Z. J. Public Health* **2010**, *34*, 620–623. [CrossRef]
73. Visscher, T.L.; Viet, A.L.; Kroesbergen, I.H.; Seidell, J.C. Underreporting of BMI in Adults and Its Effect on Obesity Prevalence Estimations in the Period 1998 to 2001. *Obesity* **2006**, *14*, 2054–2063. [CrossRef]
74. Kurina, L.M.; McClintock, M.K.; Chen, J.-H.; Waite, L.J.; Thisted, R.A.; Lauderdale, D.S. Sleep duration and all-cause mortality: A critical review of measurement and associations. *Ann. Epidemiol.* **2013**, *23*, 361–370. [CrossRef]

12

Validity of Virtual Reality Body Exposure to Elicit Fear of Gaining Weight, Body Anxiety and Body-Related Attentional Bias in Patients with Anorexia Nervosa

Bruno Porras-Garcia [1], Marta Ferrer-Garcia [1], Eduardo Serrano-Troncoso [2], Marta Carulla-Roig [2], Pau Soto-Usera [2], Helena Miquel-Nabau [1], Nazilla Shojaeian [1], Isabel de la Montaña Santos-Carrasco [3], Bianca Borszewski [3], Marina Díaz-Marsá [3], Isabel Sánchez-Díaz [4], Fernando Fernández-Aranda [4] and José Gutiérrez-Maldonado [1,*]

1 Department of Clinical Psychology and Psychobiology, University of Barcelona, Passeig de la Vall d'Hebron 171, 08035 Barcelona, Spain; brporras@ub.edu (B.P.-G.); martaferrerg@ub.edu (M.F.-G.); helena.mn29@gmail.com (H.M.-N.); nazila.shojaeian@gmail.com (N.S.)
2 Department of Child and Adolescent Psychiatry and Psychology, Hospital Sant Joan de Déu of Barcelona; Passeig de Sant Joan de Déu, 2, 08950 Esplugues de Llobregat, Spain; eserrano@sjdhospitalbarcelona.org (E.S.-T.); mcarulla@sjdhospitalbarcelona.org (M.C.-R.); psoto@sjdhospitalbarcelona.org (P.S.-U.)
3 Department of Psychiatry and Mental Health, Hospital Clínico San Carlos, Madrid, Calle del Prof Martín Lagos, s/n, 28040 Madrid, Spain; isabelmsc.is@gmail.com (I.d.l.M.S.-C.); biancbor@ucm.es (B.B.); marinadiaz.marsa@salud.madrid.org (M.D.-M.)
4 Department of Psychiatry and Mental Health, Hospital Universitario de Bellvitge- IDIBELL and CIBEROBN, Barcelona; Carrer Feixa Llarga s/n, 08907 Hospitalet del Llobregat, Spain; isasanchez@bellvitgehospital.cat (I.S.-D.); ffernandez@bellvitgehospital.cat (F.F.-A.)
* Correspondence: jgutierrezm@ub.edu

Abstract: Fear of gaining weight (FGW), body image disturbances, associated anxiety and body-related attentional bias are the core symptoms of anorexia nervosa (AN) and play critical roles in its development and maintenance. The aim of the current study is to evaluate the usefulness of virtual reality-based body exposure software for the assessment of important body-related cognitive and emotional responses in AN. Thirty female patients with AN, one of them subclinical, and 43 healthy college women, 25 with low body dissatisfaction (BD) and 18 with high BD, owned a virtual body that had their silhouette and body mass index. Full-body illusion (FBI) over the virtual body was induced using both visuo-motor and visuo-tactile stimulation. Once the FBI was induced, the FBI itself, FGW, body anxiety and body-related attentional bias toward weight-related and non-weight-related body areas were assessed. One-way analyses of covariance (ANCOVA), controlling for age, showed that AN patients reported higher FGW, body anxiety and body-related attentional bias than healthy controls. Unexpectedly, patients with AN reported significantly lower FBI levels than healthy participants. Finally, Pearson correlations showed significant relationships between visual analog scales and body-related attentional bias measures, compared to other eating disorder measures. These results provide evidence about the usefulness of virtual reality-based body exposure to elicit FGW and other body-related disturbances in AN patients. Thus, it may be a suitable intervention for reducing these emotional responses and for easing weight recovery.

Keywords: anorexia nervosa; virtual reality; fear of gaining weight; body anxiety; body image disturbances; body-related attentional bias

1. Introduction

Anorexia nervosa (AN) is considered one of the most serious eating disorders (ED), affecting women worldwide [1]. Although the age of onset of AN is established at around 14 to 19 years old [2,3], this condition has been progressively diagnosed in younger patients [4,5], making early preventive interventions in AN a public health priority.

According to the Diagnostic and Statistical Manual of Mental Disorders, 5th Edition [6], individuals with AN show severe restriction of food intake that leads to a significantly low body weight. In addition, they usually feel an intense fear of gaining weight (FGW) and disturbances in the way they experience their body weight and shape, also referred to as body image disturbances [7]. Greater FGW has also been related to more severe ED symptoms [8,9], and it is considered as one of the strongest predictors of ED symptomatology (e.g., dietary restraint and compulsive exercise) in AN patients [10]. In fact, it has been suggested that AN patients are more susceptible to learning fear associations than healthy individuals [11] (Strober, 2004); for instance, they are more likely to develop an intense FGW after starting a low-fat diet. Another psychopathological model has highlighted the importance of the anxiety symptomatology that AN patients usually experience as a direct reinforcement of their fears and behaviors [12]. The subjective feelings of tension, worried thoughts and physical changes that AN patients present are sometimes focused on their own body or toward specific body areas (i.e., weight-related body areas), a phenomenon known as body anxiety [13]. Previous studies have suggested that the core fears in AN (such as FGW) elicit high anxiety levels, which, in turn, lead to a progressive increase in ritualistic eating- and activity-related behaviors (e.g., the initiation of noncaloric diets or doing intense physical exercise). Over time, this allows the reinforcement of undereating and other dysfunctional behavioral disturbances [12].

Other theories have focused on the study of the mechanisms underlying the information processing biases typically found among individuals with EDs: biases in memory, interpretation and attention of body-related information, which, in turn, influence and maintain body image disturbances and ED symptomatology [14,15]. Among these cognitive biases, the dysfunctional role of attention has received increasing consideration over the last decades. Previous research suggests that ED patients pay more attention to disorder-relevant information (e.g., food- and body-related stimuli) than to other sorts of information [16,17]. Furthermore, dysfunctional body-related attention presumably maintains body image disturbances by processing only body information that is consistent with dysfunctional cognitive schema content (such as my thighs or stomach are getting fatter), while schema-inconsistent information tends to be visually neglected [16]. When considering patients with AN, body-related attentional bias seems to be especially pronounced in restrictive-type AN patients [18].

Therefore, these body-related constructs and underlying cognitive mechanisms may play a critical differential role in the development and maintenance of AN symptomatology. Consequently, the implementation of specific, tailored interventions targeting them is needed in AN.

Mirror exposure therapy aims to decrease body- and weight-related fears and is used to improve cognitive behavioral therapy (CBT) [19]. Several studies support the use of mirror exposure therapy to reduce body image disturbances in ED patients [20,21] and high body-dissatisfied individuals [22,23]. However, mirror exposure therapy frequently elicits a highly negative initial reaction in patients [24], which increases the probability of treatment rejection and the risk of dropout [25]. Furthermore, mirror exposure therapy is usually conducted in controlled settings (e.g., a laboratory or therapist's office), and the generalization of positive changes learned during exposure is impaired [26].

These limitations can be overcome by the application of virtual reality (VR) techniques. For instance, VR technology is proposed as a good complement to in vivo exposure, especially in the initial stages of the intervention, since it is perceived as safer by participants and reduces the rates of withdrawal [27]. In addition, although VR is also conducted in a controlled setting, it allows researchers to create real-size 3D simulations of participants' bodies with their physical characteristics and place them in immersive environments that reproduce real life situations related to their body image concerns (e.g., a dressing room, a beach or a bathroom), thus enhancing the generalization of positive results [26,28]. Another advantage of using VR is that it allows certain stimuli or environments to be manipulated in ways that may not be possible in mirror exposure therapy. For instance, it allows patients with AN to increase/decrease the weight (or the body mass index (BMI)) of the virtual avatar until it reaches a target weight, thus helping to confront their core fears (i.e., the fear of gaining weight).

VR technology has evolved notably over the last few years. For instance, the newest VR systems can achieve a full-body motion tracking that captures the individual's body silhouette and movements using a head-mounted display, VR controllers and a series of body trackers that can be attached to different body areas (e.g., the feet and the waist). These technological advances have allowed the development of countless applications for improving health-related problems in a new transdisciplinary research field known as embodied medicine or embodied technology (for an extensive review, see [29,30]). This paradigm allows individuals to perceive and feel a virtual body as their real body by activating predicting neurological brain circuits to elicit the feelings of ownership over a virtual avatar [29,30]. Specifically, the subjective experience in which individuals feel an artificial body to be their own is known as full-body illusion (FBI) [31]. To accomplish this, different types of information (visual, acoustic, proprioceptive and vestibular) must be combined into multisensory representations [32].

One of the most widely studied and best-known paradigms for eliciting feelings of ownership over a specific body area is the rubber hand illusion [33], in which the participant's nonvisible real hand is synchronously touched by the experimenter while the participants see the same touches delivered to a fake rubber hand. Following the rubber hand illusion paradigm, a previous study found that ED patients tend to experience a stronger illusion over a fake hand than healthy individuals [34]. Alternatively, a large number of studies have investigated the effects of the FBI on the whole body to assess body image disturbances, for a review, see [28], finding that the perception of body size and weight may be changed in nonclinical samples [35–38] and ED patients [39–41]. Specifically, among AN patients, Keizer et al. [39] found that owning a skinny virtual body significantly reduced the perceived body size in AN patients, as well as in healthy participants. These results were later replicated by two case report studies, which showed that VR embodiment-based techniques (e.g., using a visuo-tactile stimulation procedure) allowed the modification of body image disturbances either in the short term [40] or over several sessions [41].

Curiously, while most body exposure-based therapies, such as mirror exposure therapy, focus on treating body image disturbances, little information is available about the use of body exposure techniques, with or without VR, to treat FGW. Levinson, Rapp and Riley [42] proposed an imaginal exposure procedure that consisted of five sessions in which the patient had to visualize her own weight gain and the possible associated adverse consequences. The authors reported a clinically significant change in ED symptomatology from pretherapy to one-month follow-up and a steady increase in weight throughout the exposure sessions, which was maintained at follow-up. Imaginal exposure therapy directly targeting the FGW seems to be an interesting approach in AN treatments. However, its effectiveness must be explored in controlled clinical studies. Furthermore, imagery exposure may have some significant limitations—for example, difficulty in achieving or maintaining visualization and the risk of avoidance of the most feared stimulus during visualization. These limitations can be overcome by the application of VR techniques that do not rely on the patient's visualization ability and reduce the possibility of avoidance behaviors. Therefore, VR exposure therapy provides a useful approach to targeting FGW [41].

The aim of the current study was to assess the usefulness of a VR-based body exposure software to elicit FGW and other important body-related cognitive and emotional responses, such as body anxiety or body-related attentional bias among patients with AN. Specifically, the objective was to assess levels of FBI, body anxiety, FGW and body-related attentional bias when healthy women with high and low body dissatisfaction (BD) and AN patients owned a virtual body (VB) with their real silhouette and body mass index (BMI). In addition, the relationship between FGW, body anxiety and body-related attentional bias experienced during VR exposure and ED measures, collected prior to entering the VR, were assessed. Based on previous research, it was expected that: (i) AN patients would report higher levels of FBI, body anxiety and FGW than healthy women when they owned their real-size VB; (ii) AN patients would show higher body-related attentional bias, specifically in weight-related body areas, than healthy participants; (iii) healthy women with high BD would show higher FBI, body anxiety, FGW and body-related attentional bias than women with low BD; (iv) and there would be positive relationships between the measures assessed during VR exposure and the ED measures.

2. Materials and Methods

2.1. Participants

Forty-three female college students from the University of Barcelona, Spain and 30 AN female patients from different ED units in Barcelona participated in the study. College women were recruited through campus flyers and advertisements in social network groups. The exclusion criteria were a self-reported diagnosis of a current ED, a body mass index (BMI) of less than 17 (moderate thinness) or over 30 (obesity, according to the World Health Organization, 2004) or a self-reported current severe mental disorder diagnosis (e.g., schizophrenia or bipolar disorder).

The inclusion criteria were patients with a primary diagnosis of AN (DSM-5 criteria) over 13 years of age with a BMI < 19. Furthermore, one subsyndromal patient who met all anorexia criteria but two was also included. Visual deficits that prevent exposure, epilepsy, pregnancy and clinical cardiac arrhythmia were considered exclusion criteria for the nonclinical and clinical samples.

Nineteen adolescents with AN were diagnosed at the ED Unit of Hospital Sant Joan de Déu of Barcelona, while 11 adults with AN were diagnosed at the ED Unit of Bellvitge Hospital and Hospital Clínico San Carlos of Madrid, Spain. All patients underwent a day-patient treatment for adolescents and young adults with ED. This was an intensive day-patient treatment program conducted at the ED Unit in 11-h periods, with permission to sleep at home.

2.2. Measures

2.2.1. ED Symptomatology Measures

- BMI = weight (in kilograms)/ height (in m)^2.
- Eating Disorder Inventory (EDI-3) [43]. The EDI-3 is a self-reported inventory consisting of 12 scales and 91 items, in which the answers are provided on a 6-point Likert scale. In the current study, only the 10-item body dissatisfaction scale (EDI-BD) and 7-item drive for thinness (EDI-DT) scales were used. EDI-BD measures body dissatisfaction with the whole body and specific body parts. EDI-DT measures the desire to be thinner, concern with dieting, preoccupation with weight and FGW. The Spanish version of the EDI-3 has robust validity indices and good internal consistency, with a Cronbach's alpha ranging from 0.74 to 0.96 [44]. In the current study, Cronbach's alphas for the clinical samples were 0.76 for the EDI-BD scale and 0.84 for EDI-DT. Cronbach's alpha values for both scales were 0.77 to 0.79 in the nonclinical sample.
- Physical Appearance State and Trait Anxiety Scale (PASTAS) [13]. The PASTAS is a self-reported questionnaire that assesses body anxiety, understood as the subjective feelings of tension, worried thoughts and physical changes that patients and participants feel about their body or toward specific parts of their body. The PASTAS comprises two self-report scales measuring weight-related and non-weight-related anxiety. In this study, the weight scale (W) with 8 items was used. The questionnaire presents good reliability, with a Cronbach's alpha between 0.82 and 0.92 and good test-retest ($r = 0.87$) and convergent validity indices for the W scale ($r = 0.74$ EDI-BD and $r = 0.62$ EDI-DT) [13].
- Body Image Assessment Scale-Body Dimensions (BIAS-BD) [45]. The BIAS-BD was used to assess body image disturbances in this study. The BIAS is a figural drawing scale questionnaire, which presents the physical anthropometric dimensions of adult women in a series of human silhouettes. Participants selected the one that was perceived as their body size (perceived

silhouette) and the one they desired to have (desired body size). Then, according to their BMI, the real silhouette was also selected. The scale allows researchers to estimate the participant's body dissatisfaction (discrepancy between perceived and ideal body size) and body distortion (discrepancy between perceived and real body size). This scale shows good psychometric properties, such as good test-retest reliability (r = 0.86) with data collection before and after a two-week interval and good concurrent validity (r = 0.76) after comparing participants' perceived actual body size and self-reported BMI [45].

- Body Appreciation Scale (BAS) [46], translated by Jáuregui-Lobera and Bolaños-Ríos [47]. The BAS consists of 12 items assessing a positive attitude towards one's body on a 5-point Likert scale. It presents good internal consistency, with a Cronbach's alpha of 0.908 [47].

2.2.2. Body-Related Attentional Bias

Weight-related body parts (W-AOIs or areas of interest) were chosen based on the weight scale of body items from the PASTAS questionnaire [13] and drawn onto a picture of a female avatar in a frontal view. Body parts included in the W-AOIs were the legs, thighs, buttocks, hips, stomach (abdomen) and waist. After the separation of the W-AOIs, the remaining body parts (head, neck, chest, shoulders, arms and feet) were labeled as non-weight-related body parts (NW-AOIs) (Figure 1).

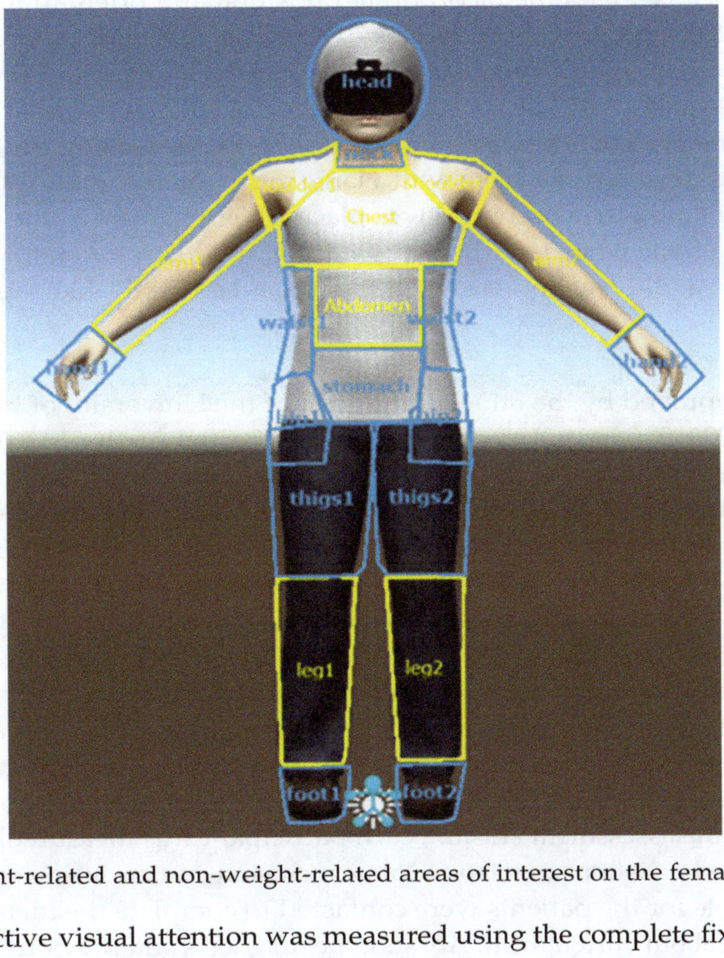

Figure 1. Weight-related and non-weight-related areas of interest on the female virtual avatar.

Participants' selective visual attention was measured using the complete fixation time and number of fixations on the areas of interest (AOIs). Visual fixation was defined by Jacob and Karn [48] as the visual act of maintaining one's gaze on a single location for a minimum duration, usually 100–200 ms. In this study, a duration of 100 ms was considered. Previous studies focusing on body-related attention used these specific gaze-behavioral measures, provided by eye-tracking (ET) technology, as reliable and continuous measures of attention allocation toward specific body areas [18,49–52].

2.2.3. Visual Analog Scales (VAS)

- Full-body illusion (FBI) was assessed by means of a VAS estimating the intensity of the illusion from 0 to 100. "On a scale of 0 to 100, indicate to what extent you felt that the virtual body was your own body, where 0 is not at all and 100 is completely."
- FGW and anxiety related to the whole body were assessed on a VAS from 0 to 100. "On a scale of 0 to 100, indicate the level of anxiety toward your body that you are feeling at this moment, where 0 is not at all and 100 is a lot." "On a scale of 0 to 100, indicate to what extent you are afraid of gaining weight at this moment, where 0 is not at all and 100 is a lot."

2.3. Hardware and Software Features

All participants were exposed to an immersive virtual scenario using a VR HTC-VIVE head-mounted display (HMD HTC VIVE, HTC Corporation, New Taipei City, Taiwan). In addition to the two controllers that HTC-VIVE usually provides, three additional body trackers were used to achieve full-body motion tracking. The VR trackers and headsets were connected to a computer with a powerful graphics card (Nvidia RTX 2080, Nvidia Corporation, Santa Clara, CA, USA) to run VR environments fluently.

HMD FOVE-Eye Tracking (FOVE, Inc., Torrance, CA, USA) was used to detect and register eye movements. The headset uses the incorporated position and orientation eye-tracking systems. The FOVE display has 2560*1440 pixels and creates 70 frames per second. Infrared eye-tracking sensors create 120 frames per second, with an accuracy level of less than 1 degree. FOVE setup 0.16.0 (FOVE, Inc., Torrance, CA, USA) and Unity 3D 3.0.0 (Unity Technologies, San Francisco, CA, USA) were used to create the virtual simulations. The virtual avatars were created using the software Blender 2.78. The virtual environment consisted of a room with a large mirror on the front wall. The mirror was large enough to reflect every limb of the body and was placed 1.5 m in front of the participants. A young female avatar wearing a basic white t-shirt with blue jeans and black trainers was created. The avatar also wore a swim cap to avoid any influence of hairstyle and an HMD, like the participants.

2.4. Procedure

This study was approved by the ethics committee of the University of Barcelona (Institutional review board IRB00003099), and all sessions were conducted at the ED units of each hospital. Furthermore, all AN patients were previously informed about the nature of the study by the clinicians responsible for their care at each ED unit. All participants signed the informed consent after being informed about the study, the data confidentiality and the possibility of withdrawing from the study at any point without consequences. When participants were under 18, informed consent was also signed by their legal guardians. Additionally, confidentiality was ensured by assigning a different identification code to each participant. Patients were previously diagnosed by senior trained clinical psychologists and psychiatrists using nonstructured clinical interviews and applying the DSM-5 criteria strictly. The Mini International Neuropsychiatric Interview (MINI) [53] was also conducted at two of the ED units. The assessment was carried out by trained clinical psychologists who had previous experience with the latest version of the MINI.

Before the start of the assessment session, each participant was measured to calculate their BMI, and the researchers asked questions in relation to the inclusion and exclusion criteria. In the ED units, the clinicians responsible for the patients were contacted to complete the identification form for the study, with information about current BMI, AN subtype diagnosis and previous history of the disorder, and to confirm that the inclusion and exclusion criteria were fulfilled.

All the participants underwent the same procedure. Firstly, the virtual avatar was generated by taking frontal and lateral photos of the participant and creating an avatar whose silhouette matched the pictures by adjusting the body parts (shoulders, arms, chest, waist, stomach, hip, thighs and legs) to the photographs. In the meantime, a second researcher administered the paper-based questionnaires.

Next, the FBI was induced using two procedures: visuo-motor and visuo-tactile stimulation. Visuo-motor stimulation consisted of synchronizing the movement of the participants and the avatar using motion capture sensors placed on the hands, feet and waist. Once inside the virtual environment, all participants could observe themselves in the first-person perspective and look at themselves in a mirror (in the third-person perspective). The movements were carried out in a structured way, and the procedure lasted one and a half minutes. The visuo-tactile stimulation consisted of synchronizing the participants' visual and tactile stimulation. When participants were touched with one of the HTC-VIVE controllers on different areas of the body (upper and lower limbs and stomach), they saw (in first and third person) how their avatars were touched in the same areas at the same time by a virtual controller. The visuo-tactile stimulation lasted one and a half minutes and was always performed by a female experimenter. Once the FBI was induced, the three VAS examining the intensity of the FBI, body-related anxiety and the FGW were assessed.

Finally, to assess the body-related attentional bias, a calibration and recording procedure was conducted using VR HMD-FOVE-Eye Tracking. The participants' gaze was tracked while they were asked to observe their virtual body in the mirror for 30 s (a similar recording time to that used in other studies) [50,54,55]. During the process, and as a cover story, the participant was told to remain still and avoid abrupt head movements while the virtual avatar position was being recalibrated.

2.5. Statistical Analysis

Ogama (Open Gaze Mouse Analyzer) software (Freie Universität, Berlin, Germany) was used to transform ET raw data into suitable quantitative data. The sum of the visual fixation times of each of the subjects was estimated using the complete fixation time and the number of fixations on the AOIs. This was achieved by summing up separate complete fixation times and the number of fixations displayed on W-AOIs vs. on NW-AOIs. Additional data transformation was conducted by calculating the difference between weight-related and non-weight-related AOIs (e.g., complete fixation time (W-AOIs: 1615 ms − NW-AOIs: 1505 ms = 110 ms)). Therefore, a positive outcome would mean that the participant looked at weight-related body parts longer than at non-weight-related body parts, while a negative outcome would mean the opposite.

Likewise, healthy women were divided into high vs. low BD levels using the median score of the EDI-BD as a cut-off point ($_{Me}$ BD = 8).

One-way analyses of covariance (ANCOVA) were run to determine if there were differences in all measures, including ED measures assessed prior to entering the VR environment, VR-VASs and ET measures between participants with high and low BD and AN patients. Given the age differences between ED and healthy participants, this variable was controlled and introduced as a covariable in the analyses. Analyses of ET measures were conducted for the groups of AOIs (e.g., the difference between W-AOIs and NW-AOIs) and for single W-AOIs (e.g., arms, shoulders and chest, etc.).

There was homogeneity of the regression slopes as the interaction terms were not statistically significant ($p > 0.05$) for any of the measures. The other assumptions were partially met. There was homogeneity of the variances, as assessed by Levene's test, in almost all measures except for BMI, EDI-BD, EDI-DT and BIAS-BD. In addition, data were not normally distributed in all the variables assessed by the Kolmogorov–Smirnov test. However, it was decided to conduct the analyses regardless, as ANCOVA is considered a robust test, even in the case of deviation from normality [56]. Finally, a few outliers were detected in some measures, as assessed by inspection of a boxplot. Statistical analyses were conducted with and without the outliers. Since the results did not differ significantly, it was decided to include them in the analyses.

Finally, Pearson correlations were run to assess the relationship between ED measures, VASs and body-related attentional bias measures in the overall sample. They were also conducted separately among healthy participants with low and high BD and patients with AN. All the analyses were conducted with the statistical software IBM SPSS Statistics v.24 (IBM Corp. Released 2016. Armonk, NY, USA).

3. Results

The demographic and clinical information of healthy controls and AN patients are summarized here. The healthy control sample consisted of 43 healthy college women (M_{age} = 21.12, SD = 1.56 and age range: 18–23 years and M_{BMI} = 21.94, SD = 2.53 and BMI range: 17.12 – 27.82), with 25 women with low BD and 18 women with high BD. The clinical sample consisted of 30 AN female patients (M_{age} = 17.73 and SD = 4.60 and M_{BMI} =17.55 and SD =1.07), with 19 adolescents (age range: 13–17 years and BMI range: 16.06–18.94 kg/m^2) and 11 adults (age range: 18–32 years and BMI range: 13.96–18.98). Of the adolescent AN patients, 18 were diagnosed with restrictive AN (AN-R) and the other one with purgative AN (AN-P). Three adolescent patients presented comorbidities with anxiety disorders: two presented mood-related disorders, and one presented both anxiety and mood-related disorders. Eight patients received pharmacological treatment: two with antidepressants, three with anxiolytics and three with a combination of antidepressants and anxiolytics.

Six of the adult patients were diagnosed with the AN-P subtype and five with the AN-R subtype. In addition, two adult patients presented comorbidities with borderline personality disorder, one presented borderline personality disorder and post-traumatic stress disorder and one presented a major depressive disorder. Five adult patients were receiving pharmacological treatment: one with antidepressants, one with anxiolytics and antidepressants and three with antidepressants or anxiolytics combined with antipsychotics.

All the descriptive results are summarized in Table 1, including ED measures assessed prior to entering the VR environment, VASs assessed within the VR environment and body-related attentional bias measures.

Table 1. Adjusted for age and unadjusted descriptive results. Mean (M), standard deviation (SD) and standard error (SE).

	Women with Low BD (*n*= 25)		Women with High BD (*n*= 18)		AN Patients (*n* = 30)	
	Unadjusted	Adjusted	Unadjusted	Adjusted	Unadjusted	Adjusted
	M (SD)	M (SE)	M (SD)	M (SE)	M (SD)	M (SE)
BMI	21.65 (2.39)	21.60 (.42)	22.38 (2.75)	22.32 (.53)	17.55 (1.07)	17.63 (0.40)
EDI-3-DT	1.88 (1.76)	2.41 (1.07)	4.89 (4.39)	5.57 (1.27)	19.23 (7.43)	18.38 (1.03)
EDI-3-BD	4.04 (1.44)	4.53 (1.32)	14.61 (6.30)	15.26 (1.56)	24.03 (10.03)	23.23 (1.27)
PASTAS	5.04 (3.77)	5.80 (1.09)	8.56 (4.77)	9.70 (1.38)	17.20 (7.18)	15.95 (1.05)
BIAS-Body distortion	9.60 (13.06)	9.93 (3.59)	18.13 (13.76)	18.61 (4.51)	39.17 (21.45)	38.63 (3.43)
BIAS-Body dissatisfaction	7.40 (9.90)	7.53 (4.02)	14.37 (19.56)	14.56 (5.07)	36.83 (24.62)	36.62 (3.86)
BAS	52.32 (5.29)	51.82 (1.57)	42.06 (7.54)	41.32 (1.98)	29.43 (9.30)	30.24 (1.51)
VAS-FBI	65.72 (23.25)	67.94 (5.05)	54.94 (19.20)	58.24 (6.38)	46.18 (29.50)	42.15 (4.86)
VAS-A	15.20 (19.12)	17.44 (5.15)	26.25 (22.97)	29.60 (6.51)	40.00 (31.15)	35.34 (4.95)
VAS-FGW	22.88 (28.80)	25.12 (5.84)	51.88 (26.39)	55.21 (7.38)	79.82 (27.70)	72.86 (5.62)
Complete fixation time (in ms) *	−2858 (10,589)	−4492 (1732)	965 (7578)	−1079 (2055)	6899 (7457)	10,198 (2014)
Number of fixations *	2.20 (15.80)	−0.45 (2.96)	5.20 (15.49)	1.90 (3.51)	22.00 (12.99)	27.25 (3.41)

Note: body mass index (BMI); Eating Disorder Inventory (EDI-3) drive for thinness (DT) and body dissatisfaction (BD) scales; Physical Appearance State and Trait Anxiety Scale (PASTAS); Body Image Assessment Test (BIAS); Body Appreciation Scale (BAS) and visual analog scales (VAS) of full body illusion (FBI), body anxiety (A) and fear of gaining weight (FGW). AN = Anorexia Nervosa. Complete fixation time in milliseconds (ms). * For eye-tracking (ET) measures, the clinical sample was comprised of 19 adolescents and 5 adults with AN.

3.1. Eating Disorder Measures Assessed Prior to Entering the VR Environment

As Table 1 shows, patients with AN reported higher levels of BD, a drive for thinness, body anxiety and body image disturbances (including body distortion and BD assessed with BIAS and EDI questionnaires, respectively) than healthy participants. Patients with AN also had lower BMI and showed lower body appreciation than healthy participants.

After adjusting for age, the ANCOVA analyses showed group differences on all ED measures. Specifically, the results showed significant group differences in BMI ($F(2,67) = 29.035$, $p < 0.001$, partial $\eta^2 = 0.464$); drive for thinness ($F(2,69) = 56.775$, $p < 0.001$, partial $\eta^2 = 0.622$); BD ($F(2,69) = 49.101$, $p < 0.001$, partial $\eta^2 = 0.587$); body anxiety ($F(2,67) = 20.600$, $p < 0.001$, partial $\eta^2 = 0.381$); body image disturbances (including body distortion: $F(2,67) = 15.703$, $p < 0.001$, partial $\eta^2 = 0.319$ and BD: $F(2,67) = 12{,}968$, $p < 0.001$, partial $\eta^2 = 0.279$, as assessed with the BIAS-BD questionnaire) and body appreciation ($F(2,67) = 45.426$, $p < 0.001$). Post-hoc analyses revealed that there were significant differences ($p < 0.05$) between patients with AN and women with high and low BD in all ED measures.

3.2. VASs of Full-Body Illusion, Body Anxiety and Fear of Gaining Weight

Once in the VR environment, and according to the VASs, AN patients reported lower values of FBI than healthy participants. Additionally, AN patients reported higher levels of body anxiety and FGW, while owning their real-size VB, than healthy participants. Women with high BD also reported higher body anxiety and FGW, as well as lower levels of FBI than women with low BD (see Table 1).

To clarify whether these differences between patients with AN and women with high and low BD were, indeed, significant, one-way ANCOVAs were run. After controlling for age, the results reported significant group differences in FBI levels ($F(2,68) = 6.252$, $p = 0.003$, partial $\eta^2 = 0.157$); FGW ($F(2,67) = 16{,}670$, $p < 0.001$, partial $\eta^2 = 0.332$) and marginally significant differences in body anxiety ($F(2,67) = 3.077$, $p = 0.053$, partial $\eta^2 = 0.084$). Effect sizes according to Cohen (1988) were medium in body anxiety, high in FBI and very high in FGW. Post-hoc analyses revealed significant differences ($p < 0.05$) between patients with AN and women with low BD in FBI and FGW VASs and marginally significant differences ($p = 0.057$) in VAS-A (see Table 2). In addition, there were also significant differences between women with high BD and low BD (see Table 2).

Table 2. Post-hoc analyses (pairwise comparison) between AN patients and women with high and low BD.

Measures	AN Patients vs. Women with Low BD			AN Patients vs. Women with High BD			Women with High vs. Low BD		
	MD	p	95% CI	MD	p	95% CI	MD	p	95% CI
VAS-FBI	−25.79	0.002	(−43.72, −7.86)	−16.10	0.179	(−36.73, 4.53)	−9.69	0.672	(−29.08, 9.70)
VAS-A	17,89	0.057	(−0.39, 36.18)	5,74	0.896	(−15.30, 26.78)	12,15	0.408	(−7.62, 31.93)
VAS-FGW	47.74	<0.001	(68.48, 27.00)	17.64	0.221	(−6.21, 41.51)	30.09	0.005	(7.66, 52.52)
Complete fixation time (in ms) *	14,722	<0.001	(7626, 21,818)	11,317	0.002	(3590, 19,045)	3404	0.568	(−2904, 9712)
Number of fixations *	27.70	<0.001	(15.66, 39.74)	25.35	<0.001	(12.24, 38.45)	2.35	0.787	(−8.34, 13.05)

Note: Mean differences (MD), p-values and 95% confidence intervals (CI) stated for each group comparison. ms = milliseconds. * For ET measures, the clinical sample was comprised of 19 adolescents and 5 adults with AN.

3.3. Body-Related Attentional Bias Measures

The descriptive results of both ET measures revealed that AN patients spent more time looking at and showed a higher number of fixations on weight-related AOIs than on non-weight-related AOIs, as indicated by a positive outcome in both ET measures. In contrast, women with high BD spent a similar time and number of fixations looking at weight- and non-weight-related AOIs. Finally, women with low BD showed a tendency to spend more time looking at NW-AOIs and a similar number of fixations on weight- and non-weight-related AOIs (see Table 1).

The one-way ANCOVA results showed statistically significant group differences in the complete fixation time ($F(2,63) = 13.114$, $p < 0.001$, partial $\eta^2 = 0.294$) and the number of fixations ($F(2,63) = 17.107$, $p < 0.001$, partial $\eta^2 = 0.352$) after controlling for age. Post-hoc analyses revealed that these differences were statically significant ($p < 0.05$) between patients with AN and women with high and low BD in both attentional bias measures (see Table 2). Finally, there were no significant differences ($p > 0.05$) between women with high and low BD.

One-way ANCOVAs were also run to assess the group differences at single W-related AOIs. After controlling for age, the results showed statistically significant group differences ($p < 0.05$) for the thighs (complete fixation time: $F(2,63) = 7707$, $p = 0.001$, partial η2 = 0.197 and number of fixations: $F(2,63) = 10.573$, $p < 0.001$, partial η2 = 0.251); hips (number of fixations: $F(2,63) = 4663$, $p < 0.013$, partial η2 = 0.129) and stomach (complete fixation time: $F(2,63) = 5239$, $p = 0.008$, partial η2 = 0.143 and number of fixations: $F(2,63) = 7078$, $p = 0.002$, partial η2 = 0.183). Post-hoc analyses revealed that patients with AN spent significantly more time looking and showed higher numbers of fixations on the stomach, hips and, particularly, the thighs in contrast to women with low and high BD (Figure 2). No significant differences were found between women with high and low BD for any of the single AOIs.

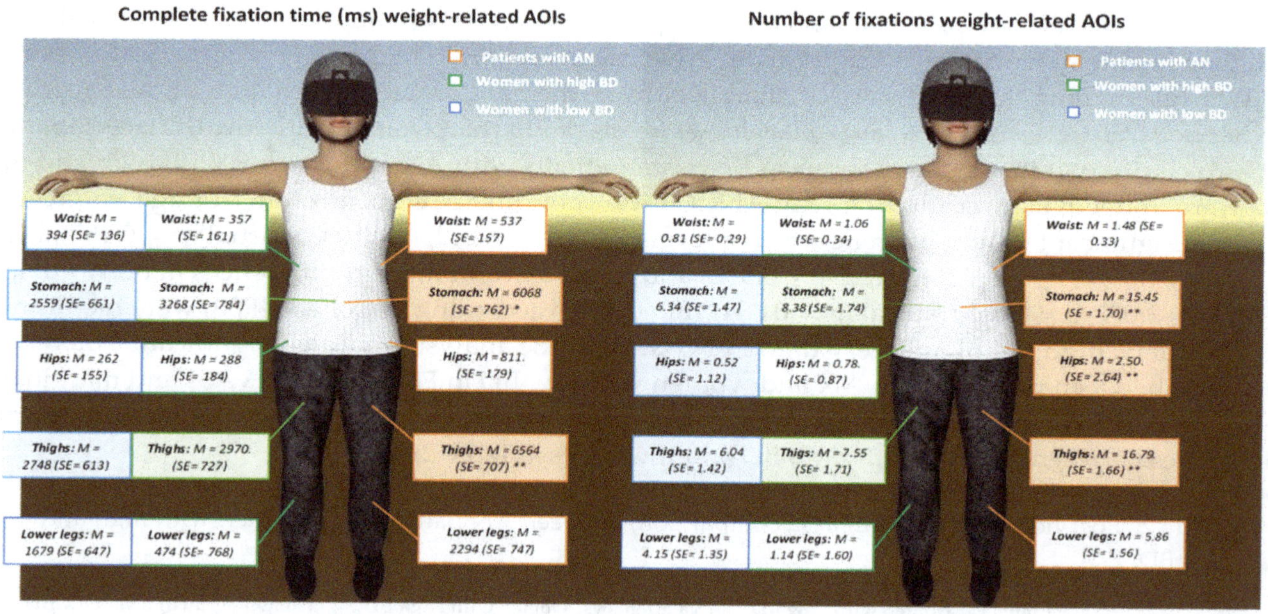

Figure 2. Differences between patients with Anorexia Nervosa (AN) and women with high and low body dissatisfaction (BD) (means and standard errors) in the complete fixation time (in milliseconds; ms) and the number of fixations on individual weight-related areas of interest (AOIs). Post-hoc analyses: ** $p < 0.01$ and * $p < 0.05$.

3.4. Pearson Correlations

According to multiple Pearson correlations, the results showed statistically significant moderate or large positive correlations between VAS-A and VAS-FGQ and all ED measures ($p < 0.05$), which were significantly larger for VAS-FGW (see Table 3). There were also moderate or large positive correlations between VAS-A/FGW and the BMI and BAS scale. Furthermore, VAS-FBI negatively correlated ($p < 0.05$) with the VAS-FGW, EDI-DT, EDI-BD, BAS and BIAS-BD measures, with moderate correlations (Cohen, 1988). There was a moderate positive correlation between the VAS-FBI and BAS. Finally, there were significant moderate positive correlations between the body-related attentional bias measures and the EDI-DT, EDI-BD and PASTAS (only for the number of fixations (NF)) scales, while there were moderate negative correlations between the body-related attentional bias measures and the BMI and BAS.

Multiple Pearson correlations were conducted separately for women with low and high BD and for patients with AN. The results among women with low BD showed that, overall, the previously reported positive and negative correlations between the VASs/attentional bias measures and other ED measures were not significant, with the exception of the VAS-FGW and PASTAS/BAS (see Table 4). Similar results were found among women with high BD, in which there were statistically significant positive/negative correlations between the VAS-FGW and BMI, EDI-DT, PASTAS and BAS (See Table 5). Finally, among patients with AN, there were statistically significant and similar positive and negative correlations to those previously reported for the entire clinical and nonclinical samples (see Table 6).

Table 3. Correlations between eating disorder (ED) measures and virtual reality (VR) body exposure responses in the entire sample.

	VAS-FBI	VAS-A	VAS-FGW	CFT	NF
VAS-FBI					
VAS-A	−0.16				
VAS-FGW	−0.24 *	0.70 **			
CFT	−0.21	0.16	0.35 **		
NF	−0.28	1.18	0.42 **	0.91 **	
BMI	0.23	−0.22	−0.38 **	−0.38 **	−0.43 **
EDI-DT	−0.37 **	0.55 **	0.72 **	0.32 **	0.41 **
EDI-BD	−0.30 **	0.53 **	0.73 **	0.35 **	0.40 **
PASTAS	−0.22	0.60 **	0.80 **	0.22	0.32 **
BIAS-Body distortion	−0.43 **	0.38 **	0.56 **	0.16	0.21
BIAS-Body dissatisfaction	−0.38 **	0.28 *	0.50 **	0.19	0.23
BAS	0.34 **	−0.58 **	−0.77 **	−0.32 **	−0.40 **

* = p-values < 0.005 or ** = p-values < 0.001. NOTE: CFT = complete fixation time. NF= number of fixations.

Table 4. Correlations between ED measures and VR body exposure responses in healthy participants with low BD.

	VAS-FBI	VAS-A	VAS-FGW	CFT	NF
VAS-FBI					
VAS-A	−0.028				
VAS-FGW	−0.209	0.778 **			
CFT	−0.290	−0.097	0.205		
NF	−0.255	0.064	0.402 *	0.938 **	1.00
BMI	−0.020	0.071	−0.013	−0.277	−0.243
EDI-DT	−0.268	0.279	0.325	0.235	0.246
EDI-BD	−0.045	0.153	0.172	0.316	0.336
PASTAS	−0.057	0.728 **	0.686 **	−0.045	0.015
BIAS-Body distortion	−0.147	0.142	−0.085	−0.155	−0.199
BIAS- Body dissatisfaction	0.239	0.195	−0.041	−0.149	−0.099
BAS	−0.201	−0.503 *	−0.593 **	−0.214	−0.322

* = p-values < 0.05 or ** = p-values < 0.01. NOTE: CFT = complete fixation time. NF = number of fixations.

Table 5. Correlations between ED measures and VR body exposure responses in healthy participants with high BD.

	VAS-FBI	VAS-A	VAS-FGW	CFT	NF
VAS-FBI					
VAS-A	0.173				
VAS-FGW	0.282	0.710 **			
CFT	0.300	0.040	0.017		
NF	0.433	0.183	0.006	0.876 **	
BMI	0.170	−0.045	0.016	−0.096	0.009
EDI-DT	0.086	0.271	0.519 *	−0.241	−0.281
EDI-BD	0.035	0.452	0.546 *	0.071	0.132
PASTAS	0.077	0.719 **	0.753 **	0.030	0.057
BIAS-Body distortion	−0.103	0.171	0.377	0.041	−0.143
BIAS-Body dissatisfaction	−0.108	−0.246	0.048	0.040	−0.093
BAS	−0.162	−0.350	−0.674 **	0.053	0.099

* = p-values < 0.05 or ** = p-values < 0.01. NOTE: CFT = complete fixation time. NF = number of fixations.

Table 6. Correlations between ED measures and VR body exposure responses in patients with AN.

	VAS-FBI	VAS-A	VAS-FGW	CFT	NF
VAS-FBI					
VAS-A	−0.093				
VAS-FGW	−0.031	0.563 **			
CFT	−0.057	−0.187	−0.191		
NF	−0.064	−0.317	−0.340	0.862 **	
BMI	0.042	0.116	0.059	0.141	0.149
EDI-DT	−0.290	0.562 **	0.620 **	−0.326	−0.263
EDI-BD	−0.107	0.442*	0.594 **	−0.211	−0.206
PASTAS	0.014	0.399 *	0.675 **	−0.527 **	−0.472 *
BIAS-Body distortion	−0.425 *	0.216	0.458 *	−0.280	−0.220
BIAS-Body dissatisfaction	−0.436 *	0.163	0.396 *	−0.164	−0.172
BAS	0.351	−0.550 **	−0.564**	0.377	0.321

* = p-values < 0.05 or ** = p-values < 0.01. NOTE: CFT = complete fixation time. NF = number of fixations.

Surprisingly, some of the strongest significant negative correlations were found in FBI levels and body image disturbance measures only among patients with AN. To explain these preliminary results, it was hypothesized that the individuals with higher body image disturbance (i.e., body distortion/body dissatisfaction) levels were those who experienced lower FBI levels once they owned their real-size virtual body. Thus, it was decided to conduct predictive post-hoc linear regression analyses. The results showed that having higher body distortion levels statistically significantly predicted experiencing lower FBI levels ($F(1,29) = 6.160$, $p = 0.019$), accounting for 18% of the explained variability in FBI levels only among patients with AN. This relationship between body distortion and FBI levels was not significant among women with high and low BD ($p > 0.05$). Similarly, experiencing higher BD levels significantly predicted experiencing lower FBI levels ($F(1, 29) = 6.561$, $p = 0.016$), which accounted for 19% of the explained variability in FBI levels only among patients with AN. Again, the relationship between body distortion and FBI levels was not significant among women with high and low BD ($p > 0.05$).

4. Discussion

The current study aimed to provide initial evidence of the usefulness of VR body exposure to elicit FGW, body anxiety and body-related attentional bias in patients with AN. For this purpose, we assessed whether there were significant differences in the levels of FBI, body anxiety, FGW and body-related attentional bias when AN patients and healthy women with high and low BD owned a virtual body with their real silhouette and body mass index (BMI). As expected, patients with AN showed higher levels of FGW, body anxiety and body-related attentional bias than healthy controls when they owned their real-size VB. Unexpectedly, patients with AN reported significantly lower levels of FBI than women with low BD. Furthermore, no significant differences were found between healthy women with high and low BD on FBI, body anxiety or body-related attentional bias. The only significant group differences were observed in the levels of FGW reported.

Furthermore, the relationship between the ED measures assessed prior to entering the VR and the responses produced during VR exposure was also assessed. As expected, there were positive relationships between some measures assessed by VR body exposure (e.g., body anxiety and FGW) software and other ED measures assessed previously. This relation was particularly strong among patients with AN. Hence, the participants and patients with higher ED symptomatology were also those who experienced higher levels of FGW, body anxiety and attentional bias during exposure. Additionally, significant negative relationships were found among FBI and body image disturbance measures, including body distortion and BD, only among patients with AN.

According to the measures assessed during the VR body exposure, patients with AN reported significantly higher FGW and body anxiety levels than women with high and low BD, with high effect sizes. Specifically, the FGW was the variable that best distinguished between AN patients and women with low BD and between women with high and low BD. Relatedly, the FGW during VR body exposure was the measure that had the largest significant correlations with the ED measures assessed before exposure, such as BD, drive for thinness, body anxiety, BMI and body appreciation. Similar tendencies were observed not only among patients with AN but, also, among women with high BD. These results support the increasing evidence in favor of the critical role that the FGW might display not only in AN [6,8–10] but, also, in healthy women with body concerns. Indeed, several studies have reported high prevalence of FGW among adult women [2,57] and young women between 16 to 25 years old [58].

Unexpectedly, patients with AN reported significantly lower FBI levels than healthy participants with low BD. Our results seem to contradict previous research that found that ED patients tend to experience a stronger illusion than healthy individuals [34]. However, those studies induced the feeling of ownership in one hand only, following the rubber hand illusion paradigm [33]. In the current study, the illusion of ownership was induced over a whole virtual body, which suggests that other body-related factors (e.g., body image disturbances) could influence these results as well. For instance, several patients with AN described their virtual body as being slimmer than their real body, while healthy women with high and low BD did not report such a phenomenon. Accordingly, there was a significant negative relationship between FBI and body image disturbances only among patients with AN, while this relationship was not significant among women with high and low BD. After further analyses, it was found that AN patients with higher body distortion and body dissatisfaction levels experienced lower FBI levels once they owned their real-size virtual body. These results provide preliminary evidence about the influence that body image disturbances have on FBI over the whole body among patients with AN. Accordingly, two interesting questions should be considered. Firstly, would these low FBI levels increase during a body exposure treatment, for instance, over several sessions? Secondly, if this were the case, would a continuous increase in FBI levels produce a change in body image disturbances in the participants or the other way around? Unfortunately, it is not possible to answer either question, since there is a lack of studies in which FBI levels were assessed over several sessions with AN patients. In fact, to the best of our knowledge, only one study has assessed FBI over a short period among healthy participants, finding that, after a synchronous visuo-motor embodiment procedure, FBI levels remained high after 30 and 55 s of synchronous or no movement [59].

Regarding body-related attentional bias measures, our results agree with previous studies that suggest that women with EDs tend to pay more attention to self-defined unattractive body areas, while healthy participants tend to show more general scanning behavior, covering the whole body [17,54,60,61]. While most of the studies assessing body-related attention have been conducted with adults, little information is available about body-related attention in youths. Therefore, our results also support studies that assessed body-related attentional bias among adolescents with EDs and showed that adolescents with AN and Bulimia Nervosa spent more time on self-reported unattractive body parts [18,62]. For instance, Bauer et al. [18] found that dysfunctional body-related attention was more marked among adolescents with AN-R than among healthy individuals and other ED patients (e.g., patients with AN-binge eating/purging subtype or Bulimia Nervosa). Since almost all our patients were diagnosed with an AN-R subtype, this study reinforced the evidence of dysfunctional body-related attention among adolescents with AN-R. When single W-related AOIs were considered, we observed that all individuals paid more attention to the thighs, stomach and lower legs. The W-AOIs that best distinguished between patients with AN and women with high and low BD were the thighs, the stomach, and the hips (only in number of fixations). This suggests that these areas might be particularly salient for patients with AN.

Nevertheless, some key methodological differences between the current study and other studies that assess body-related attentional bias should be mentioned. As described before, some previous studies used a similar free-viewing, single-body paradigm but measured the attentional bias towards self-reported attractive vs. unattractive body areas. This is a successful, well-established methodology to define the areas of interest [16,17]. Although self-reported unattractive body areas among individuals with EDs could indeed be areas related with weight, the evidence for attentional bias towards specific weight-related body areas could not be clearly established, since there might be weight-related body areas in both the self-reported attractive and unattractive body parts. In this study and in previous studies conducted by our group, a different methodology was used to define the areas of interest, in which an individual's gazing behavior was analyzed using the same definition of areas of interest for all participants e.g., weight- vs. non-weight-related body areas [50,51]. These areas of interest were defined based on well-established questionnaires that assess the same body image construct, such as the weight-related scale of the PASTAS.

Finally, no differences in body-related attentional bias were found between women with high and low BD. Women with high BD tended to pay more attention to W-related AOIs, while women with low BD showed the opposite visual tendency toward NW-related AOIs. None of these tendencies showed a clear attentional bias to weight- or non-weight-related AOIs. However, overall, both groups showed more general scanning behavior, covering the whole body. These results are in-line with a previous study conducted in our group [50] in which women with high and low BD showed similar attentional patterns toward their own virtual bodies. This previous study was conducted with a previous version of the virtual simulation. Although the results obtained were very similar, some technical improvements that were made to the current version of the simulation should be considered. For instance, a more precise method could be used to create the avatar (by taking a frontal and lateral photo and incorporating the BMI information of each participant), and the full-body tracking system could be improved to conduct a visual-motor stimulation.

Some limitations should be considered in the current study. For instance, most of the patients with AN were adolescents (19 out of 30), while the healthy women were college students between 18 and 22 years old. Although the potential effect of age between groups was controlled in this study by ANCOVAs, these statistical analyses could not control the effect that age might play within each group and, particularly, in the more heterogeneous AN sample. Future studies should try to overcome this important bias and replicate the current study with age-balanced samples.

Regarding the assessment, no screening questionnaires or structured clinical interviews were used properly to assess the presence of EDs or other mental disorders among the healthy participants. Furthermore, to diagnosticate the clinical sample, a MINI diagnostic interview was used in two of the three ED units, while, at the last ED unit, senior trained clinical psychologists and psychiatrists conducted nonstructured clinical interviews following thoroughly the DSM-5 criteria.

FBI and FGW were assessed using a VAS; even though VASs are usually considered as a valid measure to assess this sort of construct (for instance, FGW among patients with AN [63]), they should be complemented with evidence-based questionnaires. For instance, the embodiment questionnaire [64] might offer a more accurate assessment of the FBI based on the location of the body, the ownership illusion, the motor agency and the general appearance. One of the reasons for using the VAS was to assess the FBI while patients and participants were owning their real-size virtual bodies. It was important to assess the FBI levels directly in the VR environment and not later, since this bodily illusion might have been reduced once the participants left the VR (after the ET assessment task), and the results might have been affected as a consequence. However, since several questionnaires were already used in the current research, it was decided not to extend the assessment sessions (which lasted approximately 1h) any further and to refrain from applying larger tests. Future studies might try to implement evidence-based questionnaires that assess these two measures. Finally, in the current study, the average levels of BD among women labeled as "high BD" were very similar to in a previous study conducted by our group [50], corresponding to medium-to-high BD levels among nonclinical Spanish women [44]. Thus, it would have been necessary to recruit participants with higher levels of BD to provide a more exhaustive distinction of the BD levels among women with high and low BD. Relatedly, the suitability of using the median as an "artificial categorization" of a continuous variable—in this study, BD—could have some limitations. These could affect the statistical power and accuracy of the estimated relations and reduce the observed relations among the variables [65].

Some limitations in the VR software should also be considered. Although several improvements were implemented (e.g., the avatar sharing the same silhouette and BMI as the participant), the general appearance of the virtual body (clothes and skin color, etc.) was not exactly that of the individuals. The latest VR studies allow the simulation of an exact 3D biometric avatar with all the individual's features [66] using 3D body scans. This sort of technology might notably enhance the realism of VR embodiment-based techniques and, consequently, improve VR studies on body-related issues and EDs. The current study used two separate HMDs: one for conducting the visuo-tactile and visuo-motor FBI procedures (HTC-VIVE) and the other to record the body-related attentional bias measures (FOVE-VR). Having two separate devices might have reduced the FBI levels when the participants had to change from one HMD to the other. This limitation could have been overcome by using the new generation of VR HMD with ET devices all-in-one (e.g., the HTC VIVE-Pro Eye, which has a complete full-body tracking system and can be used to elicit FBI over the virtual body and measure gaze patterns).

The implications of VR embodiment-based techniques might be critical to improving evidence-based therapies in AN, such as body exposure-based techniques. For instance, instead of exposing a patient with AN to food or to her current body image, as has been done so far, what would be the result of exposing her to her core fear, i.e., weight gain? Patients with AN associate weight gain with negative consequences, and food avoidance prevents them from learning that maintaining a normal weight does not lead to such catastrophic consequences [67]. Consequently, focusing on the primary conditioned stimulus (weight gain) rather than on the secondary ones, such as eating, may be an effective strategy. As has been reported, VR embodiment-based techniques are a successful way to change body image disturbances in patients with AN [39–41]. We propose going one step further. First, we could allow the patient with AN to experience the illusion of ownership of a virtual body that reproduces their real-size silhouette, with their specific physical particularities and their exact BMI. Then, we could apply progressive increases in weight (or an increase in the BMI) of the virtual avatar, until it reaches a healthy BMI.

Furthermore, the combination of VR and ET technologies to assess body-related attentional bias might lead to new possibilities in coming years. For instance, it might improve some of the current limitations of research conducted with fixed ET, such as the lack of external validity [68]. In other words, combining ET and VR might enable the reproduction of more ecological environments, such as bathrooms and dressing rooms, to assess patient's gaze patterns while they own their real-size virtual avatars in each session or before and after the therapy.

To sum up, our results show that, while owning their real-size virtual body, patients with AN reported significantly higher FGW and body anxiety levels than women with low BD, with high effect sizes. Specifically, FGW was the variable that best distinguished between AN patients and healthy participants and between healthy participants with high and low BD. Unexpectedly, patients with AN reported significantly lower FBI levels than healthy participants with low BD. After post-hoc analyses, it was found that body image disturbances influence FBI levels among patients with AN. Furthermore, our results suggest that the patients with AN showed a body-related attentional bias. Specifically, they spent more time and looked more frequently at the weight-related body areas (e.g., thighs, stomach and hips) than healthy women. Finally, these results provide evidence about the usefulness of VR-based body exposure to elicit FGW and other body-related disturbances in AN patients. Thus, it may be a suitable intervention for reducing these emotional responses and for easing weight recovery.

Author Contributions: Conceptualization, B.P.-G., M.F.-G., M.D.-M., I.S.-D.; F.F.-A. and J.G.-M; validation, B.P.-G., M.C.-R., P.S.-U., H.M.-N., I.d.l.M.S.-C. and B.B.; formal analysis, B.P.-G.; investigation, B.P.-G., H.M.-N., N.S., I.d.l.M.S.-C. and B.B.; resources, E.S.-T., M.C.-R., P.S.-U., M.D.-M., I.S.-D.; F.F.-A. and J.G.-M.; data curation, B.P.-G., writing—original draft preparation, B.P.-G., writing—review and editing, B.P.-G., M.F.-G., N.S. and J.G.-M., visualization, B.P.-G. and M.F.-G.; supervision M.F.-G. and J.G.-M.; project coordinator; J.G.-M. and funding acquisition, J.G.-M. All authors have read and agreed to the published version of the manuscript.

Acknowledgments: CIBEROBN is an initiative of Instituto Carlos III (Spain).

References

1. Hoek, H.W. Review of the worldwide epidemiology of eating disorders. *Curr. Opin. Psychiatry* **2016**, *29*, 336–339. [CrossRef] [PubMed]
2. Micali, N.; Hagberg, K.W.; Petersen, I.; Treasure, J.L. The incidence of eating disorders in the UK in 2000–2009: Findings from the General Practice Research Database. *BMJ Open* **2013**, *3*. [CrossRef] [PubMed]
3. Herpertz-Dahlmann, B. A1dolescent Eating Disorders: Definitions, Symptomatology, Epidemiology and Comorbidity. *Child. Adolesc. Psychiatr. Clin. N. Am.* **2009**, *24*, 177–196. [CrossRef] [PubMed]
4. Favaro, A.; Caregaro, L.; Tenconi, E.; Bosello, R.; Santonastaso, P. Time trends in age at onset of anorexia nervosa and bulimia nervosa. *J. Clin. Psychiatry* **2009**, *70*, 1715–1721. [CrossRef]
5. Nicholls, D.E.; Lynn, R.; Viner, R.M. Childhood eating disorders: British national surveillance study. *Br. J. Psychiatry* **2011**, *198*, 295–301. [CrossRef]
6. American Psychiatric Association. *Diagnostic and Statistical Manual of Mental Disorders*, 5th ed.; American Psychiatric Association: Arlington, VA, USA, 2013.
7. Legenbauer, T.; Thiemann, P.; Vocks, S. Body image disturbance in children and adolescents with eating disorders: Current evidence and future directions. *Z. Kinder. Jugendpsychiatr. Psychother.* **2014**, *42*, 51–59. [CrossRef]
8. Carter, J.C.; Bewell-Weiss, C.V. Nonfat phobic anorexia nervosa: Clinical characteristics and response to inpatient treatment. *Int. J. Eat. Disord.* **2011**, *44*, 220–224. [CrossRef]
9. Calugi, S.; El Ghoch, M.; Conti, M.; Dalle Grave, R. Preoccupation with shape or weight, fear of weight gain, feeling fat and treatment outcomes in patients with anorexia nervosa: A longitudinal study. *Behav. Res. Ther.* **2018**, *105*, 63–68. [CrossRef]
10. Linardon, J.; Phillipou, A.; Castle, D.; Newton, R.; Harrison, P.; Cistullo, L.L.; Griffiths, S.; Hindle, A.; Brennan, L. The relative associations of shape and weight over-evaluation, preoccupation, dissatisfaction, and fear of weight gain with measures of psychopathology: An extension study in individuals with anorexia nervosa. *Eat. Behav.* **2018**, *29*, 54–58. [CrossRef]
11. Strober, M. Pathologic Fear Conditioning and Anorexia Nervosa: On the Search for Novel Paradigms. *Int. J. Eat. Disord.* **2004**, *35*, 504–508. [CrossRef]
12. Steinglass, J.E.; Sysko, R.; Glasofer, D.; Albano, A.M.; Simpson, H.B.; Walsh, B.T. Rationale for the application of exposure and response prevention to the treatment of anorexia nervosa. *Int. J. Eat. Disord.* **2011**, *44*, 134–141. [CrossRef] [PubMed]
13. Reed, D.L.; Thompson, J.K.; Brannick, M.T.; Sacco, W.P. Development and validation of the physical appearance state and trait anxiety scale (PASTAS). *J. Anxiety Disord.* **1991**, *5*, 323–332. [CrossRef]
14. Williamson, D.A.; White, M.A.; York-Crowe, E.; Stewart, T.M. Cognitive-behavioral theories of eating disorders. *Behav. Modif.* **2004**, *28*, 711–738. [CrossRef] [PubMed]
15. Lee, M.; Shafran, R. Information processing biases in eating disorders. *Clin. Psychol. Rev.* **2004**, *24*, 215–238. [CrossRef] [PubMed]
16. Rodgers, R.F.; DuBois, R.H. Cognitive biases to appearance-related stimuli in body dissatisfaction: A systematic review. *Clin. Psychol. Rev.* **2016**, *46*, 1–11. [CrossRef]
17. Kerr-Gaffney, J.; Harrison, A.; Tchanturia, K. Eye-tracking research in eating disorders: A systematic review. *Int. J. Eat. Disord.* **2019**, *52*, 3–27. [CrossRef]
18. Bauer, A.; Schneider, S.; Waldorf, M.; Braks, K.; Huber, T.J.; Adolph, D.; Vocks, S. Selective Visual Attention Towards Oneself and Associated State Body Satisfaction: An Eye-Tracking Study in Adolescents with Different Types of Eating Disorders. *J. Abnorm. Child. Psychol.* **2017**, *45*, 1647–1661. [CrossRef]
19. Forrest, L.N.; Jones, P.J.; Ortiz, S.N.; Smith, A.R. Core psychopathology in anorexia nervosa and bulimia nervosa: A network analysis. *Int. J. Eat. Disord.* **2018**, *51*, 668–679. [CrossRef]
20. Hildebrandt, T.; Loeb, K.; Troupe, S.; Delinsky, S. Adjunctive mirror exposure for eating disorders: A randomized controlled pilot study. *Behav. Res. Ther.* **2012**, *50*, 797–804. [CrossRef]
21. Key, A.; George, C.L.; Beattie, D.; Stammers, K.; Lacey, H.; Waller, G. Body image treatment within an inpatient program for anorexia nervosa: The role of mirror exposure in the desensitization process. *Int. J. Eat. Disord.* **2002**, *31*, 185–190. [CrossRef]

22. Moreno-Domínguez, S.; Rodríguez-Ruiz, S.; Fernández-Santaella, M.C.; Jansen, A.; Tuschen-Caffier, B. Pure versus guided mirror exposure to reduce body dissatisfaction: A preliminary study with university women. *Body Image* **2012**, *9*, 285–288. [CrossRef] [PubMed]
23. Jansen, A.; Voorwinde, V.; Hoebink, Y.; Rekkers, M.; Martijn, C.; Mulkens, S. Mirror exposure to increase body satisfaction: Should we guide the focus of attention towards positively or negatively evaluated body parts? *J. Behav. Ther. Exp. Psychiatry* **2016**, *50*, 90–96. [CrossRef] [PubMed]
24. Vocks, S.; Legenbauer, T.; Wächter, A.; Wucherer, M.; Kosfelder, J. What happens in the course of body exposure? Emotional, cognitive, and physiological reactions to mirror confrontation in eating disorders. *J. Psychosom. Res.* **2007**, *62*, 231–239. [CrossRef] [PubMed]
25. Delinsky, S.S.; Wilson, G.T. Mirror exposure for the treatment of body image disturbance. *Int. J. Eat. Disord.* **2006**, *39*, 108–116. [CrossRef]
26. Gutiérrez-Maldonado, J.; Wiederhold, B.K.; Riva, G. Future directions: How virtual reality can further improve the assessment and treatment of eating disorders and obesity. *Cyberpsychol. Behav. Soc. Netw.* **2016**, *19*, 148–153. [CrossRef]
27. Garcia-Palacios, A.; Botella, C.; Hoffman, H.; Fabregat, S. Comparing acceptance and refusal rates of virtual reality exposure vs. in vivo exposure by patients with specific phobias. *Cyberpsychol. Behav.* **2007**, *10*, 722–724. [CrossRef]
28. Gutiérrez-Maldonado, J.; Ferrer-García, M.; Dakanalis, A.; Riva, G. Virtual reality: Applications to eating disorders. In *The Oxford Handbook of Eating Disorders*; Oxford University Press: Oxford, UK, 2018.
29. Riva, G.; Serino, S.; Di Lernia, D.; Pavone, E.F.; Dakanalis, A. Embodied medicine: Mens sana in corpore virtuale sano. *Front. Hum. Neurosci.* **2017**, *11*, 120. [CrossRef]
30. Riva, G.; Wiederhold, B.K.; Mantovani, F. Neuroscience of Virtual Reality: From Virtual Exposure to Embodied Medicine. *Cyberpsychol. Behav. Soc. Netw.* **2019**, *22*, 82–96. [CrossRef]
31. Maselli, A.; Slater, M. The building blocks of the full body ownership illusion. *Front. Hum. Neurosci.* **2013**, *7*, 83. [CrossRef]
32. Piryankova, I.V.; Wong, H.Y.; Linkenauger, S.A.; Stinson, C.; Longo, M.R.; Bülthoff, H.H.; Mohler, B.J. Owning an overweight or underweight body: Distinguishing the physical, experienced and virtual body. *PLoS ONE* **2014**, *9*, e103428.
33. Botvinick, M.; Cohen, J. Rubber hands 'feel' touch that eyes see. *Nature* **1998**, *391*, 756. [CrossRef] [PubMed]
34. Eshkevari, E.; Rieger, E.; Longo, M.R.; Haggard, P.; Treasure, J. Increased plasticity of the bodily self in eating disorders. *Psychol. Med.* **2012**, *42*, 819–828. [CrossRef] [PubMed]
35. Serino, S.; Pedroli, E.; Keizer, A.; Triberti, S.; Dakanalis, A.; Pallavicini, F.; Chirico, A.; Riva, G. Virtual reality body swapping: A tool for modifying the allocentric memory of the body. *Cyberpsychol. Behav. Soc. Netw.* **2016**, *19*, 127–133. [CrossRef] [PubMed]
36. Preston, C.; Ehrsson, H.H. Illusory changes in body size modulate body satisfaction in a way that is related to non-clinical eating disorder psychopathology. *PLoS ONE* **2014**, *9*, e85773.
37. Preston, C.; Ehrsson, H.H. Illusory obesity triggers body dissatisfaction responses in the insula and anterior cingulate cortex. *Cereb. Cortex* **2016**, *26*, 4450–4460. [CrossRef]
38. Porras Garcia, B.; Ferrer Garcia, M.; Olszewska, A.; Yilmaz, L.; González Ibañez, C.; Gracia Blanes, M.; Gültekin, G.; Serrano Troncoso, E.; Gutiérrez Maldonado, J. Is this my own body? Changing the perceptual and affective body image experience among college students using a new virtual reality embodiment-based technique. *J. Clin. Med.* **2019**, *8*, 925. [CrossRef]
39. Keizer, A.; Van Elburg, A.; Helms, R.; Dijkerman, H.C. A virtual reality full body illusion improves body image disturbance in anorexia nervosa. *PLoS ONE* **2016**, *11*, e0163921. [CrossRef]
40. Serino, S.; Polli, N.; Riva, G. From avatars to body swapping: The use of virtual reality for assessing and treating body-size distortion in individuals with anorexia. *J. Clin. Psychol.* **2019**, *75*, 313–322. [CrossRef]
41. Porras-Garcia, B.; Serrano-Troncoso, E.; Carulla-Roig, M.; Soto-Usera, P.; Ferrer-Garcia, M.; Figueras-Puigderrajols, N.; Yilmaz, L.; Onur Sen, Y.; Shojaeian, N.; Gutiérrez-Maldonado, J. Virtual Reality Body Exposure Therapy for Anorexia Nervosa. A Case Report with Follow-Up Results. *Front. Psychol.* **2020**, *11*, 956. [CrossRef]
42. Levinson, C.A.; Rapp, J.; Riley, E.N. Addressing the fear of fat: Extending imaginal exposure therapy for anxiety disorders to anorexia nervosa. *Eat. Weight Disord. Stud. Anorex. Bulim. Obes.* **2014**, *19*, 521–524. [CrossRef]

43. Garner, D. *Eating Disorder Inventory-3: Professional Manual*; Psychological Assessment Resources: Lutz, FL, USA, 2004.
44. Elosua, P.; López-Jaúregui, A.; Sánchez-Sánchez, F. *EDI-3, Inventario de Trastornos de la Conducta Alimentaria-3, Manual*; Tea Ediciones: Madrid, Spain, 2010.
45. Gardner, R.M.; Jappe, L.M.; Gardner, L. Development and validation of a new figural drawing scale for body-image assessment: The BIAS-BD. *J. Clin. Psychol.* **2009**, *65*, 113–122. [CrossRef] [PubMed]
46. Avalos, L.; Tylka, T.L.; Wood-Barcalow, N. The body appreciation scale: Development and psychometric evaluation. *Body Image* **2005**, *2*, 285–297. [CrossRef] [PubMed]
47. Lobera, I.J.; Ríos, P.B. Spanish Version of the Body Appreciation Scale (BAS) for Adolescents. *Span. J. Psychol.* **2011**, *14*, 411–420. [CrossRef] [PubMed]
48. Jacob, R.J.K.; Karn, K.S. Eye Tracking in Human-Computer Interaction and Usability Research. Ready to Deliver the Promises. In *The Mind's Eye: Cognitive and Applied Aspects of Eye Movement Research*; Elsevier: Amsterdam, The Netherlands, 2003; pp. 573–605.
49. Jiang, M.Y.W.; Vartanian, L.R. A review of existing measures of attentional biases in body image and eating disorders research. *Aust. J. Psychol.* **2018**, *70*, 3–17. [CrossRef]
50. Porras-Garcia, B.; Ferrer-Garcia, M.; Ghita, A.; Moreno, M.; López-Jiménez, L.; Vallvé-Romeu, A.; Serrano-Troncoso, E.; Gutiérrez-Maldonado, J. The influence of gender and body dissatisfaction on body-related attentional bias: An eye-tracking and virtual reality study. *Int. J. Eat. Disord.* **2019**, *52*, 181–1190. [CrossRef]
51. Porras-Garcia, B.; Ferrer-Garcia, M.; Yilmaz, L.; Sen, Y.O.; Olszewska, A.; Ghita, A.; Serrano-Troncoso, E.; Treasure, J.; Gutiérrez-Maldonado, J. Body-related attentional bias as mediator of the relationship between body mass index and body dissatisfaction. *Eur. Eat. Disord. Rev.* **2020**. [CrossRef]
52. Porras-Garcia, B.; Exposito-Sanz, E.; Ferrer-Garcia, M.; Castillero-Mimenza, O.; Gutiérrez-Maldonado, J. Body-Related Attentional Bias among Men with High and Low Muscularity Dissatisfaction. *J. Clin. Med.* **2020**, *9*, 1736. [CrossRef]
53. Sheehan, D.V.; Lecrubier, Y.; Sheehan, K.H.; Amorim, P.; Janavs, J.; Weiller, E.; Dunbar, G.C. The Mini-International Neuropsychiatric Interview (MINI): The development and validation of a structured diagnostic psychiatric interview for DSM-IV and ICD-10. *J. Clin. Psychiatry* **1998**, *9*, 1736.
54. Jansen, A.; Nederkoorn, C.; Mulkens, S. Selective visual attention for ugly and beautiful body parts in eating disorders. *Behav. Res. Ther.* **2005**, *50*, 90–96. [CrossRef]
55. Roefs, A.; Jansen, A.; Moresi, S.; Willems, P.; van Grootel, S.; van der Borgh, A. Looking good. BMI, attractiveness bias and visual attention. *Appetite* **2008**, *51*, 552–555. [CrossRef]
56. Schminder, E.; Ziegler, M.; Danay, E.; Beyer, L.; Bühner, M. Is it really robust? Reinvestigating the robustness of ANOVA against violations of the normal distribution. *Methodology* **2010**, *6*, 147–151. [CrossRef]
57. Gagne, D.A.; Von Holle, A.; Brownley, K.A.; Runfola, C.D.; Hofmeier, S.; Branch, K.E.; Bulik, C.M. Eating disorder symptoms and weight and shape concerns in a large web-based convenience sample of women ages 50 and above: Results of the gender and body image (GABI) study. *Int. J. Eat. Disord.* **2012**, *45*, 832–844. [CrossRef] [PubMed]
58. Slof-Op 't Landt, M.C.T.; van Furth, E.F.; van Beijsterveldt, C.E.M.; Bartels, M.; Willemsen, G.; de Geus, E.J.; Ligthart, L.; Boomsma, D.I. Prevalence of dieting and fear of weight gain across ages: A community sample from adolescents to the elderly. *Int. J. Public Health* **2017**, *62*, 911–919. [CrossRef] [PubMed]
59. Keenaghan, S.; Bowles, L.; Crawfurd, G.; Thurlbeck, S.; Kentridge, R.W.; Cowie, D. My body until proven otherwise: Exploring the time course of the full body illusion. *Conscious. Cogn.* **2020**, *78*, 102882. [CrossRef] [PubMed]
60. Freeman, R.; Touyz, S.; Sara, G.; Rennie, C.; Gordon, E.; Beumont, P. In the eye of the beholder: Processing body shape information in anorexic and bulimic patients. *Int. J. Eat. Disord.* **1991**, *10*, 709–714. [CrossRef]
61. Tuschen-Caffier, B.; Bender, C.; Caffier, D.; Klenner, K.; Braks, K.; Svaldi, J. Selective visual attention during mirror exposure in anorexia and bulimia nervosa. *PLoS ONE* **2015**, *10*, e0145886. [CrossRef] [PubMed]
62. Heinrich, H.; Moll, G.H.; Horndasch, S.; Hönig, F.; Nöth, E.; Kratz, O.; Holczinger, A. "Looks do matter"—Visual attentional biases in adolescent girls with eating disorders viewing body images. *Psychiatry Res.* **2012**, *198*, 321–323.

63. Rushford, N. Fear of gaining weight: Its validity as a visual analogue scale in anorexia nervosa. *Eur. Eat. Disord. Rev.* **2006**, *14*, 104–110. [CrossRef]
64. Gonzalez-Franco, M.; Peck, T.C. Avatar embodiment. Towards a standardized questionnaire. *Front. Robot. AI* **2018**, *5*, 74. [CrossRef]
65. MacCallum, R.C.; Zhang, S.; Preacher, K.J.; Rucker, D.D. On the practice of dichotomization of quantitative variables. *Psychol. Methods* **2002**, *7*, 19–40. [CrossRef]
66. Mölbert, S.C.; Thaler, A.; Mohler, B.J.; Streuber, S.; Romero, J.; Black, M.J.; Zipfel, S.; Karnath, H.O.; Giel, K.E. Assessing body image in anorexia nervosa using biometric self-avatars in virtual reality: Attitudinal components rather than visual body size estimation are distorted. *Psychol. Med.* **2018**, *48*, 642–653. [CrossRef] [PubMed]
67. Murray, S.B.; Loeb, K.L.; Le Grange, D. Dissecting the core fear in anorexia nervosa: Can we optimize treatment mechanisms? *JAMA Psychiatry* **2016**, *73*, 891–892. [CrossRef] [PubMed]
68. Kredel, R.; Vater, C.; Klostermann, A.; Hossner, E.J. Eye-tracking technology and the dynamics of natural gaze behavior in sports: A systematic review of 40 years of research. *Front. Psychol.* **2017**, *8*, 1845. [CrossRef] [PubMed]

13

Exploring Patterns of Disturbed Eating in Psychosis

Nicolette Stogios [1,2,†], Emily Smith [1,2,†], Roshanak Asgariroozbehani [1,2,†], Laurie Hamel [1], Alexander Gdanski [3], Peter Selby [1,4,5,6], Sanjeev Sockalingam [1,2,6,7], Ariel Graff-Guerrero [1,2,6], Valerie H. Taylor [8], Sri Mahavir Agarwal [1,2,6,‡] and Margaret K. Hahn [1,2,6,*,‡]

1 Centre for Addiction and Mental Health (CAMH), Toronto, ON M6J 1H3, Canada; nicolette.stogios@mail.utoronto.ca (N.S.); emilycc.smith@mail.utoronto.ca (E.S.); roshanak.asgariroozbehani@mail.utoronto.ca (R.A.); laurie.hamel@camh.ca (L.H.); peter.selby@camh.ca (P.S.); sanjeev.sockalingam@camh.ca (S.S.); ariel.graff@camh.ca (A.G.-G.); mahavir.agarwal@camh.ca (S.M.A.)
2 Institute of Medical Science (IMS), University of Toronto, Toronto, ON M5S 1A8, Canada
3 Department of Human Biology, University of Toronto, Toronto, ON M5S 3J6, Canada; alexander.gdanski@mail.utoronto.ca
4 Department of Family and Community Medicine, University of Toronto, Toronto, ON M5G 1V7, Canada
5 Dalla Lana School of Public Health, University of Toronto, Toronto, ON M5T 3M7, Canada
6 Department of Psychiatry, University of Toronto, Toronto, ON M5T 1R8, Canada
7 Bariatric Surgery Program, University Health Network, Toronto, ON M5T 2S8, Canada
8 Department of Psychiatry, University of Calgary, Calgary, AB T2N 1N4, Canada; valerie.taylor3@albertahealthservices.ca
* Correspondence: margaret.hahn@camh.ca
† These authors contributed equally to this work.
‡ These authors contributed equally to this work.

Abstract: Disturbed eating behaviours have been widely reported in psychotic disorders since the early 19th century. There is also evidence that antipsychotic (AP) treatment may induce binge eating or other related compulsive eating behaviours. It is therefore possible that abnormal eating patterns may contribute to the significant weight gain and other metabolic disturbances observed in patients with psychosis. In this scoping review, we aimed to explore the underlying psychopathological and neurobiological mechanisms of disrupted eating behaviours in psychosis spectrum disorders and the role of APs in this relationship. A systematic search identified 35 studies that met our eligibility criteria and were included in our qualitative synthesis. Synthesizing evidence from self-report questionnaires and food surveys, we found that patients with psychosis exhibit increased appetite and craving for fatty food, as well as increased caloric intake and snacking, which may be associated with increased disinhibition. Limited evidence from neuroimaging studies suggested that AP-naïve first episode patients exhibit similar neural processing of food to healthy controls, while chronic AP exposure may lead to decreased activity in satiety areas and increased activity in areas associated with reward anticipation. Overall, this review supports the notion that AP use can lead to disturbed eating patterns in patients, which may contribute to AP-induced weight gain. However, intrinsic illness-related effects on eating behaviors remain less well elucidated, and many confounding factors as well as variability in study designs limits interpretation of existing literature in this field and precludes firm conclusions from being made.

Keywords: food intake; eating behaviour; diet; overconsumption; binge eating; weight gain; obesity; hedonic pathway; homeostatic pathway

1. Introduction

Psychosis is the hallmark feature of various psychiatric illnesses, including schizophrenia (SCZ), schizoaffective disorder, schizophreniform disorder and bipolar disorder [1]. It is a severely debilitating condition with an estimated worldwide prevalence of approximately 4.6 per 1000 people [2]. The American Psychiatric Association and World Health Organization have conceptualized psychosis as consisting of altered perception and impaired reality testing, including positive symptoms such as hallucinations and delusions [3]. Severe mental illnesses additionally are associated with cognitive deficits and negative symptoms, which can drive functional impairment and illness associated disability [4,5].

Antipsychotic (AP) medications are currently the cornerstone treatment for psychotic disorders [6]. Unfortunately, APs are associated with serious metabolic adverse effects [7], which increase patients' risk of developing metabolic syndrome, type 2 diabetes, and cardiovascular disease (CVD). Notably, CVD is the leading cause of premature mortality in severe mental illness, reducing life expectancy by 11–20 years [8–10]. While clozapine and olanzapine carry the greatest metabolic liability [11], all AP medications cause weight gain in younger patients with limited previous AP exposure [12]. Similarly, these medications have been shown, independently of class or individual agent, to increase risk of type 2 diabetes in patients with SCZ [10].

Weight gain, a common consequence of AP treatment, occurs when there is a positive energy balance, meaning that energy intake exceeds energy expenditure [13]. Beyond the metabolic effect of APs, weight gain in psychotic disorders is also, in part, explained by unfavorable behaviours. For instance, patients with SCZ may have higher intake of calorie dense foods and lower intake of healthy foods than the general population [14]. Other contributing factors include lower levels of physical activity and significantly higher rates of smoking and alcohol consumption [15]. All these behaviours are also associated with lower socioeconomic status and higher unemployment among patients with SCZ [15,16]. Furthermore, epidemiological reviews have suggested that approximately 10% of patients with SCZ suffer from binge eating disorder (BED) or night eating syndromes, which is five times higher than in the general population [17]. Thus, disturbed eating behaviour may also contribute to the significant weight gain and metabolic disturbances experienced by these patients.

Looking beyond social, environmental and behavioural factors, energy homeostasis is controlled by intricate physiological pathways. Patients with SCZ may have subclinical metabolic dysregulations including dyslipidemia [18], hyperglycemia and insulin resistance [19] present at the earliest stages of the illness, which are further exacerbated by AP therapy [20,21]. Furthermore, impaired regulation of appetite related hormones including elevated insulin (linked with insulin resistance) and low leptin and adiponectin (secreted by adipose tissue) levels are also implicated in the pathophysiology of weight gain in psychosis spectrum disorders [18,22]. Ghrelin, which stimulates hunger, does not appear to be altered in AP-naïve or largely unmedicated first episode psychosis (FEP) patients [18]; however, olanzapine use may be associated with decreased ghrelin levels, which is a similar phenomenon to what is observed in obesity [23].

While the physiological homeostatic mechanisms underlying altered eating patterns in this population have been the subject of recent meta-analyses and reviews [18,20], less is known about the psychopathological and neurobiological mechanisms that may be implicated in the non-homeostatic regulation of food intake. Non-homeostatic eating behaviour involves the hedonic and reward aspects of food intake that is separate from the physiological drive stimulated by energy requirement [24]. This aspect of eating behaviour is regulated by the reward system, which includes the mesolimbic dopamine circuit (involving the ventral tegmental area and nucleus accumbens), as well as nuclei in the amygdala and hippocampus that are interconnected to the hypothalamus and brainstem (the latter implicated in homeostatic feeding regulation) [25]. Disruption at any level of these complex neural networks regulating eating behaviour may be implicated in the weight gain and metabolic sequalae associated with SCZ. Moreover, these disruptions are likely to involve aspects intrinsic to

SCZ, and/or associated with AP treatment [26]. The reward and limbic pathways involved in eating behavior and appetite are depicted in Figure 1 in more detail.

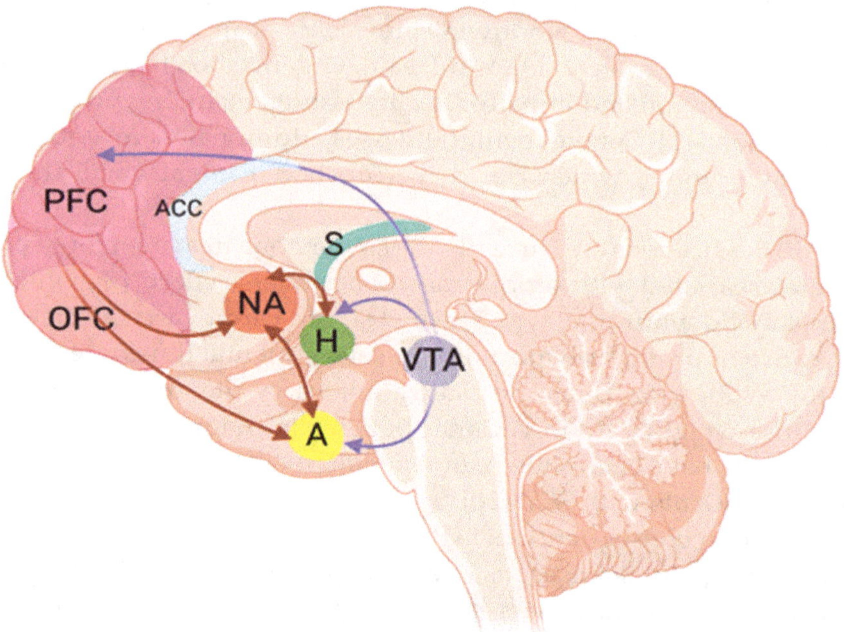

Figure 1. Limbic and reward pathways involved in eating behaviour and appetite. Eating behavior is closely associated with activity of the reward circuitry of the brain, which involves a group of neuronal structures that become activated and release dopamine when exposed to rewarding stimuli like food [27]. The pathway most associated with reward circuitry of the brain is referred to as the mesolimbic dopamine pathway, which starts with production and release of dopamine in the ventral tegmental area (VTA). The mesolimbic dopamine pathway then relays VTA signaling to the nucleus accumbens (NA), an area associated with motivation. The other aspect of the reward system is known as the mesocortical pathway which connects the VTA to the prefrontal cortex (PFC). This region also includes the orbitofrontal cortex (OFC), a key area involved in cognitive processes, such as decision making and memory. The PFC additionally forms connections with sensory and limbic pathways as well. Importantly, the reward pathway is activated, both before and after receipt of a reward suggesting that dopamine increases reward seeking behavior. Thus, any disruption of these pathways could potentially lead to disordered eating behavior. The VTA is also functionally and anatomically connected to the hypothalamus (H), primarily the lateral hypothalamus. The hypothalamus integrates homeostatic signals from various peripheral organs along with reward responses to modulate food intake and energy expenditure according to changes in metabolic state [28]. The arcuate nucleus of the hypothalamus (not shown), where neuropeptide Y (orexigenic) and proopiomelanocortin (anorexigenic) producing neurons reside, is the main area responsible for energy sensing and eating behavior. VTA, ventral tegmental area; NA, nucleus accumbens; H, hypothalamus; PFC, prefrontal cortex; OFC, orbitofrontal cortex; A, amygdala; ACC, anterior cingulate gyrus; S, striatum.

Given the high metabolic comorbidity observed in psychosis spectrum disorders, elucidating the psychopathological and neurobiological mechanisms underlying disrupted eating behaviours is crucial in helping to improve both the physical and psychological well-being of patients. In this scoping review, we aim to provide a comprehensive overview of disordered eating behaviours observed in psychosis spectrum disorders. We synthesize evidence from clinical studies employing self-report questionnaires and surveys to measure changes in food intake, craving and appetite, as well as behavioural neuroimaging studies to further explore the neurobiological mechanisms underlying these disturbances in eating patterns. In an attempt to distinguish illness intrinsic effects from those caused by treatment with APs, we present separately, when possible, results from studies examining

AP-naïve patients (vs. matched healthy controls), and healthy controls (HCs) or AP-naïve patients beginning APs.

2. Methods

Our protocol was developed using the scoping review methodological framework proposed by the Joanna Briggs Institute [29]. The objectives, inclusion criteria and methods for this scoping review were specified in advance and documented in a protocol.

2.1. Search Strategy

An a priori search strategy was developed and tested in consultation with the Education and Liaison Librarian for the Institute of Medical Science at the University of Toronto. Databases searched included Ovid MEDLINE, Ovid EMBASE, Ovid PsychINFO, EBSCO's CINAHL, CENTRAL on Wiley and Scopus. A grey literature search was also performed by mining references from relevant articles and review papers identified in the search, as well as searching SCOPUS for conference proceedings. Vocabulary and syntax were adjusted across databases. There were no language, date or methodology restrictions, with the exception of case studies and opinion pieces, which were excluded from the results. The specific search string for each database can be found in Supplementary Table S1.

2.2. Source of Evidence Screening and Study Selection

Article screening, including automatic duplicate removal, was completed using Covidence [30]. Two authors independently screened and assessed titles and abstracts (NS and AG), while another two independently completed the full-text screening (ES and RA). Conflicts were resolved by discussion and consensus between the authors and in consultation with the senior authors (SMA and MH). At all stages, screening decisions were made according to prespecified inclusion and exclusion criteria which are outlined in Table 1.

Table 1. List of inclusion and exclusion criteria for selected studies.

Inclusion Criteria	Exclusion Criteria
1. Schizophrenia or other Schizophrenia Spectrum Disorders a. First episode patients (FEP) b. Chronic c. AP-naïve 2. Psychosis, psychotic disorders 3. Bipolar disorder 4. Eating disorders a. Bulimia nervosa b. Binge eating disorder c. Night eating syndrome 5. Food addiction 6. Behavioral studies a. Neuroimaging b. Questionnaires 7. Antipsychotics a. First Generation Antipsychotics (FGA)/typical b. Second Generation Antipsychotics (SGA)/atypical	1. Any psychiatric diagnosis not listed in the inclusion criteria (e.g., major depression disorder, anxiety disorders) included as the primary population of interest 2. Off-label AP use 3. Opinion pieces, letters 4. Treatment studies of APs for Anorexia Nervosa 5. At-risk/subclinical psychosis/psychotic-like experiences included as primary population of interest 6. Purely physiological studies (i.e., no behavioural/appetite measures) 7. Pre-clinical studies (mice/rodent, other non-human animals)

2.3. Charting the Data

A data extraction template was created and piloted among study authors (NS, ES, RA) and was refined and finalized based on data extracted from a sample of studies. The information displayed in Table 2 was extracted from each included full-text article.

Table 2. List of information extracted from each full-text article meeting inclusion criteria.

	Extracted Data
1.	Author(s)
2.	Year of publication
3.	Origin/country or ethnicity of participants
4.	Aims/purpose
5.	Type of study
6.	Population and sample size within the source of evidence (if applicable)
7.	Population demographics (Sex/gender, age)
8.	Methodology/methods
9.	Intervention type, comparator and details of these (e.g., duration of the intervention) (if applicable). Duration of the intervention (if applicable)
10.	Outcomes and details of these (e.g., how measured) (if applicable)
11.	Key findings that relate to the scoping review question/s and concepts

2.4. Synthesis and Presentation of Results

Studies were summarized and presented according to their relevant category: (1) Studies describing eating patterns, food preferences and diet composition using dietary recall, food diaries and food frequency questionnaires; (2) studies measuring self-reported appetite, hunger and/or satiety using a mix of validated questionnaires and semi-structured interviews (see Table 3); and (3) studies using neuroimaging methodologies to assess neurobiological changes in relation to aspects of eating or food intake. A narrative summary of each study is reported in its respective subsection, with overlap in other subsections if applicable. Where appropriate, tables were created to concisely summarize characteristics of included studies and relevant findings (see Tables 4–6).

3. Results

3.1. Search Results

Our initial search revealed 3545 results, which was reduced to 2654 after removal of duplicates. Following title and abstract screening, 94 studies were assessed for full-text eligibility. A total of 35 studies that considered dietary composition, food preference and cravings and/or eating patterns in patients with SCZ or HCs exposed to APs were deemed eligible and included in our qualitative synthesis (Figure 2; preferred reporting items for systematic reviews and meta-analyses (PRISMA) flow diagram).

The studies identified in our search used a number of validated methodologies and questionnaires to examine different aspects of eating behavior. The most commonly employed subjective dietary assessments include food diaries, 24-h dietary recall, the Three Factor Eating Questionnaire (TFEQ), the Dutch Eating Behavior Questionnaire (DEBQ), visual analog scales (VAS), the Food Craving Inventory (FCI), the Food Craving Questionnaire (FCQ) and the Food Frequency Questionnaire (FFQ). The TFEQ addresses three aspects of eating behaviour including restriction of food intake, loss of control of food intake and responsivity to internal hunger cues. Previous studies in the general population indicate that increased body weight is positively associated with TFEQ scores [31–33], particularly disinhibition and susceptibility to hunger [34–36]. The DEBQ is a self-report questionnaire designed to assess different factors regulating eating behaviour including desire to restrict food intake, tendency to eat in response to emotions and responsivity to external cues. Overweight and obese individuals generally display greater scores in all DEBQ domains compared to normal weight individuals [37–39], with the most robust relationship found for the emotional eating factor [37,39,40]. General hunger and appetite rating scales (VAS, and Likert scales) are also frequently employed to assess eating behaviour [41], while the FCQ and FCI are used to measure general and specific food cravings, respectively. A more detailed description of these questionnaires can be found in Table 3.

Table 3. Description of self-report questionnaires used to measure subjective appetite and eating behaviour; 'Original Source' indicates the authors who originally developed the questionnaire.

Name	Original Source	Description	Subscales and Other Relevant Information
Three-Factor Eating Questionnaire (TFEQ)	Stunkard and Messick, 1985 [42]	51-item questionnaire measuring three aspects of eating behaviour (cognitive restraint, disinhibition, hunger)	• Cognitive dietary restraint: active attempt to restrict caloric intake and control body weight • Disinhibition: likelihood of overeating when exposed to a favorable environment (e.g., palatable food) or stress • Susceptibility to hunger: susceptibility of individuals to perceive hunger and ingest food as a result; can be triggered by internal and external stimuli • High disinhibition and hunger scores associated with increased weight, obesity [34,35] and overconsumption/binge-eating (DSM-IV/DSM 5 criteria) [43,44])
Dutch Eating Behaviour Questionnaire (DEBQ)	Van Strien et al., 1986 [40]	33-item questionnaire measuring three factors that regulate eating behaviour (restraint, emotion, external factors)	• Restrained eating: the desire or intention to restrict food intake; correlated with TFEQ cognitive restraint • Emotional eating: the tendency to eat in response to negative emotions; associated with overconsumption and obesity; positively correlated with TFEQ disinhibition [35,38,45] • External eating: the tendency to eat in response to environmental triggers and food cues; differs between overweight and normal weight individuals but does not appear to be predictive of weight gain [37,39,45]
Visual Analog Scale (VAS)	Stubbs et al., 2000 (review) [46]	Psychometric tool used to quantify subjective appetite	• The most common method used in appetite research includes a horizontal (100-mm) line anchored by two extremes such as "not at all hungry/as hungry as I've ever felt" • Sensitive to experimental manipulations (e.g., dietary composition, levels of food intake, medication effects) • Best used in conjunction with more objective measures such as calorie intake or physiological changes
Food Craving Questionnaire (FCQ)	Cepeda-Benito et al., 2000 [47]	Questionnaire measuring general food cravings (trait and state version)	• FCQ-Trait (FCQ-T): 9 factors measuring general food cravings and tendencies • FCQ-State (FCQ-S): 5 factors measuring food cravings in response to situational factors • Higher cravings are associated with binge eating and overconsumption • FCQ scores are positively correlated with TFEQ disinhibition and hunger scores

Table 3. *Cont.*

Name	Original Source	Description	Subscales and Other Relevant Information
Food Craving Inventory (FCI)	White et al., 2002 [48]	Questionnaire measuring specific food cravings (carbohydrates, sweets, fats, fast-food fats)	• Considers both intensity and frequency of food cravings, where craving is defined as "an intense desire to consume a particular food (or food type) that is difficult to resist" • Fat craving associated with increased BMI • Positively correlated with TFEQ disinhibition and hunger scores (stronger effect for hunger)
Drug-Related Eating Behavior Questionnaire (DR-EBQ)	Lim et al., 2008 [49]	14-item questionnaire that quantifies changes in appetite, craving and eating behaviour after beginning antipsychotic treatment	• Statements cover feelings of hunger, pre-occupations with food, desire to eat, control of eating and food cravings [50] • For each statement, patients indicate whether the frequency of behaviour/cravings have increased since starting AP therapy using a Likert scale
Questionnaire on Eating and Weight Patterns (QEWP)	Spitzer et al., 1993 [51]	Questionnaire used to evaluate the presence of binge-eating symptomatology and binge-eating related disorders	• Developed using DSM-IV criteria for BED/BN and validated using clinical assessments • Can be used to diagnose BED and BN (purging or non-purging type) • Statements cover social impairment, body image, history of dieting, comorbidities (e.g., depression, alcohol/drug abuse, sexual abuse), compensatory behaviours
Mizes Anorectic Cognitions Questionnaire—Revised (MAC-R)	Mizes et al., 2000 [52]	24-item questionnaire used to assess eating disorder-related cognitions (anorexia nervosa, bulimia nervosa, binge eating disorder)	• Covers three aspects: weight regulation, approval and self-control; statements rated on a 5-point Likert scale (higher scores represent greater dysfunction)

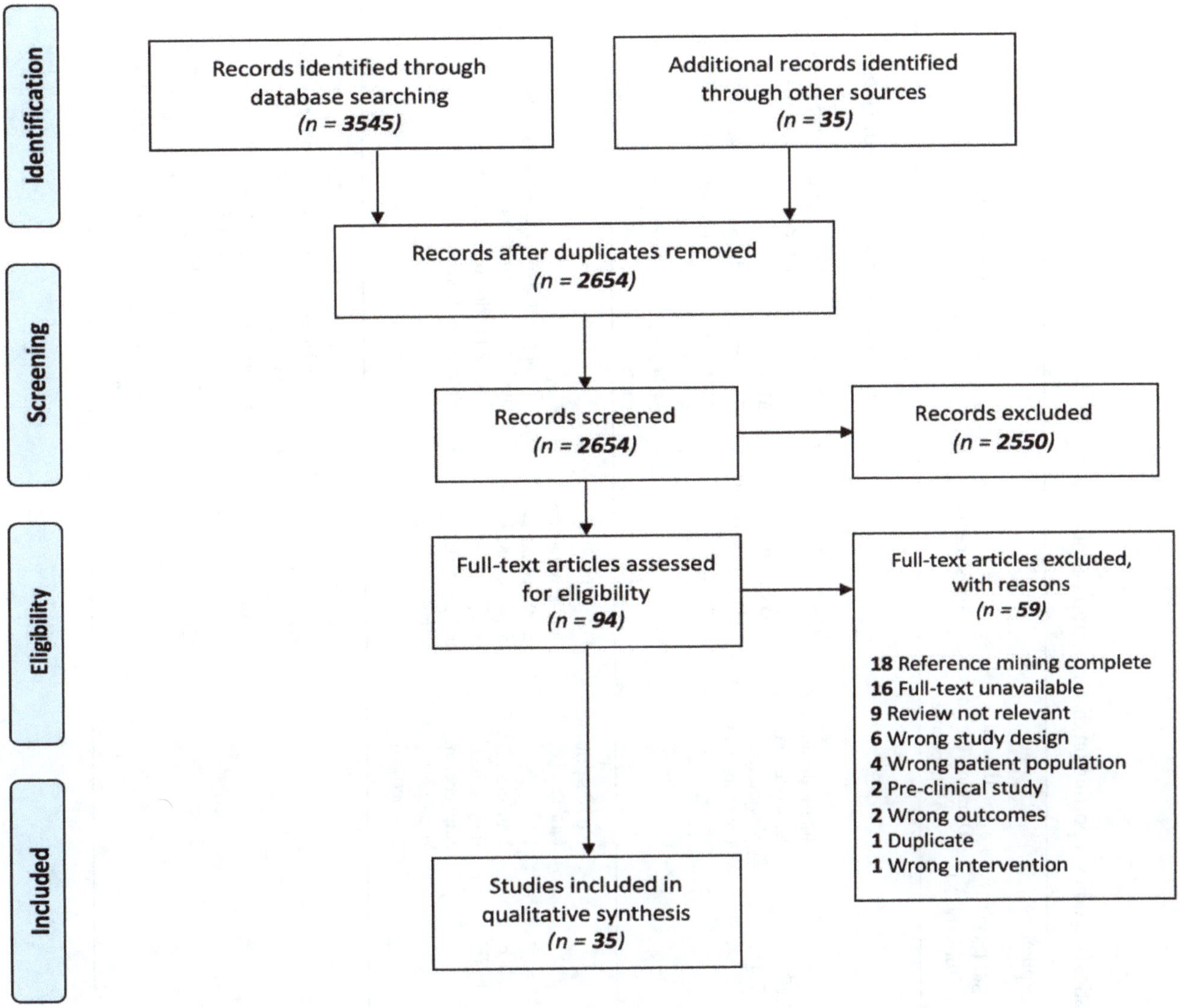

Figure 2. Preferred reporting items for systematic reviews and meta-analyses (PRISMA) flowchart. Literature search and selection process of included studies.

Our search yielded 9 studies that described dietary composition (summarized in Section 1 below); 19 studies that looked at eating patterns and food-related cognitions (summarized in Section 2 below); and 7 studies that used neuroimaging methodologies (summarized in Section 3 below). In order to facilitate elucidation of the specific effects of illness vs. APs, we have divided the results within each of the three methodology-based sections into three subsections based on population type: Patients only, patients (specifying AP-naïve cohorts) vs. controls and HCs exposed to APs.

3.2. *Findings from Subjective Food Preference and Dietary Composition Studies*

We retrieved nine studies that measured dietary composition and food preference using 24-h dietary recall, food diaries and the Food Frequency Questionnaire (FFQ) [53]. Only two studies indicated that part of the patient population studied were AP-naïve, although no subgroup analyses for these patients were available [54]. Table 4 summarizes the characteristics of included studies in this section, along with main findings.

Table 4. Characteristics of studies reporting on dietary composition.

Study	Study Description					Main Significant Results
	Design/Aim	Sample (Size, Diagnosis), Mean Age (Years), Mean BMI (kg/m^2)	Sex (% F), Race/Ethnicity (%)	Illness Duration/Previous AP Exposure	Assessments	
Amani 2007 [55]	Cross-sectional (case-control) Dietary preference in patients with SCZ compared to HC	30 SCZ inpatients, 16–76 years Age: 32.3 (M), 32.5 (F) BMI: 22 (M), 26 (F) 30 HCs (matched for age, sex) Age: 35.6 (M), 36.6 (F) BMI: 25.6 (M), 25.4 (F)	SCZ: 37% F HC: 47% F	Illness duration: at least one year; previous AP exposure not stated	Dietary recall (FFQ) Food Guide Pyramid to calculate dietary scores	Females: • Dietary scores ↓ and percent body fat ↑ for patients than HCs. • Consumed ↑ carbonated drinks, but ↓ milk, vegetables and nuts daily than the HCs Males: • Patients ate ↑ hydrogenated fats and full-fat cream, but ↓ red meats, vegetable oils and nuts servings per day than HCs • Male patients ate ↑ vegetables, eggs, cream and chocolate than female patients
Eder 2001 [56]	Longitudinal (8 weeks) Association of olanzapine induced weight gain with an increase in body fat	10 SCZ in patients treated with OLA monotherapy Dose range: 7.5–20 mg/d Age: 30.4 BMI: 22.4 10 HCs (matched for age, sex) Age: 35.2 BMI: 22.1	SCZ: 20% F HC: 20% F	No APs prior to OLA: 5 Previous APs: 5 (flupentixol, fluphenazine, risperidone, or haloperidol)	Semi-standardized structured interview to assess changes in eating behaviour and physical activity	• 70% of patients reported they ingested a significantly greater amount of food than usual during a period of time throughout the study • No change in physical activity
Fountaine 2010 [53]	Randomized, placebo controlled, two treatment crossover study (15 + 15 days, 12-day washout between arms) Comparing food intake and energy expenditure following olanzapine vs. placebo in healthy men	30 male HCs (21 completers) Age: 27 (range: 18–49) BMI: 22.6	All Males	N/A	Food intake monitored and weighed REE, daily activity level	• Mean total food intake in OLA group ↑ 18% (from 3860 kcal to 4230 kcal) relative to PBO • Mean weight change with OLA: 4.1 kg • 43.9% of patients experienced clinically significant weight gain (≥ 7%) • Early significant weight gain after 2 months of therapy occurred in 23.4% of the patients • ↑ REE and respiratory quotient with OLA compared to PBO

Table 4. *Cont.*

Study	Study Description					Main Significant Results
	Design/Aim	Sample (Size, Diagnosis), Mean Age (Years), Mean BMI (kg/m^2)	Sex (% F), Race/Ethnicity (%)	Illness Duration/Previous AP Exposure	Assessments	
Gattere 2018 [57]	Cross-sectional Dietary intake in early psychosis	124 early psychotic disorder (PD), 82 (66.1%) FEP patients with <5 years from illness onset Schizophreniform: $n = 22$ Schizoaffective: $n = 12$ Psychotic disorder NOS: $n = 70$ Age: 24.7 BMI: 24.3 36 at-risk mental state (ARMS) Age: 22.2 BMI: 22.2 62 HCs (not matched) Age: 23.5 BMI: 22.2	PD: 34.7% F; 76.6% Caucasian, 9.7% Latino American, 8.1% Arabian, 4.0% Gypsy, 0.8% Black, 0.8% Asian ARMS: 27.8% F; 88.9% Caucasian, 8.3% Latino American, 2.8 Arabian HC: 48.4% F; 95.2% Caucasian, 3.2% Latino America, 1.6% Arabian	PD: Monotherapy: 72 (58.1%) RIS = 31 PAL = 13 OLA = 17 QUE = 1 ARI = 10 Combination: 33 (26.6%) No APs: 19 (15.3%) ARMS: Monotherapy: 7 (19.4%) RIS = 1 OLA = 3 ARI = 3 Combination: 3 (8.3%) No APs: 27 (75%)	24-h dietary recall Food Craving (FCQ-State) IPAQ-short form	• Patients consumed ↑ calories/day and % of calories from saturated fatty acids than HCs • Patients consumed ↓ protein than HCs • Trend towards increased food craving scores (Food Craving Questionnaire; FCQ) with increasing psychopathology (psychotic disorders > at risk mental states > controls) • Both patient groups (PD and ARMS) reported reduced physical activity compared to HCs
Gothelf 2002 [54]	Longitudinal (4 weeks) Food intake and weight gain in adolescent males with SCZ treated with OLA vs. HAL	20 male SCZ inpatients OLA: $n = 10$ (MD: 14 mg/d) HAL: $n = 10$ (MD: 6.5 mg/d) Age (both): 17 BMI (OLA only): 24.5	All Males	OLA: mean washout period = 17.6 days Drug naïve = 1 Clomipramine = 1 AP other than OLA = 8	Dietary Evaluation (2-day monitoring of food intake by dietician; food weighed) Daily energy expenditure, REE, physical activity	• BMI ↑ greater for OLA than HAL • ↑ caloric intake (27.7%) in OLA group. • No changes in dietary composition (carbohydrates, fats, or proteins), REE or physical activity levels

Table 4. *Cont.*

Study	Study Description					Main Significant Results
	Design/Aim	Sample (Size, Diagnosis), Mean Age (Years), Mean BMI (kg/m^2)	Sex (% F), Race/Ethnicity (%)	Illness Duration/Previous AP Exposure	Assessments	
Nunes 2014 [58]	Cross-sectional (case-control) Evaluating nutritional status, food intake and cardiovascular disease risk in SCZ patients	25 SCZ outpatients Age: 40.5 (range: 18–59) BMI: 29.09 25 HCs (matched for age, sex, BMI) Age: 37.2 BMI: 26.91 Total sample Age: 38.9 BMI: 28.0	SCZ: 40% F HC: 48% F	SGA = 68% FGA = 28% Both = 4%	Dietary recall (FFQ)	• Patients consumed ↑ total calories, calories per kg body weight, protein per kg body weight, and % of carbohydrates and trans fatty acids • Patients consumed ↓ saturated fat, unsaturated fat and omega−6
Strassnig 2003 [59]	Cross-sectional (case-control) Exploring potential causes of weight gain in SCZ patients compared to general population (NHANES III)	146 outpatients with psychosis SCZ, paranoid type: $n = 69$ Schizoaffective: $n = 53$ Psychotic disorder NOS: $n = 24$ Age: 43 BMI: 32.7 Patient data compared to general population (NHANES III)	47% F 54% White, 46% Black	NR	24-h dietary recall	• Patients consumed ↑ total calories, fats and carbohydrates compared to general population (NHANES III). • Relative proportion of each food group (carbohydrates, fat, protein) did not differ between groups.
Stefanska 2017 [60]	Cross-sectional Eating habits and nutritional status in patients with SCZ and affective disorders	60 SCZ, 18–67 years Age: 34.1 (M), 41.3 (F) BMI: 27.6 (M), 27.2 (F) 61 recurrent depressive disorder, 18–67 years Age: 38.0 (M), 46.4 (F) BMI: 26.1 (M), 26.7 (F) 98 HCs (not matched), Age: 33.0 (M), 43.0 (F) (range: 18–69 years) BMI: 27.3 (M), 25.8 (F)	SCZ: 53.3% F Depression: 54.1% F HCs: 61.2% F	AP treatment (FGA or SGA) for at least one year (AP type not specified) Age at onset: 23.3 (M), 30.1 (F) Illness duration (years): 9.5 (M), 10.4 (F)	24-h dietary recall Resting metabolic rate (RMR)	• Patients consumed ↑ fat (with a predominance of saturated fatty acids over polyunsaturated fatty acids), and ↓ protein than HCs • Lower energy intake promoted lower BMI, waist circumference, waist-to-hip ratio and body fat • Female SCZ patients consumed ↑carbohydrates and % of energy from carbohydrates compared to female HCs • Male SCZ patients consumed ↑ fat, particularly saturated fatty acids compared to male HCsb

Table 4. *Cont.*

Study	Study Description					Main Significant Results
	Design/Aim	Sample (Size, Diagnosis), Mean Age (Years), Mean BMI (kg/m^2)	Sex (% F), Race/Ethnicity (%)	Illness Duration/Previous AP Exposure	Assessments	
Stefanska 2018 [61]	Cross-sectional (case-control) Assessing the nutritional value males consumed by patients with SCZ	85 SCZ outpatients, 18–65 years Age: 37.8 (M), 39.0 (F) BMI: 25.0 (M), 25.1 (F) 70 HCs (not matched) Age: 35.9 (M), 38.2 (F) BMI: 25.9 (M), 24.4 (F)	SCZ: 52.9% F HC: 57.1% F	AP treatment (FGA or SGA) for at least one year (AP type not specified) 1 AP = 39% 2 or 3 APs = 61% Age at onset: 26.7 (M), 273 (F) Illness duration (years): 10.0 (M), 12.3 (F)	24-h dietary recall	• ↑ snacking in patients than HCs • Female SCZ patients consumed ↑ calories and showed an ↑preference for sweets than HCs • Male SCZ patients had ↓ energy intake and content of the majority of assessed nutrients compared to HCs

Note: All main findings reported in this table are statistically significant unless otherwise indicated. SCZ = Schizophrenia, BP = Bipolar Disorder. HC = Healthy controls, FEP: First episode psychosis, AMI = amisulpride, PBO = Placebo, OLA = olanzapine, PAL = Paliperidone, HAL = Haloperidol, RIS = Risperidone, QUE = Quetiapine, ZIP = Ziprasidone, CPZ = Chlorpromazine, FGA = First generation antipsychotics, SGA = Second generation antipsychotic, NR = Not reported, TFEQ = Three-Factor Eating Questionnaire, FCQ = Food Craving Questionnaire, FCI = Food Craving Inventory, VAS = visual analog scale, DR-EBQ = Drug-Related Eating Behaviour Questionnaire, FFQ = Food Frequency Questionnaire, EBA = Eating Behaviour Assessment, DEBQ = Dutch Eating Behaviour Questionnaire, QEWP = Questionnaire on Eating and Weight Patterns, MD = Mean Dose.

3.2.1. Patients vs. Healthy Controls

Seven of the included dietary composition studies compared patients with healthy controls [55–61]; of these studies, only three matched patients to HCs according to key baseline features, such as age, sex and BMI [55,56,58].

Three cross-sectional studies [57–59] revealed that patients consumed significantly more total calories per day than HCs. However, results regarding specific dietary composition (carbohydrates, fat, protein) were less consistent, with the authors reporting either increased protein consumption and decreased saturated fat consumption by patients [58], decreased protein consumption and a trend towards increased saturated fat [57] or no difference between patients and controls [59]. Gattere et al. (2018) noted a trend towards increased scores on the FCQ with increasing psychopathology (psychotic disorders > at risk mental states > controls), suggestive of a relationship between food cravings and disease state, while Nunes et al. (2014) found no significant association between body mass index (BMI) and antipsychotic type (FGA, SGA).

The three remaining case-control studies also noted differences in nutritional patterns between patients and HCs, including increased fat consumption and more frequent snacking in patients [57,62]. Interestingly, these studies also stratified their results by sex, revealing differences in dietary composition and eating behaviour such as snack preference and calorie intake. Details of the differences between males and females are reported in Table 4. Beyond sex effects, Stefanska et al. (2017) also found that in the patient group, lower caloric intake was associated with lower BMI, waist circumference, waist-to-hip ratio and body fat content [60].

The final study included in this section explored eating behaviour differences between HCs and patients with SCZ on OLA treatment. This study revealed that that 70% of the OLA-treated patients reported ingesting a significantly greater amount of food than usual, with no compensatory increase in physical activity levels [56].

3.2.2. Patients Only

Only one dietary composition study explored the effects of APs on food intake and energy expenditure in patients [54]. The study was conducted in males only and compared patients treated with olanzapine to those treated with haloperidol. After four weeks, the olanzapine group experienced a significant increase in BMI and caloric intake, but no difference in dietary composition, energy expenditure or physical activity level. Important to note is that, similar to the aforementioned study by Eder et al. (2001) [56], physical activity levels were low [54], suggesting that olanzapine may lead to weight gain through a combination of increased caloric intake and decreased physical activity.

3.2.3. Healthy Controls Only

Consistent with the patient-only studies discussed above, an HC study conducted by Fountaine et al. revealed that volunteers randomized to receive olanzapine gained more weight and consumed significantly more calories than those randomized to placebo [53]. Interestingly, this weight gain was accompanied by an increase in resting energy expenditure and a trend towards increased physical activity in the olanzapine group, which the authors hypothesize may have occurred to compensate for the increase in caloric intake.

3.3. Findings from Subjective/Self-Report Questionnaires on Appetite, Satiety and Craving

In total, there were 19 studies [50,62–79] that examined differences in eating behaviour, subjective appetite and food craving using self-reported questionnaires and interviews. Table 5 presents a detailed summary of these studies. Seven studies specifically considered DSM-IV diagnostic and research criteria for eating disorders (EDs) including binge eating disorder (BED); Section 2.1) [62–68], while the remainder of the studies assessed subjective appetite and/or eating-related cognitions (Section 2.2) [50,69–74,76,77].

Table 5. Characteristics of studies reporting on subjective ratings of appetite, craving and hunger.

Study	Study Description					Main Significant Results
	Design/Aim	**Sample (Size, Diagnosis), Mean Age (Years), Mean BMI (kg/m^2)**	**Sex (% F), Race/Ethnicity**	**Mean Illness Duration/Previous AP Exposure (*n*)**	**Assessments**	
Bromel 1998 [63]	Longitudinal (10 weeks) Effect of CLZ on food craving in patients with SCZ	12 SCZ in patients treated with CLZ (MD: 273 mg/d; range: 81–475 mg/d) SCZ: $n = 9$ FGA: $n = 3$ Age: 31 (range: 18–65) BMI: 25.8	50% F	Nine patients treated with psychotropic medication (including APs) prior to starting CLZ (type/duration of previous exposure not specified)	Binge eating/ED symptomatology (DSM-IV) Binary appetite/craving scale	• CLZ treatment ↑ weight, BMI and adiposity • 75% (9/12) of patients reported ↑ appetite/hunger and specific food cravings • 17% (2/12) of patients reported onset of binge eating behaviour • One patient saw remittance and re-occurrence of binge eating after discontinuing and then restarting CLZ
Gebhardt 2007 [64]	Longitudinal (retrospective) Binge-eating symptomatology associated with CLZ and OLA use in patients with psychosis	64 patients being treated for psychotic symptoms with CLZ or OLA SCZ: 52.3% SCZ spectrum disorder: 12.3% Mood disorder: 18.5% Substance abuse: 7.7% Personality disorder: 3.1% Other diagnoses: 7.7% Age: 30.7 (range: 13.3–64.6)	47% F	Patients were treated with CLZ or OLA for at least 4 weeks prior to inclusion in study CLZ: $n = 33$ OLA: $n = 31$	QEWP (DSM-IV binge-eating) Adverse drug reaction (ADR) scale Appetite (4-point Likert-type scale)	• 69% of patients experienced an increase in appetite after starting CLZ/OLA, with a stronger effect for CLZ • Post-CLZ/OLA weight gain was associated with ↑ appetite • 14% of patients met DSM-IV criteria for BED or bulimia nervosa • ED onset was "definitely" or "probably" linked to CLZ/OLA exposure (Naranjo probability) • Post-CLZ/OLA EDs were more common in patients with a history of EDs
Kluge 2007 [65]	Randomized, double blind, parallel (6 weeks) Effect of CLZ and OLA on food craving and binge eating in patients with SCZ spectrum disorders	30 SCZ ($n = 26$), Schizoaffective ($n = 3$), Schizophreniform ($n = 1$) inpatients, 18–65 years CLZ: $n = 15$ OLA: $n = 15$ Age: 36.7 (CLZ), 32.8 (OLA) BMI: 25.4 (CLZ), 24.4 (OLA) Dosing (last 4 weeks of study): mean modal dose = 266.7 mg (CLZ), 21.2 mg (OLA)	CLZ: 53% F OLA: 67% F	Age of illness onset: 30 (CLZ), 28 (OLA)	Binge eating/ED symptomatology (DSM-IV) Binary appetite/craving scale	• CLZ/OLA treatment ↑ body weight and BMI • 97% (29/30) of patients reported ↑ appetite and 90% (27/30) reported ↑ food intake • Patients experienced ↑ binge eating and craving for sweet and fatty foods, with no significant effect of gender

Table 5. *Cont.*

Study	Study Description					Main Significant Results
	Design/Aim	Sample (Size, Diagnosis), Mean Age (Years), Mean BMI (kg/m^2)	Sex (% F), Race/Ethnicity	Mean Illness Duration/Previous AP Exposure (*n*)	Assessments	
Theisen 2003 [66]	Cross-sectional (BE vs. non-BE) with an exploratory retrospective analysis Comparing binge eating symptomatology in patients with SCZ treated with clozapine and olanzapine	74 SCZ inpatients CLZ: $n = 57$ OLA: $n = 17$ Age: 19.8 (range: 15.6–26.6) Two sub-groups based on prevalence of binge eating behaviour Binge eating (BE): $n = 37$ Non-binge eating (non-BE): $n = 37$	36% F	Illness duration (years): 2.4 (range = 0.3–7.1)	QEWP (DSM-IV binge-eating)	• 26% (7/27) of females and 11% (5/47) of males met lifetime criteria for full BED or BN • In the BE group, 54% (20/37) of patients reported onset of binge eating episodes during the current CLZ/OLA regime • Patients in the BE group had ↑ current BMI and experienced ↑ weight gain from medication onset to time of study compared to those in the non-BE group
Treuer 2009 [67]	Longitudinal (6 months) Food intake and nutritional factors associated with weight gain in patients with SCZ and BD treated with OLA	622 SCZ or BD outpatients (589 completers) treated with OLA (MD: 11.4 mg/d; mean duration during study: 5.4 months) SCZ: 85% of sample BD: 15% of sample Age: 32.6 years BMI: 23.2	56% F Multinational (China, Romania, Mexico, Taiwan) 61% East Asian, 25% Caucasian, 14% Hispanic	Lifetime AP exposure: 74.5% of sample (duration not specified) Past 6 months: 45.2% of sample	Interview to assess appetite (5-point Likert), frequency of food consumption, subjective energy levels and physical activity	• 44% of patients experienced clinically significant weight gain (≥ 7%) • 49% of patients experienced ↑ appetite relative to baseline and 35% required more food to reach satiety • Weight gain was associated with ↑ frequency and quantity of food intake, ↑ preoccupation with food, and ↓ vigorous physical activity
Khazaal 2006a * [62]	Cross-sectional (case-control) Eating and weight related cognitions in patients with SCZ vs. HCs	40 SGA-treated SCZ outpatients Age: 33.8 40 HCs (matched for BMI) Age: 35.5 Two subgroups ($n = 20$) for each group: Overweight = BMI > 28 Comparison = BMI < 28	SCZ: 47.5% F HC: 52.5% F	Previous AP exposure (mean duration = 8.3 years): OLA, CLZ, QUE, RIS	Revised version of the Mizes Anorectic cognitive questionnaire (MAC-R)	• Patients had ↑ total MAC-R and weight regulation subscale scores relative to controls • Patients with BMI < 28 had ↑ MAC-R scores on all sub-scales compared to weight-matched controls • Females had ↑ MAC-R scores than men

Table 5. *Cont.*

Study	Study Description					Main Significant Results
	Design/Aim	Sample (Size, Diagnosis), Mean Age (Years), Mean BMI (kg/m^2)	Sex (% F), Race/Ethnicity	Mean Illness Duration/Previous AP Exposure (n)	Assessments	
Khazaal 2006b * [68]	Cross-sectional (case-control) Binge eating symptomatology in overweight and obese patients with SCZ vs. HCs	40 SGA-treated SCZ outpatients Age: 33.8 40 HCs (matched for BMI) Age: 35.5 Two subgroups (n = 20) for each group: Overweight = BMI > 28 Comparison = BMI < 28	SCZ: 47.5% F HC: 52.5% F	NR	Binge eating/ED symptomatology (DSM-IV)	• ↑ prevalence of binge-eating symptoms and full BED in SCZ patients with BMI > 28 compared to weight-matched controls
Garriga 2019 [69]	Longitudinal (18 weeks) Effect of CLZ on food craving and consumption in patients with SMI	34 SMI patients SCZ: n = 27 Schizoaffective: n = 5 BD: n = 2 Age: 36.8 (range: 18–65) BMI: 27.3 Dosing: CLZ was initiated with a dose of 12.5–25 mg in the first day of treatment, followed by weekly upward adjustments of 25–50 mg (i.e., standard titration) Two subgroups: Normal weight (NW) = BMI < 25, n = 13 Overweight/obese (OWO) = BMI > 25, n = 21	38% F	Previous AP exposure (mean duration = 8.5 years): SGA = 28 (82.4%) FGA = 3 (8.8%) None = 3 (8.8%)	Food Craving (FCI, Spanish version) Cuestionario de Frecuencia de Consumo de Alimentos (CFCA)	• No significant longitudinal changes in food craving or consumption, however moderating effects of baseline BMI and gender were observed • In the NW group, ↑ cravings for "complex carbohydrates/proteins" and "simple sugar/trans fat" were associated with male gender and recent onset psychosis • NW males had ↑ craving for "fast-food fats" at both time points compared to NW females • In the OWO group, ↑ "fast-food fats" craving at Week 18 was associated with recent onset of psychosis • In both groups, craving scores (FCI) were positively correlated with frequency of consumption (CFCA)

Table 5. *Cont.*

Study	Study Description					Main Significant Results
	Design/Aim	Sample (Size, Diagnosis), Mean Age (Years), Mean BMI (kg/m^2)	Sex (% F), Race/Ethnicity	Mean Illness Duration/Previous AP Exposure (n)	Assessments	
Karagianis 2009 [70]	Randomized, double blind, double dummy study (16 weeks) Effect of OLA on BMI, efficacy scores, weight and subjective appetite in patients with SMI	149 OLA-treated outpatients (115 completers) SCZ: n = 82 BD: n = 41 Schizoaffective: n = 15 Schizophreniform: n = 9 Other related disorder: n = 2 Age: 39 (range: 18–65) BMI: 28.1 Two treatment groups: Orally disintegrating OLA (ODO): n = 84 (MD: 13.87 mg/d) Standard OLA tablets (SOT): n = 65 (MD: 13.23 mg/d)	46% F 52.3% Caucasian, 33.6% Hispanic, 10.1% Black, 2.0% Asian, 1.3% First-nation, 0.7% Other	Previous AP exposure: 5–20 mg/day SOT (duration 4–52 weeks)	Hunger/appetite scale (VAS)	• Patients in both groups experienced ↑ BMI, • Patients in both groups experienced a non-significant trend towards ↓ hunger/appetite
Ryu 2013 [50]	Longitudinal (12 weeks) Effect of SGA treatment on eating behaviour in patients with SCZ	45 SCZ patients treated with SGA monotherapy OLA: n = 13 RIS: n = 24 ARI: n = 8 Age: 32.1 (range: 18–50)	50% F	Treated with current AP for 4–12 weeks (AP-free for 4 weeks prior to starting medication)	Binge eating/ED symptomatology (DSM-IV) Binary appetite/craving scale Food Craving (FCQ) DR-EBQ	• BMI ↑ over time • DR-EBQ total score was positively associated with weight gain and FCQ scores (“pre-occupation with food”, “loss of control”)
Smith 2012 [71]	Randomized trial (5 months) Effect of OLA and RIS on appetite in patients with chronic SCZ	46 SCZ inpatients OLA: n = 13 (MD: 25.2 mg/d) RIS: n = 17 (MD: 6.1 mg/d) Age: 41.2 (OLA), 42.5 (RIS)	2% F	All patients had been treated with multiple antipsychotics in the past	Hunger/appetite scale (VAS from 0–100) Eating Behavior Assessment (EBA)	• Neither medication had a significant effect on appetite, with a non-significant trend towards ↓ appetite • Both medications resulted in weight gain which was not correlated with changes in appetite (VAS) or eating behaviour (EBA)

Table 5. *Cont.*

Study	Study Description					Main Significant Results
	Design/Aim	Sample (Size, Diagnosis), Mean Age (Years), Mean BMI (kg/m^2)	Sex (% F), Race/Ethnicity	Mean Illness Duration/Previous AP Exposure (n)	Assessments	
Sentissi 2009 [72]	Cross-sectional (medication type) Effect of SGAs on eating behaviours and motivation in patients with SCZ	153 SCZ in- and outpatients SGA: $n = 93$ FGA: $n = 27$ Untreated: $n = 33$ Age: 33.1 (range: <50) BMI: 25.6 Among the untreated patients, 23 were AP-naïve, and 10 were AP-free for >3 months (mean duration: 7 months; range: 3–29 months)	38.6% F	SGA monotherapy: CLZ = 20 (MD: 374 mg/d) OLA = 23 (MD: 12 mg/d) AMI = 14 (MD: 571.4 mg/d) RIS = 20 (MD: 3.7 mg/d) ARI = 16 (MD: 11.9 mg/d) FGA: mainly HAL (n = 16, 59% of sample) or phenothiazines; MD = 289 mg/d (CPZ equivalents) Mean treatment duration (months): 36.2 (range = 3–86) Illness duration: 9.6 years	TFEQ DEBQ	• ↑ BMI was associated with ↑ TFEQ disinhibition (significant) and susceptibility to hunger (nearing significance) • SGA-treated patients displayed ↑ reactivity to external eating cues (DEBQ) compared to FGA-treated, but not untreated patients • Patients with both high restraint and high disinhibition were more likely to be overweight (significant) and to be treated with SGAs (nearing significance)

Table 5. *Cont.*

Study	Study Description					Main Significant Results
	Design/Aim	Sample (Size, Diagnosis), Mean Age (Years), Mean BMI (kg/m^2)	Sex (% F), Race/Ethnicity	Mean Illness Duration/Previous AP Exposure (*n*)	Assessments	
Abbas 2013 [73]	Cross-sectional (case-control) Food craving in OLA- or FGA-treated patients with SCZ vs. HCs	40 SCZ in- and outpatients OLA: n = 20 FGA: n = 20 Age (both): 39.4 (range: 18–65) BMI: 29.5 (OLA), 27.3 (FGA) 20 HCs (un-matched) Age: 40.9 BMI: 25.8	OLA: 45% F FGA: 55% F HC: 55% F	OLA (n = 20) or FGA (n = 20) for at least one month Flupentixol = 6 Zuclopenthixol acetate = 5 CPZ = 3 HAL = 2 Fluphenazine decanoate = 1 Pipotiazine palmitate = 1 Stelazine = 1 Trifluperazine = 1 Mean treatment duration (months): 15.1 (OLA), 19.7 (FGA)	Food Craving (FCI)	• No significant difference in food craving between patients and controls
Blouin 2008 [74]	Cross-sectional (case-control) Adiposity and post-meal challenge eating behaviours in SGA-treated patients with SCZ vs. HCs	18 SCZ outpatients Age: 30.5 (range: 18–65) BMI: 28.8 20 HCs (matched for age and physical activity) Age: 29.5 BMI: 25.0	All Males	Previous AP exposure: FGA or SGA (mean duration = 35.3 months) Current SGA treatment: at least 3 months (mean duration = 24.6 months) OLA = 9 QUE = 3 CLZ = 2 RIS = 2 ZIP = 2	TFEQ Hunger/Appetite Scale (150-mm VAS) Food preference test and spontaneous intake (food weighed) 12 h fast prior to standardized breakfast, followed by an ad libitum buffet-type meal ~3 h later	• Compared to HCs, patients reported ↑ subjective hunger and ↓ satiation following a standardized meal • Compared to HCs, patients displayed ↑ TFEQ scores in all three domains which remained significant after controlling for BMI • Among patients, susceptibility to hunger was positively associated with emotional susceptibility to disinhibition • No significant group differences in spontaneous intake or food preference during ad libitum conditions

Table 5. *Cont.*

Study	Study Description					Main Significant Results
	Design/Aim	Sample (Size, Diagnosis), Mean Age (Years), Mean BMI (kg/m^2)	Sex (% F), Race/Ethnicity	Mean Illness Duration/Previous AP Exposure (n)	Assessments	
Folley 2010 [75]	Cross-sectional (case-control) Relative food preferences and hedonic judgements in SGA-treated patients with SCZ vs. HCs	18 SCZ outpatients treated with SGAs (MD: 93.6 mg/d) Age: 40.5 (range: 21–58) 18 HCs (matched for education and intelligence scores) Age: 38.9 (range: 20–52)	SCZ: 33% F HC: 44% F	Illness duration: 16.4 years	Food preference and food ratings task (Extra scanner task, 5-point Likert scale); participants tested prior to eating lunch	• No significant group differences in response time or food preference during preference task • Both patients and controls were more likely to give positive vs. neutral or negative ratings to food stimuli • In patients, ↓ positive ratings were associated with ↑ anhedonia
Knolle-Veentjer 2008 [76]	Cross-sectional (case-control) Role of eating behaviour in body weight regulation in patients with SCZ vs. HCs	29 SCZ patients Paranoid subtype: n = 27 Disorganized subtype: n = 2 Age: 34 (range: 21–56) BMI: 26.8 23 HCs (matched for age, sex, educational level) Age: 32 (range: 20–58) BMI: 23.9	SCZ: 34.5% F HC: 26.1% F	QUE = 9 (MD: 600 mg/d) RIS = 8 (MD: 5.3 mg/d) OLA = 6 (MD: 15.83 mg/d) AMI = 4 (MD: 700 mg/d) ARI = 1 (MD: 20 mg/d) Flupentixol = 1 (MD: 10 mg/d)	FEV (German version of the TFEQ) Author-developed board game to assess delay of gratification using food reward Behavioral assessment of the dysexecutive syndrome (BADS)	• Patients had ↓ delay of gratification, ↓ executive functioning (BADS), and ↑ BMI compared to controls • In patients, ↑ FEV scores (disinhibition, restraint) were associated with ↓ executive functioning and ↑ BMI • No significant difference in subjective appetite between patients and controls
Schanze 2008 [77]	Cross-sectional Comparing eating behaviours in patients with SCZ and MDD vs. HCs	42 SCZ inpatients Age: 33.6 BMI: 27.28 83 MDD inpatients Age: 40.42 BMI: 26.01 46 HCs (un-matched) Age: 35.7 BMI: 23.51	SCZ: 40.5% F MDD: 47% F HC: 47.8% F	SCZ (last 4 weeks): QUE = 6 RIS = 5 ZIP = 4 OLA = 2 CLZ = 1 SSRI = 1 None = 23 MDD (last 4 weeks): QUE = 1 RIS = 1 SSRI = 15 Mirtazapine = 10 None = 56	TFEQ	• No significant group differences (patients vs. HCs, MDD vs. SCZ) for all TFEQ domains • No significant effect of medication class (antidepressant, antipsychotic, no medication) on TFEQ scores

Table 5. *Cont.*

Study	Study Description					Main Significant Results
	Design/Aim	Sample (Size, Diagnosis), Mean Age (Years), Mean BMI (kg/m^2)	Sex (% F), Race/Ethnicity	Mean Illness Duration/Previous AP Exposure (*n*)	Assessments	
Roerig 2005 [78]	Randomized, double blind, parallel (2 weeks) Effect of OLA and RIS vs. placebo on eating behaviours in HCs	48 HCs, 18–60 years OLA: *n* = 16 (MD: 8.75 mg/d) RIS: *n* = 16 (MD: 2.875 mg/d) PLA: *n* = 16 Age: 33.6 (OLA), 36.2 (RIS), 32.7 (PBO) BMI: 23.6 (OLA), 25.0 (RIS), 24.1 (PBO)	OLA: 87.5% F RIS: 75% F PBO: 68.75% F	N/A	Hunger/appetite scale (100-mm VAS) Feeding laboratory (standardized breakfast, liquid lunch, ad libitum dinner where food was weighed) Resting energy expenditure (REE)	• Participants in both AP groups gained weight, however only the OLA group reached statistical significance • In the OLA group, weight gain was associated with a non-significant ↑ in food intake (kcal/day) and appetite compared to RIS or PBO • None of the groups (OLA, RIS, PBO) showed a significant change in REE
Teff 2015 [79]	Randomized trial (12 days; 9 days of SGA exposure) Effect of acute SGA exposure on hunger and food intake in HCs	30 HCs OLA: *n* = 10 RIS: *n* =10 PBO: *n* = 10 Age: 26.1 (OLA), 25.9 (ARI), 29.9 (PBO) BMI: 22.1 (OLA), 22.4 (ARI), 21.8 (PBO) reported in [80]	30% F	N/A	Hunger/appetite scale (9-point Likert) Food intake weighed (objective) Activity level (number of steps)	• Neither medication had a significant effect on weight, subjective hunger/fullness or calorie intake compared to PBO • No significant change in physical activity levels in any group

Note: All main findings reported in this table are statistically significant unless otherwise indicated. SCZ = Schizophrenia, BD = Bipolar Disorder, MDD = Major Depressive Disorder, SMI = Severe Mental Illness, HCs = Healthy Controls, FEP = First Episode Psychosis, AMI = amisulpride, OLA = olanzapine, HAL = Haloperidol, RIS = Risperidone, QUE = Quetiapine, ZIP = Ziprasidone, CPZ = Chlorpromazine, PBO = Placebo, FGA = First generation antipsychotics, SGA = Second generation antipsychotic, NR = Not reported, TFEQ = Three-Factor Eating Questionnaire, FCQ = Food Craving Questionnaire, FCI = Food Craving Inventory, VAS = visual analog scale, DR-EBQ = Drug-Related Eating Behaviour Questionnaire, FFQ = Food Frequency Questionnaire, EBA = Eating Behaviour Assessment, DEBQ = Dutch Eating Behaviour Questionnaire, QEWP = Questionnaire on Eating and Weight Patterns, MD = Mean Dose, * = studies from the same cohort (Khazaal 2006a, 2006b).

3.3.1. Binge Eating and Other Eating Disorder-Related Behaviours

Seven studies [62–68] explored the occurrence of binge-eating symptomatology in patients being treated with SGAs. In all cases, binge eating symptomatology was determined based on DSM-IV research criteria for BED unless otherwise specified.

3.3.2. Patients Only

Consistent with the dietary composition studies discussed above, all five patient studies [63–67] found that treatment with clozapine or olanzapine increased appetite, food intake, food craving and/or risk of weight gain in non-FEP patients. Interestingly, the studies further suggest that these changes may be related to AP-mediated induction of binge eating. For example, one study [63] found that 17% of patients reported episodes of binge eating after starting clozapine, with one patient seeing remittance and re-occurrence of binge eating after discontinuing and then restarting treatment. In another study, the authors found that half of all included clozapine- and olanzapine-treated patients screened positively for binge eating behaviour (BE group), with over half reporting *onset* of episodes of binge eating during the current medication regime [66]. A similar retrospective clozapine/olanzapine study [64], found that 14% of patients met DSM-IV diagnostic criteria for an ED, specifically eating disorders not otherwise specified (including BED) or bulimia nervosa. Subsequent comparison of scores from the Questionnaire on Eating and Weight Patterns QEWP [51] and adverse drug reaction (ADR) scale [81] revealed that ED onset was "definitely" or "probably" linked to AP exposure. Prospective studies also appear to support a relationship between clozapine/olanzapine treatment and binge eating, with one showing a significant increase in binge eating episodes from baseline to endpoint [65], and another identifying a positive correlation between olanzapine-induced appetite increases and behaviours similar to DSM-IV BED criteria such as "preoccupation with food" and "eating until uncomfortably full" [67].

3.3.3. Patients vs. Controls

Similar to the findings mentioned above, two case-control studies conducted by Khazaal et al. found evidence of a link between psychosis and disordered eating. In their first study [62], the authors observed altered self-esteem and self-control, greater fear of weight gain, and a greater desire to control weight in patients with SCZ compared to controls as determined by a revised version of the Mizes Anorectic Cognitive Questionnaire (MAC-R). They also found that females had higher MAC-R scores than men, suggestive of sex and/or gender effects. In the second study [68], they found a significantly higher prevalence of DSM-IV binge eating symptoms and BED in overweight/obese patients with SCZ compared to weight-matched controls.

3.4. Subjective Appetite, Hunger and Satiety

Our search identified 12 studies [50,69–74,76,77] that used self-report measures including visual analog scales (VAS), the TFEQ and the DEBQ to measure subjective appetite/hunger and eating-related cognitions.

3.4.1. Patients Only

Conclusions from longitudinal studies regarding the effects of AP medications (particularly SGAs) on appetite were mixed. For example, two studies, one in which patients were randomized to receive olanzapine or risperidone [71], and another where patients were randomized to either disintegrating or standard olanzapine tablets [70] found no significant effect of AP treatment on appetite (Eating Behaviour Assessment and VAS) with a non-significant trend towards decreased appetite. In contrast, two different studies found significant weight-related changes in eating behaviour following AP exposure. In particular, Ryu et al. found that SGA treatment increased weight as well as subjective hunger, appetite and food craving (Drug-Related Eating Behaviour Questionnaire; DR-EBQ) [50].

On the other hand, despite failing to report overall longitudinal changes, Garriga et al. (2019) observed interesting moderating effects of baseline BMI, stage of illness and sex in clozapine-treated patients [69] (see Table 5). The authors also found a significant positive correlation between specific food cravings (FCI) and subsequent consumption (Cuestionario de Frecuencia de Consumo de Alimentos; CFCA), suggesting that psychological desire may translate into behavioural changes.

In the only cross-sectional study identified, Sentissi et al. compared eating behaviour between AP-naïve or AP-free, FGA-treated and SGA-treated patients with SCZ [72]. They found that BMI status was positively associated with TFEQ disinhibition (significant) and hunger (nearing significance) scores. Furthermore, SGA-treated patients showed greater reactivity to external eating cues (DEBQ) than the FGA-treated, but not the untreated patients.

3.4.2. Patients vs. Healthy Controls

All five studies comparing patients and controls were cross-sectional studies. Generally, there were mixed results regarding group differences in appetite/satiety, which highlights a need for longitudinal studies in this area.

In one study, although patients experienced increased hunger (VAS) and decreased satiation compared to HCs following a standardized meal [74], the groups did not differ in spontaneous intake and food preference during a buffet-type meal three hours later. The authors also found that patients had increased TFEQ scores in all three domains (cognitive restraint, disinhibition, susceptibility to hunger), a finding that remained significant after controlling for BMI. A separate study exploring executive functioning (which is known to be impaired in SCZ), found that patients displayed significantly worse delay of gratification and executive functioning than HCs in a task involving food reinforcement [76]. These impairments were associated with increased restrained eating behaviour and disinhibition, as well as increased BMI, suggesting that disease-related dysfunction in the dorsolateral prefrontal cortex (DLPFC) and dorsal anterior cingulate cortex (ACC) (prefrontal-ACC network) may increase susceptibility to overeating, thereby promoting weight gain.

In contrast to the studies discussed above, Schanze et al. (2008) found no group differences between patients with SCZ, patients with major depressive disorder, and HCs in any of the TFEQ domains [77]. Furthermore, they observed no effect of medication class (AP, antidepressant, no medication) on TFEQ scores [77]. Similarly, Abbas et al. (2013) found no significant difference in food craving (FCI) between AP-treated patients with SCZ and HCs [73]. Finally, Folley et al. (2010) found that patients and HCs did not differ in their response time or food preference when asked to choose between two food images [75]. Interestingly, although patients generally gave higher positive ratings to food stimuli than HCs, instances when they gave lower ratings were correlated with increased anhedonia. This led the authors to suggest that while preference judgements appear to be intact in patients, the hedonic value they place on food may be altered.

3.4.3. Controls Only

Our search retrieved two randomized, double-blind, placebo-controlled studies in HCs examining subjective appetite/hunger following short-term SGA exposure. In the first study, Roerig et al. (2005) found that two weeks of either olanzapine or risperidone exposure led to weight gain compared to placebo, although only olanzapine reached statistical significance [78]. The authors also observed a trend towards both greater food intake (kcal/day) and an increase in appetite (measured using a 100 mm VAS) in the olanzapine group relative to the other groups. In contrast, Teff et al. (2015) observed no significant change in weight, subjective hunger/fullness or calorie intake following nine days of SGA exposure [79]. Importantly, in contrast to the aforementioned HC study by Fountaine (2010), neither study reported significant changes in physical activity or energy expenditure in association with AP treatment.

3.5. *Findings from Neuroimaging and Brain Structure Studies*

Our search yielded seven studies that used neuroimaging methodologies to study food preference and eating behavior in patients with SCZ. The characteristics of these studies and a summary of their main findings can be found in Table 6. Six studies used functional magnetic resonance imaging (fMRI) along with visual analog scales (VAS) and/or eating questionnaires [82–87] and one study used structural MRI to study brain morphology [88]. One study was conducted on AP-naïve (n = 22) patients [88], and one was conducted on patients who were AP-naïve (n = 9) or had been medication free for at least six weeks (n = 20) [86] (Section 3.2).

3.5.1. Patients Only

A study by Stip (2015) and colleagues compared brain activity (fMRI) in response to videos of food in patients with SCZ before and after initiating or switching to olanzapine therapy [84]. The authors found that 16 weeks of olanzapine exposure led to significantly decreased neuronal activation in the salience network (SN), an important network involved in reward processing and reward anticipation. Specific regions affected by olanzapine included the anterior fronto-insular (aFI) cortex, amygdala, thalamus and anterior cingulate cortex (ACC). The decrease in SN activation was associated with a decrease in dietary restraint (TFEQ), leading the authors to suggest that AP-mediated disruptions of the SN may promote changes in eating behaviour.

3.5.2. Patients vs. Healthy Controls

In an earlier publication (conducted in the same cohort as the 2015 study [84], but including a HC comparator), Stip et al. (2012) used static food images and examined subjective appetite (VAS) and TFEQ scores in patients with SCZ before and after starting olanzapine [85]. Using fMRI, they found that 16 weeks of olanzapine treatment led to a significant increase in activation in the supplementary motor area, right fusiform gyrus, insular cortex, amygdala and parahippocampal regions in response to static food images. Comparing these changes in activation to controls, it was found that neural activity in the premotor area, somatosensory cortices and bilaterally in the fusiform gyri of patients with SCZ was normalized, while activity in the insular cortices, amygdala and cerebellum was 'overshot'. Interestingly, this hyperactivation was positively correlated with disinhibition (TFEQ), suggestive of an association between OLA-induced increases in brain activity and dysfunctional processing of food-related stimuli.

An earlier study, using the same patient cohort (but pre-switch to olanzapine) as the two aforementioned studies by Stip and colleagues [84,85], similarly assessed brain activity (fMRI) in response to food cues [83]. Relative to HCs, patients with SCZ showed increased activation in brain regions involved in action planning and regulation of homeostatic signals including the red thalamic nucleus, left parahippocampal gyrus and left middle frontal gyrus. Furthermore, the authors found that activity in the red thalamic nucleus was positively correlated with cognitive restraint (TFEQ Factor 1), while activity in the left middle frontal gyrus was associated with increased disinhibition (TFEQ Factor 2). This led them to suggest that cortical processes may disrupt or override sub-cortical hypothalamic appetite regulation signals in patients with SCZ. Additional correlational analyses controlling for either AP dose (chlorpromazine CPZ equivalents) or disease severity (Positive and Negative Syndrome Scale; PANSS) revealed a significant positive correlation between AP dose and susceptibility to hunger (TFEQ Factor 3) and a significant negative correlation between PANSS score and cognitive restraint. This led to the conclusion that both SCZ and AP medications may contribute to appetite dysregulation in patients, but through different mechanisms.

Table 6. Characteristics of studies with neuroimaging methodologies.

Study	Design/Aim	Sample (Size, Diagnosis), Mean Age (Years), Mean BMI	Sex (% F), Race/Ethnicity	Mean Illness Duration/Previous AP Exposure (n)	Assessments	Main Significant Results
Stip 2015 * [84]	Longitudinal (16 week) study, pre- post with OLA administration Examining the salience network in SCZ patients on OLA treatment	15 SCZ patients not previously exposed to OLA switching to OLA Same cohort as 2012 study (authors did not specify switchers vs. AP-naïve, fasted)	NR	NR	fMRI (BOLD) during neutral vs. dynamic appetitive stimuli Hunger/appetite scale (VAS from 0–5) TFEQ	• ↓ Activation of SN (including ACC, aFI, and amygdala) in response to dynamic appetitive stimuli • ↓ ACC and aFI activity were associated with ↑ ghrelin levels and ↓ dietary restraint (TFEQ)
Lungu 2013 * [83]	Cross sectional (case-control) Neuronal correlates of appetite regulation in patients with SCZ vs. HC (3 h since last meal)	25 SCZ (20 completers) AP (OLA excluded): n = 21 AP-naïve: n = 3 Age: 34.5 BMI: 26.62 11 HCs (10 included) Age: 35.2 BMI: 25.07	48% F SCZ: 24% F HC: 20% F	RIS = 12 QUE = 6 HAL = 2 CLZ = 1 Perphenazine = 1 No medication = 3	fMRI (BOLD) during neutral vs. static appetitive stimuli Hunger/appetite scale (VAS from 0–5) TFEQ	• Common neuronal networks activated in both groups (left insula, primary sensory motor areas, and inferior temporal and parietal cortices) • ↑ Responses to appetitive cues in areas of action planning and homeostatic signals (red thalamic nucleus, left parahippocampus, and left middle frontal gyrus) in SCZ group • PANSS positive symptom scores positively correlated with activity in left middle frontal gyrus (action planning) and TFEQ disinhibition scores • TFEQ restraint scores correlated positively with thalamic activity and negatively with disease severity (PANSS score) • TFEQ hunger scores correlated negatively with parahippocampal activity and positively with AP dose (CPZ equivalents)
Stip 2012 * [85]	Longitudinal intervention (16 weeks) vs. HCs Evaluating neural changes associated with appetite in SCZ patients pre, and post OLA treatment vs. HCs (3 h since last meal)	24 SCZ patients not previously exposed to OLA (15 completers) Switch (no washout): n = 19 AP-naïve: n = 3 Age: 30.04 10 HCs Age: 33.9 Same cohort as Lungu 2013	SCZ: 21% F; 91.66% Caucasians, 8.33% Caribbean HC: 20% F; 100% Caucasian	RIS = 12 QUE = 6 HAL = 2 CLZ = 1 Perphenazine = 1 No medication = 3	fMRI (BOLD) during neutral vs. static appetitive stimuli Hunger/appetite scale (VAS from 0–5) TFEQ	• OLA treatment ↑ weight gain significantly • OLA treatment ↑ BOLD signal in response to appetitive stimuli in supplementary motor area, right fusiform gyrus, insular cortex, amygdala and parahippocampus • OLA ↑ Neural activity in premotor area, somatosensory cortices and bilaterally in the fusiform gyri of patients to the same levels as HCs • Hyperactivation (vs. HC) in 4 regions (insular cortices, amygdala, and cerebellum) in response to appetitive stimuli • OLA-induced ↑ brain activity in response to appetitive stimuli was negatively corelated with TFEQ (dietary restraint) scores

Table 6. *Cont.*

Study	Design/Aim	Sample (Size, Diagnosis), Mean Age (Years), Mean BMI	Sex (% F), Race/Ethnicity	Mean Illness Duration/Previous AP Exposure (n)	Assessments	Main Significant Results
Grimm 2012 [82]	Cross sectional (case-control) Striatal activation during appetitive cues (fasting state)	23 fasted (6h) chronic SCZ in- and outpatients on stable AP medication (MD: 346 mg/d CPZ equivalents) Age: 30.3 23 fasted HCs (matched for age, gender, parental SES, handedness) Age: 28.9	74% F	No change in the medication dose >25% or a switch to a different medication was allowed in the last 4 weeks SGA: n = 22 RIS = 4 OLA = 3 CLZ = 4 AMI = 3 QUE = 3 ARI = 3 ZIP = 1 FGA: n = 1 Flupenthixol = 1 Illness duration: 4.1 years	fMRI (BOLD) during neutral vs. static appetitive stimuli Hunger/appetite scale (VAS)	• ↓ Activation in the dorsal striatal region in patients • Reduced activity remained significant after controlling for AP dose (CPZ equivalents) and body weight • Patients and controls were similar in appetite ratings evoked by presentation of neutral or appetite stimuli
Emsley 2015 [88]	Prospective (13 weeks of AP treatment vs. HC) Morphological changes in brain regions associated with food intake regulation, metabolic parameters (BMI, fasting glucose, lipids) (fasting not specified)	22 AP-naïve FEP in- and outpatients randomized to receive RIS or flupenthixol decanoate long-acting injections (n not specified) SCZ: n = 13 Schizophreniform: n = 9 Age: 24.6 (range: 16–45) BMI: 22.1 23 untreated HCs (matched for age, sex, ethnicity, educational status) Age: 27	24% F FEP: 14% F; 64% mixed descent, 36% Black HC: 35% F; 70% mixed descent, 30% Black	No previous AP exposure; mean duration of untreated psychosis: 41 weeks Mean endpoint dose: 31.66 mg 2-weekly (RIS), 13.07 mg 2-weekly (flupenthixol)	Structural MRI changes in prespecified brain regions associated with hedonic and homeostatic body weight regulation	• ↑ Baseline left vDC volumes in patients compared to HCs • Medicated FEP patients had ↓ vDC size (homeostatic), but no difference in prefrontal cortex (hedonic) size • This volume change was also associated with ↑ BMI, dyslipidemia and elevated glucose in patients • ↓ Volumes were not significant following post-hoc testing and were accompanied by ↑ volumes in control group

Table 6. *Cont.*

Study	Design/Aim	Sample (Size, Diagnosis), Mean Age (Years), Mean BMI	Sex (% F), Race/Ethnicity	Mean Illness Duration/Previous AP Exposure (n)	Assessments	Main Significant Results
Borgan 2019 [86]	Cross-sectional (case-control) Neural responsivity to food cues in unmedicated first episode psychosis (fasting state used)	29 fasted (>12 h), untreated FEP patients SCZ: $n = 27$ Schizoaffective: $n = 2$ Age: 26.1 (range: 18–65) BMI: 25.2 28 fasted HCs (matched for age) Age: 26.4 BMI: 24.7	17% F FEP: 14% F; 12 White, 9 Black African or Black Caribbean, 6 Asian, 2 Mixed HC: 21% F; 10 White, 3 Black African or Black Caribbean, 11 Asian, 4 Mixed	Patients were AP-naïve or free from all psychotropic medication for at least 6 weeks Prior use = 20 AP-naïve = 9 Duration of prior treatment: 4.74 months Illness duration: 21.5 months	fMRI (BOLD signal) during neutral vs. static food cue (low and high calorie) IPAQ Dietary Instrument for Nutrition Education	• ↑ BOLD response in HCs vs. patients in the right insula, right anterior, posterior, medial and inferior orbitofrontal gyrus to food cues • Comparing ROIs: ↑ Response to food cues in HCs in nucleus accumbens, but not in insula or hypothalamus • In HCs, BMI was inversely correlated with mean BOLD signal in nucleus accumbens in response to food cues • No group differences in neural responses to food cues between patients and HCs • ↑ Fat consumption in patients than HCs in neural response to food cues
Mathews 2012 [87]	Interventional (pre- post 1-week OLA administration) open-label prospective design Neural activity associated with anticipation and receipt of food rewards after 1 week of OLA (in fasting state)	19 fasted (overnight) HCs Age: 27.5 (range = 18–50) BMI: 25.78 Dosing: 5 mg of OLA on the first night and 10 mg on the subsequent 6 nights	47.4% F 73.7% White, 10.5% African American, 10.5% Hispanic, 5.3% Mixed	N/A	fMRI (BOLD) during appetitive visual stimuli, and in response to receipt of cued food or water control (chocolate milk, tomato juice) Consumption of "liquid breakfast" measured post scan Hunger/appetite scale (5-point Likert) TFEQ	• OLA ↑ Weight (1.1kg) • OLA ↑ activation in regions for anticipatory reward (inferior frontal cortex, striatum, ACC) in response to visual food cues; ↑ activation of reward receipt regions (caudate, putamen); and ↓ activation in regions of inhibitory control of feeding (lateral orbital frontal cortex) • OLA was associated with ↑ consumption of breakfast, and ↑ in disinhibited eating behavior (TFEQ)

Note: All main findings reported in this table are statistically significant unless otherwise indicated. SCZ = Schizophrenia, BP = Bipolar Disorder. HC = Healthy controls, FEP: First episode psychosis, AMI = amisulpride, OLA = olanzapine, HAL = Haloperidol, RIS = Risperidone, QUE = Quetiapine, ZIP = Ziprasidone, CPZ = Chlorpromazine, FGA = First generation antipsychotics, SGA = Second generation antipsychotic, NR = Not reported, TFEQ = Three-Factor Eating Questionnaire, FCQ = Food Craving Questionnaire, FCI = Food Craving Inventory, VAS = visual analog scale, DR-EBQ = Drug-Related Eating Behaviour Questionnaire, FFQ = Food Frequency Questionnaire, EBA = Eating Behaviour Assessment, DEBQ = Dutch Eating Behaviour Questionnaire, QEWP = Questionnaire on Eating and Weight Patterns; BOLD= blood oxygen level dependent response; ACC= anterior cingulate cortex, aFI= Anterior Fronto-insular, vDC= ventral Diencephalon, MD = Mean Dose, * = studies from the same cohort (Lungu 2013, Stip 2012, Stip 2015).

In a similar but independent fMRI study, Grimm et al. (2012) asked chronic patients with SCZ and HCs to rate their appetite levels on a VAS following presentation of neutral or appetitive stimuli [82]. Even after adjusting for body weight and AP dose (CPZ equivalents), patients were found to have significantly weaker activation in the dorsal striatal region (post appetitive stimulus vs. neutral images) compared to controls. In keeping with the findings by Stip et al. 2012 [84], these results led the authors to suggest that SCZ may involve intrinsic disruptions in the SN, leading to altered reward anticipation and eating behavior. However, despite these functional differences (and in contrast to some of the studies already discussed), Grimm et al. found no significant difference in appetite between patients and controls.

3.5.3. First Episode Patients vs. Controls

In a structural MRI study, Emsley and colleagues [88] investigated morphological brain changes after 13 weeks of AP treatment (risperidone or flupentixol injections) in AP-naïve FEP patients with SCZ, in relation to changes in BMI and metabolic indices. Regions of interest included the ventral diencephalon (vDC) and prefrontal cortex (PFC), which respectively represent key homeostatic and hedonic food intake regulatory areas. As there were no differences in MRI or metabolic outcomes between AP treatment groups, patients from both groups were pooled together for analysis. The authors found that compared to HCs, patients experienced a volume reduction in the vDC (a region containing the hypothalamus), which was strongly correlated with BMI and glucose increases and dyslipidemia. In contrast, no changes were observed in the PFC region, leading the authors to suggest that acute AP treatment primarily results in disruption of homeostatic functions (and not reward pathways). However, following post-hoc testing, these volume reductions were no longer significant and increased volumes in the control group were reported, which the authors attributed to random fluctuations due to small sample size.

In a recent fMRI study, Borgan et al. (2019) investigated neural responsiveness to appetitive stimuli in untreated FEP patients and HCs [86]. Comparing fMRI blood oxygen level dependent (BOLD) signaling response to appetitive stimuli between groups, the authors found that patients consistently exhibited the same regional patterns of neural activity observed in controls, indicative of normal neural responses to food cues. This led them to suggest that neural processing of food may be unaltered in the early stages of the illness and may instead be influenced by AP treatment.

3.6. Healthy Controls Only

We retrieved one neuroimaging study in HCs, which examined the effects of seven days of olanzapine administration on fMRI responses to visual stimuli (appetitive and neutral) as well as to receipt of an actual food reward [87]. Olanzapine treatment resulted in increased appetite as measured by both liquid breakfast intake and TFEQ scores (particularly disinhibition). This was accompanied by increased activation in brain regions involved in the reward pathway in response to both anticipation (inferior frontal cortex, striatum and ACC) and receipt (caudate, putamen) of appetitive stimuli. Interestingly, they also observed a concurrent decrease in activation in the lateral orbitofrontal cortex, which is thought to be involved in satiety.

4. Discussion

We performed a scoping review, which aimed to explore associations between psychosis spectrum disorders, food consumption, and disruptions in appetite and eating behaviors. Our search retrieved 35 studies, which we subsequently organized into three sections based on main theme or methodology: (1) Food composition and dietary preference, (2) patterns of eating behaviour and subjective appetite and (3) neural correlates of appetite and eating behavior. These sections are discussed individually, followed by a discussion of postulated mechanisms, and a more general discussion of limitations and future directions of this field.

4.1. *Food Composition and Dietary Preference*

The studies identified in our search provide evidence that overconsumption, in the form of both increased frequency and quantity of food consumption, differs between patients and HCs [57–60], which may contribute to the high rates of obesity in patient populations. In keeping with the general population, lower calorie intake among patients is associated with lower BMI, waist circumference, waist-to-hip ratio and body fat content [60]. Furthermore, dietary preference appears to be sex-specific [55,60,61], which could explain the differential propensity for weight gain among male and female SCZ spectrum disorder patients [89].

Disentangling the extent to which observed differences in caloric intake and dietary composition relate to biological factors intrinsic to the illness and/or AP treatment is challenging. While work in AP-naïve FEP populations can be helpful in delineating intrinsic illness related factors, only two of the dietary composition studies we retrieved included AP-naïve individuals [56,57]. However, subgroup analyses comparing HCs and AP-naïve patients were not performed, precluding inferences on dietary alterations that may primarily result from intrinsic illness effects. Unfortunately, it is similarly difficult to delineate the relative effects of APs on diet as studies in HCs indicate either no significant difference [78,79] or a significant increase in caloric intake [53] following SGA exposure.

It is also important to consider socioeconomic, environmental, and lifestyle factors that may precipitate a snowball effect on unhealthy dietary patterns among patients. Patients with psychosis spectrum disorders tend to belong to lower socioeconomic status (SES) groups [15,90]. This in turn relates to their ability to afford or have access to a nutritious diet. Notably, none of the dietary composition studies we reviewed matched patients to HCs in terms of SES, including income and education level. Three cross-sectional studies did, however, report significant differences in socio-demographic variables of patients vs. controls [58,60,61]. As such, it is possible that psychosocial stress related to socioeconomic factors, or symptoms of psychosis, may influence food intake in patients. Chronic stress has also been associated with hyperphagia [91] and preference for palatable foods [92]. Thus, failure to match patients to HCs according to key demographic features such as SES is a potential source of variation and should be considered in future studies.

4.2. *Eating Behaviour, Cravings and Subjective Appetite*

Synthesis of the studies identified in our search revealed a positive association between BMI/weight and altered appetite, hunger and/or food cravings in patients with psychosis spectrum disorders [50,64,65,69,72], as well as between SGA treatment and binge eating symptomatology [62–66,68]. Similar to what is observed in the ED literature [93,94], two studies also noted a relationship between restrictive eating behaviour (high restraint and high disinhibition scores) and increased consumption and weight gain among patients [72,74]. This may potentially suggest a common mechanism between EDs and the disordered eating patterns seen in psychosis patients.

In addition, APs may increase appetite and response to both internal and external hunger cues (as assessed by the TFEQ), putting patients at higher risk of overeating and subsequent weight gain [54,56,74,83,89]; however, the literature appears quite contradictory [70,71,73,82]. Potential explanations for these discrepancies could be choice of rating scale or questionnaire [95] and experimental conditions (i.e., fasting state, meal challenge and type), which differed widely across studies. As such, it is difficult to determine the relative contribution of illness vs. AP drugs on appetite.

Longitudinal HC studies also provide mixed evidence regarding the effects of APs on appetite and eating behaviors. Some studies indicate increased appetite, body weight and food intake following olanzapine treatment, indicative of a potential causal link [53,87], while other studies indicate SGA exposure does not significantly affect appetite or food intake despite inducing weight gain [78] and metabolic changes such as insulin resistance [79]. The latter point may suggest that central insulin and/or leptin resistance resulting from AP-induced weight gain and increases in adiposity may lead to appetite change, rather than appetite driving weight change [79].

4.3. Neural Correlates of Appetite and Eating Behavior

A variety of neuroimaging strategies have been employed to examine neurobiological mechanisms implicated in food intake patterns in patients, with a majority of the work (six out of seven retrieved studies) focusing on functional changes captured by fMRI in response to appetitive cues. Unfortunately, though, the different behavioural paradigms and brain regions of interest of each study made it difficult to draw any broad conclusions or generalizations. Two studies suggest that APs may contribute to disrupted appetite regulation and eating behaviour by increasing activation in areas involved in action planning and homeostatic signals [85], and regions implicated in cognitive and motivational processing of food [83]. However, these findings appear limited to static appetitive stimuli as dynamic stimuli led to decreased activation of the SN [84]. Interestingly, changes in regional activation correlated with disinhibition (TFEQ) scores across all three studies [83–85]. Similarly, AP treatment in HCs appears to [87] enhance activation in the brain reward circuitry, and decrease activation in the lateral orbital frontal cortex, consistent with loss of inhibitory effects on eating behaviour.

In determining the relative effects of illness vs. AP treatment, one AP-naïve study did not report any neural differences between patients or controls, indicating that food-related neural processing is not intrinsically dysregulated in SCZ [86]. In contrast, a different study found that chronic patients with SCZ on stable AP therapy exhibited significantly reduced activation in striatal regions involved in reward processing, an association that persisted even after controlling for AP dose. This suggests that the neural alterations involved in appetite regulation may be related to factors intrinsic to SCZ, which become more prominent as the illness progresses, and further exacerbated by AP therapy. This is consistent with structural MRI findings, which found that AP treatment reduced the volume of the vDC, but not the PFC in AP-naïve FEP patients [88].

4.4. Postulated Neurobiological Mechanisms Involved in Appetite/Feeding Regulation

While the contributing effects of intrinsic illness related factors vs. those of AP medications remain difficult to separate, existing theoretical frameworks may provide a neurobiological rationale for the differences in eating behaviours and appetite between patients with pychosis spectrum disorders and HCs. The postulated disruptions in hedonic/motivational and homeostatic mechanisms in patients with pyschosis spectrum disorders are summarized in Figure 3.

4.5. Hedonic Reward Mechanisms

The mesolimbic dopamine reward system is instantiated by a network of brain structures innervated by dopaminergic projections from the ventral tegmental area (VTA), including the nucleus accumbens (NAc), hypothalamus, amygdala, and PFC regions [96,97] (see Figure 1). Mesolimbic dopamine has primarily been implicated in the incentive motivational dimension of reward, including reward prediction [98], and the attribution of motivational salience to reward-related cues (associated with the concept of 'wanting' or 'craving') [99].

In turn, increased dopaminergic transmission in the striatum is a core neurobiological feature of SCZ that responds to first line AP treatment [100,101]. The striatum integrates inputs received from the majority of the cortex and projects to the mesolimbic dopamine system and cortical salience networks [102]. Its role has been associated with making inferences about the current state of the environment [103], whereas abnormal dopaminergic reactivity in the striatum may lead to misattribution of salience to external or internal cues relating to food or appetite.

Moreover, reward hypoactivity, which is related to negative symptoms of SCZ [104,105], may result in compensatory responses such as increased food consumption to achieve sufficient rewarding stimulation [82,106]. Furthermore, as function in the dorsal striatum is believed to be modulated by body weight, metabolic dysregulations accumulated throughout the course of the illness and perturbated by AP therapy may also be implicated in reduced striatal activity, similar to what is seen in obese individuals [106].

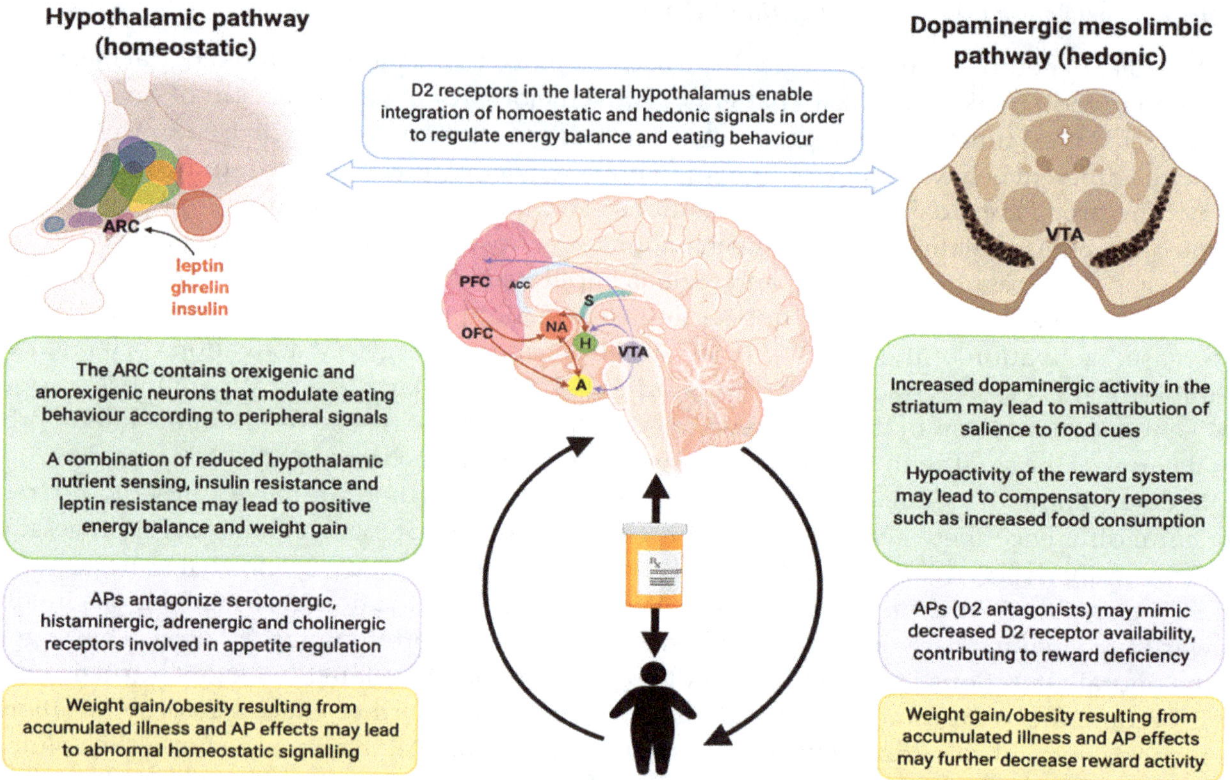

Figure 3. Overview of the homeostatic and hedonic pathways regulating appetite and eating behaviour. Text in green boxes describe the function of each pathway and implications for regulation of eating behaviour; text in purple boxes describes antipsychotic-induced effects; text in yellow boxes describes how weight gain affects pathway function. Abbreviations: VTA, ventral tegmental area; NA, nucleus accumbens; H, hypothalamus; PFC, prefrontal cortex; OFC, orbitofrontal cortex; A, amygdala; ACC, anterior cingulate gyrus; S, striatum; AP, antipsychotic; D2 = dopamine 2.

Additionally, disrupted function in the DLPFC, ACC and mediodorsal nucleus of the thalamus has been associated with impaired executive function in SCZ [107]. Analogous to observations of diminished executive function in the obese population, this may lead to poorer choices in food selection or difficulty in inhibiting responses to cravings. Consistent with this, several studies included in this review suggest that patients with SCZ have increased disinhibition [72,74,83–85], and an increased incidence of binge eating [59,67,68,72,81,108], which may reflect deficits in executive function related to prefrontal-ACC dysfunction [107].

The limited body of literature reporting on AP-naïve FEP patients precludes direct attribution of any dysregulations to inherent illness factors. However, APs share the uniting property of dopamine 2 (D2) receptor antagonism, which may mimic decreased D2 receptor availability, and thus contribute to the reward deficiency/overcompensation phenotype. Indeed, a relationship between reduced D2 receptor function and reward dysfunction has already been observed in obesity [109]. Beyond their effects on the dopamine system, APs also interact with serotonergic, histaminergic, adrenergic, muscarinic and cholinergic receptors, all of which are differentially involved in appetite modulation [84,110]. As such, the role of APs in disturbed eating behaviours is likely complex, involving widespread regions of the brain and signaling networks, with additional interfaces with illness-related disruptions in these pathways.

4.6. Homeostatic Mechanisms

Homeostatic mechanisms of food regulation are thought to be primarily regulated by the hypothalamus, a region anatomically situated to confer accessibility to hormones (leptin, ghrelin, insulin) and nutrients (glucose, fatty acids) in the blood and cerebral spinal fluid (CSF) to relay information about the body's energy stores to the brain [28] (see Figure 3). The topic of impaired hormonal regulation of feeding in SCZ has been the subject of a recent comprehensive review, supporting that early disruptions in these pathways likely progress over the course of illness and are further exacerbated by APs [20]. These homeostatic pathways are also thought to interact with dopamine reward circuits to regulate eating behavior and energy balance [111], potentially mediated by the high concentration of D2 receptors in the lateral hypothalamus [20] Thus, it is possible that the connections between these pathways may be altered in SCZ. For example, Stip et al. (2012) found evidence of increased signaling in the amygdala, a key limbic structure responsible for integrating homeostatic signals with extrinsic influences to modulate eating behavior [85]. However, this field of research is not well developed and is likely further complicated by the interaction between intrinsic aspects of psychosis spectrum disorders, AP treatment and psychological or environmental factors [112,113]. Interestingly, one study included in our review demonstrated volume reductions in the hypothalamus of AP-naïve patients following olanzapine treatment [88]. However, the relevance of changes in hypothalamic size in relation to obesity and metabolic disorders as well as the effects of AP treatment in relation to brain volume changes are controversial [114,115]. Further research combining advanced neuroimaging approaches (functional and structural) with food cues and stimuli relevant to hedonic and non-hedonic aspects of eating and assessments of hormonal activity is needed.

4.7. Strengths, Limitations and Future Directions

A key strength of this scoping review is that the search was broad, allowing for a comprehensive overview of the current state of the literature pertaining to eating behaviours and food consumption in psychosis spectrum disorders. Moreover, to the best of our knowledge, this is the first review to summarize the findings of neuroimaging studies that sought to elucidate the neurobiological mechanisms underlying eating behaviours among psychosis spectrum patients.

Nevertheless, there are some limitations which must be addressed. First, our search revealed high heterogeneity in both study design and questionnaires employed, which made comparing studies difficult and precluded conclusions from being made. Second, the majority of studies used subjective self-report measures of appetite/craving, results of which may be influenced by factors outside of hunger [58]. Additionally, the use of patient recall, as in the case of food diaries or during retrospective interviews, may lead to inaccurate estimations of food intake [57]. This is particularly relevant given that recall is known to be impaired in SCZ [58]. As alluded to by others, future studies that use both subjective and objective measures of appetite (e.g., calorie intake) [71], complemented by neuroimaging approaches [82] are required to move the field forward. Furthermore, only one fMRI study examined the effect of somatosensory (gustatory) stimuli on appetite and eating preferences [87]; the remaining five studies focused solely on visual processing of food-related cues, potentially missing key mediators of altered eating behaviour [116].

Importantly, very few of the studies identified in our search considered AP-naïve FEP patients, with the vast majority involving patients who had previously been exposed to AP therapy. This makes it difficult to determine whether any abnormal eating patterns observed in patients are intrinsic to the illness or secondary to the effects of APs. Additionally, while HC studies are a good way to remove the confounding effect of illness, they preclude identification of any interaction between intrinsic dysfunction in eating and AP effects. Prospective studies in which AP-naïve patients are exposed to APs would be particularly useful in exploring this illness-treatment interaction. Moreover, it should also be considered that studies in chronic patients with SCZ are confounded by cumulative illness associated lifestyle factors and treatments, which may affect both eating patterns and weight gain [7,117]. Further to this point, once obesity and other metabolic comorbidity is established, this may have secondary effects on physiology of feeding regulation [28]. Finally, metabolic consequences of AP treatment are known to be most pronounced in AP-naïve or FEP patients, suggesting that this may represent the critical period to capture early changes in eating behavior and appetite, which drive early weight gain [118]. Unfortunately, at present, the temporal course or trajectory of disordered eating in psychosis cannot be determined as most studies did not report trends over multiple timepoints. This would be a point worth considering when designing future longitudinal studies.

Finally, many of the studies comparing patients with HCs did not match groups on key sociodemographic and physiological (i.e., BMI, gender/sex) factors (see Tables 4–6), constituting a significant confound. To this last point, while sex emerged as an important mediator of appetite and feeding disruptions in some of the studies included in this review, the majority of studies did not account for sex. This is highly relevant given that in the general population, global obesity rates differ for males and females (10% and 18%, respectively [119]), as do TFEQ and DEBQ scores [36,120,121]. Furthermore, in SCZ, females seem to be more at risk for AP-induced metabolic disturbances than males [122,123]. Further investigation is therefore warranted to determine whether sex-related differences in eating behaviors can explain this increased vulnerability.

5. Conclusions

While disruptions in hormones involved in homeostatic mechanisms of appetite control in patients with pychosis spectrum disorders have been the subject of several reviews and meta-analyses, our scoping review highlights the behavioral and neurobiological underpinnings of altered eating behaviour in this population. Our synthesis of evidence from food surveys and self-report questionnaires generally supports the notion that patients with pychosis spectrum disorders exhibit increased appetite and craving for fatty food, increased caloric intake and increased frequency of (over) consumption, which may be associated with increased disinhibition. Early evidence also suggests that disturbed eating behaviours in this population could be mediated by abnormal processing of food-related stimuli within neural systems related to the mesolimbic reward circuit. In addition, it is possible that impaired cognitive restraint and executive functioning intrinsic to psychosis may make patients more susceptible to developing disordered eating patterns in response to weight gain and/or increased appetite and cravings. Future prospective studies with larger samples and AP-naïve populations are needed to improve the evidence base in this field and help dissect the intrinsic and extrinsic illness factors involved in disturbed appetite regulation. This will have important implications for development of pharmacological and behavioral interventions which, by targeting cardiometabolic comorbidities, may have the potential to increase patient life span and improve overall quality of life.

Author Contributions: Conceptualization, N.S., E.S. and R.A.; methodology, N.S., E.S. and R.A.; screening, N.S., E.S., R.A. and A.G.; data curation, N.S., E.S. and R.A.; investigation, N.S., E.S. and R.A.; writing—original draft preparation, N.S., E.S., R.A., L.H. and A.G.; writing—review and editing, N.S., E.S., R.A., L.H., P.S., S.S., A.G.-G., V.H.T., S.M.A. and M.K.H.; visualization, N.S., E.S. and R.A.; supervision, S.M.A. and M.K.H. All authors have read and agreed to the published version of the manuscript.

Acknowledgments: All figures were created using BioRender.com. N.S. is supported by the CIHR Canada Graduate Scholarship Master's Program (CGS-M) and the Banting and Best Diabetes Centre (BBDC) Novo-Nordisk Graduate Studentship. E.S. is supported by the CIHR Canada Graduate Scholarship Master's Program (CGS-M) and the Banting and Best Diabetes Centre (BBDC) Novo-Nordisk Graduate Studentship. R.A. is supported by the Banting & Best Diabetes Centre-Novo Nordisk Studentship and the Cleghorn Award. P.S. reports receiving grants and/or salary and/or research support from the Centre for Addiction and Mental Health, Health Canada, Ontario Ministry of Health and Long-term care (MOHLTC), Canadian Institutes of Health Research (CIHR), Canadian Centre on Substance Use and Addiction, Public Health Agency of Canada (PHAC), Ontario Lung Association, Medical Psychiatry Alliance, Extensions for Community Healthcare Outcomes, Canadian Cancer Society Research Institute (CCSRI), Cancer Care Ontario, Ontario Institute for Cancer Research, Ontario Brain Institute, McLaughlin Centre, Academic Health Sciences Centre, Workplace Safety and Insurance Board, National Institutes of Health (NIH), and the Association of Faculties of Medicine of Canada. PS also reports receiving funding and/or honoraria from the following commercial organizations: Pfizer Inc./Canada, Shoppers Drug Mart, Bhasin Consulting Fund Inc., Patient-Centered Outcomes Research Institute, ABBVie, and Bristol-Myers Squibb. Further, PS reports receiving consulting fees from Pfizer Inc./Canada, Evidera Inc., Johnson & Johnson Group of Companies, Medcan Clinic, Inflexxion Inc., V-CC Systems Inc., MedPlan Communications, Kataka Medical

Communications, Miller Medical Communications, Nvision Insight Group, and Sun Life Financial. Through an open tender process Johnson & Johnson, Novartis, and Pfizer Inc. are vendors of record for providing smoking cessation pharmacotherapy, free or discounted, for research studies in which PS is the principal investigator or co-investigator. S.M.A is supported in part by an Academic Scholars Award from the Department of Psychiatry, University of Toronto and has grant support from the Canadian Institutes of Health Research, PSI foundation, Ontario, and the CAMH Discovery Fund. M.K.H. is supported in part by an Academic Scholars Award from the Department of Psychiatry, University of Toronto and has grant support from the Banting and Best Diabetes Center (BBDC) through the New Investigator Award, Canadian Institutes of Health Research (PJT–153262) (CIHR), PSI foundation, Ontario, and holds the Kelly and Michael Meighen Chair in Psychosis Prevention and Cardy Schizophrenia Research Chair. M.K.H. has also received consultant fees from Alkeremes.

References

1. Prentice, P. Psychosis and schizophrenia. *Arch. Dis. Child. Educ. Pract. Ed.* **2013**, *98*, 128–130. [CrossRef]
2. Moreno-Küstner, B.; Martín, C.; Pastor, L. Prevalence of psychotic disorders and its association with methodological issues. A systematic review and meta-analyses. *PLoS ONE* **2018**, *13*, e0195687. [CrossRef] [PubMed]
3. Arciniengas, D.B. Psychosis. *Continuum* **2015**, *21*, 715–736.
4. Bowie, C.R.; Harvey, P.D. Cognition in schizophrenia: Impairments, determinants, and functional importance. *Psychiatr. Clin. N. Am.* **2005**, *28*, 613–633. [CrossRef] [PubMed]
5. Harvey, P.D.; Strassnig, M. Predicting the severity of everyday functional disability in people with schizophrenia: Cognitive deficits, functional capacity, symptoms, and health status. *World Psychiatry* **2012**, *11*, 73–79. [CrossRef]
6. Maric, N.P.; Jovicic, M.J.; Mihaljevic, M.; Miljevic, C. Improving current treatments for schizophrenia. *Drug Dev. Res.* **2016**, *77*, 357–367. [CrossRef]
7. De Hert, M.; Cohen, D.; Bobes, J.; Cetkovich-Bakmas, M.; Leucht, S.; Ndetei, D.M.; Newcomer, J.W.; Uwakwe, R.; Asai, I.; Möller, H.J.; et al. Physical illness in patients with severe mental disorders. II. Barriers to care, monitoring and treatment guidelines, plus recommendations at the system and individual level. *World Psychiatry* **2011**, *10*, 138–151. [CrossRef]
8. Hennekens, C.H.; Hennekens, A.R.; Hollar, D.; Casey, D.E. Schizophrenia and increased risks of cardiovascular disease. *Am. Heart J.* **2005**, *150*, 1115–1121. [CrossRef]
9. Kredentser, M.S.; Martens, P.J.; Chochinov, H.M.; Prior, H.J. Cause and rate of death in people with schizophrenia across the lifespan: A population-based study in Manitoba, Canada. *J. Clin. Psychiatry* **2014**, *75*, 154–161. [CrossRef]
10. Rajkumar, A.P.; Horsdal, H.T.; Wimberley, T.; Cohen, D.; Mors, O.; Borglum, A.D.; Gasse, C. Endogenous and antipsychotic-related risks for diabetes mellitus in young people with schizophrenia: A Danish population-based cohort study. *Am. J. Psychiatry* **2017**, *174*, 686–694. [CrossRef]
11. Musil, R.; Obermeier, M.; Russ, P.; Hamerle, M. Weight gain and antipsychotics: A drug safety review. *Expert Opin. Drug Saf.* **2015**, *14*, 73–96. [CrossRef] [PubMed]
12. Alvarez-Jiménez, M.; González-Blanch, C.; Crespo-Facorro, B.; Hetrick, S.; Rodríguez-Sánchez, J.M.; Pérez-Iglesias, R.; Vázquez-Barquero, J.L. Antipsychotic-induced weight gain in chronic and first-episode psychotic disorders: A systematic critical reappraisal. *CNS Drugs* **2008**, *22*, 547–562. [CrossRef] [PubMed]
13. Hill, J.O.; Wyatt, H.R.; Peters, J.C. The importance of energy balance. *Eur. Endocrinol.* **2013**, *9*, 111–115. [CrossRef] [PubMed]
14. Dipasquale, S.; Pariante, C.M.; Dazzan, P.; Aguglia, E.; McGuire, P.; Mondelli, V. The dietary pattern of patients with schizophrenia: A systematic review. *J. Psychiatr. Res.* **2013**, *47*, 197–207. [CrossRef]
15. Heald, A.; Pendlebury, J.; Anderson, S.; Narayan, V.; Guy, M.; Gibson, M.; Haddad, P.; Livingston, M. Lifestyle factors and the metabolic syndrome in Schizophrenia: A cross-sectional study. *Ann. Gen. Psychiatry* **2017**, *16*, 12. [CrossRef]
16. Suvisaari, J.; Keinänen, J.; Eskelinen, S.; Mantere, O. Diabetes and Schizophrenia. *Curr. Diabetes Rep.* **2016**, *16*, 16. [CrossRef]
17. Kouidrat, Y.; Amad, A.; Lalau, J.D.; Loas, G. Eating disorders in schizophrenia: Implications for research and management. *Schizophr. Res. Treat.* **2014**, *2014*, 791573. [CrossRef]

18. Misiak, B.; Stańczykiewicz, B.; Łaczmański, Ł.; Frydecka, D. Lipid profile disturbances in antipsychotic-naive patients with first-episode non-affective psychosis: A systematic review and meta-analysis. *Schizophr. Res.* **2017**, *190*, 18–27. [CrossRef]
19. Greenhalgh, A.M.; Gonzalez-Blanco, L.; Garcia-Rizo, C.; Fernandez-Egea, E.; Miller, B.; Arroyo, M.B.; Kirkpatrick, B. Meta-analysis of glucose tolerance, insulin, and insulin resistance in antipsychotic-naïve patients with nonaffective psychosis. *Schizophr. Res.* **2017**, *179*, 57–63. [CrossRef]
20. Lis, M.; Stanczykiewicz, B.; Liskiewicz, P.; Misiak, B. Impaired hormonal regulation of appetite in schizophrenia: A narrative review dissecting intrinsic mechanisms and the effects of antipsychotics. *Psychoneuroendocrinology* **2020**, *119*, 104744. [CrossRef] [PubMed]
21. Benarroch, L.; Kowalchuk, C.; Wilson, V.; Teo, C.; Guenette, M.; Chintoh, A.; Nesarajah, Y.; Taylor, V.; Selby, P.; Fletcher, P.; et al. Atypical antipsychotics and effects on feeding: From mice to men. *Psychopharmacology* **2016**, *233*, 2629–2653. [CrossRef] [PubMed]
22. Bartoli, F.; Crocamo, C.; Clerici, M.; Carrà, G. Second-generation antipsychotics and adiponectin levels in schizophrenia: A comparative meta-analysis. *Eur. Neuropsychopharmacol.* **2015**, *25*, 1767–1774. [CrossRef] [PubMed]
23. Goetz, R.L.; Miller, B.J. Meta-analysis of ghrelin alterations in schizophrenia: Effects of olanzapine. *Schizophr. Res.* **2019**, *206*, 21–26. [CrossRef] [PubMed]
24. Matafome, P.; Seiça, R. The role of brain in energy balance. *Adv. Neurobiol.* **2017**, *19*, 33–48. [CrossRef] [PubMed]
25. Yu, Y.H.; Vasselli, J.R.; Zhang, Y.; Mechanick, J.I.; Korner, J.; Peterli, R. Metabolic vs. hedonic obesity: A conceptual distinction and its clinical implications. *Obes. Rev.* **2015**, *16*, 234–247. [CrossRef]
26. Teff, K.L.; Kim, S.F. Atypical antipsychotics and the neural regulation of food intake and peripheral metabolism. *Physiol. Behav.* **2011**, *104*, 590–598. [CrossRef]
27. Adinoff, B. Neurobiologic processes in drug reward and addiction. *Harv. Rev. Psychiatry* **2004**, *12*, 305–320. [CrossRef]
28. Roh, E.; Song, D.K.; Kim, M.S. Emerging role of the brain in the homeostatic regulation of energy and glucose metabolism. *Nat. Publ. Group* **2016**, *48*, 216. [CrossRef]
29. Peters, M.D.; Godfrey, C.M.; Khalil, H.; McInerney, P.; Parker, D.; Soares, C.B. Guidance for conducting systematic scoping reviews. *Int. J. Evid. Based Healthc.* **2015**, *13*, 141–146. [CrossRef]
30. Covidence Systematic Review Software. Available online: www.covidence.org (accessed on 10 June 2020).
31. Lindroos, A.-K.; Lissner, L.; Mathiassen, M.E.; Karlsson, J.; Sullivan, M.; Bengtsson, C.; Sjöström, L. Dietary intake in relation to restrained eating, disinhibition, and hunger in obese and nonobese Swedish women. *Obes. Res.* **1997**, *5*, 175–182. [CrossRef]
32. Westenhoefer, J.; Stunkard, A.J.; Pudel, V. Validation of the flexible and rigid control dimensions of dietary restraint. *Int. J. Eat. Disord.* **1999**, *26*, 53–64. [CrossRef]
33. Provencher, S.W. Automatic quantitation of localized in vivo 1H spectra with LCModel. *NMR Biomed.* **2001**, *14*, 260–264. [CrossRef] [PubMed]
34. Löffler, A.; Luck, T.; Then, F.S.; Sikorski, C.; Kovacs, P.; Böttcher, Y.; Breitfeld, J.; Tönjes, A.; Horstmann, A.; Löffler, M.; et al. Eating behaviour in the general population: An analysis of the factor structure of the German version of the Three-Factor-Eating-Questionnaire (TFEQ) and its association with the body mass index. *PLoS ONE* **2015**, *10*, e0133977. [CrossRef] [PubMed]
35. Bohrer, B.K.; Forbush, K.T.; Hunt, T.K. Are common measures of dietary restraint and disinhibited eating reliable and valid in obese persons? *Appetite* **2015**, *87*, 344–351. [CrossRef]
36. Bryant, E.J.; Rehman, J.; Pepper, L.B.; Walters, E.R. Obesity and eating disturbance: The role of TFEQ restraint and disinhibition. *Curr. Obes. Rep.* **2019**, *8*, 363–372. [CrossRef]
37. Sung, J.; Lee, K.; Song, Y.M. Relationship of eating behavior to long-term weight change and body mass index: The Healthy Twin study. *Eat. Weight Disord. Stud. Anorex. Bulim. Obes.* **2009**, *14*, e98–e105. [CrossRef]
38. Van Strien, T.; Herman, C.P.; Verheijden, M.W. Eating style, overeating, and overweight in a representative Dutch sample. Does external eating play a role? *Appetite* **2009**, *52*, 380–387. [CrossRef]
39. Koenders, P.G.; van Strien, T. Emotional eating, rather than lifestyle behavior, drives weight gain in a prospective study in 1562 employees. *J. Occup. Environ. Med.* **2011**, *53*, 1287–1293. [CrossRef]

40. Van Strien, T.; Frijters, J.E.R.; Bergers, G.P.A.; Defares, P.B. The Dutch Eating Behavior Questionnaire (DEBQ) for assessment of restrained, emotional, and external eating behavior. *Int. J. Eat. Disord.* **1986**, *5*, 295–315. [CrossRef]
41. Gibbons, C.; Hopkins, M.; Beaulieu, K.; Oustric, P.; Blundell, J.E. Issues in measuring and interpreting human appetite (satiety/satiation) and its contribution to obesity. *Curr. Obes. Rep.* **2019**, *8*, 77–87. [CrossRef]
42. Stunkard, A.J.; Messick, S. The three-factor eating questionnaire to measure dietary restraint, disinhibition and hunger. *J. Psychosom. Res.* **1985**, *29*, 71–83. [CrossRef]
43. Vinai, P.; Da Ros, A.; Speciale, M.; Gentile, N.; Tagliabue, A.; Vinai, P.; Bruno, C.; Vinai, L.; Studt, S.; Cardetti, S. Psychopathological characteristics of patients seeking for bariatric surgery, either affected or not by binge eating disorder following the criteria of the DSM IV TR and of the DSM 5. *Eat. Behav.* **2015**, *16*, 1–4. [CrossRef] [PubMed]
44. Bas, M.; Bozan, N.; Cigerim, N. Dieting, dietary restraint, and binge eating disorder among overweight adolescents in Turkey. *Adolescence* **2008**, *43*, 635–648. [PubMed]
45. Van Strien, T.; Peter Herman, C.; Verheijden, M.W. Eating style, overeating and weight gain. A prospective 2-year follow-up study in a representative Dutch sample. *Appetite* **2012**, *59*, 782–789. [CrossRef]
46. Stubbs, R.J.; Hughes, D.A.; Johnstone, A.M.; Rowley, E.; Reid, C.; Elia, M.; Stratton, R.; Delargy, H.; King, N.; Blundell, J.E. The use of visual analogue scales to assess motivation to eat in human subjects: A review of their reliability and validity with an evaluation of new hand-held computerized systems for temporal tracking of appetite ratings. *Br. J. Nutr.* **2000**, *84*, 405–415. [CrossRef] [PubMed]
47. Cepeda-Benito, A.; Gleaves, D.H.; Williams, T.L.; Erath, S.A. The development and validation of the state and trait food-cravings questionnaires. *Behav. Ther.* **2000**, *31*, 151–173. [CrossRef]
48. White, M.A.; Whisenhunt, B.L.; Williamson, D.A.; Greenway, F.L.; Netemeyer, R.G. Development and validation of the food-craving inventory. *Obes. Res.* **2002**, *10*, 107–114. [CrossRef]
49. Lim, M.; Noh, J.; Nam, H.; Kim, J.; Lee, D.; Hong, K. Development and validation of drug-related eating behavior questionnaire in patients receiving antipsychotic medications. *Korean J. Schizophr. Res.* **2008**, *11*, 39–44.
50. Ryu, S.; Nam, H.J.; Oh, S.; Park, T.; Lim, M.; Choi, J.S.; Baek, J.H.; Jang, J.H.; Park, H.Y.; Kim, S.N.; et al. Eating-behavior changes associated with antipsychotic medications in patients with schizophrenia as measured by the Drug-Related Eating Behavior Questionnaire. *J. Clin. Psychopharmacol.* **2013**, *33*, 120–122. [CrossRef]
51. Spitzer, R.L.; Yanovski, S.; Wadden, T.; Wing, R.; Marcus, M.D.; Stunkard, A.; Devlin, M.; Mitchell, J.; Hasin, D.; Horne, R.L. Binge eating disorder: Its further validation in a multisite study. *Int. J. Eat. Disord.* **1993**, *13*, 137–153.
52. Mizes, J.S.; Christiano, B.; Madison, J.; Post, G.; Seime, R.; Varnado, P. Development of the mizes anorectic cognitions questionnaire-revised: Psychometric properties and factor structure in a large sample of eating disorder patients. *Int. J. Eat. Disord.* **2000**, *28*, 415–421. [CrossRef]
53. Fountaine, R.J.; Taylor, A.E.; Mancuso, J.P.; Greenway, F.L.; Byerley, L.O.; Smith, S.R.; Most, M.M.; Fryburg, D.A. Increased food intake and energy expenditure following administration of olanzapine to healthy men. *Obesity* **2010**, *18*, 1646–1651. [CrossRef] [PubMed]
54. Gothelf, D.; Falk, B.; Singer, P.; Kairi, M.; Phillip, M.; Zigel, L.; Poraz, I.; Frishman, S.; Constantini, N.; Zalsman, G.; et al. Weight Gain Associated With Increased Food Intake and Low Habitual Activity Levels in Male Adolescent Schizophrenic Inpatients Treated With Olanzapine. *Am. J. Psychiatry* **2002**, *159*, 1055–1057. [CrossRef] [PubMed]
55. Amani, R. Is dietary pattern of schizophrenia patients different from healthy subjects? *BMC Psychiatry* **2007**, *7*. [CrossRef] [PubMed]
56. Eder, U.; Mangweth, B.; Ebenbichler, C.; Weiss, E.; Hofer, A.; Hummer, M.; Kemmler, G.; Lechleitner, M.; Fleischhacker, W.W. Association of olanzapine-induced weight gain with an increase in body fat. *Am. J. Psychiatry* **2001**, *158*, 1719–1722. [CrossRef] [PubMed]
57. Gattere, G.; Stojanovic-Perez, A.; Monseny, R.; Martorell, L.; Ortega, L.; Montalvo, I.; Sole, M.; Algora, M.J.; Cabezas, A.; Reynolds, R.M.; et al. Gene-environment interaction between the brain-derived neurotrophic factor Val66Met polymorphism, psychosocial stress and dietary intake in early psychosis. *Early Interv. Psychiatry* **2018**, *12*, 811–820. [CrossRef] [PubMed]

58. Nunes, D.; Eskinazi, B.; Camboim Rockett, F.; Delgado, V.B.; Schweigert Perry, I.D. Nutritional status, food intake and cardiovascular disease risk in individuals with schizophrenia in southern Brazil: A case–control study. *Rev. Psiquiatr. Salud Ment.* **2014**, *7*, 72–79. [CrossRef] [PubMed]
59. Strassnig, M.; Singh Brar, J.; Qanguli, R. Nutritional assessment of patients with schizophrenia: A preliminary study. *Schizophr. Bull.* **2003**, *29*, 393–397. [CrossRef]
60. Stefanska, E.; Lech, M.; Wendołowicz, A.; Konarzewska, B.; Waszkiewicz, N.; Ostrowska, L. Eating habits and nutritional status of patients with affective disorders and schizophrenia. *Psychiatr. Pol.* **2017**, *51*, 1107–1120. [CrossRef]
61. Stefańska, E.; Wendołowicz, A.; Lech, M.; Wilczyńska, K.; Konarzewska, B.; Zapolska, J.; Ostrowska, L. The assessment of the nutritional value of meals consumed by patients with recognized schizophrenia. *Rocz. Państwowego Zakładu Hig.* **2018**, *69*, 183–192.
62. Khazaal, Y.; Fresard, E.; Zimmermann, G.; Trombert, N.M.; Pomini, V.; Grasset, F.; Borgeat, F.; Zullino, D. Eating and weight related cognitions in people with Schizophrenia: A case control study. *Clin. Pract. Epidemiol. Ment. Health CP EMH* **2006**, *2*, 29. [CrossRef] [PubMed]
63. Brömel, T.; Blum, W.F.; Ziegler, A.; Schulz, E.; Bender, M.; Fleischhaker, C.; Remschmidt, H.; Krieg, J.C.; Hebebrand, J. Serum leptin levels increase rapidly after initiation of clozapine therapy. *Mol. Psychiatry* **1998**, *3*, 76–80. [CrossRef] [PubMed]
64. Gebhardt, S.; Haberhausen, M.; Krieg, J.C.; Remschmidt, H.; Heinzel-Gutenbrunner, M.; Hebebrand, J.; Theisen, F.M. Clozapine/olanzapine-induced recurrence or deterioration of binge eating-related eating disorders. *J. Neural Transm.* **2007**, *114*, 1091–1095. [CrossRef] [PubMed]
65. Kluge, M.; Schuld, A.; Himmerich, H.; Dalal, M.; Schacht, A.; Wehmeier, P.M.; Hinze-Selch, D.; Kraus, T.; Dittmann, R.W.; Pollmächer, T. Clozapine and olanzapine are associated with food craving and binge eating: Results from a randomized double-blind study. *J. Clin. Psychopharmacol.* **2007**, *27*, 662–666. [CrossRef]
66. Theisen, F.M.; Linden, A.; König, I.R.; Martin, M.; Remschmidt, H.; Hebebrand, J. Spectrum of binge eating symptomatology in patients treated with clozapine and olanzapine. *J. Neural Transm.* **2003**, *110*, 111–121. [CrossRef]
67. Treuer, T.; Hoffmann, V.P.; Chen, A.K.-P.; Irimia, V.; Ocampo, M.; Wang, G.; Singh, P.; Holt, S. Factors associated with weight gain during olanzapine treatment in patients with schizophrenia or bipolar disorder: Results from a six-month prospective, multinational, observational study. *World J. Biol. Psychiatry* **2009**, *10*, 729–740. [CrossRef]
68. Khazaal, Y.; Frésard, E.; Borgeat, F.; Zullino, D. Binge eating symptomatology in overweight and obese patients with schizophrenia: A case control study. *Ann. Gen. Psychiatry* **2006**, *5*, 15. [CrossRef]
69. Garriga, M.; Mallorqui, A.; Serrano, L.; Rios, J.; Salamero, M.; Parellada, E.; Gomez-Ramiro, M.; Oliveira, C.; Amoretti, S.; Vieta, E.; et al. Food craving and consumption evolution in patients starting treatment with clozapine. *Psychopharmacology* **2019**, *236*, 3317–3327. [CrossRef]
70. Karagianis, J.; Grossman, L.; Landry, J.; Reed, V.A.; de Haan, L.; Maguire, G.A.; Hoffmann, V.P.; Milev, R. A randomized controlled trial of the effect of sublingual orally disintegrating olanzapine versus oral olanzapine on body mass index: The PLATYPUS Study. *Schizophr. Res.* **2009**, *113*, 41–48. [CrossRef]
71. Smith, R.C.; Rachakonda, S.; Dwivedi, S.; Davis, J.M. Olanzapine and risperidone effects on appetite and ghrelin in chronic schizophrenic patients. *Psychiatry Res.* **2012**, *199*, 159–163. [CrossRef]
72. Sentissi, O.; Viala, A.; Bourdel, M.C.; Kaminski, F.; Bellisle, F.; Olie, J.P.; Poirier, M.F. Impact of antipsychotic treatments on the motivation to eat: Preliminary results in 153 schizophrenic patients. *Int. Clin. Psychopharmacol.* **2009**, *24*, 257–264. [CrossRef] [PubMed]
73. Abbas, M.J.; Liddle, P.F. Olanzapine and food craving: A case control study. *Hum. Psychopharmacol.* **2013**, *28*, 97–101. [CrossRef] [PubMed]
74. Blouin, M.; Tremblay, A.; Jalbert, M.E.; Venables, H.; Bouchard, R.H.; Roy, M.A.; Alméras, N. Adiposity and eating behaviors in patients under second generation antipsychotics. *Obesity* **2008**, *16*, 1780–1787. [CrossRef] [PubMed]
75. Folley, B.S.; Park, S. Relative food preference and hedonic judgments in schizophrenia. *Psychiatry Res.* **2010**, *175*, 33–37. [CrossRef] [PubMed]
76. Knolle-Veentjer, S.; Huth, V.; Ferstl, R.; Aldenhoff, J.B.; Hinze-Selch, D. Delay of gratification and executive performance in individuals with schizophrenia: Putative role for eating behavior and body weight regulation. *J. Psychiatr. Res.* **2008**, *42*, 98–105. [PubMed]

77. Schanze, A.; Reulbach, U.; Scheuchenzuber, M.; Groschl, M.; Kornhuber, J.; Kraus, T. Ghrelin and eating disturbances in psychiatric disorders. *Neuropsychobiology* **2008**, *57*, 126–130. [CrossRef] [PubMed]
78. Roerig, J.L.; Mitchell, J.E.; de Zwaan, M.; Crosby, R.D.; Gosnell, B.A.; Steffen, K.J.; Wonderlich, S.A. A comparison of the effects of olanzapine and risperidone versus placebo on eating behaviors. *J. Clin. Psychopharmacol.* **2005**, *25*, 413–418.
79. Teff, K.L.; Rickels, K.; Alshehabi, E.; Rickels, M.R. Metabolic impairments precede changes in hunger and food intake following short-term administration of second-generation antipsychotics. *J. Clin. Psychopharmacol.* **2015**, *35*, 579–582. [CrossRef]
80. Teff, K.L.; Rickels, M.R.; Grudziak, J.; Fuller, C.; Nguyen, H.-L.; Rickels, K. Antipsychotic-induced insulin resistance and postprandial hormonal dysregulation independent of weight gain or psychiatric disease. *Diabetes* **2013**, *62*, 3232–3240. [CrossRef]
81. Naranjo, C.A.; Busto, U.; Sellers, E.M.; Sandor, P.; Ruiz, I.; Roberts, E.A.; Janecek, E.; Domecq, C.; Greenblatt, D.J. A method for estimating the probability of adverse drug reactions. *Clin. Pharmacol. Ther.* **1981**, *30*, 239–245. [CrossRef]
82. Grimm, O.; Vollstadt-Klein, S.; Krebs, L.; Zink, M.; Smolka, M.N. Reduced striatal activation during reward anticipation due to appetite-provoking cues in chronic schizophrenia: A fMRI study. *Schizophr. Res.* **2012**, *134*, 151–157. [CrossRef] [PubMed]
83. Lungu, O.; Anselmo, K.; Letourneau, G.; Mendrek, A.; Stip, B.; Lipp, O.; Lalonde, P.; Ait Bentaleb, L.; Stip, E. Neuronal correlates of appetite regulation in patients with schizophrenia: Is there a basis for future appetite dysfunction? *Eur. Psychiatry J. Assoc. Eur. Psychiatr.* **2013**, *28*, 293–301. [CrossRef] [PubMed]
84. Stip, E.; Lungu, O.V. Salience network and olanzapine in schizophrenia: Implications for treatment in anorexia nervosa. *Can. J. Psychiatry Rev. Can. Psychiatr.* **2015**, *60*, S35–S39.
85. Stip, E.; Lungu, O.V.; Anselmo, K.; Letourneau, G.; Mendrek, A.; Stip, B.; Lipp, O.; Lalonde, P.; Bentaleb, L.A. Neural changes associated with appetite information processing in schizophrenic patients after 16 weeks of olanzapine treatment. *Transl. Psychiatry* **2012**, *2*, e128. [CrossRef]
86. Borgan, F.; O'Daly, O.; Hoang, K.; Veronese, M.; Withers, D.; Batterham, R.; Howes, O. Neural responsivity to food cues in patients with unmedicated first-episode psychosis. *JAMA Netw. Open* **2019**, *2*, e186893. [CrossRef]
87. Mathews, J.; Newcomer, J.W.; Mathews, J.R.; Fales, C.L.; Pierce, K.J.; Akers, B.K.; Marcu, I.; Barch, D.M. Neural correlates of weight gain with olanzapine. *Arch. Gen. Psychiatry* **2012**, *69*, 1226–1237. [CrossRef]
88. Emsley, R.; Asmal, L.; Chiliza, B.; du Plessis, S.; Carr, J.; Kidd, M.; Malhotra, A.K.; Vink, M.; Kahn, R.S. Changes in brain regions associated with food-intake regulation, body mass and metabolic profiles during acute antipsychotic treatment in first-episode schizophrenia. *Psychiatry Res.* **2015**, *233*, 186–193. [CrossRef] [PubMed]
89. Gebhardt, S.; Haberhausen, M.; Heinzel-Gutenbrunner, M.; Gebhardt, N.; Remschmidt, H.; Krieg, J.C.; Hebebrand, J.; Theisen, F.M. Antipsychotic-induced body weight gain: Predictors and a systematic categorization of the long-term weight course. *J. Psychiatr. Res.* **2009**, *43*, 620–626. [CrossRef] [PubMed]
90. Vancampfort, D.; Rosenbaum, S.; Schuch, F.B.; Ward, P.B.; Probst, M.; Stubbs, B. Prevalence and predictors of treatment dropout from physical activity interventions in schizophrenia: A meta-analysis. *Gen. Hosp. Psychiatry* **2016**, *39*, 15–23. [CrossRef] [PubMed]
91. Kyrou, I.; Tsigos, C. Chronic stress, visceral obesity and gonadal dysfunction. *Hormones* **2008**, *7*, 287–293. [CrossRef]
92. Dallman, M.F.; Pecoraro, N.; Akana, S.F.; La Fleur, S.E.; Gomez, F.; Houshyar, H.; Bell, M.E.; Bhatnagar, S.; Laugero, K.D.; Manalo, S. Chronic stress and obesity: A new view of "comfort food". *Proc. Natl. Acad. Sci. USA* **2003**, *100*, 11696–11701. [CrossRef] [PubMed]
93. Burger, K.S.; Stice, E. Relation of dietary restraint scores to activation of reward-related brain regions in response to food intake, anticipated intake, and food pictures. *NeuroImage* **2011**, *55*, 233–239. [CrossRef] [PubMed]
94. Spinella, M.; Lyke, J. Executive personality traits and eating behavior. *Int. J. Neurosci.* **2004**, *114*, 83–93. [CrossRef] [PubMed]
95. Case, M.; Treuer, T.; Karagianis, J.; Hoffmann, V.P. The potential role of appetite in predicting weight changes during treatment with olanzapine. *BMC Psychiatry* **2010**, *10*. [CrossRef] [PubMed]

96. Cardinal, R.N.; Parkinson, J.A.; Hall, J.; Everitt, B.J. Emotion and motivation: The role of the amygdala, ventral striatum, and prefrontal cortex. *Neurosci. Biobehav. Rev.* **2002**, *26*, 321–352. [CrossRef]
97. Le Moal, M.; Simon, H. Mesocorticolimbic dopaminergic network: Functional and regulatory roles. *Physiol. Rev.* **1991**, *71*, 155–234. [CrossRef] [PubMed]
98. Schultz, W. Dopamine neurons and their role in reward mechanisms. *Curr. Opin. Neurobiol.* **1997**, *7*, 191–197. [CrossRef]
99. Berridge, K.C. The debate over dopamine's role in reward: The case for incentive salience. *Psychopharmacology* **2007**, *191*, 391–431. [CrossRef]
100. Amato, D.; Vernon, A.C.; Papaleo, F. Dopamine, the antipsychotic molecule: A perspective on mechanisms underlying antipsychotic response variability. *Neurosci. Biobehav. Rev.* **2018**, *85*, 146–159. [CrossRef]
101. Kapur, S. Psychosis as a state of aberrant salience: A framework linking biology, phenomenology, and pharmacology in schizophrenia. *Am. J. Psychiatry* **2003**, *160*, 13–23. [CrossRef]
102. McCutcheon, R.A.; Abi-Dargham, A.; Howes, O.D. Schizophrenia, dopamine and the striatum: From biology to symptoms. *Trends Neurosci.* **2019**, *42*, 205–220. [CrossRef] [PubMed]
103. Nour, M.M.; Dahoun, T.; Schwartenbeck, P.; Adams, R.A.; FitzGerald, T.H.B.; Coello, C.; Wall, M.B.; Dolan, R.J.; Howes, O.D. Dopaminergic basis for signaling belief updates, but not surprise, and the link to paranoia. *Proc. Natl. Acad. Sci. USA* **2018**, *115*, E10167–E10176. [CrossRef] [PubMed]
104. Blanchard, J.J.; Cohen, A.S. The structure of negative symptoms within schizophrenia: Implications for assessment. *Schizophr. Bull.* **2006**, *32*, 238–245. [CrossRef] [PubMed]
105. Strauss, G.P.; Waltz, J.A.; Gold, J.M. A review of reward processing and motivational impairment in schizophrenia. *Schizophr. Bull.* **2014**, *40*, S107–S116. [CrossRef]
106. Stice, E.; Spoor, S.; Bohon, C.; Veldhuizen, M.G.; Small, D.M. Relation of reward from food intake and anticipated food intake to obesity: A functional magnetic resonance imaging study. *J. Abnorm. Psychol.* **2008**, *117*, 924–935. [CrossRef]
107. Minzenberg, M.J.; Laird, A.R.; Thelen, S.; Carter, C.S.; Glahn, D.C. Meta-analysis of 41 functional neuroimaging studies of executive function in schizophrenia. *Arch. Gen. Psychiatry* **2009**, *66*, 811–822. [CrossRef]
108. Khazaal, Y.; Billieux, J.; Fresard, E.; Huguelet, P.; van der Linden, M.; Zullino, D. A Measure of dysfunctional eating-related cognitions in people with psychotic disorders. *Psychiatr. Q.* **2010**, *81*, 49–56. [CrossRef]
109. Benton, D.; Young, H.A. A meta-analysis of the relationship between brain dopamine receptors and obesity: A matter of changes in behavior rather than food addiction? *Int. J. Obes.* **2016**, *40*, S12–S21. [CrossRef]
110. Hahn, M.; Chintoh, A.; Giacca, A.; Xu, L.; Lam, L.; Mann, S.; Fletcher, P.; Guenette, M.; Cohn, T.; Wolever, T.; et al. Atypical antipsychotics and effects of muscarinic, serotonergic, dopaminergic and histaminergic receptor binding on insulin secretion in vivo: An animal model. *Schizophr. Res.* **2011**, *131*, 90–95. [CrossRef]
111. Ahima, R.S.; Antwi, D.A. Brain regulation of appetite and satiety. *NIH Public Access* **2008**, *37*, 811–823. [CrossRef]
112. Agarwal, S.M.; Caravaggio, F.; Costa-Dookhan, K.A.; Castellani, L.; Kowalchuk, C.; Asgariroozbehani, R.; Graff-Guerrero, A.; Hahn, M. Brain insulin action in schizophrenia: Something borrowed and something new. *Neuropharmacology* **2020**, *163*, 107633. [CrossRef] [PubMed]
113. MacKenzie, N.E.; Kowalchuk, C.; Agarwal, S.M.; Costa-Dookhan, K.A.; Caravaggio, F.; Gerretsen, P.; Chintoh, A.; Remington, G.J.; Taylor, V.H.; Mueller, D.J.; et al. Antipsychotics, metabolic adverse effects, and cognitive function in schizophrenia. *Front. Psychiatry* **2018**, *9*, 622. [CrossRef] [PubMed]
114. Thomas, B.L.; Claassen, N.; Becker, P.; Viljoen, M. Validity of commonly used heart rate variability markers of autonomic nervous system function. *Neuropsychobiology* **2019**, *78*, 14–26. [CrossRef]
115. Turkheimer, F.E.; Selvaggi, P.; Mehta, M.A.; Veronese, M.; Zelaya, F.; Dazzan, P.; Vernon, A.C. Normalizing the abnormal: Do antipsychotic drugs push the cortex into an unsustainable metabolic envelope? *Schizophr. Bull.* **2020**, *46*, 484–495. [CrossRef] [PubMed]
116. Lemon, C.H. It's all a matter of taste: Gustatory processing and ingestive decisions. *MO Med.* **2010**, *107*, 247–251. [PubMed]
117. Vancampfort, D.; Knapen, J.; Probst, M.; van Winkel, R.; Deckx, S.; Maurissen, K.; Peuskens, J.; de Hert, M. Considering a frame of reference for physical activity research related to the cardiometabolic risk profile in schizophrenia. *Psychiatry Res.* **2010**, *177*, 271–279. [CrossRef] [PubMed]

118. Mitchell, A.J.; Vancampfort, D.; Sweers, K.; van Winkel, R.; Yu, W.; de Hert, M. Prevalence of metabolic syndrome and metabolic abnormalities in schizophrenia and related disorders—A systematic review and meta-analysis. *Schizophr. Bull.* **2013**, *39*, 306–318. [CrossRef]
119. Garawi, F.; Devries, K.; Thorogood, N.; Uauy, R. Global differences between women and men in the prevalence of obesity: Is there an association with gender inequality? *Eur. J. Clin. Nutr.* **2014**, *68*, 1101–1106. [CrossRef]
120. Burton, P.; Smit, H.J.; Lightowler, H.J. The influence of restrained and external eating patterns on overeating. *Appetite* **2007**, *49*, 191–197. [CrossRef]
121. Bellisle, F.; Clément, K.; Le Barzic, M.; Le Gall, A.; Guy-Grand, B.; Basdevant, A. The eating inventory and body adiposity from leanness to massive obesity: A study of 2509 adults. *Obes. Res.* **2004**, *12*, 2023–2030. [CrossRef]
122. Castellani, L.N.; Costa-Dookhan, K.A.; McIntyre, W.B.; Wright, D.C.; Flowers, S.A.; Hahn, M.K.; Ward, K.M. Preclinical and clinical sex differences in antipsychotic-induced metabolic disturbances: A narrative review of adiposity and glucose metabolism. *J. Psychiatry Brain Sci.* **2019**, *4*. [CrossRef]
123. Seeman, M.V. Men and women respond differently to antipsychotic drugs. *Neuropharmacology* **2020**, *163*, 107631. [CrossRef] [PubMed]

Permissions

All chapters in this book were first published by MDPI; hereby published with permission under the Creative Commons Attribution License or equivalent. Every chapter published in this book has been scrutinized by our experts. Their significance has been extensively debated. The topics covered herein carry significant findings which will fuel the growth of the discipline. They may even be implemented as practical applications or may be referred to as a beginning point for another development.

The contributors of this book come from diverse backgrounds, making this book a truly international effort. This book will bring forth new frontiers with its revolutionizing research information and detailed analysis of the nascent developments around the world.

We would like to thank all the contributing authors for lending their expertise to make the book truly unique. They have played a crucial role in the development of this book. Without their invaluable contributions this book wouldn't have been possible. They have made vital efforts to compile up to date information on the varied aspects of this subject to make this book a valuable addition to the collection of many professionals and students.

This book was conceptualized with the vision of imparting up-to-date information and advanced data in this field. To ensure the same, a matchless editorial board was set up. Every individual on the board went through rigorous rounds of assessment to prove their worth. After which they invested a large part of their time researching and compiling the most relevant data for our readers.

The editorial board has been involved in producing this book since its inception. They have spent rigorous hours researching and exploring the diverse topics which have resulted in the successful publishing of this book. They have passed on their knowledge of decades through this book. To expedite this challenging task, the publisher supported the team at every step. A small team of assistant editors was also appointed to further simplify the editing procedure and attain best results for the readers.

Apart from the editorial board, the designing team has also invested a significant amount of their time in understanding the subject and creating the most relevant covers. They scrutinized every image to scout for the most suitable representation of the subject and create an appropriate cover for the book.

The publishing team has been an ardent support to the editorial, designing and production team. Their endless efforts to recruit the best for this project, has resulted in the accomplishment of this book. They are a veteran in the field of academics and their pool of knowledge is as vast as their experience in printing. Their expertise and guidance has proved useful at every step. Their uncompromising quality standards have made this book an exceptional effort. Their encouragement from time to time has been an inspiration for everyone.

The publisher and the editorial board hope that this book will prove to be a valuable piece of knowledge for researchers, students, practitioners and scholars across the globe.

List of Contributors

Emma Kinnaird, Zhuo Li and Katherine Smith
King' s College London, Department of Psychological Medicine, Institute of Psychology, Psychiatry and Neuroscience, London SE5 8AZ, UK

Caroline Pimblett and Rafiu Agbalaya
National Eating Disorders Service, South London and Maudsley NHS Foundation Trust, London BR3 3BX, UK

Yasemin Dandil
King' s College London, Department of Psychological Medicine, Institute of Psychology, Psychiatry and Neuroscience, London SE5 8AZ, UK
National Eating Disorders Service, South London and Maudsley NHS Foundation Trust, London BR3 3BX, UK

Catherine Stewart
Child and Adolescent Eating Disorders Service, South London and Maudsley NHS Foundation Trust, London SE5 8AZ, UK

Kerry S. O'Brien, Jessica D. Reid, Zarina Vakhitova and Ayoub Bouguettaya
School of Social Sciences, Faculty of Arts, Monash University, Melbourne 3800, Australia

Rebecca M. Puhl
Department of Human Development and Family Sciences, Rudd Center for Food Policy & Obesity, University of Connecticut, Storrs, CT 06269, USA

Janet D. Latner
Department of Psychology, College of Social Sciences, University of Hawaii, Manoa, HI 96822, USA

Dermot Lynott
Department of Psychology, Faculty of Science and Technology University of Lancaster, Lancaster LA1 4YW, UK

John A. Hunter and Damian Scarf
Division of Sciences, Department of Psychology, University of Otago, Dunedin 9016, New Zealand

Ruth Jeanes
Curriculum & Pedagogy, Faculty of Education, Monash University, Melbourne 3800, Australia

Adrian Carter
School of Psychology, Faculty of Medicine, Nursing, and Health Sciences, Monash University, Melbourne 3800, Australia

Thorsten Koerner, Julia Heese, Matislava Karacic and Elmar Ngo
Schon Clinic Roseneck; Am Roseneck 6, 83209 Prien am Chiemsee, Germany

Verena Haas
Clinic for Psychiatry, Psychosomatics and Psychotherapy of childhood and adolescence, Charité - University Berlin, corporate member of Free University Berlin, Humboldt-University Berlin, and Berlin Institute of Health, 13353 Berlin, Germany

Christoph U. Correll
Clinic for Psychiatry, Psychosomatics and Psychotherapy of childhood and adolescence, Charité - University Berlin, corporate member of Free University Berlin, Humboldt-University Berlin, and Berlin Institute of Health, 13353 Berlin, Germany
Department of Psychiatry and Molecular medicine, Donald and Barbara Zucker School of Medicine at Hofstra/Northwell, Hempstead, NY 11549, USA
Department of Psychiatry, the Zucker Hillside Hospital, Glen Oaks, NY 11004, USA

Ulrich Voderholzer
Schon Clinic Roseneck; Am Roseneck 6, 83209 Prien am Chiemsee, Germany
Department of Psychiatry and Psychotherapy, Ludwig-Maximilians-Universitat Munchen (LMU), 80336 Munchen, Germany

Ulrich Cuntz
Schon Clinic Roseneck; Am Roseneck 6, 83209 Prien am Chiemsee, Germany
Research program for the evaluation of psychotherapy in complex therapeutic settings, PMU Paracelsus Medical University Salzburg, 5020 Salzburg, Austria

María Lozano-Madrid, Isabel Sánchez and Nadine Riesco
Department of Psychiatry, Bellvitge University Hospital-IDIBELL, 08907 L'Hospitalet de Llobregat, Barcelona, Spain
Psychiatry and Mental Health Group, Neuroscience Program, Institut d'Investigació Biomèdica de Bellvitge – IDIBELL, 08907 L'Hospitalet de Llobregat, Barcelona, Spain
Ciber Fisiopatologia Obesidad y Nutrición (CIBERobn), Instituto Salud Carlos III, 28029 Madrid, Spain

Núria Mallorquí-Bagué
Ciber Fisiopatologia Obesidad y Nutrición (CIBERobn), Instituto Salud Carlos III, 28029 Madrid, Spain
Department of Psychiatry, Addictive Behavior Unit, Hospital de la Santa Creu i Sant Pau, Biomedical Research Institute Sant Pau, 08001 Barcelona, Spain

Susana Jiménez-Murcia and Fernando Fernández-Aranda
Department of Psychiatry, Bellvitge University Hospital-IDIBELL, 08907 L'Hospitalet de Llobregat, Barcelona, Spain
Psychiatry and Mental Health Group, Neuroscience Program, Institut d'Investigació Biomèdica de Bellvitge—IDIBELL, 08907 L'Hospitalet de Llobregat, Barcelona, Spain
Ciber Physiopathology, Obesity and Nutrition (CIBERObn), Instituto de Salud Carlos III, 08907 Barcelona, Spain
Department of Clinical Sciences, School of Medicine and Health Sciences, University of Barcelona, 08907 L'Hospitalet de Llobregat, Barcelona, Spain

Giulia Testa, Isabel Baenas, Cristina Vintró-Alcaraz, Isabel Sánchez and Nadine Riesco
Ciber Physiopathology, Obesity and Nutrition (CIBERObn), Instituto de Salud Carlos III, 08907 Barcelona, Spain
Department of Psychiatry, Bellvitge University Hospital-IDIBELL, 08907 Barcelona, Spain

Roser Granero
Ciber Physiopathology, Obesity and Nutrition (CIBERObn), Instituto de Salud Carlos III, 08907 Barcelona, Spain
Department of Psychobiology and Methodology of Health Sciences, Universitat Autònoma de Barcelona, 08193 Barcelona, Spain

Zaida Agüera
Ciber Physiopathology, Obesity and Nutrition (CIBERObn), Instituto de Salud Carlos III, 08907 Barcelona, Spain
Department of Psychiatry, Bellvitge University Hospital-IDIBELL, 08907 Barcelona, Spain
Department of Public Health, Mental Health and Maternal-Child Nursing, School of Nursing, University of Barcelona, 08907 Barcelona, Spain

Jess Kerr-Gaffney
Department of Psychological Medicine, Institute of Psychiatry, Psychology and Neuroscience, King's College London, London SE5 8AB, UK

Luke Mason and Emily Jones
Centre for Brain & Cognitive Development, Birkbeck, University of London, London WC1E 7JL, UK

Hannah Hayward, Eva Loth and Declan Murphy
Department of Forensic & Neurodevelopmental Sciences, Institute of Psychiatry, Psychology and Neuroscience, King's College London, London SE5 8AB, UK

Jumana Ahmad
School of Human Sciences, University of Greenwich, London SE10 9LS, UK

Amy Harrison
Department of Psychology and Human Development, University College London, London WC1H 0AA, UK
South London and Maudsley NHS Trust, National Eating Disorders Service, Psychological Medicine Clinical Academic Group, London SE5 8AZ, UK

Kate Tchanturia
Department of Psychological Medicine, Institute of Psychiatry, Psychology and Neuroscience, King's College London, London SE5 8AB, UK
South London and Maudsley NHS Trust, National Eating Disorders Service, Psychological Medicine Clinical Academic Group, London SE5 8AZ, UK
Department of Psychology, Ilia State University, Tbilisi 0162, Georgia

Janet Treasure, Daniel Willmott, Valentina Cardi, Danielle Clark Bryan, Katie Rowlands and Ulrike Schmidt
Section of Eating Disorders, Department of Psychological Medicine, Institute of Psychiatry, Psychology and Neuroscience, King's College London, SE5 8AF London, UK

Suman Ambwani
Department of Psychology, Dickinson College, Carlisle, PA17013, USA

Philibert Duriez and Philip Gorwood
GHU Paris Psychiatry and Neuroscience, Clinique des Maladies Mentales et de l'Encéphale (CMME), Sainte-Anne Hospital, 75014 Paris, France
Institute of Psychiatry and Neurosciences of Paris (IPNP), UMR_S1266, INSERM, Université de Paris, 102-108 rue de la Santé, 75014 Paris, France

Yara Chamoun
Department of Psychiatry, Hotel Dieu de France- Saint Joseph University, 166830 Beirut, Lebanon

Rami Bou Khalil
Department of Psychiatry, Hotel Dieu de France- Saint Joseph University, 166830 Beirut, Lebanon
Neuropsychiatry: Epidemiological and Clinical Research, Université Montpellier, INSERM, CHU de Montpellier, 34295 Montpellier, France

Redwan Maatoug
Sorbonne Université, AP-HP, Service de Psychiatrie Adulte de la Pitié-Salpêtrière, Institut du Cerveau, ICM, 75013 Paris, France

Robertas Strumila
Faculty of Medicine, Institute of Clinical Medicine, Psychiatric Clinic, Vilnius University, 03101 Vilnius, Lithuania

Maude Seneque, Philippe Courtet and Sébastien Guillaume
Neuropsychiatry: Epidemiological and Clinical Research, Université Montpellier, INSERM, CHU de Montpellier, 34295 Montpellier, France
Department of Emergency Psychiatry and Post-Acute Care, CHRU Montpellier, 34295 Montpellier, France

Isabel Sánchez and Nadine Riesco
Department of Psychiatry, University Hospital of Bellvitge-IDIBELL, 08907 Barcelona, Spain

María Lozano-Madrid, Giulia Testa and Cristina Vintró-Alcaraz
Department of Psychiatry, University Hospital of Bellvitge-IDIBELL, 08907 Barcelona, Spain
CIBER Fisiopatologia Obesidad y Nutrición (CIBERobn), Instituto de Salud Carlos III, 28029 Madrid, Spain

José Antonio Fernández-Formoso
CIBER Fisiopatologia Obesidad y Nutrición (CIBERobn), Instituto de Salud Carlos III, 28029 Madrid, Spain

Nuria Mallorquí-Bagué
Department of Psychiatry, University Hospital of Bellvitge-IDIBELL, 08907 Barcelona, Spain
CIBER Fisiopatologia Obesidad y Nutrición (CIBERobn), Instituto de Salud Carlos III, 28029 Madrid, Spain
Addictive Behavior Unit, Department of Psychiatry, Hospital de la Santa Creu i Sant Pau, 08001 Barcelona, Spain

José César Perales and Alberto Megías
Department of Experimental Psychology, Mind, Brain, and Behavior Research Centre, University of Granada 18071 Granada, Spain

Juan Francisco Navas
Department of Basic Psychology, Autonomous University of Madrid, 28049 Madrid, Spain
Universitat Oberta de Catalunya, 08018 Barcelona, Spain

Alexander Gdanski
Department of Human Biology, University of Toronto, Toronto, ON M5S 3J6, Canada

Ignacio Martínez-Zalacaín
Department of Psychiatry, University Hospital of Bellvitge-IDIBELL, 08907 Barcelona, Spain
Clinical Sciences Department, School of Medicine, University of Barcelona, 08907 Barcelona, Spain

Misericordia Veciana De Las Heras
Neurophysiology Unit, Neurology Department, Hospital Universitari de Bellvitge, 08907 Barcelona, Spain

Rayane Chami
Section of Eating Disorders, Institute of Psychiatry, Psychology & Neuroscience (IoPPN), King's College London, London SE5 8AF, UK

Julia Philipp, Stefanie Truttmann, Michael Zeiler, Claudia Franta, Tanja Wittek, Gabriele Schöfbeck, Michaela Mitterer, Dunja Mairhofer, Gudrun Wagner and Andreas F. K. Karwautz
Eating Disorders Unit, Department of Child and Adolescent Psychiatry, Medical University of Vienna, 1090 Vienna, Austria

Annika Zanko and Hartmut Imgart
Parkland Clinic, Clinic for Psychosomatic Medicine and Psychotherapy, 34537 Bad Wildungen, Germany

Marzena Jezewska-Zychowicz, Aleksandra Małachowska and Marta Plichta
Institute of Human Nutrition Sciences, Warsaw University of Life Sciences (SGGW-WULS), 159C Nowoursynowska Street, 02-787 Warsaw, Poland

Bruno Porras-Garcia, Marta Ferrer-Garcia, Eduardo Serrano-Troncoso, Helena Miquel-Nabau, Nazilla Shojaeian and José Gutiérrez-Maldonado
Department of Clinical Psychology and Psychobiology, University of Barcelona, Passeig de la Vall d'Hebron 171, 08035 Barcelona, Spain

Marta Carulla-Roig and Pau Soto-Usera
Department of Child and Adolescent Psychiatry and Psychology, Hospital Sant Joan de Déu of Barcelona; Passeig de Sant Joan de Déu, 2, 08950 Esplugues de Llobregat, Spain

Isabel de la Montaña Santos-Carrasco, Bianca Borszewski and Marina Díaz-Marsá
Department of Psychiatry and Mental Health, Hospital Clínico San Carlos, Madrid, Calle del Prof Martín Lagos, s/n, 28040 Madrid, Spain

Laurie Hamel
Centre for Addiction and Mental Health (CAMH), Toronto, ON M6J 1H3, Canada

Isabel Sánchez-Díaz and Fernando Fernández-Aranda
Department of Psychiatry and Mental Health, Hospital Universitario de Bellvitge- IDIBELL and CIBEROBN, Barcelona; Carrer Feixa Llarga s/n, 08907 Hospitalet del Llobregat, Spain

Nicolette Stogios, Emily Smith and Roshanak Asgariroozbehani
Centre for Addiction and Mental Health (CAMH), Toronto, ON M6J 1H3, Canada
Institute of Medical Science (IMS), University of Toronto, Toronto, ON M5S 1A8, Canada

Peter Selby
Centre for Addiction and Mental Health (CAMH), Toronto, ON M6J 1H3, Canada
Department of Family and Community Medicine, University of Toronto, Toronto, ON M5G 1V7, Canada
Dalla Lana School of Public Health, University of Toronto, Toronto, ON M5T 3M7, Canada
Department of Psychiatry, University of Toronto, Toronto, ON M5T 1R8, Canada

Ariel Graff-Guerrero, Sri Mahavir Agarwal and Margaret K. Hahn
Centre for Addiction and Mental Health (CAMH), Toronto, ON M6J 1H3, Canada
Institute of Medical Science (IMS), University of Toronto, Toronto, ON M5S 1A8, Canada
Department of Psychiatry, University of Toronto, Toronto, ON M5T 1R8, Canada

Sanjeev Sockalingam
Centre for Addiction and Mental Health (CAMH), Toronto, ON M6J 1H3, Canada
Institute of Medical Science (IMS), University of Toronto, Toronto, ON M5S 1A8, Canada
Department of Psychiatry, University of Toronto, Toronto, ON M5T 1R8, Canada
Bariatric Surgery Program, University Health Network, Toronto, ON M5T 2S8, Canada

Valerie H. Taylor
Department of Psychiatry, University of Calgary, Calgary, AB T2N 1N4, Canada

Index

www.ingramcontent.com/pod-product-compliance
Lightning Source LLC
LaVergne TN
LVHW082215200926
848484LV00008B/2257
9798887401140